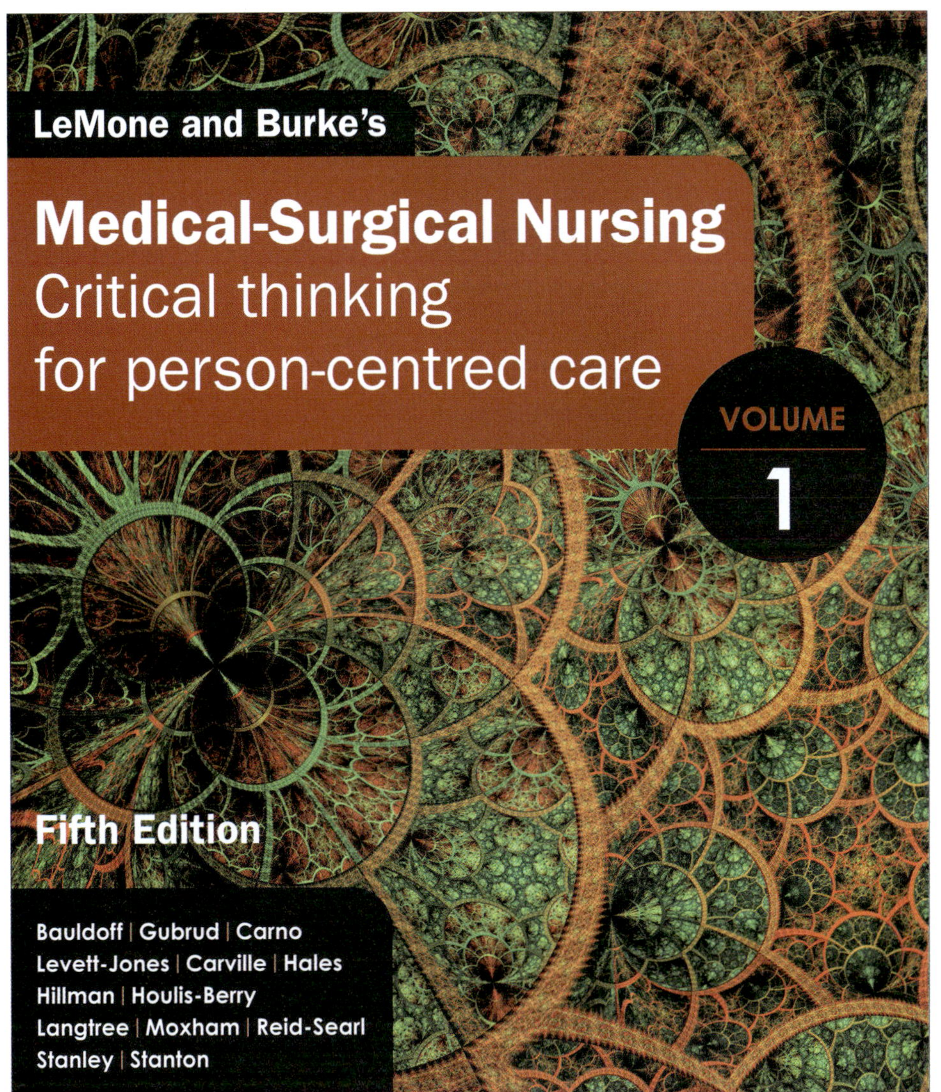

LeMone and Burke's
Medical-Surgical Nursing
Critical thinking
for person-centred care
VOLUME
1
Fifth Edition
Bauldoff | Gubrud | Carno
Levett-Jones | Carville | Hales
Hillman | Houlis-Berry
Langtree | Moxham | Reid-Searl
Stanley | Stanton

AF583883

Pearson Australia
Building B, Level 1
459–471 Church Street
Richmond Victoria 3121

www.pearson.com.au

Authorised adaptation from the United States edition entitled *LeMone's Medical–Surgical Nursing: Clinical Reasoning in Patient Care*, 7th edition, by LeMone, Priscilla; Burke, Karen; Bauldoff, Gerene, Gubrud, Paula, published by Pearson Education, Inc., Copyright © 2020.

Fifth adaptation edition published by Pearson Australia Group Pty Ltd, Copyright © 2024

Pearson respects and honours Aboriginal and Torres Strait Islander Elders past, present and future. We acknowledge the stories, traditions and living cultures of the Traditional Custodians of the lands on which our company is located and where we conduct our business. Pearson is committed to honouring Australian Aboriginal and Torres Strait Islander peoples' unique cultural and spiritual relationships to the land, waters and seas and their rich contribution to society.

Aboriginal and Torres Strait Islander peoples are advised that this text may contain images, voices and names of deceased persons.

Links to National Patient Safety Standards reproduced with permission from *National Safety and Quality Health Service Standards* (second edition), developed by the Australian Commission on Safety and Quality in Health Care (ACSQHC). ACSQHC: Sydney 2021.

Senior Commercial Product Manager: Mandy Sheppard
Development Editor: Anna Carter
Senior Project Manager: Bernadette Chang
Content Producer: Linda Chryssavgis
Digital Media Production Manager: Paul Ryan
Assistant Manager Rights and Permissions: Samantha Russell-Tulip
Lead Editor/Copy Editor: Katie Millar
Indexer: Integra Software Services
Cover and internal design by Natalie Bowra
Cover image by Sabena Jane Blackbird/Alamy Stock Photo
Typeset by Integra Software Services

Printed in Malaysia (CTP-VVP)

Etext ISBN: 9780655709152
Print ISBNs: 9780655709145 (Vol 1), 9780655709275 (Vol 2), 9780655709282 (Vol 3)
ePUB ISBN: 9780655709169

1 2 3 4 5 28 27 26 25 24

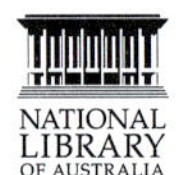

A catalogue record for this
work is available from the
National Library of Australia

Pearson Australia Group Pty Ltd ABN 40 004 245 943

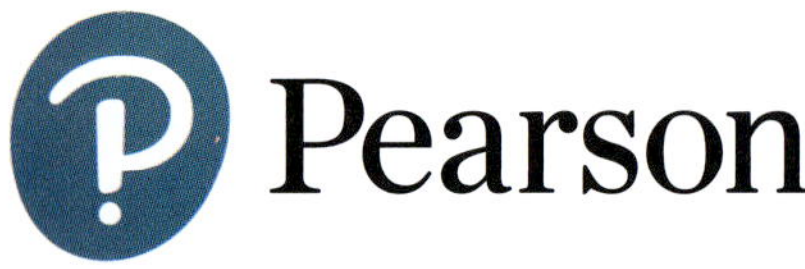

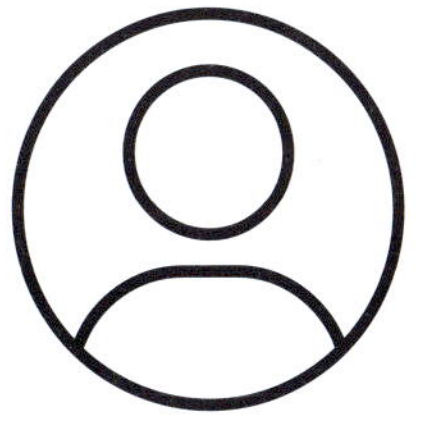

Pearson's Commitment to Diversity, Equity, and Inclusion

Pearson is dedicated to creating bias-free content that reflects the diversity, depth, and breadth of all learners' lived experiences.

We embrace the many dimensions of diversity, including but not limited to race, ethnicity, gender, sex, sexual orientation, socioeconomic status, ability, age, and religious or political beliefs.

Education is a powerful force for equity and change in our world. It has the potential to deliver opportunities that improve lives and enable economic mobility. As we work with authors to create content for every product and service, we acknowledge our responsibility to demonstrate inclusivity and incorporate diverse scholarship so that everyone can achieve their potential through learning. As the world's leading learning company, we have a duty to help drive change and live up to our purpose to help more people create a better life for themselves and to create a better world.

Our ambition is to purposefully contribute to a world where:

- Everyone has an equitable and lifelong opportunity to succeed through learning.
- Our educational content accurately reflects the histories and lived experiences of the learners we serve.
- Our educational products and services are inclusive and represent the rich diversity of learners.
- Our educational content prompts deeper discussions with students and motivates them to expand their own learning (and worldview).

Accessibility

We are also committed to providing products that are fully accessible to all learners. As per Pearson's guidelines for accessible educational Web media, we test and retest the capabilities of our products against the highest standards for every release, following the WCAG guidelines in developing new products for copyright year 2022 and beyond.

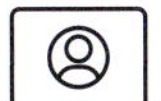

You can learn more about Pearson's commitment to accessibility at **https://www.pearson.com/us/accessibility.html**

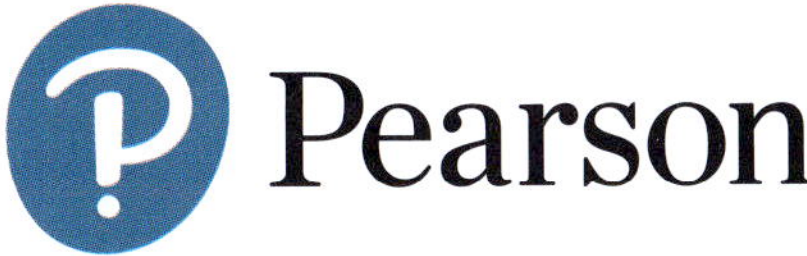

Contact Us

While we work hard to present unbiased, fully accessible content, we want to hear from you about any concerns or needs with this Pearson product so that we can investigate and address them.

Please contact us with concerns about any potential bias at **https://www.pearson.com/report-bias.html**

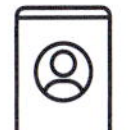

For accessibility-related issues, such as using assistive technology with Pearson products, alternative text requests, or accessibility documentation, email the Pearson Disability Support team at **disability.support@pearson.com**

Brief contents

VOLUME 1

VOLUME 2

Detailed contents

VOLUME 2

About the authors

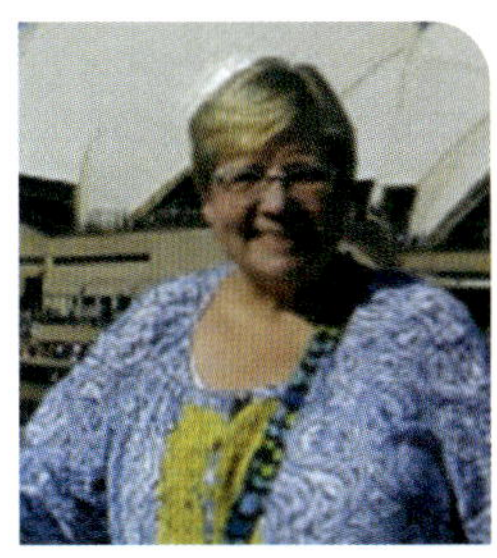

GERENE BAULDOFF RN, PhD, FAAN

Gerene Bauldoff is a Professor of Clinical Nursing at The Ohio State University College of Nursing in Columbus, Ohio. She has been a nurse educator for 19 years, teaching medical–surgical nursing, clinical and research methods and measurement, and evidence-based practice courses at the baccalaureate, master's and doctoral levels. Prior to her nursing educator role, her clinical background included home health nurse, lung transplant coordinator and pulmonary rehabilitation coordinator. Dr Bauldoff has a diploma from the Western Pennsylvania Hospital School of Nursing in Pittsburgh, Pennsylvania, and a BSN from LaRoche College in Pittsburgh. Her graduate education is from the University of Pittsburgh, with an MSN in medical–surgical nursing (cardiopulmonary clinical nurse specialist) and PhD in nursing in 2001, training under Leslie Hoffman, PhD, RN, FAAN.

Dr Bauldoff is an active member of multiple professional organisations including the American Academy of Nursing (AAN), Sigma Theta Tau International Honor Society of Nursing, the American Association of Cardiovascular and Pulmonary Rehabilitation (AACVPR), the American Thoracic Society Nursing Assembly and the American College of Chest Physicians (ACCP). She is a recognised expert in medical–surgical nursing, focusing on the care of the patient with chronic pulmonary disease, serving on committees focusing on international standards for and patient-centred outcomes in pulmonary rehabilitation. She has been honoured with fellowships in AAN and ACCP, and is a master fellow in AACVPR. Dr Bauldoff has conducted several international presentations related to evidence-based practice and clinical outcomes.

Dr Bauldoff considers nursing as the greatest profession, using scientific evidence to provide the highest quality of care while maintaining the personal relationship with patients and their families. Her experiences provide her with insights and lessons that she shares with her students.

I dedicate this book to the memory of my parents, to my sisters and to my friends, especially Vicki von Sadovszky, Linda Daley, Patty Orndoff and Eileen Collins—you are my touchstones to the world and are my greatest sounding boards. You help me keep my feet on the ground and my face turned towards new opportunities. You mean the world to me!

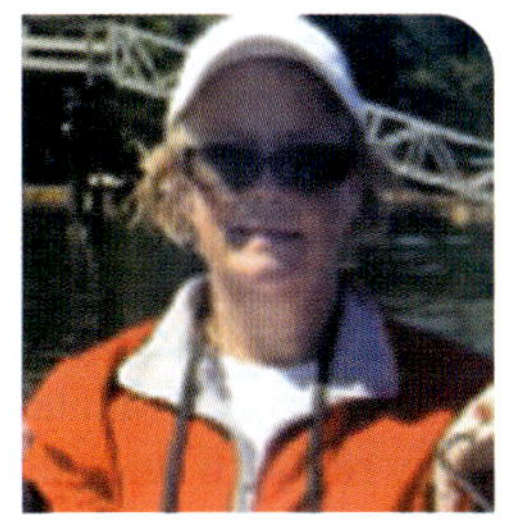

PAULA GUBRUD RN, MS, EdD, FAAN

Paula Gubrud is Senior Associate Dean for Academic Affairs and an Associate Professor at Oregon Health and Science University (OHSU) School of Nursing. She has more than 25 years of experience as a nurse educator, involving multiple levels of programs from LPN to doctoral education. Dr Gubrud is a founding leader and co-director of the Oregon Consortium for Nursing Education, an award-winning consortium that includes the five campuses of OHSU and nine community colleges. She also has more than 20 years of experience in medical–surgical nursing, critical care, home health and hospice. Dr Gubrud earned a baccalaureate degree in nursing from Walla Walla University (1980), an MS in community-based nursing from OHSU (1993) and an EdD in post-secondary education from Portland State University (2008). She is a frequent invited speaker at national and international nursing education/conferences and consults with other states and countries on the development of competency-based curriculum and nursing education consortiums designed to promote academic progression in nursing education. Her research activity is focused on clinical education redesign and the integration of simulation into nursing curriculum.

Dr Gubrud is passionate about nursing and the opportunities it provides members of the profession. She values the sacred relationship nurses experience with patients as they promote health, treat illness and provide comfort and palliative care. She believes the nation's health depends on highly qualified nurses who are dedicated to lifelong learning in pursuit of evidence-based, patient-centred care.

Dr Gubrud lives in the Pacific Northwest and enjoys reading, camping, hiking and fishing. She catches really big salmon year round!

I dedicate this book to my husband, Leland Howe, and my children, Elizabeth Gubrud-Howe, Gabriel Howe and Caleb Howe, for encouraging me to pursue my professional passions and goals. I also dedicate this book to my father, Allan Gubrud, who instilled insatiable curiosity, a love of learning and a passion to teach.

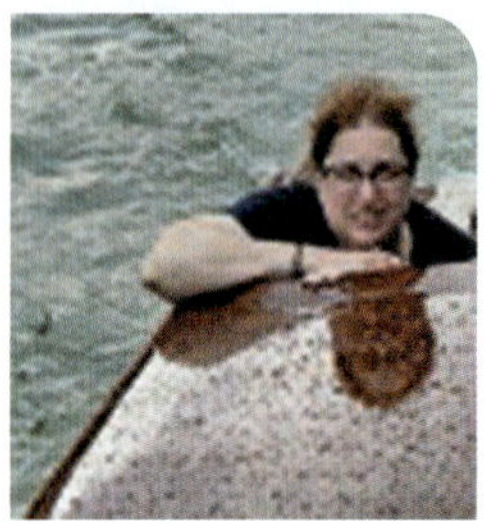

MARGARET-ANN CARNO PhD, MBA, MJ, RN, CPNP, D, ABSM, ATSF, FAAN

Margaret-Ann Carno is Professor of Clinical Nursing and Pediatrics as well as Co-Director of Baccalaureate Programs at the University of Rochester, School of Nursing. Dr Carno has over 20 years of teaching across baccalaureate, master's and doctoral levels of nursing education in medical–surgical nursing, paediatrics, ethics, health law, sleep across the lifespan and research. Seeing students be successful gives Dr Carno the greatest joy.

Dr Carno earned her baccalaureate in nursing at Syracuse University and then went on to complete an MBA in Operations Management and an MS in Nursing (Pediatric Critical Care), also from Syracuse University. She received her PhD from the University of Pittsburgh under the guidance of Leslie Hoffman, PhD, RN, FAAN. Dr Carno also holds a Master of Jurisprudence in Health Law from University of Loyola–Chicago and a post-Master's certification as a Pediatric Nurse Practitioner from the University of Rochester, School of Nursing. She is a Fellow of the American Academy of Nursing and of the American Thoracic Society. Dr Carno is a Diplomate of the American Board of Sleep Medicine.

When she is not teaching or working on other duties, Dr Carno enjoys travelling the world with her beloved cousins.

I dedicate this book to my father, Joseph, who while in my life only for a short time, instilled the idea I could be anything I wanted and to never stop learning. Also to my mother, Libera, who has been my champion and support throughout my life.

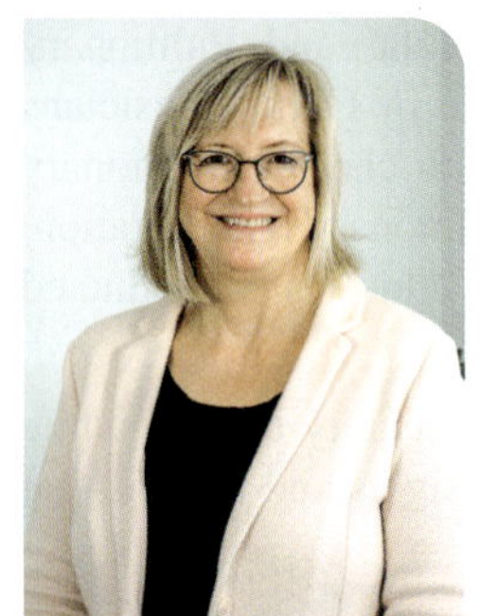

TRACY LEVETT-JONES RN, PhD, MEd & Work, BN, DipAppSc(Nur)

Tracy Levett-Jones is a Distinguished Professor in the School of Nursing & Midwifery at the University of Technology Sydney. Her program of research focuses on patient safety, empathy, belongingness, clinical reasoning and simulation. Tracy has authored or edited 10 books, the most recent being *Clinical Reasoning: Learning to Think Like a Nurse* and *Critical Conversations for Patient Safety*, as well as over 200 book chapters and journal articles. She has been the recipient of multiple research and teaching awards and was inducted into the Sigma Theta Tau International Honor Society of Nursing Researcher Hall of Fame in 2022. Tracy has been awarded over $7 million of Category 1 funding for projects designed to improve healthcare students' capacity to practise safely and empathically.

Twitter: @Prof_TLJ

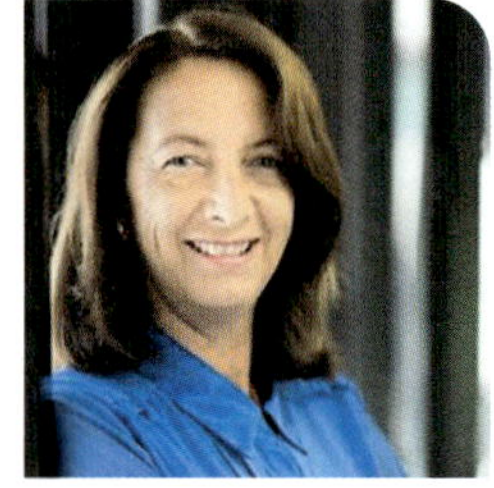

LORNA MOXHAM RN, PhD (CQU), MHN, DAS(Nsg) (MIHE), MEd (UNSW), GCOH&S (CQU), GCQualMgmt (CQU), BHSc (UWS), Cert IV (Training & Assessment) (CQIT), FACMHN, FACN

Professor Lorna Moxham started nursing in 1980 at Concord Hospital, Sydney, and then completed a 3-year specialist hospital-trained psychiatric nurse certificate at Rozelle Hospital. Lorna is passionate about the nursing profession, particularly mental health nursing, and is actively contributing at regional, state, national and international levels. Lorna has spent time living and working in regional Queensland, regional New South Wales and metropolitan New South Wales and has served on many ministerial committees as both a member and chair. In addition, she has held several leadership and governance roles within the tertiary education sector, at Board level and in nursing. Lorna is currently Professor of Mental Health Nursing at the University of Wollongong. Lorna has successfully supervised numerous higher degrees by research students to on-time completion, all of whom have published their work. She is a well-published researcher and clinical educator and thinks that being a mental health nurse is 'the very best job in the world'. Lorna is recognised nationally for co-founding 'Recovery Camp'—a mental health clinical placement for nursing and health students and a psychosocial intervention for people with a lived experience of mental illness. Lorna describes this program as the best professional thing she ever did.

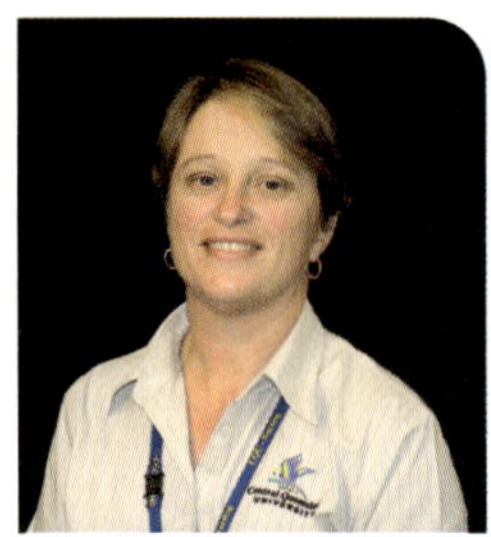

KERRY REID-SEARL RN, RM, PhD, BHSc (Nsg), MClinEdu, MRCNA, FCN

Kerry Reid-Searl is currently a Professor of Innovation and Simulation in the School of Nursing and Midwifery at the University of Tasmania. Kerry is also an Emeritus Professor at CQUniversity, Australia, and a consultant to Massey University in New Zealand. Kerry has been involved in nursing education for more than 30 years and, over this time, she has remained clinically current. Kerry's research interests include patient safety, simulation, paediatrics and wound care. She has been the recipient of 10 teaching awards, including two Australian Learning and Teaching Citations for her outstanding contribution to student learning and an Australian University Teaching Excellence Award. She was named Pearson/Australian Nurse Teacher Society Nurse Teacher of the Year in 2009, and in 2013, received the Simulation Australia Achievement award. Kerry is recognised nationally and internationally for her pioneering work in creating, designing and researching two innovative simulation strategies called Mask Ed (KRS Simulation) and Pup Ed (KRS Simulation).

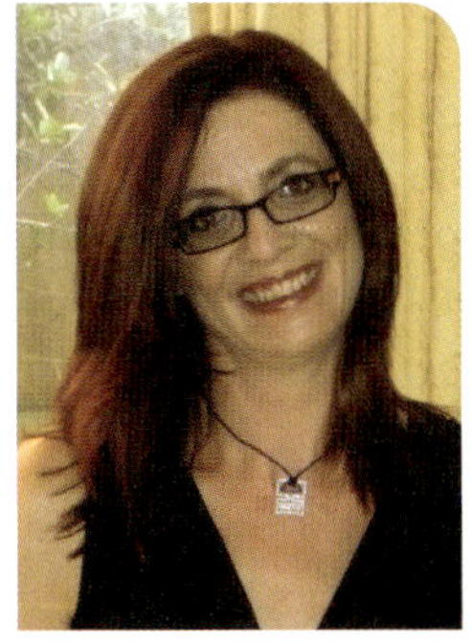

KAMAREE HOULIS-BERRY PhD, MEd Stds (Hon), PGDip Clinical Nursing (Perioperative), RN, BN, MACN, MAHRI, GAICD, MIML

Kamaree's career spans more than 25 years and commenced with the Australian Army, where she trained as a medic and then became a nursing officer at the rank of lieutenant. She has been employed in the public, private and academic sectors in a number of roles, spanning from an RN, senior lecturer and academic undergraduate chair to General Manager Learning, Director Operational Capability and now Founder and Director/CEO of her own advisory and consulting company drK & Co.

A successful career has provided her with the opportunity to teach at both undergraduate and postgraduate levels, along with employment within the corporate and commercial sector at a national level. Underpinning Kamaree's philosophy and values of learning, development and professional education is her strong conviction of innovative leadership and direction for both staff and students. She values the importance of continuing professional education and development; this has been acknowledged by her peers making use of her extensive expertise and contemporary approach to teaching and learning, curriculum development and review, program designs, staff and student mentorship, and currency on educational trends within the nursing profession across a number of specialties. She has been awarded a Bachelor of Nursing, Postgraduate Diploma Clinical Nursing—Perioperative, a Master of Educational Studies (Hons) and has completed her doctoral thesis.

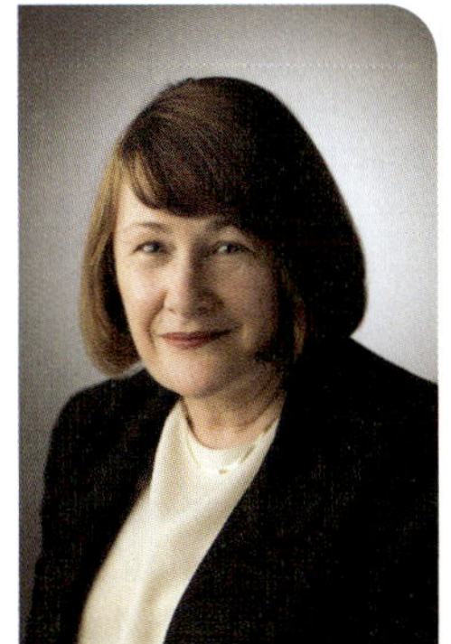

KERYLN CARVILLE PhD, RN, STN (Cred), Professor Primary Health Care & Community Nursing, Silver Chain Group and Curtin University, Western Australia

Keryln has extensive clinical experience and is committed to research and education within the domains of wound and ostomy care. She was appointed a Fellow of the Australian Wound Management Association (now Wounds Australia) in 2006. She is Chair of the Australian Pressure Injury Advisory Panel and Chair Pan Pacific Pressure Injury Alliance, Chair of the Wounds Australia Wound Standards Committee and sits on the International Wound Infection Institute Committee. Keryln was awarded the Western Australia Health Lifetime Achievement Award for Nursing in 2010.

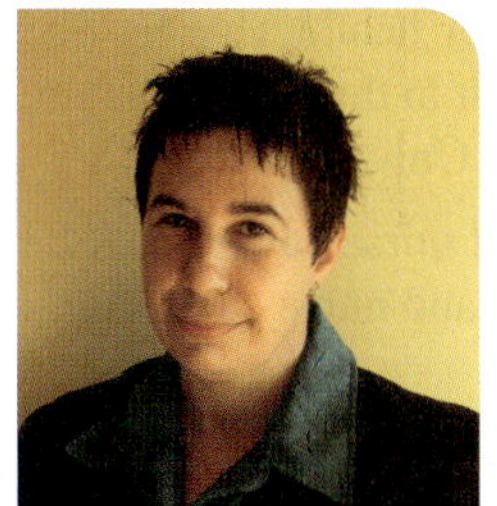

MAJELLA HALES RN, MAppSci, GCHE, BN

Majella Hales works as a casual academic at the Australian Catholic University in Brisbane. Originally hospital trained, she has worked in nursing for over 25 years. She maintains her clinical experience by undertaking agency shifts in critical care units across South-East Queensland and provides clinical facilitation for undergraduate nursing students for various local universities. Majella authored several chapters of Kozier and Erb's *Fundamentals of Nursing* Volumes 1–3 and co-authored *Principles of Pathophysiology* with Associate Professor Shane Bullock. Along with journal articles and conference presentations, she has also produced the skills DVD for Tollefson's *Clinical Psychomotor Skills* text and adapted the American case study resource *The Neighbourhood*. Majella is a co-owner of Sciencopia, a company producing informative, novel and fun educational resources for academics, students and healthcare professionals. One of Sciencopia's first products—*Essential Aussie Drugs: A Little Pocket Book of Common Aussie Drug Facts*—is a great resource for assisting individuals to improve their drug knowledge and safety in the ever-changing and complex world of pharmacology and drug administration.

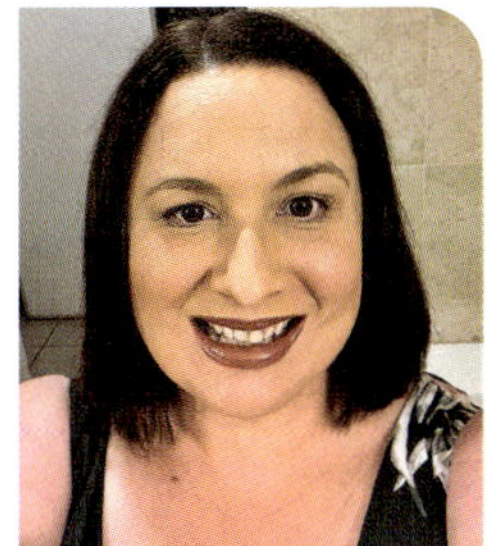

TANYA LANGTREE RN, PhD, MNSt, PGDipAdvClinN(NeuroSC), PGCERTNsc(INTCARE), GCertHEdlLearnTeach, BNSc, CHIA, JP(QUAL.)

Tanya Langtree has been a Registered Nurse since 2000. Tanya has worked in both public and private sectors, with her main areas of clinical expertise being neurosciences and critical care nursing. She has a keen interest in nursing history, psychomotor skill development and clinical simulation and has been teaching undergraduate nursing students in the simulated environment since 2005. In 2010, Tanya joined the discipline of Nursing and Midwifery at James Cook University (JCU). Since then, she has held a variety of roles including subject coordinator, Director of Clinical Simulation, Deputy Director of the Centre for Nursing and Midwifery Research and remote site coordinator. Tanya's PhD examined the progression of early nursing theory and praxis prior to nursing's professionalisation in the mid-19th century.

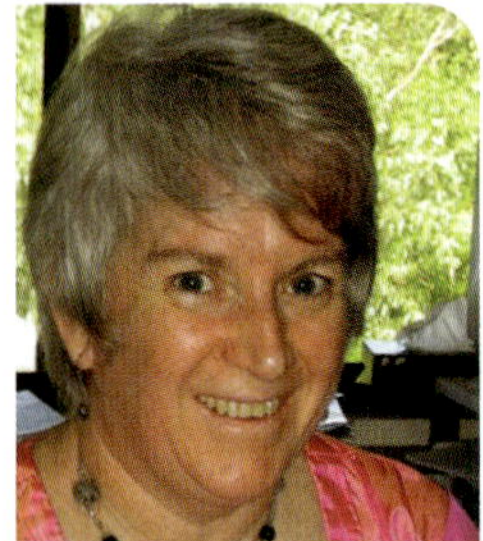

ELSPETH HILLMAN RN, BN, MN

Elspeth Hillman is Academic Lead: Professional Practice in nursing at James Cook University, with an interest in nursing education research. Elspeth has extensive clinical experience in a range of clinical situations from rural to critical care nursing. Her experience includes facilitation of both undergraduate nursing students in various clinical facilities and postgraduate nursing students in high-dependency units.

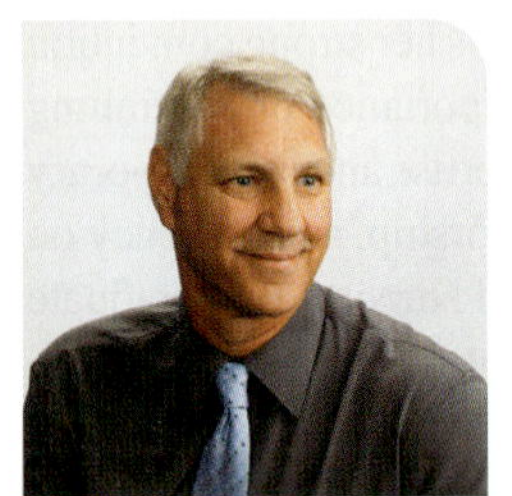

DAVID STANLEY NURSD, MSC HS, BA NG, DIP HE (NURSING), RN, RM, TF, GERONTIC CERT, GRAD CERT HPE

David Stanley began his nursing career in the days when nurses wore huge belt buckles and funny hats. He 'trained' as a Registered Nurse and midwife in South Australia and worked through his formative career in a number of hospitals and clinical environments in Australia. In 1993, he completed a Bachelor of Nursing at Flinders University, Adelaide (for which he was awarded the University Medal) and, after a number of years of volunteer work in Africa, he moved to the UK and worked as the Coordinator of Children's Services and as a Nurse Practitioner. He completed a Master of Health Science degree at Birmingham University.

For a short time he worked in Central Australia for Remote Health Services before returning to the UK to complete his nursing doctorate, researching in the area of clinical leadership. He retains a research interest in clinical leadership, men in nursing and the role of the media in nursing. He is currently in the process of retiring but retains his research interests and is an avid poet and writer of children's books and fiction.

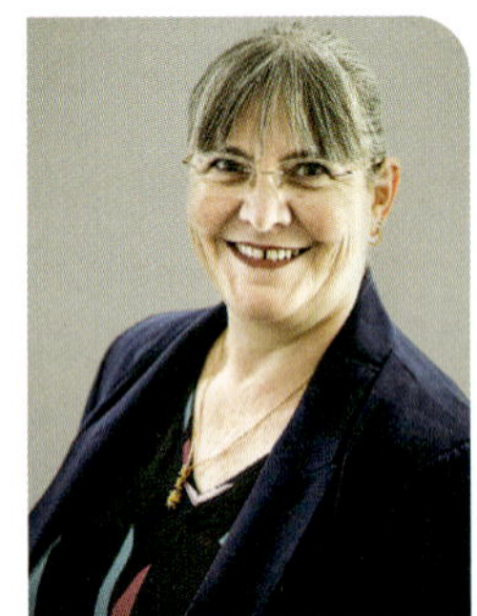

SHARON STANTON BN, RN, MN (Urological and Continence), GCTAE, Cert IV TAE, ANZUP (Member), CNSA (Assoc. Member), NSWUNS/ANZUNS (Member), MACN

Sharon has been involved in an undergraduate nursing degree across several Australian universities for over 10 years. She has also taught in the private sector with a Registered Training Organisation. She completed a Bachelor of Nursing at University of New England in 2007. After commencing her Master of Nursing in 2010, Sharon successfully became CNS Urology on the surgical unit where she was employed. As part of a team, in 2012, Sharon successfully applied for funding from the Prostate Cancer Foundation of Australia to secure a Prostate Cancer Specialist Nurse role for her health service. She subsequently was successful in applying for the position and became one of the first in the pilot program. Sharon graduated her Master of Nursing (Urological and Continence) at La Trobe University in 2013.

Sharon has a research interest in prostate cancer, specifically patient support needs, and is passionate about nurse education. She has presented at a number of Australian and International Conferences across topics of prostate cancer care and nurse education.

Sharon is now working as a Lecturer in Nursing at the University of Canberra.

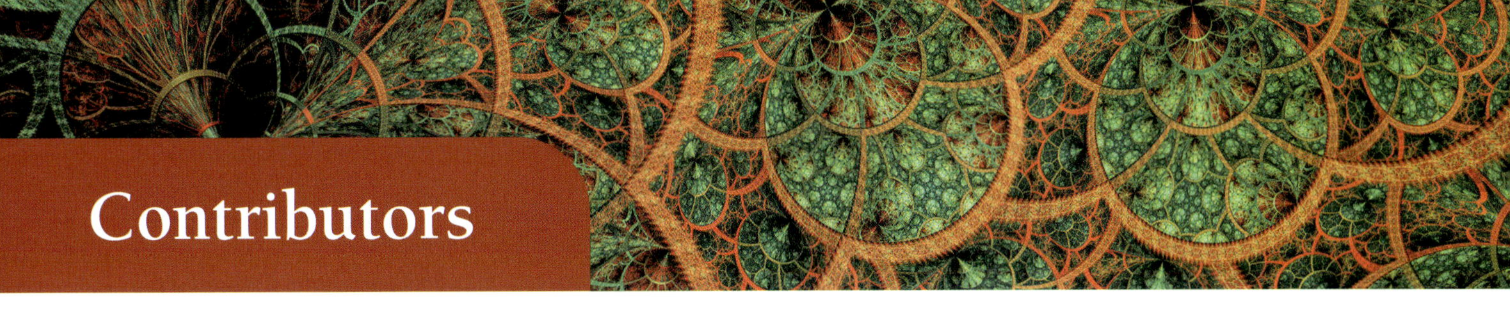

Contributors

We extend deep, sincere thanks to our contributors who gave their time, effort and expertise so willingly to the development and writing of chapters and resources that will help foster our goal of achieving nursing excellence through building clinical competence.

AUSTRALIAN CONTRIBUTORS

Chapter 1 Medical–Surgical Nursing

5th edition: Tracy Levett-Jones, University of Technology Sydney, and Aimee Lamb, University of Western Sydney

4th edition: Tracy Levett-Jones, University of Technology Sydney, and Lorinda Palmer, University of Newcastle

Chapter 2 Health and Illness in Adults

4th and 5th editions: Amanda Wilson, University of Technology Sydney, and Tracy Levett-Jones, University of Technology

Chapter 3 Nursing Care of People Having Surgery

5th edition: Judith Smith, Australian College of Nursing

4th edition: Judith Smith, Australian College of Nursing, and Natalie Govind, University of Technology Sydney

Chapter 4 Nursing Care of People Experiencing Loss, Grief and Death

5th edition: Natalie Govind, University of Technology Sydney

4th edition: Pamela van der Riet, University of Newcastle, Victoria Pitt, University of Newcastle, and Greg Blyton, University of Newcastle

Chapter 5 Nursing Care of People with Substance Misuse Problems

4th and 5th editions: Anna Treloar, University of Newcastle

Chapter 6 Nursing Care of People in the Emergency Department or Experiencing Disasters

5th edition: Julia Morphet, Monash University

4th edition: Joy Lynham, University of Newcastle, and Julia Morphet, Monash University

Chapter 7 Genetic Implications of Adult Health Nursing

5th edition: Kamaree Houlis-Berry, drK & Co

4th edition: Deborah McDonough, Cairns Hospital, Queensland Health

Chapter 8 Nursing Care of People in Pain

5th edition: Adam Burston, ACU

4th edition: Adam Burston, ACU, and Floraidh Corfee, NHS

Chapter 9 Nursing Care of People with Altered Fluid, Electrolyte and Acid–Base Balance

5th edition: Kamaree Houlis-Berry, drK & Co

4th edition: Deborah McDonough, Cairns Hospital, Queensland Health

Chapter 10 Nursing Care of People Experiencing Trauma and Shock

5th edition: Kamaree Houlis-Berry, drK & Co

4th edition: Lisa Gatzonis, ADON Nursing Workforce Unit

Chapter 11 Nursing Care of People with Infections

5th edition: Kamaree Houlis-Berry, drK & Co

4th edition: Lisa Gatzonis, ADON Nursing Workforce Unit

Chapter 12 Nursing Care of People with Altered Immunity

5th edition: Kamaree Houlis-Berry, drK & Co

4th edition: Catherine Bethell, Western Health Victoria

Chapter 13 Nursing Care of People with Cancer

5th edition: Kamaree Houlis-Berry, drK & Co

4th edition: Catherine Bethell, Western Health Victoria

Chapter 14 Assessing the Integumentary System

4th and 5th editions: Keryln Carville, Silver Chain Group, Kerry Reid-Searl, University of Tasmania, and Joy Sears, Curtin University

Chapter 15 Nursing Care of People with Integumentary Disorders

4th and 5th editions: Keryln Carville, Silver Chain Group and Curtin University, Kerry Reid-Searl, University of Tasmania, Kate Crowley, CQUniversity, and Joy Sears, Curtin University

Chapter 16 Nursing Care of People with Burns

5th edition: Kamaree Berry, drK & Co, and Sharon Rowe, State Adult Burn Unit, Fiona Stanley Hospital Perth

4th edition: Sharon Rowe, State Adult Burn Unit, Fiona Stanley Hospital Perth, Dr Fiona Wood, Director of the Burns Service of Western Australia and Winthrop, Dr Dale Edgar, The University of Notre Dame, and Rosemary Kendell, State Adult Burn Unit, Fiona Stanley Hospital Perth

Chapter 17 A Person-Centred Approach to Assessing the Endocrine System

5th edition: Tanya Langtree, James Cook University

4th edition: Nicole Knox, Western Sydney University

Chapter 18 Nursing Care of People with Endocrine Disorders

5th edition: Tanya Langtree, James Cook University

4th edition: Nicole Knox, Western Sydney University

Chapter 19 Nursing Care of People with Diabetes Mellitus

5th edition: Tanya Langtree, James Cook University, and Jane Medved, Western Sydney University

4th edition: Jane Medved, Western Sydney University

Chapter 20 A Person-Centred Approach to Assessing the Gastrointestinal System

5th edition: Elspeth Hillman, James Cook University

4th edition: Nicole Knox, Western Sydney University

Chapter 21 Nursing Care of People with Nutritional Disorders

5th edition: Elspeth Hillman, James Cook University

4th edition: Daniel Van Vorst, Western Sydney University

Chapter 22 Nursing Care of People with Upper Gastrointestinal Disorders

5th edition: Jane Medved, Western Sydney University, and Elspeth Hillman, James Cook University

4th edition: Jane Medved, Western Sydney University

Chapter 23 Nursing Care of People with Bowel Disorders

4th and 5th editions: Elspeth Hillman, James Cook University

Chapter 24 Nursing Care of People with Gallbladder, Liver and Pancreatic Disorders

4th and 5th editions: Jane Medved, Western Sydney University

Chapter 25 A Person-Centred Approach to Assessing the Renal System

5th edition: Sharon Stanton, University of Canberra, and Amanda McKie, University of Canberra

4th edition: Trudy Dwyer, CQUniversity, and Jennifer Borg RN, MidCert, GradCert Diabetes

Chapter 26 Nursing Care of People with Urinary Tract Disorders

5th edition: Sharon Stanton, University of Canberra

4th edition: Trudy Dwyer, CQUniversity, Jennifer Borg RN, MidCert, GradCert Diabetes, and Sharon Stanton, BN, RN, MN (Urol. & Cont.) CQUniversity

Chapter 27 Nursing Care of People with Kidney Disorders

5th edition: Sharon Stanton, University of Canberra, and Leanne Sharples, Barwon Health

4th edition: Tracy Flenady, CQUniversity RN PhD, Sharon Stanton, CQUniversity BN, RN, MN (Urol. & Cont.), and Monica Schoch, Deakin University

Chapter 28 A Person-Centred Approach to Assessing the Cardiovascular and Lymphatic Systems

4th and 5th editions: Alicia J. Perkins, Federation University

Chapter 29 Nursing Care of People with Coronary Heart Disease

5th edition: Adam Burston, ACU

4th edition: Adam Burston, ACU, and Floraidh Corfee, NHS

Chapter 30 Nursing Care of People with Cardiac Disorders

5th edition: Adam Burston, ACU

4th edition: Adam Burston, ACU, and Floraidh Corfee, ACU

Chapter 31 Nursing Care of People with Vascular and Lymphatic Disorders

4th and 5th editions: Majella Hales

Chapter 32 Nursing Care of People with Haematological Disorders

4th and 5th editions: Liz Ryan, University of New England

Chapter 33 A Person-Centred Approach to Assessing the Respiratory System

4th and 5th editions: Alison Kloehs, ACU, and Majella Hales

Chapter 34 Nursing Care of People with Upper Respiratory Disorders

4th and 5th editions: Sam Serginson, Queensland Health

Chapter 35 Nursing Care of People with Ventilation Disorders

4th and 5th editions: Sam Serginson, Queensland Health

Chapter 36 Nursing Care of People with Gas Exchange Disorders

5th edition: Kamaree Houlis-Berry, drK & Co

4th edition: Majella Hales

Chapter 37 A Person-Centred Approach to Assessing the Musculoskeletal System

4th and 5th editions: David Stanley

Chapter 38 Nursing Care of People with Musculoskeletal Trauma

4th and 5th editions: David Stanley

Chapter 39 Nursing Care of People with Musculoskeletal Disorders

5th edition: David Stanley

4th edition: Liz Ryan, University of New England

Chapter 40 A Person-Centred Approach to Assessing the Nervous System

5th edition: David Stanley

4th edition: Zach Byfield, University of New England

Chapter 41 Nursing Care of People with Intracranial Disorders

5th edition: David Stanley

4th edition: Zach Byfield, University of New England

Chapter 42 Nursing Care of People with Cerebrovascular and Spinal Cord Disorders

4th and 5th editions: David Stanley

Chapter 43 Nursing Care of People with Neurological Disorders

4th and 5th editions: David Stanley

Chapter 44 A Person-Centred Approach to Assessing the Eye and Ear

4th and 5th editions: Kamaree Houlis-Berry, drK & Co

Chapter 45 Nursing Care of People with Eye and Ear Disorders

4th and 5th editions: Kamaree Houlis-Berry, drK & Co

Chapter 46 A Person-Centred Approach to Assessing the Male and Female Reproductive Systems

5th edition: Maria Mackay, University of Wollongong, and Kelly Marriott-Statham, University of Wollongong

4th edition: Dr Rebekkah Middleton, University of Wollongong

Chapter 47 Nursing Care of Men with Reproductive System and Breast Disorders

5th edition: Suzi Russell, University of Wollongong, and Peter Thomas, University of Wollongong

4th edition: Peter Thomas, University of Wollongong

Chapter 48 Nursing Care of Women with Reproductive System and Breast Disorders

4th and 5th editions: Shahla Meedya, University of Wollongong

Chapter 49 Nursing Care of People Who Have Sexually Transmitted Infections

5th edition: Heidi Green, NWS Health

4th edition: Susan McInnes, University of Wollongong

Chapter 50 Mental Healthcare in the Australian Context

4th and 5th editions: Lorna Moxham, University of Wollongong, Paul Robson, Illawarra Shoalhaven Mental Health Service, and Christopher Patterson, University of Wollongong

Chapter 51 Community Care

5th edition Gemma McEarlean, University of Wollongong, Catherine Stephen, University of Wollongong, and Elizabeth Halcomb, University of Wollongong

4th edition: Ann Clare Thorington Taylor, University of Newcastle, and Sharyn Hunter, University of Newcastle

Chapter 52 Nursing Care of People in Regional and Remote Areas of Australia

5th edition: Helen Pratt, University of Wollongong, and Heidi Green, NWS Health

4th edition: Ms Leeanne Heaton, CQUniversity

Preface

The landscape of healthcare in Australia has shifted significantly over the past 3 years. Along with this, the journey to becoming a nurse has also changed, with students having to adapt to new ways of learning and unprecedented clinical challenges.

Howard Catton, International Council of Nurses Chief Executive Officer, stated that:

The pandemic has exposed the weaknesses in our health systems and the enormous pressures our nurses are working under, as well as shining a light on their incredible commitment and courage. What the pandemic has also done is given us the opportunity to call for a reset and the opportunity to explore new models of care where nurses are at the centre of our health systems. (Catton, 2020. International Council of Nurses announces International Nurses Day theme for 2022 International Nurses Day 2021)

Today's nursing students are tomorrow's nursing leaders, and this presents exciting opportunities and new responsibilities. Committed nurses whose practice is based on a strong foundation of knowledge, clinical skills and the ability to think critically in challenging and complex situations will be needed to usher in new models of care. The fifth Australian edition of *LeMone and Burke's Medical–Surgical Nursing: Critical Thinking for Person-centred Care* has been written to help you develop the professional attributes and skills you will need on your career journey.

Our goal—helping you to excel as a nurse

In writing this text, our commitment has been to provide students with a strong knowledge base, an understanding of contemporary practice issues in Australia and the capacity for sound clinical reasoning. These professional attributes will allow you to provide nursing care that is safe and effective. Throughout this text, we also demonstrate how competent nurses provide person-centred care that is empathic, holistic and respectful of each person's age, ethnicity, culture, needs and values.

This text has been designed to:

- emphasise a person-centred philosophy whereby the person who is the recipient of care is seen as an integral member of the team and consideration of their needs and wishes is paramount
- foster critical-thinking and clinical reasoning skills as the basis for safe clinical practice and nursing excellence
- recognise the nurse's role as an essential member of the interprofessional healthcare team.

We are confident that this text will support your learning and professional practice, and we wish you well as you undertake your nursing journey.

Organisation

This easily understood, straightforward Australian text uses effective design principles and learning strategies such as advanced organisers, special features, colourful illustrations and critical-thinking exercises to help you transfer your learning to practice. The text contains 52 chapters in 14 units. Units 1 and 2 provide an overview of medical–surgical nursing, the meaning of health and illness, and alterations in patterns of health in particular populations, contexts and situations. The remaining units are based on alterations in human structure and function. Each unit has a focus on altered health states and opens with an assessment chapter, which draws upon the student's prerequisite knowledge and serves to reinforce basic principles of anatomy and physiology as applied to assessment in both health and illness. Following the assessment chapter, each nursing care chapter focuses on major conditions and diseases and includes three key components:

1. ***Pathophysiology*** The discussion of each major illness or condition begins with incidence and prevalence, an overview of pathophysiology, and disease manifestations and complications.
2. ***Interprofessional care*** The role of both nurses and the other members of the healthcare team in managing illness is then profiled. This section includes information about specific tests necessary for diagnosis, medications, surgery and treatments, fluid management, dietary management, and complementary and alternative therapies.
3. ***Nursing care*** Nursing care within a context of priority nursing diagnoses and interventions is then provided and rationales outlined for each intervention. This section also takes into account that health promotion and illness prevention are critical nursing roles in contemporary healthcare.

Finally, for each major disorder or condition, a narrative *Nursing care plan* is provided with a brief case study, followed by the steps of the nursing process.

Chapter highlights This end-of-chapter section concludes with multiple-choice revision questions to reinforce comprehension of the chapter content. (The correct answers with rationales are found in the Instructors' Manual.)

Language and terminology

In developing this text, we have used terminology that is familiar and applicable to most Australians. While person-centred care is most often used to reflect our philosophical stance, the term 'patient' is also used as appropriate throughout the text and according to the context of care being described.

Culturally competent nursing

Chapter 1 introduces the concept of culturally competent healthcare with particular attention to the culture and history of Indigenous peoples in Australia. Throughout the text, *Focus on cultural diversity* boxes present cultural nursing in context and highlight the importance of acknowledging the dignity, culture, values, beliefs and rights of not only Indigenous Australians but also people from all cultural and ethnic backgrounds.

We acknowledge the importance of using non-discriminatory and appropriate language to describe groups of people, policies and events, and have thus followed the guidelines set out by NSW Health in its publication *Communicating Positively: A Guide to Appropriate Aboriginal Terminology*.

Nursing diagnoses

In this updated edition of *LeMone and Burke's Medical–Surgical Nursing*, we refer to the well-known nursing process as a logical approach to managing nursing care. Within this process we refer to diagnostic terminologies that are typical of those used by Australian nurses.

The Patient Safety Competency Framework

The evidence-based Patient Safety Competency Framework (PSCF) is referred to throughout this text and will help you focus on the skills and knowledge that are directly relevant to safe and effective patient care.

Competency frameworks constitute a blueprint for optimal performance in a given area of practice; competency statements refer to the specific outcomes of learning. The knowledge and skill statements included in the PSCF were structured with reference to Miller's pyramid of competence (see Figure 1). In the PSCF, knowledge statements are conceptualised as the foundation for competence. To practise safely, nursing students must have a requisite level of *knowledge*. Next, they must *know how* to apply their knowledge using cognitive skills such as analysis, interpretation and evaluation. The third level of the pyramid refers to skills and behaviours, in particular *showing how* or demonstration of skills (e.g. in a simulated setting). The fourth level of the pyramid refers to what the learner *does* with their knowledge and skills in a real-life clinical setting.

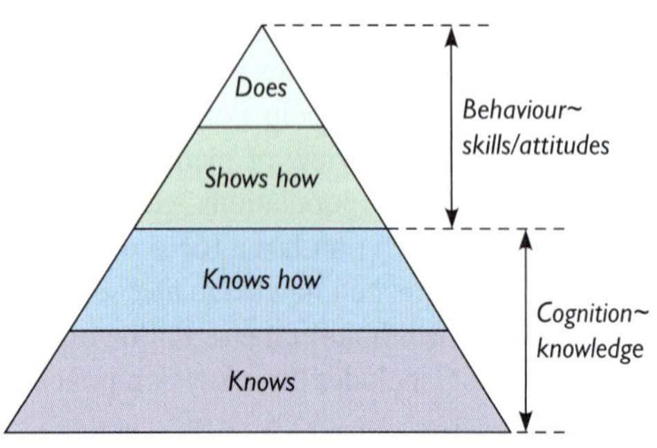

FIGURE 1 ***Miller's pyramid of competence***

Source: G. Miller (1990). The assessment of clinical skills/competence/performance. *Academic Medicine*, 65(9), s63–s67, Figure 1.

The nine overarching domains of the PSCF are:

1. Person-centred care
2. Therapeutic communication
3. Cultural competence
4. Teamwork and collaborative practice
5. Clinical reasoning
6. Evidence-based practice
7. Preventing, minimising and responding to adverse events
8. Infection prevention and control
9. Medication safety

The full PSCF document can be accessed at the end of the Prelims.

Source: Levett-Jones, T., Dwyer, T., Reid-Searl, K., Heaton, L., Flenady, T., Applegarth, J., Guinea, S. & Andersen, P. (2017). *Patient Safety Competency Framework (PSCF) for Nursing Students*. Sydney. Retrieved from http://psframework.wpengine.com/.

Australian Commission on Safety and Quality in Health Care's National Patient Safety Standards

These are included in the relevant chapters to link key content with key patient safety initiatives.

What's new in the fifth edition

A new section, *Essentials for Nurses: COVID-19*, has been included as an Appendix in the text. It provides relevant information on the pandemic in Australia. Where relevant, there are COVID-19 icons in the main text which show the reader that they should make reference to the COVID Primer in the Appendix.

Visual engagement and accuracy

The authors understand the importance of not only making the text visually engaging but also ensuring that any visual representations accurately reflect nursing in Australia. For this reason, the photographs featured in *LeMone and Burke's Medical–Surgical Nursing* have been carefully selected to ensure that they accurately depict Australian nursing equipment, uniforms, clinical settings, processes and procedures.

Guided tour

Key features of the Australian edition include:

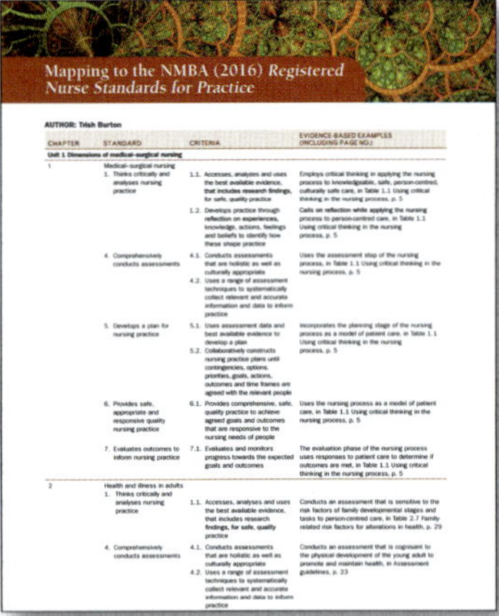

Mapping to the NMBA (2016) *Registered Nurse Standards for Practice*

AUTHOR: Trish Burton

CHAPTER	STANDARD	CRITERIA	EVIDENCE-BASED EXAMPLES (INCLUDING PAGE NO.)
Unit 1 Dimensions of medical-surgical nursing			
1	Medical–surgical nursing 1. Thinks critically and analyses nursing practice	1.1. Accesses, analyses and uses the best available evidence, that includes research findings, for safe, quality practice	Employs critical thinking in applying the nursing process to knowledgeable, safe, person-centred, culturally safe care, in Table 1.1 Using critical thinking in the nursing process, p. 5
		1.2. Develops practice through reflection on experiences, knowledge, actions, feelings and beliefs to identify how these shape practice	Calls on reflection while applying the nursing process to person-centred care, in Table 1.1 Using critical thinking in the nursing process, p. 5
	4. Comprehensively conducts assessments	4.1. Conducts assessments that are holistic as well as culturally appropriate 4.2. Uses a range of assessment techniques to systematically collect relevant and accurate information and data to inform practice	Uses the assessment step of the nursing process, in Table 1.1 Using critical thinking in the nursing process, p. 5
	5. Develops a plan for nursing practice	5.1. Uses assessment data and best available evidence to develop a plan 5.2. Collaboratively constructs nursing practice plans until contingencies, options, priorities, goals, actions, outcomes and time frames are agreed with the relevant people	Incorporates the planning stage of the nursing process as a model of patient care, in Table 1.1 Using critical thinking in the nursing process, p. 5
	6. Provides safe, appropriate and responsive quality nursing practice	6.1. Provides comprehensive, safe, quality practice to achieve agreed goals and outcomes that are responsive to the nursing needs of people	Uses the nursing process as a model of patient care, in Table 1.1 Using critical thinking in the nursing process, p. 5
	7. Evaluates outcomes to inform nursing practice	7.1. Evaluates and monitors progress towards the expected goals and outcomes	The evaluation phase of the nursing process uses responses to patient care to determine if outcomes are met, in Table 1.1 Using critical thinking in the nursing process, p. 5
2	Health and illness in adults 1. Thinks critically and analyses nursing practice	1.1. Accesses, analyses and uses the best available evidence, that includes research findings, for safe, quality practice	Conducts an assessment that is sensitive to the risk factors of family developmental stages and tasks to person-centred care, in Table 2.7 Family-related risk factors for alterations in health, p. 29
	4. Comprehensively conducts assessments	4.1. Conducts assessments that are holistic as well as culturally appropriate 4.2. Uses a range of assessment techniques to systematically collect relevant and accurate information and data to inform practice	Conducts an assessment that is cognisant to the physical development of the young adult to promote and maintain health, in Assessment guidelines, p. 23

Mapping to the NMBA (2016) ***Registered Nurse Standards for Practice*** *maps examples from the text to relevant* Registered Nurse Standards for Practice, *thereby aligning the content to contemporary professional practice in Australia.*

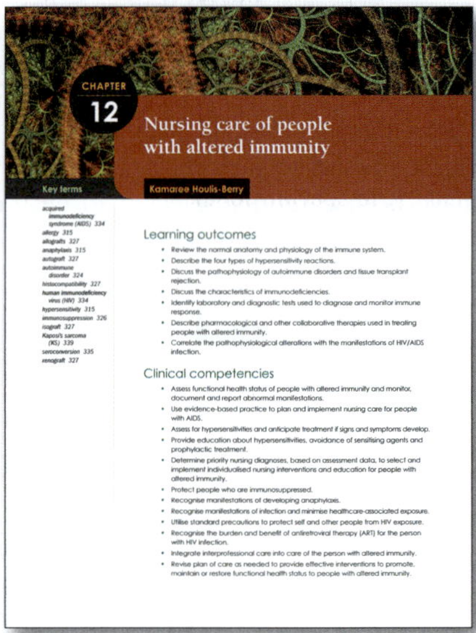

CHAPTER 12

Nursing care of people with altered immunity

Kamaree Houlis-Berry

Key terms

acquired immunodeficiency syndrome (AIDS) 334
allergy 315
allografts 327
anaphylaxis 315
autograft 327
autoimmune disorder 324
histocompatibility 327
human immunodeficiency virus (HIV) 334
hypersensitivity 315
immunosuppression 326
isograft 327
Kaposi's sarcoma (KS) 339
seroconversion 335
xenograft 327

Learning outcomes

- Review the normal anatomy and physiology of the immune system.
- Describe the four types of hypersensitivity reactions.
- Discuss the pathophysiology of autoimmune disorders and tissue transplant rejection.
- Discuss the characteristics of immunodeficiencies.
- Identify laboratory and diagnostic tests used to diagnose and monitor immune response.
- Describe pharmacological and other collaborative therapies used in treating people with altered immunity.
- Correlate the pathophysiological alterations with the manifestations of HIV/AIDS infection.

Clinical competencies

- Assess functional health status of people with altered immunity and monitor, document and report abnormal manifestations.
- Use evidence-based practice to plan and implement nursing care for people with AIDS.
- Assess for hypersensitivities and anticipate treatment if signs and symptoms develop.
- Provide education about hypersensitivities, avoidance of sensitising agents and prophylactic treatment.
- Determine priority nursing diagnoses, based on assessment data, to select and implement individualised nursing interventions and education for people with altered immunity.
- Protect people who are immunosuppressed.
- Recognise manifestations of developing anaphylaxis.
- Recognise manifestations of infection and minimise healthcare-associated exposure.
- Utilise standard precautions to protect self and other people from HIV exposure.
- Recognise the burden and benefit of antiretroviral therapy (ART) for the person with HIV infection.
- Integrate interprofessional care into care of the person with altered immunity.
- Revise plan of care as needed to provide effective interventions to promote, maintain or restore functional health status to people with altered immunity.

Learning Outcomes *show you the knowledge you'll gain, while*

Clinical Competencies *demonstrate how you will apply that knowledge.*

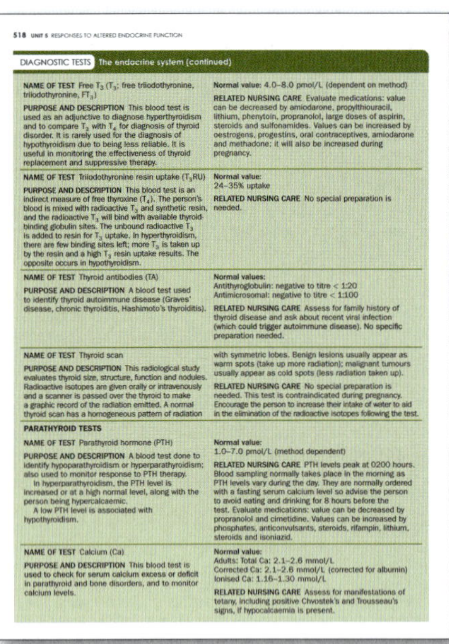

518 UNIT 5 RESPONSES TO ALTERED ENDOCRINE FUNCTION

DIAGNOSTIC TESTS The endocrine system (continued)

NAME OF TEST Free T_3 (T_3: free triiodothyronine, triiodothyronine, FT_3) **PURPOSE AND DESCRIPTION** This blood test is used as an adjunctive to diagnose hyperthyroidism and to compare T_3 with T_4 for diagnosis of thyroid disorder. It is rarely used for the diagnosis of hypothyroidism due to being less reliable. It is useful in monitoring the effectiveness of thyroid replacement and suppressive therapy.	**Normal value:** 4.0–8.0 pmol/L (dependent on method) **RELATED NURSING CARE** Evaluate medications: value can be decreased by amiodarone, propylthiouracil, lithium, phenytoin, propranolol, large doses of aspirin, steroids and sulfonamides. Values can be increased by oestrogens, progestins, oral contraceptives, amiodarone and methadone; it will also be increased during pregnancy.
NAME OF TEST Triiodothyronine resin uptake (T_3RU) **PURPOSE AND DESCRIPTION** This blood test is an indirect measure of free thyroxine (T_4). The person's blood is mixed with radioactive T_3 and synthetic resin, and the radioactive T_3 will bind with available thyroid-binding globulin sites. The unbound radioactive T_3 is added to resin for T_3 uptake. In hyperthyroidism, there are few binding sites left; more T_3 is taken up by the resin and a high T_3 resin uptake results. The opposite occurs in hypothyroidism.	**Normal value:** 24–35% uptake **RELATED NURSING CARE** No special preparation is needed.
NAME OF TEST Thyroid antibodies (TA) **PURPOSE AND DESCRIPTION** A blood test used to identify thyroid autoimmune disease (Graves' disease, chronic thyroiditis, Hashimoto's thyroiditis).	**Normal values:** Antithyroglobulin: negative to titre < 1:20 Antimicrosomal: negative to titre < 1:100 **RELATED NURSING CARE** Assess for family history of thyroid disease and ask about recent viral infection (which could trigger autoimmune disease). No specific preparation needed.
NAME OF TEST Thyroid scan **PURPOSE AND DESCRIPTION** This radiological study evaluates thyroid size, structure, function and nodules. Radioactive isotopes are given orally or intravenously and a scanner is passed over the thyroid to make a graphic record of the radiation emitted. A normal thyroid scan has a homogeneous pattern of radiation	with symmetric lobes. Benign lesions usually appear as warm spots (take up more radiation); malignant tumours usually appear as cold spots (less radiation taken up). **RELATED NURSING CARE** No special preparation is needed. This test is contraindicated during pregnancy. Encourage the person to increase their intake of water to aid in the elimination of the radioactive isotopes following the test.
PARATHYROID TESTS	
NAME OF TEST Parathyroid hormone (PTH) **PURPOSE AND DESCRIPTION** A blood test done to identify hypoparathyroidism or hyperparathyroidism; also used to monitor response to PTH therapy. In hyperparathyroidism, the PTH level is increased or at a high normal level, along with the person being hypercalcaemic. A low PTH level is associated with hypothyroidism.	**Normal value:** 1.0–7.0 pmol/L (method dependent) **RELATED NURSING CARE** PTH levels peak at 0200 hours. Blood sampling normally takes place in the morning as PTH levels vary during the day. They are normally ordered with a fasting serum calcium level so advise the person to avoid eating and drinking for 8 hours before the test. Evaluate medications: value can be decreased by propranolol and cimetidine. Values can be increased by phosphates, anticonvulsants, steroids, rifampin, lithium, steroids and isoniazid.
NAME OF TEST Calcium (Ca) **PURPOSE AND DESCRIPTION** This blood test is used to check for serum calcium excess or deficit in parathyroid and bone disorders, and to monitor calcium levels.	**Normal value:** Adults: Total Ca: 2.1–2.6 mmol/L Corrected Ca: 2.1–2.6 mmol/L (corrected for albumin) Ionised Ca: 1.16–1.30 mmol/L **RELATED NURSING CARE** Assess for manifestations of tetany, including positive Chvostek's and Trousseau's signs, if hypocalcaemia is present.

Diagnostic Tests *include diagnostic test tables and a narrative summary. The tables include the name of the test, the purpose and description of the test, and related nursing care.*

Pathophysiology Illustrated *art brings physiological processes to life.*

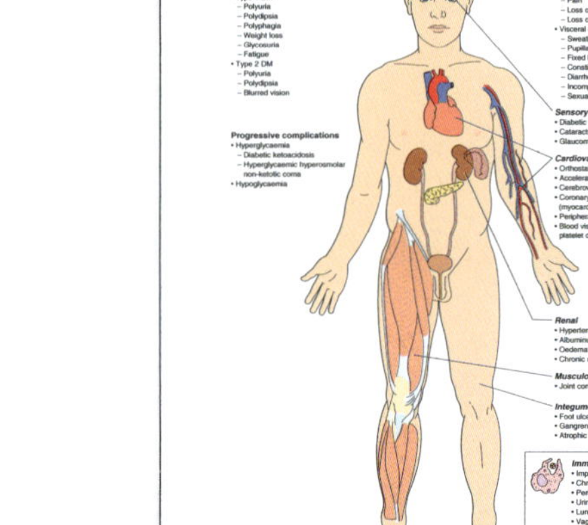

FOCUS ON CULTURAL DIVERSITY Diabetes in Aboriginal and Torres Strait Islander communities

Type 2 DM represents a serious public health problem for Aboriginal and Torres Strait Islander communities, occurring at a much higher rate than in the non-Indigenous population, and with a much earlier age of onset of the disease and its micro- and macrovascular complications. It is likely that type 2 DM is an important contributor to the considerably higher circulatory disease mortality rate among Aboriginal and Torres Strait Islander communities at younger ages. Thus, type 2 DM imposes significant financial and human costs on Australian society, which are disproportionately borne by Aboriginal and Torres Strait Islander communities.

The National Aboriginal and Torres Strait Islander Health Survey of 2018–2019 found that 8% of Aboriginal and Torres Strait Islander people reported they had DM (ABS, 2019), the most common being type 2 DM. The prevalence of DM is almost three higher in Aboriginal and Torres Strait Islander communities than in the rest of the population across all age groups. In 2021, diabetes was the second leading cause of death for Aboriginal and Torres Strait Islander people (ABS, 2022). The incidence of GDM in pregnancy is also two to three times higher among Aboriginal and Torres Strait Islander women than in the general Australian population. Living in remote areas also increases the prevalence rates for Aboriginal and Torres Strait Islander groups to six times higher than non-remote areas.

Focus on Cultural Diversity boxes *demonstrate how culture, age and gender produce differences in incidence, prevalence and mortality.*

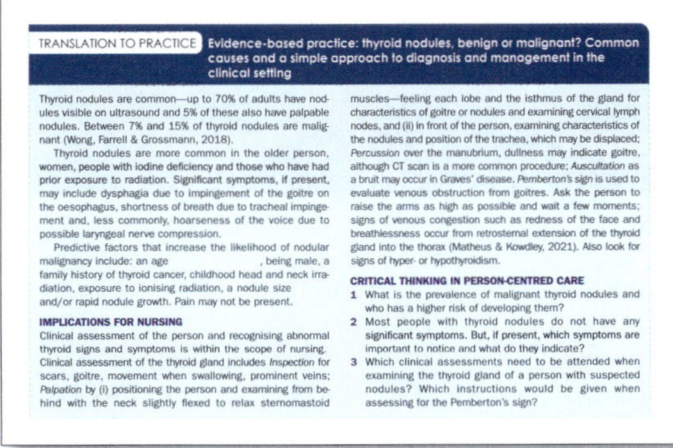

TRANSLATION TO PRACTICE **Evidence-based practice: thyroid nodules, benign or malignant? Common causes and a simple approach to diagnosis and management in the clinical setting**

Thyroid nodules are common—up to 70% of adults have nodules visible on ultrasound and 5% of these also have palpable nodules. Between 7% and 15% of thyroid nodules are malignant (Wong, Farrell & Grossmann, 2018).

Thyroid nodules are more common in the older person, women, people with iodine deficiency and those who have had prior exposure to radiation. Significant symptoms, if present, may include dysphagia due to impingement of the goitre on the oesophagus, shortness of breath due to tracheal impingement and, less commonly, hoarseness of the voice due to possible laryngeal nerve compression.

Predictive factors that increase the likelihood of nodular malignancy include: an age , being male, a family history of thyroid cancer, childhood head and neck irradiation, exposure to ionising radiation, a nodule size and/or rapid nodule growth. Pain may not be present.

IMPLICATIONS FOR NURSING

Clinical assessment of the person and recognising abnormal thyroid signs and symptoms is within the scope of nursing. Clinical assessment of the thyroid gland includes *Inspection* for scars, goitre, movement when swallowing, prominent veins; *Palpation* by (i) positioning the person and examining from behind with the neck slightly flexed to relax sternomastoid muscles—feeling each lobe and the isthmus of the gland for characteristics of goitre or nodules and examining cervical lymph nodes, and (ii) in front of the person, examining characteristics of the nodules and position of the trachea, which may be displaced; *Percussion* over the manubrium, dullness may indicate goitre, although CT scan is a more common procedure; *Auscultation* as a bruit may occur in Graves' disease. *Pemberton's sign* is used to evaluate venous obstruction from goitres. Ask the person to raise the arms as high as possible and wait a few moments; signs of venous congestion such as redness of the face and breathlessness occur from retrosternal extension of the thyroid gland into the thorax (Matheus & Kowdley, 2021). Also look for signs of hyper- or hypothyroidism.

CRITICAL THINKING IN PERSON-CENTRED CARE

1 What is the prevalence of malignant thyroid nodules and who has a higher risk of developing them?
2 Most people with thyroid nodules do not have any significant symptoms. But, if present, which symptoms are important to notice and what do they indicate?
3 Which clinical assessments need to be attended when examining the thyroid gland of a person with suspected nodules? Which instructions would be given when assessing for the Pemberton's sign?

Translation to Practice boxes *focus on how research relates to current nursing care and application of evidence in clinical settings.*

Nursing care

Health promotion

Because of the large stores of calcium in bones, most healthy adults have a very low risk of developing hypocalcaemia. However, a deficit of total body calcium is often associated with ageing, increasing the risk of osteoporosis, fractures and disability. Women have a higher risk of developing osteoporosis than men, due to lower bone density and hormonal influences. Educate women of all ages about the importance of maintaining adequate calcium intake through diet and, as needed, calcium supplements. Stress the relationship between weight-bearing exercise and bone density and encourage women to engage in a regular aerobic and weight-training exercise regimen. Discuss hormone replacement therapy and its potential benefits during and after menopause. See the chapter 'Nursing care of people with musculoskeletal disorders' for more information about osteoporosis.

inspiratory sound indicative of upper airway obstruction), or increased respiratory rate or effort, to the doctor. *These changes may indicate laryngeal spasm due to tetany.*

- Monitor cardiovascular status, including heart rate and rhythm, blood pressure and peripheral pulses. *Hypocalcaemia decreases myocardial contractility, causing reduced cardiac output and hypotension. It also can cause bradycardia or ventricular arrhythmias. Cardiac arrest may occur in severe hypocalcaemia.*
- Continuously monitor ECG in the person receiving intravenous calcium preparations, especially if the person also is taking digitalis. *Rapid administration of calcium salts can lead to hypercalcaemia and cardiac arrhythmias. Calcium administration increases the risk of digitalis toxicity and resultant arrhythmias.*
- Provide a quiet environment. Institute seizure precautions such as raising the side rails and keeping an airway at the bedside. *A quiet environment reduces central nervous system stimuli and the risk of convulsions in the person with tetany.*

Community-based care

In preparing the person with hypocalcaemia for discharge and home care, consider the circumstances leading to low serum

Nursing Care *sections detail the assessment and planning aspects relating to specific conditions and outline potential pain and risks.*

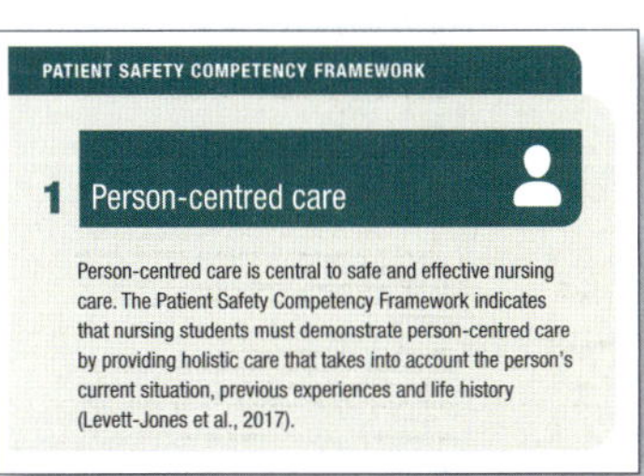

PATIENT SAFETY COMPETENCY FRAMEWORK

1 Person-centred care

Person-centred care is central to safe and effective nursing care. The Patient Safety Competency Framework indicates that nursing students must demonstrate person-centred care by providing holistic care that takes into account the person's current situation, previous experiences and life history (Levett-Jones et al., 2017).

Patient Safety Competency Framework *boxes appear in the chapters where applicable to demonstrate how concepts relate back to the skills and knowledge that underpin patient safety.*

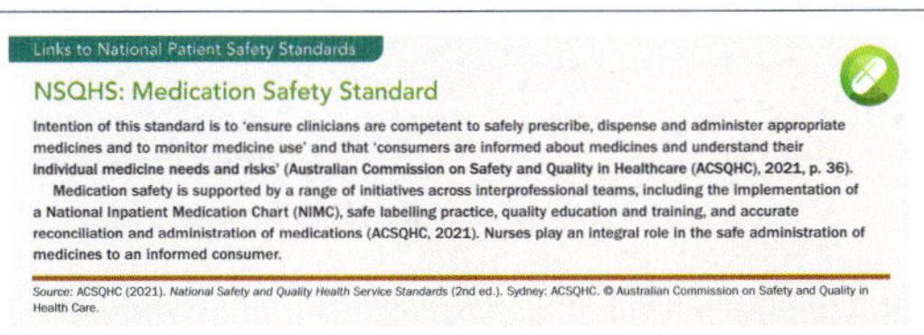

Links to National Patient Safety Standards

NSQHS: Medication Safety Standard

Intention of this standard is to 'ensure clinicians are competent to safely prescribe, dispense and administer appropriate medicines and to monitor medicine use' and that 'consumers are informed about medicines and understand their individual medicine needs and risks' (Australian Commission on Safety and Quality in Healthcare (ACSQHC), 2021, p. 36).

Medication safety is supported by a range of initiatives across interprofessional teams, including the implementation of a National Inpatient Medication Chart (NIMC), safe labelling practice, quality education and training, and accurate reconciliation and administration of medications (ACSQHC, 2021). Nurses play an integral role in the safe administration of medicines to an informed consumer.

Source: ACSQHC (2021). *National Safety and Quality Health Service Standards* (2nd ed.). Sydney: ACSQHC. © Australian Commission on Safety and Quality in Health Care.

Links to National Patient Safety Standards *boxes appear in the chapters where applicable to demonstrate how concepts relate back to patient safety standards.*

FAST FACTS

- Older people have the highest rate of illness and surgical procedures associated with pain; they also have the highest rate of complications associated with surgical interventions.
- Persistent pain is common in older adults. For those over 70 years of age, 50% of those living in the community and 80% of those in residential care suffer persistent pain.
- Musculoskeletal pain affecting major joints and back, or neuropathic pain from diabetic neuropathy and post-herpetic neuralgia have an increased prevalence in the ageing population.
- Concurrent illnesses are common in the elderly, making clinical presentation complex and sometimes difficult.
- Cognitive impairment enhances the risk of poor pain control, negatively influencing the individual's quality of life.

Sources: ANZCA (2020). *Acute pain management: Scientific evidence* (5th ed.). Melbourne: Australian and New Zealand College of Anaesthetists; Youngcharoen (2022). A cross-sectional study of factors associated with nurses' postoperative pain management practices for older patients. *Nursing Open*. https://doi.org/10.1002/nop2.1281

Fast Facts boxes *highlight and summarise important data about the prevalence and incidence of selected disorders in Australia, and of other featured content.*

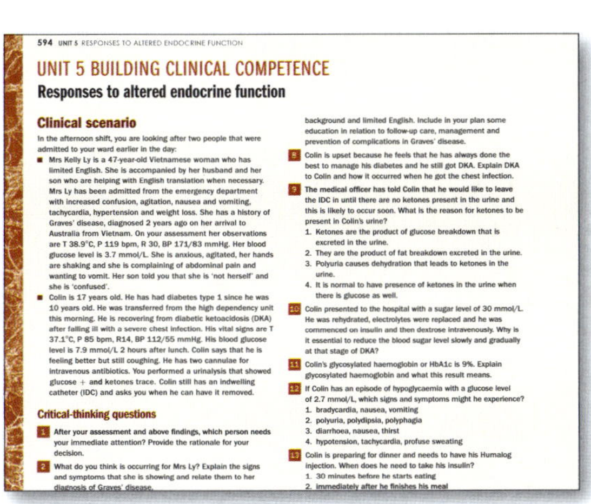

594 UNIT 5 RESPONSES TO ALTERED ENDOCRINE FUNCTION

UNIT 5 BUILDING CLINICAL COMPETENCE

Responses to altered endocrine function

Clinical scenario

In the afternoon shift, you are looking after two people that were admitted to your ward earlier in the day:

- Mrs Kelly Ly is a 47-year-old Vietnamese woman who has limited English. She is accompanied by her husband and her son who are helping with English translation when necessary. Mrs Ly has been admitted from the emergency department with increased confusion, agitation, nausea and vomiting, tachycardia, hypertension and weight loss. She has a history of Graves' disease, diagnosed 2 years ago on her arrival to Australia from Vietnam. On your assessment her observations are T 38.9°C, P 119 bpm, R 30, BP 171/83 mmHg. Her blood glucose level is 3.7 mmol/L. She is anxious, agitated, her hands are shaking and she is complaining of abdominal pain and wanting to vomit. Her son told you that she is 'not herself' and she is 'confused'.
- Colin is 17 years old. He has had diabetes type 1 since he was 10 years old. He was transferred from the high dependency unit this morning. He is recovering from diabetic ketoacidosis (DKA) after falling ill with a severe chest infection. His vital signs are T 37.1°C, P 85 bpm, R14, BP 112/55 mmHg. His blood glucose level is 7.9 mmol/L 2 hours after lunch. Colin says that he is feeling better but still coughing. He has two cannulae for intravenous antibiotics. You performed a urinalysis that showed glucose + and ketones trace. Colin still has an indwelling catheter (IDC) and asks you when he can have it removed.

Critical-thinking questions

1 After your assessment and above findings, which person needs your immediate attention? Provide the rationale for your decision.

2 What do you think is occurring for Mrs Ly? Explain the signs and symptoms that she is showing and relate them to her diagnosis of Graves' disease.

background and limited English. Include in your plan some education in relation to follow-up care, management and prevention of complications in Graves' disease.

8 Colin is upset because he feels that he has always done the best to manage his diabetes and he still got DKA. Explain DKA to Colin and how it occurred when he got the chest infection.

9 The medical officer has told Colin that he would like to leave the IDC in until there are no ketones present in the urine and this is likely to occur soon. What is the reason for ketones to be present in Colin's urine?
1. Ketones are the product of glucose breakdown that is excreted in the urine.
2. They are the product of fat breakdown excreted in the urine.
3. Polyuria causes dehydration that leads to ketones in the urine.
4. It is normal to have presence of ketones in the urine when there is glucose as well.

10 Colin presented to the hospital with a sugar level of 30 mmol/L. He was rehydrated, electrolytes were replaced and he was commenced on insulin and then dextrose intravenously. Why is it essential to reduce the blood sugar level slowly and gradually at that stage of DKA?

11 Colin's glycosylated haemoglobin or HbA1c is 9%. Explain glycosylated haemoglobin and what this result means.

12 If Colin has an episode of hypoglycaemia with a glucose level of 2.7 mmol/L, which signs and symptoms might he experience?
1. bradycardia, nausea, vomiting
2. polyuria, polydipsia, polyphagia
3. diarrhoea, nausea, thirst
4. hypotension, tachycardia, profuse sweating

13 Colin is preparing for dinner and needs to have his Humalog injection. When does he need to take his insulin?
1. 30 minutes before he starts eating
2. immediately after he finishes his meal

An end-of-unit review for each of the units, called **Building Clinical Competence**, *synthesises what you have learned in the unit and applies the knowledge to specific cases. The feature includes:*

- *A* **clinical scenario** *involving a priority issue reflection piece that synthesises the underlying concepts and includes a variety of questions that allow students to apply different skills.*
- *A* **case study** *with concept map that further synthesises material using the nursing process.*

Educator support

A suite of resources is provided to assist with delivery of the text, as well as to support teaching and learning.

Solutions Manual

The Solutions Manual provides educators with detailed, accuracy-verified solutions to in-chapter and end-of-chapter problems in the text.

Test Bank

The Test Bank provides a wealth of accuracy-verified testing material. Updated for the new edition, each chapter offers a wide variety of question types, arranged by learning objective and tagged by NMBA Standards.

Questions can be integrated into Blackboard, Canvas and Moodle Learning Management Systems.

Digital Image Powerpoint slides

All the diagrams and tables from the text are available for lecturer use.

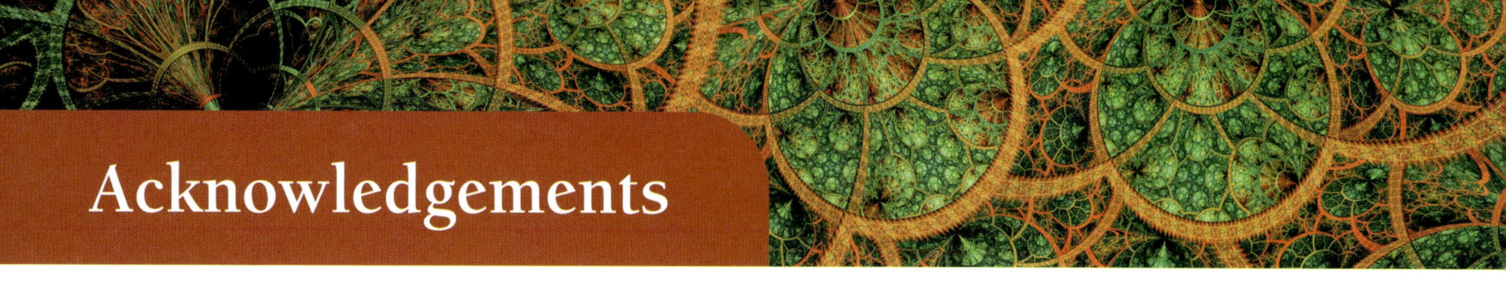

Acknowledgements

A collaborative adventure

LeMone and Burke's Medical–Surgical Nursing: Critical Thinking for Person-centred Care, fifth Australian edition, is the result of an exciting and productive collaboration between academic staff and clinicians across Australia. Authors and reviewers alike have been generous in sharing their expertise and crafting a text that is uniquely Australian and directly relevant to contemporary practice. The following people are to be acknowledged for carefully reviewing the chapters and providing a thoughtful and constructive critique:

Academic reviewers

Nitasha Narayan, Notre Dame University

Lyn Taylor, Australian Catholic University

Rachel Euler, CQUniversity

Renee Stone, Griffith University

Katherine Riley, University of Wollongong

We would also like to thank Trish Burton for updating the Mapping to the NMBA Registered Nurse Standards for Practice.

We also thank the editorial team at Pearson, including Mandy Sheppard, our Senior Commercial Product Manager; Anna Carter, our Development Editor; Samantha Russell-Tulip, Rights and Permissions Editor; Linda Chryssavgis, Content Producer; and Katie Millar, Copy Editor.

Tracy Levett-Jones, Lorna Moxham, Kerry Reid-Searl, Kamaree Houlis-Berry, Keryln Carville, Majella Hales, David Stanley, Sharon Stanton, Tanya Lantgree, Elspeth Hillman

Mapping to the NMBA (2016) *Registered Nurse Standards for Practice*

AUTHOR: Trish Burton

CHAPTER	STANDARD	CRITERIA	EVIDENCE-BASED EXAMPLES (INCLUDING PAGE NO.)
Unit 1 Dimensions of medical–surgical nursing			
1 Medical–surgical nursing	1. Thinks critically and analyses nursing practice	1.1. Accesses, analyses and uses the best available evidence, that includes research findings, for safe, quality practice	Employs critical thinking in applying the nursing process to knowledgeable, safe, person-centred, culturally safe care, in Table 1.1 Using critical thinking in the nursing process, p. 5
		1.2. Develops practice through reflection on experiences, knowledge, actions, feelings and beliefs to identify how these shape practice	Calls on reflection while applying the nursing process to person-centred care, in Table 1.1 Using critical thinking in the nursing process, p. 5
	4. Comprehensively conducts assessments	4.1. Conducts assessments that are holistic as well as culturally appropriate 4.2. Uses a range of assessment techniques to systematically collect relevant and accurate information and data to inform practice	Uses the assessment step of the nursing process, in Table 1.1 Using critical thinking in the nursing process, p. 5
	5. Develops a plan for nursing practice	5.1. Uses assessment data and best available evidence to develop a plan 5.2. Collaboratively constructs nursing practice plans until contingencies, options, priorities, goals, actions, outcomes and time frames are agreed with the relevant people	Incorporates the planning stage of the nursing process as a model of patient care, in Table 1.1 Using critical thinking in the nursing process, p. 5
	6. Provides safe, appropriate and responsive quality nursing practice	6.1. Provides comprehensive, safe, quality practice to achieve agreed goals and outcomes that are responsive to the nursing needs of people	Uses the nursing process as a model of patient care, in Table 1.1 Using critical thinking in the nursing process, p. 5
	7. Evaluates outcomes to inform nursing practice	7.1. Evaluates and monitors progress towards the expected goals and outcomes	The evaluation phase of the nursing process uses responses to patient care to determine if outcomes are met, in Table 1.1 Using critical thinking in the nursing process, p. 5
2 Health and illness in adults	1. Thinks critically and analyses nursing practice	1.1. Accesses, analyses and uses the best available evidence, that includes research findings, for safe, quality practice	Conducts an assessment that is sensitive to the risk factors of family developmental stages and tasks to person-centred care, in Table 2.7 Family-related risk factors for alterations in health, p. 29
	4. Comprehensively conducts assessments	4.1. Conducts assessments that are holistic as well as culturally appropriate	Conducts an assessment that is cognisant to the physical development of the young adult to promote and maintain health, in Assessment guidelines, p. 23
		4.2. Uses a range of assessment techniques to systematically collect relevant and accurate information and data to inform practice	Conducts an assessment that addresses the physical changes in the middle adult years to detect cancer and promote, restore and maintain health, in Assessment guidelines, p. 25

CHAPTER	STANDARD	CRITERIA	EVIDENCE-BASED EXAMPLES (INCLUDING PAGE NO.)
			Conducts an assessment that is sensitive to the physical changes in the older adult years to promote, restore and maintain health, in Assessment guidelines, p. 27
Unit 2 Alterations in patterns of health			
3 Nursing care of people having surgery	1. Thinks critically and analyses nursing practice	1.1. Accesses, analyses and uses the best available evidence, that includes research findings, for safe, quality practice	Addresses patient safety by identifying risks and providing targeted nursing care, in Table 3.2 Nursing implications for surgical risk factors, p. 36
			Patient safety of the older adult in the postoperative phase is promoted by targeted nursing interventions to prevent complications, in Table 3.7 Nursing interventions for older people having surgery, p. 60
		1.4. Complies with legislation, regulations, policies, guidelines and other standards or requirements relevant to the context of practice when making decisions	Recognises laboratory test values as part of patient safety in the perioperative phase, in Table 3.4 Laboratory tests for perioperative assessment, p. 39
			Complies with the legal requirement of patient safety in the preoperative phase by identifying medication management implications, in Table 3.5 Preoperative medications, p. 41
		1.5. Uses ethical frameworks when making decisions	Is aware of advocate role in relation to person-informed consent, in Legal requirements, p. 35
	2. Engages in therapeutic and professional relationships	2.5. Advocates on behalf of people in a manner that respects the person's autonomy and legal capacity	Facilitates informed consent for the person, in Legal requirements, p. 35
		2.6. Uses delegation, supervision, coordination, consultation and referrals in professional relationships to achieve improved health outcomes	In collaboration with the surgeon and dietitian, promotes weight gain for a malnourished person, in Table 3.2 Nursing implications for surgical risk factors, p. 36
			Notifies anaesthetist of all prescribed and over-the-counter drugs as surgical risk factors in care of the person, in Table 3.2 Nursing implications for surgical risk factors, p. 36
			Works with the surgeon to maintain patient safety in the preoperative phase by implementing glycaemic control for the person with diabetes, in Consideration for practice, p. 38
			Notifies surgeon of abnormal urinalysis findings, in Table 3.4 Laboratory tests for perioperative assessment, p. 39
			Promotes patient safety in the preoperative phase by working with the surgeon, anaesthetist and pain team to implement pain control for the person in the postoperative period, in Consideration for practice, p. 43
	4. Comprehensively conducts assessments	4.1. Conducts assessments that are holistic as well as culturally appropriate	Considers the assessment required for surgical risk factors in person-centred care, in Table 3.2 Nursing implications for surgical risk factors, p. 36
		4.2. Uses a range of assessment techniques to systematically collect relevant and accurate information and data to inform practice	Identifies risks of abnormal laboratory test results and provides targeted nursing care, in Table 3.4 Laboratory tests for perioperative assessment, p. 39
			Patient safety in the preoperative phase includes identifying medication management implications, in Table 3.5 Preoperative medications, p. 41

CHAPTER	STANDARD	CRITERIA	EVIDENCE-BASED EXAMPLES (INCLUDING PAGE NO.)
	5. Develops a plan for nursing practice	5.1. Uses assessment data and best available evidence to develop a plan	Plans for the nursing implications for surgical risk factors in person-centred care, in Table 3.2 Nursing implications for surgical risk factors, p. 36 Devises a teaching plan for the person in the postoperative phase to prepare them for discharge, in Community-based care, p. 60
	6. Provides safe, appropriate and responsive quality nursing practice	6.1. Provides comprehensive, safe, quality practice to achieve agreed goals and outcomes that are responsive to the nursing needs of people	Implements appropriate nursing interventions, in Table 3.2 Nursing implications for surgical risk factors, p. 36 Complies with the legal requirement of patient safety in the preoperative phase by identifying risks and providing targeted nursing care, in Table 3.4 Laboratory tests for perioperative assessment, p. 39 Adheres to safety guidelines and completes checklists in the preoperative phase, in Links to National Patient Safety Standards, NSQHS Communicating for Safety Standard, p. 53 Nursing interventions are in response to the older adult having an increased risk of complications in the postoperative period, in Table 3.7 Nursing interventions for older people having surgery, p. 60
	7. Evaluates outcomes to inform nursing practice	7.1. Evaluates and monitors progress towards the expected goals and outcomes	Evaluates patient responses to medications, inTable 3.5 Preoperative medications, p. 41 Evaluates interventions to reduce the increased risk of complications in the postoperative period, in Table 3.4 Laboratory tests for perioperative assessment, p. 39, Table 3.7 Nursing interventions for older people having surgery, p. 60
4 Nursing care of people experiencing loss, grief and death	2. Engages in therapeutic and professional relationships	2.2. Communicates effectively and is respectful of a person's dignity, culture, values, beliefs and rights	Promotes trust in the therapeutic relationship with the person experiencing loss and grief, in Nursing care plan, p. 80
	4. Comprehensively conducts assessments	4.1. Conducts assessments that are holistic as well as culturally appropriate	Makes assessments for appropriate nursing interventions, in Box 4.3 Providing comfort for the person nearing death, p. 74 Provides comprehensive nursing care for the person experiencing loss and grief, in Nursing care plan, p. 80
	5. Develops a plan for nursing practice	5.1. Uses assessment data and best available evidence to develop a plan	Plans for appropriate nursing interventions, in Box 4.3 Providing comfort for the person nearing death, p. 74 Devises a teaching plan for individuals and families who will experience loss, in Meeting individualised needs, p.78 Plans for comprehensive nursing care for the person experiencing loss and grief, in Nursing care plan, p. 80

CHAPTER	STANDARD	CRITERIA	EVIDENCE-BASED EXAMPLES (INCLUDING PAGE NO.)
	6. Provides safe, appropriate and responsive quality nursing practice	6.1. Provides comprehensive, safe, quality practice to achieve agreed goals and outcomes that are responsive to the nursing needs of people	Implements appropriate nursing interventions, in Box 4.3 Providing comfort for the person nearing death, p. 74 Provides comprehensive nursing care for the person experiencing loss and grief, in Nursing care plan, p. 80
	7. Evaluates outcomes to inform nursing practice	7.1. Evaluates and monitors progress towards the expected goals and outcomes	Evaluates appropriate nursing interventions, in Box 4.3 Providing comfort for the person nearing death, p. 74 Evaluates comprehensive nursing care for the person experiencing loss and grief, in Nursing care plan, p. 80
5 Nursing care of people with substance misuse problems	1. Thinks critically and analyses nursing practice	1.1. Accesses, analyses, and uses the best available evidence, that includes research findings, for safe, quality practice	Uses evidence-based research to plan and implement nursing care for people experiencing withdrawal symptoms of tobacco use, in Box 5.1 Management of alcohol withdrawal in hospital, p. 97
	2. Engages in therapeutic and professional relationships	2.6. Uses delegation, supervision, coordination, consultation and referrals in professional relationships to achieve improved health outcomes	As part of collaborative care, consults and plans interventions in conjunction with the doctor for alcohol withdrawal, in Box 5.1 Management of alcohol withdrawal in hospital, p. 97 Refers person to healthcare professionals to assist with nicotine withdrawal, in Table 5.5 Guide for the management of nicotine-dependent inpatients, p. 98
	4. Comprehensively conducts assessments	4.1. Conducts assessments that are holistic as well as culturally appropriate	Assesses for alcohol withdrawal, in Box 5.1 Management of alcohol withdrawal in hospital, p. 97 Assesses for nicotine withdrawal, in Table 5.5 Guide for the management of nicotine-dependent inpatients, p. 98
	5. Develops a plan for nursing practice	5.2. Collaboratively constructs nursing practice plans until contingencies, options, priorities, goals, actions, outcomes and time frames are agreed with the relevant people	Plans specific interventions for alcohol withdrawal, in Box 5.1 Management of alcohol withdrawal in hospital, p. 97 Plans interventions for nicotine withdrawal, in Table 5.5 Guide for the management of nicotine-dependent inpatients, p. 98
	6. Provides safe, appropriate and responsive quality nursing practice	6.1. Provides comprehensive, safe, quality practice to achieve agreed goals and outcomes that are responsive to the nursing needs of people	Provides needs-specific nursing interventions for alcohol abuse and medical conditions, in Box 5.1 Management of alcohol withdrawal in hospital, p. 97 Provides interventions for nicotine withdrawal, in Table 5.5 Guide for the management of nicotine-dependent inpatients, p. 98
	7. Evaluates outcomes to inform nursing practice	7.1. Evaluates and monitors progress towards the expected goals and outcomes	Evaluates interventions for alcohol withdrawal, in Box 5.1 Management of alcohol withdrawal in hospital, p. 97 Evaluates interventions for nicotine withdrawal, in Table 5.5 Guide for the management of nicotine-dependent inpatients, p. 98
6 Nursing care of people in the emergency department or experiencing disasters	2. Engages in therapeutic and professional relationships	2.6. Uses delegation, supervision, coordination, consultation and referrals in professional relationships to achieve improved health outcomes	Organises orthopaedic review for management of limb fractures for the person with trauma, in Nursing care plan, p. 120

CHAPTER	STANDARD	CRITERIA	EVIDENCE-BASED EXAMPLES (INCLUDING PAGE NO.)
	4. Comprehensively conducts assessments	4.2. Uses a range of assessment techniques to systematically collect relevant and accurate information and data to inform practice	Assesses the person with trauma, in Nursing care plan, p. 120
	5. Develops a plan for nursing practice	5.2. Collaboratively constructs nursing practice plans until contingencies, options, priorities, goals, actions, outcomes and time frames are agreed with the relevant people	Provides comprehensive nursing care for a person with trauma, in Nursing care plan, p. 120
		5.5. Coordinates resources effectively and efficiently for planned actions	In the disaster setting, plans the use of resources, in Table 6.3 Disaster triage system, by category, p. 110
	6. Provides safe, appropriate and responsive quality nursing practice	6.1. Provides comprehensive, safe, quality practice to achieve agreed goals and outcomes that are responsive to the nursing needs of people	Provides comprehensive nursing care for a person with trauma, in Nursing care plan, p. 120
	7. Evaluates outcomes to inform nursing practice	7.1. Evaluates and monitors progress towards the expected goals and outcomes	Evaluates comprehensive nursing care for a person with trauma, in Nursing care plan, p. 120
Unit 3 Pathophysiology and patterns of health			
7 Genetic implications of adult health nursing	4. Comprehensively conducts assessments	4.1. Conducts assessments that are holistic as well as culturally appropriate	Conducts a health assessment and maps pedigree, in Box 7.11 Adult indicators for a referral to a genetic specialist, p. 145 Assesses cultural and religious beliefs of genetic concepts for people and their families, in Education, pp. 146–147
	5. Develops a plan for nursing practice	5.2. Collaboratively constructs nursing practice plans until contingencies, options, priorities, goals, actions, outcomes and time frames are agreed with the relevant people	Develops a nursing care plan, in Box 7.11 Adult indicators for a referral to a genetic specialist, p. 145 Develops a nursing care plan, including integrating genetic concepts into education for people and their families, in Education, pp. 146–147
	6. Provides safe, appropriate and responsive quality nursing practice	6.1. Provides comprehensive, safe, quality practice to achieve agreed goals and outcomes that are responsive to the nursing needs of people	Delivers nursing care, in Box 7.11 Adult indicators for a referral to a genetic specialist, p. 145, and Education, pp. 146–147
	7. Evaluates outcomes to inform nursing practice	7.1. Evaluates and monitors progress towards the expected goals and outcomes	Evaluates a nursing care plan, in Box 7.11 Adult indicators for a referral to a genetic specialist, p. 145, and Education, pp. 146–147
8 Nursing care of people in pain	1. Thinks critically and analyses nursing practice	1.5. Uses ethical frameworks when making decisions	Ensures the person is an active participant in planning nursing care for their persistent pain, in Nursing care plan, p. 172
	2. Engages in therapeutic and professional relationships	2.2. Communicates effectively and is respectful of a person's dignity, culture, values, beliefs and rights	Conducts education to promote pain relief, in Medication administration, p. 163 Conducts education to familiarise the person with pain control methods, in Nursing care plan, p. 172

CHAPTER	STANDARD	CRITERIA	EVIDENCE-BASED EXAMPLES (INCLUDING PAGE NO.)
		2.6. Uses delegation, supervision, coordination, consultation and referrals in professional relationships to achieve improved health outcomes	In collaboration with the doctor, determines appropriate non-opioid analgesic, in Nursing care plan, p. 172
	4. Comprehensively conducts assessments	4.1. Conducts assessments that are holistic as well as culturally appropriate	Conducts assessments as part of medication management, in Medication administration, p.163 Conducts a nursing assessment for pain, in Nursing care plan, p. 171
	5. Develops a plan for nursing practice	5.1. Uses assessment data and best available evidence to develop a plan	Plans for administering medication safely and effectively, in Medication administration, p. 163
		5.2. Collaboratively constructs nursing practice plans until contingencies, options, priorities, goals, actions, outcomes and time frames are agreed with the relevant people	Develops a nursing care plan for pain management, in Nursing care plan, p. 172
		5.3. Documents, evaluates and modifies plans accordingly to facilitate the agreed outcomes	Revises plan of care according to the person's response to interventions and need for control, in Nursing care plan, p. 172
	6. Provides safe, appropriate and responsive quality nursing practice	6.1. Provides comprehensive, safe, quality practice to achieve agreed goals and outcomes that are responsive to the nursing needs of people	Administers medication safely and effectively, in Medication administration, p. 163 Administers medication safely and effectively, in Nursing care plan, p. 172 Implements nursing care plan for persistent pain management, in Nursing care plan, p. 172
	7. Evaluates outcomes to inform nursing practice	7.1. Evaluates and monitors progress towards the expected goals and outcomes	Evaluates effectiveness of pain medication, in Medication administration, p. 163 Evaluates the person's response to pain relief measures throughout the nursing process, in Nursing care plan, p. 172
9 Nursing care of people with altered fluid, electrolyte and acid–base balance	2. Engages in therapeutic and professional relationships	2.2. Communicates effectively and is respectful of a person's dignity, culture, values, beliefs and rights	Employs effective communication processes to facilitate education of the person with fluid volume excess, in Nursing care plan, p. 194
	4. Comprehensively conducts assessments	4.1. Conducts assessments that are holistic as well as culturally appropriate	When caring for a person with hyperkalaemia, carries out the processes involved in the assessment phase that specifically address the multidisciplinary team, in Nursing care plan, p. 209 Conducts assessment of a person with respiratory acidosis, in Nursing care plan, p. 234

CHAPTER	STANDARD	CRITERIA	EVIDENCE-BASED EXAMPLES (INCLUDING PAGE NO.)
	5. Develops a plan for nursing practice	5.2. Collaboratively constructs nursing practice plans until contingencies, options, priorities, goals, actions, outcomes and time frames are agreed with the relevant people	Devises a teaching plan for the person with a fluid volume deficit, in Community-based care, p. 191 Devises a teaching plan for diuretic administration, which includes a healthy diet, in Medication administration, p. 193 Plans comprehensive nursing care for a person with hypokalaemia, in Nursing care plan, p. 205 Determines priority nursing diagnosis, based on assessment data, to select and implement individualised nursing interventions for hyperkalaemia, in Nursing care plan, p. 209 Determines priority nursing diagnosis, based on assessment data, for individualised nursing interventions for respiratory acidosis, in Nursing care plan, p. 234
	6. Provides safe, appropriate and responsive quality nursing practice	6.1. Provides comprehensive, safe, quality practice to achieve agreed goals and outcomes that are responsive to the nursing needs of people	Delivers focused nursing care for a person with a fluid deficit, in Box 9.3 Fluid restriction guidelines, p. 192 Delivers a teaching plan for diuretic administration, in Medication administration, p. 193 Implements nursing care plan for fluid volume excess management, in Nursing care plan, p. 194 Monitors urine output and positive fluid balance to prevent complications, in Consideration for practice, p. 195 Monitors vital signs, CVP, heart sounds and lung sounds to prevent complications during the administration of hypertonic saline, in Consideration for practice, p. 198 Administers fluids and medications knowledgeably and safely for hypokalaemia, in Medication administration, p. 204 When caring for a person with hypokalaemia, carries out the processes involved in the implementation phase that specifically address the person's needs, in Nursing care plan, p. 205 When caring for a person with hyperkalaemia, carries out the processes involved in the intervention phase that specifically address the multidisciplinary team and nutrition, in Nursing care plan, p. 209 Administers calcium salts medications knowledgeably and safely, and provides health education, in Medication administration, p. 213 Administers magnesium sulphate knowledgeably and safely, in Medication administration, p. 218 When caring for a person with respiratory acidosis, monitoring physiological parameters indicates responses to care, in Nursing care plan, p. 234

CHAPTER	STANDARD	CRITERIA	EVIDENCE-BASED EXAMPLES (INCLUDING PAGE NO.)
	7. Evaluates outcomes to inform nursing practice	7.1. Evaluates and monitors progress towards the expected goals and outcomes	Evaluates responses to nursing interventions for fluid volume excess, in Nursing care plan, p. 194 Evaluates responses to nursing interventions for hypokalaemia, in Medication administration, p. 205 Evaluates individualised nursing care for the person with hyperkalaemia, in Nursing care plan, p. 209 Evaluates assessment findings and monitors progress of respiratory acidosis, in Nursing care plan, p. 234
		7.3. Determines, documents and communicates further priorities, goals and outcomes with the relevant persons.	Reports low urine output, in Consideration for practice, p. 195 Communicates nursing assessment of serum potassium levels and ECG findings in relation to hyperkalaemia to the doctor, in Nursing care plan, p. 209 Establishes additional goals in relation to assessment findings and monitors progress of respiratory acidosis, in Nursing care plan, p. 234
10 Nursing care of people experiencing trauma and shock	4. Comprehensively conducts assessments	4.2. Uses a range of assessment techniques to systematically collect relevant and accurate information and data to inform practice	Conducts assessment of a person with multi-trauma within the emergency department, in Nursing care plan, pp. 253–254 Conducts assessment of a person with septic shock, in Nursing care plan, p. 269
	5. Develops a plan for nursing practice	5.1. Uses assessment data and best available evidence to develop a plan	Devises a plan for a blood transfusion, to ensure safe administration, in Medication administration, p. 251 Determines priority nursing diagnosis, based on assessment data, and plans comprehensive nursing care for a person with multi-trauma within the emergency department, in Nursing care plan, pp. 253–254 Devises a plan for the infusion of colloid solutions, in Medication administration, p. 266 Determines priority nursing diagnosis, based on assessment data, and plans comprehensive nursing care for a person with septic shock, in Nursing care plan, p. 269
	6. Provides safe, appropriate and responsive quality nursing practice	6.1. Provides comprehensive, safe, quality practice to achieve agreed goals and outcomes that are responsive to the nursing needs of people	Administers the blood transfusion and monitors the individual's reaction, in Medication administration, p. 251 Demonstrates comprehensive nursing care for a person with multi-trauma within the emergency department, in Nursing care plan, pp. 253–254 Administers colloid solutions and monitors the individual's reaction, in Medication administration, p. 266 Demonstrates comprehensive nursing care for a person with septic shock, in Nursing care plan, p. 269

CHAPTER	STANDARD	CRITERIA	EVIDENCE-BASED EXAMPLES (INCLUDING PAGE NO.)
	7. Evaluates outcomes to inform nursing practice	7.1. Evaluates and monitors progress towards the expected goals and outcomes	Evaluates response to medical and nursing interventions for the person with multi-trauma, in Nursing care plan, p. 254
			Evaluates assessment findings and monitors progress of septic shock, in Nursing care plan, p. 269
		7.3. Determines, documents and communicates further priorities, goals and outcomes with the relevant persons	Communicates abnormal assessment findings in relation to blood administration to the doctor, in Medication administration, p. 251
			Establishes additional goals in relation to assessment findings and monitors progress of the person with multi-trauma, in Nursing care plan, p. 254
			Communicates abnormal assessment findings in relation to the administration of colloids to the doctor, in Medication administration, p. 266
11 Nursing care of people with infections	2. Engages in therapeutic and professional relationships	2.6. Uses delegation, supervision, coordination, consultation and referrals in professional relationships to achieve improved health outcomes	Conducts education for taking antibiotic medication for an infection, which includes the person notifying the care provider about adverse effects, in Medication administration, pp. 303–306
	4. Comprehensively conducts assessments	4.1. Conducts assessments that are holistic as well as culturally appropriate	When caring for a person who requires immunisation, carries out the processes involved in the assessment, that specifically address the person's needs, in Nursing care plan, p. 290
			Assesses for a history of hypersensitivity to antibiotics, in Medication administration, pp. 303–306
	5. Develops a plan for nursing practice	5.1. Uses assessment data and best available evidence to develop a plan	Determines nursing diagnosis, based on assessment data, to select and implement nursing interventions for immunisation, in Nursing care plan, p. 290
			Devises a teaching plan for the person with wound healing, in Community-based care, p. 296
			Devises a teaching plan for the person with an infection, in Community-based care, pp. 309–310
		5.4. Plans and negotiates how practice will be evaluated and the time frame of engagement 5.5. Coordinates resources effectively and efficiently for planned actions	Plans for antibiotic administration, which includes fluid dilution, length of administration and compatibility with other medications, in Medication administration, pp. 303–306
	6. Provides safe, appropriate and responsive quality nursing practice	6.1. Provides comprehensive, safe, quality practice to achieve agreed goals and outcomes that are responsive to the nursing needs of people	When caring for a person who requires immunisation, carries out the processes involved in the implementation phase that specifically address the person's needs, in Nursing care plan, p. 290
			At the intervention stage, monitors the response of the person for adverse effects, including administration site and allergic reactions, and laboratory results, with targeted health education, in Medication administration, pp. 303–306

CHAPTER	STANDARD	CRITERIA	EVIDENCE-BASED EXAMPLES (INCLUDING PAGE NO.)
	7. Evaluates outcomes to inform nursing practice	7.1. Evaluates and monitors progress towards the expected goals and outcomes	Evaluates the person's responses to immunisation, in Nursing care plan, p. 290 At the evaluation stage, monitors the response of the person for adverse effects, including health assessment findings, administration site and allergic reactions, and laboratory results, in Medication administration, pp. 303–306
12 Nursing care of people with altered immunity	1. Thinks critically and analyses nursing practice	1.1. Accesses, analyses and uses the best available evidence, that includes research findings, for safe, quality practice	Recognises that taking antiretroviral nucleoside analogues can induce adverse reactions, as well as prolonging life, in Medication administration, pp. 342–343
	4. Comprehensively conducts assessments	4.1. Conducts assessments that are holistic as well as culturally appropriate	When caring for a person with HIV, carries out the processes involved in the assessment phase, in Nursing care plan, pp. 348–349
	5. Develops a plan for nursing practice	5.1. Uses assessment data and best available evidence to develop a plan	Devises a teaching plan for the person with a hypersensitivity, in Community-based care, p. 324 Plans for safe nursing and medication management of immunosuppressive agents, in Medication administration, pp. 330–331 Devises a teaching plan for the person with an organ/tissue transplant, in Community-based care, p. 333 Plans for safe medication management of antiretroviral agents, in Medication administration, pp. 342–343 Uses assessment findings to plan nursing care for the person with HIV, in Nursing care plan, pp. 348–349
	6. Provides safe, appropriate and responsive quality nursing practice	6.1. Provides comprehensive, safe, quality practice to achieve agreed goals and outcomes that are responsive to the nursing needs of people	Provides appropriate and safe nursing management, including health education, of immunosuppressive agents, in Medication administration, pp. 330–331 Provides appropriate and safe nursing management, including health education, of antiretroviral agents, in Medication administration, pp. 342–343 When caring for a person with HIV, carries out the processes involved in the intervention phase, in Nursing care plan, p. 349
	7. Evaluates outcomes to inform nursing practice	7.1. Evaluates and monitors progress towards the expected goals and outcomes	Evaluates the person's responses to nursing care, including health education, in Nursing care plan, p. 349
13 Nursing care of people with cancer	2. Engages in therapeutic and professional relationships	2.6. Uses delegation, supervision, coordination, consultation and referrals in professional relationships to achieve improved health outcomes	Works together with the healthcare team to provide optimal care for the person with cancer, in Nursing care plan, pp. 389–390

CHAPTER	STANDARD	CRITERIA	EVIDENCE-BASED EXAMPLES (INCLUDING PAGE NO.)
	4. Comprehensively conducts assessments	4.1. Conducts assessments that are holistic as well as culturally appropriate	Conducts a comprehensive health assessment for a person with cancer and provides ongoing monitoring of status, in Assessment, Focused interview and Physical assessment, pp. 387–388
			When caring for a person with cancer, carries out the processes involved in the assessment phase that specifically address the person's needs, in Nursing care plan, p. 389
	5. Develops a plan for nursing practice	5.1. Uses assessment data and best available evidence to develop a plan	Plans for safe nursing and medication management of chemotherapeutic drugs and adjunct agents, in Table 13.10 Classification of chemotherapeutic drugs, pp. 378–379
			Safely administers chemotherapeutic medications and other medications for pain, nausea and vomiting, mucositis or anaemia, in Table 13.10 Classification of chemotherapeutic drugs, pp. 378–379
			Prioritises nursing diagnosis based on assessment data and implements appropriate nursing interventions for the person with cancer, in Nursing care plan, p. 389
			Uses the nursing process as a framework for planning individualised care and integrating interprofessional care for people with cancer to meet their healthcare needs, in Nursing care plan, pp. 389–390
	6. Provides safe, appropriate and responsive quality nursing practice	6.1. Provides comprehensive, safe, quality practice to achieve agreed goals and outcomes that are responsive to the nursing needs of people	Safely administers chemotherapeutic medications and other medications for pain, nausea and vomiting, mucositis or anaemia, in Table 13.10 Classification of chemotherapeutic drugs, pp. 378–379
			Demonstrates comprehensive nursing care, including health education, for a person receiving radiation therapy, in Nursing care of the person, p. 383
			Demonstrates comprehensive nursing care, including health education, for a person receiving immunotherapy, in Nursing care of the person, p. 384
			When caring for a person with cancer, carries out the processes involved in the intervention phase that specifically address the person's and carer's needs, in Nursing care plan, p. 390
	7. Evaluates outcomes to inform nursing practice	7.1. Evaluates and monitors progress towards the expected goals and outcomes	Evaluates individualised nursing care for the person and family, in nursing care plan, p. 390
Unit 4 Responses to altered integumentary structure and function			
14 Assessing the integumentary system	4. Comprehensively conducts assessments	4.1. Conducts assessments that are holistic as well as culturally appropriate	Conducts a health history for a person with an alteration or at risk of alterations in the integument, in Functional health pattern interview, pp. 412–413
		4.2. Uses a range of assessment techniques to systematically collect relevant and accurate information and data to inform practice	Conducts a health history for a person with an alteration in the integument, in Functional health pattern interview, pp. 412–413
			Conducts and/or assists in the collection of skin, blood and tissue samples, in Diagnostic tests, pp. 421–422

CHAPTER	STANDARD	CRITERIA	EVIDENCE-BASED EXAMPLES (INCLUDING PAGE NO.)
	6. Provides safe, appropriate and responsive quality nursing practice	6.1. Provides comprehensive, safe, quality practice to achieve agreed goals and outcomes that are responsive to the nursing needs of people	Provides related nursing care and monitors the results of diagnostic tests, in Diagnostic tests, pp. 421–422
15 Nursing care of people with integumentary disorders	1. Thinks critically and analyses nursing practice	1.1. Accesses, analyses and uses the best available evidence, that includes research findings, for safe, quality practice	Recognises that people who are at risk of a pressure injury or have a pressure injury require specific nursing management protocols, in Box 15.13 Nursing care of the person at risk of a pressure injury and the person with a pressure injury, p. 464, and Nursing care plan, pp. 465–466
	2. Engages in therapeutic and professional relationships	2.2. Communicates effectively and is respectful of a person's dignity, culture, values, beliefs and rights	Provides information on how to manage dry skin and pruritus, in Box 15.1 Teaching to reduce dry skin and relieve pruritus, p. 427
		2.6. Uses delegation, supervision, coordination, consultation and referrals in professional relationships to achieve improved health outcomes	Works together with the healthcare team to provide optimal care for a person with a pressure injury, in Nursing care plan, pp. 465–466
	4. Comprehensively conducts assessments	4.2. Uses a range of assessment techniques to systematically collect relevant and accurate information and data to inform practice	When caring for a person with a pressure injury, carries out the processes involved in the assessment phase that specifically address the person's needs, in Box 15.13 Nursing care of the person at risk of a pressure injury and the person with a pressure injury, p. 464, and Nursing care plan, p. 465
	5. Develops a plan for nursing practice	5.1. Uses assessment data and best available evidence to develop a plan of care	Plans an education session to promote the reduction of dry skin and relieving pruritus, in Box 15.1 Teaching to reduce dry skin and relieve pruritus, p. 427
			Devises a teaching plan for the person with psoriasis, in Community-based care, p. 431
			Plans for the safe nursing management of antifungal agents, in Medication administration, p. 436
			Uses evidence-based research to plan nursing care for people with pressure injuries and skin tears, in Box 15.13 Nursing care of the person at risk of a pressure injury and the person with a pressure injury, p. 464
			When caring for a person with a pressure injury, carries out the processes involved in the assessment phase, in Nursing care plan, p. 465
		5.2. Collaboratively constructs nursing practice plans until contingencies, options, priorities, goals, actions, outcomes and time frames are agreed with the relevant people	When planning care for a person with a pressure injury, integrates interprofessional care, in Nursing care plan, p. 465

CHAPTER	STANDARD	CRITERIA	EVIDENCE-BASED EXAMPLES (INCLUDING PAGE NO.)
	6. Provides safe, appropriate and responsive quality nursing practice	6.1. Provides comprehensive, safe, quality practice to achieve agreed goals and outcomes that are responsive to the nursing needs of people	Conducts education to promote the self-care of pruritus, in Box 15.1 Teaching to reduce dry skin and relieve pruritus, p. 427 Administers topical and oral antifungal medications used to treat integumentary disorders knowledgeably and safely, in Medication administration, p. 436 When caring for a person with a pressure injury, carries out the processes involved in the intervention phase that specifically address the person's needs, in Box 15.13 Nursing care of the person at risk of a pressure injury and the person with a pressure injury, p. 464, and Nursing care plan, pp. 465–466
	7. Evaluates outcomes to inform nursing practice	7.1. Evaluates and monitors progress towards the expected goals and outcomes	When caring for a person with a pressure injury, carries out the processes involved in the evaluation phase that specifically address the multidisciplinary team, in Nursing care plan, p. 466
16 Nursing care of people with burns	4. Comprehensively conducts assessments	4.2. Uses a range of assessment techniques to systematically collect relevant and accurate information and data to inform practice	When caring for a person with a major burn, carries out the processes involved in the assessment phase that specifically address the person's needs, in Nursing care plan, p. 500
	5. Develops a plan for nursing practice	5.1. Uses assessment data and best available evidence to develop a plan	When caring for a person with a major burn, carries out the processes involved in the planning phase that specifically address the person's needs, in Nursing care plan, p. 500 Devises a teaching plan for the person with burns, in Community-based care, pp. 501–502
		5.2. Collaboratively constructs nursing practice plans until contingencies, options, priorities, goals, actions, outcomes and time frames are agreed with the relevant people	When caring for a person with a major burn, carries out the processes involved in the planning phase that specifically address the person's needs, in Nursing care plan, p. 500
	6. Provides safe, appropriate and responsive quality nursing practice	6.1. Provides comprehensive, safe, quality practice to achieve agreed goals and outcomes that are responsive to the nursing needs of people	When caring for a person with a major burn, carries out the processes involved in the intervention phase that specifically address the person's needs, in Nursing care plan, pp. 500–501
	7. Evaluates outcomes to inform nursing practice	7.1. Evaluates and monitors progress towards the expected goals and outcomes	When caring for a person with a major burn, carries out the processes involved in the evaluation phase that specifically address physiological stabilisation as part of burn management, in Nursing care plan, p. 501
Unit 5 Responses to altered endocrine function			
17 A person-centred approach to assessing the endocrine system	4. Comprehensively conducts assessments	4.1. Conducts assessments that are holistic as well as culturally appropriate	Conducts a health history for a person with an alteration in the endocrine system, in Functional health pattern interview, pp. 514–515

CHAPTER	STANDARD	CRITERIA	EVIDENCE-BASED EXAMPLES (INCLUDING PAGE NO.)
		4.2. Uses a range of assessment techniques to systematically collect relevant and accurate information and data to inform practice	Conducts and/or assists in the collection of blood and urine samples and radiographical studies, in Diagnostic tests, pp. 516–521
			Conducts a physical assessment for a person with an alteration in the endocrine system, in Endocrine assessments, pp. 522–524
	6. Provides safe, appropriate and responsive quality nursing practice	6.1. Provides comprehensive, safe, quality practice to achieve agreed goals and outcomes that are responsive to the nursing needs of people	Provides related nursing care and monitors the results of diagnostic tests, in Diagnostic tests, pp. 516–521
18 Nursing care of people with endocrine disorders	4. Comprehensively conducts assessments	4.1. Conducts assessments that are holistic as well as culturally appropriate	When caring for a person with hyperthyroidism, carries out the processes involved in the assessment phase that specifically address the person's needs, in Nursing care plan, p. 534
			When caring for a person with hypothyroidism, carries out the processes involved in the assessment phase that specifically address the person's needs, in Nursing care plan, p. 540
			When caring for a person with Cushing's syndrome, carries out the processes involved in the assessment phase that specifically address the person's needs, in Nursing care plan, p. 547
		4.2. Uses a range of assessment techniques to systematically collect relevant and accurate information and data to inform practice	Assesses respiratory function and wound status, in Nursing care of the person, p. 532
			When caring for a person with Addison's disease, carries out the processes involved in the assessment phase that specifically address the person's needs, in Nursing care plan, p. 552
	5. Develops a plan for nursing practice	5.1. Uses assessment data and best available evidence to develop a plan	Plans for the safe nursing management of anti-thyroid agents, in Medication administration, p. 531
			Determines priority nursing diagnoses, based on assessed data, to select and implement individualised nursing interventions for a person with hyperthyroidism, in Nursing care plan, p. 534
			Plans for the safe nursing management of thyroid agents, in Medication administration, p. 538
			Plans education to ensure the person knows that hormone replacement is for life and knows how to take medications, in Medication administration, p. 538
			Determines priority nursing diagnoses, based on assessed data, to select and implement individualised nursing interventions for a person with hypothyroidism, in Nursing care plan, p. 540

CHAPTER	STANDARD	CRITERIA	EVIDENCE-BASED EXAMPLES (INCLUDING PAGE NO.)
			Determines priority nursing diagnoses, based on assessed data, to select and implement individualised nursing interventions for a person with Cushing's syndrome, in Nursing care plan, p. 547
			Determines priority nursing diagnoses, based on assessed data, to select and implement individualised nursing interventions for a person with Addison's disease, in Nursing care plan, p. 552
	6. Provides safe, appropriate and responsive quality nursing practice	6.1. Provides comprehensive, safe, quality practice to achieve agreed goals and outcomes that are responsive to the nursing needs of people	When caring for a person with hyperthyroidism, carries out the processes involved in the intervention phase that specifically address the person's needs, in Nursing care plan, p. 534
			Monitors wound management, vital signs, laboratory results and pain scale of the person having an adrenalectomy, in Nursing care of the person, p. 546
			When caring for a person with Cushing's syndrome, carries out the processes involved in the intervention phase that specifically address the person's pre-post-surgical needs, in Nursing care plan, p. 547
			When caring for a person with Addison's disease, carries out the processes involved in the intervention phase that specifically address the person's needs, in Nursing care plan, p. 552
	7. Evaluates outcomes to inform nursing practice	7.1. Evaluates and monitors progress towards the expected goals and outcomes	When caring for a person with hyperthyroidism, carries out the processes involved in the evaluation phase that specifically address physiological stabilisation as part of nursing management, in Nursing care plan, p. 534
			When caring for a person with hypothyroidism, carries out the processes involved in the evaluation phase that address stabilisation as part of nursing management, in Nursing care plan, p. 540
			When caring for a person with Cushing's syndrome, carries out the processes involved in the evaluation phase that address the pre-postoperative phases as part of nursing management, in Nursing care plan, p. 547
		7.3. Determines, documents and communicates further priorities, goals and outcomes with the relevant persons	Communicates abnormal electrolyte levels to the doctor, in Nursing care plan, p. 552
19 Nursing care of people with diabetes mellitus	4. Comprehensively conducts assessments	4.1. Conducts assessments that are holistic as well as culturally appropriate	Make assessments for appropriate nursing care for the person with type 1 diabetes, in Nursing care plan, p. 587

CHAPTER	STANDARD	CRITERIA	EVIDENCE-BASED EXAMPLES (INCLUDING PAGE NO.)
	5. Develops a plan for nursing practice	5.1. Uses assessment data and best available evidence to develop a plan	Plans for education to promote administration of: insulin via injection, in Medication administration, p. 568, and oral hypoglycaemic agents, in Medication administration, pp. 574–575
			Determines priority nursing diagnoses, based on assessed data, to select and implement individualised nursing interventions for the person with type 1 diabetes, in Nursing care plan, pp. 587–588
			Devises a teaching plan for the relationship of hygiene, neuropathy and impaired microcirculation to infection, teaches the principles and procedures of effective foot care, in Meeting individualised needs, p. 589
	6. Provides safe, appropriate and responsive quality nursing practice	6.1. Provides comprehensive, safe, quality practice to achieve agreed goals and outcomes that are responsive to the nursing needs of people	Conducts education to promote administration of: insulin via injection, in Medication administration, p. 568, and oral hypoglycaemic agents, in Medication administration, pp. 574–575
			Administers medication safely and effectively, and monitors patient response, in Medication administration, p. 582
			Provides safe and appropriate nursing care for the person with type 1 diabetes, in Nursing care plan, p. 588
			Conducts education to promote effective foot care in diabetics, in Meeting individualised needs, p. 589
	7. Evaluates outcomes to inform nursing practice	7.1. Evaluates and monitors progress towards the expected goals and outcomes	Evaluates nursing care for the person with type 1 diabetes, in Nursing care plan, p. 588

Source: Nursing and Midwifery Board of Australia (NMBA) (2016). *Registered Nurse Standards for Practice*. © Nursing and Midwifery Board of Australia, www.nursingmidwiferyboard.gov.au/.

The Patient Safety Competency Framework for Nursing Students

For a full explanation of the Patient Safety Competency Framework (PSCF), please see the Preface.

1 Person-centred care[2]

The nursing student demonstrates the ability to plan and provide care that is respectful of the person's individual needs, values and life experiences.

KNOWLEDGE

The nursing student:

1. Discusses the meaning of person-centred care
2. Describes how person-centred care impacts patient safety and wellbeing
3. Outlines interpersonal skills that are consistent with a person-centred approach
4. Describes strategies that can be used to support people to take responsibility for their own health and wellbeing
5. Describes when it is or is not appropriate to advocate for people

SKILLS

The nursing student:

1. Demonstrates an ability to provide holistic care that takes into account the person's current situation, previous experiences and life history
2. Works in partnership with the person by including them in decisions and plans related to their healthcare
3. Considers the person's rights, preferences, needs and values when planning and providing care
4. Supports the person to make informed choices about their healthcare
5. Provides care with the person's informed consent
6. Demonstrates empathy by seeking to understand the person's perspectives, views and feelings
7. Demonstrates respect by maintaining the person's dignity and privacy
8. Advocates for people, if required, to ensure that their values, needs and preferences are upheld

Person-centred care is the central tenet underpinning the delivery of safe and effective nursing care. It is a holistic approach that is grounded in a philosophy of personhood [7]. Person-centred care means treating each person as an individual, protecting their dignity, respecting their rights and preferences, and developing a therapeutic relationship that is built on mutual trust and empathic understandings [8].

2. The term 'person' in this context refers to the patient, their family and/or significant others. In the case of a child, person-centred care also denotes family-centred care.

2 Therapeutic communication

The nursing student demonstrates the ability to use verbal and non-verbal communication skills to convey respect and empathy, and to encourage the person to express their feelings and needs, while at the same time maintaining professional boundaries.

KNOWLEDGE

The nursing student:

1. Discusses the meaning and principles of therapeutic communication
2. Describes the relationship between therapeutic communication and patient safety
3. Outlines interpersonal and environmental factors that can interfere with therapeutic communication
4. Discusses the importance of maintaining professional boundaries
5. Describes strategies to evaluate and improve people's health literacy
6. Outlines the principles of effective patient education

SKILLS

The nursing student:

1. Demonstrates the ability to develop therapeutic relationships while maintaining professional boundaries
2. Uses verbal and nonverbal communication techniques effectively
3. Asks the person for their understanding of the situation, issue, or problem
4. Responds to the person's requests and concerns courteously, kindly and in a timely manner
5. Shares information with the person in a way that is understandable and that encourages participation in decision-making
6. Communicates in a way that is appropriate to the person's level of health literacy and avoids jargon and complex terms
7. Provides education that is appropriate and meets the needs of the person and their family/carer
8. Ensures privacy and confidentiality when communicating with and about patients
9. Ensures relevant family/significant others are included in discussions about healthcare decision-making (as appropriate)

Therapeutic communication occurs when nurses use verbal and nonverbal communication techniques in a goal-directed way, ensuring that the healthcare needs of the person remain the central focus. Therapeutic communication is built on trust, authenticity, empathy and self-awareness. Nurses who communicate therapeutically listen to understand, maintain a non-judgmental stance, and are 'fully present' with the person [9].

3 Cultural Competence

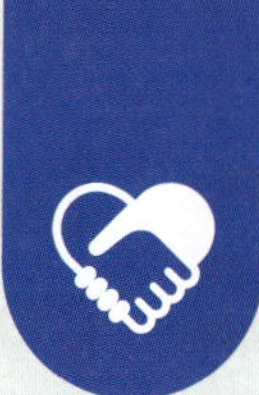

The nursing student demonstrates respect for each person's cultural values, beliefs, life experiences and health practices.

KNOWLEDGE

The nursing student:

1. Defines the terms culture, cultural awareness, cultural humility, cultural competence and cultural safety
2. Discusses the history and principles of cultural safety
3. Discusses the relationship between cultural competence and patient safety
4. Discusses when and how interpreting and translation services should be used
5. Describes how to work collaboratively with a Cultural Liaison Officer[3]
6. Discusses how the life experiences of migrants and refugees can impact their health and wellbeing
7. Discusses how colonisation and racism has impacted the health and wellbeing of Aboriginal and Torres Strait Islander Peoples
8. Articulates personal views about caring for people from different cultural backgrounds
9. Openly discusses own cultural values, attitudes, biases and preconceptions

SKILLS

The nursing student:

1. Demonstrates the ability to conduct a cultural assessment
2. Demonstrates cultural empathy by seeking to understand the person's cultural and spiritual values, needs, practices and perspectives
3. Adapts practice to accommodate the person's cultural needs and values (where appropriate)
4. Avoids generalisations and stereotypes when discussing people from different cultural groups
5. Demonstrates how to access an interpreter (if required)
6. Demonstrates how to access an appropriate Cultural Liaison Officer /community support representative (if required)
7. Seeks to understand whether the person feels culturally safe

Cultural competence is integral to safe and effective clinical practice. The term cultural competence refers to behaviours and attitudes that enable systems, organisations, professions and individuals to work effectively in cross-cultural situations [10]. Cultural competence refers to the willingness to adapt practice to meet the needs of people from diverse cultures, and the ability to interact with persons from cultures and/or belief systems different to one's own [11]. Cultural safety is as important to quality care as clinical safety; however, the presence or absence of cultural safety is determined by the recipient of care, rather than the caregiver [12].

3. Cultural Liaison Officer in this context refers to Aboriginal and Torres Strait Islander Liaison Officers and Refugee and Migrant Health Officers etc

4 Teamwork and collaborative practice

The nursing student demonstrates the ability to collaborate and communicate effectively with members of the healthcare team in ways that facilitate mutual respect and shared decision-making.

KNOWLEDGE

The nursing student:

1. Describes the characteristics of effective healthcare teams
2. Discusses how effective intraprofessional and interprofessional communication and collaboration can improve patient safety
3. Outlines differences in the scope of practice, roles and responsibilities of different members of the nursing profession
4. Describes the roles and responsibilities of other healthcare professionals
5. Discusses the impact of effective leadership and followership on team dynamics
6. Discusses own strengths and limitations as a team member
7. Discusses the influence of hierarchy and power differentials on assertive communication

SKILLS

The nursing student:

1. Recognises that the patient and their significant others are integral members of the healthcare team
2. Works in partnership with other healthcare professionals towards common goals that prioritise the patient's perspectives, values and needs
3. Communicates and collaborates confidently and respectfully with all members of the healthcare team
4. Seeks and values the perspectives of all team members
5. Engages in collaborative goal setting and decision-making when planning person-centred care
6. Provides clear and accurate handover reports to members of the healthcare team
7. Communicates effectively using ISBAR (or other appropriate communication tool)
8. Documents clearly, accurately and contemporaneously in patient records
9. Uses only recognised terms and abbreviations when communicating
10. Raises concerns about patient care in a timely manner and with clarity and confidence
11. Manages conflict effectively and, when required, escalates concerns using graded assertiveness
12. Responds to all forms of overt and covert horizontal or vertical violence using appropriate strategies and reporting processes

Teamwork and collaborative practice refers to healthcare professionals working together using complementary knowledge and skills to provide patient care, based on trust, respect and understanding of each other's expertise [13]. Collaborative practice prioritises the patient's needs, requires well developed intra and interprofessional communication skills, and the ability to speak up if one has concerns [14].

5 Clinical Reasoning

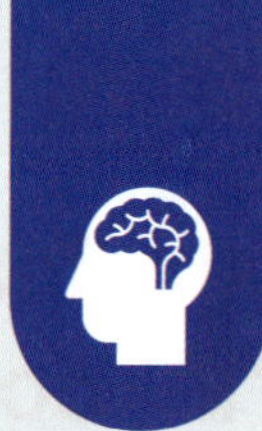

The nursing student demonstrates the ability to accurately assess, interpret and respond to individual patient data in a systematic and timely way.

KNOWLEDGE

The nursing student:

1. Discusses the relationship between patient safety and clinical reasoning
2. Identifies examples of assessment frameworks that can be used to systematically collect patient data and inform clinical reasoning
3. Differentiates between normal and abnormal vital signs and other critical patient data
4. Outlines the pathophysiology underpinning abnormal patient data
5. Discusses the impact of situational awareness on clinical reasoning and patient safety
6. Discusses the importance of lifelong learning to safe and effective clinical reasoning
7. Reflects on and discusses how cognitive biases can influence clinical reasoning

SKILLS

The nursing student:

1. Uses a systematic and logical process for clinical reasoning
2. Conducts a comprehensive and focused nursing assessment using appropriate frameworks and techniques
3. Refers to a range of patient data including handover reports, medical records, the person's social and medical history and evidence-based guidelines
4. Elicits the person's concerns and understanding of the situation
5. Differentiates between normal and abnormal vital signs and other critical patient data
6. Analyses, synthesises and interprets assessment data accurately and systematically
7. Notices subtle changes in a patient's condition that signal the need for further investigation, immediate clinical review or rapid response
8. Uses early warning charts and systems appropriately
9. Anticipates, recognises and responds appropriately to clinical deterioration
10. Matches the features of the person's presentation with other similar or previous patient encounters
11. Identifies priority patient problems based on accurate and complete interpretation of available patient data
12. Plans and implements nursing care both autonomously and in consultation with other members of the healthcare team
13. Evaluates progress towards expected outcomes by re-assessing the person's condition
14. Critically reflects on and learns from previous experiences to improve clinical reasoning skills

Clinical reasoning is a cyclical process by which nurses collect cues, interpret the information, come to an understanding of a patient problem or situation, plan and implement interventions, evaluate outcomes, and reflect on and learn from the process [15]. Clinical reasoning requires a critical thinking disposition and is influenced by the nurse's assumptions, attitudes and cognitive biases [16].

6 Evidence-based practice

The nursing student demonstrates the ability to provide care that takes into account best available evidence, clinical expertise and patient's individual needs, values and preferences.

KNOWLEDGE

The nursing student:

1. Describes different sources of evidence (e.g. empirical studies, clinical expertise, patient values and preferences)
2. Outlines and discriminates between different levels of evidence
3. Describes different approaches used to collect and collate data to inform evidenced-based practice
4. Explains the terms validity, reliability, trustworthiness and credibility in reference to healthcare studies
5. Explains how evidence-based practice influences the choice of interventions in the provision of effective patient care
6. Describes personal strategies used to access nursing evidence to inform and improve patient care

SKILLS

The nursing student:

1. Plans and provides healthcare based on the best available evidence
2. Accesses, appraises and critiques multiple sources of evidence
3. Uses information and communication technologies to access valid sources of evidence
4. Considers clinical expertise as a valuable source of evidence
5. Includes patient's values and preferences as valid sources of evidence
6. Provides rationales for patient care that are informed by the best available evidence
7. Demonstrates ethical standards in the collection, interpretation and use of data

Evidence-based practice is the conscientious and explicit use of contemporary research, current evidence, clinical expertise and patient values to make decisions about patient care [17]. Evidence-based practice requires the ability to search for, critically appraise, utilise and translate research into practice.

7 Preventing, minimising and responding to adverse events

The nursing student demonstrates the ability to anticipate and respond to human and systems factors that have the potential to jeopardise patient safety, and take appropriate actions to prevent reoccurrence of errors and near misses.

KNOWLEDGE

The nursing student:

1. Defines the terms error, adverse event, near miss and violation
2. Describes human and system factors that lead to potential high risk clinical situations and errors in healthcare
3. Discusses professional factors (e.g staffing levels, skill mix, training opportunities, workload, leadership styles etc) that impact on patient safety
4. Discusses environmental factors (e.g. lighting, noise, clutter etc) that impact on patient safety
5. Discusses personal factors (e.g fatigue, stress, substance use) that impact on patient safety
6. Discusses factors that contribute to a culture of workplace safety (e.g. open communication, teamwork, and error reporting systems)
7. Identifies how vulnerable individuals and groups are at increased risk of adverse outcomes and discusses preventive strategies
8. Analyses the benefits and limitations of technologies designed to reduce risk (e.g. barcodes, infusion pumps)
9. Describes the importance and process of continuous quality improvement as a strategy to improve patient safety
10. Describes the process for reporting errors and near misses
11. Describes the process and purpose of open disclosure
12. Describes how healthcare professionals can learn from errors and near misses
13. Discusses strategies to minimise the risk of injury to self and others (e.g. safe patient moving and use of PPE)
14. Discusses strategies for self-care and to enhance resilience and coping skills
15. Acknowledges, takes responsibility, reflects on and learns from own mistakes

SKILLS

The nursing student:

1. Uses appropriate patient identifiers and seeks consent prior to initiating care
2. Practices within legal and ethical frameworks, relevant guidelines, policies and evidence-based resources
3. Conducts regular and appropriate risk assessments (e.g. falls, pressure area, cognitive and nutrition etc.)
4. Recognises particular risks associated with vulnerable individuals and groups and initiates actions to prevent adverse outcomes
5. Implements appropriate nursing actions to address identified risks to patient safety or wellbeing
6. Encourages patients and family members to speak up if they identify factors that may compromise safety
7. Responds appropriately to people's concerns and complaints with reference to organisational protocols and within own scope of practice
8. Notices, anticipates and addresses human and system factors that may lead to errors
9. Uses strategies to reduce reliance on memory such as checklists, cue cards, algorithms and mnemonics
10. Uses technologies designed to improve patient safety accurately and effectively
11. Contributes to the prevention and management of agitation, aggression and violence in the workplace
12. Reports concerns related to hazards, errors and near misses in a timely manner using organisational reporting systems
13. Seeks to understand the cause of an error or near miss rather than attributing blame
14. Maintains own capability to practice and takes responsibility for personal factors (mental, physical or emotional) that have the potential to negatively impact patient safety
15. Raises concerns about other healthcare professionals' capability to practice and factors that have the potential to negatively impact patient safety (e.g fatigue, stress, substance use) confidentially and using appropriate channels
16. Acknowledges, takes responsibility, reflects on and learns from own mistakes

Preventing and minimising adverse events refers to the ability to anticipate and effectively manage human and systems factors that have the potential to impact patient safety [18]. **Responding appropriately to adverse events** encompasses the ability to recognise and manage patient deterioration, to participate in analysis of the events in order to identify system failures and appropriate solutions, and to provide honest and timely communication about the facts of the adverse event [19].

8 Infection prevention and control

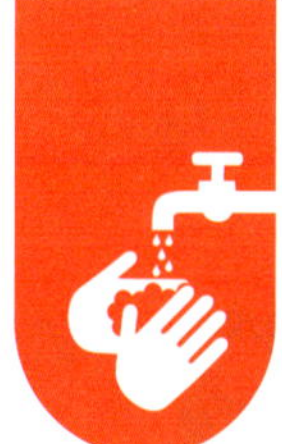

The nursing student demonstrates the ability to reduce the risk of patients acquiring healthcare-associated infections and effectively manage infections if they occur.

KNOWLEDGE

The nursing student:

1. Describes the chain of infection and the different modes of transmission of infection in healthcare
2. Describes how different types of microorganisms spread
3. Defines the terms colonisation, infection and antimicrobial resistance
4. Outlines the principles of standard and transmission-based precautions
5. Identifies people who are at particular risk of healthcare-associated infections (e.g. people who are immunocompromised) and advocates on their behalf when required (e.g. by ensuring hand hygiene practices are maintained)
6. Explains the principles of antimicrobial stewardship
7. Outlines procedures for informing authorities of notifiable diseases

SKILLS

The nursing student:

1. Educates patients, visitors and colleagues about infection control practices and prevention strategies
2. Demonstrates effective hand hygiene
3. Demonstrates the use of standard and transmission-based precautions for infection prevention and control
4. Demonstrates aseptic and non-touch techniques
5. Uses and removes personal protective equipment in a way that minimises cross contamination
6. Demonstrates correct use and disposal of sharps and waste
7. Cleans or discards used equipment appropriately
8. Manages blood and body fluid spills appropriately
9. Raises concerns about inappropriate antimicrobial use
10. Complies with organisational requirements for immunisation

Infection prevention and control refers to the use of effective, evidence-based strategies to prevent and manage healthcare-associated infections. It also focuses on minimising the risk of transmission by effectively using standard and transmission-based precautions and reducing the development of resistant organisms [20, 21].

9 Medication safety

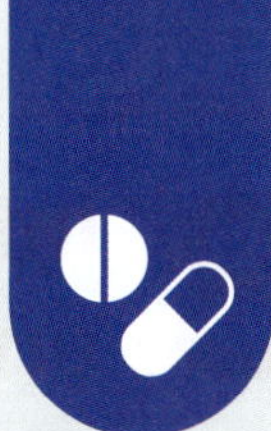

The nursing student demonstrates the ability to administer and monitor the therapeutic use of medications; and respond appropriately to medication errors and adverse drug reactions.

KNOWLEDGE

The nursing student:

1. Outlines key principles of safe medication management
2. Identifies factors that have the potential to compromise safe medication practices
3. Defines and differentiates between a medication error, adverse drug reaction, drug sensitivity, side effect and drug allergy
4. Describes the roles and responsibilities of members of the medication team responsible for prescribing, dispensing and administering medications
5. Outlines legislative and organisational requirements for medication prescription, storage, use and administration
6. Describes how to report medication incidents including adverse drug reactions, medication errors and near misses

Medication safety refers to the safe use of medicines to achieve therapeutic outcomes and improve people's quality of life, while minimising risks and responding to errors [22]. Medication safety is dependent upon the nurses' ability to manage the human and systems factors that have the potential to adversely impact the accuracy of medication prescribing, dispensing and administration, and to educate patients to self-manage medications appropriately [23].

SKILLS

The nursing student:

1. Demonstrates the ability to take an accurate medication history
2. Identifies previous drug allergies, sensitivities or adverse reactions
3. Uses evidence-based sources of information when administering medications
4. Includes the person as an active member of the medication team
5. Consults with members of the medication team responsible for prescribing and dispensing medications (e.g. medical officers and pharmacists)
6. Takes medication orders via telephone in accordance with legislation and organisational policies
7. Complies with legislative and organisational requirements related to safe and appropriate handling, storage administration and disposal of medications (including S4D and S8)
8. Works within own scope of practice with regards to medication administration
9. Uses only recognised and approved abbreviations related to medication administration
10. Administers medications only when a valid medication order is provided
11. Demonstrates safe and accurate medication administration using 6 rights and 3 checks
12. Prevents and manages interruptions while administering medications
13. Takes appropriate precautions with high risk medications such as:

    Anti-infectives
    Potassium and other electrolytes
    Insulin
    Narcotics and other sedatives
    Chemotherapeutic agents
    Heparin and other anticoagulants
14. Accurately documents medication administration and medications that are refused or withheld
15. Provides appropriate patient education about medication use, side-effects, storage and disposal
16. Responds to, reports and documents adverse drug reactions, medication errors and near misses in accordance with legislation and organisational policies

References

1. Yanhua, C. & Watson, R. (2011). A review of clinical competence assessment in nursing. *Nurse Education Today.* 31(8), 832-836
2. The Bristol Royal Infirmary Inquiry. (2001). *Learning from Bristol: the report of the public inquiry into children's heart surgery at the Bristol Royal Infirmary 1984-1995. Bristol Royal Infirmary Inquiry, July 2001.* Accessed 5.10.17 at www.bristol-inquiry.org.uk
3. Australian Commission of Safety and Quality in Health Care (2016). National Safety and Quality Health Service Standards Accessed 5.10.17 at https://www.safetyandquality.gov.au/wp-content/uploads/2011/09/NSQHS-Standards-Sept-2012.pdf
4. Nursing and Midwifery Board of Australia (NMBA) (2016). Registered nurse standards for practice Accessed 5.10.17 at http://www.nursingmidwiferyboard.gov.au/Codes-Guidelines-Statements/Professional-standards.aspx
5. Thistlethwaite, J., Forman, D., Matthews, L., Rogers, G., Steketee, C. & Yassine, T. (2014). Competencies and frameworks in interprofessional education: A comparative analysis. *Academic Medicine* 89(6), 1-7
6. Miller, G. (1990). The assessment of clinical skills/competence/performance. *Academic Medicine.* 65(9), s63-s67
7. Kitwood, T. (1997). *Dementia Reconsidered: The person comes first.* Buckingham: Open University Press
8. Australian College of Nursing. (2014). *Person-centred care position statement.* Accessed 5.10.17 at https://www.acn.edu.au/sites/default/files/advocacy/submissions/PS_Person-centered_Care_C2.pdf
9. Rossiter, R., Scott, R & Walton, C. (2014). Key attributes of therapeutic communication. T Levett-Jones (ed). *Critical conversations for patient safety: An essential guide for health professionals.* Sydney, Pearson.
10. National Health and Medical research Council. (2006). *Cultural competency in health: A guide for policy, partnerships and participation.* Accessed 5.10.17 at http://www.mhahs.org.au/images/cald/CulturalCompetencyInHealth.pdf
11. Australian Indigenous Doctors Association. (2014). *An introduction to cultural competency.* Accessed 5.10.17 at https://www.racp.edu.au/docs/default-source/advocacy-library/an-introduction-to-cultural-competency.pdf
12. Congress of Aboriginal and Torres Strait Islander Nurses and Midwives (CATSINaM). (2014), *Towards a shared understanding of terms and concepts: Strengthening nursing and midwifery care of Aboriginal and Torres Strait Islander peoples*, Canberra. Accessed 5.10.17 at http://catsinam.org.au/policy/cultural-safety
13. Rogers, G., Thistlethwaite, J., Anderson, E., Abrandt Dahlgren, M., Grymonpre, R., Moran, M. & Samarasekera, D. (2107). International consensus statement on the assessment of interprofessional learning outcomes. *Medical Teacher.* 39(40), 347-357
14. Stone, J. (2009). *Interprofessional collaborative practice - definitions and terminology: attempting to speak the same language.* ACT, Australia: ACT Health.
15. Levett-Jones, T. (2018). Clinical reasoning – What it is and why it matters. T Levett-Jones (ed.) *Clinical Reasoning: Learning how to think like a nurse.* (2nd Ed). Frenchs Forrest: Pearson
16. Croskerry, P., Singhal, G. & Mamede, S. (2013). Cognitive debiasing 1: origins of bias and theory of debiasing. *BMJ Quality & Safety,* 22, ii58-ii64.
17. Sackett, D., Straus, S., Richardson, W., Rosenberg, W. & Haynes, R. (2000). *Evidence-based medicine: How to practice and teach EBM* (2 ed.). New York: Churchill Livingstone.
18. Endacott, R., Kidd, T., Chaboyer, W. & Edington, J. (2007). Recognition and communication of patient deterioration in a regional hospital: a multi-methods study. *Australian Critical Care.* 20, 100-105
19. Canadian Institute of Patient Safety. (2008). The safety competencies. Enhancing patient safety across disciplines. Accessed 5.10.17 at www.patientsafetyinstitute.ca
20. National Health and Medical research Council. (2010) *Australian Guidelines for the prevention and control of infection in healthcare.* Commonwealth of Australia, Sydney. Accessed 24.10.17 at https://www.nhmrc.gov.au/guidelines-publications/cd33
21. Australian Commission on Safety and Quality in Health Care. (2014). *Antimicrobial Stewardship Clinical Care Standard,* Sydney. Accessed 5.10.17 at https://www.safetyandquality.gov.au/wp-content/uploads/2014/11/Antimicrobial-Stewardship-Clinical-Care-Standard-web.pdf
22. Roughhead, E., Semple, S. & Rosenfeld, E. (2013). *Literature Review: Medication Safety in Australia.* Australian Commission on Safety and Quality in Health Care, Sydney. Accessed 5.10.17 at https://safetyandquality.gov.au/wp-content/uploads/2014/02/Literature-Review-Medication-Safety-in-Australia-2013.pdf
23. Lapkin, S., Levett-Jones, T. Johnson, M & Chenoweth, L. (2016). The effectiveness of interventions designed to reduce medication administration errors: A synthesis of findings from systematic reviews. *Journal of Nursing Management.* 24(7), 845-858

Acknowledgments

We are grateful to the content experts and expert panel members who participated in this study and without whom the Patient Safety Competency Framework would not have eventuated.

Support for this project has been provided by the Australian Government Office for Learning and Teaching. The views expressed in the project do not necessarily reflect the views of the Australian Government Office for Learning and Teaching.

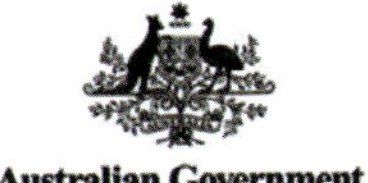

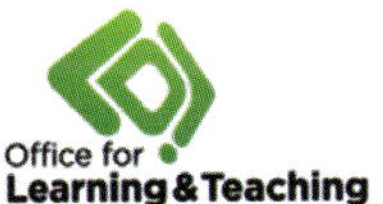

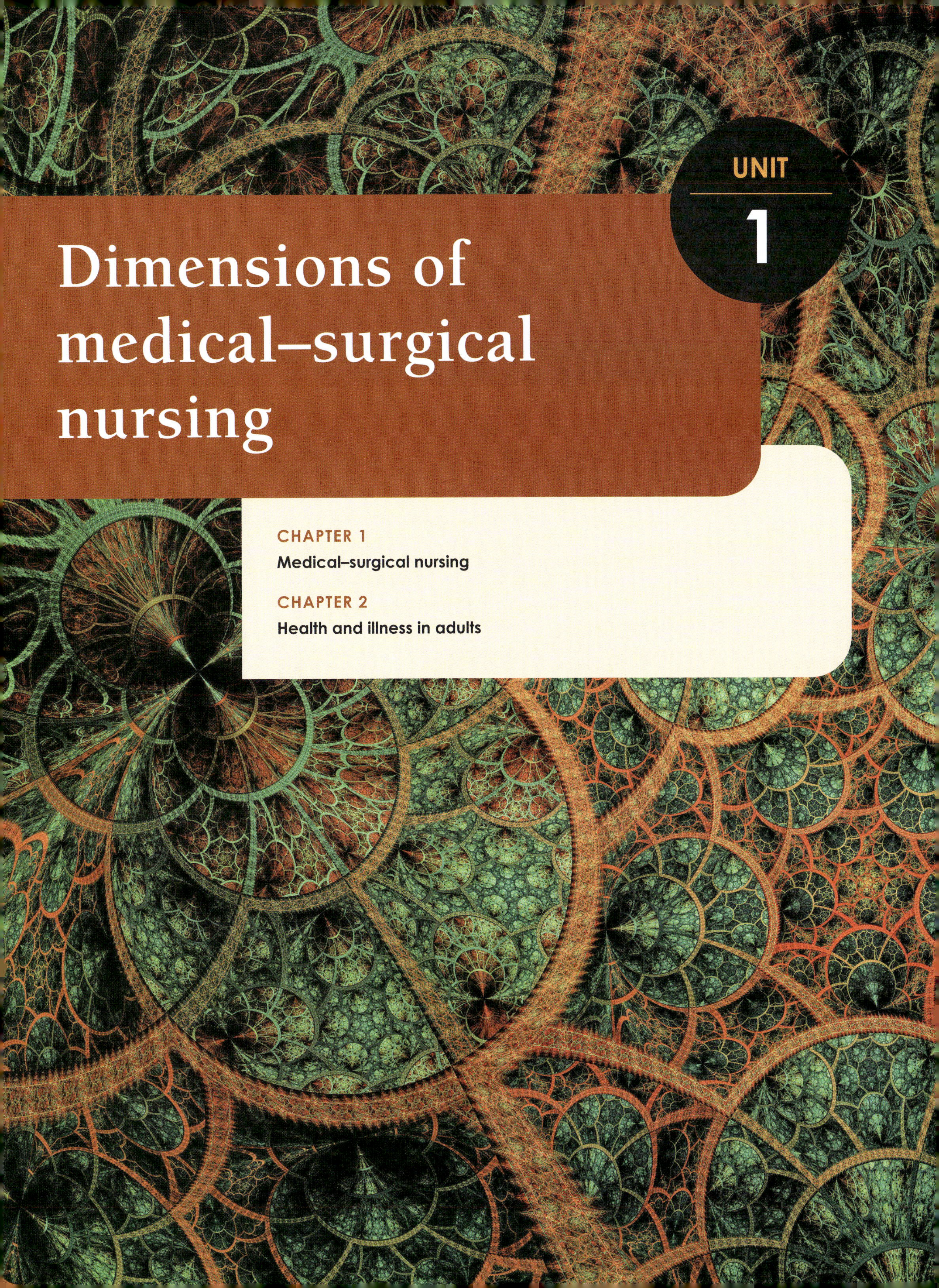

UNIT 1

Dimensions of medical–surgical nursing

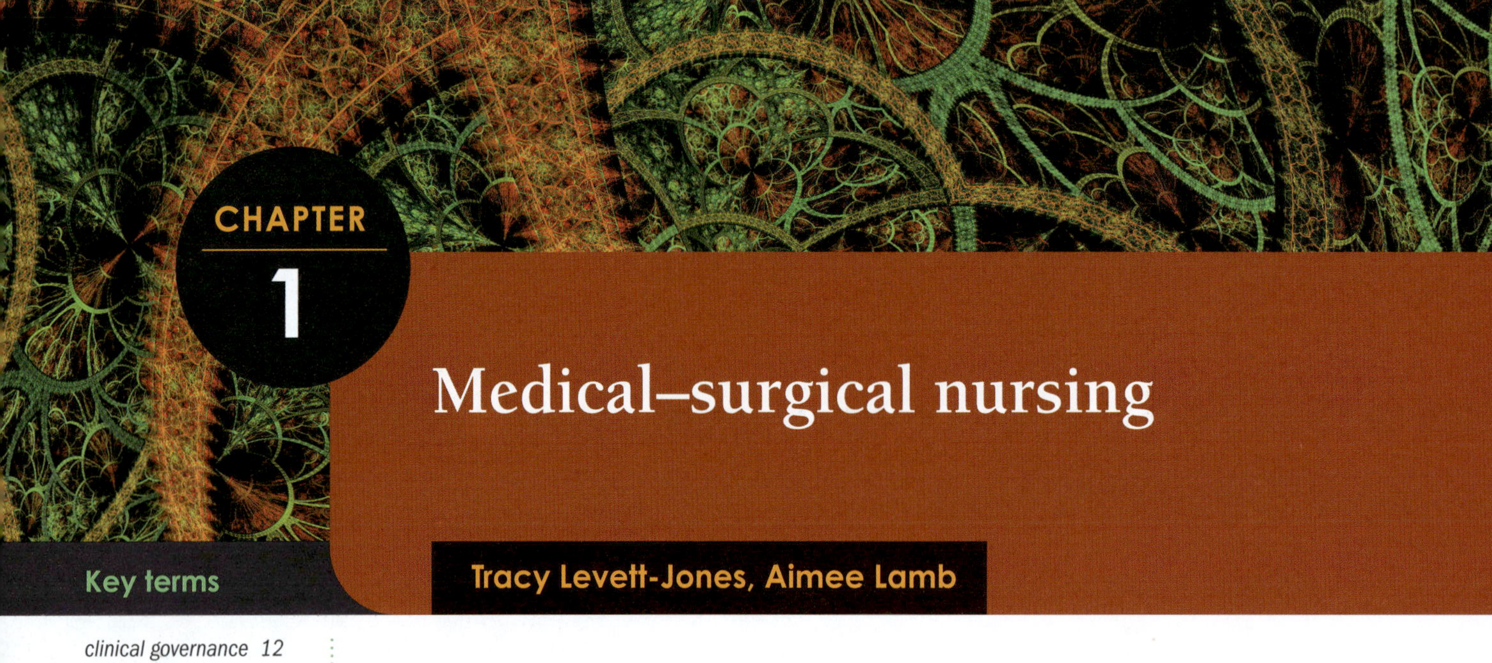

CHAPTER 1

Medical–surgical nursing

Tracy Levett-Jones, Aimee Lamb

Key terms

clinical governance 12
clinical pathway 12
clinical reasoning 6
critical thinking 3
cultural competence 9
cultural safety 9
culture 9
delegation 12
dilemma 10
electronic medical records (EMRs) 6
medical–surgical nursing 3
nursing process 4
person-centred care 3
scope of practice 12

Learning outcomes

- Define and discuss the importance of person-centred care.
- Describe the attitudes, attributes and skills necessary for critical thinking when providing nursing care.
- Outline the stages of the nursing process.
- Outline the stages of the Clinical Reasoning Cycle and how it was designed to positively impact on patient safety.
- Describe the importance of standards for practice, codes of ethics and codes of professional conduct as guidelines for accountable and professional nursing practice.
- Outline the concept of cultural competence as an integral component of nursing care.
- Discuss some of the legal and ethical dilemmas evident in medical–surgical nursing.
- Discuss the roles and functions of the nurse as caregiver, educator, advocate, leader/manager and researcher.

Clinical competencies

- Demonstrate critical thinking and clinical reasoning when providing evidence-based, professional, safe, person-centred and culturally competent nursing care.
- Provide clinical care within a framework that integrates, as appropriate, the medical–surgical nursing roles of caregiver, educator, advocate, leader/manager and researcher.

Medical–surgical nursing is one type of specialty nursing practice. However, within this area of practice there are also many sub-specialty areas; for example, acute care, day surgery, general practice, community nursing and renal dialysis. Medical–surgical nurses focus on the promotion of health, prevention of illness and the care of ill, disabled and dying people across the lifespan and in diverse practice contexts. Medical–surgical nurses are responsible for the provision of safe, empathic, person-centred, evidence-based care. They communicate and collaborate with patients, families and other healthcare professionals, and their care is informed by professional, ethical and legal frameworks. This chapter provides a broad overview of medical–surgical nursing, including the roles and functions of the medical–surgical nurse.

PERSON-CENTRED CARE

The terms '*person*' and '*patient*' denote the individual who is the recipient of care and are often used interchangeably, depending on the context of care. In this book, we generally use the term 'person' as this aligns with the concept of person-centred care.

Person-centred care means seeing the *person*, not just the patient or their disease process. That is, we speak of a *person* with a disease; for example, 'In bed 4 is Mr Johns who has had an appendectomy' rather than 'the appendectomy in bed 4', or 'Joanne requires assistance with her meals' rather than 'Joanne is a feed'.

Person-centred nurses are empathic, respectful, ethical, open-minded and self-aware. They have a profound sense of personal responsibility for actions (moral agency) and consider the person's needs and wishes as paramount (Australian College of Nursing, 2020). Integral to person-centred care is therapeutic communication and the nurse's commitment to understanding the person's beliefs and values, life history and cultural needs. There is a body of evidence indicating that person-centred care results in improved patient outcomes; for example, decreased mortality, fewer medication errors, decreased infection and readmission rates and improved quality of life for people with dementia (Rossiter, Levett-Jones & Pich, 2020).

PATIENT SAFETY COMPETENCY FRAMEWORK

1 Person-centred care 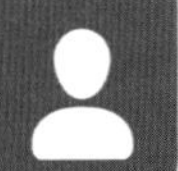

Person-centred care is central to safe and effective nursing care. The Patient Safety Competency Framework indicates that nursing students must demonstrate person-centred care by providing holistic care that takes into account the person's current situation, previous experiences and life history (Levett-Jones et al., 2017).

CRITICAL THINKING

Critical thinking is a complex collection of cognitive skills and affective habits of the mind and has been described as the process of analysing and assessing thinking with a view to improving it. Critical thinking includes the ability to reflect on and think about one's own thinking; this is called metacognition.

To make sound clinical decisions, nurses require critical-thinking skills built on clinical reasoning (Christianson, 2020). Critical thinking requires practice so that it becomes integral to your clinical decision making. Thinking critically involves more than just cognitive (knowledge) skills. It is strongly influenced by one's attitudes and mental habits. These attitudes and mental habits include the following:

- Being able to think independently so that you make clinical decisions based on sound thinking and judgment. This means, for example, that you are not influenced by negative comments from other healthcare professionals about a person.
- Being willing to listen to and be fair in your evaluation of others' ideas and beliefs. This involves listening carefully to other people's ideas and views and making decisions based on what you have learned instead of how you feel.
- Having empathy and practising in a person-centred way by being able to put yourself in the place of another to better understand that person. For example, if you put yourself in the place of the person with severe pain, you are better able to understand why they are so upset when pain medications are late.
- Being fair minded, just and considerate of all viewpoints before making a decision. This means you consider the viewpoints of others that may be different from your own before reaching a conclusion. You also realise that you are constantly learning from others. You are not afraid to say, 'I don't know the answer to that question, but I will find out and let you know.'
- Being disciplined so that you do not stop at easy answers but continue to consider alternatives.
- Being creative and self-confident. Nurses often need to consider different ways of providing care and constantly look for improved and more cost-effective methods.

The major critical-thinking skills are divergent thinking, reasoning, clarifying and reflection. A description of each follows.

Divergent thinking is having the ability to weigh the importance of information. This means that when you collect data (information/cues) from a person, you can sort out the data that are relevant for the care of that person from the data that are not relevant and then explore alternatives before reaching a conclusion. Abnormal data are usually considered relevant; normal data are helpful but may not change the care you provide.

Reasoning is having the ability to discriminate between facts and guesses. By using known facts, problems are solved and decisions are made in a systematic, logical way. For example, when you take a pulse you must know the parameters of the normal pulse rate for a person of this age, the types of medications the person is taking that may alter their pulse rate, and the emotional and physical state of the person. Based on these facts, you are able to decide if the pulse rate is normal or abnormal.

Clarifying involves noting similarities and differences and sifting out unnecessary information to help focus on the present situation. For example, when caring for a person with persistent (chronic) pain, you must know the definition of persistent pain and the similarities and differences between acute pain and persistent pain.

Reflection is a crucial professional activity and one that is intrinsic to learning. It is not simply introspection but is a deliberate, orderly and structured intellectual activity. It allows nurses to process their experiences and explore their understanding of what they are doing, why they are doing it and the impact it has on themselves and others. When this skill is developed and enhanced in relation to personal and professional practice, reflection becomes a purposeful activity that leads to improvement in practice and better patient outcomes.

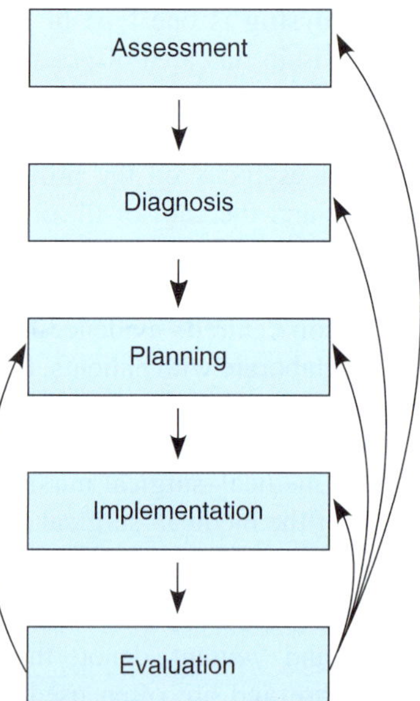

FIGURE 1.1 ***The nursing process. Steps of the nursing process. Notice that the steps are interrelated and interdependent. For example, evaluation of the person might reveal the need for further assessment, additional nursing diagnoses and/or a revision of the plan of care***

THE NURSING PROCESS

The **nursing process** has been described as a tool that helps nurses to think critically in order to provide a competent level of care (Movlavi & Salehi, 2021). The activities within the nursing process differentiate nursing from other healthcare professions. The nursing process can be used in any healthcare setting and is aimed at promoting wellness, maintaining health, restoring health or facilitating coping with disability or death. The nursing process allows for the inclusion of holistic and person-centred care. The five steps or phases in the nursing process are assessment, diagnosis, planning, implementation and evaluation. These steps are interrelated and interdependent (see Figure 1.1).

This text assumes that students already have a basic understanding of the nursing process and are now ready to expand and apply that knowledge to people with medical–surgical health problems. Table 1.1 articulates the links between the steps of the nursing process and the corresponding critical-thinking applications.

Assessment

Assessment is usually listed as the first step of the nursing process, but it is a critical element in each of the steps. It begins with the person's first encounter with the healthcare system and continues as long as the person requires care. During assessment, data (cues or pieces of information) about the person's health status are collected, validated, organised, clustered into patterns and communicated either verbally or in written form. Assessment serves as the basis for developing an accurate nursing diagnosis, for planning and implementing both initial and ongoing care, and for evaluating the effectiveness of the care provided.

The data that the nurse collects must be holistic; that is, the nurse must carefully consider all dimensions of an individual (physical, mental, social, emotional and spiritual). The data collected are both objective and subjective. Information that the nurse perceives by the senses is *objective data*; it is seen, heard, touched or smelled, and can be verified by another person (e.g. blood pressure, temperature, pulse or the presence of infected drainage). Information that is perceived only by the person experiencing it (e.g. pain, dizziness or anxiety) is *subjective data*.

Nurses assess people in two ways: through an initial assessment and through focused assessments. The initial assessment of the person, conducted through a nursing history and physical assessment, is necessary to obtain comprehensive base-line data about health responses, to identify specific factors that contribute to these responses and to facilitate mutually established goals and outcomes of care.

Focused assessments (e.g. respiratory assessment) enable the nurse to evaluate nursing actions and make decisions about whether to continue or change interventions. They also provide structure for the documentation of nursing care. In addition, focused assessments enable the nurse to identify responses to a disease process or treatment modality not present during the initial assessment, or to monitor the status of an actual or potential problem previously identified.

To make accurate and holistic assessments, nurses must use a wide range of knowledge and skills. The ability to assess the physical, emotional and mental status of the person is essential, as is the ability to use effective communication techniques.

Nurses must be knowledgeable in pathophysiology and pharmacology, and be able to identify abnormal pathology and diagnostic test data. Finally, nurses must have a solid foundation of nursing knowledge and skills that will enable them to interpret assessment data and to use that interpretation as the basis for individualised care.

TABLE 1.1 Using critical thinking in the nursing process

NURSING PROCESS STEP	CRITICAL-THINKING SKILLS	QUESTIONS TO CHECK YOUR THINKING
Assessment	Selecting the correct assessment instrument Making reliable observations Distinguishing relevant from irrelevant data Distinguishing important from unimportant data Validating data Organising data Categorising data according to a framework Recognising assumptions	What assumptions am I making about the person? Are my data correct and accurate? How reliable are my sources? What data are important? What data are relevant? What biases do I have that might cause me to miss important information? Am I listening carefully to get the person's and family's perspective? Do I have all the facts? What other data might I need?
Diagnosis	Finding patterns and relationships among cues Identifying gaps in the data Making inferences Suspending judgment when lacking data Making interdisciplinary connections Stating the problem Examining assumptions Comparing patterns with norms Identifying factors contributing to the problem	Do I know what is within normal limits for the data? Do I have enough data to make a valid inference? What biases might I have that could affect how I see the person's problems? Do I have enough data to make a nursing diagnosis or should I make a 'possible' diagnosis? What other problems might this data suggest other than the one that seems most obvious to me?
Planning	Forming valid generalisations Transferring knowledge from one situation to another Developing evaluative criteria Hypothesising Making interprofessional connections Prioritising the person's problems Generalising principles from other sciences	Do I need help to plan interventions or am I qualified to do it? Did I remember to give high priority to the problems the person and family identified as important? What are the most important problems we need to address? What interventions worked in similar situations? Is this situation similar enough to merit using them with this person? Are there other plans that might be more agreeable to the person and therefore more likely to work? Why do I expect these interventions to be effective? Based on what knowledge?
Implementation	Applying knowledge to perform interventions Using interventions to test hypotheses	Has the person's condition changed since the plan was made? Have I overlooked any new developments? What is the person's initial response to the intervention? Are there any safety issues I have overlooked?
Evaluation	Deciding whether hypotheses are correct Making criterion-based evaluations	What are the person's responses after the interventions? Have I overlooked anything? Do the data indicate that goals were met? Does the person feel their goals were met? Does the person trust me enough to give honest answers? Am I sure the problem is really resolved? What might we have done that would have been more effective? What nursing care is still needed, if any?

Source: Wilkinson (2011). *Nursing process and critical thinking* (5th ed., pp. 325–327). Electronically reproduced by permission of Pearson Education, Inc., Upper Saddle River, NJ.

Diagnosis

The nurse examines each cluster of data (or pattern) derived from the assessment to develop appropriate nursing diagnoses. Nursing diagnoses are clinical judgments about a person's actual or potential health problems. Nursing diagnoses provide the basis for determining nursing interventions to achieve outcomes for which the nurse is accountable. Nurses then develop and implement a plan of care to address health concerns and prevent illness.

Writing a nursing diagnosis

A nursing diagnosis is generally written as a two- or three-part statement. The first part is the issue or problem that has been identified from the examination of the data collected during the patient assessment. The second part is the physical, psychosocial, cultural, spiritual and/or environmental factors (aetiologies) that cause or contribute to the occurrence of the problem. The final part is the cluster of cues (signs and/or symptoms) that provide evidence of the problem.

Examples of nursing diagnoses include:

- *Faecal incontinence* (part 1: problem) related to loss of sphincter control (part 2: cause), manifested by frequent and involuntary passage of stool (part 3: evidence).
- *Acute pain* related to inadequate education about patient-controlled analgesia (PCA) use, manifested by withdrawal, grimacing, restlessness and guarded positioning.
- *Fatigue* related to the side effects of chemotherapy, evidenced by exhaustion when undertaking activities of daily living.

A risk nursing diagnosis is a clinical judgment about a potential problem where the presence of risk factors indicates that a problem may develop unless nurses intervene appropriately.

A risk diagnosis is written in two parts and does not include signs and symptoms.

Examples of risk diagnoses include:

- risk of infection related to skin tear and type 2 diabetes
- risk of falls related to confusion.

Planning

During the planning step, the nurse identifies appropriate evidence-based nursing interventions (actions) and outcomes to improve health and/or to prevent or ameliorate ill health. These outcomes are usually developed collaboratively by the person, nurse and, at times, other healthcare professionals. They identify what the person will be able to do as a result of the care provided. For example, '30 minutes following administration of analgesic medication the person will report a reduction in pain from 8 to 3 on the numeric rating scale'.

Implementation

The implementation step is the action phase of the nursing process during which the nurse carries out planned interventions. Ongoing assessment of the person before, during and after the intervention is an essential component of implementation. Although the plan may be appropriate, many factors can influence how the person responds, making a revision to the plan necessary. For example, the nurse would not be able to encourage fluid intake if the person became nauseous. Additionally, the nurse should be aware of the interrelated nature of nursing interventions. For example, while giving a bed bath the nurse can assess the person's skin condition and at the same time use therapeutic communication to provide comfort.

Documentation is the final component of implementation and is a legal requirement. Many different methods are used to document care, including problem-oriented charting, charting by exception and electronic documentation. Additionally, systems assessments are becoming increasingly common for documentation of progress notes and the development of nursing care plans.

In Australia and internationally, documentation is increasingly being undertaken using **electronic medical records (EMRs)**. EMRs allow patient data to be stored in a structured, online form, supported by real-time active decision support. EMRs are seen as a way to increase efficiency and reduce duplication and healthcare errors (Patterson, Anders & Moffatt-Bruce, 2017).

Evaluation

The evaluation step allows the nurse to determine whether the actions taken were effective and whether to continue, revise or terminate the plan of care. The outcome criteria (goals) that were established during the planning step provide the basis for evaluation. Although evaluation is listed as the last part of the nursing process, it takes place continuously throughout each person's care. To evaluate a plan, the nurse collects data from the person and their clinical records. If the outcomes have not been accomplished, the nurse must modify the nursing diagnoses, outcomes or plan.

The nursing process in clinical practice

Experienced nurses may not consciously stop and consider each step of the nursing process. For example, when caring for a person who is haemorrhaging, the nurse would use all five steps simultaneously to meet critical, life-threatening needs. In contrast, when considering long-term needs for a person with a chronic illness or disability, the nurse undertakes in-depth assessments, mutually determines goals with the person, and provides a documented plan of care that can be developed over time and revised as necessary by all nurses providing care. As a nurse becomes an expert clinician, the nursing process becomes so much a part of their practice that they may not even consciously consider it while providing care.

CLINICAL REASONING

Clinical reasoning is often used interchangeably with the terms 'clinical judgment', 'problem solving', 'decision making' and 'critical thinking'. While in some ways the terms are similar, clinical reasoning is a cyclical process that often leads to a series of linked clinical encounters. **Clinical reasoning** can be defined as 'the process by which nurses (and other clinicians) collect cues, process the information, come to an understanding of a person's problem or situation, plan and implement interventions, evaluate outcomes, and reflect on and learn from the process' (Levett-Jones, 2023). Clinical reasoning can be influenced by the nurse's assumptions, perspectives, attitudes and preconceptions, and the capacity for self-awareness of one's cognitive biases is essential to patient safety.

Over the past decade, research has identified the need for an explicit and sophisticated model both to explain how expert nurses think and as a foundation for nursing education

Links to National Patient Safety Standards

NSQHS: Communicating for Safety Standard

The use of EMRs to improve the quality of healthcare is recognised by the Australian Commission on Safety and Quality in Health Care (ACSQHC) in the National Safety and Quality Health Service Standards. The Communicating for Safety Standard states that computerised healthcare records should be used across the organisation to enable electronic data entry and retrieval by clinicians, but high levels of security and access should be ensured.

Source: ACSQHC (2021). *National Safety and Quality Health Service Standards* (2nd ed.). Sydney: ACSQHC. © Australian Commission on Safety and Quality in Health Care.

(Levett-Jones, 2023; Vierula et al., 2020). A model titled the Clinical Reasoning Cycle (CRC) was developed by Australian nurse researchers to clearly articulate how nurses use sophisticated thinking skills to inform their practice decisions and enhance patient safety (see Figure 1.2). The CRC builds upon the nursing process framework and represents the multi-faceted and increasingly complex nature of nursing care, and the necessity to respond appropriately to patients' needs, particularly in emergent, non-routine and unpredictable clinical situations. The CRC is integral to students' developing ability to 'think like a nurse' and its explicit meta-cognitive and reflective processes aim to identify and prevent cognitive errors that may lead to adverse patient outcomes. A body of evidence has identified that clinical reasoning skills have a positive impact on patient outcomes and that nurses with poor clinical reasoning skills often fail to detect and appropriately respond to patient deterioration (Liaw, Cooper & Levett-Jones, 2018). Clinical reasoning errors have also been implicated as a key factor in the majority of adverse patient outcomes (Institute of Medicine, 2016).

The Clinical Reasoning Cycle consists of eight main stages or steps: *consider the patient situation, collect cues, process information, identify problems and priorities, establish goals, take action, evaluate outcomes* and *reflect on process and new learning.*

ACCOUNTABLE AND RESPONSIBLE NURSING PRACTICE

The Australian Nursing and Midwifery Accreditation Council (ANMAC) is responsible for accreditation of nursing and midwifery programs, while the Nursing and Midwifery Board of Australia (NMBA) has responsibility for professional registration, professional codes, standards and competency issues.

In Australia, there are three key documents that form the basic framework for accountable and responsible practice as a Registered Nurse. These are:

1. Nursing and Midwifery Board of Australia (NMBA), *Registered Nurse Standards for Practice* (2016).
2. The International Council of Nurses (ICN), *Code of Ethics for Nurses* (2012).
3. Nursing and Midwifery Board of Australia (NMBA), *Code of Conduct for Nurses* (2018).

Nursing and Midwifery Board of Australia (NMBA) *Registered Nurse Standards for Practice*

The *Registered Nurse Standards for Practice* (2016) were developed to promote a national approach to nursing in Australia. These standards are an integral component of the

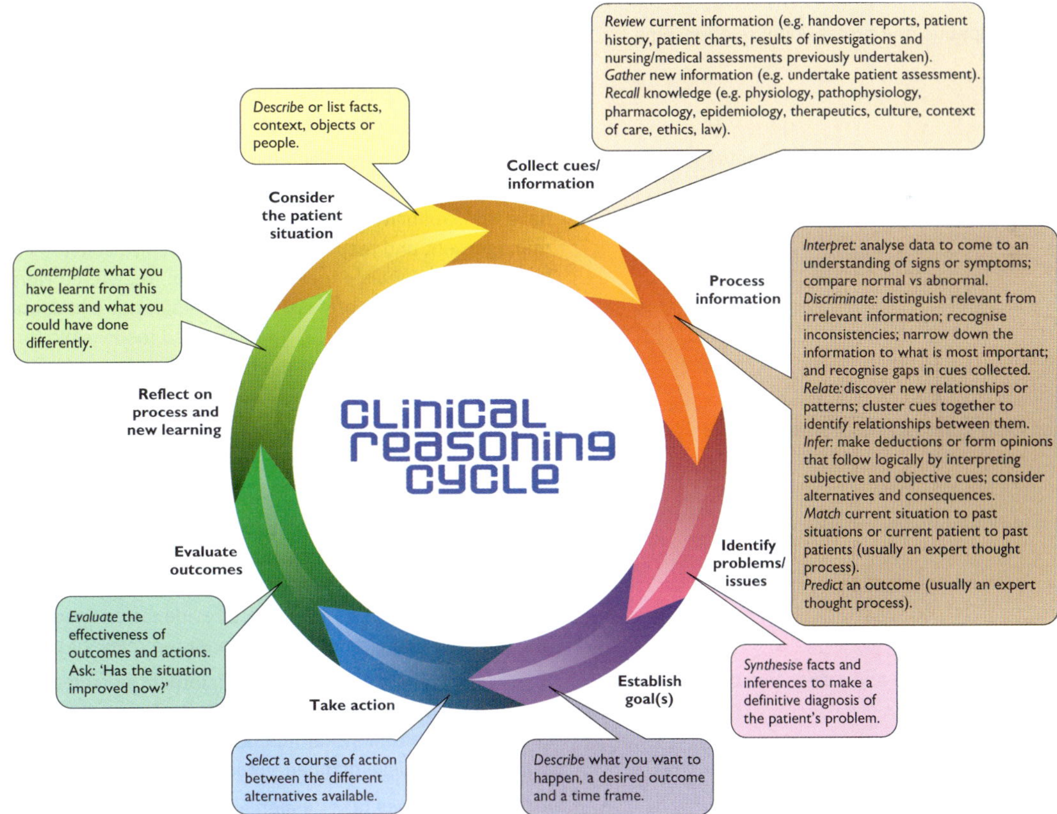

FIGURE 1.2 *The clinical reasoning process with descriptors*

Source: Levett-Jones (2023). *Clinical reasoning: Learning to think like a nurse*, p. 7; adapted from Levett-Jones et al. (2010). The 'five rights' of clinical reasoning: An educational model to enhance nursing students' ability to identify and manage clinically 'at risk' patients. *Nurse Education Today, 30*(6), 515–520.

nursing regulatory framework that assists nurses to deliver safe and competent care. They are the standards by which a nurse's performance is assessed to obtain and retain registration to practise as a nurse in Australia. As the ever-changing healthcare needs and expectations of Australians impact on quality and safety within the healthcare system, so must practice standards be regularly reviewed by the nursing profession. The NMBA standards for practice were reviewed and updated during 2015 and were published early in 2016. The standards are organised into domains, as illustrated in Box 1.1.

Code of Ethics for Nurses

In March 2018, the NMBA adopted the International Council of Nurses (ICN) *Code of Ethics for Nurses* (2012) as the guiding document for ethical decision making for nurses in Australia. The ICN Code of Ethics is a guide for action based on social values and needs, and is premised on the understanding that nurses have four fundamental responsibilities: (1) to promote health, (2) to prevent illness, (3) to restore health, and (4) to alleviate suffering. The Code includes respect for human rights, including cultural rights, the right to life and choice, and the right to dignity and to be treated with respect. It also emphasises that nursing care must be unrestricted by considerations of age, colour, creed, culture, disability or illness, gender, sexual orientation, nationality, politics, race or social status (ICN, 2012).

Code of Conduct for Nurses

The *Code of Conduct for Nurses* (NMBA, 2018) sets out the legal requirements, professional behaviours and conduct expectations for nurses in Australia, and underpins the delivery of safe, kind and compassionate nursing care. The principles of the Code apply to all types of nursing practice in all contexts. This includes any work where a nurse uses nursing skills and

BOX 1.1 Domains of the Nursing and Midwifery Board of Australia (NMBA) *Registered Nurse Standards for Practice*

1. Thinks critically and analyses nursing practice	Nurses use a variety of thinking strategies, research and best available evidence in making decisions and providing safe, quality nursing practice within a person-centred framework.
2. Engages in therapeutic and professional relationships	Nursing practice is based on purposefully engaging in the formation and maintenance of effective therapeutic and professional relationships. This includes collegial generosity in the context of interdisciplinary and professional relationships.
3. Maintains fitness for practice and participates in lifelong learning	Registered Nurses, as regulated health professionals, are responsible and accountable for ensuring they are safe and have the capability for practice. This includes ongoing self-management and responding when there are concerns about other health professionals' fitness for practice. Registered Nurses are responsible for their professional development and contribute to the development of others. They are also responsible for providing information and education to enable people to make decisions and take action in relation to their health.
4. Comprehensively conducts assessments	Registered Nurses accurately conduct comprehensive and systematic assessments, analyse information and data and communicate outcomes as the basis of practice.
5. Develops a plan for nursing practice	Registered Nurses are responsible for the planning and communication of nursing practice. Agreed plans are developed in partnership. They are based on the Registered Nurse's comprehensive assessment, use of evidence and judgment that is documented and communicated to all the relevant people.
6. Provides safe, appropriate and responsive quality nursing practice	Registered Nurses delegate and implement person-centred, quality and ethical goal-directed actions. These are based on comprehensive and systematic assessment, and the best available evidence to achieve planned outcomes.
7. Evaluates outcomes to inform nursing practice	Registered Nurses take responsibility for the evaluation of practice based on agreed outcomes to plan and revise practice accordingly.

Source: Nursing and Midwifery Board of Australia (NMBA) (2016). *Registered Nurse Standards for Practice*. © Nursing and Midwifery Board of Australia, www.nursingmidwiferyboard.gov.au/.

BOX 1.2 NMBA *Code of Conduct for Nurses*

Domain: Practise legally

1. **Legal compliance**
   Nurses respect and adhere to their professional obligations under the National Law, and abide by relevant laws.

Domain: Practise safely, effectively and collaboratively

2. **Person-centred practice**
   Nurses provide safe, person-centred and evidence-based practice for the health and wellbeing of people and, in partnership with the person, promote shared decision making and care delivery between the person, nominated partners, family, friends and health professionals.
3. **Cultural practice and respectful relationships**
   Nurses engage with people as individuals in a culturally safe and respectful way, foster open and honest professional relationships, and adhere to their obligations about privacy and confidentiality.

Domain: Act with professional integrity

4. **Professional behaviour**
   Nurses embody integrity, honesty, respect and compassion.
5. **Teaching, supervising and assessing**
   Nurses commit to teaching, supervising and assessing students and other nurses in order to develop the nursing workforce across all contexts of practice.
6. **Research in health**
   Nurses recognise the vital role of research to inform quality healthcare and policy development, conduct research ethically and support the decision making of people who participate in research.

Domain: Promote health and wellbeing

7. **Health and wellbeing**
   Nurses promote health and wellbeing for people and their families, colleagues, the broader community and themselves, and in a way that addresses health inequality.

Source: NMBA (2018). *Code of Conduct for Nurses.* © Nursing and Midwifery Board of Australia, www.nursingmidwiferyboard.gov.au/.

knowledge, whether paid or unpaid, clinical or non-clinical. The code of conduct includes seven principles of conduct, grouped into four domains (see Box 1.2).

CULTURALLY COMPETENT NURSING

The primary focus of nursing care is the person and how they respond to their environment and experiences or situations related to health or illness. These experiences are given shape and personal meaning by **culture**—the socially inherited characteristics of a human group. The healthcare system encompasses many people (staff and patients) who are culturally diverse. This diversity includes differences in country of origin, health beliefs, sexual orientation, race, socioeconomic level and age.

Culture influences us all in our work, home and social lives. We therefore need to understand what the term 'culture' means. Rosenjack-Burcham (2002) defines culture as 'a learned world viewpoint or paradigm shared by a population or group and transmitted socially. It influences values, beliefs, customs and behaviours, and is reflected in the language, dress, food, materials and social interactions of a group' (p. 7). In Leininger's seminal work (1991), culture is described as 'the learned and transmitted values, beliefs and practices … the blueprint for living, remaining healthy, or for dying' (p. 36). Culture is primarily learned in our family or community life and can be shared with others. Our own culture can be experienced by us in an unconscious way and can change over time. Culture is therefore different from ethnicity, which is determined at birth. Interacting across cultures requires us to be aware of our own culture and requires an understanding of and skill in interpersonal and group communication.

Increasing cultural and ethnic diversity in most regions of the world over the past 40 years has made provision of culturally competent care essential for nurses and other health professionals (Everson et al., 2015). However, studies indicate that people from non-English-speaking backgrounds experience significantly more adverse health events than English-speaking people do and that misunderstandings, miscommunication and culturally unsafe care by health professionals are frequently reported (Johnstone & Kanitsaki, 2008). Many factors account for culturally unsafe care, including lack of awareness, skills and empathy, as well as ethnocentrism (people's belief that their own cultural group's beliefs and values are the only acceptable ones) and prejudice.

People of every culture have the right to have their cultural values known, respected and addressed appropriately in nursing and other healthcare services (Leininger, 1991). To provide nursing care that is culturally competent, nurses must develop sensitivity to personal fundamental values about health and illness, must accept the existence of differing values and must be respectful of, interested in and empathetic towards people from different cultures without being judgmental. **Cultural competence** is essential to quality care. According to Betancourt et al. (2003), cultural competence 'entails understanding the importance of social and cultural influences on patients' health beliefs and behaviours, considering how these factors interact at multiple levels of the health care delivery system, and devising interventions that take these issues into account' (p. 294).

A related concept, **cultural safety**, was developed in a First Nations' context and is a philosophy of practice that takes into account people's unique needs. Cultural safety refers to how people are treated in society, and its focus is on systemic and structural issues that influence the social determinants of health. Unsafe cultural practice comprises any action that 'diminishes, demeans or disempowers the cultural identity and wellbeing of an individual' (Nursing Council of New Zealand, 2012, pp. 32–33). Importantly, the 'presence or absence of cultural safety is determined by the recipient of care not by the caregiver' (Congress of Aboriginal and Torres Strait Islander Nurses and Midwives, 2014, p. 9).

Standard 2 of the NMBA *Registered Nurse Standards for Practice* (2016) refers to therapeutic relationships and indicates that Registered Nurses must 'establish, sustain and conclude therapeutic relationships in a way that is respectful and acknowledges the dignity, culture, values and beliefs and rights of a person'.

While developing a growing appreciation of the various cultural groups you come into contact with in your many nursing roles is essential, developing an appreciation and understanding of the history and culture of Aboriginal and Torres Strait Islander peoples (Australia's First Peoples) is fundamental to the development of professional nurses and to nursing practice which is experienced as culturally safe. In order to be effective in delivering appropriate care to Aboriginal and Torres Strait Islander people, nurses need:

- awareness of important Aboriginal and Torres Strait Islander issues, such as cultural differences, and specific aspects of Indigenous history and their impact on Indigenous peoples in contemporary Australian society
- the skills to interact and communicate sensitively and effectively with Indigenous peoples
- the motivation to interact successfully with Indigenous peoples in order to improve access, service delivery and patient outcomes (Farrelly & Lumby, 2009).

Undertaking this journey into the history and culture of Indigenous Australians is likely to challenge your understanding of your own culture and how your cultural values impact on the way you provide nursing care to all people.

In the chapters that follow, the cultural implications of the various clinical situations are discussed and expanded upon, and you will be presented with opportunities to apply and contextualise your learning about cultural safety.

LEGAL AND ETHICAL DILEMMAS IN NURSING

A **dilemma** is a choice between two unpleasant, ethically troubling alternatives. Nurses face dilemmas almost daily—so many, in fact, that a complete discussion of them is impossible here. However, many commonly experienced dilemmas involve confidentiality, human rights and issues of dying and death. The nurse must use ethical and legal guidelines to make decisions about moral actions when providing care in these and many other situations.

The rights of each individual can result in dilemmas for nurses in the clinical setting. For example, the right to refuse treatment (including surgery, medication, nutrition and hydration) is an example of a person's rights that can conflict with a nurse's personal and professional values and may cause ethical dilemmas. The situation, the alternatives and the potential consequences of refusal must be carefully explored with the person.

The issues surrounding dying and death have become increasingly topical as advances in technology extend the lives of people with chronic debilitating illness and major trauma. These changes have altered concepts of living and dying, resulting in ethical dilemmas regarding quality of life and death with dignity versus technological preservation of life. Additionally, difficulties in establishing a person's competence to make informed decisions about withholding and withdrawing treatment, and use of opioids at the end of life are some of the issues that nurses will encounter in their practice.

ROLES OF THE NURSE IN MEDICAL–SURGICAL NURSING PRACTICE

Healthcare today is a vast and complex system. It reflects changes in society, changes in the populations requiring nursing care and a philosophical shift towards health promotion rather than illness care. The roles of the medical–surgical nurse have broadened and expanded in response to these changes. Medical–surgical nurses are not only caregivers, but also educators, advocates, leaders, managers, and researchers. The nurse assumes these various roles to promote and maintain health, to prevent illness and to facilitate coping with disability or death for people in a range of healthcare settings.

The nurse as caregiver

Nurses have always been caregivers. However, the activities carried out within the caregiver role have changed tremendously in the 21st century. From 1900 to the 1960s, the nurse was almost always female and was regarded primarily as the person who gave personal care and carried out doctors' orders. This dependent role has changed as a result of the increased education of nurses, research into and the development of nursing knowledge, a strong evidence base and the recognition that nurses are autonomous and well-informed professionals.

The caregiver role for the nurse today is both independent and collaborative. Nurses independently make assessments and plan and implement patient care based on nursing knowledge and skills. Nurses also collaborate with other members of the interprofessional healthcare team to implement and evaluate care (see Figure 1.3).

In providing comprehensive and person-centred care, the nurse uses critical-thinking skills to analyse and synthesise knowledge from the arts, the sciences, and nursing research and theory. The science (knowledge base) of nursing is translated into the art of nursing through caring. Caring is the means by which the nurse is connected with and concerned for the person who is the recipient of care. Thus, the nurse as caregiver is knowledgeable, skilled and empathic. Nursing care must address not only the physical needs but also the psychosocial, cultural, spiritual and environmental needs of each person and their family. Considering all aspects of a person's being ensures a holistic approach to nursing. Subsumed within the concept of 'holistic healthcare' is the concept of caring for the mind, body and spirit.

The nurse as educator

The nurse's role as educator is becoming increasingly important for several reasons. There is much greater emphasis on health promotion and illness prevention, hospital stays are becoming shorter and the number of people with chronic illnesses in our society is increasing. Early discharge of people from the hospital

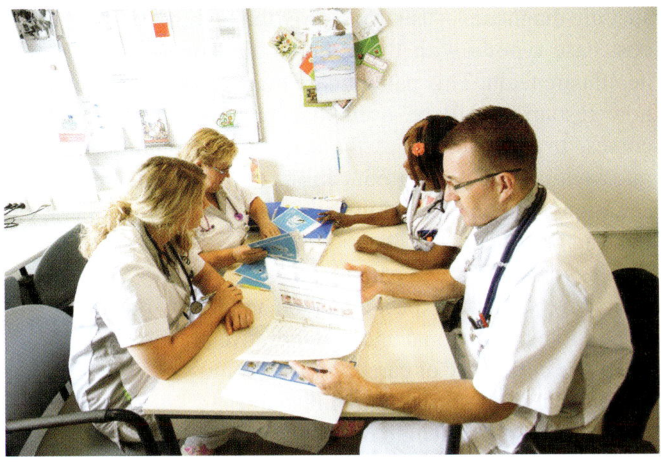

FIGURE 1.3 ***The healthcare team discusses the individualised plan of care and outcomes***

Source: Arno Massee/Science Photo Library/Alamy.

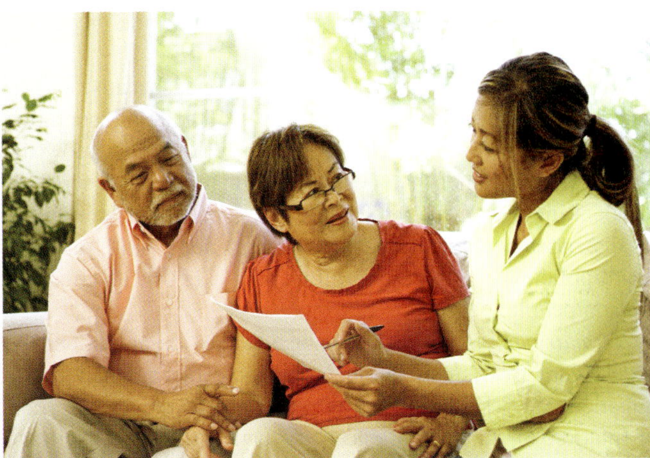

FIGURE 1.4 ***The nurse's role as educator is an essential component of care. As part of the discharge planning process, the nurse is responsible for teaching for self-care at home***

Source: © Monkey Business Images/Shutterstock.com.

setting to the home means that family caregivers must learn how to perform complex skills. All these factors make the educator role essential to maintaining people's health and wellbeing.

The framework for the role of educator is the teaching–learning process. Within this framework the nurse assesses learning needs, plans and implements teaching methods to meet those needs, and evaluates the effectiveness of the teaching. To be effective educators, nurses need effective interpersonal skills and familiarity with adult learning principles (see Figure 1.4).

A major component of the educator role today is discharge planning. Discharge planning, which begins on admission to a healthcare setting, is a systematic method of preparing the person and their family for departure from the healthcare facility and for maintaining continuity of care after they leave the setting. Discharge planning also involves making referrals, identifying community and personal resources, and arranging necessary equipment and supplies for home care.

The nurse as advocate

The person entering the healthcare system may not always be prepared to make independent decisions. However, nurses need to be aware that today's healthcare consumer is better educated about options for care and may have very definite opinions. The nurse as patient advocate actively promotes the patient's right to autonomy and free choice. The nurse as advocate speaks for the person if needed, mediates between the person and other people, and/or protects the person's right to self-determination. The goals of the nurse as advocate are to:

- assess the need for advocacy
- communicate with other healthcare team members
- assist and support decision making
- serve as a change agent in the healthcare system
- participate in health policy formulation.

The nurse must practise advocacy while maintaining the belief that people have the right to choose treatment options, based on information about the results of accepting or rejecting the treatment, without coercion. The nurse must also accept and respect the decisions of the person, even though they may differ from the decisions the nurse would make.

The nurse as leader and manager

All nurses are leaders and managers. They practise leadership and they manage time, people, resources and the environment in which they provide care. Nurses carry out these roles by directing, delegating and coordinating nursing activities. Nurses must be knowledgeable about how and when to delegate, as well as the legal requirements of delegation. As leaders and managers, nurses also evaluate the quality of care provided.

Models of care delivery

Nurses are leaders and managers of patient care within a variety of models of care delivery. Models of care may include:

- task-oriented nursing
- team nursing
- patient allocation or total patient care
- primary nursing
- case management.

Task-oriented nursing refers to a model in which nurses undertake specific tasks related to nursing care across a group of people. Some examples of task allocation may be when a nurse showers all the people in a ward while another nurse administers medications for the same group of people. In this model of care delivery, nursing care relates to discrete sets of activities that are performed by nurses.

Team nursing is a model that 'teams' experienced nurses with less experienced or casual staff to achieve nursing goals using a group-based approach. A team may consist of a Registered Nurse, an Enrolled Nurse and an Assistant in Nursing. The Registered Nurse is the team leader. The team leader is responsible for delegating care activities and has overall responsibility for patient care by team members.

All team members work together, each performing the activities for which they are best prepared.

Patient allocation models were developed because nurses recognised the need for total patient care. The implementation of these types of models results in nurses getting to know the whole person, rather than people being cared for as a series of tasks. A nurse will be allocated to their patients (the number is dependent on factors such as patient need, staff mix and ward policies) and undertake all nursing care for the allocated person/people.

Primary nursing allows the nurse to provide individualised direct care to a small number of people during their entire inpatient stay. This model was developed to reduce the fragmentation of care experienced by patients and to facilitate continuity of care. In primary nursing, the nurse provides care; communicates with the person, families and other healthcare providers; and carries out discharge planning.

Case management focuses on management of a caseload (group) of patients. The purpose of case management is to maximise positive outcomes and contain costs. The nurse who is case manager is usually a clinical specialist, and the caseload consists of people with similar healthcare needs. As case manager, the nurse makes appropriate referrals to other healthcare providers and manages the quality of care provided, including accuracy, timeliness and cost. The case manager is also in contact with patients after discharge, ensuring continuity of care and health maintenance.

The model of care delivery implemented on a ward will depend on a range of factors, including the degree of innovation and commitment by the people involved. Some models work better when there are sufficient numbers of experienced Registered Nurses to deliver care; others may focus on supporting less experienced staff using a team approach.

Delegation

Delegation is carried out when the nurse assigns appropriate work activities to other members of the healthcare team. When the nurse delegates nursing care activities to another person, that person is authorised to act in the place of the nurse, although the nurse retains the accountability for the activities performed. Delegation depends on knowing one's own scope of practice and that of the person to whom one plans to delegate.

Nurses' **scope of practice** refers to the roles, functions, responsibilities, activities and decision-making capacity that they are educated, competent and authorised to perform. One's scope of practice is influenced by the wider environment, the specific setting, legislation, policy, education, standards and the health needs of the population. Registered Nurses have a key role in the coordination and supervision of others who assist them in the provision of care to people.

Evaluating outcomes of nursing care

CLINICAL PATHWAYS A **clinical pathway** is a plan designed to provide healthcare, often within a multidisciplinary team. Such pathways are generally developed for specific diagnoses—usually high-volume, high-risk and high-cost case types—with the collaboration of members of the healthcare team. This patient care management tool describes how resources will be used to achieve predetermined outcomes. It also establishes the sequence of multidisciplinary interventions, including education, discharge planning, consultations, medication administration, diagnostics, therapeutics and treatments.

The goals of clinical pathways are to:

- achieve realistic, expected person and family outcomes
- promote professional and collaborative practice and care
- ensure continuity of care
- guarantee appropriate use of resources
- reduce costs and length of stay
- provide the framework for continuous improvement.

Clinical pathways are often used in conjunction with case management models and/or quality improvement efforts. The overall goal is to design pathways that facilitate a reproducible standard of care for specific patient populations and improve the quality and proficiency of that care.

The healthcare facility determines the process for developing a clinical pathway. Information imperative to the development of any clinical pathway includes literature reviews, chart reviews and expert opinion. A typical approach is to first identify high-cost, high-volume and high-risk case types for the agency. Next, a multidisciplinary team develops a consensus around the management of the case type and a clinical pathway. The pathway is then piloted with a designated group of people and revised based on the number and types of variances. The goal is to develop a pathway that best meets the needs of people in the particular practice setting.

When people do not achieve expected outcomes, variances (deviations from the established plan) from the clinical pathways are recorded and studied by the multidisciplinary team. In many facilities, clinical pathways are designed so that interventions and variances can be easily documented. Most documentation systems require a check-off when interventions are performed or variances occur.

In many facilities, clinical pathways are replacing traditional nursing care plans. The advantages of clinical pathways are that they are outcome driven and provide a timeline to achieve specified goals. Additionally, clinical pathways provide opportunities for healthcare workers to collaborate and establish dynamic plans of care that consider all of the people's needs. Although initially developed for acute hospitalisations, clinical pathways are now being developed to manage people in the home, outpatients and those in long-term settings.

Clinical governance

Clinical governance is defined as a systematic and integrated approach that improves quality and safety and results in optimal patient outcomes. Clinical governance places the responsibility for the quality of care jointly on organisations and on individuals within organisations. As a leader and manager within a

Links to National Patient Safety Standards

NSQHS: Clinical Governance Standard

The Clinical Governance Standard of the National Safety and Quality Health Service Standards specifies that there is the set of relationships and responsibilities established by a health service organisation to ensure that systems are in place to deliver safe and high-quality healthcare and to continuously improve services.

Source: ACSQHC (2021). *National Safety and Quality Health Service Standards* (2nd ed.). Sydney: ACSQHC.

healthcare organisation, the nurse has an important role in promoting continuous quality improvement through governance structures such as:

- clinical risk management
- clinical quality and safety frameworks
- consumer participation
- clinical effectiveness
- clinical audit
- evidence-based practice
- credentialling/professional development
- research and development.

The medical–surgical nurse is well placed to contribute to the evaluation of the quality of clinical practice through peer review, clinical audit and external accreditation processes.

The nurse as researcher

The science of nursing is established through clinical research and then published so that the findings can be used by all nurses to provide evidence-based, person-centred care. This means that all nurses must consider the researcher role as integral to nursing practice and are expected to use the best clinical evidence available to inform their patient care decisions. Nursing care that is based on high-quality research evidence is more likely to be cost effective and result in positive patient outcomes (Chien, 2019).

This text is informed by and based on nursing research, with summaries of relevant studies included throughout many chapters. These include discussions about each study and a critical-thinking section that encourages students to apply the findings to their clinical practice.

CHAPTER HIGHLIGHTS

- Safe and effective nursing care focuses on the provision of person-centred care, working in interprofessional teams, using evidence-based practice and working within legal and ethical frameworks.
- The nursing process is an approach used by nurses to provide care to promote wellness, maintain health, restore health or facilitate coping with disability or death. The five steps of the nursing process are assessment, diagnosis, planning, implementation and evaluation.
- Clinical reasoning is a dynamic process in which nurses collect cues, process this information, come to an understanding of the situation (or patient's problem), plan and implement care, evaluate outcomes, and reflect on and learn from the process. The questioning of assumptions and the avoidance of clinical reasoning errors are integral to this process.
- The clinical practice of nurses is guided by codes of conduct, codes of ethics and standards for practice.
- Nurses function as caregivers, educators, advocates, leaders and managers, and researchers to promote and maintain health, prevent illness and facilitate coping with disability or death for the adult person.

CONCEPT CHECK

1 The Nursing and Midwifery Board of Australia (NMBA) has developed a set of standards for practice. What is the primary purpose of these standards?
1 to make all nurses equal
2 to promote safe and effective nursing care
3 to reduce the number of legal actions
4 to provide a set of ethical guidelines

2 What does the nurse use in the clinical setting to make clinical judgments and decisions?
1 nursing process
2 standards of care
3 clinical reasoning skills
4 all of the above

3 Which of the following statements is true of outcomes developed during the planning phase of the nursing process?
1 Outcomes are mutually established by the person and the nurse.
2 Outcomes are mutually established by the nurse and the doctor.
3 Outcomes are mandated by institutional policies and standards.
4 Outcomes are written by the person receiving care and their family members.

4 The steps of the nursing process are used when providing care. From the list below, select the order in which the steps are most often used.
1 diagnosis
2 assessment
3 evaluation
4 implementation
5 planning

5 When nurses discuss the 'science of nursing', what does this phrase mean?
1 clinical competency
2 holistic care
3 evidence-based practice
4 practice component

6 What role does the nurse demonstrate when appraising health information?
1 advocate
2 caregiver
3 researcher
4 educator

7 What goal is a component of the nurse's role as advocate?
1 assisting and supporting the person in their decision making
2 conducting research about the effects of exercise
3 delegating responsibilities for care to others
4 performing range-of-motion exercises

8 A nurse assigns appropriate work activities to other members of her team. What role is being illustrated?
1 advocate
2 leader/manager
3 researcher
4 caregiver

9 A method of establishing a standard of care and evaluating outcomes of that standard involves:
1 writing a dress-code policy for a healthcare agency
2 creating a clinical pathway for a specific type of person
3 establishing clinical governance approaches
4 implementing a new procedure to change dressings

10 A Registered Nurse delegates vital signs assessment to an Assistant in Nursing. Who is accountable for the assessment findings?
1 the Assistant in Nursing
2 the person receiving care
3 the nurse
4 the doctor

BIBLIOGRAPHY

Australian College of Nursing (2020). *Person-centred care position statement*. Reviewed May 2020. Retrieved from https://www.acn.edu.au

Australian Commission on Safety and Quality in Health Care (2021). *National Safety and Quality Health Service Standards* (2nd ed.). Sydney: ACSQHC.

Betancourt, J. R., Green, A. R., Carrillo, J. E. & Ananeh-Firempong, O. (2003). Defining cultural competence: A practical framework for addressing racial/ethnic disparities in health and health care. *Public Health Reports*, *118*, 293–302.

Chien L. Y. (2019). Evidence-based practice and nursing research. *The Journal of Nursing Research*, *27*(4), e29. https://doi.org/10.1097/jnr.0000000000000346

Christianson, K. L. (2020). Emotional intelligence and critical thinking in nursing students: Integrative review of literature. *Nurse Educator*, *45*, E62–E65. https://doi.org/10.1097/NNE.0000000000000801

Congress of Aboriginal and Torres Strait Islander Nurses and Midwives (2014). *Towards a shared understanding of terms and concepts: Strengthening nursing and midwifery care of Aboriginal and Torres Strait Islander peoples*. Canberra. Retrieved from http://catsinam.org.au/

Everson, N., Levett-Jones, T., Lapkin, S., Pitt, V., van der Riet, P., Rossiter, R., Courtney-Pratt, H., Gilligan, C. & Jones, D. (2015). Measuring the impact of a 3D simulation experience on nursing students' cultural empathy using a modified version of the Kiersma-Chen Empathy Scale. *Journal of Clinical Nursing*, *24*(19–20), 2849–2858.

Farrelly, T. & Lumby, B. (2009). A best practice approach to cultural competence training. *Aboriginal and Islander Health Worker Journal*, *33*(5), 14–22.

Institute of Medicine (2016). *The future of nursing: Focus on education*. Retrieved from http://www.nursingworld.org

International Council of Nurses (ICN) (2012). *The ICN Code of Ethics for Nurses*. Geneva. Retrieved from http://www.icn.ch/

Johnstone, M. J. & Kanitsaki, O. (2008). Cultural racism, language prejudice and discrimination in hospital contexts: An Australian study. *Diversity in Health and Social Care*, *5*, 19–30. Retrieved from www.ingentaconnect.com/

Leininger, M. (1991). Transcultural care principles, human rights, and ethical considerations. *Journal of Transcultural Nursing*, *3*(1), 21–23.

Levett-Jones, T. (2023). Clinical reasoning: What it is and why it matters. In T. Levett-Jones (ed.), *Clinical reasoning: Learning how to think like a nurse* (3rd ed.). Frenchs Forest: Pearson.

Levett-Jones, T., Dwyer, T., Reid-Searl, K., Heaton, L., Flenady, T., Applegarth, J., Guinea, S. & Andersen, P. (2017). *Patient Safety Competency Framework (PSCF) for Nursing Students*. Sydney. Retrieved from http://psframework.wpengine.com/

Levett-Jones, T., Hoffman, K., Dempsey, Y., Jeong, S., Noble, D., Norton, C., Roche, J. & Hickey, N. (2010). The 'five rights' of clinical reasoning: An educational modelto enhance nursing students' ability to identify and manage clinically 'at risk' patients. *Nurse Education Today*, *30*(6), 515–520.

Liaw, S., Cooper, S. & Levett-Jones, T. (2018). Development and psychometric testing of a Clinical Reasoning Evaluation Simulation Tool (CREST) for assessing ability to recognize and respond to clinical deterioration. *Nurse Education Today*, 62, 74–79. https://doi.org/10.1016/j.nedt.2017.12.009

Movlavi, S. & Salehi, S. (2021). Examining the effect of implementation of the nursing process on students' health behaviors. *International Journal of Adolescent Medicine and Health*, *33*(5). https://doi.org/10.1515/ijamh-2018-0244

Nursing and Midwifery Board of Australia (NMBA) (2016). *Registered Nurse Standards for Practice*. Retrieved from https://www.nursingmidwiferyboard.gov.au/

Nursing and Midwifery Board of Australia (NMBA) (2018). *Code of Conduct for Nurses*. Retrieved from https://www.nursingmidwiferyboard.gov.au/

Nursing Council of New Zealand (2012). *Competencies for registered nurses*. Retrieved from https://www.nursingcouncil.org.nz/

Patterson, E., Anders, S. & Moffatt-Bruce, S. (2017). Clustering and prioritizing patient safety issues during EHR implementation and upgrades in hospital settings. *Proceedings of the International Symposium on Human Factors and Ergonomics in Health Care*, 6(1), 125–131.

Rosenjack-Burcham, J. L. (2002). Cultural competence: An evolutionary perspective. *Nursing Forum*, *37*(4), 5–16.

Rossiter, C., Levett-Jones, T. & Pich, J. (2020). The impact of person-centred care on patient safety: An umbrella review of systematic reviews. *International Journal of Nursing Studies*, *109*, 103658.

Vierula, J., Hupli, M., Talman, K. & Haavisto, E. (2020). Identifying reasoning skills for the selection of undergraduate nursing students: A focus group study. *Contemporary Nurse*, *56*(2), 120–131.

Wilkinson, J. M. (2011). *Nursing process and critical thinking* (5th ed.). Upper Saddle River, NJ: Pearson Education, Inc.

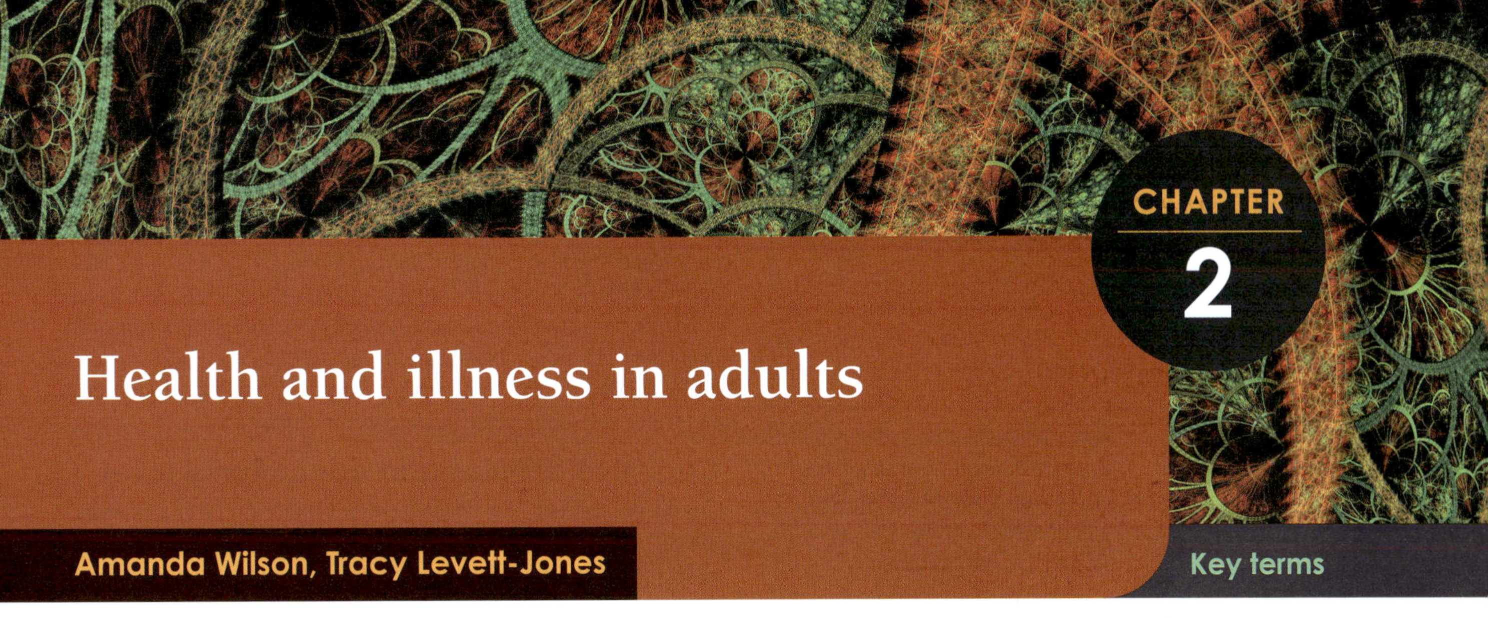

CHAPTER 2

Health and illness in adults

Amanda Wilson, Tracy Levett-Jones

Learning outcomes

- Define health, including the concepts of the illness–wellness continuum and high-level wellness.
- Explain what determinants of health are and how they influence health, disease and illness.
- Discuss the nurse's role in promoting healthy lifestyles and preventing illness and injury.
- Describe the different behaviours and needs of people with acute and chronic illness.
- Describe the primary, secondary and tertiary levels of illness prevention.
- Compare and contrast the physical status, changes in health, assessment guidelines and healthy behaviours of the young adult, middle adult and older adult.
- Explain the definitions, functions and developmental stages and tasks of the family.

Clinical competencies

- Include knowledge of developmental levels and of activities to promote, restore and maintain health when planning and implementing care for adults.
- Include family members in teaching to promote and maintain health of the adult.

Key terms

DEFINING HEALTH

The Constitution of the World Health Organization (WHO) defines **health** as 'a state of complete physical, mental, and social well-being, and not merely the absence of disease or infirmity' (WHO, 1948, p. 1). This definition is fundamental to contemporary healthcare perspectives and can be expanded to encompass the various levels of health people experience throughout their life. However, the concept of health is subjective and reflects an individual's perspective of quality of life. For example, someone with a terminal diagnosis can still enjoy life and feel 'well', although their definition of health may be very different to that of a person without that diagnosis. All these factors are important influences on how we provide nursing care and reflect the illness–wellness continuum and the concept of high-level wellness.

The illness–wellness continuum

The **illness–wellness continuum** represents health as a dynamic process. At one extreme of the continuum is high-level wellness, while death is at the opposite extreme. During our lifetime, we traverse different points on this continuum. The continuum of health and illness was expanded from its original form to include the concept of high-level wellness, with 'good health' differentiated from 'wellness' in the following way:

> *Good health can exist as a relatively passive state of freedom from illness in which the individual is at peace with… (their)… environment… Wellness is an integrated method of functioning, which is oriented toward maximising the potential of which the individual is capable, within the environment where he [or she] is functioning.* (Dunn 1959, p. 4)

The philosophy of **holistic healthcare** includes physical, psychosocial, cultural, spiritual and intellectual aspects of the person. Similarly, elements of wellness include self-perception, environment, culture and philosophical values. To promote, maintain or restore health, both the nurse and the person receiving care need to recognise and address these wellness factors.

DETERMINANTS OF HEALTH

Australia has a population of approximately 25.75 million people (Australian Bureau of Statistics (ABS), 2021a). Australians today are living 25 years longer than their great-grandparents, who were born a century ago. Females born in 2016–2018 have a life expectancy of 85 years; males born in that period have a life expectancy of 81 years (Australian Institute of Health and Welfare (AIHW), 2020a). Many different factors affect health and wellness; these are referred to as **determinants of health**. Determinants of health can influence good health or be risk factors for poor health. The following sections describe some of the major determinants of health and their impact.

Genetic make-up

Genetic make-up is composed of inherited features from generations of family members and provides a blueprint for health throughout life. Genetic make-up determines eye colour, and affects personality, temperament and intellectual potential; it also makes us susceptible to developing hereditary conditions. Cystic fibrosis (CF), haemophilia, type 2 diabetes, hypercholesterolaemia (elevated levels of cholesterol in the blood) and some types of cancer are examples of genetic diseases and disorders. Research into genetic make-up, referred to as genomics, is providing insights into ways to diagnose, treat and even prevent these conditions. Research has also shown how quickly genetic structure changes and how our health choices can influence the genetic health of our children.

Cognitive abilities and educational level

Cognitive abilities are developed in childhood, which is why school education is considered to be an important determinant of health. Our level of cognitive development affects our perceptions of health and illness and may also affect health practices. Educational levels affect our ability to understand and follow guidelines for health—this is called health literacy. If a person cannot read well, written materials such as brochures or handouts on health behaviours and resources are of little value. In Australia, people in major cities are more likely to complete Year 12 or equivalent than those living in regional, rural or remote areas (AIHW, 2021a).

Race, ethnicity and cultural background

Ethnicity and cultural background influence health values and behaviours, lifestyle and illness behaviours. Every culture defines health and illness uniquely and every culture has different health beliefs and practices. Certain diseases occur at different rates in some races and ethnic groups. For example, the blood disease beta thalassaemia is a genetic disease that occurs more often in people of Italian or Greek descent. For this reason, it is also known as Mediterranean anaemia.

Indigenous health

Many Aboriginal and Torres Strait Islander people experience disability and reduced quality of life due to poor health, and die earlier than the general Australian population. They also have disproportionately higher rates of chronic disease, such as diabetes and heart disease, which occur at much younger ages. Indigenous Australians die on average 10 years earlier than non-Indigenous Australians. In 2020, only 5% of the Indigenous population was aged over 65 years, compared with 16% of non-Indigenous Australians (AIHW, 2021b). Aboriginal and Torres Strait Islander people carry a higher burden of emotional distress and mental illness than that experienced by the wider community. The major contributing factors to these problems include persistent social and economic disadvantages, limited access to healthcare and low levels of nutrition. Nursing care of Aboriginal and Torres Strait Islander people is covered in the chapter 'Nursing care of people in regional and remote areas of Australia'.

A major national initiative called Close the Gap was developed at the 2008 Indigenous Health Summit. This initiative included a Statement of Intent between the Australian Government and Indigenous peoples of Australia 'to work together to achieve equality in health status and life expectancy between Aboriginal and Torres Strait Islander peoples and non-Indigenous Australians by the year 2030' (Australian Human Rights Commission, 2008). Close the Gap aimed to reduce Indigenous disadvantage in terms of life expectancy, child mortality, access to early childhood education, educational achievement and employment outcomes. However, a 10-year review by the Close the Gap Campaign Steering Committee for Indigenous Health Equality found that 'Australian governments have not yet succeeded in closing the health gap to date, with the latest Closing the Gap report stating that, 'The target to close the life expectancy gap by 2031 is not on track' (Department of the Prime Minister and Cabinet, 2020). In fact, a December 2017 AIHW report found that mortality and life expectancy gaps are actually widening due to accelerating non-Indigenous population gains (Holland, 2018).

Age, gender and developmental level

Age, gender and developmental level are key factors in health and illness. Chronic conditions vary with age. For example, asthma and hay fever are common in the younger age groups, whereas arthritis and hypertensive diseases are more prevalent among people aged 55 years and over. Some diseases occur only in one gender; for example, prostate cancer in men and cervical cancer in women. The older adult is more likely to experience chronic illnesses and is more at risk of serious illness or death from infectious diseases such as influenza and pneumonia.

Lifestyle and environment

The way we live directly affects our health. What we eat and how much, alcohol and smoking rates, use of illegal drugs, exercise patterns, stress, grief and happiness all contribute to our health and wellbeing. Too much of the wrong food can result in obesity, diabetes and hypertension. Smoking causes cancers and respiratory diseases as well as contributing to heart disease and stroke. Lack of exercise is linked to multiple health problems including cardiovascular problems and mental health issues.

The environment we live and work in also impacts our health. Occupational exposure to toxic substances, such as asbestos or coal dust, increases the risk of pulmonary disorders. Air, water and food pollution increase the risk of respiratory disorders, infectious diseases and cancers. Environmental temperature variations can result in hypothermia or hyperthermia, especially in the older adult.

The United Nations has developed the Sustainable Development Goals (SDGs), which call for all countries to address a range of essential social needs including health, education and environmental protection, with a focus on climate change and recovery from the COVID-19 pandemic (United Nations, 2022).

Socioeconomic background

Socioeconomic status is mainly linked to income and has a major impact on health status. Socially and economically disadvantaged Australians are more likely to have shorter lives, higher levels of disease and lower use of preventive healthcare than those who are better off. This population tends to smoke more, exercise less, weigh more and eat less fresh food and more processed food high in fat and sugar. These are all risk factors for chronic health conditions including respiratory diseases, cancers and endocrine and cardiovascular diseases. The socioeconomic disadvantage experienced by Aboriginal and Torres Strait Islander peoples makes them more vulnerable to health risk factors such as smoking, alcohol misuse and domestic violence (AIHW, 2020a).

Geographical area

The geographical area in which a person lives influences their health status as access to healthcare services varies greatly between regional, rural and remote areas of Australia. For example, factors such as larger catchment areas, smaller populations and fewer general and specialist health professionals can affect healthcare services in rural and remote areas. Rural and remote area residents generally have poorer health than people living in major cities, with higher levels of mortality, disease and health risk factors. For example, the prevalence of chronic conditions such as coronary heart disease, stroke, chronic kidney disease and diabetes in people living in rural and remote areas is higher than in people living in metropolitan areas (AIHW, 2020a). Residents of the more remote regions of Australia are also more disadvantaged in their educational and employment opportunities, income and access to goods and services. In some areas, they also have limited access to basic necessities such as fresh fruit and vegetables.

Compared with those in major urban centres, Australians living in rural and remote areas generally have less infrastructure, including primary healthcare services and staff, more driving risks (such as poorer road conditions and longer travelling times), longer patient transport times and jobs with higher risks, such as primary production and mining. Preventable cancers, such as those associated with sun exposure (melanoma) or smoking (lung, head and neck) and those detectable through screening (cervix, prostate and breast), have significantly higher incidence rates in rural and remote areas. Higher rates of morbidity and mortality in rural and remote areas are also partly influenced by the larger proportion of Indigenous Australians living in these areas (AIHW, 2020a).

PROMOTION OF HEALTH AND PREVENTION OF ILLNESS AND INJURY

For many years, the emphasis in nursing was on the care of acutely ill people in the hospital setting. Changes in society and healthcare have seen this emphasis shift towards public health, preventive and community-based care. The importance of the nurse's role in health protection and promotion, as well as teaching illness prevention behaviours, is an essential component of medical–surgical nursing. Community nursing is discussed more fully in the chapter 'Community care'. Nurses promote health by teaching activities that maintain wellness, providing information about the characteristics and consequences of diseases when risk factors have been identified, and by supplying specific information about decreasing risk factors (Murdaugh, Parsons & Pender, 2018).

Australian public health programs such as the National Immunisation Program provide widespread immunisation against a large number of communicable diseases (see Table 2.1). This initiative aims to increase national immunisation rates by funding free vaccination programs and

TABLE 2.1 National Immunisation Program (NIP) Schedule

AGE	VACCINE
Under 4 years	Vaccines for the following diseases are free under the NIP: • chickenpox (varicella) • diphtheria • flu (influenza) • hepatitis B • *Haemophilus influenzae* type B (Hib) • measles • meningococcal C • mumps • pneumococcal • polio • rotavirus • rubella • tetanus • whooping cough (pertussis) • hepatitis A (Aboriginal and Torres Strait Islander people in high-risk areas) • pneumococcal (Aboriginal and Torres Strait Islander people in high-risk areas)
12–13 years	• human papillomavirus (HVP)
5–19 years	All children aged 5 to 19 years should receive any missed routine childhood vaccinations.
15–49 years	Pneumococcal (Aboriginal and Torres Strait Islander people in high-risk areas)
50 years and over	Shingles (herpes zoster) for all adults aged 70–79 years if not previously vaccinated against varicella or shingles. Flu (influenza) Boosters: • diphtheria, tetanus and whooping cough (pertussis) Pneumococcal (Aboriginal and Torres Strait Islander people)

Source: Adapted from Department of Health (2022). *National immunisation program schedule*. Retrieved from https://www.health.gov.au/health-topics/immunisation/when-to-get-vaccinated/national-immunisation-program-schedule. © National Immunisation Program Schedule 2020, Australian Government Department of Health and Aged Care. Refer to the website (www.health.gov.au) for the most up-to-date version of the Schedule.

providing information about immunisation to the general public and health professionals (Department of Health, 2020). Nurses play an integral role in educating the public about the effectiveness of immunisation to save lives and prevent serious illness. The occupational nature of healthcare workers, including nursing students, places them at risk of acquiring vaccine-preventable diseases, and health department policies generally require students and non-immune workers to be immunised.

ACUTE AND CHRONIC ILLNESS

Previously, governments focused on developing management and treatment strategies that targeted specific conditions in Australia. These include conditions with high mortality, such as cardiovascular, cancer and respiratory, and those with highest burden of disease (years of healthy life lost), which include mental health, cancer and injuries. But this approach has not been successful, so the focus has now shifted to prevention. The National Preventive Health Strategy 2021–2030 (see Figure 2.1) is a program that focuses on providing all Australians with the best start in life in order to keep them in the best possible health for as long as possible. There are seven specific focus areas including reducing smoking and alcohol intake, increasing healthy diet and activity, cancer screening, immunisation and protecting mental health.

Chronic conditions include cardiovascular disease, cancer, diabetes, arthritis and asthma (AIHW, 1997). Coronary heart disease is the leading cause of disease burden in Australia, followed by anxiety and mental health disorders. The rate of deaths due to heart attacks has decreased over the past decade; however, coronary heart disease is still the leading cause of premature death. Survival rates are improving for cancer due to improvements in treatments, knowledge and screening programs. One in 10 Australians have asthma, and while it is one

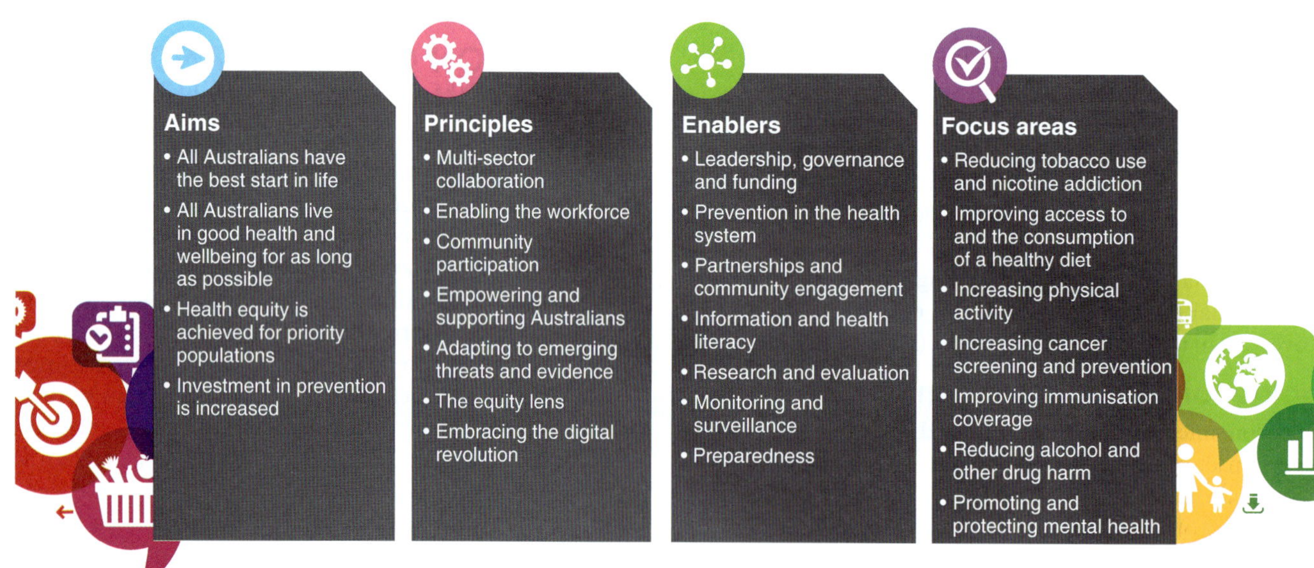

FIGURE 2.1 ***National Preventive Health Strategy 2021–2030***

Source: Department of Health (2021). *National Preventive Health Strategy 2021–2030*. Retrieved from https://www.health.gov.au/resources/publications/national-preventive-health-strategy-2021-2030. Commonwealth of Australia Department of Health and Aged Care, 2021. Current version online on the Department's website (www.health.gov.au).

of the most common chronic health conditions in children, it is most common among females aged 55 years and over. Around 1 in 20 Australians have diabetes: the prevalence increases with age and is higher in males than females. Each year, over 25,000 Australians received kidney replacement therapy (53% on dialysis and 47% with a transplant) (AIHW, 2020a).

Box 2.1 discusses incidence and prevalence. See Figure 2.2 for the most recent available overview of the burden of disease in Australia.

Disease and illness

Disease and illness are terms that are often used interchangeably, but they do have different meanings. In general, nursing is concerned with illness, whereas medicine is concerned with disease.

Disease

Disease (literally meaning 'without ease') is a medical term describing alterations in the structure and function of the body or mind. Diseases usually have mechanical, biological or normative causes. Mechanical causes of disease result in damage to the structure of the body, such as trauma or extremes of temperature. Biological causes of disease impact on body function and can result from a variety of reasons including the normal ageing process. Normative causes are psychological but involve a mind–body interaction, so physical manifestations occur in response to the psychological disturbance.

The causes of many diseases are still unknown but common causes include:

- genetic defects
- fetal exposure to viruses, chemicals or drugs
- biological agents or toxins (including viruses, bacteria, fungi, protozoa and helminths)
- physical agents such as temperature, radiation and electricity
- chemical agents such as alcohol, drugs, strong acids or bases, and heavy metals
- generalised response of tissues to injury or irritation
- changes in antibody productions, resulting in allergies or hypersensitivities
- faulty metabolic processes where production of hormones or enzymes is above or below normal.

Diseases may be classified as acute or chronic, infectious (communicable), congenital, degenerative, functional, malignant, psychosomatic, idiopathic or iatrogenic. These classifications are defined in Table 2.2. In all diseases, alterations in structure or function cause signs and symptoms (manifestations). These warning signs often prompt a person to seek health advice.

Symptoms are subjective in that the person perceives them: 'I feel nauseous and have a headache.' Signs are objective in that they can be seen and measured; for example, bleeding, vomiting, diarrhoea, limitation of movement, swelling. Pain (a subjective symptom) is the most common reason people seek healthcare.

Chronic conditions cause the greatest health problems in the world today, and the number of people with chronic conditions is rising steadily as people live longer and more populations are impacted by lifestyle, behaviour and environmental factors. See AIHW (2020a, pp. 13 and 14) for more information: https://www.aihw.gov.au/getmedia/2aa9f51b-dbd6-4d56-8dd4-06a10ba7cae8/aihw-aus-232.pdf.aspx?inline=true.

BOX 2.1 Incidence and prevalence

- *Incidence* refers to the number of new cases of an illness, disease or event occurring during a given period. Example: The number of new cases of type 1 diabetes in Australia in 2018 was 2,800.
- *Prevalence* is the number of cases of a disease that exist at any given time. This includes new cases, ongoing cases and people who died during this period. Example: An estimated 1.2 million Australians had diabetes in 2017–2018.

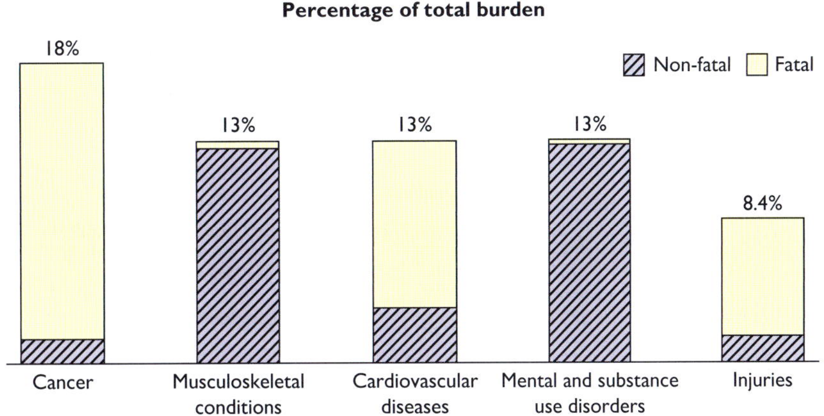

FIGURE 2.2 *Proportion (%) of total burden by disease group in 2018*

Source: AIHW (2021c). *Australian burden of disease study: Impact and causes of illness and death in Australia 2018*. Retrieved from https://www.aihw.gov.au/. Licensed under the Creative Commons Attribution 4.0 International License, https://creativecommons.org/licenses/by/4.0/.

TABLE 2.2 Disease classifications and definitions

CLASSIFICATION	DEFINITION
Acute	Rapid onset, lasts a relatively short time and is self-limiting.
Chronic	Has one or more of the following: (1) is ongoing or permanent, (2) leaves permanent disability, (3) causes irreversible pathophysiology, (4) requires rehabilitation, (5) requires a long period of care.
Communicable	Can spread from one person to another.
Congenital	Existing at or before birth.
Degenerative	Resulting from deterioration or impairment of organs or tissues.
Functional	Affects function or performance but does not have manifestations of organic illness.
Malignant	Tends to become worse and cause death.
Psychosomatic	A psychological disease, causing physiological symptoms.
Idiopathic	Unknown cause.
Iatrogenic	Unintended or unnecessary harm or suffering arising from healthcare management.

Chronic conditions are a major health problem in all developed countries, accounting for a high proportion of deaths, disability and illness. Yet many of these conditions are preventable, or their onset can be delayed, by relatively simple measures. Chronic conditions:

- have complex and multiple causes
- can occur alone or with comorbidities (other diseases)
- usually have a gradual onset but can occur suddenly, and have acute stages
- occur at any age but are more prevalent in older age
- compromise quality of life, cause limitations and disability
- are long-term, usually leading to deterioration of health and loss of independence
- are not usually immediately life threatening but are the leading underlying cause of premature death (see Figure 2.3) (AIHW, 2022).

More than 50% of Australians report having at least one chronic condition, and 23% have two or more chronic conditions. As people age, they are more likely to have one or more chronic conditions (AIHW, 2022).

Chronic conditions range from mild to severe and are usually characterised by periods of remission and exacerbation. During periods of remission, the person may be symptom free; however, in periods of exacerbation, the symptoms reappear. Each person with a chronic condition has a unique set of responses and needs. The response of the person to the disease is influenced by the following factors:

- when in their life cycle the condition occurs
- the type and degree of limitations imposed by the condition
- the visibility of impairment or disfigurement
- the pathophysiology causing the condition
- the relationship between the impairment and functioning in social roles
- pain and fear.

These factors are highly complex. They are interrelated and result in individualised responses. Because there are so many different chronic conditions, and because every person will have a unique response, it is difficult to generalise about needs. However, most people with a chronic condition will need to:

- live as normally as possible—symptoms and treatment can make the person feel alienated, lonely and different
- adapt activities of daily living and self-care
- grieve the loss of physical function and structure, income, status, roles and dignity
- comply with a treatment plan
- maintain a positive self-concept and a sense of hope
- maintain a feeling of being in control
- confront the inevitability of death (Miller, 2000).

Some people with chronic conditions successfully meet health-related needs whereas others do not. Nursing interventions for the person with a chronic condition focus on education and support to promote independent functioning, reduce healthcare costs and improve quality of life.

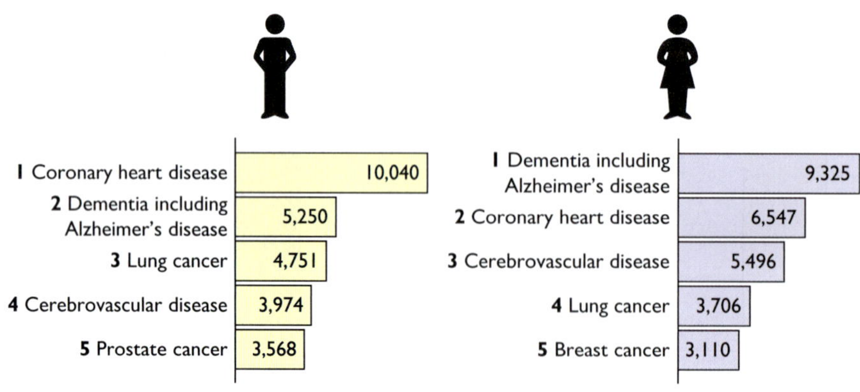

FIGURE 2.3 ***Leading underlying causes of death, 2020***

Source: AIHW (2021b). *Deaths in Australia*. Based on AIHW National Mortality Database (Table S3.1) released 9 June 2022. Licensed under the Creative Commons Attribution 4.0 International License, https://creativecommons.org/licenses/by/4.0/.

Illness

Illness is the response a person has to a disease or condition. This response is highly individualised, because the person responds with their own perceptions of the condition as well as those of others. The concept of illness combines pathophysiological changes and psychological effects of these and the impact on the individual's roles, relationships and values, and cultural and spiritual beliefs. A person may have a disease but not see themself as ill or they may validate feelings of illness through the comments of others: 'You look pale, do you feel okay?'

An **acute illness** occurs rapidly, lasts for a relatively short time and is usually self-limiting (it will resolve itself). The condition may respond to self-treatment or to medical–surgical intervention. People with uncomplicated acute illnesses usually have full recovery and return to normal pre-illness functioning.

Illness behaviours are the way people cope with the changes caused by a condition. Illness behaviours are highly individualised and are influenced by age, gender, family values, economic status, culture, educational level and mental status. The concept of a sequence of illness behaviour was first defined in 1972 (Suchman, 1972):

1. *Experiencing symptoms*. The first stage of an acute illness is when someone experiences signs or symptoms that alert them to a change in their health. The most significant example is pain but other signals of illness include bleeding (haemorrhage), swelling (oedema), fever (pyrexia) or difficulty with breathing (dyspnoea). If the signs and symptoms are mild or are familiar (coughing and nasal congestion), the person will often self-medicate. It is only if the symptoms are prolonged or become more severe that the person moves to the second-stage illness behaviour. Most people would not define this stage to be an illness as they consider it a normal part of the fluctuating status of health: 'It's nothing, just a sniffle.'
2. *Assuming the sick role*. At this stage the individual accepts that their symptoms are proof of illness. They may seek external health advice and take steps to rest by not attending work or school. They may cautiously admit to illness: 'I am feeling a bit unwell.' Self-preoccupation is characteristic of this stage, so the person focuses on changes in function and ability caused by the illness. As the illness resolves, the individual resumes normal activities and may retrospectively admit to illness: 'I was feeling sick but I'm much better now.' However, if the signs and symptoms persist or become worse, the person moves to the next stage by seeking medical care.
3. *Seeking medical care*. In our society, a general practitioner or other healthcare provider usually provides the initial validation of illness. People who believe they are ill, or are encouraged to contact a healthcare provider, seek help in finding out the cause of the illness (diagnosis), how long it will last (prognosis) and the best way of treating it. If the diagnosis requires interventions, the person moves to the next stage. If the diagnosis does not require support, the person may return to normal functioning or, if dissatisfied with this answer, may seek validation from a different healthcare provider.
4. *Assuming a dependent role*. At this stage the person accepts the diagnosis, trajectory and planned treatment of the illness. As the severity of the illness increases, so does their dependent role. During this stage the person may enter a hospital for treatment and care. How an individual responds to care depends on many factors: severity of the illness, anxiety or fear about the outcome, loss of roles, their support systems available, their reaction to stress and their previous experiences with illness care.
5. *Recovery and rehabilitation*. The final stage of acute illness is recovery and rehabilitation. Institutional healthcare sees recovery begin in the hospital but completed at home. This process means education for the person and continuity of care as a major goal for nursing. The shift in settings means nursing care continues outside the hospital in community settings and the home. The person now relinquishes their dependent role and resumes normal roles and responsibilities. The experience and knowledge gained during treatment and care may place the person on a higher level of wellness after recovery is complete. Recovery time is flexible as the severity of the illness and the method of treatment will affect this, as will the person's compliance and motivation.

ILLNESS PREVENTION

Prevention includes any measures that limit the progression of an illness at any point of its course. Three levels of illness prevention were first defined in 1965. Each level of prevention occurs at a distinct point in the development of a disease process and requires specific nursing interventions (Edelman & Kudzma, 2022):

1. *Primary level of prevention*. Generalised health promotion activities as well as specific actions that prevent or delay a disease occurring, including:
   - protecting against environmental risks, such as air and water pollution
   - eating nutritious foods
   - protecting against industrial hazards
   - wearing seat belts and helmets
   - sex counselling and practising safe sex
   - being immunised
   - genetic screenings
   - not smoking and reducing alcohol intake.
2. *Secondary level of prevention*. Interventions around early diagnosis and treatment if an illness is already present. Stopping or slowing the pathological process and helping the person to return to health as soon as possible. These include:
   - screenings for diseases such as hypertension, diabetes and glaucoma
   - physical examinations and diagnostic tests for cancer
   - specific treatments; for example, the treatment of streptococcal infections of the throat will prevent secondary infections of the heart and/or kidneys.

3. *Tertiary level of prevention*. Stopping the disease process and rehabilitating the person back to their normal place in society. Tertiary prevention measures include:
   - medical or surgical treatment for an illness
   - specific rehabilitation programs for cardiovascular problems, head injuries and strokes
   - work training programs following illness or injury
   - educating the public to employ rehabilitated people to the fullest possible extent.

STAGES OF ADULTHOOD

The adult years of life can be divided into three major stages: the young adult (18 to 40 years), the middle adult (40 to 65 years) and the older adult (over 65 years). Adult developmental markers are not as clearly delineated as in the infant or child; however, specific changes do occur with ageing in intellectual, psychosocial and spiritual development, along with physical structures and functions.

The developmental theories specific to the adult, with related stages and tasks, are listed in Table 2.3. Applying a variety of developmental theories is important to the holistic care of the adult as nurses perform assessments, implement care and provide teaching.

The young adult

In Australia, an adult is considered to be aged 18 years or over. A 'young adult' is someone aged between 18 and 25 years. A young adult is typically at the peak of physical development with all body systems functioning at maximum efficiency.

TABLE 2.3 Theories of adult development

	THEORIST	AGE	TASK
Psychosocial development	Erikson	18-25	Identity versus role confusion • Establishing an intimate relationship with another person • Committing to work and relationships
		25-65	Generativity versus stagnation • Accepting one's own life as creative and productive • Having concern for others
		65-death	Integrity versus despair • Accepting worth of one's own life • Accepting inevitability of death
Spiritual development	Fowler	After 18	• Having a high degree of self-consciousness • Constructing one's own spiritual system
		After 30	• Being aware of truth from a variety of viewpoints
	Westerhoff	Young adult	Searching faith • Acquiring a cognitive and an affective faith through questioning one's own faith
		Middle-older adult	Owned faith • Putting faith into action and standing up for beliefs
Moral development	Kohlberg	Adult	Post-conventional level Social contract/legalistic orientation • Defining morality in terms of personal principles • Adhering to laws that protect the welfare and rights of others Universal-ethical principles • Internalising universal moral principles • Respecting others; believing that relationships are based on mutual trust
Developmental tasks	Havighurst	18-35	• Selecting and learning to live with a mate • Starting a family and rearing children • Managing a home • Starting an occupation • Taking on civic responsibility • Finding a congenial social group
		35-60	• Achieving community and social responsibility • Establishing and maintaining an economic standard of living • Assisting teenage children in becoming responsible and happy adults • Developing relaxation-time activities • Relating to one's spouse as a person • Accepting and adjusting to the physiological changes of middle age • Adjusting to ageing parents
		60 and over	• Meeting community and social obligations • Establishing an affiliation with one's own age group • Establishing satisfactory physical living arrangements • Adjusting to decreasing physical strength, health, retirement, reduced income, death of spouse

Sources: Data from Erikson (1963). *Childhood and society* (2nd ed.). New York: Norton; Fowler (1981). *Stages of faith: The psychology of human development and the quest for meaning*. New York: Harper & Row; Havighurst (1972). *Human development and education* (3rd ed.). New York: Longman; Kohlberg (1979). *The meaning and measurement of moral development*. New York: Clark University; and Westerhoff (1976). *Will our children have faith?* New York: Seabury Press.

TABLE 2.4 Physical status and changes in the young adult years

ASSESSMENT	TWENTIES	THIRTIES
Skin	Smooth and even	Wrinkles begin to appear
Hair	Slightly oily, shiny Balding may begin	Greying may begin Balding may begin
Vision	Snellen 20/20	Some loss of visual acuity and accommodation
Musculoskeletal	Strong, coordinated	Some loss of strength and muscle mass
Cardiovascular	Maximum cardiac output	Slight decline in cardiac output
Functional	60-90 beats/min Mean BP: 120/80	60-90 beats/min Mean BP: 120/80
Respiratory	Rate: 12-20 Full vital capacity	Rate: 12-20 Decline in vital capacity

During the thirties, normal physiological changes begin to occur. Table 2.4 gives a comparison of physical status for young adults during their twenties and thirties.

Risks for alterations in health

The young adult is at risk of accidents, sexually transmitted infections, substance abuse, and physical or psychosocial stressors. These risk factors may be interrelated.

INJURIES Injury causes a range of physical, cognitive and psychological disabilities that seriously affect the quality of life of individuals and their families. Factors that increase the risk of injury are age, gender, alcohol use, place of residence, ethnicity, socioeconomic status and occupation. Suicide is the leading cause of death in Australian young adults (15–44 years) followed by accidental poisoning, land transport accidents, assault (15–24 years) and coronary heart disease (25–44 years) (AIHW, 2020a).

SEXUALLY TRANSMITTED INFECTIONS Sexually transmitted infections include chlamydia, genital herpes, human papillomavirus (HPV), gonorrhoea, syphilis and HIV/AIDS. Young adults who are sexually active with a variety of partners and who do not use protection such as condoms are at greatest risk of these diseases. Nursing care of people with sexually transmitted infections is discussed in the chapter 'Nursing care of people who have sexually transmitted infections'.

SUBSTANCE ABUSE The 2019 *National Drug Strategy Household Survey* found that 11% of Australians smoked tobacco, 24% drank alcohol at risky levels and 16% had used an illicit drug in the past 12 months. Compared with people in the same age group in 2001, young adults were less likely to drink, smoke or use illicit drugs (AIHW, 2020b).

Alcohol and nicotine are the drugs most commonly used by Australians. With the exception of marijuana/cannabis, the proportion of the population who have used illicit drugs at some time in their life is relatively low. However, nicotine, alcohol and illicit drug use contributes to significant illness and disease, injury, workplace concerns, violence, crime and breakdowns in families and relationships in Australia.

The most commonly reported illicit drugs used are marijuana/cannabis, followed by ecstasy, meth/amphetamine and cocaine. Although alcohol abuse occurs at all ages, males in their forties were the most likely group to drink at risky levels (AIHW, 2020b). Alcohol contributes to motor vehicle accidents and physical violence and damages the developing fetus in pregnant women. It can cause liver disease and nutritional deficits. Nursing care of people with substance abuse issues is discussed in the chapter 'Nursing care of people with substance misuse problems'.

PHYSICAL AND PSYCHOSOCIAL STRESSORS
Physical stressors that increase the risk of illness in young adults include environmental pollutants and work-related risks such as falls, electrical hazards, mechanical injuries or exposure to toxins or infectious agents. Other physical stressors include exposure to the sun and ingestion of chemical substances such as caffeine, alcohol and nicotine.

Many different and individualised psychosocial stressors may affect young adults, including the pressure to make choices regarding education, occupation, relationships, independence and lifestyle. The young adult without adequate education or job skills may face unemployment, poverty and homelessness. Divorce is another psychological stressor that often results in loneliness, feelings of failure, financial difficulties, domestic violence and child abuse. In 2020, the divorce rate in Australia was 1.9 per 1,000 people. The average time from marriage to divorce was 12 years, and the median age at divorce was 46 years for men and 43 years for women (ABS, 2021b).

Assessment guidelines

The following guidelines are useful in assessing the achievement of significant developmental tasks in the young adult.

Does the young adult:

- feel independent from parents?
- have a realistic self-concept?
- like themself and the direction in which their life is going?
- interact well with family?
- cope with the stresses of constant change and growth?
- have well-established bonds with significant others, such as marriage partners or close friends?
- have a meaningful social life?
- have a career or occupation?
- demonstrate emotional, social and economic responsibility for their own life?
- have a set of values that guide behaviour?
- have a healthy lifestyle?

Physical assessment of the young adult includes height and weight, blood pressure and vision. During the health history, the nurse should ask specific questions about substance use, sexual activity and concerns, exercise, eating habits, menstrual history and patterns, coping mechanisms, any familial chronic illnesses and family changes.

Promoting healthy behaviours in the young adult

Health information for the young adult is primarily provided in community settings including:

- Health-related courses and seminars at community colleges and universities provide information on exercise, alcohol and drug abuse, smoking cessation, mental health and sexual health.
- Workplace programs emphasise blood pressure monitoring, exercise, smoking cessation, nutrition guidelines and stress reduction activities.
- Community programs provide information on media, support groups, and risk factors for disease and injury.

The middle adult

Many physical status and function changes take place between ages 40 and 65. Table 2.5 lists the physical changes that normally occur in the middle years.

Risks for alterations in health

The middle adult is at risk of obesity, cardiovascular disease, cancer, substance abuse, and physical and psychosocial stressors. These factors may be interrelated.

OBESITY The middle adult often has a problem maintaining a healthy weight. Weight gain at this age is the result of consuming the same number of kilojoules/calories while physical activity decreases and basal metabolic rate falls. Obesity affects all major organ systems, increasing the risk of atherosclerosis, hypertension, elevated cholesterol and triglyceride levels, and diabetes. Obesity is also associated with heart disease, osteoarthritis and gallbladder disease.

CARDIOVASCULAR DISEASE The major risk factors, especially for coronary artery disease, include age, male gender, physical inactivity, cigarette smoking, hypertension, elevated blood cholesterol levels and diabetes. Other contributing factors include obesity, stress and lack of exercise. The middle adult is also at risk of peripheral vascular, cerebrovascular and cardiovascular disease.

CANCER Cancer is the leading cause of death and illness in Australia, closely followed by cardiovascular disease. The five most common cancers in Australia are prostate, colorectal, breast, melanoma and lung cancer. One in every 2 Australian males and 1 in every 3 Australian females will be diagnosed with cancer before age 85 (AIHW, 2020a). The AIHW's *Australia's Health 2020* report shows that of the target population:

- 1.8 million women aged 50–74 participated in Breast Screen Australia
- 3 million women aged 20–69 participated in the National Cervical Screening Program
- 42% of people aged 50–74 participated in the National Bowel Cancer Screening Program.

Nursing care of the person with cancer is discussed in the chapter 'Nursing care of people with cancer'.

SUBSTANCE ABUSE Although middle adults use a variety of substances, the most commonly abused are alcohol, nicotine and prescription drugs. Excess alcohol use in the middle adult contributes to an increased risk of liver cancer, cirrhosis, pancreatitis, hyperlipidaemia and anaemia. Alcoholism also increases the risk of accidental injury or death and disrupts careers and relationships. Tobacco smoking increases the risk of cancers of the larynx, lung, mouth, pharynx, bladder, pancreas, oesophagus and kidney, as well as chronic obstructive pulmonary disease and cardiovascular disorders.

PHYSICAL AND PSYCHOSOCIAL STRESSORS The middle adult years are ones of change and transition, frequently resulting in stress. Both men and women must adapt

TABLE 2.5 Physical changes in the middle adult years

ASSESSMENT	CHANGES
Skin	• Decreased turgor, moisture and subcutaneous fat result in wrinkles. • Fat is deposited in the abdominal and hip areas.
Hair	• Loss of melanin in hair shaft causes greying. • Hairline recedes in males and sometimes females.
Sensory	• Visual acuity for near vision decreases (presbyopia) during the 40s. • Auditory acuity for high-frequency sounds decreases (presbycusis), more commonly in men. • Sense of taste diminishes.
Musculoskeletal	• Skeletal muscle mass decreases by about age 60. • Thinning of intervertebral discs results in loss of height (about 2.5 cm). • Postmenopausal women may have loss of calcium and develop osteoporosis.
Cardiovascular	• Blood vessels lose elasticity. • Systolic blood pressure may increase.
Respiratory	• Loss of vital capacity (about 1L from age 20 to 60) occurs.
Gastrointestinal	• Large intestine gradually loses muscle tone; constipation may result. • Gastric secretions are decreased.
Genitourinary	• Hormonal changes: menopause, women (↓ oestrogen); andropause, men (↓ testosterone).
Endocrine	• Gradual decrease in glucose tolerance.

to changes and declines in physical appearance and function and accept their own mortality. The age for first-time parents has risen substantially in the past few decades, and children are living at home longer, usually due to financial reasons. The middle adult becomes part of what is known as 'the sandwich generation' (Miller, 1981), caring simultaneously for children and ageing parents. Both men and women may make career changes, and approaching retirement becomes a reality. Divorce in the middle years is also a major emotional, social and financial stressor.

Assessment guidelines

The following guidelines are useful in assessing the achievement of significant developmental tasks in the middle adult. Does the middle adult:

- accept the ageing body?
- feel comfortable with and respect themself?
- enjoy some new freedom to be independent?
- accept changes in family roles?
- enjoy success and satisfaction from work and/or family roles?
- interact well and share companionable activities with a partner?
- expand or renew previous interests?
- pursue charitable and altruistic activities?
- consider plans for retirement?
- have a meaningful philosophy of life?
- follow health promotion practices?

Physical assessment of the middle adult includes all body systems, including blood pressure, vision and hearing. Monitoring for risks and possible cancer symptoms is essential. The nurse should ask specific questions about food intake and exercise habits, substance abuse, sexual concerns, changes in the reproductive system, coping mechanisms and family history of chronic illnesses.

Promoting healthy behaviours in the middle adult

Health information for the middle adult can be provided in a variety of community settings, including outpatient clinics, occupational health clinics and private practice. Examples are as follows:

- Specific programs emphasise accepting responsibility for one's own health. This type of teaching can be through seminars or on a one-to-one basis, and includes information specific to individuals with an identified need, such as smokers, women who have re-entered the workforce or men nearing retirement.
- Community and employment agencies provide information about safety hazards in the home, workplace and community.
- There are many community resources available including programs offered at alcohol/drug abuse treatment centres, clinics and health centres, counselling services, crisis intervention centres, intimate partner violence programs, and health education and promotion agencies (e.g. the Association of Relatives and Friends of the Mentally Ill, Red Cross Australia, the Cancer Council Australia, the Heart Foundation of Australia and Diabetes Australia).

The older adult

The older adult period begins at age 65, but it can be further divided into three periods: the young-old (ages 65 to 74), the middle-old (ages 75 to 84) and the old-old (age 85 and over). With increasing age, a number of normal physiological changes occur (see Table 2.6).

The World Health Organization (WHO) is leading the global implementation of '2021–2030 the Decade of Healthy Ageing'. The WHO has called for public health interventions to decrease ageist concepts and discrimination and to increase opportunities for older people to improve health outcomes and quality of life. These include the prevention of disease and functional decline, extended longevity and enhanced quality of life (WHO, 2020).

The AIHW has developed a person-centred, socioecological framework of the determinants of health and welling (see Figure 2.4). It uses seven domains reflecting the biological, lifestyle, socioeconomic, societal and environmental factors which overlap and interact across the lifespan. Some of these can be modified while others are fixed. For older Australians, there are many gaps where interventions and developments can be instituted to improve health and wellbeing outcomes.

The increase in numbers of older adults has important implications for nursing. People needing healthcare in all settings will be older, requiring nursing interventions and teaching specifically designed to meet needs that differ from those of young

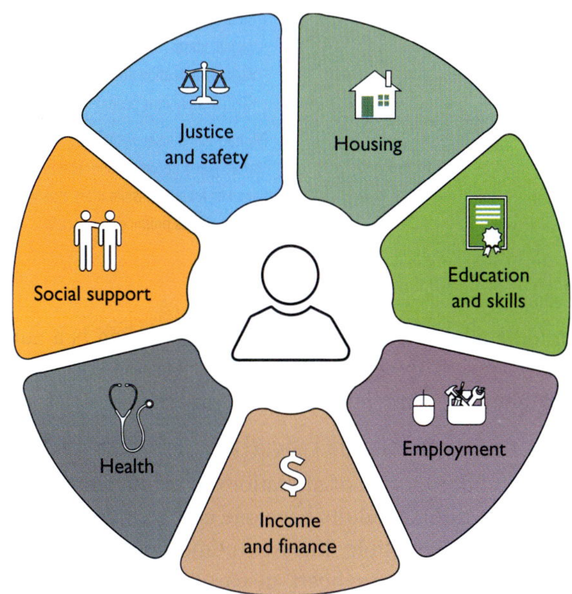

FIGURE 2.4 ***Person-centred model***

Source: AIHW (2021d). *Older Australians.* Licensed under the Creative Commons Attribution 4.0 International License, https://creativecommons.org/licenses/by/4.0/.

TABLE 2.6 Physical changes in the older adult years

ASSESSMENT	CHANGES
Skin	• Decreased turgor and sebaceous gland activity result in dry, wrinkled skin. Melanocytes cluster, causing 'age spots' or 'liver spots'.
Hair and nails	• Scalp, axillary and pubic hair thins; nose and ear hair thickens. Women may develop facial hair. • Nails grow more slowly; may become thick and brittle.
Sensory	• Visual field narrows, and depth perception is distorted. • Pupils are smaller, reducing night vision. • Lenses yellow and become opaque, resulting in distortion of green, blue and violet tones, and increased sensitivity to glare. • Production of tears decreases. • Sense of smell, taste and thirst decreases. • Age-related hearing loss progresses, involving middle- and low-frequency sounds. • Threshold for pain and touch increases. • Alterations in proprioception (sense of physical position) may occur.
Musculoskeletal	• Loss of overall mass, strength and movement of muscles occurs; tremors may occur. • Loss of bone structure and deterioration of cartilage in joints results in increased risk of fractures and limitation of range of motion.
Cardiovascular	• Systolic blood pressure rises. • Cardiac output decreases. • Peripheral resistance increases, and capillary walls thicken.
Respiratory	• Continued loss of vital capacity occurs as the lungs become less elastic and more rigid. • Anteroposterior chest diameter increases; kyphosis. • Although blood carbon dioxide levels remain relatively constant, blood oxygen levels decrease by 10–15%.
Gastrointestinal	• Production of saliva decreases, and decreased number of taste buds decrease accurate receptors for salt and sweet. • Gag reflex is decreased, and stomach motility and emptying are reduced. • Both large and small intestines have some atrophy, with decreased peristalsis. • The liver decreases in weight and storage capacity; gallstones increase; pancreatic enzymes decrease.
Genitourinary	• Kidneys lose mass and the glomerular filtration rate is reduced (by nearly 50% from young adulthood to old age). • Bladder capacity decreases and the micturition reflex is delayed. Urinary retention is more common. • Women may have stress incontinence; men may have an enlarged prostate gland. • Reproductive changes in men occur: - Testosterone decreases. - Sperm count decreases. - Testes become smaller. - Length of time to achieve an erection increases; erection is less full. • Reproductive changes in women occur: - Oestrogen levels decrease. - Breast tissue decreases. - Vagina, uterus, ovaries and urethra atrophy. - Vaginal lubrication decreases. - Vaginal secretions become alkaline.
Endocrine	• Pituitary gland loses weight and vascularity. • Thyroid gland becomes more fibrous and plasma decreases. • Pancreas releases insulin more slowly; increased blood glucose levels are common. • Adrenal glands produce less cortisol.

and middle adults. Although older person nursing is a nursing specialty area, it is also an integral component of medical–surgical nursing (see Figure 2.5).

Risks for alterations in health

The older adult is at risk of alterations in health from a variety of causes. Most older adults have one chronic health problem, while many have multiple illnesses (comorbidities). Ischaemic heart disease (coronary heart disease) and cerebrovascular diseases (notably stroke) are the two leading causes of death, accounting for about 30% of all deaths among older Australian men and women. Like the middle adult, the older adult is at risk of decreased health from obesity and a sedentary lifestyle. Other risk factors specific to this age group include accidental injuries, pharmacological effects, and physical and psychosocial stress.

INJURIES Injuries in the older adult cause many problems: illness, financial burdens, hospitalisation, self-care deficits, loss of independence and even death. The risk of injury is increased by the normal physiological changes that accompany ageing, pathophysiological alterations in health, environmental hazards and lack of support systems. The two major causes of injury in the older adult are falls and motor vehicle accidents. Of these, falls with resultant hip fractures are the most significant in terms of long-term disability and death.

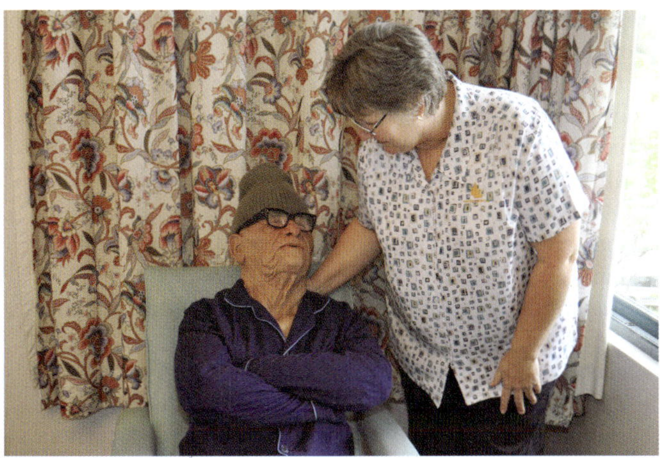

FIGURE 2.5 ***The older adult population is increasing more rapidly than any other age group, making nursing of older adults an integral component of medical–surgical nursing practice***

Source: Courtesy of Tracy Levett-Jones.

PHARMACOLOGICAL EFFECTS Medications are commonly used by older Australians to treat and manage illness and health conditions and include prescription pharmaceuticals, over-the-counter medications, vitamins and minerals and, increasingly, illegal drugs. The level of use of pharmaceuticals generally increases with age, with the majority of prescribed medication dispensed to Australians aged 65–74 years (AIHW, 2021d).

A number of risk factors predispose the older adult to experiencing drug toxicity. Age-related changes in tissue and organ structure and function alter the absorption of both oral and parenteral medications. Low nutritional levels and decreased liver function may alter drug metabolism. Ageing kidneys may not excrete drugs at the normal clearance rate. Self-administration of both prescribed and non-prescribed medications presents risks for error from confusion, forgetfulness or misreading the directions. Many older adults take multiple medications (polypharmacy), placing them at risk of drug interaction or an adverse drug event. These events are responsible for high rates of hospital admissions and mortality in older Australians (Australian Commission on Safety and Quality in Health Care (ACSQHC), 2020).

PHYSICAL AND PSYCHOSOCIAL STRESSORS The older adult is exposed to the same environmental hazards as the young and middle adult, but the accumulation of years of exposure may now appear; for example, skin cancer from many years of sun exposure and hearing loss due to long-term noise pollution. Older adults (especially males) are at increased risk of respiratory disorders as a result of smoking or from such pollutants as coal or asbestos dust. Living conditions and economic constraints may prevent the older adult from having necessary heating and cooling, contributing to thermal-related illnesses and even death. Mistreatment of older people (elder abuse) and neglect further increases the risk of injury or illness.

Psychosocial stressors for the older adult include the illness or death of a spouse, decreased or limited income, retirement, isolation from friends and family because of lack of transportation or distance, return to the home of a child or relocation to an aged care facility. A further stressor may be role loss or reversal; for example, when the wife becomes the caretaker of her chronically ill husband.

Assessment guidelines

The following guidelines are useful in assessing the achievement of significant developmental tasks in the older adult. Does the older adult:

- adjust to the physiological changes of ageing?
- manage retirement years in a satisfying manner?
- have satisfactory living arrangements and income to meet changing needs?
- participate in social and leisure activities?
- have a social network of friends and support people?
- view life as worthwhile?
- have high self-esteem?
- have the abilities to care for self or to secure appropriate help?
- gain support from a value system or spiritual philosophy?
- adapt lifestyle to their diminishing energy and ability?
- accept and adjust to their own death and that of significant others?

FOCUS ON CULTURAL DIVERSITY Diversity in older Australian adults

- Australians have one of the highest life expectancies in the world.
- Older Australians (65 and over) make up 16% of the total population.
- More than 56% of all older people in Australia are aged 65–74 years (young-old). About 31% are the middle-old (75 to 84 years) and 13% are the old-old (85 years and over).
- The number of older Australians continuing to work past the age of 65 years has doubled over the past 20 years, from 6% in 2001 to 15% in 2021.
- Most older people live in their own homes, although mortgage-free home ownership continues to decline.
- Australian women of all cultural backgrounds tend to live longer than the men.
- Older Indigenous Australians make up 1.5% of the population aged over 50. Although Indigenous life expectancy is increasing, the 'older Indigenous' population is considered to include people aged 50 years and over.

Physical assessment of the older adult includes a careful examination of all body systems. When taking a health history, the nurse should ask specific questions about dietary patterns; elimination; exercise and rest; use of alcohol, nicotine, over-the-counter medications, and prescription and non-prescription drugs; sexual concerns; financial concerns; and support systems.

Promoting healthy behaviours in the older adult

Older adults derive the same benefits from health teaching as young adults and middle adults and should never be viewed as being 'too old' for healthy living practices. However, nurses need to structure teaching activities to meet age-related physiological changes, such as using large print. Health education for the older adult is provided in hospitals, aged care facilities, retirement villages, outpatient clinics, senior citizen centres and other community settings. Examples are as follows:

- Educational seminars teach about accident prevention in the home, in cars and when using public transport.
- Health screenings that are specifically aimed at the older adult.
- Community programs provide immunisation for influenza and pneumonia.
- Literature gives information about financial assistance for healthcare, crisis hotlines, community services and resources (described earlier for the middle adult), transportation and nutrition.

THE CONCEPT OF FAMILY

Although some people are totally alone in the world, most have one or more other people who are significant in their lives. These significant others may be related or bonded to the person by birth, adoption, marriage or friendship. Although not always meeting traditional definitions, people (or even pets) significant to the person are considered the person's family. The nurse should always include the family as an integral component of care in all healthcare settings.

Definitions and functions of the family

What is a **family**? The definitions of a family are changing as society changes. The ABS defines a family as 'two or more persons, one of whom is at least 15 years of age, who are related by blood, marriage (registered or de facto), adoption, step or fostering, (who) are usually resident in the same household' (ABS, 2021a). A more comprehensive definition is that a family is composed of two or more people of any gender who are emotionally involved with each other. In a global society, it may not be possible for family members to live in close proximity, but they can remain emotionally involved.

Although every family is unique, all families have certain structural and functional features in common. Family structure (family roles and relationships) and family function (interactions among family members and with the community) provide the following:

- *Interdependence*. The behaviours and level of development of individual family members constantly influence and are influenced by the behaviours and level of development of all other members of the family.
- *Maintaining boundaries*. The family creates boundaries that guide its members, providing a distinct and unique family culture. This culture, in turn, provides values.
- *Adapting to change*. The family changes as new members are added, current members leave and the development of each member progresses.
- *Performing family tasks*. Essential tasks maintain the stability and continuity of the family. These tasks include physical maintenance of the home and the people in the home, the production and socialisation of family members and the maintenance of the psychological wellbeing of members.

Family developmental stages and tasks

The family, like the individual, has developmental stages and tasks. Each stage brings change, requiring adaptation, and each new stage also presents family-related risk factors for alterations in health. The nurse must consider the person's needs both at a specific developmental stage and within a family with specific developmental tasks. Family developmental stages and developmental tasks are described next. Related risk factors and health problems for each stage are listed in Table 2.7.

The couple

The developmental tasks of the couple include adjusting to living together, establishing a mutually satisfying relationship, relating to relatives and deciding whether to have children (for those of child-bearing age).

Family with infants and preschoolers

The family with infants or preschoolers must adjust to having and supporting the needs of more than two members. Other developmental tasks of the family at this stage include developing an attachment between parents and children, adjusting to the economic costs of having more members, coping with energy depletion and lack of privacy, and carrying out activities that enhance the growth and development of the children.

Family with school-age children

The family with school-age children has the developmental tasks of adjusting to the expanded world of children in school and encouraging educational achievement. A further task is promoting joint decision making between children and parents.

Family with adolescents and young adults

The developmental tasks of the family with adolescents and young adults focus on transition. While providing a supportive home base and maintaining open communications, parents must balance freedom with responsibility and release adult children as they seek independence.

TABLE 2.7 Family-related risk factors for alterations in health

STAGE	RISK FACTORS	HEALTH PROBLEMS
Couple or family with infants and preschoolers	• Lack of knowledge about family planning, contraception, sexual and marital roles • Inadequate antenatal care • Altered nutrition: inadequate nutrition, overweight, underweight • Smoking, alcohol/drug abuse • First pregnancy before age 16 or after age 35 • Low socioeconomic status • Lack of knowledge about child health and safety • Rubella, syphilis, gonorrhoea, HIV/AIDS	• Premature pregnancy • Low-birth-weight infant • Birth defects • Injury to infant or child • Accidents
Family with school-age children	• Unsafe home environment • Working parents with inappropriate or inadequate resources for child care • Low socioeconomic status • Child abuse or neglect • Multiple, closely spaced children • Repeated infections, accidents and hospitalisations • Unrecognised and unattended health problems • Poor or inappropriate nutrition • Toxic substances in the home	• Behaviour problems • Speech and vision problems • Learning disabilities • Communicable diseases • Physical abuse • Cancer • Developmental delay • Obesity, underweight
Family with adolescents and young adults	• Family values of aggressiveness and competition • Lifestyle and behaviour leading to chronic illness (substance abuse, inadequate diet) • Lack of problem-solving skills • Conflicts between parents and children	• Violent death and injury • Alcohol/drug abuse • Unwanted pregnancy • Suicide • Sexually transmitted infections • Domestic abuse
Family with middle adults	• High-cholesterol diet • Overweight • Hypertension • Smoking, alcohol abuse • Physical inactivity • Personality patterns related to stress • Exposure to environment: sunlight, radiation, asbestos, water or air pollution • Depression	• Cardiovascular disease (coronary artery disease and cerebral vascular disease) • Cancer • Accidents • Suicide • Mental illness
Family with older adults	• Age • Depression • Drug interactions • Chronic illness • Death of spouse • Reduced income • Poor nutrition • Lack of exercise • Past environment and lifestyle	• Impaired vision and hearing • Hypertension • Acute illness • Chronic illness • Infectious diseases (influenza, pneumonia) • Injuries from burns and falls • Depression • Alcohol abuse

Family with middle adults

The family with middle adults (in which the parents are middle aged and children are no longer at home) has the developmental tasks of maintaining ties with older and younger generations and planning for retirement. If the family consists of just the middle-aged couple, they have the developmental tasks of re-establishing their relationship as a couple and possibly taking on the role of grandparents.

Family with older adults

The older adult family has the developmental tasks of adjusting to retirement, adjusting to ageing and coping with the loss of a spouse. If a spouse dies, further tasks include adjusting to living alone and perhaps selling the family home.

The family of the person with a chronic illness

The person with a chronic illness may be hospitalised for diagnosis and treatment of acute exacerbations, but their care is primarily provided at home. Chronic illness in a family member is a major stressor that causes changes in family structure and function and performing family developmental tasks.

Many factors affect family responses to chronic illness and these responses in turn affect the person's response to and perception of the illness. Factors influencing response to chronic illness include personal, social and economic resources, as well as the nature and course of the disease and the demands of the illness as perceived by family members.

Support for the family is essential. The following information should be considered when performing any family assessment and developing a plan of care:

- cohesiveness and communication patterns within the family
- family interactions that support self-care
- friends and relatives available to help
- family values and beliefs about health and illness
- cultural and spiritual beliefs
- developmental level of the person and family.

It is important to remember that standardised teaching plans may not be effective. People with chronic illnesses and their families should be given the freedom to choose appropriate literature, self-help or support groups, and interactions with others who have the same illness.

CHAPTER HIGHLIGHTS

- Health is an ever-changing state affected by genetic make-up, cognitive abilities, education, ethnicity, cultural background, age, gender, developmental level, lifestyle, environment, socioeconomic background and geographical area.
- The emphasis of nursing has shifted from acute care in the hospital setting to preventive community-based care. An essential component of medical–surgical nursing is teaching health behaviours that promote and maintain functional health status.
- Illnesses may be acute or chronic and behaviours of illness follow a sequence of experiencing symptoms, assuming the sick role, seeking medical help, assuming a dependent role, recovery and rehabilitation.
- Young adults are at risk of alterations in health from injury, sexually transmitted infections, substance abuse, workplace exposure to pollutants, sun exposure and psychological stressors.
- Middle adults are at risk of alterations in health from obesity, cardiovascular disease, cancer, substance abuse, and the stresses of change and transition.
- Older adults are at risk of alterations in health from chronic illnesses, injuries, drug toxicities, and changes in income and marital status.
- The family is an integral component in planning and implementing nursing care for the adult.

CONCEPT CHECK

1 Which definition best describes wellness?
1 a complete absence of disease
2 depends on the number of chronic illnesses
3 never having to take medications
4 gaining the best potential functioning of an individual

2 Many different factors affect the health of an individual. Which of the following are included? (Select all that apply.)
1 genetic make-up
2 cognitive abilities
3 height
4 age
5 ethnicity

3 Which of the following diseases has a genetic basis?
1 tuberculosis
2 cystic fibrosis
3 appendicitis
4 indigestion

4 Primary levels of prevention are general health promotion actions that prevent or delay the occurrence of a disease. Which of the following is a primary preventive activity?
1 practising safer sex
2 screening for hypertension
3 breast self-examination
4 having surgery

5 You call your tutor to say you have the 'flu' and will not be in class. What level of illness behaviour are you demonstrating?
1 experiencing symptoms
2 assuming the sick role
3 seeking medical care
4 assuming a dependent role

6 Your nephew was born with a heart defect. How would this disorder be classified?
1 an acute illness
2 a malignant illness
3 an iatrogenic illness
4 a congenital illness

7 Of the following descriptors, which is specific to a chronic illness?
1 occurs rapidly
2 lasts for a long time
3 is self-limiting
4 lasts for a short time

8 Mr Jones, age 50, is 15 kg overweight, smokes and rarely exercises. As a middle adult these factors increase his risk of disorders of which body system?
1 cardiovascular
2 renal
3 gastrointestinal
4 nervous

9 You are asked to present a health-related program at the local senior citizen centre. What would be an appropriate topic?
1 the hazards of substance abuse
2 accident prevention in the home
3 family roles and tasks
4 treating acute illness

10 Which of the following developmental tasks are part of the life of a family with older adults if a spouse dies? (Select all that apply.)
1 coping with lack of privacy
2 planning for retirement
3 adjusting to ageing
4 coping with loss
5 relating to family

BIBLIOGRAPHY

Australian Bureau of Statistics (ABS) (2021a). *2900.0 Census of population and housing: Understanding the Census and Census data, Australia, 2016*. Retrieved from https://www.abs.gov.au/

Australian Bureau of Statistics (ABS) (2021b). *Marriages and divorces, 2020*. Retrieved from https://www.abs.gov.au/

Australian Commission on Safety and Quality in Health Care (ACSQHC) (2020). *Medication without harm—WHO global patient safety challenge. Australia's response*. Sydney: ACSQHC.

Australian Human Rights Commission (2008). *Close the Gap: Indigenous health equality summit, statement of intent*. Retrieved from https://www.humanrights.gov.au/

Australian Institute of Health and Welfare (AIHW) (2020a). *Australia's health 2020*. Retrieved from https://www.aihw.gov.au/

Australian Institute of Health and Welfare (AIHW) (2020b). *National drug strategy household survey 2019*. Retrieved from https://www.aihw.gov.au/

Australian Institute of Health and Welfare (AIHW) (2021a). *Australia's welfare 2021*. Retrieved from https://www.aihw.gov.au/

Australian Institute of Health and Welfare (AIHW) (2021b). *Deaths in Australia*. Retrieved from https://www.aihw.gov.au/

Australian Institute of Health and Welfare (AIHW) (2021c). *Australian burden of disease study: Impact and causes of illness and death in Australia 2018*. Retrieved from https://www.aihw.gov.au/

Australian Institute of Health and Welfare (AIHW) (2021d). *Older Australians*. Retrieved from https://www.aihw.gov.au/

Australian Institute of Health and Welfare (AIHW) (2022). *National strategic framework for chronic conditions: Reporting framework* Retrieved from https://www.aihw.gov.au/

Australian Institute of Health and Welfare (AIHW) and Commonwealth Department of Health and Family Services (1997). *First report on National Health Priority Areas 1996*. AIHW Cat. No. PHE 1. Canberra: AIHW and DHFS. Retrieved from https://www.aihw.gov.au/

Department of Health (2020). *Immunisation*. Retrieved from https://www.health.gov.au/

Department of Health (2021). *National preventive health strategy 2021–2030* Retrieved from https://www.health.gov.au/

Department of Health (2022). *National immunisation program schedule*. Retrieved from https://www.health.gov.au/

Department of the Prime Minister and Cabinet (2020). *Closing the Gap Prime Minister's report*. Canberra: Author.

Dunn, H. (1959). High-level wellness for man and society. *American Journal of Public Health*, *49*, 786–972.

Edelman, C. & Kudzma, E. (2022). *Health promotion throughout the lifespan* (10th ed.). St Louis, MO: Elsevier

Erikson, E. (1963). *Childhood and society* (2nd ed.). New York: Norton.

Fowler, J. (1981). *Stages of faith: The psychology of human development and the quest for meaning*. New York: Harper & Row.

Havighurst, R. (1972). *Human development and education* (3rd ed.). New York: Longman.

Holland, C. (2018). *Close the Gap*. Close the Gap Campaign Steering Committee for Indigenous Health Equality. Retrieved from https://www.humanrights.gov.au/

Kohlberg, L. (1979). *The meaning and measurement of moral development*. New York: Clark University.

Miller, D. (1981). The 'sandwich' generation: Adult children of the aging. *Social Work*, *26*, 419–423.

Miller, J. (2000). *Coping with chronic illness: Overcoming powerlessness* (3rd ed.). Philadelphia: F. A. Davis.

Murdaugh, C., Parsons, M. & Pender, N. (2018). *Health promotion in nursing practice* (8th ed.). New York: Pearson.

Suchman, E. (1972). Stages of illness and medical care. In E. Jaco (ed.), *Patients, physicians and illness*. New York: Free Press.

United Nations (2022). *Sustainable developments*. Retrieved https://www.un.org/

Westerhoff, J. (1976). *Will our children have faith?* New York: Seabury Press.

World Health Organization (WHO) (1948). *Constitution of the World Health Organization: Chronicle of the World Health Organization*. Geneva: Author.

World Health Organization (WHO) (2020). *Decade of healthy ageing: Baseline report*. Geneva: WHO. Retrieved from https://www.who.int/

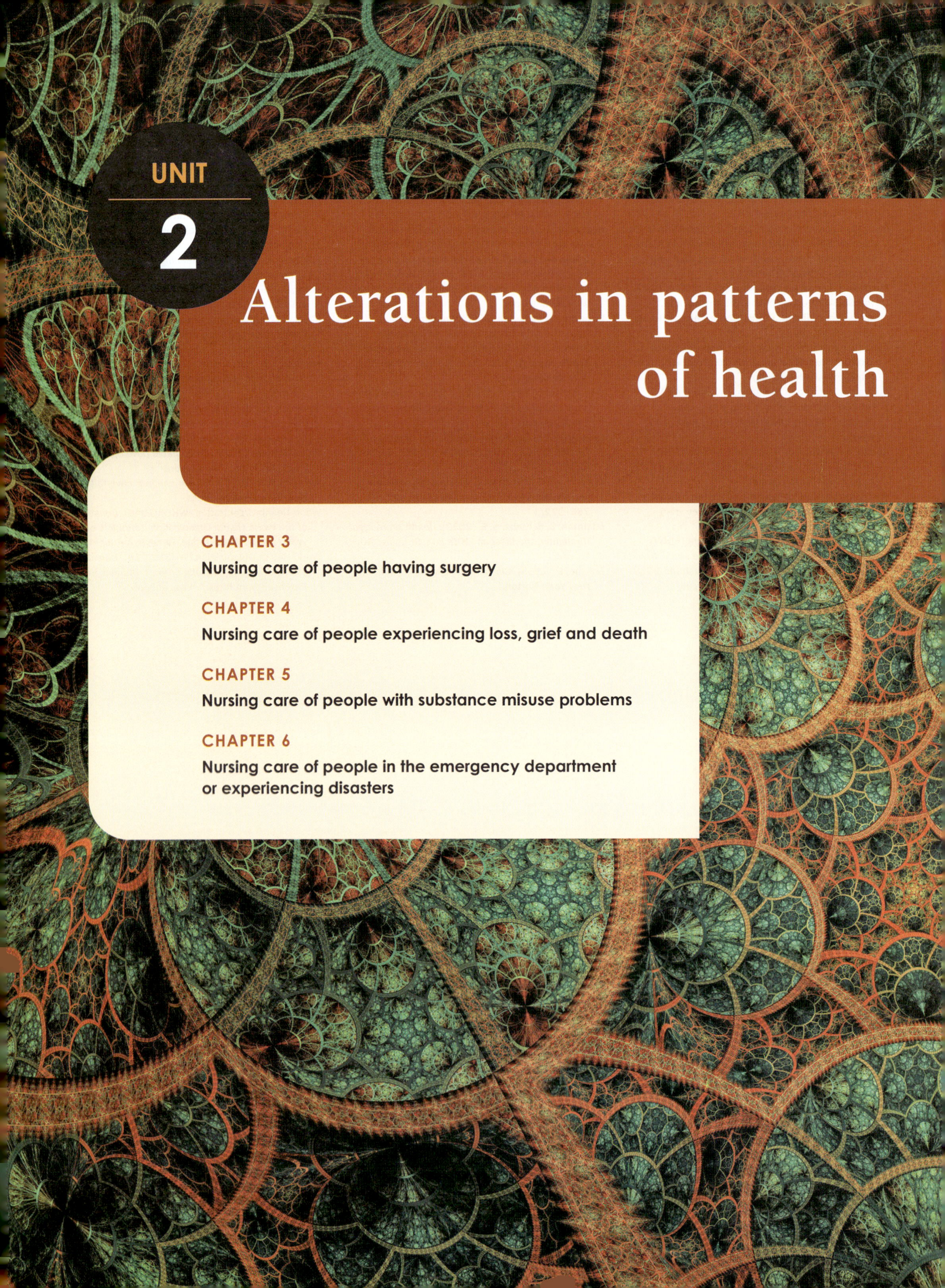

UNIT

2

Alterations in patterns of health

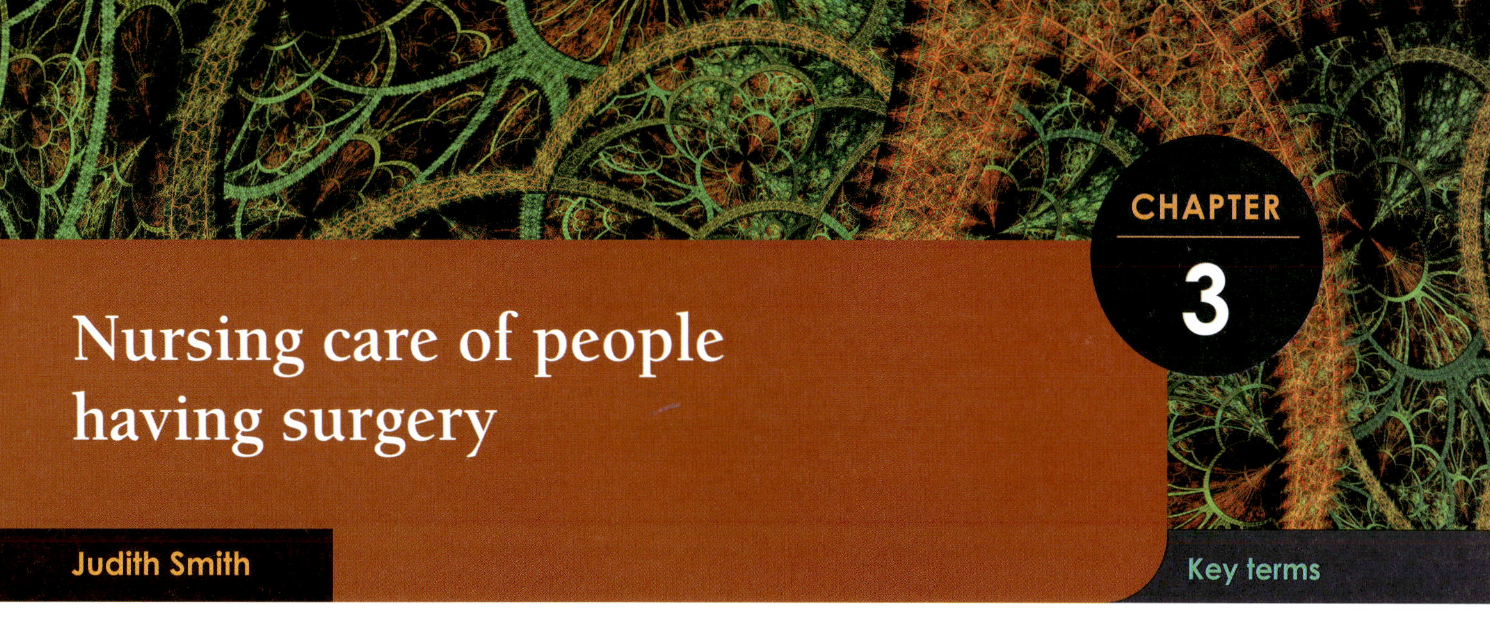

CHAPTER 3

Nursing care of people having surgery

Judith Smith

Key terms

Learning outcomes

- Discuss the differences and similarities between ambulatory/day surgery and inpatient surgery.
- Describe legal requirements and responsibilities prior to surgery.
- Describe the various classifications and risk factors of surgical procedures.
- Identify diagnostic tests used during the perioperative period.
- Describe nursing implications for medications prescribed for the person having surgery.
- Describe appropriate nursing care for people having surgery in the preoperative, intraoperative and postoperative phases of surgery.
- Identify variations in perioperative care for the older adult.
- Describe principles of pain management specific to acute postoperative pain control.
- Apply the nursing process as a framework for providing individualised care for people undergoing surgery.

Clinical competencies

- Assess the physiological health status of people having surgery to determine their ability to tolerate surgery and risks of complications.
- Assess the psychosocial health status of the person having surgery and their family.
- Ensure safety of the person having surgery within the operating theatre and throughout the postoperative period.
- Participate in education for the person and their family prior to anaesthesia and prior to discharge from the facility.
- Describe the sterile field in the operating theatre, practise aseptic technique and take occupational health and safety precautions to prevent infections and minimise hazards.
- As part of the interprofessional team, monitor and control the environment to prevent accidents or injury to the person having surgery and members of the healthcare team.
- Respect the person's rights, including privacy, at all times.

Surgery is an invasive medical procedure performed to diagnose or treat illness, injury or deformity. Although surgery is a medical treatment, the nurse assumes an active role in caring for the person before, during and after surgery. **Interprofessional care** and teamwork by nurses, surgeons, anaesthetists, pharmacists and allied health professionals can prevent complications and promote optimal recovery of the person having surgery.

Perioperative nursing is a highly skilled, specialised area of practice incorporating a number of sub-specialties. There are clearly defined nursing roles for providing patient care during the three phases of the surgical experience: preoperative, intraoperative and postoperative. The **preoperative phase** begins when the decision for surgery is made and ends when the person having surgery is transferred to the operating room. The **intraoperative phase** begins with the person's entry into the operating room and ends with transfer to the post anaesthesia care unit (PACU), or recovery room. The **postoperative phase** begins with the person's arrival at the PACU and ends with their complete recovery from the surgical intervention.

CLASSIFICATIONS OF SURGICAL PROCEDURES

Surgical procedures can be classified according to purpose, risk factor and urgency (see Table 3.1). Based on this information, nursing care can be individualised to meet the needs of the person having surgery.

Although the perioperative nurse works in collaboration with other healthcare professionals to identify and meet the needs of the person having surgery, the perioperative nurse has the primary responsibility and accountability for nursing care of the person undergoing surgery.

SETTINGS FOR SURGERY

People having surgery may be inpatients or outpatients. The complexity of the surgery and the recovery and expected condition of the person following the surgery are the major differences. Sometimes outpatients (i.e. people intending to be discharged home immediately following surgery) need to be admitted to the hospital. Cataract removal with or without lens implants, hernia repairs, tubal ligations, vasectomies, dilation and curettage (D&C), haemorrhoidectomies and biopsies are commonly performed in outpatient surgeries.

Inpatient and outpatient surgeries are performed in the same operating suites in many hospitals. There are also **day surgery units/centres** (also called *ambulatory surgery*), which are not physically connected to a hospital. Perioperative nursing roles support people having surgery irrespective of whether surgeons practise in hospitals or in freestanding surgical facilities. Some outpatient surgeries are performed in surgeons' offices rather than surgical centres. Modern day surgery has changed during the past decade, and it is estimated that over 61% of all elective surgery is carried out in day surgery settings (Australian Institute of Health and Welfare (AIHW), 2020). With advancements in minimally invasive surgical techniques, day surgery centres can now offer high-quality, safe and cost-effective alternatives to inpatient surgical services.

However, day surgery settings are often fast-paced, and patient contact is transitory. Therefore, providing safe, competent and person-centred care in this environment requires nurses to work within their full scope of practice, with additional specialist knowledge and clear communication and teamwork abilities. The increase in the number of procedures and acuity level of people having surgery in day surgery settings can present challenges for the perioperative nurse, the person having surgery and their family.

Day surgery potentially offers several advantages:

- decreased cost to the person having surgery and the hospital
- reduced risk of hospital-acquired infection
- less interruption to the person's and their family's routine
- possible reduction in time lost from work and/or other responsibilities
- less physiological stress for the person and their family.

Day surgery also presents some disadvantages:

- less time for the nurse to establish rapport with the person and their family
- less time for the nurse to assess, evaluate and teach the person and their family

TABLE 3.1 Classification of surgical procedures

	CLASSIFICATION	FUNCTION	EXAMPLES
Purpose	Diagnostic	Determine or confirm a diagnosis	Breast biopsy, bronchoscopy
	Ablative	Remove diseased tissue, organ or extremity	Appendectomy, amputation
	Constructive	Build tissue/organs that are absent (congenital anomalies)	Repair of cleft palate
	Reconstructive	Rebuild tissue/organ that has been damaged	Skin graft after a burn, total joint replacement
	Palliative	Alleviate symptoms of a disease (not curative)	Bowel resection in a person with terminal cancer
	Transplant	Replace organs/tissue to restore function	Heart, lung, liver, kidney transplant
Risk factor	Minor	Minimal physical assault with minimal risk	Removal of skin lesions, dilation and curettage (D&C), cataract extraction
	Major	Extensive physical assault and/or serious risk	Transplant, total joint replacement, cholecystectomy, colostomy, nephrectomy
Urgency	Elective	Suggested, though no foreseen ill effects if postponed	Cosmetic surgery, cataract surgery, bunionectomy
	Urgent	Necessary to be performed within 1 to 2 days	Heart bypass surgery, amputation resulting from gangrene, fractured hip
	Emergency	Performed immediately	Obstetric emergencies, bowel obstruction, ruptured aneurysm, life-threatening trauma

- lack of opportunity for the nurse to assess for the risk of postoperative complications that may occur after discharge
- less time for adequate pain control before discharge
- increased burden and stress on primary caregivers as the patient recovers at home.

Following day surgery, the person is discharged after meeting the discharge criteria of the institution with respect to the Australian Day Surgery Nurses Association (ADSNA) *Best Practice Guidelines for Ambulatory Surgery and Procedures* (2018). Prior to discharge, the person must demonstrate:

- normal vital signs for at least 1 hour post procedure
- orientation to time, place and person
- minimal nausea, vomiting or dizziness
- minimal pain minimal bleeding or wound drainage
- ability to urinate.

The day surgery nurse must also ensure that the person has a responsible caregiver, that suitable analgesia has been provided and that the patient understands the written and verbal postoperative instructions provided.

Many similarities exist between the nursing care of people admitted for inpatient and for outpatient surgery. Physical care is provided in much the same manner in the preoperative, intraoperative and postoperative phases of surgery. The major differences lie in the degree of teaching and emotional support that must be provided for people having outpatient surgical procedures and their families. In addition to the physiological insult of surgery, the person having outpatient surgery must cope with the stress of needing to learn a great deal of information in a short span of time. The nurse teaches the person and their family in both the preoperative and postoperative periods to enable the person to perform self-care following discharge and recognise the development of complications that require further clinical management. More extensive teaching and emotional support is necessary as people requiring more complex surgical procedures and experiencing more complicated health problems undergo outpatient surgery.

CONSIDERATION FOR PRACTICE

People having outpatient surgery should wear or bring clothing that will be easy to put on after surgery and accommodate any dressings or appliances. Despite fasting, people having outpatient surgery may be instructed to bring any medications such as steroids, antibiotics, anticoagulants, antivirals, diuretics, oral contraceptives, hypotensives, cardiotonics, hypoglycaemics, asthma medications, seizure medications and analgesics, as well as any herbal preparations, that they regularly use. People having surgery should consult with the surgeon and anaesthetist before taking these medications, prior to and following surgery.

LEGAL REQUIREMENTS

It is the responsibility of the surgeon who performs the procedure to obtain the person's consent for the surgical procedure. The surgeon should discuss the procedure with the person and their family in language they can understand. **Informed consent** is disclosure of the risks associated with the intended procedure or operation to the person and includes completion of a legal document required for certain diagnostic procedures or therapeutic measures, including surgery. The language of the document varies according to the statutory and common law of each state. This legal document protects the person undergoing surgery, the nurse, the surgeon and the healthcare facility.

Informed consent includes provision of the following information prior to the person signing a consent for medical procedure treatment form:

- need for the procedure in relation to the diagnoses
- description and purpose of the proposed procedure
- possible benefits and potential risks
- likelihood of a successful outcome
- alternative treatments or procedures available
- anticipated risks should the procedure not be performed
- surgeon's advice about what is needed
- the person's right to refuse treatment or withdraw consent.

The nurse may be present when the preceding information is provided. Later, the nurse can discuss the information with the person and their family, if necessary. If the person having surgery has questions or concerns that were not discussed or made clear, or if the nurse questions the person's understanding, the surgeon is responsible for supplying further information. Following a thorough discussion of the consent for operation or special procedures, the person having surgery voluntarily signs the form. The nurse will then complete the Surgical Safety Checklist, introduced by the World Health Organization (WHO) and World Alliance for Patient Safety (2009), to confirm that all components of a legal consent have been addressed and confirmed with the person. In many circumstances, the person having surgery is admitted to the surgical unit or day surgery with an already completed consent form.

PERIOPERATIVE RISK FACTORS

Prior to planning and implementing care for the person having surgery, the nurse must first assess their needs and the factors that may increase the risks associated with surgery. The type of surgical procedure directs the assessment and interventions planned by the nurse. However, a complete assessment is also necessary to identify *risk factors* and to determine the person's overall health status. Table 3.2 lists common risk factors for the person undergoing surgery and the related nursing interventions and implications. For example, when a person is admitted for surgery on the right knee, it should be of concern to the nurse if this person has diabetes, requires insulin, smokes 25 cigarettes per day and has numbness in their right foot. This information should be incorporated into a nursing care plan, using appropriate nursing diagnoses and interventions to meet all of the person's needs and to assist them towards full postoperative recovery.

There are risks are associated with all surgical interventions. For example, transporting the person to and from the operating

TABLE 3.2 Nursing implications for surgical risk factors

FACTOR	ASSOCIATED RISK	NURSING IMPLICATIONS
Advanced age	Older adults have age-related changes that affect physiological, cognitive and psychosocial responses to the stress of surgery; decreased tolerance of general anaesthesia and postoperative medications; and delayed wound healing.	Selected nursing interventions are summarised in Table 3.7.
Obesity	The obese person is at increased risk of delayed wound healing, wound dehiscence, infection, pneumonia, atelectasis, thrombophlebitis, arrhythmias and heart failure.	Promote weight reduction if time permits. Monitor closely for wound, pulmonary and cardiovascular complications postoperatively. Encourage coughing, turning, and diaphragmatic breathing exercises and early ambulation.
Malnutrition	Reserves may not be sufficient to allow the body to respond satisfactorily to the physical assault of surgery; organ failure and shock may result. Increased metabolic demands may result in poor wound healing and infection. The person's fluid balance may be impacted if they have decreased serum albumin levels caused by malnutrition.	With the surgeon and dietitian, promote weight gain by providing a well-balanced diet high in kilojoules, protein and vitamin C. Administer nutritional supplements and, if indicated, total parenteral nutrition intravenously, and tube feedings as prescribed. Daily weights and kilojoule counts also may be ordered.
Dehydration/electrolyte imbalance	Depending on the degree of dehydration and/or type of electrolyte imbalance, hypotension, cardiac arrhythmia or heart failure may occur. Liver and renal failure may also result.	Administer intravenous fluids as ordered. Monitor fluid input and output and weight. Monitor for evidence of fluid and electrolyte imbalance (see the chapter 'Nursing care of people with altered fluid, electrolyte and acid–base balance'). Closely monitor fluid intake (oral and parenteral) to prevent circulatory overload.
Renal and liver dysfunction	The person with renal or liver dysfunction may poorly tolerate general anaesthesia, have fluid/electrolyte and acid–base imbalances, decreased metabolism and excretion of drugs, increased risk of haemorrhage, and delayed wound healing.	Monitor for fluid volume overload, intake and output, and response to medication. Evaluate closely for drug side effects and evidence of acidosis or alkalosis.
Cardiovascular disorders	Presence of cardiovascular disease increases the risk of haemorrhage and shock, hypotension, thrombophlebitis, pulmonary embolism, stroke (especially in the older person) and fluid volume overload.	Diligently monitor vital signs, especially pulse rate, regularity and rhythm, and general condition of the person. Assess skin colour. Assess for chest pain, lung congestion and peripheral oedema. Observe for signs of hypoxia, and administer oxygen as ordered. Early postoperative ambulation and leg exercises reduce the risk of vascular problems such as thrombophlebitis and pulmonary embolism.
Respiratory disorders	Respiratory conditions such as asthma, bronchitis, atelectasis and pneumonia are some of the most common and serious risk factors for postoperative complications. Respiratory depression from general anaesthesia and acid–base imbalance may also occur.	Closely monitor respirations, pulse and breath sounds. Also assess for hypoxia, dyspnoea, lung congestion and chest pain. Encourage coughing, turning and diaphragmatic breathing exercises and early postoperative ambulation. Encourage the person to stop smoking or at least to reduce the number of cigarettes smoked.
Diabetes mellitus	Diabetes causes an increased risk of fluctuating blood glucose levels, which can lead to life-threatening hypoglycaemia or ketoacidosis. A history of diabetes also increases the risk of cardiovascular disease, decreased gut motility resulting in bowel obstruction, delayed wound healing and wound infection.	Monitor the person closely for signs and symptoms of hypoglycaemia and hyperglycaemia. Monitor blood glucose levels every 4 hours or as ordered. Administer insulin or oral hypoglycaemic medications as prescribed. Encourage intake of food at the designated meal and snack times.
Alcoholism	The person may be malnourished and experience alcohol withdrawal and delirium tremens. More general anaesthesia may be required. Haemorrhage and delayed wound healing can result from liver damage and poor nutritional status.	Monitor closely for signs of alcohol withdrawal and delirium tremens. Encourage well-balanced diet. Monitor for wound complications. Administer supplementary nutrients parenterally as ordered.
Nicotine use	Cigarette smokers are at increased risk of venous thrombosis, delayed wound healing and respiratory complications such as pneumonia, atelectasis and bronchitis because of increased mucous secretions and a decreased ability to expel them.	Ideally, the person having surgery should stop smoking. Be supportive of them and monitor closely for respiratory difficulties. Coughing, turning and diaphragmatic breathing exercises with early ambulation are very important. Increase daily fluid intake to 2,500–3,000 mL (unless contraindicated) to help liquefy respiratory secretions to aid expectoration. A nicotine patch may help them to tolerate withdrawal during the postoperative period.
Adolescence	Diversity in age and physical, cognitive and psychological maturation makes preparation for surgery vary in content and inclusion of significant others. Increased need for control, privacy and peer interaction poses special challenges in the acute care setting.	Adapt assessment and interventions to the developmental level of individual people, involving them in preparation and care to the extent possible. Allow for regressive and independent behaviour, including rejection of adult support.
Medications	Anaesthesia interaction with some medications can cause respiratory difficulties, hypotension and circulatory collapse. Other medications can produce side effects that may increase surgical risk.	Inform the anaesthetist of all prescribed or over-the-counter medications.
Anticoagulants (including aspirin)	May cause intraoperative and postoperative haemorrhage.	Monitor for bleeding. Assess prothrombin time (PT value) and partial thromboplastin time (PTT value).
Diuretics (particularly thiazides)	May lead to fluid and electrolyte imbalances, producing altered cardiovascular response and respiratory depression.	Monitor fluid input and output and electrolytes. Assess cardiovascular and respiratory status.
Antihypertensives (particularly phenothiazines)	Increase the hypotensive effects of anaesthesia.	Closely monitor blood pressure.
Antidepressants (particularly monoamine oxidase inhibitors)	Increase the hypotensive effects of anaesthesia.	Closely monitor blood pressure.
Antibiotics (particularly the 'mycin' group)	May cause apnoea and respiratory paralysis.	Monitor respirations.
Herbal supplements	Some may prolong the effects of anaesthesia. Others may increase the risks of bleeding or raise blood pressure.	Inquire about the use of herbs or other dietary supplements. These should be discontinued at least 2 weeks before surgery.
Temperature variations	Deviations from normothermia, either hypothermia or hyperthermia, may cause infection, cardiac morbidity, myocardial ischaemia, surgical bleeding, skin damage or discomfort for the person having surgery.	Monitor core temperatures and prevent chilling or overheating. Use warmed fluids. Remove wet drapes and ensure the person is clean and dry immediately post surgery.

suite needs to be organised in advance and be well planned, and patients need to be assessed for supplementary oxygen, intravenous therapy, cardiac monitoring and safety issues pertaining to the means of transport. Many people enter the operating suite highly anxious and may benefit from medication to help them relax prior to administration of anaesthesia. This can be discussed with the anaesthetist. Chemicals, electrical equipment and environmental hazards in the surgical area have the potential to cause harm and must be monitored and maintained carefully.

Unfortunately, there is a risk of performing the wrong surgery on the wrong person: including wrong site, wrong procedure and/or wrong person. In 2012, the Joint Commission on Accreditation of Healthcare Organizations (2012) issued a universal protocol mandating the requirement for preoperatively: (1) verifying the procedure, (2) physically marking and initialling the site, and (3) taking a 'time out' before starting any procedure. The goal of the 'time out' is to ensure the right procedure will be performed on the right person on the correct site with the necessary and correct healthcare professionals in attendance. A 'time out' is an intentional stoppage of the preparation for the operation, in the operating suite, before the person having surgery is anaesthetised. All participants are introduced and encouraged to ask any questions or express any concerns before the surgery is commenced to prevent adverse outcomes. The WHO and World Alliance for Patient Safety (2009) now recommend use of the Surgical Safety Checklist for this purpose. This checklist has been reported to significantly reduce surgical morbidity and mortality (Shear et al., 2018), and a statement on the WHO Patient Safety (2022) webpage claims that half a million deaths per annum are potentially preventable if the checklist is implemented worldwide.

Another potential error is retained foreign bodies such as instruments, needles or sponges. To prevent accidental retention of foreign objects, standardised procedures for counting objects used in surgery must be consistently applied and adhered to. The Australian College of Operating Room Nurses (ACORN) Standards (2020) provide guidelines regarding best practice on management of accountable items used during surgery and procedures. In addition, methodical wound exploration before closing the site, using x-ray-detectable materials in the wound, maintenance of optimal operating theatre environments to allow focused surgical performance and employing technological methods to ensure no unintended item remains are now the norm in surgical practice. Research indicates team attentiveness and communication as most significant in preventing retained surgical instruments. Systems approaches such as barcoding and other automated identification cannot replace the manual count procedure (Steelman et al., 2019).

People having surgery may be using medications that increase the risk of complications associated with a surgical procedure, such as increasing the risk of bleeding. Over-the-counter medicines and herbal preparations, as well as prescription medications, may interact with drugs given during surgery, putting a person at increased risk. The American Society of Anesthesiologists suggests surgical patients cease herbal products at least 1 week prior to their scheduled surgery (Dagli et al., 2016; Donoghue, 2018). A complete history of the medications the person has been taking regularly is vital information. As part of the preoperative planning and teaching, early consideration of complementary and alternative medicine is also important. This information should be obtained in a non-judgmental manner, because a judgmental attitude could cause the person to withhold information.

Anticoagulant medications are frequently discontinued by the anaesthetist in the preoperative clinic prior to surgery to prevent excessive blood loss during surgery. These include aspirin and non-steroidal anti-inflammatory drugs. If laboratory tests of clotting/bleeding time, prothrombin time (PT), partial thromboplastin time (PTT) and INR (International Normalized Ratio) are elevated, the surgery may be cancelled. Guidelines for discontinuing use vary according to the particular medication; it is generally recommended that aspirin or products containing aspirin be discontinued 5 days or longer before surgery. Similarly, herbs or nutritional supplements interfering with blood clotting have the potential to pose significant bleeding and should be discontinued prior to surgery as advised by the surgeon (Abebe, 2019). The most common self-prescribed medicines that may inhibit coagulation are vitamin E, garlic, ginkgo, ginseng and fish oil. Many plants that contain coumarins have the potential to interact with warfarin and inhibit coagulation. Others inhibit platelet aggregation or prevent the conversion of fibrinogen to fibrin. All of these create a risk of bleeding. Table 3.3 lists commonly used over-the-counter herbal and supplemental preparations that may increase the risk of complications associated with anaesthesia and surgery.

People taking warfarin for the risk of blood clots due to atrial fibrillation will be counselled about the appropriate time to withdraw warfarin. If surgery is urgent due to trauma or sudden onset of morbidity, the impact of anticoagulants needs to be evaluated, with PT, PTT and INR results required before the operation and appropriate medication administered to promote clotting.

In addition to clotting impairment, excessive consumption of herbal medicines or dietary supplements can produce levels of chemicals that interact with conventional medications, exacerbating or impairing the intended effect (see Table 3.3) (Abebe, 2019). Anaesthetic drugs often decrease hepatic blood flow and interfere with the metabolism and elimination of medications. This increases the risk of adverse drug–herbal supplement interactions during surgery. Cardiovascular instability, impaired glucose control, increased metabolism of perioperative medication, and unpredictable response to anaesthesia are categories of adverse reactions of perioperative herbal use (Dagli et al., 2016; Donoghue, 2018).

In the perioperative period, hypothermia and hyperthermia are risks. Typically, surgical suites are maintained as cooler environments; however, research shows that normothermia (core body temperature in the range of 36.0°C to 37.5°C) in the person having surgery reduces the risk of infection, cardiac

TABLE 3.3 Commonly used over-the-counter herbal and supplemental preparations that may increase the risk of complications associated with anaesthesia and surgery

INTERACTION	HERBAL PREPARATION	ASSOCIATED RISK
Coagulation The most common interactions of botanicals with coagulation include prolonged bleeding or clotting times and interference with platelet aggregation through the blocking of platelet fibrinogen receptors.	• Garlic	• Potential for irreversible inhibition of platelet function.
	• Chamomile	• Can cause an increased risk of bleeding because it contains phytocoumarins, which have additive effects with warfarin.
	• Ginger and ginseng	• Increase bleeding risk by interacting with antiplatelet drugs to inhibit platelet aggregation and fibrinolysis. They also augment the effects of warfarin.
	• Feverfew	• Increases the risk of bleeding because it individually inhibits platelet aggregation and has additive effects with other antiplatelet drugs.
	• Ginkgo	• Inhibits platelet-activating factors but also modulates neurotransmitter and receptor activity.
Sedation Some botanicals have sedative actions. They cause CNS depression through the inhibition of receptor activation and gamma-aminobutyric acid (GABA)-receptor mediation.	• St John's wort	• Has been found to inhibit the binding of naloxone.
	• Ginger	• Known to inhibit serotonergic pathways.
	• Valerian and kava	• Potentiate GABA-mediated systems, which can interfere with inhalation anaesthetics that work on GABA receptors.
	• Motherwort	• Taken with benzodiazepines, can have a synergistic sedative effect and may result in coma.
Cardiovascular Many of the herbs that interfere with coagulation can also impact on the cardiovascular system. The pharmacokinetics involved include: • SNS stimulation—hypertension, tachycardia and cardiac arrhythmias • hypokalaemia—arrhythmias • inotropic effects • reduced bioavailability of antihypertensive.	• St John's wort	• Could potentially result in serious adverse reactions because of its effect on drug metabolism, such as antihypertensive drugs (clopidogrel and amiodarone) and beta-blockers such as metoprolol. It may result in reduced bioavailability and effectiveness of these drugs with subsequent recurrence of arrhythmia, hypertension or other undesirable effects.
	• Hawthorn	• Enhances the activity of digitalis, and its concomitant use should be monitored carefully for potential toxic effects.
	• Ginseng	• Excessive use can cause hypotension.
	• Aconite	• Can cause atrial or ventricular fibrillation from the direct effect of aconite on the myocardium.

morbidity, myocardial ischaemia, surgical bleeding and personal discomfort (Collins et al., 2019). Methods to minimise the risk of hypothermia include:

- Apply warm blankets on arrival in the surgical area and after sterile drapes are removed.
- Limit the amount of skin exposed during positioning and skin preparation.
- Limit the time of skin exposure between prepping and draping.
- Prevent surgical drapes from becoming wet.
- Monitor the person's temperature to avoid overheating.
- Use heat-maintenance devices such as warming units, stockings, caps and leggings.
- Humidify the airway.
- Clean and dry the person immediately postoperatively.

An anaesthetised person loses heat intraoperatively and is unable to restore temperature through the normal mechanisms of shivering or muscle contractions (Collins et al., 2019). Hyperthermia should also be avoided. Heating of fluids or use of heating units necessitates accurate measurement of the person's temperature. Body temperature is best evaluated through core temperature monitoring, which includes oesophageal or tympanic assessment.

Interpreting and responding to identified risk factors requires adequate clinical reasoning and interprofessional communication skills. It is important to bring concerns to the attention of the surgeon and/or anaesthetist prior to surgery, so that necessary modifications can be made for the person during the perioperative period.

CONSIDERATION FOR PRACTICE

Remind people with diabetes that the stress of surgery increases, rather than decreases, blood sugar. Coordinate insulin injections and/or hypoglycaemic medication with the person, surgeon and anaesthetist.

INTERPROFESSIONAL CARE

The person undergoing surgery receives care from a number of healthcare professionals. Surgeons, nurses, anaesthetists, anaesthetic technicians, pathologists, x-ray technicians, physiotherapists and paramedical staff such as registration clerks and wardspeople/porters are often involved in securing the safety and health of people having surgery. Case managers, social workers and spiritual care providers are available based on the person's needs and preferences. This interprofessional approach focuses on maintaining the person in the best possible health status before, during and after surgery (Nursing and Midwifery Board of Australia (NMBA), 2016). For some major and frequently performed procedures, the interprofessional team can develop and map a routine clinical process of recovery. This process is described in a document called a *clinical pathway* (or critical pathway, care path or map). These are multidisciplinary maps that document the various stages of recovery, and appropriate therapeutic responses by team members, in order to assist the person to arrive safely and successfully at the point of discharge. Any divergence from a stated pathway results in variances that must be carefully documented and appropriately managed by the interprofessional team.

Diagnostic tests

The use of preoperative investigations should follow evidence-based guidelines to reduce the volume of unnecessary investigations without compromising patient safety (O'Neill et al., 2016). Diagnostic tests performed prior to surgery provide baseline data or reveal problems that may place the person at additional risk during and after surgery. Because of the trend towards shortened hospital stays, many diagnostic studies and procedures are performed in a preadmission clinic (pre-op clinic) within a week prior to elective surgery as part of the preadmission assessment process.

Complete blood counts, electrolyte studies, coagulation studies and urinalysis are the most commonly performed preoperative laboratory tests. Table 3.4 discusses the significance and nursing implications of abnormal findings for these common tests. Additional diagnostic tests may be performed as the history and physical findings indicate. For example, if the person has a low haemoglobin and haematocrit, and significant blood loss during surgery is anticipated, then the surgeon may order a type and crossmatch of the person's blood for a possible transfusion.

In addition to laboratory tests, older people or those with risk factors related to heart and lung function typically have a chest x-ray. This radiological procedure provides baseline information about the size, shape and condition of the heart and lungs. Pulmonary complications such as lung disease, tuberculosis, calcification, infiltration or pneumonia may require that surgery be postponed to allow the person to undergo further evaluation or treatment. If findings are abnormal and the surgery cannot be postponed, information from the chest x-ray study can be used to determine the safest form of anaesthesia.

Another commonly performed preoperative diagnostic procedure is the electrocardiogram (ECG). This test is ordered routinely for people undergoing general anaesthesia when they have cardiovascular disease or risk factors (O'Neill et al., 2016). The ECG provides data for the evaluation of either new or pre-existing cardiac conditions. The person's surgery may be cancelled or postponed if a life-threatening cardiac condition is discovered.

In addition to the chest x-ray study and ECG, other diagnostic tests may be performed preoperatively to gather

TABLE 3.4 Laboratory tests for perioperative assessment

TEST	SIGNIFICANCE OF INCREASED VALUES	SIGNIFICANCE OF DECREASED VALUES	NURSING IMPLICATIONS
Haematology:			
Haemoglobin (Hgb or Hb) and haematocrit (HCT)	Dehydration, excessive fluid plasma loss, polycythaemia vera	Fluid overload, excessive blood loss, anaemia	Monitor oxygenation, fluid input and output, and vital signs; assess for bleeding.
Glucose and haemoglobin-A (HbA1c)	Impaired glucose metabolism, stress or infection	Inadequate glucose intake in relation to insulin	If decreased, monitor for signs and symptoms of hypoglycaemia. Notify surgeon if < 48 mmol/mol or > 59 mmol/mol for diabetics and < 20 mmol/mol or > 42 mmol/mol for non-diabetics.
White blood cell (WBC) count	Infectious/inflammatory processes, leukaemia	Immune deficiencies	Monitor for signs of inflammation; monitor drainage, temperature and pulse. Use standard or transmission-based precautions.
Platelet count	Malignancies, polycythaemia vera	Clotting deficiency disorders, chemotherapy	If decreased, assess for bleeding at incision sites and drainage tubes, and assess for haematomas.
Blood gas analysis (pH)	Metabolic and/or respiratory alkalosis	Metabolic and/or respiratory acidosis	Monitor respiratory and renal status and arterial blood gases (ABGs).
Carbon dioxide (CO_2)	Emphysema, chronic bronchitis, asthma, pneumonia, respiratory acidosis, vomiting, nasogastric (NG) suctioning	Metabolic acidosis, hyperventilation	Monitor respiratory status and arterial blood gases (ABGs).
Oxygen (O_2)	Can be excessive for exacerbated COPD patients or CO_2 retainers	May indicate respiratory depression associated with narcotic analgesia or physiological deterioration including haemorrhage	Monitor O_2 % using pulse oximetry and ABGs if respiratory status deteriorates.
Biochemistry:			
Potassium (K^+)	Kidney dysfunction, dehydration, suctioning	Side effects of diuretics, vomiting, nasogastric (NG) suctioning	Monitor K^+ level, cardiac and neurological function, and preoperative diuretic therapy.
Sodium (Na^+)	Kidney dysfunction, normal saline-containing intravenous fluids	Side effects of diuretics, vomiting, NG suctioning	Monitor Na^+ level and fluid input and output; assess for peripheral oedema and effects of perioperative diuretic therapy.
Chloride (Cl^-)	Kidney dysfunction, dehydration, alkalosis	Side effects of diuretics, vomiting, NG suctioning	Monitor Cl^- level and fluid input and output; assess for peripheral oedema and perioperative diuretic therapy.
Coagulation studies:			
Prothrombin time (PT) and partial thromboplastin time (PTT)	Defect in mechanism for blood clotting, anticoagulant therapy (aspirin, heparin, warfarin), side effect of other drugs affecting clotting time	Hypercoagulability of the blood may lead to thrombus formation in the veins	If clotting time is elevated, monitor PT/PTT values. Assess for bleeding at incision site and drainage tubes and for haematomas. If clotting time is decreased, monitor for thrombus formation (pulmonary emboli, thrombophlebitis), and evaluate PT and PTT values.
Urinalysis	Varied	Varied	Used to detect abnormal substances (e.g. protein, glucose, red blood cells or bacteria) in the urine. Notify surgeon if abnormalities are detected.

further assessment data. For example, for people who have chronic obstructive pulmonary disease, lung function tests are often performed to determine the extent of respiratory dysfunction. This information guides the anaesthetist before and during surgery in choosing the type of anaesthetic to be used, and it guides the surgeon and nursing staff in the recovery phase.

The glomerular filtration rate is a rapid and useful indicator of renal function. A low serum creatinine is an indicator of good renal function, so the creatinine value must be confirmed in the urine; however, it is useful to know that normal values are lower in older adults due to decreased muscle mass. Older adults are especially susceptible to renal insufficiency, which puts them at risk of volume overload in the perioperative period and accumulation of metabolic by-products and medications dependent on renal clearance.

Pregnancy testing for women may also be useful prior to surgery, particularly for elective procedures.

Medications

The person having surgery receives medications before, during and after surgery to achieve specific therapeutic outcomes. Routine oral medications may be withheld during preoperative fasting periods, and the anaesthetist will normally specify medications that should be given, and those that should be withheld. People with diabetes require careful management of their medications during fasting so they don't experience extreme fluctuations in blood glucose levels and associated risks. The anaesthetist will often order pain medication, anticoagulants and antibiotics postoperatively if indicated. Generally, routine medication orders must be revised by the surgeon or anaesthetist when the person returns to the post-surgical care unit.

The person having surgery may be given preoperative medications 45 to 70 minutes before the scheduled surgery depending on medical orders. Any delay in administration should be reported promptly to the anaesthetist. Preoperative medications may also be given in the anaesthetic room to produce the desired effects.

An increasingly common strategy to prevent or minimise postoperative pain is the use of *pre-emptive analgesia*. Pre-emptive analgesia prevents sensitisation of the central and peripheral nervous system by painful stimuli, by blocking the pain pathways with local, regional or epidural analgesia prior to incision. Sensitisation to pain prolongs the painful experience; however, blocking the sensitisation throughout the perioperative period results in decreased pain in the postoperative period, shortened hospital stay, quicker return to self-care and decreased residual pain (Spofford & Hurley, 2018).

A combination of preoperative drugs may be ordered to achieve the desired outcomes with minimal side effects. Such outcomes include sedation, reducing anxiety, inducing amnesia to minimise unpleasant surgical memories, increasing comfort during preoperative procedures, reducing gastric acidity and volume, increasing gastric emptying, decreasing nausea and vomiting, and reducing the incidence of aspiration by drying oral and respiratory secretions.

Antibiotic prophylaxis is effective in the prevention of postoperative complications in many surgeries. This encompasses the principle of antimicrobial stewardship, defined as 'coordinated actions designed to promote and increase the appropriate use of antimicrobials' (Australian Commission on Safety and Quality in Health Care (ACSQHC), 2022), and is considered an important strategy for the conservation of the effectiveness of antibiotics.

Thromboprophylaxis should also be provided for many procedures. People should be assessed to identify their risk factors for developing postoperative venous thrombosis (VTE). VTE is a major cause of morbidity and mortality for people admitted to hospital, and a common preventable cause of in-hospital death. It is estimated to account for 7% of all deaths in Australian hospitals and to cost the Australian health system $1.72 billion annually (ACSQHC, 2018). People having surgery who develop postoperative venous thrombus may complain of pain, tenderness, swelling, increased heat, changes to skin colouration or enlarged veins. Adverse outcomes may lead to pulmonary embolism, sudden death or post-thrombotic syndrome (Assareh et al., 2016). In 2018, the National Institute of Care and Excellence updated its guidelines covering assessing and reducing the risk of VTE, or blood clots, and deep vein thrombosis (DVT) in people aged 16 and over in hospital. These guidelines aim to help healthcare professionals identify people most at risk and describe interventions that can be used to reduce the risk of VTE. VTE prophylaxis includes careful assessment of patient risk factors and commencement of preventive strategies in the preoperative period. These strategies include pharmacological management such as the administration of subcutaneous low-dose unfractionated heparin (LDUH), low molecular weight heparin (LMWH) and pentasaccharide fondaparinux. Other strategies include mechanical devices such as graduated compression stockings and intermittent pneumatic compression.

Links to National Patient Safety Standards

NSQHS: Preventing and Controlling Infections Standard

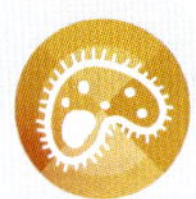

The National Safety and Quality Health Service Standards (ACSQHC, 2021) specify that health service organisations must implement systems for the safe and appropriate prescribing and use of antimicrobials as part of an antimicrobial stewardship program.

Source: ACSQHC (2021). *National Safety and Quality Health Service Standards: Second edition.* Sydney: ACSQHC.

TABLE 3.5 Preoperative medications

GENERIC	ACTION BY CATEGORY	NURSING IMPLICATIONS
Antibiotics	Prevent surgical site infections in orthopaedic and general surgeries and are associated with lower risk of mortality in elderly people	Correct timing is important for maximum effectiveness. Monitor people for reactions. Be aware of microbial resistance and responsible use of medicines.
Thromboprophylaxis: low molecular weight heparins (LMWHs)	Prevents formation of clots in the peripheral circulation which otherwise may result in deep venous thrombosis and possible emboli	Be aware of bruising and monitor bleeding.
Benzodiazepines (midazolam, diazepam, lorazepam)	Decrease anxiety and produce sedation to some extent. May induce amnesia	Monitor for respiratory depression, hypotension, drowsiness and lack of coordination.
Narcotic analgesics (morphine, fentanyl)	Decrease anxiety, provide analgesia	Monitor for respiratory depression and safety if ambulating. Anti-emetics may be needed.
Non-opioid analgesics	Provide mild to moderate analgesia. Single dose or 4-hourly administration over a short period. Sometimes referred to as NSAIDs, due to antipyretic and anti-inflammatory actions	Reassessment required if pain has not ceased. Assess for adverse effects. Cease 72 hours preoperatively and assess clotting times.
Antacids (sodium citrate)	Increase the pH and reduce volume of gastric fluid; used in people with gastro-oesophageal reflux disease and/or trauma	No significant factors in this setting.
H_2 receptor antagonists (cimetidine, famotidine, ranitidine)	Reduce gastric acid volume and concentration	Monitor for confusion and dizziness in older adults.
Gastric acid pump inhibitors (lansoprazole, pantoprazole, omeprazole)	Suppress gastric acid secretion	Monitor for dizziness and headache, rash or thirst.
Anti-emetics (metoclopramide, prochlorperazine, ondansetron)	Enhance gastric emptying. Often used with narcotic analgesics to alleviate side effects of nausea and vomiting	Monitor for sedation and extra-pyramidal reaction (involuntary movement, muscle tone changes and abnormal posture).
Anticholinergics (atropine sulfate, scopolamine)	Reduce oral and respiratory secretions to decrease risk of aspiration; decrease vomiting and laryngospasm	Monitor for confusion, restlessness and tachycardia. Prepare the person to expect a dry mouth.

Table 3.5 outlines some commonly prescribed preoperative medications.

Decisions made about which of the person's routine medications to administer prior to surgery when the person is required to be nil by mouth (NBM) are made in consultation with the surgeon and/or anaesthetist. Caution is required in relation to potential interactions between anaesthesia and medications and the effect on the person if drugs such as steroids, anti-seizure medications and tranquillisers are discontinued abruptly. It may not be necessary to cease all antihyperglycaemic agents prior to surgery and organisational policy should guide diabetic management of surgical patients (Kuzulugil et al., 2019). Under anaesthesia, the signs and symptoms of hypoglycaemia (insulin reaction) are absent, so withholding insulin the morning of surgery when the person is NBM is advisable. Plasma glucose is monitored intermittently during surgery with the goal of maintaining a normal blood sugar level (see Table 3.2). Studies have shown that high preoperative and perioperative glucose levels are associated with poor surgical outcomes and an increased risk of postoperative complications including respiratory, wound and urinary tract infections (Kuzulugil et al., 2019). It is common to manage hyperglycaemia with sliding-scale insulin. However, evidence-based practice now supports, where possible, diabetic patients being admitted on the day of surgery, with both the patient and the ward staff aware of the planned perioperative diabetes care, including a plan to manage hypo- and hyperglycaemia. Surgery should also be scheduled at the start of the theatre list to minimise disruption to the patient's glycaemic control. Variable-rate intravenous insulin infusions are preferred in most patients with diabetes requiring surgery as they maintain good glycaemic control and normal electrolyte concentrations, while optimising cardiovascular function and renal perfusion (Kuzulugil et al., 2019).

Assessment of medications that the person normally uses is vital prior to anaesthesia. In addition to medications prescribed by a doctor, assessment should include over-the-counter preparations (including aspirin and illegal drugs) and herbal medications (see Table 3.2).

INTRAOPERATIVE MEDICATIONS **Anaesthesia** is used to produce unconsciousness, analgesia, reflex loss and muscle relaxation during a surgical procedure. General anaesthesia produces these effects, whereas regional anaesthesia results in analgesia, reflex loss and muscle relaxation but does not cause the person to lose consciousness. An anaesthetist administers anaesthetics during the intraoperative phase of surgery.

General anaesthesia **General anaesthesia** can be administered by inhalation or intravenous routes. It produces central nervous system depression. As a result, the person loses consciousness and does not perceive pain, skeletal muscles relax and reflexes diminish.

Advantages of general anaesthesia include rapid excretion of the anaesthetic agent and prompt reversal of its effects when desired. Additionally, general anaesthesia can be used with all age groups and any type of surgical procedure. It produces amnesia.

Disadvantages of general anaesthesia include risks associated with circulatory, respiratory, hepatic and renal side effects. People with serious respiratory or circulatory diseases, such as emphysema or congestive heart failure, are at greater risk of complications. People with renal or hepatic disease cannot metabolise and eliminate anaesthetics safely.

General anaesthesia can be provided using total intravenous anaesthesia (TIVA) or targeted controlled infusions (TCI), also known as neuroleptanalgesia. People with a history of malignant hyperthermia (MH) must avoid inhalational agents because they can trigger this complication (see Box 3.1). With the increase in ambulatory and minimally invasive surgeries, anaesthetics that enable shorter recovery phases are used, allowing a *fast-tracking* approach with a rapid recovery phase.

General anaesthesia comprises three distinct phases: induction, maintenance and emergence. During the induction phase, the person receives the anaesthetic agent intravenously or by inhalation. During this phase, airway patency is achieved and maintained with either endotracheal intubation or laryngeal mask airway (LMA). Intubation can be difficult with some people; therefore, alternative devices such as LMA, Fastrach or oesophageal–tracheal Combitube are an option to avoid other more invasive airway alternatives such as creation of a surgical airway with a cricothyroidotomy or tracheostomy,

The next phase of general anaesthesia is maintenance. During this period, the person is positioned, the skin is prepared and surgery is performed. The anaesthetist maintains the required depth of anaesthesia while constantly monitoring physiological parameters such as heart rate, blood pressure, respiratory rate, temperature, and oxygen and carbon dioxide levels. The final phase of anaesthesia is the person's emergence from this altered physiological state. As the anaesthetic agents are withdrawn or the effects reversed pharmacologically, the person begins to awaken. The endotracheal tube or laryngeal mask is removed (extubated) once the person is able to re-establish voluntary breathing. It is critical to ensure airway patency during this period, because extubation may cause bronchospasm or laryngospasm.

BOX 3.1 Malignant hyperthermia

Malignant hyperthermia (MH) is a rare but serious reaction to volatile inhalational anaesthetic gases and succinylcholine, a depolarising neuromuscular blocker. The person who suffers this reaction manifests the following signs and symptoms: unexplained rise in end-tidal carbon dioxide that does not respond to ventilation, hyperthermia, tachypnoea, tachycardia and sustained skeletal muscle contraction. If unchecked the condition can progress to hyperkalaemia, myoglobinuria, disseminated intravascular coagulation, congestive heart failure, bowel ischaemia and compartment syndrome in the limbs. Dantrolene sodium is the drug that inhibits the muscular pathology and prevents death.

Because the condition is inherited, susceptibility testing is available but the testing is expensive and the most accurate test involves an invasive procedure. The 'gold standard' involves biopsy of thigh skeletal muscle tissue to determine sensitivity to caffeine and halothane (CHCT). Genetic testing is not as sensitive and reliable as CHCT but will be improved with the discovery of more causative mutations. People with muscle myopathies such as muscular dystrophy sometimes experience early signs of MH and respond well to dantrolene. The symptoms of MH may manifest with other pathologies, so it is important for people to know if they have a genetic susceptibility to MH, which could affect all members of their family.

MH can develop during an operation or up to 48 hours after the administration of inhalation anaesthesia and/or succinylcholine. If the early symptoms of MH (e.g. escalating temperature, increased carbon dioxide production) are suspected, immediately administer 100% oxygen with a non-rebreather mask, stay with the person, ensure good IV access and immediately call the anaesthetist, who will order dantrolene, which can be given as an IV bolus dose. Administration of dantrolene can be repeated until the signs and symptoms of MH diminish. Measures to decrease core body temperature should be started at once and continued until core temperature is 36.0°C. A urinary catheter should be placed to monitor urine output. Blood samples are taken and sent to pathology for testing. Blood gases should measure pH; and sodium bicarbonate is given to correct metabolic acidosis. Insulin may be ordered to decrease serum potassium. These people require critical care and are transferred to the intensive care unit for continued monitoring and doses of dantrolene every 4–6 hours.

Regional anaesthesia **Regional anaesthesia** is a type of local anaesthesia in which medication instilled around the nerves blocks transmission of nerve impulses in a particular area. Regional anaesthesia produces analgesia, relaxation and reduced reflexes. The person is awake and conscious during the surgical procedure but does not perceive pain. Regional anaesthesia may be classified in several ways:

- Local nerve infiltration is achieved by injecting a local anaesthetic agent such as bupivacaine around a local nerve to depress nerve sensation over a limited area of the body. This technique may be used when a skin or muscle biopsy is obtained or when a small wound is sutured.
- Nerve blocks are accomplished by injecting a local anaesthetic agent at the nerve trunk to produce a lack of sensation over a specific area, such as an extremity.
- Epidural blocks are local anaesthetic agents injected into the epidural space, outside the dura mater of the spinal cord. This type of intraspinal anaesthesia provides effective pain relief for surgeries for people of all ages, with less risk of adverse effects than general anaesthesia. It is indicated for surgeries of the arms and shoulders, thorax, abdomen, pelvis and lower extremities. The epidural catheter is often left in place for pain relief in the postoperative period.
- Spinal anaesthesia is administered similarly to epidural except the anaesthetic medication is infused in a single injection. Spinal anaesthesia is effective for approximately 90 minutes. Surgeries of the lower abdomen, perineum and lower extremities are likely to use this type of regional anaesthesia. Any leakage of cerebrospinal fluid (CSF) into the epidural space may cause reduced CSF pressure and postoperative headaches. Treatment for this headache may

include hydration, caffeine, analgesics or administration of an epidural blood patch. Hypotension is common with epidural and spinal anaesthesia. Monitor BP and, if critical hypotension occurs, alert the anaesthetist and expect to increase intravenous fluids and administer vasoactive medications.

CONSIDERATION FOR PRACTICE

The addition of adrenaline to local anaesthetic agents such as bupivacaine suppresses bleeding around the surgical site. Care must be taken to ensure that plain lignocaine is only ever used for end-digit surgery (i.e. fingers, toes, tip of nose) to ensure that tissues remain perfused. Care should also be taken using adrenaline in people with cardiovascular disease as it can cause arrhythmias.

Twilight sedation An increasing number of surgical and diagnostic procedures are being performed using **twilight sedation**. This type of anaesthesia provides analgesia, amnesia and moderate sedation. The pharmacological effects are produced by administering a combination of propofol with opioids (such as morphine sulfate and fentanyl) and/or sedatives (such as diazepam and midazolam). During twilight sedation, the person is able to independently maintain an open airway. This allows them to respond to verbal and physical stimulation. Supervision by the surgeon or anaesthetist is always required, and staff must be prepared to initiate rescue if sedation becomes too deep. This type of sedation is increasingly being used in ambulatory care for procedures such as colonoscopy and cataract surgery.

Assessment prior to twilight sedation includes evaluating the person's physical status. People with compromised circulation or airway, a history of sleep apnoea or snoring, a history of problems with anaesthesia or analgesia, or medications that would potentially interact with conscious analgesia medications require more careful assessment. People who will be managed with conscious sedation should be appropriately fasted with a patent IV line in situ, and baseline vital signs are assessed and recorded prior to administration of the sedative. Equipment to rescue the person should be available if sedation becomes too deep. Monitor oxygen saturation, blood pressure, pulse, breathing and level of consciousness throughout the procedure.

Common adverse side effects include venous thrombosis, phlebitis, local irritation, confusion, drowsiness, hypotension and apnoea. Reversal agents (naloxone hydrochloride) are used as needed to enhance the safety of conscious sedation.

POSTOPERATIVE MEDICATIONS Management of acute postoperative pain by medication improves with greater understanding of pain physiology and the development of better methods to deliver adequate pain medication. For more information on pain management, see the 'Nursing care' section later in this chapter on managing acute postoperative pain and also see the chapter 'Nursing care of people in pain'.

Established, persistent, severe pain is more difficult to treat than recently commenced pain. Therefore, postoperative analgesics should be administered pre-emptively and at regular intervals around the clock to maintain a therapeutic blood level. Administering analgesics on an 'as needed' (prn) basis lowers this therapeutic level and delays in medication administration further increase pain intensity. Therefore, regular rather than prn administration of analgesics is recommended in the first 36 to 48 hours postoperatively. People using patient-controlled analgesia (PCA) or patient-controlled epidural analgesia (PCEA) in the postoperative period need to be taught the importance of using the allowed dosages regularly to prevent increasing pain levels.

CONSIDERATION FOR PRACTICE

Nurses are responsible for assessing the pain level of people having surgery and administering pain medication. Work collaboratively with surgeons, anaesthetists and the pain team and people in the postoperative period to schedule pre-emptive and postoperative analgesics, rather than rely on prn administration orders.

Non-steroidal anti-inflammatory drugs (NSAIDs) can be used to treat mild to moderate postoperative pain. Although NSAIDs may not be sufficient to control pain completely, they allow lower doses of opioid analgesics and, therefore, fewer side effects. NSAIDs can usually be given safely to older people, but observe closely for side effects, particularly gastric and renal toxicity and bleeding. Be aware that NSAIDS are not comparable and their actions and side effects vary substantially; thus, they cannot be used interchangeably.

The Australian and New Zealand College of Anaesthetists and Faculty of Pain Medicine (Schug et al., 2020) has specific guidelines for managing acute postoperative pain. These guidelines include the administration of multimodal the concurrent use of different classes of analgesics. Drugs that may be used include opioids, NSAIDs and local anaesthetics, as well as adjuvant agents such as antidepressants and anticonvulsants.

Physical dependence and tolerance to opioid analgesics is uncommon in short-term postoperative use. Additionally, opioid analgesics, when used to treat acute pain, rarely lead to psychological dependence and addiction. Acute pain can be appropriately treated initially with opioids, and subsequently with simple analgesia as healing progresses. Management of chronic or persistent pain, in contrast, evolves from paracetamol to opioids as tolerance develops or the condition worsens. The opioid-naive person will tolerate and achieve analgesia with a lower dose of opioid than the person who is opioid tolerant and uses opioids for persistent pain.

In the immediate postoperative period, older people benefit from the same protocol for morphine titration as younger people. Intravenous morphine may be initiated at a slightly reduced dose and then titrated to the same protocol as younger people. Morphine-related adverse effects such as nausea, vomiting, respiratory depression, urinary retention, pruritus and allergy or sedation are similar among age groups. However, older adults may require fewer opioids than younger people in the later postoperative period. PCEA may be more effective for older adults and is associated with earlier improved mental status and bowel activity (Schug et al., 2020). Older people tend to be more sensitive to the analgesic effects of opioids, experiencing a higher peak effect with a longer duration of pain control.

Surgical environment

MEMBERS OF THE SURGICAL TEAM The intraoperative environment is complex and requires members of the surgical team to function as a coordinated unit. The surgeon, surgical assistant(s), anaesthetist, anaesthetic nurse, instrument nurse (scrub) (see Figure 3.1) and circulating nurse (scout) constitute the main surgical team. Each member provides specialised skills and is essential to the successful outcome of the surgery. Risks to members of the surgical team from blood-borne pathogens or injury are minimised when the surgical team is well organised and prepared.

The surgeon is the medical officer who performs the operative procedure. As head of the surgical team, the surgeon is responsible for all medical actions and judgments.

The surgical assistant works closely with the surgeon in performing the operation. The number of assistants varies according to the complexity of the procedure. The assistant may be another surgeon. The assistant performs such duties as exposing the operative site, retracting nearby tissue, sponging and/or suctioning the wound, ligating bleeding vessels and suturing or helping suture the surgical wound.

The anaesthetist evaluates the person preoperatively, administers the anaesthesia and other required medications, transfuses blood or other blood products, infuses intravenous fluids, continuously monitors the person's physiological status, alerts the surgeon to developing problems and treats them as they arise, and supervises the person's recovery in the PACU.

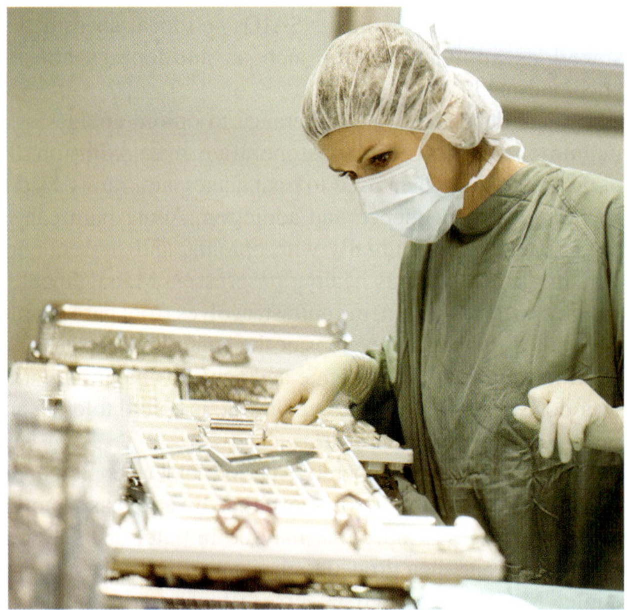

FIGURE 3.1 ***An instrument nurse in the operating room***

Source: © Westend61 GmbH/Alamy Stock Photo.

The **circulating nurse** is a highly experienced nurse who coordinates and manages a wide range of activities before, during and after the surgical procedure. For example, the circulating nurse oversees the physical aspects of the operating room itself, including the equipment. The circulating nurse also assists with transferring and positioning the person, prepares the person's skin, ensures that no break in aseptic technique occurs and records the surgical count of all accountable items, including sharps, sponges and instruments (ACORN, 2020). The handling of surgical instruments and associated accountable items must also comply with relevant state department of health policy directives. The circulating nurse assists all other team members. Thorough documentation in the surgical area is essential, and the circulating nurse is responsible for documenting intraoperative nursing activities, medications, placement of drains and catheters, and length of the procedure. The circulating nurse also formulates a care plan based on physiological and psychosocial assessments of the person. Finally, the circulating nurse is at all times an advocate for the safety and wellbeing of the person having surgery.

The role of the **instrument nurse** primarily involves manual dexterity and in-depth knowledge of the anatomical and mechanical aspects of a particular surgery. The instrument nurse handles sutures, instruments and other equipment immediately adjacent to the sterile field. The Registered Nurse ensures appropriate delegation and supervision of staff and participates in the surgical count (ACORN, 2020).

The role of nurses in surgery continues to evolve to improve the care of people having surgery. Although not participating in the surgical procedure, PACU (recovery) nurses are part of the surgical team and are responsible for assessing, monitoring and implementing care of people during the immediate recovery period from anaesthesia. Within the perioperative unit, specialty surgical teams are developing in response to the demands of increasingly complex technical surgeries. For example, a designated open-heart surgical team may be responsible for all open cardiac cases and not be routinely involved with other procedures. The use of specialty surgical teams allows nurses to become highly skilled in a particular range of procedures and communications impacting on the care of people having surgery.

SURGICAL ATTIRE Strict dress codes are necessary to provide infection control within the operating theatre, to reduce cross-contamination between the surgery department and other hospital units or departments, and to promote the health and safety of people having surgery. As per evidence-based research, guidelines for surgical attire differ from those of a general ward environment. Following the ACORN (2020) standards, all personnel in the surgical department must be in proper surgical attire. The design and composition of the surgical attire minimises bacterial shedding, thus reducing wound contamination. The area in the surgical department is divided into *unrestricted, semi-restricted* and *restricted zones*. The unrestricted zones permit access by those in hospital uniforms or street clothes. These areas may also allow limited access for communicating with operating room personnel and handover of people having surgery.

TRANSLATION TO PRACTICE Evidence-based practice: assisting older adults to communicate postoperative pain

Nurses rely heavily on people's assessments of the pain they are experiencing. Pain is a subjective experience—a symptom rather than a sign. Rating of pain intensity by the person who has had surgery is the gold standard for knowing when to provide an intervention to decrease pain, and it is considered more accurate than nurses' evaluations of behavioural manifestations of pain. Older people who believe that healthcare providers know how to manage their pain are at risk of inadequately treated pain.

Pain assessment is a fundamental process in effective pain management (Schofield, 2018). However, older people sometimes fail to report pain because they think it is a normal part of ageing or they have fears about intervention or the unwanted effects of analgesics, especially opioids. Sensory impairment and social isolation may further impair the effective treatment of pain. Compared with the younger adult with the same clinical condition, the older adult may report less pain or atypical pain, report it later or report no pain at all (Schug et al., 2020). Patient self-report is the most reliable and accurate tool to assess older patients' pain even for patients with impaired cognition. Identifying appropriate words that elicit meaningful responses and consistently using this language, supported by communication tools, are an important part of the comprehensive assessment of an older patient's pain. Pain measurement tools that have been shown to be appropriate for use in the older patient include the Verbal Numerical Rating Scale (VNRS), Faces Pain Scale—Revised (FPS-R) and Verbal Descriptor Scale (VDS). Trialling of different self-assessment scales may be warranted, including in those with severe impairment, and the patients may need more time to understand and respond to questions regarding pain (Schofield, 2018; Schug et al., 2020).

IMPLICATIONS FOR NURSING

Establishing trust between the nurse and the person receiving care is critical to relieving pain. Coaching older people to describe their pain location, intensity and sensation gives them permission to communicate in a manner with which they may feel uncomfortable at first. Coaching is necessary to dispel myths about professional expertise and to allow personal control and independence so that they are willing to ask for pain medications. Exploring with older people their perception of pain, as well as the significance it has for recovery from illness, are necessary elements in providing adequate pain relief and restoring health.

CRITICAL THINKING IN PERSON-CENTRED CARE

1 What physiological changes make pain management more difficult for an 80-year-old person following surgery than for a 30-year-old person?
2 An older person says: 'I deserved this pain, so I don't want to take anything to make it better.' What would be your response and why?
3 An Indigenous Australian man, aged 67, replies that 'Something just doesn't feel right' when asked to rate his pain on a scale of 0 to 10. His pulse is increased and he is protective of his abdominal incision. What could you ask or do to accurately assess his pain?
4 If your grandfather or grandmother were having surgery tomorrow, what would you like them to be taught about pain management?
5 An independent, 85-year-old woman has a PCA pump for analgesia following major surgery. She continuously presses the pump button, but continues to complain of severe pain. What do you do now?
6 A female, non-English-speaking Somalian refugee appears to be in pain following labiaplasty. What are the cultural issues associated with labiaplasty for these women? Would it be appropriate to ask her husband to act as a translator? How can you arrange an interpreter to assist this woman to communicate with you, so you can provide adequate pain relief for her?

CONSIDERATION FOR PRACTICE

Objects on the sterile drape are considered sterile. Remain a minimum of 30 cm away from draped tables and sterile fields to avoid contamination if you are not attired in sterile gown and gloves.

The semi-restricted zones require scrub attire, including a scrub suit and a cap or hood (see Figure 3.2). Hallways, work areas and storage areas are considered semi-restricted. Scrub attire is covered with sterile gowns in the restricted areas only if the person is 'scrubbed in' for the surgery. Only fabrics that are woven or disposable and will not harbour bacteria are allowed and all items of apparel must be covered by appropriate fabric. Nails that are chipped, varnished or artificial are not worn in surgery or in any clinical settings. These nails are associated with glove tears and even after careful handwashing can harbour potential pathogens.

CONSIDERATION FOR PRACTICE

Staff in operating theatres must be knowledgeable about the nature of hazards within the perioperative environment. Hazards include a class A electrical area due to the quantity and type of equipment (including electrosurgical equipment) used in this environment; anaesthetic gases and other chemicals such as formaldehyde and fumes from bone cement and chemical sterilising agents, and surgical plume (smoke from electrosurgical and laser equipment); latex; sharps, including needle-stick injuries; laser and x-ray exposure; assembly and transport of theatre equipment; and biological hazards, including potential for exposure to blood and body fluids and possible seroconversion for blood-borne viruses, including Creutzfeldt-Jakob disease (CJD).

Restricted zones are within operating rooms. Personnel wear masks, sterile gowns and gloves in addition to appropriate scrub attire if they are participating at the operating table. The outer sterile covering is changed between procedures or when it becomes soiled or wet.

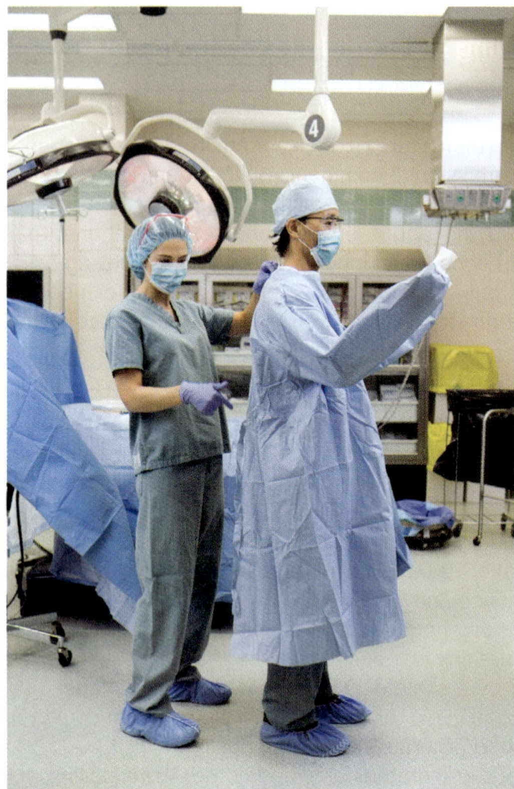

FIGURE 3.2 ***Surgical attire. Scrub attire includes scrub suit, shoe covers, and cap or hood to cover hair. Sterile attire includes scrub suit, shoe covers, and cap or hood, plus gown, gloves and mask***

Source: © Tyler Olson/Fotolia.com.

PATIENT SAFETY COMPETENCY FRAMEWORK

8 Infection prevention and control

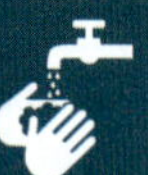

The Patent Safety Competency Framework emphasises the importance of infection prevention and control by reducing the risk of patients acquiring healthcare-associated infections and effectively managing infections if they occur. Specifically, nursing students (and Registered Nurses) must:

- demonstrate aseptic and non-touch techniques
- use and remove personal protective equipment in a way that minimises cross-contamination
- demonstrate correct use and disposal of sharps and waste
- clean or discard used equipment appropriately
- manage blood and body fluid spills appropriately (Levett-Jones et al., 2017).

THE SURGICAL SCRUB The surgical scrub is performed to render hands and arms as clean as possible in preparation for a procedure. All personnel who participate directly in the procedure must perform a surgical scrub with an approved antimicrobial solution. Skin cannot be rendered sterile, but it can be considered 'surgically clean' following the scrub. The purposes of the surgical scrub are to:

- remove dirt, skin oils and transient microorganisms from hands and forearms
- increase safety for people having surgery by reducing microorganisms on surgical personnel
- leave an antimicrobial residue on the skin to inhibit growth of microbes for several hours.

Following the 3- to 5-minute surgical scrub (ACORN, 2020), hands and arms are dried with sterile towels.

Preparation of the person having surgery

Although much preparation has taken place prior to the transfer of the person to the surgical department, additional activities such as clipping of hair or shaving and positioning may be performed. The skin preparation, which usually includes cleansing the area with a prescribed antimicrobial agent, may have been performed either by the person or by nursing personnel before the transfer to the surgical department. Additional skin cleansing is performed in the surgical department to further decrease microorganisms on the skin and thereby reduce the possibility of wound infection.

Hair at the surgical site should be left in place whenever possible as studies have found that preoperative shaving of the surgical site increases the risk of surgical site infection. However, if the surgeon requires hair to be removed, this should be performed on the day of surgery, as close to surgery time as possible and in a location outside the operating theatre or procedure room. Only hair interfering with the surgical procedure should be removed, and hair should be clipped using a single-use electric or battery-operated clipper, or a clipper with a reusable head that can be disinfected between patients. Razors should never be used as trauma to the shaved area can weaken the normal barrier that provides a defence against organisms, thus increasing the chance of surgical site infections (SSIs). Clippers or a depilatory agent should be used outside the operating room prior to entry (Sutherland-Fraser et al., 2022). The extent of hair removal for surgery varies. Generally, the area of hair removal is wider than the planned incision because of the possibility of unexpected extension of the incision (see Figure 3.3). An altered body image also may result from the psychological trauma of a surgical shave, particularly if the shave involves the head or groin area.

Preparing the person for surgery also includes **positioning** them on the operating table. Figure 3.4 shows frequently used positions and describes corresponding surgical procedures and possible adverse effects. Positioning exposes the operative site in conjunction with access for anaesthesia administration. Careful and correct positioning is imperative to prevent injury to the person. Pressure, rubbing and/or shearing forces can cause injury to the tissue over bony prominences. If positioning

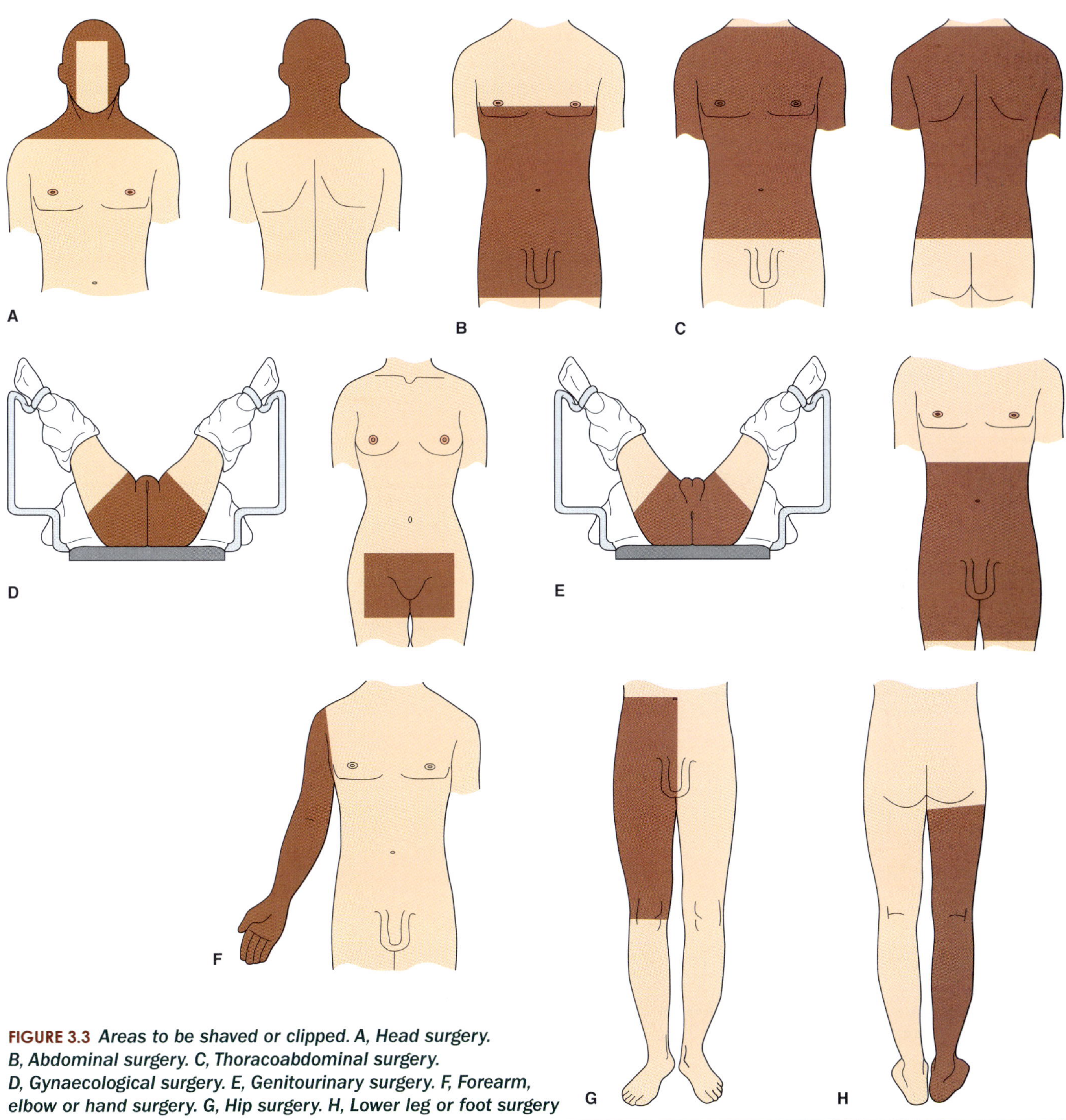

FIGURE 3.3 *Areas to be shaved or clipped. A, Head surgery. B, Abdominal surgery. C, Thoracoabdominal surgery. D, Gynaecological surgery. E, Genitourinary surgery. F, Forearm, elbow or hand surgery. G, Hip surgery. H, Lower leg or foot surgery*

causes normal joint range of motion to be exceeded, injury to muscles and joints can occur. Improper positioning also can lead to sensory and motor dysfunction, resulting in nerve damage. Pressure on peripheral blood vessels can decrease venous return to the heart and negatively affect the person's blood pressure. Additionally, oxygenation of the blood can be decreased if the person is not properly positioned to promote lung expansion.

As the anaesthetised person cannot respond to discomfort, it is the surgical team's responsibility to position them not only for the best surgical advantage but also for their safety and comfort. The circulating nurse refers to hospital policy, the surgeon's preference and the person's health history to ensure optimal positioning, and continuously assesses them during the intraoperative period as outlined in the ACORN (2020) standards.

AWARENESS UNDER ANAESTHESIA Prior to induction of anaesthesia, the anaesthetic nurse establishes rapport with the person to assess their psychological status. After anaesthetic medications have been given, the person may appear oblivious to the surroundings; however, recall of intraoperative events

POSITION AND USE	POSSIBLE ADVERSE EFFECTS AND NURSING INTERVENTIONS
(a) The *dorsal recumbent (*or *supine) position* is used for many abdominal surgeries (e.g. colostomy and herniorrhaphy), as well as for some thoracic surgeries (e.g. open-heart surgery) and some surgeries on the extremities. 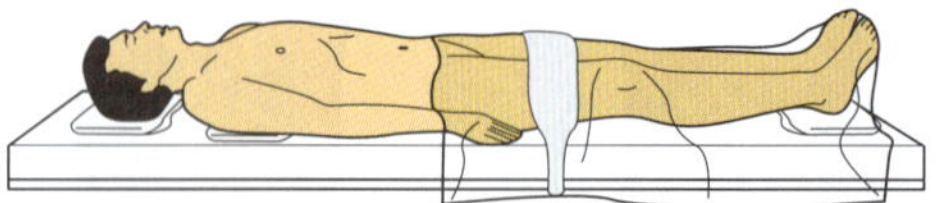 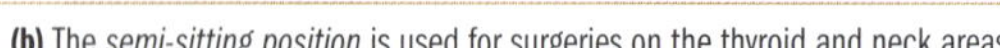	This position may cause excessive pressure on posterior bony prominences, such as the back of the head, scapulae, sacrum and heels. Pad these areas with soft materials. To avoid compression of blood vessels and sluggish circulation, ensure that the knees are not flexed. Use trochanter rolls or other padding to avoid internal or external rotation of the hips and shoulders.
(b) The *semi-sitting position* is used for surgeries on the thyroid and neck areas. 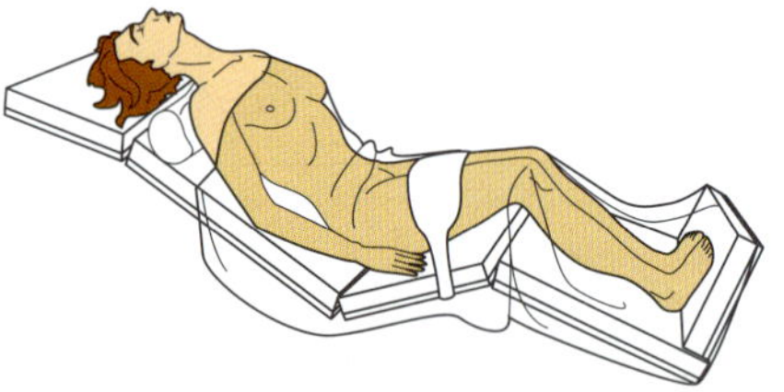	This position can lead to postural hypotension and venous pooling in the legs. It may promote skin breakdown on the buttocks. Sciatic nerve injury is possible. Assess for hypotension. Ensure that knees are not sharply flexed. Use soft padding to prevent nerve compression.
(c) The *prone position* is used for spinal fusions and removal of haemorrhoids. 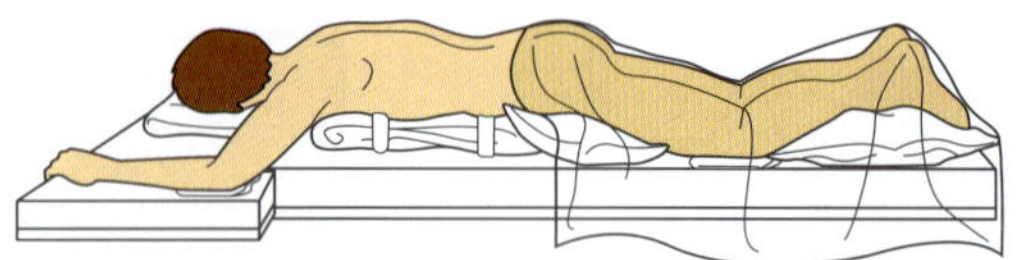	This position causes pressure on the face, knees, thighs, anterior ankles and toes. Pad bony prominences and support the feet under the ankles. To promote optimum respiratory function, raise the person's chest and abdomen, and support with padding. Corneal abrasion could occur if the eyes are not closed or are insufficiently padded.
(d) The *lateral chest position* is used for some thoracic surgeries, as well as hip replacements. 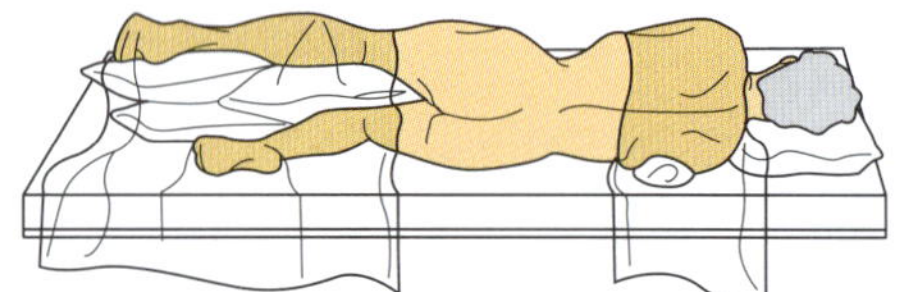	This position may cause excessive pressure on the bony prominences on the side on which the person is positioned. Ensure adequate padding and support, especially of the downside arm. The weight of the upper leg may cause peroneal nerve injury on the downside leg. Both legs must therefore be padded.
(e) The *lithotomy position* is used for gynaecological, perineal or rectal surgeries. 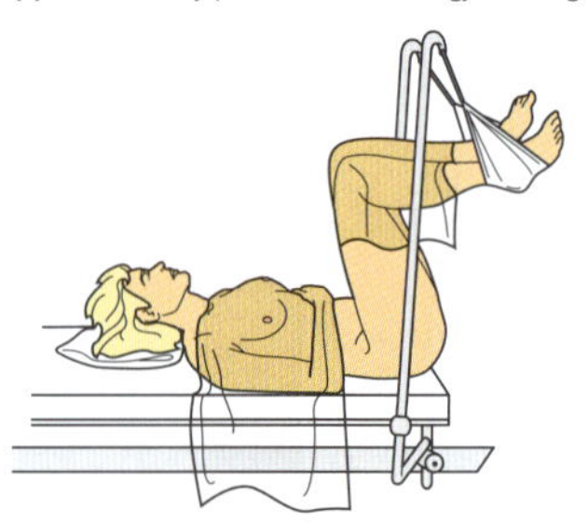	This position causes an 18% decrease (from a standing position) in vital capacity of the lungs. Monitor respirations and assess for hypoxia and dyspnoea. The lithotomy position can lead to joint damage, peroneal nerve damage and damage to peripheral blood vessels. To avoid injury, ensure adequate padding, and manipulate both legs into the stirrups simultaneously.
(f) The *jack-knife position* is used for proctological surgeries, such as removal of haemorrhoids, and for some spinal surgeries. 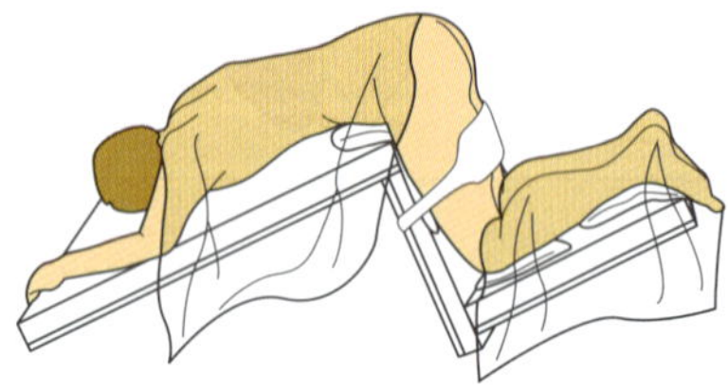	This position causes a 12% decrease (from a standing position) in vital capacity of the lungs. Monitor respirations and assess for hypoxia and dyspnoea. In this position, the greatest pressure is felt at the bends in the table. Therefore, the person is supported with pads at the groin and knees, as well as at the ankles. Padding of the chest and knees helps prevent skin breakdown. Padding and proper positioning help prevent pressure on the ear, the neck, and the nerves of the upper arm.

FIGURE 3.4 ***Common surgical positions***

has been reported. Although most people do not consciously remember what happened or what was said, psychological trauma can result. Because loss of consciousness is gradual, conversations during surgery should be professional.

SPECIAL CONSIDERATIONS FOR THE OLDER ADULT

Care of the older adult may be complicated in the postoperative period as they often have comorbidities (Sutherland-Fraser et al., 2022). Because of cardiovascular and tissue changes that result from ageing, the older adult is more prone to hypotension, hypothermia and hypoxaemia resulting from anaesthesia and the cool temperature in the operating room.

Positioning may also cause complications in the older adult. Intraoperative positioning of arthritic joints can cause postoperative joint pain unrelated to the operative site. Extended duration of surgery may increase the chance of pressure areas. The older person is at increased risk of developing pressure areas because of decreased subcutaneous fat tissue and reduced peripheral circulation.

Finally, the older adult often has some degree of hearing and/or vision impairment. These impairments combined with a strange environment can make the operating room a frightening, disorienting place. By effectively communicating with the person, the nurse can provide support and reassurance to minimise these factors. To decrease confusion and assist in communication, hearing aids and glasses should be used when appropriate and possible.

Nutrition

Wound healing after surgery depends on adequate nutritional intake. During the immediate postoperative phase, dietary intake is often withheld until evidence of peristalsis is determined and the person can tolerate liquids without nausea and vomiting. While intravenous fluids maintain hydration and electrolyte balance, they do not provide nutrition. Some people believe that intravenous fluids are the same as intravenous 'feeding', but this is a myth. Unless balanced nutrition through gastrointestinal intake can be re-established within 3–4 days, parenteral hyperalimentation is critical for homeostasis and wound healing.

- Protein, kilojoules and vitamins are needed for wound healing and recovery from surgery.
- Low-fat, high-fibre diets are important for chronic cardiovascular fitness but are contraindicated in the wound healing phase following surgery.
- Failure to use the gastrointestinal tract for more than 4–5 days allows the intestinal mucosa to atrophy, putting the person at risk of gastrointestinal tract haemorrhage and infection.

Fluid administered through peripheral veins must be isotonic, or only moderately hypertonic, to prevent sclerosing the small peripheral veins. Solutions of 10% dextrose are tolerable peripherally for a short time but do not provide adequate kilojoules for healing and maintenance. To provide adequate nutrition for people who have extended recovery periods without eating after surgery, central vein access must be established and parenteral nutrition administered. Education and counselling to support adequate nutritional intake should be ongoing throughout the preoperative and postoperative period.

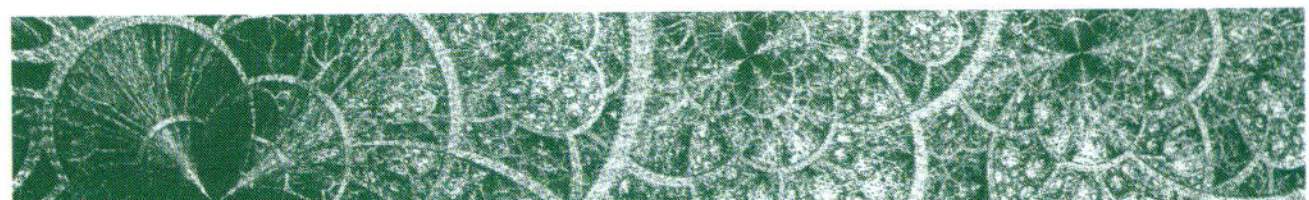

Nursing care

The following section will discuss nursing care in each of the three phases of surgery. A case study at the end of the section follows one person through the postoperative experience, bringing this information together. Perioperative nursing diagnoses are provided in Table 3.6 to assist in identifying the needs of the person having surgery. This is not an exhaustive list, but it can serve as a guide in identifying possible nursing diagnoses.

Preoperative nursing care

Each person's response to planned surgery varies greatly. When planning and implementing nursing care, consider individual psychological and physical differences, the type of surgery and the circumstances surrounding the need for surgery. A comprehensive nursing assessment is needed to determine the most appropriate care for each person undergoing surgery.

Before planning and implementing care for the person having surgery, gather assessment information by taking a nursing history and performing a physical examination. Use this

TABLE 3.6 Examples of perioperative nursing diagnoses

PREOPERATIVE	INTRAOPERATIVE	POSTOPERATIVE
• Deficient knowledge	• Deficient knowledge	• Deficient knowledge
• Anxiety	• Anxiety	• Pain
• Fear	• Fear	• Ineffective breathing pattern
• Decisional conflict	• Ineffective airway clearance	• Ineffective airway clearance
• Ineffective coping	• Risk of aspiration	• Impaired skin integrity
• Ineffective sexuality patterns	• Decreased cardiac output	• Imbalanced nutrition
• Disturbed sleep pattern	• Hypothermia	• Ineffective sexuality patterns
• Disturbed thought processes	• Risk of infection	• Disturbed sleep pattern
• Interrupted family processes	• Disturbed thought processes	• Fatigue
• Spiritual distress	• Impaired gas exchange	• Urinary retention
	• Impaired urinary elimination	• Impaired urinary elimination
	• Deficient fluid volume	• Impaired adjustment
	• Excess fluid volume	• Disturbed body image
	• Impaired communication: verbal	• Impaired mobility: physical
		• Risk of activity intolerance
		• Risk of injury
		• Ineffective health maintenance
		• Deficient diversional activity
		• Social isolation
		• Spiritual distress

information to establish baseline data, identify physical needs, determine teaching needs and psychological support for the person and their family, and prioritise nursing care. The type of surgical procedure directs the assessment and intervention planned by the nurse.

Surgery is a significant and stressful event. Regardless of the nature of the surgery (whether major or minor), the person and their family will be anxious. Some people seek care from a spiritual provider during this time. The degree of anxiety they will feel is not necessarily proportional to the magnitude of the surgical procedure. For example, a person scheduled to have a biopsy to rule out cancer, which is considered minor surgery, may be more anxious than a person undergoing gallbladder removal, which is considered major surgery.

The nurse's ability to listen actively to both verbal and non-verbal messages is imperative to establishing a trusting relationship with the person and their family. Therapeutic communication can help the person identify fears and concerns. The nurse can then plan nursing interventions and supportive care to reduce their anxiety level and assist them to cope successfully with the stressors encountered during the perioperative period.

Preoperative teaching

Teaching people is an essential nursing responsibility in the preoperative period. Education and emotional support have a positive effect on people's physical and psychological wellbeing, both before and after surgery. Previous research has determined that people who received preoperative education experienced less pain and anxiety, fewer complications, earlier discharge and increased satisfaction with their care, and returned to normal activities sooner. Positive outcomes may be attributed in part to the sense of control the person gains through the education they and their family receive.

Teaching should begin as soon as the person learns of the upcoming surgery. Teaching may begin in the surgeon's office or at the time of preadmission testing and assessment. Although education continues during postoperative care, most teaching is done before surgery because pain and the effects of anaesthesia can greatly diminish the person's ability to learn.

The amount of information desired varies for each individual. Therefore, the nurse should assess the person's need for and readiness to accept information. The teaching will be directed in part by the particular surgical procedure that is being performed and by the type of anaesthesia. The information in Box 3.2 is relevant to most people undergoing major surgery.

In addition to teaching the person and their family about measures that will decrease the risk of complications, provide other preoperative information to prepare them for surgery. This information should include the following:

- diagnostic tests—reasons and preparations
- arrival time for surgery
- preparations for surgery including: bowel preparation, skin preparation, indwelling catheter or bladder elimination, start of intravenous infusion, preoperative medication, handling of personal effects (rings, watch, money)
- sedative/hypnotic medication to be taken the night before surgery to promote rest and sleep
- education about whether to take medications on the morning of the surgery
- informed consent
- expected timetable for surgery and the recovery room
- method to inform family of progress throughout surgery
- transfer to the surgery department
- location of the surgical waiting room
- transfer to recovery room
- anticipated postoperative routine and devices or equipment (drains, tubes, equipment for IV infusions, oxygen or humidifying mask, dressings, splints, casts)
- plans for postoperative pain control
- if/when to commence fasting.

Be aware that dehydration, hypovolaemia and hypoglycaemia are recognised side effects of fasting. Thirst, worry and hunger are also reported by people having surgery and may be related to fasting. Fasting does not ensure that the stomach will be empty or that the gastric contents will be less acidic.

CONSIDERATION FOR PRACTICE

People about to undergo surgery may experience unnecessarily long preoperative fasts due to changes in surgery schedules and delays. How will this influence your management of people who are elderly, have diabetes mellitus or who may miss important medications as a result of these delays?

Preoperative preparation of people having surgery

A preoperative surgical checklist serves as a guide for preparing the person for surgery in most institutions. Complete the checklist before the person is transported to surgery. Nursing responsibilities on the day of surgery are as follows:

- Assist with bathing, grooming and changing into the operating room gown.
- Ensure that the person takes nothing by mouth. Provide additional teaching and reinforce prior teaching.
- Remove nail polish, lipstick and make-up to facilitate circulatory assessment during and after surgery.
- Ensure that identification and allergy bands are correct, legible and secure.
- Remove hair pins and jewellery; a wedding ring may be worn if it is taped to the finger.
- Complete skin or bowel preparation as ordered.
- Insert an indwelling catheter, intravenous line or nasogastric tube if ordered.
- Remove prostheses, such as artificial eyes and contact lenses, and store them in a safe place. Note that the anaesthetist may request that dentures are worn to theatre and removed immediately prior to anaesthesia.
- Leave a hearing aid in place if the person cannot hear without it and notify the operating theatre nurse.
- Verify that the informed consent has been signed prior to administering preoperative medications.

BOX 3.2 Preoperative teaching for people having surgery

Diaphragmatic breathing exercise

Diaphragmatic (abdominal) breathing exercises are taught to the person who is at risk of developing pulmonary complications, such as atelectasis or pneumonia. Risk factors for pulmonary complications include general anaesthesia, abdominal or thoracic surgery, history of smoking, chronic lung disease, obesity and advanced age.

In diaphragmatic breathing, the person inspires deeply while allowing the abdomen to expand outwards. On expiration, the abdomen contracts inwards as air from the lungs is expelled.

1. Explain to the person that the diaphragm is a muscle that makes up the floor of the thoracic cavity and assists in breathing. The purpose of diaphragmatic breathing is to promote lung expansion and ventilation and enhance blood oxygenation.
2. Position the person in a high or semi-Fowler's position (see figure below right).
3. Ask the person to place their hands lightly on their abdomen.
4. Instruct the person to breathe in deeply through their nose, allowing their chest and abdomen to expand.
5. Instruct the person to hold their breath for a count of five.
6. Tell the person to exhale completely through pursed (puckered) lips, allowing their chest and abdomen to deflate.
7. Instruct the person to repeat the exercise 5 times consecutively.

Encourage them to perform diaphragmatic breathing exercises every 1–2 waking hours, pre and postoperatively.

Coughing exercise

Coughing exercises are also taught to the person who is at risk of developing pulmonary complications. The purpose of coughing is to loosen, mobilise and remove pulmonary secretions. Splinting the incision decreases the physical and psychological discomfort associated with coughing.

1. Assist the person in following steps 1 to 4 for diaphragmatic breathing.
2. Ask them to splint the incision with hands or pillow (see figure below).
3. Tell them to take 3 deep breaths and then cough forcefully.
4. Instruct the person to repeat the exercise 5 times consecutively every 2 hours while awake, taking short rest periods between coughs, if necessary.
5. Provide fluids as appropriate following exercise.

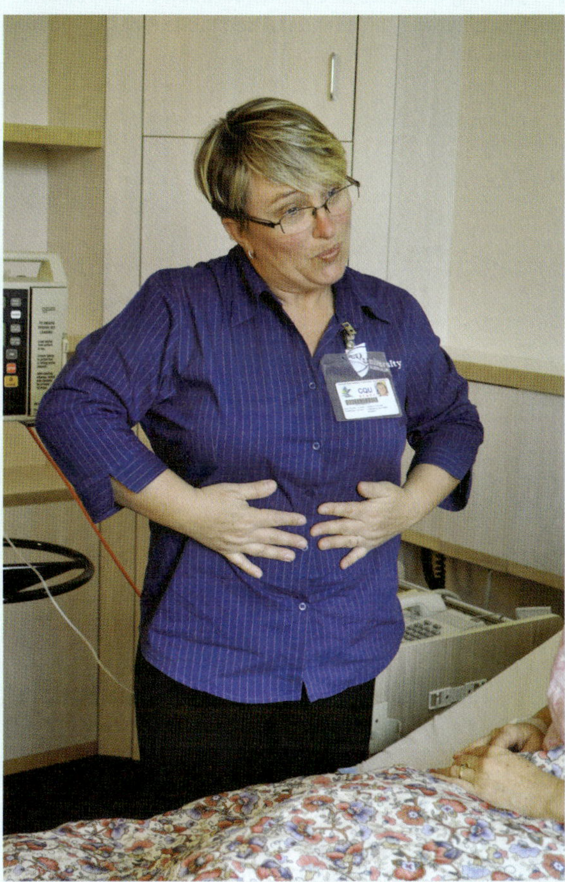

Diaphragmatic breathing exercise

Source: Courtesy of Tracy Levett-Jones.

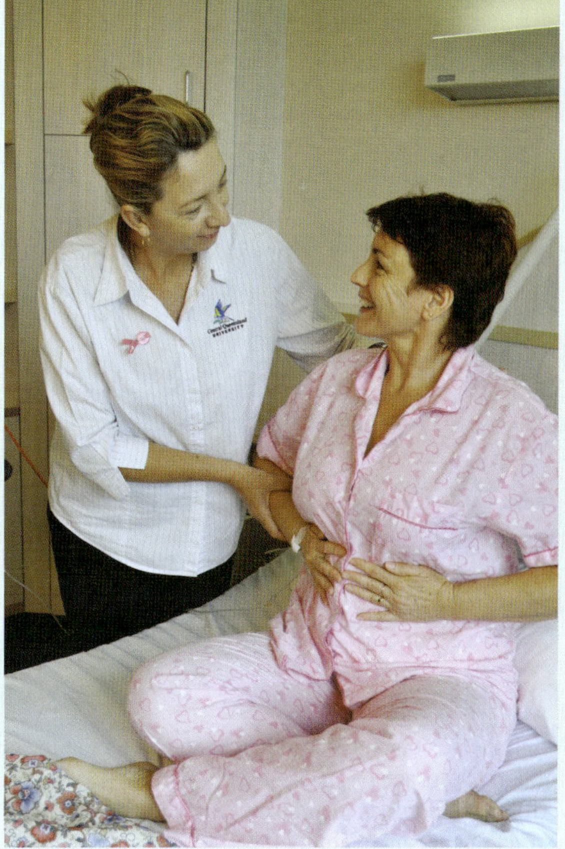

Splinting abdomen while coughing

Source: Courtesy of Tracy Levett-Jones.

(continued)

BOX 3.2 Preoperative teaching for people having surgery (continued)

Leg, ankle and foot exercises

Leg exercises are taught to people who are at risk of developing thrombophlebitis (inflammation of a vein, which is associated with the formation of blood clots). Risk factors for developing thrombophlebitis include decreased mobility preoperatively and/or postoperatively, a history of difficulties with peripheral circulation, and cardiovascular, pelvic or lower extremity surgeries.

The purpose of leg exercises is to promote venous blood return from the extremities. As the leg muscles contract and relax, blood is pumped back to the heart, promoting cardiac output and reducing venous stasis. These exercises also maintain muscle tone and range of motion, which facilitate early ambulation.

Teach the person to perform the following exercises while lying in bed:

1. Muscle pumping exercise: contract and relax calf and thigh muscles at least 10 times consecutively.
2. Leg exercises:
   a. Bend the knee and raise it towards the chest (see figure below).
   b. Straighten out leg and hold for a few seconds before lowering the leg back to the bed.
   c. Repeat exercise 5 times consecutively prior to alternating to the other foot.
3. Ankle and foot exercises:
   a. Rotate both ankles by making complete circles, first to the right and then to the left (see figure below right).
   b. Repeat 5 times and then relax.
   c. With feet together, point toes towards the head and then to the foot of the bed (see figure below right).
   d. Repeat this pumping action 10 times and then relax.

Encourage the person to perform leg, ankle and foot exercises every 1–2 hours while awake, depending on their needs and ambulatory status.

Turning in bed

The person who is at risk of circulatory, respiratory or gastrointestinal dysfunction following surgery is taught to turn in bed. Although this may be a simple task prior to surgery, after surgery (particularly after abdominal surgery) they may find it a difficult procedure. To make the procedure more comfortable, they may need to splint the incision by using the hand placed on a small pillow or blanket. Additionally, they should be taught that analgesics can be given to ease postoperative discomfort involved with turning. Encourage them to turn every 2 hours while awake.

1. Tell them to grasp the side rail towards the direction to be turned, to rest the opposite foot on the mattress and to bend the knee.
2. Instruct them to roll over in one smooth motion by pulling on the side rail while pushing off with the bent knee.
3. Pillows may need to be positioned behind their back to help them maintain a side-lying position. Older people may also need padding over pressure points between the knees and ankles to decrease the chance of decubitus ulcer formation from pressure.

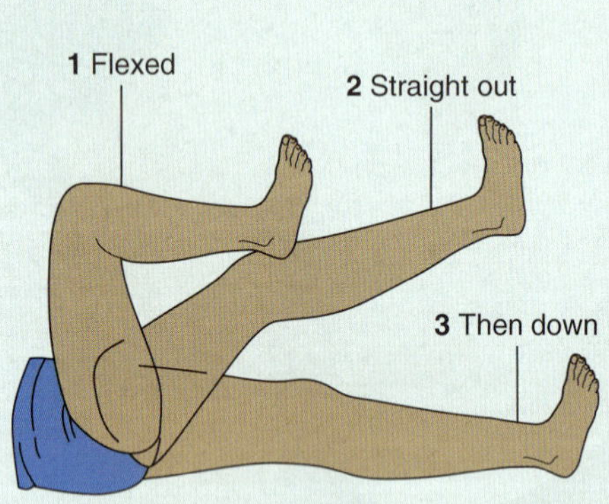

Leg exercises

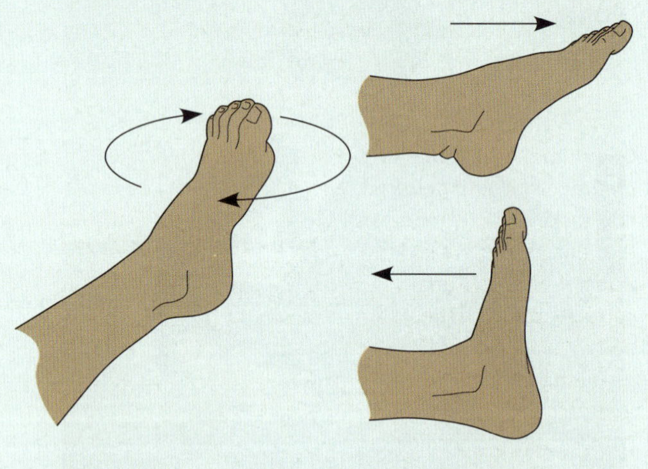

Ankle and foot exercises

- Weigh the person and record height and weight in the chart (for correct dosage of anaesthesia).
- Verify that all ordered diagnostic test reports are in the chart.
- Instruct the person to empty their bladder immediately before the preoperative medication is administered (unless an indwelling catheter is in place).
- Administer preoperative medication as scheduled (refer to 'Medications' earlier in the chapter and Table 3.5).
- Ensure the safety of the person once the medication has been given by placing them on bed rest with raised side rails and by placing the call switch within reach.
- Assess and record vital signs.

- Provide ongoing supportive care to the person and their family.
- Document all preoperative care in the appropriate location, such as the preoperative surgical checklist, the medication record and the narrative preoperative nursing notes.
- Verify with the surgical personnel the person's identity and verify that all their information is documented appropriately.
- Assist with transfer from the bed to the theatre trolley if required.
- Prepare the person's room for postoperative care, including making the surgical bed and ensuring that the anticipated supplies and equipment are in the room.

Intraoperative nursing care

The intraoperative phase of surgery begins when the person enters the operating room and ends when they are transferred to the post anaesthesia care unit (PACU). Nursing care in this phase focuses on keeping them and the environment safe and providing physiological monitoring and psychological support.

Hazards associated with surgery can be minimised for people by use of a surgical safety checklist. Preoperative checklists guide healthcare workers in the preparation of patients for surgery. Checklists have several advantages including aiding memory recall, particularly for mundane matters that can be routinely overlooked, and improved teamwork and communication (WHO, 2019). The WHO (2009) formed the World Alliance for Patient Safety, which developed a 'Safe Surgery Saves Lives' initiative. This program's Surgical Safety Checklist has been adopted in many countries, including Australia. It includes three phases—Sign in, Time out and Sign out—and requires all members of the surgical (and anaesthetic) team to contribute at critical junctures: before anaesthesia is administered, immediately before the incision and before the person is transported from the operating theatre.

Postoperative nursing care

Immediate postoperative care

Immediate postoperative care begins when the person has been transferred from the operating room to the PACU. The PACU nurse is part of the surgical team and monitors the person's vital signs and surgical site to determine the response to the surgical procedure and to detect significant changes. Assessing mental status and level of consciousness is another ongoing nursing responsibility, and the person may require repeated orientation to time, place and person. Emotional support also is essential, because the person is in a vulnerable and dependent position. Assessing and evaluating hydration status by monitoring intake and output is crucial to detecting cardiovascular or renal complications. In addition, the PACU nurse assesses the person's pain level. Careful administration of analgesics provides comfort without compounding the potential side effects from the anaesthesia.

Links to National Patient Safety Standards

NSQHS: Communicating for Safety Standard

One of the key criteria for this standard is 'correct identification and procedure matching' (ACSQHC, 2021). This refers to the importance of systems to maintain the identity of the patient and the use of documented processes to match patients and their intended care. Implementing this standard is achieved by the establishment of explicit systems and processes that ensure routine use of at least three approved patient identifiers when providing care, therapy or services, and during transfer of care. Patient/procedure matching protocols that provide guidance regarding the steps that should be taken to correctly match patients to their intended care include the WHO Surgical Safety Checklist and ensuring correct patient, correct site, correct procedure protocols (ACSQHC, 2016, p. 40).

Caring for individuals having surgery will often require multiple occasions when routine checking of patient identification and procedure matching must be undertaken, and often involves several team members checking these details together. Some examples include during the process of documenting informed consent for the surgical procedure, during use of the preoperative surgical checklist in the ward before the person is transported to the operating theatre, during the transfer of care between ward staff and operating theatre staff, at the time when the person is checked into the anaesthetic room, during the use of the Surgical Safety Checklist in the operating theatre (in particular to check the correct operative site), during transfer to the PACU, and during transfer to the ward after surgery. In addition, this standard will apply to occasions of medication administration, infusion of intravenous fluids and blood products, and diagnostic testing. When these checks are conducted it is important that they are correctly documented. The documentation of these checking processes protects clinicians from making errors such as undertaking an incorrect procedure or at an incorrect surgical site, and reduces the risk of adverse events for people having surgery.

Sources: ACSQHC (2016). *Patient identification*. Sydney: ACSQHC; ACSQHC (2021). *National Safety and Quality Health Service Standards* (2nd ed.). Sydney: ACSQHC.

Care when the person is stable

When awake and after being stabilised, the person is transferred to their hospital room. The PACU nurse communicates information about the person's condition and postoperative orders to the ward/unit nurse prior to their arrival. This prepares the ward/unit nurse for additional problems or needed equipment (see Box 3.3).

Immediate and continuing assessment is essential to detect and/or prevent complications. In documenting assessment findings, the nurse completes a flow record of the individual person's situation. Baseline data are obtained, documented and compared with preoperative data. A postoperative head-to-toe assessment includes, but may not be limited to, the following:

- general appearance
- vital signs
- level of consciousness
- emotional status
- skin colour and temperature
- discomfort/pain
- nausea/vomiting
- type of intravenous fluids and flow rate
- dressing site
- drainage on the dressing and/or bed linen
- urinary output (catheter or ability to urinate)
- ability to move all extremities.

The hospital policy or surgeon's orders dictate the frequency of follow-up assessments. After major surgery, the nurse generally assesses the person every 15 minutes during the first hour and, if they are stable, every 30 minutes for the next 2 hours, and then every hour during the subsequent 4 hours. Assessments are then carried out every 4 hours, subject to change according to the person's condition and the protocol for the particular surgical procedure. It is critical to inform the surgeon immediately if the assessment reveals any signs of impending shock or other life-threatening changes.

After carrying out the initial assessment and ensuring the person's safety by raising the side rails and placing the call switch within reach, the nurse reviews the surgeon's post-operative orders. These orders guide the nurse in the care of the postoperative person. For example, the orders specify activity level, diet, medications for pain and nausea, antibiotics, continuation of preoperative medications, frequency of vital sign assessments, administration of intravenous fluids and laboratory tests such as haemoglobin and potassium level. In most institutions, orders written prior to surgery must be reordered following surgery because the person's condition is presumed to have changed.

Nursing care of common postoperative complications

Several factors place the person at risk of postoperative complications and adverse events. Nursing care before, during and after surgery is aimed at preventing and/or minimising the effects of these complications.

Preoperative care and teaching to decrease postoperative complications have been discussed previously. The following section addresses postoperative cardiovascular, respiratory and wound complications, and problems associated with elimination.

Cardiovascular complications

Common postoperative cardiovascular complications include shock, haemorrhage, deep venous thrombosis and pulmonary embolism.

BOX 3.3 Patient handover from the PACU nurse to the ward nurse

The quality of the patient handover from the PACU nurse to the ward nurse is a critical factor in patient safety. Structured clinical handover has been shown to reduce communication errors within and between health service organisations and to improve patient safety and care because critical information is more likely to be accurately transferred and acted on. This is especially important at transitions of care, when communication errors are more likely and there is an increased risk of information being miscommunicated or lost. (ACSQHC, 2017).

Links to National Patient Safety Standards

NSQHS: Communicating for Safety Standard

This standard refers to the importance of structured clinical handover to effectively communicate about the healthcare of patients. It specifies that attention to high-quality clinical handover enhances patient safety, as critical information is more likely to be transferred and acted upon.

Source: ACSQHC (2021). *National Safety and Quality Health Service Standards* (2nd ed.). Sydney: ACSQHC. © Australian Commission on Safety and Quality in Health Care.

SHOCK Shock is a life-threatening postoperative complication. It results from an insufficient blood flow to vital organs, an inability to use oxygen and nutrients, or the inability to rid tissues of waste material. Hypovolaemic shock, the most common type in the postoperative period, results from a decrease in circulating fluid volume. Decreased fluid volume develops with blood or plasma loss or, less commonly, from severe prolonged vomiting or diarrhoea. Symptoms vary according to the severity of the shock; the greater the loss of fluid volume, the more severe the symptoms. The chapter 'Nursing care of people experiencing trauma and shock' provides a detailed discussion of nursing care of people with various types of shock.

HAEMORRHAGE Haemorrhage is an excessive loss of blood. A concealed haemorrhage occurs internally from a blood vessel that is no longer sutured or cauterised, or from a drainage tube that has eroded a blood vessel. An obvious haemorrhage occurs externally from a dislodged or ill-formed clot at the wound. Haemorrhage also may result from abnormalities in the blood's ability to clot; these abnormalities may result from a pathological condition, or they may be a side effect of medications.

Haemorrhage from a venous source oozes out quickly and is dark red, whereas an arterial haemorrhage is characterised by bright red spurts of blood pulsating with each heartbeat. Whether the haemorrhage is from a venous or an arterial source, hypovolaemic shock will occur if sufficient blood is lost from the circulation.

Common assessment findings with haemorrhage depend on the amount and rate of blood loss. Restlessness and anxiety are observed in the early stage of haemorrhage. Obvious bleeding will be present if the haemorrhage is external. The person will have symptoms characteristic of shock, such as hypotension and tachycardia (weak, thready pulse).

Care of the person who is haemorrhaging centres on stopping the bleeding and replenishing the circulating blood volume. Nursing care includes providing care for shock and one or more of the following:

- applying one or more sterile gauze pads and a firm pressure dressing to the area
- applying pressure with gloved hands (may be necessary for severe external bleeding)
- preparing the person and their family for emergency surgery (in severe situations when bleeding cannot be stopped).

DEEP VENOUS THROMBOSIS Deep venous thrombosis (DVT) is the formation of a thrombus (blood clot) in association with inflammation in deep veins. This complication most often occurs in the lower extremities of the person postoperatively. It may result from the combination of several factors, including trauma during surgery, pressure applied under the knees, sluggish blood flow during and after surgery and reduced mobility. People with a high risk of developing DVT include those who are over age 40 and who:

- have undergone orthopaedic surgery to lower extremities; urological, gynaecological or obstetric surgeries; or neurosurgery
- have a history of varicose veins
- have a history of thrombophlebitis or pulmonary emboli
- are obese
- have an infection
- have a malignancy.

Common assessment findings reveal pain or cramping in the involved calf or thigh. Redness, tenderness, warmth, discolouration of the skin and oedema (Henry & Satiani, 2014) of the entire extremity may occur along with a slightly elevated temperature. The person may have a positive Homans' sign (pain in the calf on dorsiflexion of the affected foot). Suspected DVT can be confirmed by duplex Doppler scans; however, it is important to remember that many venous thrombi are asymptomatic.

Nursing care of the person with DVT focuses on preventing a portion of the clot from dislodging and becoming an embolus (travelling blood clot) circulating to the heart, brain or lungs; preventing other clots from forming; and supporting the person's own physiological mechanism for dissolving clots. Nursing care includes the following measures:

- Administer anticoagulants and analgesics as prescribed. (NSAIDs are not usually given in combination with anticoagulants, because doing so increases the anticoagulant effects.)
- Monitor pathology results for clotting times.
- Apply thigh-high graduated compression stockings or devices to stimulate venous return.
- Ensure that the affected area is not rubbed or massaged.
- Record bilateral calf or thigh circumferences every shift.
- Teach and support the person and their family about self-management.
- Assess colour and temperature of the involved extremity every shift.

PULMONARY EMBOLISM A pulmonary embolism is a dislodged blood clot or other substance that lodges in a pulmonary artery. For the postoperative person with DVT, the threat that a portion of the thrombus may dislodge from the vein wall and travel to the lung, heart or brain is a constant concern. Early detection of this potentially life-threatening complication depends on the nurse's astute, continuing assessment of the person postoperatively.

Common assessment findings of the person experiencing a pulmonary embolism include mild to moderate dyspnoea, chest pain, diaphoresis, anxiety, restlessness, rapid respirations and pulse, arrhythmias, cough and cyanosis. The severity of the symptoms is determined by the degree of pulmonary vascular blockage. Sudden death can occur if a major pulmonary artery becomes completely blocked.

Stabilising respiratory and cardiovascular functioning while preventing the formation of additional emboli is of utmost importance in the care of the person with a pulmonary embolism. Nursing care includes the following measures:

- Immediately notify the surgeon and/or anaesthetist.
- Frequently assess and record general condition and vital signs.

- Maintain the person on bed rest and keep the head of the bed elevated.
- Provide oxygen as ordered and monitor pulse oximetry.
- Administer prescribed intravenous fluids to maintain fluid balance while preventing fluid overload.
- Administer prescribed anticoagulants.
- Maintain comfort by administering analgesics and sedatives. (Use caution to prevent respiratory depression.)
- Provide supportive measures for the person and their family.

Refer to the chapter 'Nursing care of people with upper respiratory disorders' for a detailed discussion of pulmonary embolism.

Respiratory complications

Common postoperative respiratory complications include pneumonia and atelectasis.

PNEUMONIA Pneumonia is an inflammation of lung tissue. Inflammation is *caused* either by a microbial infection or by a foreign substance in the lung, which leads to an infection. Numerous factors may be involved in the development of pneumonia, including aspiration infection, retained pulmonary secretions, failure to cough deeply and impaired cough reflex, and decreased mobility.

Common assessment findings of the person with postoperative pneumonia are as follows:

- high fever
- rapid pulse and respirations
- chills (may be present initially)
- productive cough (may be present depending on the type of pneumonia)
- dyspnoea
- hypoxia
- chest pain
- pulmonary crackles and wheezes.

Treating the pulmonary infection, supporting the person's respiratory efforts, promoting lung expansion, and preventing the organisms' spread are the goals in the care of the person with pneumonia. Nursing care includes the following measures:

- Obtain sputum specimens for culture and sensitivity testing.
- Position the person with the head of the bed elevated.
- Encourage the person to turn, cough and perform deep-breathing exercises at least every 2 hours.
- Assist with incentive spirometry, intermittent positive pressure breathing (IPPB) and/or nebuliser treatments as ordered.
- Ambulate the person as their condition permits and as prescribed.
- Administer oxygen as ordered.
- Assess vital signs, breath sounds and general condition.
- Maintain hydration so that pulmonary secretions are easier for the person to expectorate.
- Administer antibiotics, expectorants, antipyretics and analgesics as ordered.
- Provide or assist with frequent oral hygiene.
- Prevent the spread of microorganisms by teaching proper disposal of tissues, covering mouth when coughing, and good handwashing technique.
- Provide supportive measures for the person and their family.

The chapter 'Nursing care of people with upper respiratory disorders' provides a detailed discussion of pneumonia.

ATELECTASIS Atelectasis is an incomplete expansion or collapse of lung tissue resulting in inadequate ventilation and retention of pulmonary secretions. Common assessment findings include dyspnoea, hypoxia, diminished breath sounds over the affected area, anxiety, restlessness, crackles and cyanosis.

Promoting lung expansion and systemic oxygenation of tissues is a goal in the care of the person with atelectasis. Nursing care includes these tasks:

- Position the person with the head of bed elevated.
- Administer oxygen as prescribed.
- Encourage coughing, turning and deep breathing every 2 hours.
- Ambulate the person as their condition permits and as prescribed.
- Assist with incentive spirometry or other pulmonary exercises, such as inflating a balloon, as ordered.
- Administer analgesics as prescribed.
- Promote hydration.
- Provide supportive measures to the person and their family.

Wound complications

Discussion of the complications associated with surgical wounds follows an overview of wound healing, wound drainage and nursing care of wounds.

Wounds heal by *primary*, *secondary* or *tertiary* intention (see Figure 3.5). Healing by primary intention takes place when the wound is uncomplicated and clean and has sustained little tissue loss. The edges of the incision are well approximated (joined) with sutures, staples or glue for drain holes or superficial wounds. This type of surgical incision heals quickly and very little scarring is expected.

Secondary intention refers to the healing that occurs when the wound is large, gaping and irregular. Tissue loss prevents wound edges from approximating; therefore, granulation fills in the wound. This type of wound takes longer to heal, is more prone to infection, and develops more scar tissue.

If enough time passes before a wound is sutured, healing by tertiary intention occurs. Infection is more likely to take place. Because the wound edges are not approximated, tissue is regenerated by the granulation process. Closure of the wound results in a wide scar.

From the time the surgical incision is made until the wound is completely healed, all wounds progress through four stages of healing. However, healing time varies according to many factors, such as age, nutritional status, smoking, general health,

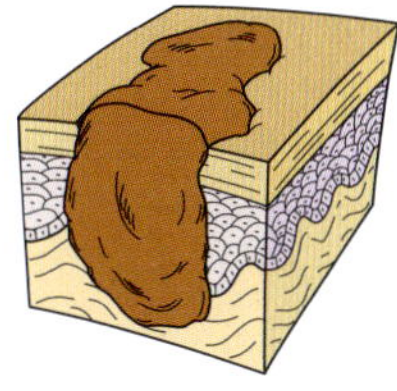
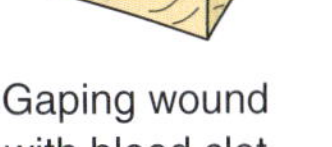
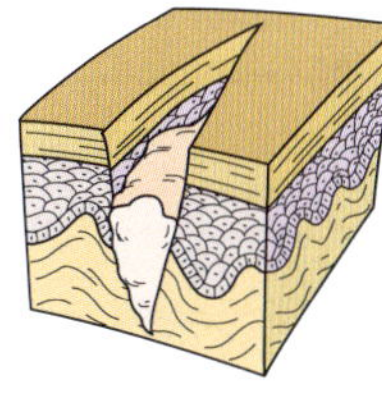
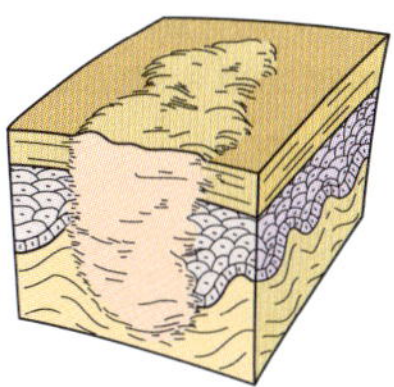

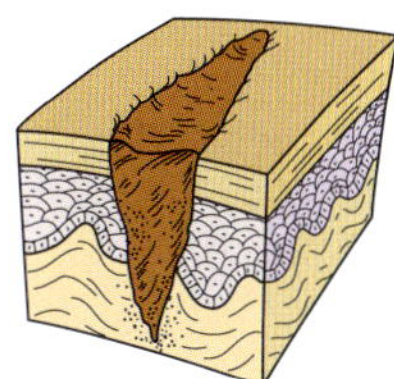
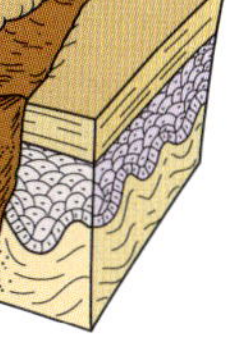
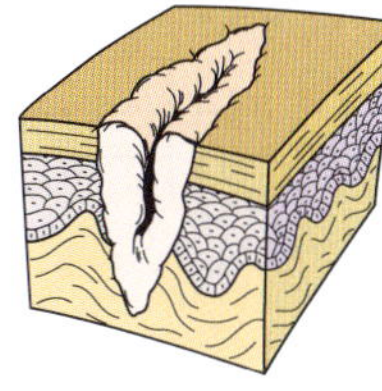
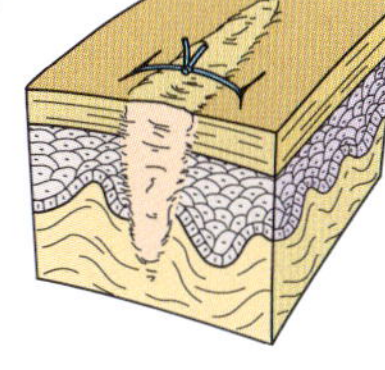

FIGURE 3.5 ***Wound healing by primary, secondary and tertiary intention***

BOX 3.4 Stages of wound healing

- *Stage I: from surgery through to day 2.* Inflammatory process occurs to prepare the surrounding tissue for healing. Blood vessels constrict, and clotting occurs. Vasodilation and increased capillary permeability follows, bringing plasma, white blood cells and fibroplastin to the wound site. Epithelial cells begin to form and re-establish blood flow in the wound tissue. A mild temperature elevation is normal.
- *Stage II: day 3 through to day 14 following surgery.* Fewer white blood cells are present. Collagen tissue forms in the wound tissue. Granulation tissue, red with a rich blood supply, is established.
- *Stage III: day 15 to week 6 following surgery.* Collagen fibres continue to strengthen the wound. As the blood supply decreases, the scar tissue appears pink and somewhat raised.
- *Stage IV: several months to a year following surgery.* As the wound tissue constricts, the scar becomes flat, smaller and white.

and the type and location of the wound. Box 3.4 provides a summary of the stages of wound healing.

Wound drainage (exudate) results from the inflammatory process in the first two stages of wound healing. The drainage is from the rich blood supply that surrounds the wound tissue and is composed of escaped fluid and cells. The drainage is described as serous, sanguineous or purulent.

- Serous drainage contains mostly the clear serous portion of the blood. The drainage appears clear or slightly yellow and is thin in consistency.
- Sanguineous drainage contains a combination of serum and red blood cells and has a thick, reddish appearance. This is the most common type of drainage from a non-complicated surgical wound.
- Purulent drainage is composed of white blood cells, tissue debris and bacteria. Purulent drainage is the result of infection and tends to be of a thicker consistency, with various colours specific to the type of organism. It also may have an unpleasant odour.

Box 3.5 describes and illustrates various types of wound drainage devices. These devices decrease pressure in the wound area by removing excess fluid, which promotes healing and decreases complications.

Nursing care of the person with a postoperative surgical wound focuses on prevention and monitoring for wound complications. The nurse assumes a leading role in supporting the wound healing process, providing emotional support to the person and teaching them wound care.

Common assessment findings of an infected wound include pain; purulent, odorous discharge and redness; warmth; tenderness; and oedema around the edges of the incision. Additionally, the person may have a fever, chills and increased respiratory and pulse rates. Nursing care includes the following measures:

- Follow the Australian Wound Management Association's (2011) *Standards for Wound Management.*
- Observe aseptic technique during dressing changes and handling of tubes and drains, including the 'Five Moments for Hand Hygiene' approach as recommended in Australia by Hand Hygiene Australia (ACSQHC, 2019).
- Assess vital signs, especially temperature.
- Evaluate the characteristics of wound discharge (colour, odour and amount).
- Assess the condition of the incision (approximation of the edges, sutures, staples or drains).
- Clean, irrigate and pack the wound in the prescribed manner. Sterile normal saline is often prescribed.
- Maintain the person's hydration and nutritional status.
- Swab the wound for a microbial culture prior to beginning antibiotic therapy (if indicated).
- Administer antibiotics and antipyretics as prescribed.

BOX 3.5 Wound drainage devices

A Penrose drain, used for passive wound drainage, promotes healing from the inside to the outside (see *Figure A* below). The use of the drain decreases the chance of abscess formation. The safety pin in the Penrose drain prevents the exposed end from slipping down into the wound and facilitates x-ray detection if necessary. Wound care focuses on cleaning around the drain with a prescribed solution, such as sterile normal saline, and replacing the pre-cut gauze dressing as necessary to keep the surrounding skin dry and encourage further drainage. An absorbent dressing is placed over the drain and gauze (not shown).

Wound suction devices promote drainage of fluid from the incision site, decreasing pressure on healing tissues and reducing abscess formation. Shown are the Jackson-Pratt and Bellovac wound suction devices (see *Figures B* and *C* below).

The frequency with which the nurse empties the device depends on the time elapsed since surgery, type of surgery, amount of drainage and hospital policy. For example, immediately after surgery the nurse may empty the device every hour. With time, as drainage decreases, the device is emptied every 2 to 4 hours (as per hospital policy). Amount, colour, consistency and odour of drainage are documented.

Usually, the drain is removed on the second to fourth day after surgery. Removal causes minor discomfort. The drain site is cleaned and a sterile dressing is applied.

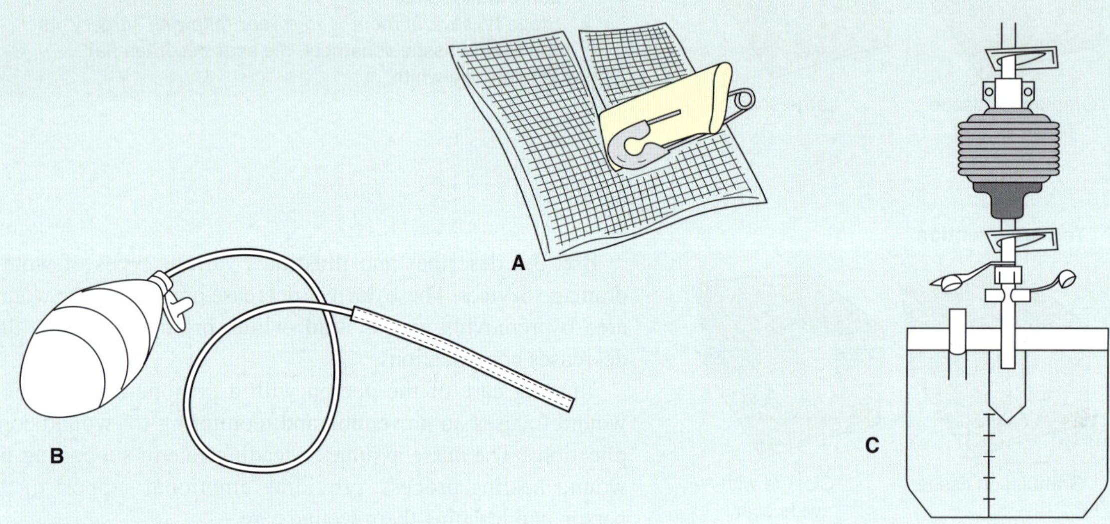

Wound drainage devices. A, Penrose passive wound drainage device. B, Jackson-Pratt wound suction device. C, Bellovac wound suction device

Source: C, © Wellspect Healthcare and Dentsply IH Pty Ltd (Australia).

Dehiscence is a separation in the layers of the incisional wound (see Figure 3.6A). Treatment depends on the extent of wound disruption. If the dehiscence is extensive, the incision must be re-sutured in surgery. **Evisceration** is the protrusion of body organs from a wound dehiscence (see Figure 3.6B). These serious complications may result from delayed wound healing or may occur immediately following surgery. They also may occur after forceful straining (coughing, sneezing or vomiting). When dehiscence occurs, immediately cover the wound with a sterile dressing moistened with normal saline. Emergency surgery is performed to repair these conditions.

The nurse or medical officer may remove sutures or staples after the wound has healed sufficiently (usually 5 to 10 days after surgery). Removal is performed using aseptic technique. Additional support may be provided to the incision by applying strips of tape (or Steri-Strips) as directed by institutional policy or by the medical officer.

Complications associated with elimination

Common postoperative complications associated with elimination include urinary retention and altered bowel elimination. The inability to urinate with urinary retention may occur postoperatively as a result of the recumbent position, effects of anaesthesia and narcotics, inactivity, altered fluid balance, nervous tension or surgical manipulation in the pelvic area. Nursing care centres on promoting normal urinary elimination and includes the following measures:

- Assess for bladder distension if the person has not voided within 7 to 8 hours after surgery or is urinating small amounts frequently. Ultrasound assessment is often used for this purpose.
- Assess the amount of urine in the bladder with a portable ultrasound scanner. This non-invasive procedure provides information to prevent unnecessary catheterisation and decreases the potential for urinary tract infections and urethral trauma from repeated catheterisations.

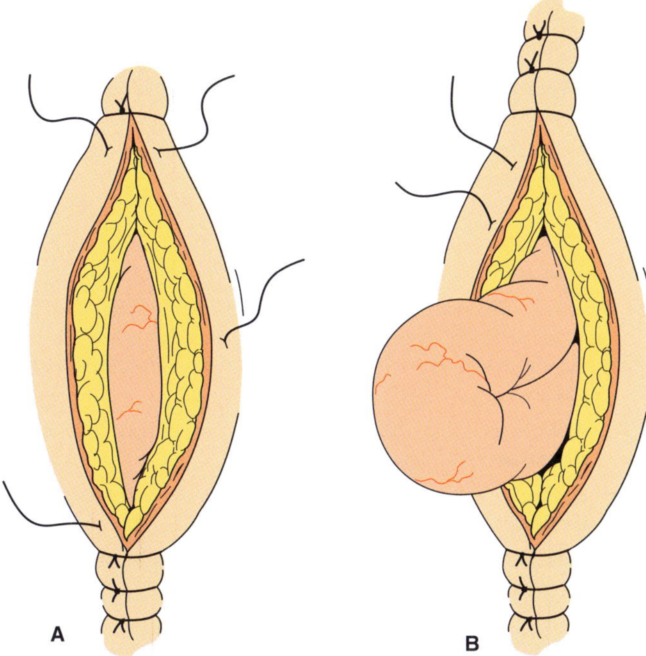

FIGURE 3.6 *Wound complications. A, Dehiscence is a disruption in the incision resulting in a separation of the layers of the wound. B, Evisceration is a protrusion of a body organ through a surgical incision*

- Monitor intake and output.
- Maintain intravenous infusion if fluids are prescribed.
- Increase daily oral fluid intake to 2,500 to 3,000 mL if the person's condition permits.
- Insert an intermittent or indwelling catheter if ordered.
- Promote normal urinary elimination by:
  a. Assisting and providing privacy when the person uses a bedpan.
  b. Helping the person to use the bedside commode or walk to the bathroom.
  c. Assisting males to stand to void.
  d. Pouring a measured amount of warm water over the perineal area (if urination occurs, subtract the amount of water from the total amount for an accurate output measurement).

Bowel elimination frequently is altered after abdominal or pelvic surgery and sometimes after other surgeries. Return to normal gastrointestinal function may be delayed by general anaesthesia, narcotic analgesia, decreased mobility or altered fluid and food intake during the perioperative period.

Nursing care centres on the return of normal bowel function and includes the following measures:

- Assess for the return of normal peristalsis:
  a. Auscultate bowel sounds every 8 hours while the person is awake.
  b. Assess the abdomen for distension. (A distended abdomen with absent or high-pitched bowel sounds may indicate paralytic ileus.)
  c. Determine whether the person is passing flatus.
  d. Monitor for passage of stool, including amount and consistency.
- Encourage early ambulation within prescribed limits.
- Facilitate a daily fluid intake of 2,500 to 3,000 mL (unless contraindicated).
- Provide privacy when the person is using the bedpan, bedside commode or bathroom.

If no bowel movement has occurred within 3 to 4 days after surgery, an aperient, suppository or an enema may be prescribed.

Special considerations for older adults

Physiological, cognitive and psychosocial changes associated with the ageing process place the older adult at increased risk of postoperative complications. These age-related changes with selected nursing interventions are summarised in Table 3.7. With an increasing population of older adults, particularly the very old, the nurse must be aware of these normal changes and modify nursing care accordingly in an effort to provide safe, supportive care.

Managing acute postoperative pain

Some pain can be expected after surgery (Schug et al., 2020). It is neither realistic nor practical to eliminate postoperative pain completely. Nevertheless, the person having surgery should receive substantial relief from and control of this discomfort. Controlling postoperative pain not only promotes comfort but also facilitates coughing, turning, deep-breathing exercises, earlier ambulation and decreased length of hospitalisation, resulting in fewer postoperative complications and therefore reducing healthcare costs. Despite the apparent benefits and methods of effective pain control and improved understanding of pain physiology, many people do not receive adequate pain relief or control postoperatively.

Managing acute postoperative pain is an important nursing role before, during and after surgery. Successful pain management involves the cooperative efforts of the person, anaesthetist and nurse (Schug et al., 2020). Preoperatively, the person should learn how much pain to anticipate and what methods are available to control pain. After discussing options with the person having surgery, healthcare providers must respect their personal preferences.

Postoperative medications were discussed earlier in the chapter. Various non-pharmacological approaches to pain management can also be used alone or in combination to control acute postoperative pain (Schug et al., 2020). Music, distraction and imagery techniques and acupuncture can decrease mild pain and anxiety. Additional information on pain management techniques is found in the chapter 'Nursing care of people in pain'.

The person's input and participation in assessing pain and pain relief is essential to a successful pain control regimen. For example, the person can rate the pain on a scale of 0 to 10 (where 0 signifies no pain and 10 signifies unbearable pain). Assess and document pain at scheduled intervals

TABLE 3.7 Nursing interventions for older people having surgery

SYSTEM	AGE-RELATED CHANGES	NURSING INTERVENTIONS
Body composition	Change in weight and fat distribution and hydration	Provide for warmth and frequent turning. Assess for dehydration and fluid imbalance. Provide comfort measures when NBM.
Integument	Diminished integrity secondary to loss of subcutaneous fat and decreased oil production and elasticity	Provide careful preoperative preparation, including hair removal, to avoid trauma. Position carefully to prevent pressure ulcers.
Sensory-perceptual	Decline in vision and hearing ability	Compensate for sensory deficits: speak low, not loud; minimise noise in environment; provide adequate room light; stay within the person's field of vision when speaking; encourage them to wear their hearing aid to the operating room.
Respiratory	Decreased efficiency of cough reflex and decreased aeration of lung fields. Reduced pulmonary functional reserve and lung function, with increased risk of infection and bronchospasm with airway obstruction	Maintain airway with positioning, provide oxygen as needed, maintain hydration and mobility. Teach and encourage coughing and diaphragmatic breathing exercises preoperatively and encourage smoking cessation. Constantly monitor lung sounds and respiratory status.
Cardiovascular	Less efficient, decreased cardiac reserve and adaptation to stress. Risk of arrhythmias and extreme blood pressure changes	Monitor for hypotension and shock. Assess for thrombus formation, cardiac arrhythmias, peripheral pulses and oedema.
Gastrointestinal	Decline in gastric motility, risk of altered drug absorption, GORD, maldigestion and bowel elimination problems	Encourage intake of adequate fluids, nutritious meals, soft diet. Assist with feeding; monitor bowel function. Encourage mobility.
Genitourinary	Decreased renal function reserve, risk of nephrotoxic injury and adverse reactions to medications, risk of volume overload, dehydration and other electrolyte imbalances; loss of bladder control and urinary tract infections. Risk for falls	Monitor fluid input and output and electrolyte levels. Assess for drug side effects. Assist with voiding as needed.
Musculoskeletal	Stiffness of joints; decrease in strength; brittleness of bones, intervertebral disc degeneration and joint erosion. Risk for falls	Carefully position on operating table with bony prominences well padded to prevent pressure sores. Move carefully and gently. Provide effective pain management. Encourage mobilisation postoperatively. Prevent falls.
Cognition and nervous system	Decreased reaction time and reflexes and slow motor skills, deficits in balance and coordination, slowed cognitive processing; risk of delirium and altered mental status while in hospital. Risk for falls	Provide ample time for making decisions. Implement safety measures. Talk to people respectfully as an adult. Orient frequently. Monitor for postoperative delirium. Provide effective pain management. Prevent falls.

Sources: Smith & Cotter (2012). *Age related changes in health. Evidence-based geriatric nursing protocols for best practice* (4th ed.). New York: Springer Publishing Company, LLC; Griffiths et al. (2014). Guidelines: Peri-operative care of the elderly 2014. *Anaesthesia, 69*(Suppl. 1), 81–98.

to determine the degree of pain control, to observe for drug side effects, and to assess the need for changes in the dosage and/or frequency of medication administration. When a range of dosage is ordered, carefully titrate opioid dosages based on individual assessments of need and response to therapy.

Community-based care

The postoperative phase does not end until the person has recovered completely from the surgical intervention. Thus, the nurse plays a vital role as they near discharge. People who have surgery are usually discharged within a few days, and many complications can develop after discharge. As people prepare to recuperate at home, the nurse provides information and support to help them successfully meet self-care demands. All aspects of teaching should be accompanied by written guidelines, directions and information. This is particularly helpful when a large amount of unfamiliar, detailed information is presented. Because the hospital stay is often brief, an organised, coordinated effort to educate the person and their family should be made. Teaching needs vary, but the most common needs include:

- Wound care. Teaching is more effective if the nurse first demonstrates and explains the procedure for the person and their family or other caregiver. They should then participate in the care. To evaluate the effectiveness of the teaching, ask them to demonstrate the procedure in return. Ideally, teaching is carried out over several days, evaluated and periodically reinforced.
- Signs and symptoms of a wound infection. The person should be able to determine what is normal and what should be reported to their doctor.
- Method and frequency of taking own temperature.
- Limitations or restrictions that may be imposed on such activities as lifting, driving, bathing, sexual activity and other physical activities.
- Control of pain. If analgesics are prescribed, instruct the person in the dosage, frequency, purpose, common side effects and other side effects to report to the surgeon. Reinforce the use of relaxation, distraction, imagery or other pain control techniques that they have found useful in controlling their postoperative pain.
- Signs and symptoms of DVT and preventative strategies.
- Recommended strategies for rehabilitation and follow-up.

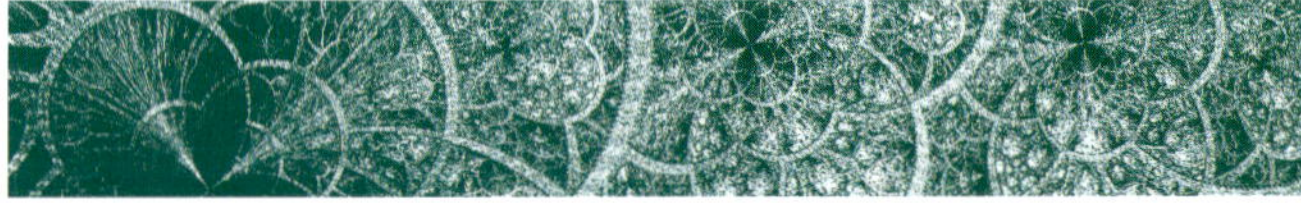

NURSING CARE PLAN A person having surgery

Martha Overbeck is a 74-year-old widow of German descent who lives alone in a retirement complex. She is active there, as well as in the Lutheran Church. She has been in good health and is independent, but she has become progressively less active as a result of arthritic pain and stiffness. Mrs Overbeck has degenerative joint changes that have particularly affected her right hip. On the recommendation of her surgeon and following a discussion with her friends, Mrs Overbeck has been admitted to the hospital for an elective right total hip arthroplasty. Her surgery has been scheduled for 8 am the following day.

Mrs Eva Jackson, a close friend and neighbour, accompanies Mrs Overbeck to the hospital. Mrs Overbeck explains that her friend will help in her home and assist her with the wound care and prescribed exercises.

ASSESSMENT

Gloria Nobis, RN, is assigned to Mrs Overbeck's care on return from surgery. Ms Nobis performs a complete physical assessment and determines that Mrs Overbeck is drowsy but oriented. Her skin is pale and slightly cool. Mrs Overbeck states that she is cold and requests additional covers. Ms Nobis places a warmed cotton blanket next to Mrs Overbeck's body, adds another blanket to her covers, and adjusts the room's thermostat to increase the room temperature. Mrs Overbeck states that she is in no pain and would like to sleep. She has even, unlaboured respirations and stable vital signs compared with preoperative readings.

Mrs Overbeck is NBM. An intravenous solution of dextrose and saline is infusing at 100 mL/h per infusion pump. No redness or oedema is noted at the infusion site. Ms Nobis notes that the antibiotic cephalothin is to be administered intravenously. Mrs Overbeck has a large secured dressing (Primapore) over her right upper lateral thigh and hip with no indications of ooze from the wound. Tubing protrudes from the distal end of the dressing and is attached to a passive suctioning device (Bellovac). Ms Nobis observes 50 mL of dark red drainage from the suctioning device and records the amount and characteristics on a wound assessment chart. Mrs Overbeck has an indwelling catheter in place with 250 mL of clear, light amber urine in the dependent gravity drainage bag.

When assessing Mrs Overbeck's lower extremities, Ms Nobis finds her feet slightly cool and pale with rapid capillary refill time bilaterally. Dorsalis pedis and posterior tibial pulses are strong and equal bilaterally. Ms Nobis notes slight pitting oedema in the right foot and ankle compared with the left extremity. She also notes sensation and ability to move both feet and toes, without numbness or tingling (paraesthesia).

Ms Nobis records these findings on the postoperative record. After ensuring that Mrs Overbeck is safely positioned and can reach her call switch, Ms Nobis gives Mrs Overbeck's friend a progress report. They then go into Mrs Overbeck's room.

DIAGNOSES

Ms Nobis makes the following postoperative nursing diagnoses for Mrs Overbeck.

- *Potential for infection:* right hip wound infection related to disruption of normal skin integrity by the surgical incision manifested by elevated temperature, redness, swelling, local pain, wound breakdown and wound exudate containing pus.
- *Injury* related to potential dislocation of right hip prosthesis secondary to hip arthroplasty manifested by acute severe pain, abnormal limb alignment and inability to mobilise.
- *Acute pain*, related to right hip incision and positioning of arthritic joints during surgery manifested by a high rating of pain on a pain scale, tachycardia, elevated blood pressure, dilated pupils, paleness, sweating, vasoconstriction, limited ability to move limb, restlessness, anxiety and shallow breathing.

PLANNING

Ms Nobis plans to use a clinical pathway to actively implement nursing strategies that will monitor the recovery of Mrs Overbeck, use evidence-based guidelines to prevent the development of potential postoperative complications, support her recovery and promote her comfort and progress during recovery. This will require using the clinical reasoning process to determine appropriate therapeutic responses, including the recognition of any indications of deterioration in physiological status. It will also include postoperative teaching to develop independence and motivate sustained self-management during hospitalisation and after discharge.

Expected outcomes

The expected outcomes established in the plan of care specify that Mrs Overbeck will:

- Regain skin integrity of the right hip incision without experiencing signs or symptoms of infection.
- Demonstrate (along with Mrs Jackson) proper aseptic technique while performing the dressing change.
- Verbalise signs and symptoms of infection to be reported to her surgeon.
- Describe measures to be taken to prevent dislocation of right hip prosthesis.
- Report control of pain at incision and in arthritic joints.
- Remain afebrile.

IMPLEMENTATION

Ms Nobis develops a care plan that includes the following interventions to assist Mrs Overbeck during her postoperative recovery.

- Provide prophylactic measures to minimise the risk of postoperative venous thromboembolism, including administration of low molecular weight heparin as ordered, early mobilisation, checking the correct application of graduated compression stockings, and/or sequential compression devices, assisting with exercises and monitoring Mrs Overbeck for potential manifestations of DVT.
- Use aseptic technique while changing dressing.
- Monitor temperature and pulse every 4 hours to assess for elevation.
- Assess wound every 8 hours for purulent drainage and odour. Assess edges of wound for approximation, oedema, redness or inflammation in excess of expected inflammatory response.

(continued)

NURSING CARE PLAN **A person having surgery (continued)**

- Teach Mrs Overbeck and Mrs Jackson how to use aseptic technique while assessing the wound and performing the dressing change.
- Teach Mrs Overbeck and Mrs Jackson the signs and symptoms of infection and when to report findings to the surgeon.
- Review and discuss with Mrs Overbeck the written materials on hip arthroplasty.
- Convey empathetic understanding of Mrs Overbeck's incisional and arthritic joint pain.
- Provide analgesia every 4 hours (or as ordered) to maintain a therapeutic blood level.

EVALUATION

Throughout Mrs Overbeck's hospitalisation, Ms Nobis works with Mrs Overbeck and Mrs Jackson to ensure that Mrs Overbeck can care for herself after discharge from the hospital. Five days after her surgery, Mrs Overbeck is discharged with a well-approximated incision with no indications of an infection. Prior to discharge, Ms Nobis is confident that with Mrs Jackson's help, Mrs Overbeck can properly assess the incision. With minimal help, Mrs Overbeck is able to replace the dressing using aseptic technique. She can state the signs and symptoms of an infection, take her own oral temperature, and describe preventive measures to decrease the chances of dislocating her prosthetic hip. Because of her reduced mobility the past 5 days, Mrs Overbeck says she can tell the arthritis in her 'old bones' is 'acting up'. She reports a lessening of pain in her right hip following surgery and a pain that is different to her arthritic pain as experienced pre-surgery. Mrs Overbeck tells Ms Nobis she will be back the following winter to have her left hip replaced.

CRITICAL THINKING IN THE NURSING PROCESS

1. Describe risk factors for Mrs Overbeck's safety; what changes in her home environment would you suggest to promote safety until she recovers more fully?
2. Why is Mrs Overbeck placed on the antibiotic cephalothin although she has no indications of an infection? What teaching would you do?
3. Mrs Overbeck's clotting time is slightly elevated as a result of an ordered anticoagulant. Why would this medication be ordered? Consider the person's age and the area of surgery.
4. Mrs Overbeck is 13.6 kg above her ideal weight and has osteoarthritis. Develop a care plan for the nursing diagnosis *Health maintenance problems* related to intake in excess of metabolic requirements and limited mobility.

REFLECTION ON THE NURSING PROCESS

1. Using the critical thinking process, identify what you have learned from this case study that you will apply to your clinical practice in the future.
2. Consider this learning in relation to the NMBA (2016) *Registered Nurse Standards for Practice.*
3. What teaching aids would be helpful to educate people recovering from hip arthroplasty surgery, during the postoperative period?

CHAPTER HIGHLIGHTS

- **Surgery takes place in traditional and non-traditional settings with increasing use of minimally invasive procedures that expedite discharge, facilitate healing and increase satisfaction for people having surgery.**
- **Surgery is an invasive procedure, and legal guidelines must be followed to protect the person having surgery and the healthcare providers. The surgical team includes surgeons, anaesthetists, nurses and anaesthetic technicians; all are responsible for the safety of the person and the progression of the surgery.**
- **The focus on safety during surgery continues to increase, with attention directed to preventing wrong site/wrong patient operations occurring. Procedures are established to verify that the right person will have the correct surgery. A team approach to safety works best; each member of the team must feel accountable for the results of the surgery and entitled to share observations and concerns as the procedure progresses.**
- **Inpatients who have surgery have relatively short stays, which are best achieved by early ambulation, pain control and proper nutrition. Providing information for self-care is challenging with the shortened stays and rate of admissions and discharges. From the time of entry to the surgical setting, the person's discharge must be planned and prepared.**
- **Teaching people prior to and following surgery empowers them to achieve successful recovery, discharge and rehabilitation. Most of the care people receive during healing is provided either by themselves or a caregiver outside the healthcare environment. People having surgery and their families need to know appropriate assessments and interventions to monitor the healing process.**
- **Pain management is offered prior to, during and after surgery with methods designed to give the best therapeutic response. While acute pain related to the surgery occurs many people also experience persistent pain that affects their response to pain management therapies.**
- **Behaviours characteristic of older adults and ethnically diverse populations increase the need for individualised care. Assessment of physical and emotional status can be more difficult when people have hearing or vision impairments or when individuals speak and understand a foreign language. Surgery can be frightening for people and their families and they need reassurance and interventions to decrease pain, relieve anxiety and promote healing.**
- **Operating room and post anaesthesia nursing care are professional specialties that require unique orientation and education. These professionals make careful assessments of the risks each person faces and make plans to ensure safe, successful surgical outcomes. Special attention is focused on early recognition and treatment of postoperative complications associated with cardiopulmonary function, respiratory function, wound healing, elimination and pain.**

CONCEPT CHECK

1 The nurse's primary responsibility relating to informed consent is:
1 defining the risks and benefits of the surgery
2 checking that the person's signature appears on the consent form and that the form is accurately completed
3 discussing alternative therapies with the person
4 advising the person and their family about what is needed for the diagnosis

2 Obtaining a preoperative blood pressure measurement serves the following purpose:
1 fulfils a legal requirement
2 provides information for the amount of anaesthetic required
3 prevents atelectasis
4 provides a baseline to compare with postoperative blood pressure levels

3 Non-steroidal anti-inflammatory drugs are given in the postoperative period to:
1 stimulate appetite
2 increase amnesia
3 potentiate analgesia
4 improve renal function

4 Discharge planning for a person following general surgery will include dietary management guidelines. Specifically, the person will eat a diet:
1 low in cholesterol, high in fat
2 high in protein, moderate in kilojoules
3 low in fat, high in fibre
4 without dairy products, but otherwise regular

5 In the immediate postoperative period for knee surgery, assessment distal to the site includes:
1 urinary pH
2 rebound tenderness
3 Chvostek's sign
4 neurovascular assessment

6 In the postoperative period, medications the person is prescribed prior to surgery must be:
1 continued after surgery
2 decreased by half for 36 hours
3 ordered anew prior to administration
4 withheld until evidence of anaesthesia is absent

7 The person with diabetes mellitus who is NBM prior to surgery:
1 has no risk of hyperglycaemia
2 should receive sliding-scale insulin prescriptions
3 will benefit from hypoglycaemia during anaesthesia
4 will fail to manifest signs of hypoglycaemia under anaesthesia

8 Acute pain management medications in the immediate postoperative period generally:
1 progress from NSAIDs to opioids
2 should include pre-emptive and multimodal analgesia
3 should be prn to promote control
4 induce a strong sedative effect to decrease the risk of nausea

9 Lengthy operative procedures can put the older person at risk of:
1 memory loss due to blood loss
2 hearing loss due to extended anaesthesia
3 weight loss due to lack of nutritional intake
4 pressure sores and joint pain from operative positioning

10 Hypothermia in the perioperative period:
1 decreases cardiac ischaemia
2 reduces the risk of wound infection
3 increases comfort and analgesia
4 requires interventions to prevent and relieve

BIBLIOGRAPHY

Abebe, W. (2019). Review of herbal medications with the potential to cause bleeding: Dental implications, and risk prediction and prevention avenues. *EPMA Journal*, *10*(1), 51–64. https://doi.org/10.1007/s13167-018-0158-2

Assareh, H., Chen, J., Ou, L., Hillman, K. & Flabouris, A. (2016). Incidences and variations of hospital acquired venous thromboembolism in Australian hospitals: A population-based study. *BMC Health Services Research*, *16*, 511.

Australian College of Operating Room Nurses (ACORN) (2020). *ACORN Standards for Perioperative Nursing* (16th ed.). Adelaide: Australian College of Operating Room Nurses Ltd.

Australian Commission on Safety and Quality in Health Care (ACSQHC) (2016). *Patient identification*. Sydney: ACSQHC.

Australian Commission on Safety and Quality in Health Care (ACSQHC) (2017). *Communication at clinical handover*. Sydney: ACSQHC.

Australian Commission on Safety and Quality in Health Care (ACSQHC) (2018). *Venous thromboembolism prevention clinical care standard*. Sydney: ACSQHC.

Australian Commission on Safety and Quality in Health Care (ACSQHC) (2019). *National Hand Hygiene Initiative*. Retrieved from https://www.safetyandquality.gov.au/

Australian Commission on Safety and Quality in Health Care (ACSQHC) (2021). *National Safety and Quality Health Service Standards* (2nd ed.). Sydney: ACSQHC.

Australian Commission on Safety and Quality in Health Care (ACSQHC) (2022). *Antimicrobial stewardship in Australian health care*. Sydney: ACSQHC.

Australian Day Surgery Nurses Association (ADSNA) (2018). *Best practice guidelines for ambulatory surgery and procedures*. Osborne Park, WA: Cambridge Publishing.

Australian Institute of Health and Welfare (AIHW) (2020). *Australian hospitals at glance 2018–19*. Cat. No. HSE 247. Canberra: Author.

Australian Wound Management Association (2011). *Standards for wound management*. West Leederville, WA: Cambridge Publishing. Retrieved from https://www.awma.com.au/

Collins, S., Budds, M., Raines, C. & Hooper, V. (2019). Risk factors for perioperative hypothermia: A literature review. *Journal of Perianesthesia Nursing*, *34*(2), 338–346.

Dagli, R., Kocoaglu, N., Bair, H., Hakki, M. & Doyan, M. (2016). Evaluation of medical drug and herbal product use before anaesthesia. *International Journal of Clinical and Experimental Medicine*, *9*(2), 4670–4674.

Donoghue, T. (2018). Herbal medication and anesthesia case management. *AANA Journal*, *86*(3), 142–248.

Griffiths, R., Beech, F., Brown, A. et al. (2014). Guidelines: Peri-operative care of the elderly 2014. *Anaesthesia*, *69*(Suppl. 1), 81–98.

Henry, J. & Satiani, B. (2014). Calf muscle venous thrombosis. *Vascular and Endovascular Surgery*, *48*(5–6), 396–401.

Joint Commission on Accreditation of Healthcare Organizations (2012). *National patient safety goals*. Retrieved from https://www.jointcommission.org/

Kuzulugil, D., Papeix, G., Luu, J. & Kerridge, R. (2019). Recent advances in diabetes treatments and their perioperative implications. *Current Opinions in Anaesthesiology*, *32*(3), 398–404.

Levett-Jones, T., Dwyer, T., Reid-Searl, K., Heaton, L., Flenady, T., Applegarth, J., Guinea, S. & Andersen, P. (2017). *Patient Safety Competency Framework (PSCF) for Nursing Students*. Sydney. Retrieved from http://psframework.wpengine.com/

Nursing and Midwifery Board of Australia (NMBA) (2016). *Registered Nurse Standards for Practice*. Retrieved from https://www.nursingmidwiferyboard.gov.au/

O'Neill, E., Carter, E., Pink, N. & Smith, I. (2016). Routine preoperative tests for elective surgery: Summary of updated NICE guidance. *British Medical Journal (Clinical Research ed.)*, *354*, i3292.

Schofield, P. (2018). The assessment of pain in older people: UK National Guidelines. *Age and Ageing*, i1–i22. doi: 10.1093/ageing/afx192

Schug, S. A., Palmer, G. M., Scott, D. A. et al. (2020). *Acute pain management: Scientific evidence* (5th ed.). Melbourne: ANZCA & FPM.

Shear, T., Deshur, M., Avram, M. et al. (2018) Procedural timeout compliance is improved with real time clinical decision making. *Journal Of Patient Safety*, *14*(3), 148–152.

Smith, C. M. & Cotter, V. T. (2012). *Age related changes in health. Evidence-based geriatric nursing protocols for best practice* (4th ed.). New York: Springer Publishing Company, LLC.

Spofford, C. & Hurley, R. (2018). Preventative analgesia. In H. T. Benzon, S. N. Raja, S. M. Fishman, S. S. Liu & S. P. Cohen, *Essentials of pain medicine* (4th ed., Chapter 11), Cambridge: Elsevier. https://doi.org/10.1016/C2014-0-03837-3

Steelman, V., Shaw, C., Shine, L. & Hardy-Fairbanks, A. (2019). Unintentionally retained foreign objects: A descriptive study of 308 sentinel events and contributing factors. *Joint Commission Journal on Quality and Patient Safety*, *45*, 249–258.

Sutherland-Fraser, S., Davies, M., Gillespie, B. & Lockwood, B. (2022). *Perioperative nursing: An introduction* (3rd ed.). Chatswood, NSW: Elsevier.

World Health Organization (WHO) (2019). *10 facts on patient safety*. Retrieved from https://www.who.int/

World Health Organization (WHO) and World Alliance for Patient Safety (2009). *Surgical safety checklist*. Retrieved from https://www.who.int/

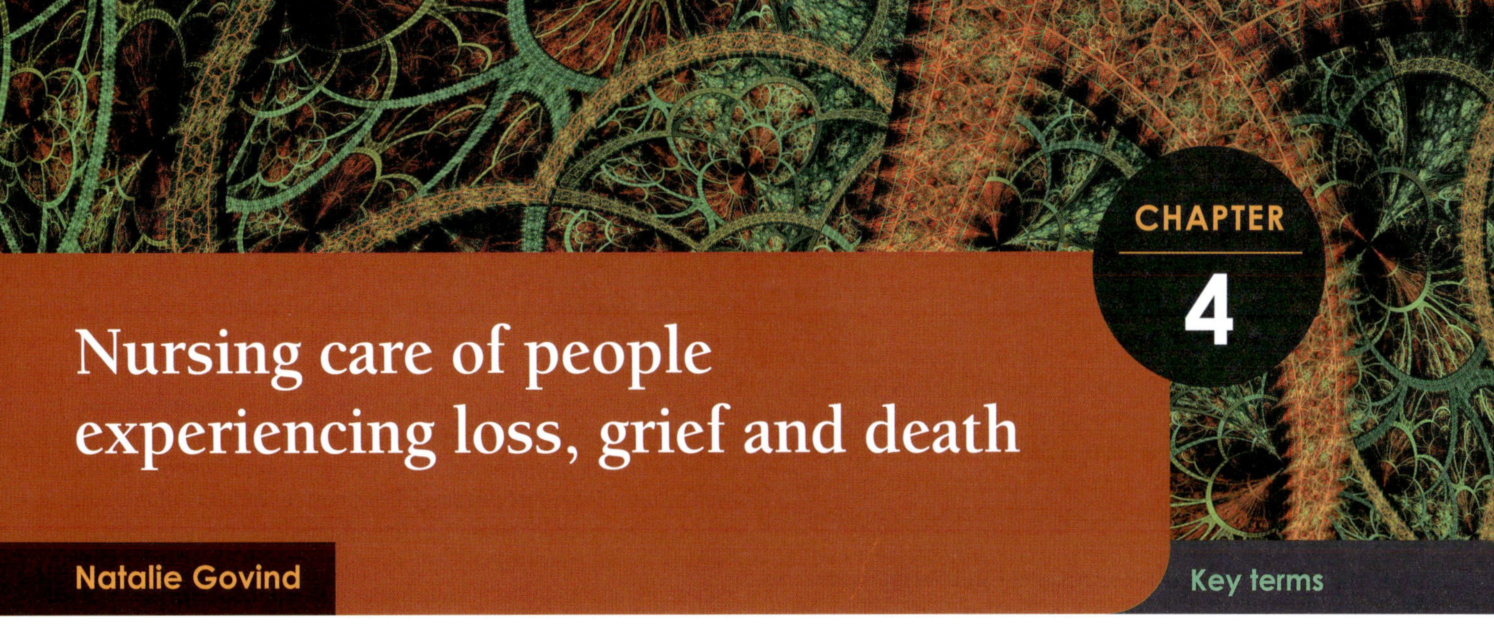

CHAPTER 4

Nursing care of people experiencing loss, grief and death

Natalie Govind

Key terms

advance directive 73
anticipatory grieving 79
chronic sorrow 79
death 66
death anxiety 79
do-not-resuscitate (DNR) directive 73
dyspnoea 74
end-of-life care 72
enduring power of attorney 73
grief 66
grieving 66
hospice care 73
life-limiting illness 66
loss 66
mourning 66
palliative care 73
voluntary assisted dying (VAD) 73

Learning outcomes

- Differentiate between loss, grief and mourning.
- Compare and contrast theories of loss and grief.
- Explain factors affecting responses to loss.
- Describe person-centred care and the role of the nurse in end-of-life care.
- Discuss legal and ethical issues in end-of-life care.
- Describe palliative care philosophy.

Clinical competencies

- Identify physiological changes in the dying person.
- Provide nursing interventions to promote a comfortable death.
- Provide person-centred care for individuals and families experiencing loss, grief or death.

LOSS, GRIEF AND MOURNING

Loss may be defined as an actual or potential situation in which a valued object, person, relationship, body part or emotion that was formerly present is lost or changed and can no longer be seen, felt, heard, known or experienced. A loss may be temporary or permanent, complete or partial, objectively verifiable or perceived, physical or symbolic. Only the person who experiences the loss can determine the meaning of the loss. Individuals experiencing health changes because of a life-limiting illness may also feel a loss of trust in their body; this is particularly so for individuals diagnosed with cancer. Although the importance of loss varies for each person, people most commonly fear the losses listed in Box 4.1.

Loss always results in change, and bereavement is considered life changing (Sadak & Weiser, 2017). The stress associated with loss may be the precipitating factor leading to physiological or psychological change in the person or family. The effective or ineffective resolution of feelings surrounding the loss determines the person's ability to deal with the resulting changes.

A **life-limiting illness** is defined as an illness:

> *where it is expected that death will be a direct consequence of the specified illness. Such illnesses may include, but are not limited to, cancer, heart disease, chronic obstructive pulmonary disease, dementia, heart failure, neurodegenerative disease, chronic liver disease and renal disease. The term 'person living with a life-limiting illness' also incorporates the concept that people are actively living with such illnesses, often for a long period of time, not simply dying.* (Palliative Care Australia, 2018a)

The word **grief** is derived from the Latin word *gravis*. Grief has been described as 'heavy, serious or burdensome' (Sadak & Weiser, 2017). It is the emotional response to loss and its accompanying changes. Grief as a response to loss is a normal and an inevitable dimension of the human experience and it should not be treated as pathological (Nyatanga, 2018). The loss of a job, a role (e.g. the loss of the role of spouse, as occurs in divorce), a goal, body integrity, a loved one, or the impending loss of one's own life may trigger grief. Loss is also integral to death. Although death is the penultimate loss, losses that occur in any phase of the life cycle may produce grief responses as intensely painful as those observed in the death experience.

BOX 4.1 Types of losses

- Death
- Health
- Body part
- Social status
- Lifestyle
- Relationship (i.e. through breakup or divorce)
- Reproductive function
- Sexual function

Grieving may be thought of as the internal process the person uses to work through the response to loss. **Mourning** describes the actions or expressions of the bereaved, including the symbols, clothing and ceremonies that make up the outward manifestations of grief. Both grieving and mourning are healthy responses to loss because they ultimately lead the person to process the loss and to invest energy in new beginnings or relationships.

A commonly used definition of **death** is an irreversible cessation of circulatory and respiratory functions or irreversible cessation of all functions of the entire brain, including the brainstem. With the current life support systems available, the most often used criterion for determining death is whole-brain death (permanent irreversible cessation of the functioning of all areas of the brain). The criteria for brain death are listed in the chapter 'Nursing care of people experiencing trauma and shock'.

Although death is an inevitable part of life, the acknowledgement of death as part of the process of a life-limiting illness is often immensely difficult for the person and their loved ones. Death may be accidental (such as from trauma), intentional (suicide) or at the end of a long and painful struggle with a life-limiting illness such as cancer or motor neurone disease.

THEORIES OF LOSS AND GRIEF

Nurses often care for individuals exhibiting responses to grieving. Highly individual in quality and duration, the grief process may range from discomforting to debilitating, and it may last a day or a lifetime, depending on what the loss means to the person experiencing it. Although each person experiences loss in a different manner, knowledge of some of the major theories of loss and grief can give nurses a framework for holistic, person-centred care of the individual and family anticipating or experiencing a loss. Table 4.1 summarises some of these theories.

TABLE 4.1 Summary of theories of loss

THEORIST	DYNAMICS
Freud (1917/1957)	Grief and mourning are reactions to loss. Grieving is the inner labour of mourning a loss. Inability to grieve a loss results in depression.
Bowlby (1973, 1980)	The successful grieving process initiated by a loss or separation during childhood ends with feelings of emancipation from the lost person or object.
Engel (1964)	After the person perceives and evaluates the loss, they adapt to it. Shock and disbelief, developing awareness and restitution occur during the first year following the loss; in the months following, the person puts the lost relationship into perspective.
Kübler-Ross (1969)	Five stages define the response to loss: denial, anger, bargaining, depression and acceptance. Stages are not necessarily sequential.
Caplan (1990)	Periods of psychological crisis are precipitated by hazardous circumstances; successful resolution of grief involves feelings of hope and engaging in activities of ordinary living.
Neimeyer (Neimeyer, Herrero & Botella, 2006)	This meaning-oriented perspective conceptualises grief as a highly individualised process that is largely influenced by the personal meanings people ascribe to a loss.

Freud: psychoanalytic theory

Freud (1917/1957) discussed grief and mourning as reactions to loss. He viewed the process of mourning as one in which the person gradually withdraws attachment from the lost object or person. Freud observed that with normal grieving, this withdrawal of attachment is followed by a readiness to make new attachments. In comparing melancholia (prolonged gloominess, depression) with the 'normal' emotions of grief and its expression in mourning, Freud observed that the 'work of mourning' is a non-pathological condition that reaches a state of completion after a period of inner labour.

Bowlby: protest, despair and detachment

Bowlby (1973, 1980) believed that the grieving process initiated by a loss or separation from a loved object or person successfully ends when the grieving person experiences feelings of emancipation. He divided the grieving process into three phases and identified behaviours characteristics of each phase.

1. *Protest.* The protest phase is marked by a lack of acceptance of the loss. All energy is directed towards protesting the loss. The person experiences feelings of anger towards self and others, and feelings of ambivalence towards the lost object or person. Crying and anger characterise this phase.
2. *Despair.* The person's behaviour becomes disorganised. Despair mounts as efforts to deny the loss compete with acceptance of permanent loss. Crying and sadness, coupled with a desire for the lost object or person to return, result in disorganised thoughts as the person recognises the reality of the loss.
3. *Detachment.* As the person realises the permanence of the loss and gradually relinquishes attachment to the lost object, a reinvestment of energy occurs. Both the positive and negative aspects of the relationship are remembered. Expressions of hopefulness and readiness to move forward are characteristic of this phase.

Engel: acute grief, restitution and long-term grief

Engel (1964) related the grief process to other methods of coping with stress: after the person perceives and evaluates the loss (the stressful event), they adapt to it. He described three main stages in the grief process: an acute stage, a restitution stage and a long-term stage. The acute stage is initiated by shock and disbelief and is manifested by denial, which may help the person to cope with their overwhelming pain. As the shock and disbelief begin to fade, the loss becomes a reality, and pain, anguish, anger, guilt and blame surface. Culturally patterned behaviour, such as maintaining a stoic pose in public or weeping openly, characterise this phase.

The acute stage is followed by a stage of restitution, in which the mourning is institutionalised. Friends and family gather to support the grieving person through rituals dictated by the culture. The mourner continues to feel a painful void and is preoccupied with thoughts of the loss. The bereaved may join a support group or seek other social support for coping with the loss. This stage lasts until the point at which the bereaved begins to come to terms with the loss and their interest in people and activities is renewed.

Kübler-Ross: stages of coping with loss

Kübler-Ross's (1969) research on death and dying identified that not all people dealing with a loss go through distinct stages, and those who do may not experience the stages in the sequence described. In identifying the stages of death and dying, Kübler-Ross (1978) repeatedly stressed the danger of prematurely labelling a 'stage' and emphasised that her goal was to describe her observations of how people come to terms with situations of loss.

Some or all of the following reactions may occur during the grieving process and may reappear as the person experiences the loss:

- *Denial.* A person may react with shock and disbelief after receiving word of an actual or potential loss. After receiving a life-limiting diagnosis, notification of a death or other serious loss, people may make such statements as 'This can't be happening to me' or 'This can't be true'.
- *Anger.* In the anger stage, the person resists the loss. The anger may be directed towards family members or healthcare providers.
- *Bargaining.* The bargaining stage serves as an attempt to postpone the reality of the loss. The person makes a secret bargain with a higher power, expressing a willingness to do anything to postpone the loss or change the prognosis.
- *Depression.* The person enters a stage of depression as the full impact of the actual or perceived loss is realised. The person prepares for the impending loss by working through the struggle of separation. While grieving over 'what cannot be', the person may either talk freely about the loss or withdraw from others.
- *Acceptance.* The person begins to come to terms with the loss and resumes activities with an air of hopefulness for the future. Some dying people, but not all, reach a stage of acceptance in which they may appear to be almost devoid of emotion. The struggle is past, and the emotional pain is gone.

Caplan: stress and loss

Caplan (1990) expanded the focus of the grief process to include not only bereavement but also other episodes of stress that people experience, such as the stress that can result from surgery or childbirth. Caplan described three factors that influence the person's ability to deal with a loss:

1. the psychic pain of the broken bond and the agony of coming to terms with the loss
2. living without the assets and guidance of the lost person or resource
3. the reduced cognitive and problem-solving effectiveness associated with the distressing emotional arousal.

He believed these factors might cause distress for a year or more following the loss.

Caplan described the process of building new attachments to replace those that have been lost. This process involves two elements: a feeling of hope and the assumption of regular activity as a form of participating in ordinary living.

Neimeyer: meaning-oriented perspective

Neimeyer's meaning-orientated approach (Holland & Neimeyer, 2010) focuses on grief as highly individualised and influenced by the personal meanings attributed to loss. Individual strategies acknowledge the meaning of the loss in ways to assist individuals cope with their grief.

FACTORS AFFECTING RESPONSES TO LOSS

A variety of factors affect a person's responses to loss. These include age, social support, families, cultural and spiritual practices, and rituals of mourning.

Age

The understanding of and reaction to loss is influenced by the age of the person experiencing the loss. In general, as people experience life transitions, their ability to understand and accept the losses associated with the transitions increases. From the age of 3 years, the development of the concept of death as a loss proceeds rapidly. However, from the toddler to older adolescents, individuals may experience difficulties expressing their emotional responses.

Social support

Grieving is painful and lonely. One's social support system is important because of its potentially positive influence on the successful resolution of grief. Some losses may lead to social isolation, placing the individual at high risk of dysfunctional grief reactions. Characteristic factors that can interfere with successful grieving include the following:

- perceived inability to share the loss
- lack of social recognition of the loss
- ambivalent relationships prior to the loss
- extreme traumatic circumstances of the loss.

The relocation of work or home, a relationship breakdown or even the death of a pet can cause a person to feel extremely isolated, yet the person experiencing these types of losses does not ordinarily receive the same social support offered to the person mourning the death of a loved one. Additionally, a woman having an abortion or giving up a child for adoption seldom receives the same social support as a mother who has lost a child at birth. It is especially important, therefore, for the nurse *not* to place a value on the individual's loss when assessing the need for support.

The painful nature of grief can cause the individual to withdraw from a previously established social support system, thereby increasing the feelings of loneliness caused by the loss. A recently widowed woman, for example, may refuse invitations involving married couples with whom she had socialised while her husband was alive. The individual's needs for social interaction, however, remain similar to those established before the loss.

Families

A well-functioning family usually rallies after the initial shock and disbelief and provides support for each other during all phases of the grieving process. After a loss, the functional family is able to shift roles, levels of responsibility and ways of communicating.

However, the family may have a negative as well as a positive impact. For example, the dying person may request that someone the family perceives as an outsider be near, and the family may respond with anger to the perceived 'intrusion'. Well-meaning family members also may try to shield the individual from the pain of grieving. It is rare for the family and the dying person to experience anger, denial and acceptance in unison. While one member is in denial, another may be angry because 'not enough is being done'.

Cultural and spiritual practices

Spirituality is at the core of human existence, involving personal authenticity and connecting oneself with nature or perhaps a God/life source (Lovgren et al., 2017). It involves a person's beliefs and values, and cannot be viewed in isolation from their culture and background (Abbas & Panjwani, 2008). When confronted by a life-limiting illness, people often ask questions of themselves, and others, as to what their life has meant, why this illness has affected them and what will happen to them when they die. Spirituality can provide structure to a person's experience, giving a sense of coherence, and can assist with coping and providing feelings of wellbeing (Vivat, 2008).

Many individuals have beliefs about their life and death, including principles and values that they have lived by, their personal philosophy and the goals they have pursued in life. These beliefs may be questioned as the individual responds to actual or perceived losses experienced in their life. If unresolved, these concerns and perceptions can lead to spiritual or existential distress, causing a sense of hopelessness, anxiety and depression. When spiritual distress is resolved, people can die more peacefully.

For some people, spirituality is about religion, while for others it is about making sense of their existence. Spirituality is a way of being and often involves multiple practices or ways of understanding experiences; it is, therefore, not necessarily the same for everyone.

Abbas and Panjwani (2008) point out that failure to provide spiritual care means failure to provide holistic care. The care of a dying person needs more than attention to physical needs; it must also take into account a holistic approach involving a spiritual dimension of care (O'Brien et al., 2019; Penman, Oliver & Harrington, 2013; Puchalski et al., 2014). Spiritual care needs to be person-centred and is central to safe and effective nursing care.

Nurses play an important role in caring for people who are experiencing a life-limiting illness (see Figure 4.1) and

PATIENT SAFETY COMPETENCY FRAMEWORK

1 Person-centred care

The Patient Safety Competency Framework indicates that nursing students must demonstrate person-centred care by providing holistic care that takes into account the person's current situation, previous experiences and life history (Levett-Jones et al., 2017).

spirituality is an important part of nursing practice. To assist with the person's spiritual needs, nurses can help them, through sensitive and empathetic responding, to accept the uncertainty that comes with their illness and possible death. Respect for the cultural and spiritual beliefs and practices of people and their families is paramount in caring for dying people. Context and environment are both an important part of a person's experience of spirituality (Rudolfsson, Berggren & da Silva, 2014). People who are religious need opportunities for prayer, devotions and religious rituals. Those without religious beliefs may find solace and achieve a sense of spirituality from meditation, guided imagery, music or art.

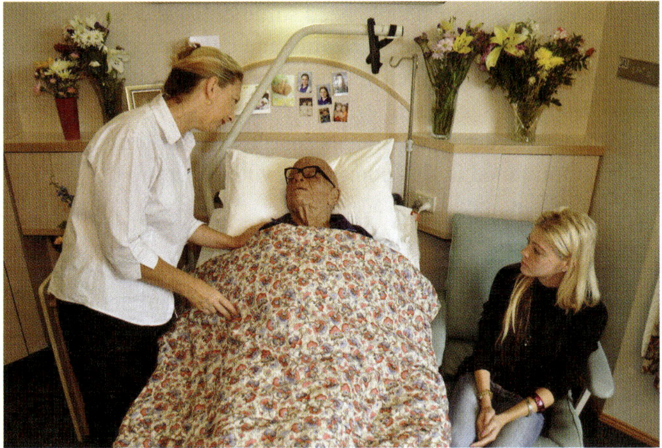

FIGURE 4.1 ***Nurses play an important role in caring for people who are experiencing a life-limiting illness.***

Source: Courtesy of Tracy Levett-Jones.

It is essential that the nurse has the ability to reflect on their own practice and actions that support the spirituality of the people they care for. For the nurse, the concept of spirituality may be captured by the sense of seeing people at peace or expressing that they feel balanced and connected again. Spirituality also encapsulates the sense of the nurse connecting with a person, having an understanding of their suffering and being privileged to see their courage and strength. It could be sharing an intimate moment with a person.

Rituals of mourning

Through participation in ceremonies such as baptisms, confirmations and weddings, people joyously celebrate progression to a new stage of life and loss of a former way of being. The funeral ceremony may serve many purposes in meeting the needs of the bereaved, as people gather to share their loss. Through the funeral preparation and ceremony, people may symbolically express triumph over death and deny the fear of death. Culture is the primary factor that dictates the rituals of mourning. It is important for health professionals to understand and respect the diversity that exists in our society in relation to grief and loss. The following section is intended to guide health professionals in developing an understanding of the diverse cultures within our society.

Death and dying in Indigenous Australian culture

There are no set rules that define how Indigenous Australians react to the loss of a loved one. However, many of the customs observed during funerals in the past are still evident in contemporary Indigenous society. Health professionals should take into account the impact of colonisation and intergenerational trauma when addressing the needs of Indigenous Australians. Christianity, assimilation and other values and beliefs adopted from colonial society have also affected how Indigenous Australians now treat death and dying. Indigenous Australian culture is an evolving social phenomenon bringing change and diversity.

Links to National Patient Safety Standards

NSQHS: Partnering with Consumers Standard

The intention of this standard is to create a health service that involves patients in their own care and provides effective communication to patients and their families (Australian Commission on Safety and Quality in Health Care (ACSQHC), 2021). Implementation of this standard is ensured through strong governance structures that reflect the importance of the cultural diversity of a population. Partnering with consumers supports the active participation of all groups in the evaluation and improvement of an organisation, especially those groups who may not always participate in providing feedback.

Patients who are dying and their grieving families are extremely vulnerable and need to feel safe and supported by compassionate and professional care. Culturally competent partnerships between healthcare systems, services, patients, families, carers and consumers are important in ensuring a sense of dignity and safety in the vulnerable state of grief and loss. Systems that support consumers as partners in planning, designing and evaluating care can strengthen the delivery of culturally competent care, ensuring that with ongoing support, patients and their families will adapt to loss.

Source: ACSQHC (2021). *National Safety and Quality Health Service Standards* (2nd ed.). Sydney: ACSQHC. © Australian Commission on Safety and Quality in Health Care.

Links to National Patient Safety Standards

NSQHS: Comprehensive Care Standard

The aim of this standard is to delivery comprehensive healthcare for patients that meets their individual needs. Comprehensive care considers the impact of their health issues on their life and wellbeing and ensures that all care is clinically appropriate.

Supporting the delivery of excellent end-of-life care is a part of delivering comprehensive care that aligns with the patient's expressed goals of care and healthcare needs, considers the impact of the patient's health issues on their life and wellbeing, and is clinically appropriate. It is important that care is provided continuously and collaboratively in line with their diagnoses and agreed goals of care. Their comprehensive care plan should reflect their individual preferences.

Source: ACSQHC (2021). *National Safety and Quality Health Service Standards* (2nd ed.). Sydney: ACSQHC. © Australian Commission on Safety and Quality in Health Care.

The following information reflects some of the history, customs and values of Indigenous Australians during times of grief, bereavement and funerals, and suggests approaches for healthcare professionals providing care for Indigenous Australians.

POST-TRAUMATIC STRESS SYNDROME Colonisation has had a major transgenerational impact on the psyche of many Indigenous Australians. As noted in Henry Reynold's seminal work, *Frontier*, the conflicts between Indigenous Australians and Europeans included massacres, dispossession, displacement and alienation, and there were many deaths and funerals (Reynolds, 1989). The socio-historical impact of these experiences on contemporary Indigenous Australians carries an intergenerational effect that should be considered when dealing with issues of death and dying.

GRIEF AND BEREAVEMENT FOR INDIGENOUS AUSTRALIANS There are fundamental issues that are critical to the provision of adequate support and comfort to Indigenous people experiencing grief and bereavement following the loss of loved ones. Even though there are commonalities in the ways in which different Indigenous groups cope with death, there are also many differences.

- *Grief counselling*. The family, extended family and friends gather around the deceased person as a collective group. This practice allows the grieving party space, connection and, most importantly, an opportunity to provide support to each other in a time of grief, loss and crisis. This support operates as a mechanism whereby the members of the group perform the roles of grief counsellor, bereavement counsellor and priest, therefore facilitating the healing process.
- *Barriers*. One of the major problems that confronts Indigenous people and healthcare professionals can result from rigid hospital policies and administrative bureaucracies. In the event that an Indigenous person dies in hospital, there may be policies that restrict visitation. For example, in some hospitals restrictions may apply that allow no more than two or three people to be with the dying or deceased person at any one time, and there may also be policies that only permit visitors between certain hours. These rules are impediments to the essence of healing in Indigenous Australian culture. They stop critical connections, respect and space, and deny the opportunity for the enactment of the healing process. Large numbers of Indigenous people faced with institutional barriers to this healing process may end up gathering inside and outside hospital areas where they can group together.
- *Space*. Indigenous people need sufficient space to gather together to facilitate the grieving and bereavement process where they can offer each other support, respect and counselling (see Figure 4.2).
- *Respect*. Health professionals should listen and understand the importance of this connection with regard to the grieving and healing process.
- *Time*. The grieving and bereavement process may take days or even weeks. It is important to respect this process and to provide space for this length of time. For example, in the early 20th century, if an Indigenous woman lost and buried her child, she grieved at the gravesite until new grass began shooting where her child was buried. During this period of

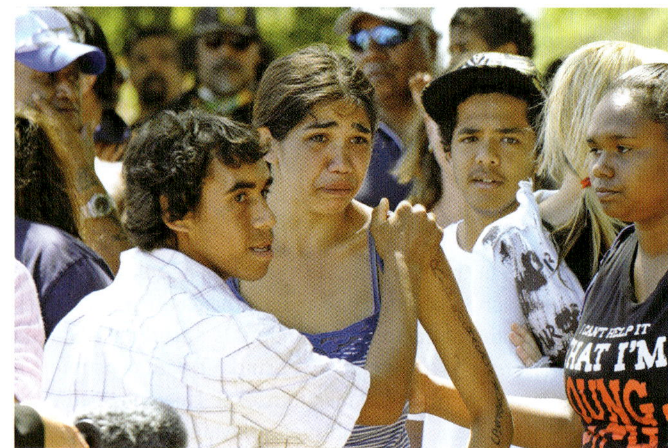

FIGURE 4.2 ***Indigenous Australians need sufficient space to gather together to facilitate the grieving and bereavement process where they can offer each other support, respect and counselling***

Source: © Dave Hunt/AAP Image.

around 2 weeks, other members of the community brought food and water to support the grieving mother.

- *Cultural safety*. Health professionals create a culturally safe environment through awareness and consideration of the Indigenous person's cultural identity and acknowledgement of their difference within a Western-orientated healthcare system. The Nursing Council of New Zealand (2002, p. 9) defines unsafe cultural practice as any actions that 'diminish, demean or disempower the cultural identity of an individual'. Listening in a non-judgmental way to Indigenous people is critical to cultural safety. As a nurse, culturally safe practice means recognising and understanding the dynamics of cultural, personal and professional power (Richardson & Carryer, 2005).

Notifying the designated Aboriginal Liaison Coordinator attached to the hospital about the death is critical, as this is often a link to the deceased person and their family.

The following quote provides some insight into the meaning of death, and the connection to life and land, for the Indigenous person: 'Tree the same as me, When he get old he'll die. He'll be dead and burn. He'll leave his ashes behind. Tree becomes earth' (Neidjie, 1985).

There may well be diversity and cultural variances that differ from a nurse's own practices and beliefs. If Indigenous Australians are able to facilitate their own healing mechanisms and engage in mutual respect, connection and group support, then these practices will often minimise the need for ongoing support or bereavement counselling.

Cultural diversity in the care of individuals with a life-limiting illness

Cultural factors shape patients' preferences around decision making, receiving bad news and end-of-life care. As Rosenblatt (2017) points out, a perspective on grief needs to be open and respectful of cultural diversity. Rituals and practices within society are fluid and diverse, and are affected by changes within the society, and community and family groups. Asking a series of respectful open-ended questions about an individual's culture provides critical insights into the person's values, beliefs and needs in the context of end-of-life care.

The following 'Focus on cultural diversity' box provides some insights into the practices of major cultural groups present in Australia. This is not a prescription for caring for individuals within these cultures with a life-limiting illness and it is important not to make assumptions about people's values and beliefs. Nurses should focus on the individual and provide respect and care in response to their particular needs.

FOCUS ON CULTURAL DIVERSITY Cultural aspects of caring for people nearing the end of life

CULTURE	NURSING CONSIDERATIONS
Arabic	Arabic-speaking people tend to come from the Middle East, Asia and north-east Africa and follow the Muslim culture. In this culture, prior to death, suffering should be relieved (administration of pain medication is acceptable). Patients who are too ill to perform *wudu* (ritual washing) may use a dry ablution kit, which can be sand or stone. After death, the patient's eyes should be closed and the patient's body covered. A final prayer may be recited by family and friends. The body of the deceased should be handed over as soon as possible to the Muslim community as burial within 24 hours is almost always requested (Leong et al., 2016).
Chinese	Within Chinese culture, traditional philosophies such as Confucianism and ancestor worship, as well as the religions of Taoism and Buddhism, influence how death and dying are perceived. These beliefs can lead to cultural avoidance towards death and dying for fear of bad luck and misfortune. Cultural aspects relating to autonomy and the importance of family also affect how death and dying are perceived, particularly in decision making. Chinese culture does not view autonomy as necessary, with families taking a more significant role than the individual in the decision-making process of illnesses (Huang et al., 2015; Zheng et al., 2015).
Indian	Hinduism, the main religion of India, views death as transition to another life by reincarnation. There is a notion of a good death, and a bad death is greatly feared. Good karma is said to lead to good birth and bad karma to bad rebirth, with suffering explained in terms of past karma. People may attempt to detach themselves from material and emotional concerns and prepare for death through prayer, scripture reading and meditation. A dying person may refuse medications so as to die with a clear and unclouded mind (Sharma et al., 2013). Nurses need to check with the family as to what they can or cannot do before the person has died. For example, if a person dies when no family member is present, the nurses need to find out if they can touch the body before a member of the family arrives.
Greek	In the past, the family may have controlled information related to an individual's condition and not provided the person with that information. However, this approach has changed over time, although the family is still significantly involved in care and decision making. Home is a significant place and is the preferred care environment. Nurses should offer to contact the family priest who may give communion, rather than 'last rites', as this has a more positive connotation.
Italian	The family is usually involved when the person's condition is discussed and may wish to shelter the person from discussions of diagnosis and prognosis. Home is the preferred place for care. Prayer may be an important part of end-of-life care and it is important to offer attendance by a priest.
Korean	The eldest son in the family should be involved in discussions concerning the individual's condition. The hospital tends to be the preferred place to die, especially if there are young children living at home. Many Koreans follow a Buddhist or Confucianist doctrine of religion and the family may have sought help from a herbal doctor called a '*Hanui*'.
Polish	Family is a significant part of healthcare; however, not all individuals have family present in Australia. Home is the preferred place for care although hospital and hospice environments are also considered acceptable. Many Polish people are involved in the Catholic Church, and respect for the church and a belief in God is a significant aspect of life.
Vietnamese	The head of the family should be present when illness and dying is discussed. The entire family may be involved in end-of-life decisions, often with assistance from spiritual leaders such as a priest or monk. Individuals often prefer to die at home. The family should have extra time with the body, and vocal expressions of grief are not uncommon. After the person has died, the family might request to open all the windows and outside doors of the room to allow the person's spirit to leave their body.

Source: Adapted from Palliative Care Victoria (2016). *Cultural perspectives and values from ten culturally and linguistically diverse communities in Victoria*. Retrieved from https://www.pallcarevic.asn.au/page/102/culturally-linguistically-diverse-people.

END-OF-LIFE CARE

End-of-life care includes physical, spiritual and psychosocial assessment, and care and management delivered by health professionals and support staff. It also includes support of families and carers and care of the person's body after their death. People are 'approaching the end of life' when they are likely to die within the next 12 months. This includes people whose death is imminent (expected within a few hours or days) and those with:

- advanced, progressive, incurable conditions
- general frailty and coexisting conditions that mean that they are expected to die within 12 months
- existing conditions if they are at risk of dying from a sudden acute crisis in their condition
- life-threatening acute conditions caused by sudden catastrophic events (Department of Health, 2018).

The ACSQHC (2020) has developed a series of fact sheets to support clinicians providing care to people who are nearing the end of life. Key points include:

- Deliver care with kindness and compassion and maintain patient dignity.
- Share decision making about end-of-life care.
- Communicate openly and honestly with patients and families about prognosis.
- Prioritise comfort measures, pain control and symptom management.
- Ensure appropriate access to subcutaneous opioids and palliative medications.
- Review medication.
- Consider time limits for trial therapies.
- Avoid unnecessary monitoring and interventions.
- Be aware of common risks of harm for patients at the end of life.
- The unique needs of dying people are considered, their comfort maximised and their dignity preserved.
- Staff and volunteers reflect on practice and initiate and maintain effective self-care strategies.

Nursing considerations for palliative and end-of-life care

Nurses care for people who are dying in many environments, including acute hospital settings such as intensive care and emergency departments; sub-acute settings such as geriatric, psychogeriatric and palliative care; residential aged care facilities; hospices; and the home. Regardless of the setting, the individual's wishes about death should be respected. (See the 'Translation to practice' box for research on intensive care nurses' experiences with end-of-life care.)

Legal and ethical issues

Decision making and consent are issues that are often debated strongly when considering end-of-life care. The legal and ethical issues surrounding advance care directives, enduring power of attorney or guardianship, and do-not-resuscitate (DNR) directives and quality of life are especially important to nurses in upholding each person's specific care requests. Types of advance directives are shown in Box 4.2.

TRANSLATION TO PRACTICE — **Challenges providing end-of-life care in acute care settings**

Patterns of dying and death are changing worldwide. Most patients state that their preference is to die at home. However, in developed countries, the majority of deaths occur in acute care settings such as medical and surgical wards, emergency departments and intensive care units (Gardiner et al., 2013). Symptom management, carer fatigue, feelings of uncertainty and limited access to resources contribute to the decision to seek hospital admission at the end of life (Gerber et al., 2019). Although studies show that death occurs more frequently in hospitals, providing end-of-life care in an acute care setting can be challenging because hospital care is typically focused on prolonging life and modifying disease. Lack of clinical knowledge; limited access to training; communication barriers across the interprofessional team and with patients and families; insufficient organisational support, including adequate staffing levels; and care environment can all impact on the delivery of quality end-of-life care (Saunders et al., 2021).

IMPLICATIONS FOR NURSING

Kirchhoff et al. (2000) advocate that, regardless of the setting for end-of-life care, nurses need to ensure that individuals are as free from pain as possible, and that their comfort and dignity are maintained. In addition, family members should be given time to begin to accept the dying process. This may be facilitated by having the family member involved in care and providing the time and space for family rituals and saying goodbye.

CRITICAL THINKING IN PERSON-CENTRED CARE

1. What environmental differences are present in the emergency department of an acute care hospital that might make quality end-of-life care more difficult for nurses?
2. The family of a person in the intensive care unit says to you, 'My son is going to die, isn't he?' What would you need to know before responding? How would you respond?
3. A person in the surgical ward, who previously had been improving, suddenly dies. Staff are saddened and several are in tears. A more experienced nurse says, 'Oh, you just have to go on. There's nothing else to do.' Do you agree? Why or why not?

BOX 4.2 Types of advance directives

Advance directives, sometimes referred to as 'living wills', are legal documents that allow a person to plan their healthcare or provide insights into treatment preferences in the event of incapacity (Weathers et al., 2016). Advance directives may be formally written legal documents, including living wills or enduring powers of attorney, or informal orally communicated requests expressed to loved ones, carers or health professionals. Advocating for the person's treatment preferences is an aspect of care that many nurses will face, and the nurse must always ensure that they are aware of the preferences stated in the patient's directives. The legislation across Australia concerning advance directives varies, so it is essential that the nurse is familiar with the approach taken by the state or territory in which they are practising.

Advanced care planning has evolved in the face of limitations associated with advance directives. An advanced care plan should support the advance directive, in that it further documents communications on the person's preferences as to future care and/or the withdrawal of care and treatment.

An **enduring power of attorney** is a document that can delegate the authority to make health, financial and/or legal decisions on a person's behalf. It must be provided in writing and state that the designated person is authorised to make healthcare decisions.

A **do-not-resuscitate (DNR) directive** or *not for resuscitation (NFR) order* is written by the doctor for the individual for whom it is believed that cardiopulmonary resuscitation (CPR) would be of no benefit. This order is usually based on the wishes of the individual and family that no CPR be performed for respiratory or cardiac arrest. However, this directive does not extend to all treatment and care, and the nurse must ensure that other treatments should be offered and discussed with the person if applicable. The nurse must ensure that current, clear verbal and written communication of the directive is established within the multidisciplinary team, the person and the family.

Source: Based on Johnstone (2019). *Bioethics: A nursing perspective* (7th ed.) Sydney: Elsevier.

Voluntary assisted dying (VAD) refers to the assistance provided to a person by a health practitioner to end their life. It includes:

- *self-administration*, where the person takes the VAD medication themselves
- *practitioner administration*, where the person is given the medication by a doctor (or in some Australian states, a Nurse Practitioner or Registered Nurse).

'Voluntary' indicates that the practice is a choice of the person. They must be competent (have capacity) to decide to access VAD and meet the eligibility criteria outlined in the relevant legislation (QUT, 2022).

VAD is a difficult and complex legal and ethical issue. In Australia, VAD laws have been passed in all states. Nurses need to be aware that there are differences across all passed VAD state laws. It is important to note that Palliative Care Australia holds the view that VAD is not part of palliative care practice.

Settings for palliative and end-of-life care

Settings and services for the provision of end-of-life care range from residential aged care facilities, hospitals and hospices to the person's own home. **Palliative care** is a term used within Australia to describe an approach that improves the quality of life of patients and their families facing the problems associated with life-limiting illness, through the prevention and relief of suffering by means of early identification and impeccable assessment and treatment of pain and other physical, psychosocial and spiritual problems.

In the literature, the term '**hospice care**' may be used to refer to the philosophy of care; however, in Australia, the term 'hospice' more often refers to a setting where palliative care is provided. The philosophy of palliative care is outlined in this section, followed by a brief description of the settings in which this philosophy may be integrated into care.

Philosophy of palliative care

Palliative care is a philosophy of care, rather than a program of care. It is person centred, comprehensive and coordinated care for individuals with a life-limiting illness, provided where possible in a setting of the person's choice (Department of Health, 2018). Palliative care reaffirms the right of every person and family to fully participate in the final stages of life. It is provided by nurses, doctors, allied health professionals and volunteers. Palliative care:

- provides relief from pain and other distressing symptoms
- affirms life and regards dying as a normal process
- intends neither to hasten nor postpone death
- integrates the psychological and spiritual aspects of patient care
- offers a support system to help patients live as actively as possible until death
- offers a support system to help the family cope during the patient's illness and in their own bereavement
- uses a team approach to address the needs of patients and their families, including bereavement counselling, if indicated
- will enhance quality of life and may also positively influence the course of illness
- is applicable early in the course of illness, in conjunction with other therapies that are intended to prolong life, such as chemotherapy or radiation therapy, and includes those investigations needed to better understand and manage distressing clinical complications (Department of Health, 2018).

HOME/RESIDENTIAL AGED CARE FACILITY/COMMUNITY LIVING An individual often prefers to die at their permanent living environment, which may include a private home or residential aged care facility. Community or hospital/hospice outreach program-based nurses working within the palliative care philosophy are usually the main care providers for individuals in this setting. It is essential that care provided to individuals in their home includes ongoing comprehensive assessment involving the person, the family and the support services that are available, including general medical and palliative care specialist teams.

HOSPICE/INPATIENT PALLIATIVE CARE UNIT The hospice or inpatient palliative care setting is not restricted to the end of life and is often used earlier in the illness experience. Individuals may seek admission for assessment, symptom management, carer's stress, respite or end-of-life care. The hospice or inpatient palliative care unit environment may be separate from or connected to a hospital setting and is focused on the relief of physical, emotional and spiritual distress for individuals who have a life-limiting illness. Its goal is to prevent and relieve suffering by early assessment and treatment of pain and other physical, psychosocial and spiritual needs to improve the person's quality of life.

The team providing care to individuals in this setting has a well-defined palliative care philosophy and usually includes doctors, nurses, allied health professionals (including social workers, physiotherapists, occupational therapists and dietitians), pastoral care, community liaison nurses and volunteers. If it is the individual's wish to return to their home environment, this is supported by the team with continued assessment and involvement of a community outreach hospice/palliative care team. The expected outcomes of care are directed by interventions to manage current manifestations of the illness and to prevent new manifestations from occurring.

ACUTE HOSPITAL SETTING Individuals with a life-limiting illness who are receiving palliative care often move between hospice/palliative environments and the acute care setting. In recognition of this, acute care nurses need to understand the palliative care philosophy in order to facilitate and support people's individual care needs.

Symptom management for the person with palliative care needs

Death is a highly individualised process and may occur rapidly or slowly. Physiological changes are a part of the dying process. Although each person responds differently, certain manifestations are common in the dying process, regardless of the trauma or illness process that is causing death. Managing symptoms is core business for palliative care. Nurses have a role in helping to achieve the best symptom control and optimum quality of life for patients with palliative care needs. The following sections outline common symptoms in palliative care.

Pain

Pain is a common problem for individuals with a life-limiting illness and people can experience unacceptably and often preventable levels of pain related to the illness or the treatment. Pain is what individuals often say they fear the most. It is a subjective experience influenced by the person's emotions, previous experiences with pain, and family and culture. Comprehensive ongoing pain assessment and treatment is essential and it is of utmost importance to keep the individual comfortable through general comfort measures (see Box 4.3). Both pharmacological and non-pharmacological approaches are available as part of effective pain management. Opioids are the first-line analgesia, along with simple analgesics or adjuvants, which may improve analgesic efficacy and reduce total opioid doses. For neuropathic pain, two groups of medications are suggested as first-line adjuvant treatment: (1) antidepressants (tricyclics, or duloxetine or venlafaxine), and (2) anticonvulsants (either gabapentin or pregabalin). The pathophysiology, treatment and nursing care of people experiencing pain are fully described in the chapter 'Nursing care of people in pain'.

BOX 4.3 Providing comfort for the person nearing death

- Maintain clean skin and bed linens.
- Use a slide sheet to turn the person as often as required to keep them comfortable.
- Position the person to promote comfort and protect bony areas with padding. Reposition the person and raise the head of the bed if fluids accumulate in the upper airways and back of the throat.
- Use incontinence pads or insert an indwelling catheter (only if ordered) for urinary incontinence.
- Use gentle massage to reduce anxiety, improve circulation and shift oedema.
- Provide small, frequent sips of fluids or ice chips.
- Provide oral care, using a soft moist brush or moistened swabs (do not use glycerine swabs as they dry out the mouth). Keep lips moist with balm such as lanoline.
- Clean secretions from the eyes and nose.
- Administer prescribed pain medications as needed to maintain comfort.

CONSIDERATION FOR PRACTICE

Pain in palliative care patients should be actively identified, carefully assessed and treated promptly.

Discussing the pain management plan with the person and their family/caregivers is an important process which can improve overall symptom management and quality of life.

Dyspnoea

Dyspnoea is the symptom of breathlessness. Although it may be experienced by some individuals with lung disease throughout their illness trajectory, it is a common symptom for many people in the terminal stage. Dyspnoea is a subjective experience and individuals may report feelings of suffocation, shortness of breath or tightness in the chest, which increase their anxiety and distress.

As death nears, respirations often become fast or slow, shallow and laboured. The person may have apnoea or Cheyne-Stokes respirations (regular periods of deep, rapid breathing followed by no breaths for 5 to 30 seconds). Secretions often gather at the back of the throat, which may cause an audible sound as the person breathes through them (Nuccio & Nuccio, 2009). This can be very distressing for family members and they should be reassured that these symptoms are normal for a person close to death. Fluid may also accumulate in the lungs, causing rales and rhonchi, especially in people who are well hydrated and are having difficulty swallowing or coughing. These sounds are not usually distressing for the person, but they may be treated by changing their position and administering oxygen and opioids (to improve respirations and decrease anxiety). Anticholergic drugs provided early in care, prior to the build-up of secretions, can also be helpful for people at the end of life (Nuccio & Nuccio, 2009).

Note that oxygen and suctioning are only temporary measures and may even be traumatic for the person. Nursing care that may improve respiration includes keeping the head of the bed elevated and regular position changes. Agents that are being studied include hyoscine hydrobromide, hyoscine butylbromide and glycopyrronium bromide. These agents inhibit salivary secretions more than bronchial secretions. At this stage, no particular medication is recommended. If used, the choice should also include consideration of the potential side effects of the various drugs available including delirium/agitation, sedation, dry mouth, urinary retention and palpitations. Side effects are presumed to be less distressing in an unconscious patient.

For individuals experiencing dyspnoea earlier in their illness, the breeze from a fan may provide some benefit.

Nausea, anorexia and dehydration

Typically, people at the end stage of life will be drinking and eating very little, if at all. This reduction in food and fluid intake may occur for a number of reasons, including symptoms of nausea and vomiting, dysphagia (difficulty swallowing) or as a result of fatigue. It may also be related to a reduced level of consciousness, a bowel obstruction or simply anorexia (the absence of appetite) (van der Riet, 2009).

Nausea, with or without vomiting, is a common problem experienced by dying people. Nausea and vomiting may be caused by reduced gastric emptying, constipation or bowel obstruction, or be a side effect of morphine, uraemia or hypercalcaemia. The following list includes anti-emetic medications that may be used for nausea and vomiting at the end stage of life: prochlorperazine (Phenergan) or odansetron (Zofran), metoclopramide (Maxalon), levomepramazine, methotrimeprazine (Nozinan), cyclizine and haloperidol (Serenace). As with all medications, those used as anti-emetics may cause further complications or compound present health issues, such as increased constipation or drowsiness. It is essential that the nurse conduct a comprehensive assessment prior to and following the initiation of any medication regimens ordered.

Anorexia is another issue faced by many people at the end of life. However, anorexia may be a protective mechanism by the body. The breakdown of body fats results in ketosis, which leads to a sense of wellbeing and helps decrease pain. This is one reason that parenteral or enteral feeding is not advocated at the end of life as it does not improve symptoms or prolong life, and may actually cause discomfort (Good et al., 2011).

Anorexia and a decrease in food and fluid intake are normal in the dying person; however, the family may view the practice of not enforcing fluids and food as 'giving up'. They may feel that their loved one is being abandoned if nurses and doctors are not intervening by providing intravenous fluids (van der Riet et al., 2008). All people at the end of life should be offered food and drink, but intravenous fluids are not routinely given (Carter, 2020).

Families need to be aware that dehydration is less of a problem than over-hydration. Forcing fluids or initiating intravenous fluids for hydration may in turn have adverse affects such as pulmonary oedema (increased fluid in the lungs), peripheral oedema, ascites, excessive wound or fistula drainage, and increased gastrointestinal secretions leading to vomiting.

Dehydration in the person nearing death primarily causes discomfort from dry mouth and thirst. The person should be given small sips of water, or an atomiser can be used to spray the inside of the mouth. Mouth care should be provided at least every 2 hours, and more often if the person is breathing through their mouth. Good mouth care should involve moistening swabs with water (not glycerine swabs, as they dry mucous membranes), an oral gel or oral spray. It is important to avoid any drying agents such as lollies (sugar-free are fine), coffee and high-sugar drinks. When cleaning the person's teeth, there is no need to rinse the toothpaste away. Mouthwashes may be used if tolerated and might include the following: salt and soda bicarbonate, Difflam and chlorhexidine.

CONSIDERATION FOR PRACTICE

Intravenous tubing may affect communication and physical contact between the person who is dying and their loved ones. In a study by van der Riet et al. (2008), nurses reported that having tubes or lines in place, such as intravenous lines, affected the intimacy and their relationship with family members.

Altered levels of consciousness

Neurological dysfunction may result from any or all of the following: decreased cerebral perfusion, hypoxaemia, metabolic acidosis, sepsis, an accumulation of toxins from liver and renal failure, the effects of medications and disease-related factors. These changes may result in a decreased level of consciousness or agitated delirium (Bush et al., 2014). People with terminal delirium may be confused, restless or agitated. Moaning, groaning and grimacing often accompany the agitation and may be misinterpreted as pain. The level of consciousness often decreases to the point where the person cannot be aroused. Although decreased consciousness and agitation are both normal states at the end of life, they can be very distressing to the individual's family.

If possible, treatment for confusion or agitation is based on its cause—for example, pain or dyspnoea. Other medications include low doses of neuroleptics, anti-psychotics or anti-anxiety medications. A person near death often has altered cerebral function, so the nurse must stand near the bedside and speak clearly and gently. Hearing is believed to be the last sense a dying person loses, so the nurse should never whisper or engage in conversation with the family as if the person were not there.

Hypotension

As death nears, cardiac output decreases, as does intravascular blood volume. As a result, the person's blood pressure gradually decreases, and the pulse is often rapid and irregular. The extremities are cooler, and cyanosis is present in nail beds, skin and lips. The skin on the legs and in dependent areas may become mottled in colour. Renal perfusion decreases, the kidneys cease to function and anuria occurs.

Complementary therapies: their use in end-of-life care

Complementary therapy is a broad term that recognises the link between the individual's mind, body and soul as fundamental to their health and wellbeing (Zeng et al., 2018). Complementary therapies at the end of life have the potential to promote relaxation and comfort. The most frequently used complementary therapies for people requiring palliative care include aromatherapy, meditation, visualisation and massage (Zeng et al., 2018). Nowadays, in a hospital setting it is not uncommon to see family members or carers practising therapies such as Reiki or therapeutic touch on a dying person. Reiki has been described as an art in which the practitioner transfers life energy between the practitioner and person in a compassionate way to bring balance, strength and harmony to both body and mind (Bossi, Ott & DeCristofare, 2008). For dying patients Reiki has the benefit of an improved sense of wellbeing and a positive sense of spiritual renewal (Viliotti, 2013). Throughout the trajectory of an illness it is important for the nurse to adequately assess, inform, educate and support the person through the process of investigation, trial and use of complementary therapies. These therapies may also contribute to a nurse's self-care strategies, especially modalities such as yoga and meditation.

Support for the person and family

As the person's condition deteriorates, the nurse's knowledge of the person and family guides the care provided. It may be necessary to provide opportunities for individuals to express personal preferences about where they want to die and about funeral and burial arrangements. If the family feels that this is morbid, the nurse may explain that it helps the person to keep a sense of control as they approach death.

People who are dying need the opportunity to say goodbye to others as a necessary part of the grief process. Family members are often afraid to be present at the moment of death, yet dying alone is the greatest fear expressed by people at end of life. It is essential during times of loss and grief that families and carers have access to bereavement support services and are provided with information about loss and grief (Palliative Care Australia, 2018b).

Death

Nurses sometimes fear being present at the moment of the person's death, and research suggests nurses and other health professionals can have difficulty dealing with death and dying (Zheng et al., 2015). In fact, Kübler-Ross (1969) noted that the nurse's fear of death frequently interferes with their ability to provide support for the dying person and family. Thoughts such as 'Please don't let him die on my shift' are common, and they express the nurse's emotional turmoil in dealing with the task. Nurses who have worked through their own feelings about death and dying with effective self-care strategies are more at ease in assisting the dying person towards a peaceful death.

After the death, the nurse should be attentive to the needs of the family and significant others and acknowledge that grief reactions and needs vary for individuals. The nurse should allow the bereaved to express their sorrow, anger or guilt, which may help them begin to resolve their grief. By accepting variations in the expression of grief, the nurse supports the family's grief reactions and helps prevent dysfunctional grieving. Dysfunctional grieving is an extended and unsuccessful resolution of grief.

Resolution of grief begins with acceptance of the loss. The nurse can encourage this by respecting the bereaved person's needs by maintaining open, honest dialogue and by providing the family with the opportunity to view, touch, hold, wash, kiss or visit with the person's body as long as is needed. As family members realise the finality of the death, they are often comforted by the presence of the nurse who cared for the person during the final days. Open and honest communication can ensure that the nurse is aware whether their presence is required.

Care after a person dies

The nurse should document the time of death (which is required for the death certificate and all official records), notify the doctor and support the family. Once a person dies, it is important that all infusion pumps and pressure mattresses are turned off. Experiencing machine alarms or noticing a deceased loved one's body move (from the rise and fall of a pressure mattress) can cause unnecessary distress for the bereaved person.

If the person dies at home, death must be pronounced before the body is removed from the home. Jewellery may be removed from the deceased and given to the family unless they ask that it be left on. Nurses should document the removal of valuables or jewellery and record who takes possession of the items, especially if the death occurs in a hospital or residential aged care facility. All tubing may be removed from the deceased unless otherwise indicated, such as in cases requiring a coroner's inquest. The body of the deceased person is kept in place until the family is ready and gives permission for the body to be removed; this may be minutes, hours or days.

Acknowledgement of death in a hospital setting

Part of the philosophy of palliative care is the acknowledgement that death is a normal part of the life cycle. However, in hospitals or residential aged care facility settings, a person's death is not always acknowledged or discussed with the other residents of the facility/setting. Nurses in acute settings must acknowledge that a person may witness the death of another person and may need an opportunity to share their experience and express their feelings. There is a changing culture in Australian residential aged care facilities, where the deceased person's life may be celebrated with the other residents, allowing them to gain closure and acknowledgement of the death of a fellow resident.

Nurses' grief

The nurse who has developed a close relationship with the person who has died may experience strong feelings of grief. Sharing grief with the family after the death of a loved one helps both the nurse and family to cope with their feelings about the loss. Taking time to grieve after the person's death provides a release that can help prevent 'blunting' of feelings, a problem often experienced by nurses who care for individuals with a life-limiting illness.

> **CONSIDERATION FOR PRACTICE**
>
> **Crying with families, at one time considered unprofessional, is now recognised as simply an expression of empathy and caring.**

Nurses working with individuals who are critically ill or have a life-limiting illness should be aware that witnessing a person's death and the family's grief may reactivate feelings about some unresolved grief in their own lives. In these cases, nurses may need to reflect on their responses to their own losses. Also, nurses who work with individuals who are dying need support from peers and other professionals to work through the often overwhelming feelings that result from dealing with death, grief and loss.

INTERPROFESSIONAL CARE

Interventions for loss and grief may be planned and implemented by any or all members of the healthcare team. Nurses and social workers provide interventions to help individuals or families adapt to a loss. They also make referrals to mental health professionals (grief counsellors, social services), support groups, chaplains/pastoral care or legal agencies.

Grieving individuals may enter the healthcare system with significant somatic symptoms. Somatic symptoms are physical symptoms caused by the distress of grief. In some cases, the symptoms of grief and loss are overlooked until the person reaches a crisis state requiring psychiatric medical intervention. Collaborative care by the doctor and the nurse early in the normal grieving process can help the person achieve an early and effective resolution of grief and avoid physical or psychiatric health problems.

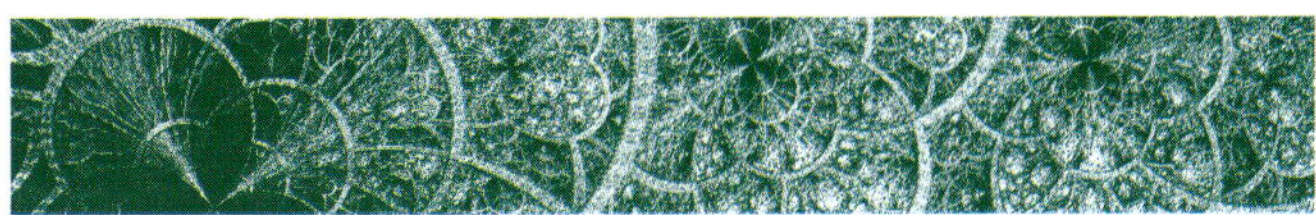

Nursing care

Nurses practising in all types of settings care for individuals who are in various stages of the grieving process. Like pain, grief is highly individual. The grief process may range from uncomfortable to debilitating, and it may last for a day or a lifetime, depending on what the loss means to the person experiencing it. The following section provides nurses with insights into the assessment and exploration of grief and loss for individuals for whom they care. It is acknowledged that this information is not exhaustive. Nurses should always maintain open communication with the person, significant others and multidisciplinary team; this will ensure individualised assessment and inquiry that has the person's needs as the main focus. Effective communication is central to person-centred care and effective therapeutic relationships and is paramount in caring for dying patients and grieving families. The Nursing and Midwifery Board of Australia (NMBA, 2016) *Registered Nurse Standards for Practice* state that Registered Nurses must communicate effectively and be respectful of each person's dignity, culture, values, beliefs and rights.

Health promotion

In planning a grief assessment of an individual, acknowledgement that the experience of loss can be associated with a range of factors is essential. It is also important that the nurse considers the individual's response, which may vary greatly from others' responses. In the rapid patient turnover in acute care hospitals, nurses may feel that an elaborate grief assessment is impossible or, at the least, impractical. However, research and clinical experience suggest that individuals who delay the grieving process after a loss are prone to have health problems that may last a lifetime.

Assessment

Grief reactions are personal and individual. However, knowledge of the expected physical reactions to loss provides the nurse with a basis for identifying reactions that require further assessment. To assess the extent of somatic distress—that is, physical symptoms caused by distress—the nurse observes for changes in sensory processes and asks questions about the individual's sleeping and eating patterns, activities of daily living, general health status and pain.

Physical assessment

Individuals may experience one or more predictable somatic symptoms as they become aware of a loss. Gastrointestinal symptoms occur frequently and may include indigestion, nausea or vomiting, anorexia, weight gain or loss, constipation or diarrhoea. The shock and disbelief that accompany a loss may cause shortness of breath, a choking sensation, hyperventilation or loss of strength. Some individuals also report insomnia, preoccupation with sleep, fatigue and decreased or increased activity level.

Crying and sadness are observed during normal grief states. Crying may make the individual feel exhausted and interfere with carrying out activities of daily living. However, a person who is unable to cry may have difficulty completing the mourning process. If the person does not express feelings of grief, somatic symptoms may increase. If a person is experiencing pain, it is imperative that their concerns are assessed, especially if the person has cancer or another painful illness. Knowledge of pain theories and pain assessment can help the nurse assess the need for pain medication (see the chapter 'Nursing care of people in pain').

Reactions to loss are not always obvious. For example, in individuals who experience an illness following a serious loss, assessment may reveal somatic complaints related to the grief state as well as the illness. When a person who has been healthy begins to develop patterns of increased illness, the nurse should be aware that this may signal dysfunctional grieving. This is especially common in the loss and grieving associated with a change in body image. In addition to making a physical assessment, assess the person's perception of the alteration in body image. The loss of a body part, weight gain or loss, and scars from surgery or trauma can be difficult for the person to accept. For example, many people may grieve hair loss that accompanies chemotherapy used in cancer treatment.

Spiritual assessment

Spiritual beliefs and practices greatly influence people's reaction to loss, and it is important for nurses to use sensitivity and skill when assessing a person's spiritual needs. Nurses need to establish rapport and trust with the person before they assess their spirituality. Nurses do not have a right to ask deeply personal questions about spirituality unless they have established trust and a connection with the person. The word 'spirituality' can have many different interpretations. As Roy (2011) reminds us, spirituality has an elusive and perplexing quality. Some people might find the word 'spiritual' quite confronting because of possible judgments and may use metaphors such as 'peace' to describe their sense of spirituality.

Assessing the person's spiritual life and its significance to the person and family helps identify spiritual support systems. However, assessment needs to be explored within the context of the individual and their culture. Areas that might be explored include beliefs and meaning, experience and emotion, ritual and practice, courage and hope.

Psychosocial assessment

When working through the grief process, individuals can be overwhelmed by the fears associated with the loss and the changes it will produce. Individuals diagnosed with cancer can also experience a lack of trust in their body, especially if their diagnosis was not prompted by specific symptoms. The individual responding to an actual or perceived loss commonly expresses anxiety (fear of the unknown). An extreme level of anxiety can threaten the individual's wellbeing. Assessment includes helping individuals openly acknowledge their fears. Some individuals may fear the feelings they experience while proceeding through the grief process more than the loss itself. The most common fear expressed by individuals facing a loss is that of losing self-control.

Focusing on the meaning of the loss to the person is more important than attempting to place the person in a sequence or phase of grief. The degree of caring and sensitivity shown when asking questions that consider the meaning of the loss influences the amount of information the person will be willing to reveal. Asking questions such as 'Why do you feel this way?' or 'What does this loss mean to you?' is less helpful than making a statement such as 'This must be difficult for you.' The latter more effectively conveys empathy and a genuine interest in hearing how the person feels about the loss.

Awareness of the altered sensorium observed during the stage of shock and disbelief provides parameters for assessment. The nurse may note that the person experiences feelings of numbness, unreality, emotional distance, intense preoccupation with the loss, helplessness, loneliness and disorganisation. As awareness of the loss begins to develop, preoccupation with the person who has died or the object that has been lost may increase, and self-accusation and ambivalence towards the person or object may follow.

Exploring grief

Anticipatory grieving, chronic sorrow and death anxiety are issues that individuals experiencing loss and grief, as well as the person who is nearing death, may experience. Nurses may

MEETING INDIVIDUALISED NEEDS Teaching suggestions for individuals experiencing a loss

- Encourage both children and adults to discuss expected or impending loss and to express their feelings.
- Encourage problem-solving skills: define what possible changes and problems may be related to the predicted loss, develop potential strategies for dealing with problems, list pros and cons of each strategy and decide which strategies might be most useful to try first to solve potential problems associated with loss.
- Talk to individuals and families about how to support a person who is dealing with an impending loss.
- Explain what to expect with a loss: sadness, fear, rejection, anger, guilt, loneliness.
- Develop strategies for goal setting and future-orientated planning.
- Discuss signs of grief resolution:
  - Individuals and families need to understand that the acute stage of grief has no set timeline and, as discussed previously, grief reactions may vary for each individual.
  - Explain that 'triggers' such as photographs, events, songs or memories and especially the anniversary of the loss may potentially cause painful 'waves' of grief.

find that the following information will assist in the assessment and exploration of anticipatory grieving, chronic sorrow and death anxiety.

Anticipatory grieving

Anticipatory grieving is a combination of intellectual and emotional responses and behaviours by which people adjust their self-concept in the face of a potential loss. Anticipatory grieving may be a response to one's own future death; to potential loss of body parts or functions; to potential loss of a significant person, animal or possession; or to potential loss of a social role. When communicating with people in a way designed to assist with grief resolution, consider the following:

- Assess for factors causing or contributing to the grief. Ask about support systems, how many losses have occurred, relationship with the lost person and previous experiences with loss and grief. *Grief and mourning occur when a person experiences any type of loss.*
- Use open-ended questions to encourage the person to share concerns and the possible effect on the family. *Grief resolution cannot occur until the individual acknowledges the loss.*
- Promote a trusting nurse–patient relationship: allow enough time for communication; speak clearly, simply and concisely; listen; be honest in responses to questions; do not give unrealistic hope; offer support; and demonstrate respect for the person's age, culture, religion, ethnicity and values. *An effective nurse–patient relationship begins with acceptance of the individual's feelings, attitudes and values related to the loss. If the person is ready to talk, listening and being present are the most appropriate interventions.*
- Discuss with the person and their family the stages of grief. *This helps them to be aware of their emotions in each stage and reassures them that their reactions are normal.*
- Provide time for decision making. *In periods of stress, people may need extra time to make informed decisions.*
- Provide information about appropriate resources, including support from family, friends and support groups, community resources and legal/financial aid. *Support from others decreases feelings of loneliness and isolation and facilitates grief work.*

Chronic sorrow

Chronic sorrow is a cyclical, recurring and potentially progressive pattern of pervasive sadness experienced in response to continual loss, throughout the trajectory of an illness or disability. It is triggered by situations that bring to mind the person's losses, disappointments or fears. It may be experienced by a patient, parent or caregiver, or a person with a chronic illness or a disability. Support the person experiencing grief or sorrow by:

- Explaining the difference between chronic sorrow and chronic grieving. *Grieving is time limited and ends in adaptation to the loss. Chronic sorrow may vary in intensity, but it persists as long as the person with the disability or chronic sorrow condition lives.*
- Encouraging verbalisation of feelings about the loss and about the personal relevance of changes to hopes for the future. *Expressing feelings is normal and necessary to decrease the emotional pain.*
- Helping to identify triggers that intensify the sorrow, such as birthdays, anniversaries and holidays. *When triggers have been identified, role-playing may make the events less painful.*
- Referral to appropriate community support groups. *Participating in support groups with others experiencing grief is helpful in coping with loss.*
- Encouraging use of personal, family, significant other and spiritual support systems to facilitate coping with loss.

Death anxiety

Death anxiety is worry or fear related to death or dying. It may be present in individuals who have an acute life-threatening illness, who have a life-limiting illness, who have experienced the death of a family member or friend, or who have experienced multiple deaths in the same family. When communicating with people about their anxiety, consider the following:

- Explore the person's knowledge of the situation. For example, ask, 'What has your doctor told you about your condition?' *This informs you of the person's knowledge base about the condition and about their ability to make informed decisions.*
- Ask them to identify their specific fears about death. *This provides data about any unrealistic expectations or misperceptions.*
- Ask the person to identify needed help. *This determines whether available resources are adequate.*
- Encourage independence and control in decisions about treatment and care. *This promotes self-esteem, decreases feelings of powerlessness and allows the person to retain dignity in dying.*
- Facilitate access to culturally appropriate spiritual rituals and practices. *This provides spiritual comfort.*
- Explain advance directives and assist with them if necessary. *Advance directives help ensure that the individual's wishes for end-of-life care are carried out.*
- Encourage life review and reminiscence. *Life review is self-affirming.*
- Encourage activities that may bring comfort such as listening to music, aromatherapy, massage or relaxation exercises. *These activities decrease anxiety.*
- Suggest keeping a journal or leaving a written legacy. *A written document provides continuing support to others after death.*

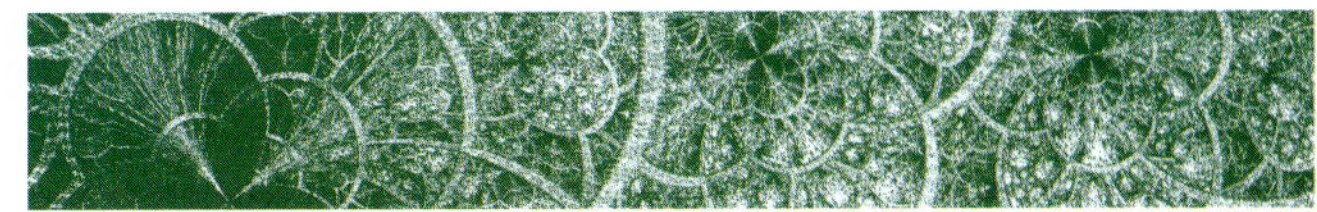

NURSING CARE PLAN A person experiencing loss and grief

Mrs Sandra Bell is an 87-year-old widow recently admitted to a residential aged care facility following her husband Allan's death 12 months ago. Mr Bell had suffered from dementia and his wife was his carer until 2 years prior to his death, when he had been admitted to a dementia unit of the local rural hospital. Mrs Bell visited her husband regularly even when he could no longer recognise her. She has lived all her life in a country town and had established a strong network of friends through membership of the golf club and local services club. However, her social contacts with friends have diminished because of their poor health. Mrs Bell has a daughter and son who both live in the city. Although they keep in regular contact by telephone, they are only able to visit on special family occasions.

Knowing the strain of maintaining a home and losing contact with close friends, Mrs Bell's family felt it would be best for her to move to the city to be closer to her children and grandchildren. Mrs Bell sold her home and entered a residential aged care facility in the city, near her family.

After several visits, Mrs Bell's daughter notices that her mother has become less social, not wanting to mix with the other residents or participate in community activities, and is more and more upset about her situation. Mrs Bell complains that the other residents are unfriendly and that she misses her home and friends. She does not like the community dining room and says that her back and hips are painful. Mrs Bell also tells her daughter she is not sleeping and is constipated. Her daughter speaks to the nurse and is told that her mother is very quiet, does not mix well with the other residents, seems resentful when approached by the staff and does not volunteer that she is unwell. The nurse reports to Mrs Bell that during her admission to the aged care facility, her medical tests showed arthritis but no other pathological disorder.

ASSESSMENT

On assessment, Mrs Bell says, 'I'm a sick woman and no one will listen to me! I can't walk, I'm so weak, my head hurts and I'm always sick in my stomach. I haven't had a bowel movement in a week and I never sleep more than three hours a night.' Physical assessment findings include swollen knees and ankles, with limited mobility of the lower extremities.

DIAGNOSES

- *Grieving* related to death of husband, lost contact with friends, and recent move from a country town to a residential aged care facility in the city.
- *Disturbed sleep pattern* related to grieving.
- *Constipation* related to inactivity.

PLANNING

- A multidisciplinary team planning meeting was organised by the Nursing Unit Manager (NUM) to review and identify Mrs Bell's issues. The following goals/outcomes, implementation and evaluation activities were identified.

Expected outcomes

- Engage in normal grief work: work through grief process with Mrs Bell. Discuss reality of losses, use non-destructive coping mechanisms, and discuss positive and negative aspects of the loss.
- Experience adequate and restful sleep.
- Have a bowel movement with soft formed stools at least every other day.

IMPLEMENTATION

- Promote trust: show empathy and caring, demonstrate respect for Mrs Bell's culture and values, offer support and reassurance, be honest and engage in active listening.
- Assist in identifying Mrs Bell's feelings: anger, fear, loneliness, guilt, isolation.
- Explore previous losses and the ways in which Mrs Bell has coped.
- Encourage review of Mrs Bell's relationship with her deceased husband.
- Reinforce expressions of behaviours associated with normal grieving.
- Encourage Mrs Bell's participation in usual spiritual practices.
- Encourage participation in a grief group that meets at the facility.
- Consult with the physical and recreational therapist to help the nursing staff provide afternoon activities tailored to Mrs Bell's interests.
- Provide measures that assist in bowel evacuation: Encourage exercise as tolerated, including walks. Offer fluids foods that stimulate bowel movement (e.g. fresh fruit). Offer privacy: close the door, ensuring that the buzzer is within reach, and do not interrupt. Administer a mild laxative and/or stool softener, if necessary, but discontinue as soon as possible.
- Provide measures to assist sleep (e.g. offer warm milk drink with honey, chamomile tea, quiet environment). Offer gentle back massage, use of aromatherapy oils such as lavender.

EVALUATION

After 4 weeks at the residential aged care facility, Mrs Bell states, 'I don't feel any better, but I know I have to accept my situation.' Although Mrs Bell says she doesn't feel better, she is walking the length of the hall, sleeping better and having regular bowel movements. She is also less withdrawn and has openly discussed her feelings related to her husband's death and the loss of her social contacts. She has attended the grief group once and has attended pastoral care services on Sunday for the past 2 weeks. Her children visit her each Saturday and take her in a wheelchair to the shopping centre.

CRITICAL-THINKING QUESTIONS

1. What common physical manifestations of grief did Mrs Bell experience?
2. Outline what you have learned from Mrs Bell's case study/story.
3. What communication strategies and education would you use if Mrs Bell told you she does not want any help and that she just wants to be left alone to die?

REFLECTION ON THE NURSING PRACTICE

1. How would you respond to Mrs Bell if she says to you, 'Please help me die'?
2. How might you broach the topic of advance directives with Mrs Bell? Do you feel comfortable about talking to people about advanced care planning?

CHAPTER HIGHLIGHTS

- Grief is the emotional response to a loss, experienced by a person as grieving. Bereavement, a form of depression accompanied by anxiety, is a common response to loss of a loved one by death. Death, although inevitable, is an immensely difficult loss.
- There are many different theories of how individuals respond to loss, and grief. These theories are useful when providing nursing care to individuals and their families.
- A person's response to loss is influenced by age, social support, family members, cultural and spiritual beliefs, and rituals of mourning. Nurses need to assess the way in which they respond to loss, to better care for people.
- Legal and ethical issues involved in end-of-life care include advance directives, advanced care planning, enduring power of attorney, do-not-resuscitate directives and euthanasia.
- Palliative care is a philosophy of care that supports a dignified and peaceful death when individuals and their families are faced with limited life expectancy. Palliative care is focused on the relief of physical, mental and spiritual distress for people with a life-limiting illness.
- To provide knowledgeable and compassionate care at the end of life, nurses must recognise symptoms that may be present as the individual nears death, support the person and their family, provide care to the individual and family immediately after death, and resolve their own grief.
- Nursing care of individuals experiencing an actual or potential loss includes accurate individualised physical, spiritual and psychosocial assessment, and awareness of responses of anticipatory grieving, chronic sorrow and/or death anxiety.

CONCEPT CHECK

1 Which of the following statements best describes loss?
1 It is determined by one's cultural values.
2 It is largely dependent on support of family and friends.
3 It can be determined only by the person who experiences it.
4 It is the same as grief and mourning.

2 Kübler-Ross believed that people's first response to a situation of loss is:
1 anger
2 bargaining
3 depression
4 denial

3 What is an important factor in the successful resolution of grief?
1 social isolation
2 support systems
3 triggers of grief
4 loss acknowledgement

4 What is the primary factor that dictates the rituals of mourning?
1 culture
2 age
3 gender
4 religion

5 What document expresses a person's wishes in relation to the planning of treatment in the event of their inability to communicate their wishes because of a life-limiting illness?
1 enduring power of attorney
2 advanced care planning
3 do-not-resuscitate directive
4 living will

6 Which of the following statements is true of a hospice?
1 A hospice is a special place of care.
2 Hospice care is a lifelong type of care.
3 A hospice is a model of care rather than a place of care.
4 A hospice is designed for individuals with serious chronic illness.

7 A person nearing death requests that no medication be given that would cause a loss of consciousness, including pain medication. What would a nurse do to provide the best end-of-life care in this situation?
1 Give the medication; comfort is the highest priority.
2 Give half the ordered dose to provide compassionate care.
3 Discuss this with family members and follow their wishes.
4 Respect the person's wishes and withhold pain medications.

8 Which of the senses is believed to be the last one lost as a person nears death?
1 hearing
2 vision
3 touch
4 smell

9 Which of the following statements best describes the treatment of pain at the end of life?
1 As an individual nears death, no pain is perceived and no medications are necessary.
2 It is important to withhold pain medications if the individual has respiratory changes.
3 There is no maximum allowable dose for opioids during end-of-life care.
4 Nurses should not administer opioids to the dying person.

10 A woman, recently widowed, tells the nurse, 'I just can't even get out of bed in the morning anymore.' What response would be most helpful in resolving her grief?
1 'I don't know why you feel that way.'
2 'This must be a difficult time for you.'
3 'Why do you think you feel this way?'
4 'After you get up, you will feel better.'

BIBLIOGRAPHY

Abbas, S. & Panjwani, S. (2008). The necessity of spiritual care towards the end of life. *Ethics and Medicine, 24*(2), 113–118.

Australian Commission on Safety and Quality in Health Care (ACSQHC) (2020). *End-of-life care*. Sydney: ACSQHC.

Australian Commission on Safety and Quality in Health Care (ACSQHC) (2021). *National Safety and Quality Health Service Standards* (2nd ed.). Sydney: ACSQHC.

Bossi, L. M., Ott, M. J. & DeCristofare, S. (2008). Reiki as a clinical intervention in oncology nursing practice. *Clinical Journal of Oncology Nursing, 12*(3), 489–494.

Bowlby, J. (1973). *Attachment and loss: Separation, anxiety, and anger* (Vol. 2). New York: Basic Books.

Bowlby, J. (1980). *Attachment and loss: Loss, sadness, and depression* (Vol. 3). New York: Basic Books.

Bush, S. H., Leonard, M. M., Agar, M., Spiller, J. A., Hosie, A., Wright, D. K. & Lawlor, P. G. (2014). End-of-life delirium: Issues regarding recognition, optimal management, and the role of sedation in the dying phase. *Journal of Pain and Symptom Management, 48*(2), 215–230.

Caplan, G. (1990). Loss, stress, and mental health. *Community Mental Health Journal, 26*(1), 27–48.

Carter, A. N. (2020). To what extent does clinically assisted nutrition and hydration have a role in the care of dying people? *Journal of Palliative Care, 35*(4), 209–216. https://doi.org/10.1177/0825859720907426

Department of Health (2018). *National palliative care strategy 2018*. Canberra: Author.

Engel, G. (1964). Grief and grieving. *American Journal of Nursing*, *64*, 93.

Freud, S. (1917/1957). Mourning and melancholia. In J. Strachey & A. Tyson (eds), *The complete psychological works of Sigmund Freud* (Vol. 14). London: Hogarth Press.

Gardiner, C., Gott, M., Ingleton, C. et al. (2013). Extent of palliative care need in the acute hospital setting: A survey of two acute hospitals in the UK. *Palliative Medicine*, *27*, 76–83.

Gerber, K., Hayes, B., Bryant, C. et al. (2019). 'It all depends!': A qualitative study of preferences for place of care and place of death in terminally ill patients and their family caregivers. *Palliative Medicine*, *33*, 802–811. doi: 10.1177/026921 6319845794

Good, P., Higgins, I., van der Riet, P. & Sneesby, L. (2011). Medical officers in acute care settings: Their views on medically assisted nutrition and hydration at the end of life. *Journal of Palliative Care*, *27*(4), 303–309.

Holland, J. & Neimeyer, R. (2010). An examination of stage theory of grief among individuals bereaved by natural and violent causes: A meaning-oriented contribution. *Omega*, *61*(2), 103–120.

Huang, H., Liu, H., Zeng, T. & Pu, X. (2015). Preference of Chinese general public and healthcare providers for a good death. *Nursing Ethics*, *22*(2), 217–227. doi: 10.1177/0969733014524760

Johnstone, M. (2019). *Bioethics: A nursing perspective* (7th ed.). Sydney: Elsevier.

Kirchhoff, K., Spuhler, V., Walker, L. et al. (2000). Intensive care nurses' experiences with end of life care. *American Journal of Critical Care*, *9*(1), 35–42.

Kübler-Ross, E. (1969). *On death and dying*. New York: Macmillan.

Kübler-Ross, E. (1978). *To live until we say goodbye*. Englewood Cliffs, NJ: Prentice Hall.

Leong, M., Olnick, S., Akmal, T., Copenhaver, A. & Razzak, R. (2016). How Islam influences end-of-life care: Education for palliative care clinicians. *Journal of Pain and Symptom Management*, *52*(6), 771–774.e3. https://doi.org/10.1016/j.jpainsymman.2016.05.034

Levett-Jones, T., Dwyer, T., Reid-Searl, K., Heaton, L., Flenady, T., Applegarth, J., Guinea, S. & Andersen, P. (2017). *Patient Safety Competency Framework (PSCF) for Nursing Students*. Sydney. Retrieved from http://psframework.wpengine.com/

Lovgren, M., Sveen, J., Steineck, G., Wallin, A., Eilertsen, M. & Kreicbergs, U. (2017). Spirituality and religious coping are related to cancer-bereaved siblings' long-term grief. *Palliative and Supportive Care*, December, 1–5. https://doi.org/10.1017/S1478951517001146

Neidjie, B. (1985). *Australia's Kakudu Man, Bill Neidjie*. Darwin: Mybrood.

Neimeyer, R. A., Herrero, O. & Botella, L. (2006). Chaos to coherence: Psychotherapeutic integration of traumatic loss. *Journal of Constructivist Psychology*, *19*, 127–145.

Nuccio, T. & Nuccio, P. (2009). Give them comfort: Controlling COPD symptoms at the end-of-life. *RT: The Journal of Respiratory Care Practitioners*, February, 30–33.

Nursing and Midwifery Board of Australia (NMBA) (2016). *Registered Nurse Standards for Practice*. Retrieved from https://www.nursingmidwiferyboard.gov.au/

Nursing Council of New Zealand (2002). *Guidelines for cultural safety, the Treaty of Waitangi, and Maori health in nursing and midwifery education and practice*. Wellington: Nursing Council of New Zealand.

Nyatanga, B. (2018). Loss, grief and bereavement: An inescapable link in palliative care. *British Journal of Community Nursing*, *23*(2), 70.

O'Brien, M. R., Kinloch, K., Groves, K. E. & Jack, B. A. (2019). Meeting patients' spiritual needs during end-of-life care: A qualitative study of nurses' and healthcare professionals' perceptions of spiritual care training. *Journal of Clinical Nursing*, *28*(1–2), 182–189. https://doi.org/10.1111/jocn.14648

Palliative Care Australia (2018a). *Palliative care service development guidelines*. Retrieved from http://palliativecare.org.au/

Palliative Care Australia (2018b). *National Palliative Care Standards* (5th ed.). Palliative Care Australia. Retrieved from http://palliativecare.org.au/

Palliative Care Victoria (2016). *Cultural perspectives and values from ten culturally and linguistically diverse communities in Victoria*. Retrieved from https://www.pallcarevic.asn.au/

Penman, J., Oliver, M. & Harrington, A. (2013). The relational model of spiritual engagement depicted by palliative care clients and caregivers. *International Journal of Nursing Practice*, *19*(1), 39–46.

Puchalski, C. M., Vitillo, R., Hull, S. K. & Reller, N. (2014). Improving the spiritual dimension of whole person care: Reaching national and international consensus. *Journal of Palliative Medicine*, *17*(6), 642–656. https://doi.org/10.1089/jpm.2014.9427

QUT (2022). *Voluntary assisted dying*. Retrieved from https://end-of-life.qut.edu.au/

Reynolds, H. (1989). *Frontier*. Sydney: Allen & Unwin.

Richardson, F. & Carryer, J. (2005). Teaching cultural safety in a New Zealand nursing education program. *Journal of Nursing Education*, *44*(5), 201–208.

Rosenblatt, P. (2017). Researching grief: Cultural relational and individual possibilities. *Journal of Loss and Trauma*, *22*(8), 617–630.

Roy, D. (2011). Editorial: Does 'spiritual' indicate a limit to palliative care? *Journal of Palliative Care*, *27*(4), 259–260.

Rudolfsson, G., Berggren, I. & da Silva, A. B. (2014). Experiences of spirituality and spiritual values in the context of nursing – An integrative review. *The Open Nursing Journal*, *8*, 64–70. https://doi.org/10.2174/1874434601408010064

Sadak, B. & Weiser, L. (2017). Acknowledging the archetypal elements of grief. *Psychological Perspectives*, *60*(4), 434–444.

Saunders, R., Glass, C., Seaman, K. et al. (2021). Clinical staff perceptions on the quality of end-of-life care in an Australian acute private hospital: A cross-sectional survey. *Australian Health Review*, *45*(6), 771. https://doi.org/10.1071/ah20329

Sharma, H., Jagdish, V., Anusha, P. & Bharti, S. (2013). End-of-life care: Indian perspective. *Indian Journal of Psychiatry*, *55*(Suppl 2), S293–S298.

van der Riet, P. (2009). Palliative care professionals' perception of nutrition and hydration at the end of life. Podcast interview: International Program for Psycho-Social Health Research (IPP-SHR), Central Queensland University.

van der Riet, P., Good, P., Higgins, I. et al. (2008). Palliative care professionals' perceptions of nutrition and hydration at the end of life. *International Journal of Palliative Nursing*, *14*(3), 145–151.

Viliotti, M. (2013). Complementary therapy: Comfort for those in need of palliative care. *End-of-life Journal*, *3*(4), 1–4.

Vivat, B. (2008). Measures of spiritual issues for palliative care patients: A literature review. *Palliative Medicine*, *22*, 859–868.

Weathers E., O'Caoimh, R., Cornally, N. et al. (2016). Advance care planning: A systematic review of randomised controlled trials conducted with older adults. *Maturitas*, *91*, 101–109.

Zeng, Y. S., Wang, C., Ward, K. E. & Hume, A. L. (2018). Complementary and alternative medicine in hospice and palliative care: A systematic review. *Journal of Pain and Symptom Management*, *56*(5), 781–794.e4. https://doi.org/10.1016/j.jpainsymman.2018.07.016

Zheng, R. S., Guo, Q. H., Dong, F. Q. & Owens, R. G. (2015). Chinese oncology nurses' experience of caring for dying patients who are on their final days: A qualitative study. *International Journal of Nursing Studies*, *52*(1), 288–296. doi: 10.1016/j.ijnurstu.2014.09.009

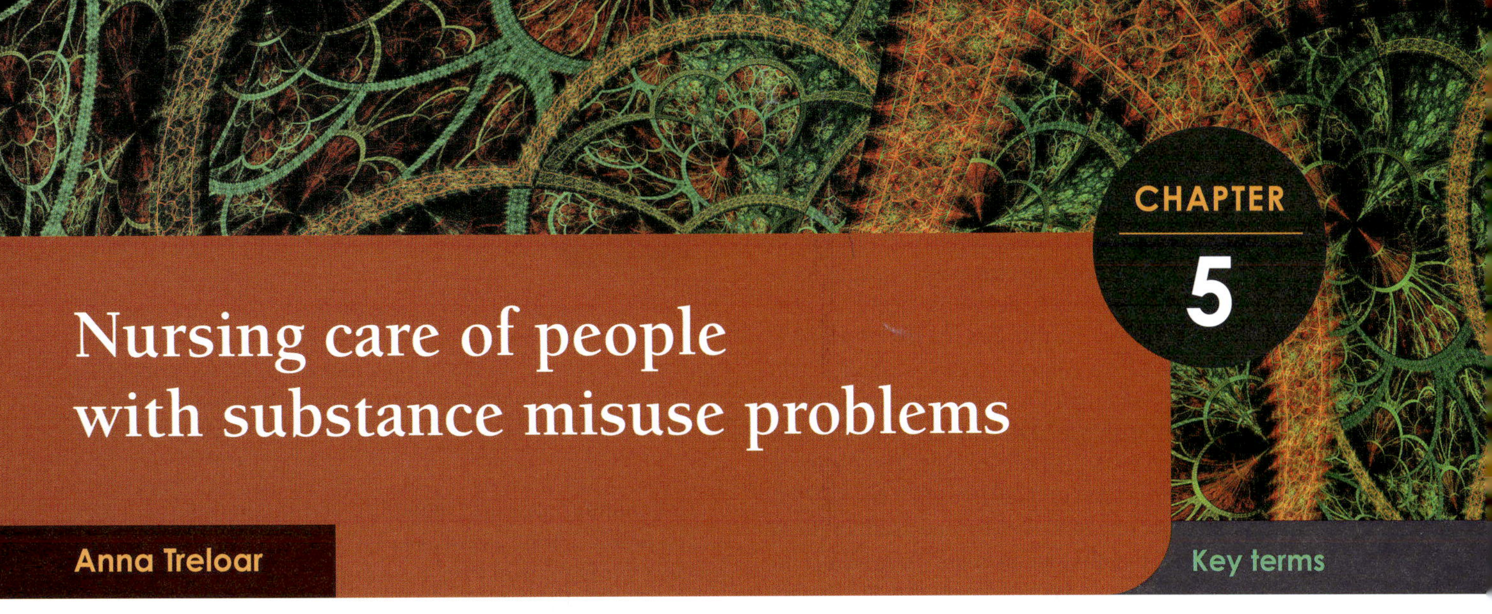

CHAPTER 5

Nursing care of people with substance misuse problems

Anna Treloar

Key terms

Learning outcomes

- Distinguish between substance use disorders and substance-induced disorders.
- Explain risk factors associated with substance misuse and possible causes.
- Classify major addictive substances and explain effects of addictive substances on physiological, cognitive, psychological and social wellbeing.
- Communicate effectively with people who misuse substances.
- Support interprofessional care in the provision of individualised care for people living with substance use problems, including comprehensive assessment, brief interventions, diagnostic tests, emergency care for intoxication and overdose, managed withdrawal and residential rehabilitation.
- Identify some common therapies used for substance use problems.
- Develop awareness of current policy, both national and international.
- Understand the difference between health education, harm minimisation and health promotion.
- Provide nursing care to special populations.

Clinical competencies

- Assess health status of people living with substance use disorders.
- Monitor, document and report physical manifestations of substance misuse.
- Plan and implement nursing care for people experiencing withdrawal symptoms.
- Plan and implement individualised nursing interventions for people living with substance use disorders.
- Collaborate with other disciplines when caring for people with substance use disorders.
- Educate people about harm minimisation and relapse prevention.

INTRODUCTION

Use and misuse of legal and illegal substances is common in Australia, although we are less likely than in the past to drink alcohol at lifetime risky levels and smoke tobacco. However, in 2020–2021, alcohol was the substance for which people most commonly sought treatment through the public health system (37%) (Australian Institute of Health and Welfare (AIHW), 2022a). This was followed by cannabis (24%), cocaine and ecstasy, with analgesics and opioids used for non-medical purposes coming next after these. Methamphetamine use has declined since its peak in 2001 (AIHW, 2022b). The National Drug Strategy Household Survey 2019 (AIHW, 2020a) reported that 16.4% of people 14 and older had used an illicit drug in the previous 12 months, an increase from 2007. In 2021, the Illicit Drug Reporting System found that the impact of COVID-19 resulted in difficulties accessing clean needles and syringes for injecting drug users, and 49% of those surveyed experienced disruption in their drug treatment services (AIHW, 2022b). Attitudes to consumption vary widely, so while misuse of prescribed medications or legal drugs is often considered acceptable, misuse of illegal substances can be heavily stigmatised, with the result that people who are known to be substance dependent can find it hard to access healthcare.

Substance use is a general term; substance misuse or abuse implies some associated problems; **substance dependence** refers to a physiological dependence, although psychological dependence can often be added to it.

Consider the people in the following scenario:

The neighbours are enjoying a backyard barbecue. Wayne and Wendy have lived next door to Kevin and Karla for 30 years. They are discussing the students who have moved into the rental house over the road.

'Probably all on drugs', says Wendy, looking in her bag for her cigarettes. It's her second pack for the day, but she can afford them, so why worry. She coughs. 'I'll give up one day', she tells herself.

Wayne goes inside to get another bottle of whisky. He gets a discount at work, so doesn't need to restrict his intake. Anyway, Kevin will probably have one or two with him. There's not that much in a bottle really, and he can make one last two days usually. It's just that lately the bottle doesn't seem to be lasting that long.

'I heard those students just live on V and Mother', says Karla, kicking her empty one litre bottle of Coke under the chair. 'Too lazy to cook, I suppose.' She checks in her bag for her packet of No-Doz. She will need those to get through night duty tonight. Good thing there's a coffee machine at work too.

Kevin excuses himself for a moment. He goes to the bathroom and takes another couple of codeine tablets. It's not his fault if his back aches after a day at work. His doctor is pretty good about prescriptions. Actually, he sees several doctors, though of course he doesn't say anything about this. And when he runs out of codeine he can get stuff from a mate or when he's at the pub after work. He looks in the bathroom cabinet and notices a box of Panadeine Forte. He takes a card of tablets and puts it in his pocket.

'It's disgusting what young people today get up to', he says as he comes back to the others. (Treloar, McMillan & Stone, 2015. Reproduced with permission)

The people in this scenario are all misusing substances. However, all of their preferred drugs are legal, and none of the people consider the use of the drugs to be problematic. In fact, they are speculating about the students and their drug use with no grounds for this whatever.

ACTIVITY

Can you calculate likely regular daily use for each substance (in milligrams, standard drinks or number of cigarettes) mentioned above and, based on that, decide whose use is most likely to lead to major health problems, both short term and long term?

Community ignorance, prejudice and stigmatising attitudes can impede accurate assessment and timely referrals to appropriate services for people with a substance misuse problem.

ACTIVITY

Kevin runs out of codeine and none of his mates can help out this week. He rings his doctor and gets an appointment straight away. When he arrives, another patient is at the reception desk. This young woman is leading a toddler by the hand. The young woman, who has been injecting street methadone and other opioids, is worried about an abscess in her left antecubital fossa. The receptionist notices it and tells her the practice is not able to take new patients at this time. The young woman says nothing and turns to leave. The child is hungry and starts to cry.

What might happen if the receptionist were to find an appointment for the young woman and if she and her child were assessed and referred to appropriate services? What might happen if the GP were to accurately calculate Kevin's total daily intake of codeine, including all the non-prescribed pills?

Many factors contribute to substance use and to the risk of substance misuse and dependence; no single element can cause one individual to develop a pattern of drug use while another does not. Some people experiment, some use recreationally, and a few become dependent. Risk factors can only help identify those who are most vulnerable. Thorough assessment is necessary in order to understand the whole person and plan appropriate interventions. A variety of healthcare professionals may be involved in these interventions, and what they can and cannot offer will be partially influenced by current national policy on alcohol and other drugs. All nurses need to be able to provide simple health education to people about their substance misuse, to recommend harm minimisation strategies and to be aware of how health promotion activities in the wider community can be planned and implemented.

In this chapter, you will learn about classes of drugs; risk factors for dependence; effective communication with the person who misuses substances; brief interventions and diagnostic tests; assessment and referrals; intoxication; withdrawal and rehabilitation, including some common therapies used; interprofessional care; national and international drug policies; health education; harm minimisation and health promotion related to substance misuse; and special populations, including

TABLE 5.1 Terminology associated with substance misuse

Abstinence	Voluntarily refraining from drugs or alcohol
Addiction	A disease process characterised by the continued use of a specific chemical substance despite physical, psychological or social harm (formerly used interchangeably with substance dependence; dependence is the preferred term)
Co-dependence	Maladaptive behaviour by a partner of a person misusing substances, tending to perpetuate the alcohol or drug dependence
Comorbidity	Concurrent diagnosis of a substance use disorder and a psychiatric disorder. One can precede and cause the other, as in the relationship between alcoholism and depression. Also called dual diagnosis
Cross-tolerance	Tolerance of one drug confers tolerance of another
Delirium tremens	A medical emergency usually occurring 3 to 5 days after start of alcohol withdrawal and lasting 2 to 3 days; characterised by paranoia, disorientation, delusions, visual hallucinations, elevated vital signs, vomiting, diarrhoea and diaphoresis
Detoxification	The process of helping an individual who is substance dependent safely through withdrawal (now called managed withdrawal)
Dual diagnosis	The coexistence of substance misuse/dependence and a psychiatric disorder in one individual (also described as comorbidity)
Harm reduction	A strategy recommended by NSW Health (2008a) which emphasises the use of realistic and practical approaches to harm reduction, focusing on reducing the negative effects of drug and alcohol use (also called harm minimisation)
Kindling	Brain sensitisation to events such as stress, trauma or the effects of substance use
Korsakoff's psychosis	Secondary dementia caused by thiamine (B_1) deficiency which may be associated with chronic alcoholism; characterised by progressive cognitive deterioration, confabulation, peripheral neuropathy and myopathy
Physical dependence	A state in which withdrawal syndrome will occur if drug use is discontinued
Polysubstance misuse	Simultaneous use of many substances
Prescription medication misuse	Non-medical use of pharmaceuticals or use for genuine medical purposes but without a valid prescription, or when prescribed in excessive quantities or frequencies, or when an iatrogenic dependence has developed
Problematic drug and alcohol use	Patterns of drug and alcohol use warranting intervention (NSW Health, 2008a)
Psychological dependence	An intensive subjective need for a particular psychoactive drug
Risk factor	Any attribute, characteristic or exposure that increases the likelihood of developing a disease or condition; may include behavioural, environmental, biomedical or genetic factors
Steroids	Often used illegally to build muscles and enhance exercise performance; also known as performance- and image-enhancing drugs (PIEDs)
Substance-induced disorder	A reversible substance-specific syndrome related to the type of drug used
Substance-related disorder	Continued use of a substance in spite of cognitive, behavioural and physiological symptoms
Tolerance	State in which a particular dose elicits a smaller response than formerly. With increased tolerance, higher and higher doses are needed to obtain the desired response
Wernicke's encephalopathy	Caused by thiamine (B_1) deficiency, characterised by nystagmus, ptosis, ataxia, confusion, coma and possible death; thiamine deficiency is common in chronic alcoholism
Withdrawal syndrome	Constellation of signs and symptoms occurring in physically dependent individuals when they discontinue drug use

adolescents, pregnant women, older people, Indigenous people, the LGBTQIA+ community and healthcare workers. Table 5.1 defines key terms associated with substance misuse.

DSM-5 AND SUBSTANCE USE DISORDERS

Substance use and psychiatric diagnoses are categorised in the *Diagnostic and Statistical Manual of Mental Disorders* (5th ed.) (DSM-5-TR) published by the American Psychiatric Association (APA) (2022). The APA currently divides **substance-related disorders** into two groups: **substance use disorders** (e.g. alcohol use disorder, opioid use disorder) and **substance-induced disorders** (e.g. substance-induced delirium, substance-induced psychotic disorder). With the substance use disorders, the person continues to use despite experiencing a cluster of cognitive, behavioural and physiological symptoms, while with the substance-induced disorders, the person develops a reversible substance-specific syndrome which is related to the type of drug used—these disorders may be intoxication and withdrawal, or a mental disorder (Dziegielewski, 2015).

Physiological dependence, including tolerance and withdrawal, is a normal response to repeated doses of many prescribed medications, including opioids, sedatives and stimulants; people should not be diagnosed with a substance use disorder solely on the basis of this (APA, 2022). Substance use disorders are seen as a pathological pattern of behaviours related to substance use (APA, 2022).

Diagnostic criteria are described in more detail in Table 5.2. A mild disorder is suggested by two or three of the points, a moderate disorder by four or five, and a severe disorder by six or more. The APA's DSM-5-TR criteria deal with

TABLE 5.2 Substance use disorders

1. Substance is taken in larger amounts or for longer periods than is intended.
2. Unsuccessful or persistent desire to cut down or control substance use.
3. More time occupied in getting, taking and recovering from the substance.
4. Intense craving.
5. Failure to fulfil important obligations.
6. Continued use of substance despite persistent problems.
7. Important activities given up or reduced because of use.
8. Continued use in hazardous situations.
9. Continued use despite knowledge of physical or psychological problems caused by use.
10. Presence of tolerance to the drug.
11. Presence of withdrawal symptoms.

Source: Adapted from American Psychiatric Association (2022). *Diagnostic and statistical manual of mental disorders* (5th ed.) (DSM-5-TR). Washington, DC: Author.

Agonistic effects

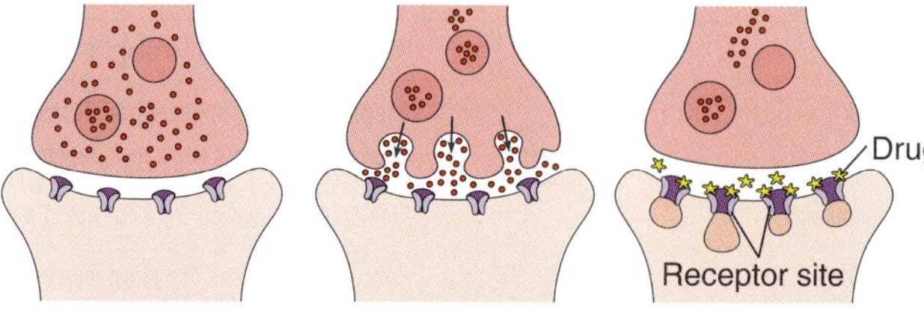

Antagonistic effects

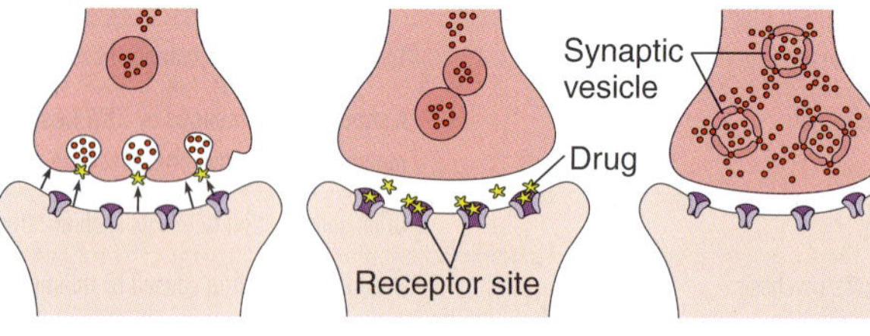

FIGURE 5.1 *Action of abusive substances at brain receptor sites*

behavioural aspects and maladaptive patterns of substance use, emphasising the physical symptoms of tolerance and withdrawal. **Tolerance** occurs when the initial dose of a substance loses its effectiveness over time. As tolerance increases, higher and higher doses are needed to obtain the desired effect. Ceasing to take a drug on which a person is physically dependent can produce withdrawal symptoms within hours—an uncomfortable state lasting several days, manifested by a range of signs and symptoms depending on which drug is involved.

RISK FACTORS AND CAUSES

Various **risk factors** help explain why one person becomes dependent while another does not. Genetic, biological and psychosocial causes may all be implicated to varying degrees. Many things can lead to continued problematic use of alcohol and/or other drugs, resulting in substance misuse and substance dependence; these include a history of abuse or trauma, and mental health problems such as antisocial personality disorder, depression and anxiety disorders including social anxiety.

- Genetic causes include an apparent hereditary factor, especially with alcohol use and dependence. Twin, adoption and family studies have demonstrated that genetic factors are responsible for 50–60% of variance in risk of developing alcoholism (Foroud, Edenberg & Crabbe, 2010). Alcohol dependence is also associated with a number of comorbid psychiatric disorders (Rietschel & Treutlein, 2013). However, no single gene causes addiction (Agrawal & Lynskey, 2008).
- Biological factors were first identified by Jellinek (1946) in his disease model of alcoholism; he hypothesised that addiction to alcohol might have a biochemical basis (see Figure 5.1), and noted specific phases of the disease. The hypothesis today is that the dopaminergic and opioid systems play different roles in the development of addictive behaviour. The dopaminergic pathway is associated with the incentive, preparatory aspects of reward (i.e. thrill, urgency, craving). The opioid system is associated with the hedonic aspects of reward (i.e. the enjoyment that follows drug use) (Teesson et al., 2012).

  Seven major neurotransmitters are involved in the response to drugs:

  1. dopamine—cocaine, amphetamines, alcohol
  2. serotonin—LSD, alcohol
  3. endorphins—opioids, alcohol
  4. gamma-aminobutyric acid (GABA)—benzodiazepines, alcohol
  5. glutamate—alcohol
  6. acetylcholine—nicotine, alcohol
  7. endocannabinoids—marijuana, alcohol (Brick & Erickson, 2012).

  Note: The drug-induced release of dopamine triggers neuroplastic changes fundamental to memory and learning (Volkow, Koob & McLellan, 2016).

  The following link shows how drugs work in the brain: http://thebrain.mcgill.ca/flash/i/i_03/i_03_cr/i_03_cr_par/i_03_cr_par.html.
- Psychosocial factors attempt to explain substance misuse through a combination of psychoanalytic, behavioural and family system theories, as well as through sociocultural and environmental issues. Psychoanalytic theorists may view substance misuse as a fixation at the oral stage of development, whereas behavioural theorists see addiction as a learned, maladaptive behaviour. Family system theory

focuses on the pattern of family relationships through several generations. Higher levels of distress have been associated in young adults with hazardous or harmful alcohol or illicit drug consumption (AIHW, 2020b), especially those in the LGBTQIA+ community (AIHW, 2022a). Sociocultural factors may influence individuals' decisions as to when and how they use which substances, as well as cultural norms about drug and alcohol. Environmental factors, such as quality of urban planning, housing, availability of public transport, cohesion of neighbourhood and community, and socioeconomic disadvantage, may also influence patterns of use (Commonwealth of Australia, Department of the Prime Minister and Cabinet, 2015).

Trauma exposure increases risk among both young males and young females (Danielson et al., 2009). Catalano et al. (2011) list many risk factors including availability of drugs; laws making it easy to access drugs; media depictions of alcohol use; communities with high rates of mobility and transitions; low neighbourhood attachment and disorganisation; extreme economic deprivation; families with a history of substance misuse and dependence; family conflict; families where there are no rules, limits or expectations for the children (or very harsh punishments); parents who misuse substances; early antisocial behaviour; starting drug use early and believing this is the norm; academic failure; low commitment to school; rebelliousness; drug-using friends; and personal characteristics such as sensation seeking, risk taking and impulsivity. Protective factors are high intelligence, resilience, social/emotional competence, prosocial behaviour, praise, bonding and healthy beliefs (Catalano et al., 2011). Epidemiological studies show that across different countries, men are more likely than women to have a substance use problem, and those under 30 are more likely than those in older age groups to experience a dependence on alcohol; however, there are higher remission rates with this group (Teesson et al., 2012). In the past 20 years, research has increasingly supported the idea that addiction is a disease of the brain; this idea includes the decreased ability to feel pleasure and the decreased motivation to get on with everyday activities, as well as increased cravings followed by negative feelings when these cravings cannot be satisfied, and the diminished decision making, control of inhibitions and self-regulation that leads to repeated relapses. Added to these significant problems are social environments, developmental stages and the role of genetics (Volkow et al., 2016). However, an alternative view is that addiction is a 'disorder of choice' (Heather, 2017) or a learned disorder, where normal learning pathways are hijacked by the pharmacological effects of the drugs used (Lamb, Stark & Ginsburg, 2021).

Reasons for use include enjoyment; added confidence; improved physical appearance; enhanced work performance; weight loss; a need to be a rule-breaker or to be part of a subculture; curiosity; availability; avoidance of boredom, pain, stress or unpleasant emotions; reduction of cravings or avoidance of withdrawal and/or to counteract withdrawal from another drug (Rassool, 2010). Substance users come from all ages and social, economic and cultural groups, with no particular personality style or traits.

CLASSIFICATION OF SUBSTANCES

CNS depressants

Alcohol is a **central nervous system (CNS) depressant** and acts on the main inhibitory neurotransmitter, GABA. It is the most commonly used drug in Australia and New Zealand because of its broad social acceptance and entrenchment in cultural norms; however, it can cause a wide range of harm (Shield, Parry & Rehm, 2013). The main psychoactive ingredient in alcohol is ethyl alcohol, which contributes to changes in mood, thinking and behaviour. Alcohol is rapidly absorbed from the small bowel (about 80%) and stomach (about 20%). It reaches the brain within 5 minutes of ingestion, with blood plasma concentrations peaking at between 30 and 90 minutes. Alcohol readily crosses the blood–brain barrier and placenta; 95% is metabolised by the liver into carbon dioxide and water, and 1–5% is excreted unchanged in saliva, urine, faeces and sweat (National Centre for Education and Training on Addiction (NCETA), 2004).

Alcohol abuse can cause severe neurological and psychiatric disorders, and damage to the liver can progress from fatty liver to other diseases such as hepatitis; chronic alcoholism is the major cause of fatal cirrhosis. Damaging effects on many other systems include myocardial disease, erosive gastritis, acute and chronic pancreatitis, sexual dysfunction and an increased risk of breast cancer. Malnutrition, another serious complication, can result in neurological impairments; in particular, thiamine (B_1) deficiency is thought to cause the severe cognitive impairment which is a principal feature of Wernicke's encephalopathy and Korsakoff's psychosis observed in people with chronic alcohol dependence (NCETA, 2004). Sometimes considered to be two distinctive disorders, these are actually different phases of the same disease, commonly called Wernicke–Korsakoff syndrome: *Wernicke's encephalopathy* describes the 'acute' stage of the illness and *Korsakoff's psychosis* describes the 'chronic' stage. Although alcohol is a CNS depressant, it actually disrupts and alters the sleep cycle, decreasing the quality, intensifying obstructive apnoea and reducing total sleeping time. Heavy drinkers have a higher mortality rate and many fatalities result from alcohol-related accidents. Chronic consumption of alcohol produces tolerance. Cross-tolerance occurs when alcohol and other CNS depressants such as benzodiazepines and opioids are used in combination; taken together they have a mutually enhancing effect, thereby increasing the possibility of respiratory depression and death (Department of Health and Ageing, 2009).

Generally, one standard alcoholic drink takes approximately 1 hour to metabolise; low doses induce a decrease in inhibitions, a feeling of comfort and relaxation, flushing of the skin and mild impairment of thinking and judgment. With rising blood alcohol levels (BALs), speech becomes slurred and is accompanied by increasing loss of motor control, including development of ataxia. At higher levels memory is affected, with potential for blackouts; the person becomes stuporous and unable to be aroused, and coma and death can occur (NSW Ministry of Health, 2021). BALs are highly predictive of CNS effects: euphoria, reduced inhibitions, impaired judgment and increased confidence are seen at 0.05%; toxic levels in excess of 0.5% can cause coma, respiratory depression, peripheral collapse and death (Brighton & Smith, 2018).

Moderate use of certain types of alcohol can have positive physiological effects in reducing coronary artery disease and protecting against stroke, but in excess it can diminish ability to function and lead ultimately to life-threatening conditions. In 2019, fewer people were drinking alcohol at risky levels and more were abstaining, with young people most likely to drink at levels exceeding single occasion risk guidelines at least once a month. Alcohol accounted for 53% of drug-related hospitalisations in 2019–2020 (AIHW, 2022a).

Benzodiazepines, minor tranquillisers belonging to the sedative–hypnotic group of drugs, have a CNS depressant effect through action at the GABA receptor sites. Prescribed for sedation, such as premedication for hospital procedures, for their muscle relaxant and amnestic properties, for relief of anxiety (anxiolytic) and as anticonvulsants, benzodiazepines also negatively affect some areas of performance, including memory, motor skills and reaction times (NCETA, 2004), and have been linked to increased falls in the elderly. Often referred to as 'benzos', they are also widely used for illicit or non-prescribed purposes. Benzodiazepines were first marketed in 1959 as a safe alternative to barbiturates and in the 1970s and 1980s, they became the most commonly prescribed class of drugs. With increasing doses the level of sedation progresses, extending to unconsciousness. The respiratory depression caused by benzodiazepines is minimal, but combination with other CNS depressants (e.g. alcohol and opioids) may have life-threatening consequences.

Opioids such as morphine (Kapanol, Anamorph, MS Contin), pethidine, codeine, methadone (Physeptone, Biodone), hydromorphone (Dilaudid, Jurnista), buprenorphine (Subutex, Suboxone, Buvidal), oxycodone (Oxycontin, Endone), fentanyl and heroin (diacetylmorphine) are narcotic analgesics. While opioids have many therapeutic uses, they also have abuse potential. Heroin has historically been the primary illicitly used opioid, but over the past decade its availability in Australia (and worldwide) has fluctuated, and abuse of pharmaceutical opioids has significantly increased. Narcotic analgesics are a pain reliever derived from natural or synthetic opioids. They interact with the endogenous opioid receptors, producing a depressant effect on the CNS, causing nausea, drowsiness, respiratory depression, reduced pain perception and euphoria, the last effect being highly reinforcing. Prolonged use of opioid drugs leads to the development of tolerance and physical dependence. Tolerance to the analgesic effects of opioids manifests itself in lowering the pain threshold: apparently mild pain may be perceived as more severe, which may inadvertently be misinterpreted by the treating nurse as drug-seeking behaviour, rather than inadequately relieved pain.

Solvents produce a CNS depressant effect. They include gases (e.g. nitrous oxide) and highly volatile compounds or mixtures (petrol, chrome-based paints, glues, aerosol spray cans, butane gas and paint thinners) giving off vapours to be inhaled through the nose or mouth, which may cause feelings of intoxication and lead to an altered state of consciousness. They can be sprayed into a plastic bag ('bagging'), soaked on a cloth or sleeve ('huffing') or inhaled directly from the container or a drink bottle ('sniffing'). Solvents are rapidly absorbed from the lungs, so small amounts quickly take effect. Brain damage or 'sudden sniffing death' can occur the first, tenth or hundredth time of use; another peril is the wide assortment of organic solvents available to and potentially inhaled by young children. Effects usually clear within a few hours. A sustained effect can be achieved by repeated use. High doses can result in coma and death.

Stimulants

Caffeine is a CNS stimulant, which increases the heart rate and acts as a diuretic. Although commonly consumed daily in soft drinks, energy drinks, coffee, tea, chocolate, guarana and some prescription and over-the-counter medicines, an excessive amount can cause negative physiological effects, especially cardiac-related risks. Approximately 400 mg per day is safe for most people, but more than 600 mg is considered excessive and is not recommended; it may cause insomnia, anxiety, depression and stomach upsets. An average cup of instant coffee may contain 60 mg of caffeine per cup; brewed coffee 80–107 mg; tea 27 mg; 375 ml of cola 48.75 mg; and 60 mg of chocolate contains 10 mg of caffeine (NSW Health, 2018). People with a history of cardiac disease are advised to reduce caffeine intake or eliminate it altogether; large quantities can cause higher total cholesterol levels. Abrupt withdrawal is likely to cause headaches, irritability and generalised feelings of tiredness in a caffeine-addicted person.

Nicotine is found in tobacco (cigarettes and cigars) and enters the system via the lungs and oral mucous membranes; in low doses, it stimulates nicotinic receptors in the brain to release noradrenaline and adrenaline, causing vasoconstriction. As a result, the heart rate accelerates and the force of ventricular contractions increases. Gastrointestinal (GI) effects include an increase in gastric acid secretion, tone and motility of GI smooth muscle, and promotion of vomiting. Nicotine acts on the CNS as a stimulant, binding to acetylcholine receptors in the brain and causing the release of dopamine and noradrenaline. Initially, nicotine increases respiration, mental alertness and cognitive ability, but eventually it depresses these responses (Brighton & Smith, 2018). Nicotine in cigarettes has a half-life of 1 to 4 hours.

Tobacco smoking is the single most preventable cause of ill health and death, being a major risk factor for coronary heart disease, stroke, peripheral vascular disease, cancer and a variety of other diseases and conditions. However, smoking rates in Australia are falling (AIHW, 2020a). Rates are higher in remote areas and for those of the lowest socioeconomic status. For women, unique health concerns arise: second-hand effects from smoking have been demonstrated, especially on the fetus during pregnancy, leading to increased risks such as low birth weight, spontaneous abortion, perinatal mortality and sudden infant death.

Psychostimulants, or CNS stimulants, comprise a diverse group of natural and synthetic drugs with a wide range of actions and effects. Psychostimulants include amphetamine-type substances such as amphetamine (speed), methamphetamine (crystal meth, ice) and dexamphetamine; methylphenidate (Ritalin®); synthetic amphetamine derivatives such as methylenedioxymethamphetamine (MDMA—ecstasy), paramethoxyamphetamine (PMA) and methylenedioxyamphetamine (MDA); cocaine; phentermine and diethylpropion, which are both prescribed appetite suppressants; ephedrine and pseudoephedrine, contained in various prescribed cold and flu preparations; and khat (Hulse, White & Cape, 2002). The amphetamines increase synaptic concentrations of the neurotransmitters dopamine, serotonin and noradrenaline. CNS or psychoactive effects include euphoria, increased alertness, increased talkativeness, sense of wellbeing, increased energy and confidence, improved mental and physical performance, loss of appetite and insomnia. Physiological effects include increased blood pressure, tachycardia or irregular heartbeat, and increased temperature (Hulse et al., 2002). Methamphetamine, MDMA (ecstasy) and cocaine are types of psychostimulants more commonly available in Australia.

Crystal methamphetamine ('crystal', 'crystal meth', 'ice') appears as crystals or coarse crystalline powder, white or translucent in colour. The most pure and potent form of methamphetamine, it is usually smoked in a glass pipe or injected, but can be snorted, swallowed or inserted rectally. Crystal methamphetamine use in Australia, as a proportion of stimulant use, more than doubled from 22% in 2010 to 50% in 2013 (AIHW, 2015), but overall, use of any methamphetamine has been declining since reporting began in 2003 (Sutherland et al., 2021).

Cocaine is a white, odourless, crystalline powder which is extracted from the coca leaf and imported into Australia. Cocaine is snorted, injected or swallowed. Crack cocaine, which is smoked, has been reported in Australia but is rare. Cocaine is less available and more expensive than amphetamines.

Stimulant drugs are used by a diverse group of people from a wide variety of socio-demographical backgrounds. Long-distance transport drivers and shift workers use them for their wakefulness-promoting effects, nightclub and dance/music festival patrons for increased energy, and others for potential weight loss, sexual enhancement and to self-medicate otherwise untreated attention-deficit and hyperactivity disorders. The range of users extends from younger age groups experimenting with drugs to polydrug users and long-term injectors.

Hallucinogens

Hallucinogens work on the brain to cause hallucinations, which can affect any of the senses—visual (sight), auditory (hearing), olfactory (smell), gustatory (taste) and tactile (touch)—and distort thoughts and moods. Sometimes called 'psychedelic drugs', they include naturally occurring and synthetic (man-made) compounds. Hallucinogenic drugs include d-lysergic acid diethylamide (LSD), ('trips', 'acid'), psilocybin ('magic mushrooms'), anticholinergics such as datura or angel's trumpet, dimethyltryptamine (DMT), phenethylamines such as mescaline and phencyclidine (PCP or 'angel dust'). Some drugs, such as cannabis and ecstasy, can cause hallucinogen-like effects in high doses. Harm (especially behavioural and psychiatric consequences) is more likely to arise from acute drug effects than from regular or dependent patterns of use.

Mixed

Cannabis is the general name given to the psychoactive substances found in the marijuana plant, cannabis sativa, the main active constituent being delta 9-tetra-hydrocannabinol (THC). The psychoactive properties are mostly of a CNS depressant nature; in high doses hallucinogenic properties can occur, affecting some of the senses (e.g. distortion of lights, sounds and music), but full hallucinations are rare (NSW Ministry of Health, 2021). THC activates specific cannabinoid receptors in the brain. Evidence indicates effects similar to those of opioids and cocaine, producing a pleasurable sensation, probably through release of endogenous opioids and then dopamine. Adverse effects include paranoia, increased appetite, anxiety, depression and sedation (Brighton & Smith, 2018). Cannabis can cause drug-induced psychosis (but usually only in people with a genetic predisposition or susceptibility); this can be difficult to distinguish from other psychotic illnesses, such as schizophrenia. Marijuana use can also trigger relapse in people living with schizophrenia. Drug-induced psychoses tend to resolve relatively quickly (within a week) with cessation of drug use (NSW Ministry of Health, 2021). A World Health Organization (WHO) study found cannabis use in the US and New Zealand (both 42%) to be far higher than in any other country surveyed (Degenhardt et al., 2008). In Australia, the National Wastewater Drug Monitoring Program showed that the population-weighted average consumption of cannabis increased in both regional (reaching record levels there) and metropolitan areas from August 2019 to August 2020 (Australian Criminal Intelligence Commission, 2021).

Steroids

Anabolic androgenic **steroids** are drugs used to build muscles and enhance exercise performance. Users tend to be men in their mid-twenties to mid-thirties. These drugs belong to a group of drugs called 'performance- and image-enhancing drugs' and are favoured by elite athletes and bodybuilders, but also by adolescents, gym attenders, professionals and students (Seear et al., 2015). Griffiths, Murray and Mond (2016) found that anabolic androgenic steroid users tend to be heavily stigmatised. Prolonged use can cause a variety of unwanted physical and psychological effects including atherosclerosis and cardiomyopathy, prolonged suppression of testicular function, major mood disorders and dependence on the drug (Kanayama, Hudson & Pope, 2008). Long-term use may also result in an effect on dopamine, serotonin and opioid pathways, and produce a hedonic effect (van Amsterdam, Opperhuizen & Hartgens, 2010).

Prescription medication

Alarmingly, **prescription medication misuse** was on the rise in Australia (AIHW, 2015), but this trend was reversed when codeine products could no longer be bought over the counter from 2018 (AIHW, 2022a). The most commonly misused prescribed drugs are oxycodone and other opioids, and the benzodiazepines.

Misuse is taken to mean the non-medical use of pharmaceuticals or use for genuine medical purposes but without a valid prescription, or when prescribed in excessive quantities or frequencies, or when an iatrogenic dependence has developed. Iatrogenic dependence occurs when a substance is prescribed for a legitimate reason and the person then becomes physically dependent on the substance, requiring higher and higher doses to achieve the desired effect. Oxycodone, fentanyl and alprazolam all have high potential for abuse and dependence, and alprazolam, which used to be a Schedule 4 drug, has now been made a Schedule 8 along with oxycodone and fentanyl. From February 2018, codeine was no longer available over the counter. The rate of dispensed opioids has climbed, with oxycodone and oxycodone/naloxone going up by 60% from 2010–2011 to 2014–2015. In 2016, the non-medical use of pharmaceuticals (pharmaceuticals include both prescribed drugs and over-the-counter drugs) was higher than of all other drugs except cannabis. Internationally (e.g. in the US and Canada), these trends are similar. Sadly, among people who misuse pharmaceuticals, the rates of chronic pain and mental illness are higher and in the past 10 years, pharmaceuticals have been responsible for more drug-induced deaths than illicit drugs. Groups at most risk for pharmaceutical misuse are those in remote and disadvantaged socioeconomic areas, those who are unable to participate in the workforce, Aboriginal and Torres Strait Islander people, injecting drug users and people in the criminal justice system (AIHW, 2017a).

Another prescription medication that is also misused is the antipsychotic quetiapine ('quell', 'Susie-Q', 'baby heroin', 'Q-ball'), with reported misuse in prisons and psychiatric units (Sansone & Sansone, 2010). This drug is increasingly prescribed 'off label' for a wide range of conditions, so it is important to be aware of its potential for misuse (Reddel et al., 2013). Pregabalin is also misused (Schifano, 2014).

Dissociative anaesthetics

Ketamine (ketamine hydrochloride) is a CNS depressant, best described as a dissociative anaesthetic agent. It is one of the newer drugs to migrate into the illicit drug-using world and was developed in the 1970s as a medical anaesthetic for both humans and animals. Illicitly, ketamine can be used as the primary drug, but also mixed with drugs such as methamphetamine and ecstasy to mimic or supplement their effects. It is pharmaceutically produced in liquid form but is converted to powder and tablet forms for illicit purposes. Commonly swallowed, snorted, smoked or injected, it has a rapid onset but short duration of action (1–6 hours). The half-life is 3 hours (Hulse et al., 2002) and it can be 24 to 48 hours before the user feels completely 'normal' again. Ketamine's effects appear to be subjective, depending on the user and the setting. Rarely in Australia do people need treatment because of ketamine, which tends to be used experimentally or socially. Whether it will become a bigger problem is not clear.

At low doses, ketamine can produce a state that has some stimulant effects and other sedating effects resembling alcohol intoxication. Larger doses can induce emesis, seizures and respiratory depression. Doses of 1 g or more can cause death. Ketamine is extremely dangerous when combined with other CNS depressants such as alcohol, benzodiazepines or gamma hydroxybutyrate because of the potentiating effects, whereby each drug increases the effect of the other drug.

Gamma hydroxybutyrate (GHB) is another CNS depressant and, although it has some mixed properties, it is essentially a dissociative anaesthetic agent. It is another of the newer drugs diverted to illicit use. Occurring naturally in the brain, GHB was first manufactured and studied in the 1960s, and used in several countries as a general anaesthetic. However, it was withdrawn from use in most countries, including Australia, because of unwanted side effects such as vomiting and seizures. GHB has a narrow dosage range between stages of a therapeutic effect, the desired effect if used illicitly, and overdose. Like most drugs, it can have a potentiating effect in combination with drugs of the same or similar class. GHB comes in the form of liquid, capsules, powder or crystals. The effects of GHB are experienced usually within 15 minutes of use and last for approximately 3 hours.

New psychoactive substances

New psychoactive substances supplement the usual range of illegal drugs but do not replace them. They are natural or synthetic drugs which mimic the traditional drugs of misuse, yet, unlike these, they are not internationally controlled. These drugs are initially produced in bulk in countries such as India or China, then sent by air or sea to Europe, where they may be sold on the illegal drug market or cut and packaged as 'research chemicals', food supplements or branded substances. In the early stages of their development, they will be used and promoted by 'psychonauts'—people interested in experimenting with new mind-altering drugs. Their experiences will be shared in online forums. However, there is no quality assurance in production or clinical testing; instead, these new psychoactive substances are tested directly by those who buy and choose to use them. They are popular because it is assumed that they are legal, and also because they are easy to acquire, cheap and difficult to detect. Patients presenting to the emergency department for help may not know exactly what they have taken; nurses need to be aware of the chemistry of this multitude of new drugs, their pharmacology, their duration of action, the route of administration, formulation and potential physical and psychological effects (Guirguis, 2017). It is also important to know which are preferred by users (Matthews et al., 2017).

The National Drug and Alcohol Research Centre at the University of NSW reports regularly on new psychoactive substances such as synthetic cannabis, which is a synthetic cannabinoid. Other classes of drugs among these new psychoactive substances are synthetic cathinones, synthetic piperazines, substituted phenethylamines, dissociative anaesthetics and substituted tryptamines (Department of Health, 2014).

ACTIVITY

Think about all classes of drugs described above. Which are legal and which are illegal? Are there any that have been made prescription only in recent years? Are there any legal drugs among them that are commonly used illegally?

COMMUNICATING EFFECTIVELY WITH PEOPLE WHO MISUSE SUBSTANCES

The key to effective work with people who misuse substances is therapeutic communication and person-centred care (Levett-Jones et al., 2017). Without good communication skills, the nurse will be unable to make comprehensive and accurate assessments and will not know which are the most appropriate referrals to offer. The importance of effective communication to patient safety is emphasised in the National Safety and Quality Health Service Communicating for Safety Standard (Australian Commission on Safety and Quality in Health Care (ACSQHC), 2021), where it is specified that health professionals must facilitate effective communication with patients, carers and families; between multidisciplinary teams; and across health service organisations.

There may be many barriers to good communication, including the nurse's personal beliefs or deeply held attitudes, the person's previous experiences with health staff or the person's intoxication, anxiety or fear of being reported or of being refused care. The person seeking care may have a sophisticated knowledge of street drugs not matched by the nurse's own knowledge. On the other hand, the nurse will have sophisticated knowledge of the health problems that can follow from unsafe drug use, and the person seeking help may be unaware of these.

A friendly, relaxed and helpful approach is a useful start. The nurse can make it clear that the person's health status and health needs are what is important. If the person uses expressions that are not clear or mentions drugs that the nurse has not heard of, asking for an explanation will show that the nurse is committed to making an accurate assessment. Responding in a matter-of-fact way to information that may surprise will allow the conversation to continue. It is important to avoid medical or nursing jargon and to keep the language fairly simple. The person seeking healthcare may not have a large vocabulary or may be intoxicated or minimally brain damaged from repeated overdoses and periods of unconsciousness, as well as from assaults.

If the person is heavily intoxicated, a full assessment will not be possible. Similarly, if the person is abusive or intimidating, the interview will be terminated, with an explanation why and an offer to continue at another time.

COMPREHENSIVE DRUG AND ALCOHOL ASSESSMENT

The ability to conduct a comprehensive health assessment is one of the seven *Registered Nurse Standards for Practice* (Nursing and Midwifery Board of Australia, 2016). It is particularly important when working with people who misuse substances because substance misuse may affect all parts of a person's life. Therefore, a full drug and alcohol assessment needs to look at all these aspects and not just focus on the current drug being used. Adopting a matter-of-fact approach to the questions that need to be asked, and avoiding being judgmental, will help encourage full disclosure and also build rapport between nurse and the person seeking help. However, assessment is not an end in itself; gathering a large amount of information has little point if nothing happens after it. The aim of this comprehensive assessment is to be able to refer the person to some appropriate treatment (Ghodse, 2010).

A helpful attitude and even a helpful start to the assessment is, 'We're interested in your health—how can we help you with that?' It is important to start with an assessment of all drugs ever used, legal and illegal. Starting with the legal ones can 'normalise' the assessment and minimise embarrassment about use of illegal drugs or excessive use. Assuring the person that the assessment is part of the medical record and remains confidential may also encourage full disclosure and effective help seeking. Many people give up one type of drug, only to develop a problem with a different one, and asking about all drugs ever used can reveal this pattern, as well as recording age when first used and how long the period of use lasted. It is very important to quantify amount used daily; writing down 'social' or 'just a couple' when estimating daily alcohol use can lead to inaccurate assessment, which may then proceed to an unmanaged withdrawal if the person is admitted to hospital and staff are unaware of preceding heavy use. Route of use and time and amount of last dose are also important.

Open questions will encourage detailed responses, although some questions only require 'yes' or 'no' as answers. Useful models for questions are: 'On a typical day when you are using alcohol or your drug of choice, how much would you have?'; 'What is the greatest number of drinks (or pills or hits or pipes) you have had at any one time during the past month?'; 'What kind of problems has substance use caused for you, your family, friends, finances and health?'

While you are completing this part of the assessment, you can also observe the patient for signs of drug use; for example, ataxia, weight loss, scars on the head, slurred speech, lacrimation, nystagmus, meiosis or mydriasis, conjunctival jaundice, dilatation of conjunctival blood vessels, rhinorrhoea, ulceration or perforation of the nasal septum, dental caries, breath odour, skin abscesses or old scars from healed abscesses, thrombophlebitis, oedema of the extremities from venous obstruction, pigmentation of the skin over the veins, sweating, piloerection, hepatomegaly, tremor, muscle twitching, muscle wasting, enlarged lymph nodes in axilla and groin, agitation or somnolence (Ghodse, 2010).

Previous experiences of withdrawal and of rehabilitation give an indication of severity of dependence and also predict likelihood of another withdrawal in this episode of care.

A comprehensive physical examination should be undertaken and should include the existence of any concomitant physical conditions likely to be drug related (e.g. HIV, hepatitis, cirrhosis, oesophageal varices, pancreatitis, gastritis, Wernicke–Korsakoff syndrome) and any relevant pathology ordered. Note allergies and all prescribed medications, especially if these are not taken as recommended, perhaps in excessive amounts or by unintended routes. Psychosocial issues are important, and an overview of the person's significant relationships including dependent children, job skills, employment, housing, legal matters pending and debts provides a picture of the total situation. Asking about family

TABLE 5.3 Stages of change model

STAGE	DESCRIPTION	STRATEGIES AND CONSIDERATIONS
Precontemplation: 'I don't have a problem.'	The person is unaware, or barely aware, that there is a problem; the cons of giving up outweigh the pros, and there is no intent to change substance using in the foreseeable future. There may also be a lack of hope because of previous failures.	Prescriptive advice can be counterproductive, creating resistance, and arousing a range of defence mechanisms which prevent people from hearing/understanding the need for change. Provide information and feedback to raise problem awareness and the possibility of change, and raise doubt to increase the perception of the risks and problems of their current behaviour.
Contemplation: 'I do have a problem and I really think I should work on it.'	The existence of a problem is acknowledged, and the person may exhibit visible signs of distress. At this stage people are open to information and education, are contemplating change but are not quite ready, and are considering the positives and negatives of giving up.	Using the person's language and goals, examine the reasons for both changing and not changing, and tip the balance in favour of change.
Preparation: 'I might cut down a bit.'	The person is beginning to set goals and make plans, and strategies are developed.	Suggest choices and probe the person's thinking about options.
Action: 'Now I am really doing something about it.'	Behavioural change has clearly begun, and significant efforts have been made to stop using alcohol or drugs. The action stage on average lasts 6 months.	Give support to take steps towards change. Raise awareness of the psychological, cognitive, behavioural and emotional events that can work against best efforts, and plan strategies to overcome potential triggers.
Relapse: 'Oh no, I mucked up everything.'	Alcohol or drugs are used again.	Treat this as a learning opportunity—a chance to ascertain which strategies and which part of the plan did not work. Help the person to identify and use strategies to prevent relapse, but to prepare for and expect it. Urge them not to give up, and to continue on the wheel of change.
Maintenance: 'I need a booster although I'm on the way.'	Continued abstention from alcohol or drugs, and intent to sustain and strengthen improvements made. It can take a few years to feel 'secure'.	

Source: Based on DiClemente (2005). Blueprint to build strong foundations for change *Addiction Today*. Retrieved from https://www.addictiontoday.org/addictiontoday/2010/08/stages-of-change-carlo-diclemente.html.

background, schools attended and highest level of education adds to this picture. A mental state examination and listing of any psychiatric treatment, current or in the past, also needs to be documented, along with an assessment of any suicidal ideation or risk of harm to others. Hazardous behaviours related to drug use should be inquired about with a view to education and harm minimisation interventions. A note can be made of the person's readiness to change. Here, the stages of change model is useful (Prochaska, Norcross & diClemente, 2013) (see Table 5.3).

ACTIVITY

A GP sends a patient (Ruelle, 27) to the community health centre (where you are on placement) with a letter requesting an AOD assessment and admission for management of prescription opioid withdrawal. Ruelle seems very agitated, fidgeting in the waiting room and regularly crossing the road to the park opposite to have a cigarette. You have been told to wait with her until the RN can 'get to her'. Ruelle takes a call on her mobile and becomes distressed. She tells you there is nobody to collect her child from preschool and she does not have a car herself. You ask the receptionist what to do, but he just shrugs. The RN sends a message that she is delayed and Ruelle will have to wait another hour. There are tears in Ruelle's eyes as she mouths, 'Sorry' to you and leaves the building.

How could Ruelle's presentation have been managed more efficiently and more compassionately? Is there a role for a student nurse in a presentation like this?

IMMEDIATE MANAGEMENT AND BRIEF INTERVENTIONS

Opportunistic intervention

Nurses are well placed to perform opportunistic interventions, which means that when they see a chance or an opportunity to raise the issue of problematic alcohol or other drug use they can do this, simply, briefly and with a focus on health education and potential referrals. At other times, the provision of factsheets, print material, cards or websites may be useful. The Alcohol and Drug Foundation (https://adf.org.au) and the Your Room website (https://yourroom.health.nsw.gov.au) provide clear and easy-to-read information that is regularly updated. The AUDIT and the CAGE screen for alcohol misuse may surprise some people, who may then move on to address the problem. The website https://hellosundaymorning.org/daybreak could be a first step, especially for younger people. The QUIT program is easy to access through www.icanquit.com.au. Larger centres may have specialist cannabis or stimulant clinics. Smaller centres usually have an alcohol and other drug (AOD) service, even if it is part time. In most places, it is easy to find an Alcoholics Anonymous or Narcotics Anonymous meeting. It is important to know what services are accessible in the area where you are working.

FRAMES is a useful mnemonic for a brief intervention. It stands for Feedback, Responsibility, Advice, Menu of change strategies, Empathy, Self-efficacy. Barriers to effective use of a brief intervention are the person's readiness to change, the person's attitude to treatment, intoxication, physical and emotional state, cultural background and literacy (Swan, Sciacchitano & Berends, 2008). The WHO developed a screening instrument called ASSIST, which screens for all psychoactive substances and is reliable and valid; this can be followed by the ASSIST-linked Brief Intervention, which is based on the FRAMES model (Ali, Gowing & Harland, 2015).

Referral

Sometimes the only referral necessary is to the person's GP. At other times the local drug and alcohol service at the community health centre (or in the hospital if the hospital is large enough) may be the appropriate source of help. The nurse may recommend quality websites, apps or online supports. The person may need to know where suitable managed withdrawal services can be found, or benefit from a referral to a mental health nurse, counsellor or psychologist to address related mental health issues. For people who have a substance misuse problem and a diagnosed mental illness, the most helpful referral will be to a comorbidity or dual diagnosis service. Integrated care has been shown to be more effective (Morley et al., 2016). A recent large-scale study of Australians living with psychosis found that alcohol and illicit drug use was very common (51% were diagnosed with alcohol dependence, 51% with cannabis misuse or dependence, and 32% with other illicit misuse or dependence), and that there has been a substantial increase in substance use among Australians living with psychosis since the last large-scale study in 1997–1998 (Moore et al., 2012). The person will be more likely to make the appointment and attend if the nurse explains the purpose of the referral and what sort of assistance will be provided. Simply thrusting a form or a card into somebody's hand and expecting the person to take all necessary steps from there without understanding the purpose, the cost or what to expect is not likely to help the person make any changes at all.

Diagnostic tests

Blood and urine are the body fluids most often tested for drug content; saliva, perspiration and hair also may be tested. More invasive procedures such as serum drug levels to treat drug overdoses or complications are useful in the emergency department and other hospital settings. Urine drug screens (UDS) may be a rapid assay test via 'dip-stick' products or sent away for laboratory analysis; UDS is non-invasive and is the preferred method for detecting substances in the body. Companies often require a precautionary UDS of prospective employees, some amateur and professional athletes have to submit to random drug testing, and determination of drug use arises in the legal system in connection with criminal activity and family court proceedings.

The period in which drugs can be found in blood and urine varies according to dosage and the metabolic properties of the drug; traces may disappear within 24 hours, or still be detectable 30 days later. The psychoactive substance found in marijuana, THC, is stored in fatty tissues (especially the brain and reproductive system) and can be detected in the body for up to 6 weeks (Brighton & Smith, 2018).

A breathalyser provides the simplest method of detecting blood alcohol content; knowledge of the BAL is helpful in ascertaining levels of intoxication and tolerance, and whether recent drinking has been accurately reported. At 0.10% (after five to six drinks in 1 to 2 hours), voluntary motor action becomes clumsy and reaction time is impaired to a degree that varies with gender, weight and food ingestion. Intoxication will occur more rapidly in small women drinking alcohol on an empty stomach than in large males who have eaten a full meal. At 0.20% (after 10 to 12 drinks in 2 to 4 hours), function of the motor area in the brain is depressed, causing staggering and ataxia (Brighton & Smith, 2018). An obtunded state does not always signify intoxication. Biological markers useful in assessing alcohol consumption include serum GGT (gamma-glutamyl transferase), AST (aspartate aminotransferase), ALT (alanine aminotransferase), HDL-cholesterol, uric acid, mean corpuscular volume and carbohydrate-deficient transferrin (CDT). Serum GGT, a liver enzyme, is the most useful of the current available tests (Department of Health and Ageing, 2009).

Intoxication

Nurses need to rule out other possible causes for the presentation that suggests intoxication. It is important not to assume the level of sedation to be due solely to intoxication if there is any possibility of a concomitant or contributing factor; conditions that can mimic aspects of intoxication include post-ictal states, hypoglycaemia, head injury, hepatic failure, stroke and other cerebrovascular events, infection, respiratory failure and hypoxia (NCETA, 2004).

ACTIVITY

Rixon (53) staggers into ED and collapses on to the floor. Rixon is well known to the staff as a heavy user of alcohol. A wardsperson is called to assist Rixon into a side room to 'sleep it off again'. ED is busy and the triage nurse says she will get to him 'when she can'. You are on placement in ED; the triage nurse tells you to do a set of observations and start an alcohol withdrawal chart. You record a full set of vital signs, fill in a first reading on the alcohol withdrawal chart and include a blood sugar level. This is below normal limits. Alcohol can lower the blood sugar (Quigley et al., 2015)*; the old notes do not mention that Rixon has diabetes or pancreatitis. What is the reason for this low blood sugar tonight? Then you notice blood on the pillow. On closer inspection you discover a wound at the base of Rixon's skull. You alert the nurse in charge of the shift who then asks one of the doctors to do an urgent physical review* (Monds & van Golde, 2017).

What might have happened if the nurse in charge of the shift had not been alerted to Rixon's deterioration? What are the implications of assuming that Rixon's condition was related to withdrawal from alcohol?

Overdose

Care of people who have overdosed on any substance is a serious medical emergency. Alcohol, opioids and sedatives are particularly dangerous, as are unusual drugs or combinations of drugs. Anyone who presents as incoherent, drowsy or disoriented should be treated as having a head injury until proved otherwise (de Crespigny & Talmet, 2012). The person may become severely sedated and difficult to arouse, requiring determined efforts to maintain wakefulness, but stupor and coma may nevertheless occur. Respiratory depression may require mechanical ventilation, while a seizure is another serious complication needing emergency treatment. Cases of intentional overdose necessitate constant monitoring for further signs of suicidal ideation—an actively suicidal person must never be left alone.

Alcohol overdose may show as altered mental state; stupor or coma; lowered temperature and blood pressure; bradycardia or tachycardia; and slow, stertorous breathing (NCETA, 2004). Benzodiazepines used alone are unlikely to result in overdose (NSW Ministry of Health, 2021). Most opioid deaths are a result of combining an opioid with other sedating drugs such as alcohol or benzodiazepines. Sudden death can occur from ventricular fibrillation and cardiac arrhythmia after sniffing solvents (NCETA, 2004). Methamphetamine overdose can cause psychosis, arrhythmias, stroke and cerebral haemorrhage (Lee et al., 2007). Ecstasy can cause life-threating hyperthermia and hyponatraemia. Toxic amounts of cocaine produce a multitude of symptoms, including cardiac, respiratory, neurological and renal. Hallucinogens in overdose may produce active hallucinations or dysphoria ('a bad trip'), while overdoses of anticholinergics such as datura and brugmansia are life threatening, with effects lasting for several days. Cannabis is not associated with fatal overdoses (NCETA, 2004). Steroids in high doses for long periods may cause irreversible heart damage (State Library of NSW, 2018). Prescription medication overdoses will be managed based on the class the drug belongs to. GHB has a narrow therapeutic index, and overdose usually occurs within 15 minutes of ingestion and is more likely when combined with alcohol (NCETA, 2004).

ACTIVITY

Rella (54) has been admitted to the medical ward (where you work as RN) for a managed withdrawal from polysubstances, including prescribed, over the counter and illegally acquired. Some of the staff whisper about her, having found out that she has a prominent position in the community. One says to you, 'She should know better; it's disgusting at her age. She'll just have to get through as best she can. I don't want to look after her.'

What can you do to assist Rella with all aspects of her managed withdrawal?

Determining which new psychoactive substance has been ingested can be challenging as the person may not know exactly what has been taken or what mixture of substances has been taken, and standard urine drug screens show only the most common classes of drugs, and standard breath tests are only used for alcohol.

Withdrawal

Many people choose to enter a facility to undertake managed **withdrawal** (sometimes called detoxification); others are admitted unexpectedly to hospital and begin to withdraw without proper monitoring or management if their admission has not included a brief drug and alcohol use screen.

Withdrawal is not pleasant, but the discomfort can be minimised by good nursing care and the use of appropriate medications. Some drugs commonly used for a managed withdrawal are listed in Table 5.4. A common belief is that withdrawal from heroin is protracted and dangerous; however, it is alcohol withdrawal and withdrawal from benzodiazepines that are the most risky if not managed carefully. Polysubstance misuse complicates withdrawal, as do concomitant medical or psychiatric issues. It is vital that the environment is safe for care delivery, both with regard to patient and staff safety, and with regard to ensuring the area is welcoming to all people, particularly that staff show cultural competence when working with Indigenous people. Without these things, and without some partnership with patients in their own care, the process of managed withdrawal may be both disappointing to the person and unsuccessful overall (ACSQHC, 2021).

Complicated alcohol withdrawal carries a significant risk of further morbidity and is potentially life threatening. Proper assessment and monitoring procedures, in combination with early and adequate institution of the necessary medical treatment, should prevent the development of complicated withdrawal syndrome in a hospital setting. Withdrawal scales provide an objective method of assessing a person at risk and the course of the syndrome. The most validated and widely used scale is the Clinical Institute Withdrawal Assessment for Alcohol—revised version (CIWA-Ar) (Sullivan et al., 1989) (see Figure 5.2). A BAL above 0.10% without associated behavioural symptoms indicates the presence of tolerance; high tolerance is a sign of physical dependence. Assessing for withdrawal symptoms is important when the BAL is high and the person shows significant tolerance; medication for treatment of withdrawal from alcohol is usually not started until the BAL is below a set norm (usually 0.10%) unless withdrawal symptoms become severe. BAL may be repeated several times, several hours apart, to assess the body's metabolism of alcohol and determine when it is safe to administer medication to minimise the withdrawal symptoms. Management of alcohol withdrawal in hospital is shown in Box 5.1.

Withdrawal scales do not diagnose withdrawal; they monitor the severity of the range of signs and symptoms of those experiencing or at risk of developing alcohol withdrawal. It is important to start the monitoring as soon as possible after admission to hospital. Supportive care alone is often effective in minor alcohol withdrawal. Early and adequate pharmacological intervention can prevent development of a complicated alcohol withdrawal syndrome carrying significant risk of added morbidity. Caution is required in treating the elderly or people

TABLE 5.4 Drugs used in the treatment of substance withdrawal/abuse

DRUG	DOSE	PURPOSE
Benzodiazepines		
1. Midazolam	Individualised, IMI, IV	Diminishes anxiety and has anticonvulsant qualities to provide safe withdrawal. May be ordered q4h or prn to manage adverse effects from withdrawal, then dose is tapered to zero.
2. Diazepam (Valium)	4-120 mg/day	
3. Oxazepam (Serepax)	30-120 mg/day	
4. Lorazepam (Ativan)	2-6 mg/day	
Vitamins		
1. Thiamine (vitamin B_1)	100 mg/day	Prevents Wernicke's encephalopathy
2. Folic acid	1 mg/day	Corrects vitamin deficiency caused by heavy long-term alcohol abuse
3. Multivitamins	1 tab/cap daily	
Anticonvulsants		
1. Phenytoin (Dilantin)	Individualised as per bodyweight	Seizure prophylaxis
2. Magnesium sulfate	1 g q6h	Reduces post-withdrawal seizures
Abstinence medications		
1. Disulfiram (Antabuse)	250 mg/day	Prevents breakdown of alcohol
2. Naltrexone (ReVia)	50 mg/day	Diminishes cravings for alcohol and opioids
3. Acamprosate (Campral)	133.3-199.8 mg/day	Decreases alcohol craving
Antidepressants		
1. Fluoxetine (Prozac)	20-80 mg/day	Enhances and stabilises mood and diminishes anxiety
2. Sertraline (Zoloft)	50-200 mg/day	Enhances and stabilises mood and diminishes anxiety
Symptomatic treatment for individual withdrawal symptoms		
Metoclopramide (Maxolon)	30 mg/day	Nausea and vomiting
Prochlorperazine (Stemetil)	10-30 mg/day	Nausea and vomiting
Paracetamol	Up to 4 g/day	Headache, generalised aches and pains
Ibuprofen (or other non-steroidal anti-inflammatory agents)	Up to 1.6 g/day	Headache, generalised aches and pains
Kaomagma	80 mg/day	Diarrhoea
Hyoscine butylbromide (Buscopan)		GIT spasm
Opioid agonists		
Methadone	Individualised	Opioid substitution agent for maintenance treatment
Buprenorphine	Individualised	Opioid substitution agent for maintenance treatment or opioid withdrawal management
Buprenorphine-naloxone	Individual dosage up to 32 mg/day	Opioid substitution agent for maintenance treatment

with respiratory compromise. Diazepam, a long-acting benzodiazepine, is widely recognised as the pharmaceutical agent of choice. Contraindications to diazepam include respiratory failure, significant liver impairment and possible head injury or cerebrovascular accident. In these situations, specialist consultation is essential (NSW Health, 2008b).

Risk factors for severe alcohol withdrawal include previous episodes of alcohol withdrawal, previous seizures during withdrawal, history of delirium tremens, CIWA-Ar score above 10, advanced age, comorbidities, detectable BAL on admission, high daily intake of alcohol, abnormal liver function, prior benzodiazepine use, male sex, previous blackouts and concomitant use of CNS depressants or illicit substances (Carlson et al., 2012; Maldonado et al., 2014).

The rate of developing benzodiazepine dependence varies. After 3 to 12 months' usage, 10–20% of users will become dependent, rising to 20–45% when duration of use exceeds 12 months. Heavy users can experience such medical complications of withdrawal as seizures, hallucinations and delirium if dosage is reduced too rapidly; gradual reduction is therefore recommended (NSW Health, 2008b). Depending on the half-life of the particular benzodiazepine, onset of benzodiazepine withdrawal occurs 2 to 5 days after stopping or significantly reducing the usual intake; the peak is usually reached on days 7 to 10, and most signs and symptoms usually abate by the end of the second or third week (NSW Health, 2008b). It is important to ask about a history of benzodiazepine use at admission as part of the AOD assessment, or as soon as practicable. Heavy users or polydrug users should be stabilised before admission on a long-acting preparation (preferably diazepam) at a dose about 40–50% of their regular intake (or 80 mg/day, whichever is lower) (NSW Health, 2008b). However, a hospital admission, during an acute illness, may not be the appropriate time to undertake an elective withdrawal; this may best be managed in an outpatient setting.

Unlike alcohol withdrawal, the syndrome associated with cessation of opioid use is not medically serious except in pregnant women. Opioid withdrawal is potentially life threatening for the fetus, as is naltrexone (an opioid antagonist) precipitated withdrawal. Opioid withdrawal can be viewed as a flu-like syndrome with major and minor symptoms: Opioid-dependent people are often admitted to hospitals and develop unplanned withdrawal. While the syndrome is not medically dangerous, the symptoms can cause considerable discomfort and may lead to resumption of use to avoid or abate the symptoms. Early discharge and thus poor intervention outcomes are probable results. The Clinical Opiate

Clinical Institute Withdrawal Assessment of Alcohol Scale, Revised (CIWA-Ar)

Patient:________________________ **Date:** _______________ **Time:** ______________ (24 hour clock, midnight = 00:00)

Pulse or heart rate, taken for one minute:_______________________ **Blood pressure:**______

NAUSEA AND VOMITING -- Ask 'Do you feel sick to your stomach? Have you vomited?' Observation.
0 no nausea and no vomiting
1 mild nausea with no vomiting
2
3
4 intermittent nausea with dry heaves
5
6
7 constant nausea, frequent dry heaves and vomiting

TACTILE DISTURBANCES -- Ask 'Have you any itching, pins and needles sensations, any burning, any numbness, or do you feel bugs crawling on or under your skin?' Observation.
0 none
1 very mild itching, pins and needles, burning or numbness
2 mild itching, pins and needles, burning or numbness
3 moderate itching, pins and needles, burning or numbness
4 moderately severe hallucinations
5 severe hallucinations
6 extremely severe hallucinations
7 continuous hallucinations

TREMOR -- Arms extended and fingers spread apart. Observation.
0 no tremor
1 not visible, but can be felt fingertip to fingertip
2
3
4 moderate, with patient's arms extended
5
6
7 severe, even with arms not extended

AUDITORY DISTURBANCES -- Ask 'Are you more aware of sounds around you? Are they harsh? Do they frighten you? Are you hearing anything that is disturbing to you? Are you hearing things you know are not there?' Observation.
0 not present
1 very mild harshness or ability to frighten
2 mild harshness or ability to frighten
3 moderate harshness or ability to frighten
4 moderately severe hallucinations
5 severe hallucinations
6 extremely severe hallucinations
7 continuous hallucinations

PAROXYSMAL SWEATS -- Observation.
0 no sweat visible
1 barely perceptible sweating, palms moist
2
3
4 beads of sweat obvious on forehead
5
6
7 drenching sweats

VISUAL DISTURBANCES -- Ask 'Does the light appear to be too bright? Is its color different? Does it hurt your eyes? Are you seeing anything that is disturbing to you? Are you seeing things you know are not there?' Observation.
0 not present
1 very mild sensitivity
2 mild sensitivity
3 moderate sensitivity
4 moderately severe hallucinations
5 severe hallucinations
6 extremely severe hallucinations
7 continuous hallucinations

ANXIETY -- Ask 'Do you feel nervous?' Observation.
0 no anxiety, at ease
1 mildly anxious
2
3
4 moderately anxious, or guarded, so anxiety is inferred
5
6
7 equivalent to acute panic states as seen in severe delirium or acute schizophrenic reactions

HEADACHE, FULLNESS IN HEAD -- Ask 'Does your head feel different? Does it feel like there is a band around your head?' Do not rate for dizziness or lightheadedness. Otherwise, rate severity.
0 not present
1 very mild
2 mild
3 moderate
4 moderately severe
5 severe
6 very severe
7 extremely severe

AGITATION -- Observation.
0 normal activity
1 somewhat more than normal activity
2
3
4 moderately fidgety and restless
5
6
7 paces back and forth during most of the interview, or constantly thrashes about

ORIENTATION AND CLOUDING OF SENSORIUM -- Ask 'What day is this? Where are you? Who am I?'
0 oriented and can do serial additions
1 cannot do serial additions or is uncertain about date
2 disoriented for date by no more than 2 calendar days
3 disoriented for date by more than 2 calendar days
4 disoriented for place/or person

Total **CIWA-Ar** Score ______
Rater's Initials ______
Maximum Possible Score 67

The ***CIWA-Ar*** *is not* copyrighted and may be reproduced freely. This assessment for monitoring withdrawal symptoms requires approximately 5 minutes to administer. The maximum score is 67 (see instrument). Patients scoring less than 10 do not usually need additional medication for withdrawal.

FIGURE 5.2 ***Assessment tool for alcohol withdrawal***

Source: Sullivan et al. (1989). Assessment of alcohol withdrawal: The revised Clinical Institute Withdrawal Assessment for Alcohol scale (CIWA-Ar). *British Journal of Addiction, 84*, 1353–1357.

BOX 5.1 Management of alcohol withdrawal in hospital

- Start with a comprehensive alcohol and other drug use history.
- Consider the possibility of alcohol withdrawal if clinical symptoms are already occurring in a patient, as some patients may minimise how much alcohol they consume when initially asked or may not be able to provide accurate information on arrival.
- Identify those at risk of alcohol withdrawal (for men, daily consumption of 80–100 g or 8–10 standard drinks, and for women 80 g or 8 standard drinks—sometimes less depending on the person's physical or psychiatric condition).
- Explain withdrawal management simply and clearly. Reassure.
- Start an alcohol withdrawal scale such as CIWA-Ar and record observations at least every 4 hours or more often if scores warrant this. If the person is intoxicated on admission, begin these observations as soon as the BAL goes below 0.10%.
- Seek medical advice and, if medicated treatment for withdrawal is indicated, commence it early and follow the local clinical guidelines strictly. The usual drug is diazepam.
- Provide a quiet, softly lit, pleasant environment.
- Even if observations are not yet due, check the person regularly.
- Reassure and re-orient when you do this.
- Give thiamine according to local clinical guidelines.
- Monitor hydration.
- Ensure adequate nutrition. Adjust diet if the person is nauseated.
- Treat symptoms such as nausea, vomiting, headache or altered mental state as they arise.

Withdrawal Scale is helpful in monitoring the progress of the syndrome (Wesson & Ling, 2003). Another method of assessment is that withdrawal signs and symptoms will usually begin around the time of the user's expected next dose. The short half-life of heroin produces onset at 6 to 24 hours after last use, and duration is 5 to 10 days. Withdrawal from methadone, which has a longer half-life, occurs 24 to 48 hours after the last dose and lasts for 10 to 20 days. People who have been treated for opioid withdrawal should be advised of the increased risk of overdose if they resume using because they have lost their tolerance; even lesser amounts than those previously used could result in overdose.

Confusion and hallucinations can occur after chronic solvent use (NSW Health, 2008b). Abrupt withdrawal from caffeine is likely to cause headaches, irritability and generalised feelings of tiredness. The difficulty of quitting smoking is thought to be caused by dopamine release, which in turn reinforces the addictive craving for more. Nicotine in cigarettes has a half-life of 1 to 4 hours, so withdrawal symptoms become evident within a few hours after the last cigarette; withdrawal peaks during days 2 and 3, and tends to resolve at about 2 to 4 weeks. According to DSM-5-TR (APA, 2022), nicotine withdrawal can be diagnosed if four or more of the following symptoms are present within the first 24 hours of nicotine reduction or cessation: depressed mood, insomnia, irritability, frustration or anger, anxiety, difficulty concentrating, restlessness and increased appetite. A guide for the management of nicotine-dependent inpatients is shown in Table 5.5.

Management of psychostimulant withdrawal is mostly supportive—understanding, patience, encouragement and positive affirmation. Medical treatment might involve judicious, short-term use of benzodiazepines to alleviate some of the anxiety and agitation and help with disturbed sleep. If protracted low mood or more severe depression exists, or psychotic features do not resolve within a couple of days, further assessment will be required. Medical complications, usually resulting from injecting drug use, may need further investigation and treatment. A primary aim of health services contact is to educate people about the risks of continued use, discuss harm minimisation options, offer referral or arrange engagement in some sort of relapse prevention support. The medical and psychiatric complications of stimulant use are listed in Table 5.6.

Hallucinogens are typically used experimentally, occasionally or irregularly, so hallucinogen withdrawal treatment is not required; few people present to treatment centres because of hallucinogen use. One of the few known long-term effects of hallucinogen use is 'flashbacks'—times when feelings similar to those caused by the drug arise intermittently some days, weeks or years after last use. Flashbacks can be precipitated by other drug use, stress, anxiety and fatigue. Other effects include difficulties with memory and concentration, and precipitation or worsening of mental health problems (NSW Ministry of Health, 2021).

Cannabis withdrawal is marked by three or more of the following: sleep disturbance (insomnia and vivid dreams), reduced appetite or weight loss, irritability, anger or aggression, anxiety or nervousness, restlessness, depressed mood and at least one of abdominal pain, shakiness, sweating, fever, chills or headaches (APA, 2022). The major part of the management approach for cannabis withdrawal should be supportive counselling, provision of accurate information about signs and symptoms, and relapse prevention planning. Medications may be appropriate for some people; most commonly prescribed are benzodiazepines, to be used with discretion and in the short term.

Steroid withdrawal is mild (van Amsterdam et al., 2010).

Prescription medication withdrawal will depend on the class of drug that has been misused. Benzodiazepine and opioid withdrawal are discussed previously.

A ketamine withdrawal syndrome involving fear, tremors, facial twitches and craving can occur after cessation of long-term daily use of ketamine (NSW Health, 2008b).

Abrupt cessation may cause a user who has developed tolerance to and dependence on GHB to suffer GHB withdrawal symptoms, which usually start about 12 hours after the last dose and can continue for approximately 2 weeks (NCETA, 2004). Management of GHB withdrawal may require use of both short- and long-acting benzodiazepines. Some users may require further sedation with a short-acting anaesthetic agent (e.g. propofol) (NSW Health, 2008b).

TABLE 5.5 Guide for the management of nicotine-dependent inpatients

1. Identify every tobacco user on admission

Use Substance Use History form or include smoking status on existing admission forms
Ex-smokers–encourage continuing abstinence
Daily/occasional smokers–follow steps 2 to 5

2. Manage inpatient nicotine dependence

Inform people of the policy for smoking in your facility and specify contra-indications to their treatment regimen if they leave the ward/facility to smoke
Discuss options for management of nicotine dependence while in hospital, such as:

- abstinence
- abstinence supported by nicotine replacement therapy (NRT), unless contra-indicated
- smoking offsite in outdoor designated areas, if available

If a person has a history of mental health problems, consult treating clinician–adjustment of medications may be necessary.

3. Prescribe nicotine therapy

Arrange prescriptions for NRT (with the person's consent)
Record:

- type (patch/inhaler/gum) and dose on medication chart
- 'Nicotine dependent' in person's notes

4. Monitor person's withdrawal symptoms

If a person is still experiencing withdrawal symptoms:

- review NRT dose/product (person may benefit from combination therapy)

5. Discharge

Ask all smokers: 'Do you plan to smoke when you go home?'

'Yes.'

- Encourage future quit attempt: 'The best thing you can do for your health is to stop smoking. When you're ready, phone the Quitline or talk to your doctor.'

'No.'

- Arrange 3-day post-discharge NRT
- Include treatment summary in discharge plan
- Advise person to seek cessation support from GP/pharmacist/Quitline 137 848
- Provide brochures on smoking cessation.

Source: Adapted from NSW Health (2015). *Managing nicotine dependence: A guide for NSW Health staff.* Reproduced by permission, NSW Ministry of Health © 2015.

TABLE 5.6 Medical and psychiatric complications of stimulant use

SYSTEM	COMPLICATIONS
Cardiovascular	Arrhythmias: tachycardia, bradycardia, ventricular tachycardia. Hypertension: may lead to cerebrovascular accidents. Spasm of arteries: leading to myocardial infarcts or cerebrovascular accidents. (Myocardial infarcts can occur during first weeks of withdrawal.) Cardiomyopathy and congestive heart failure.
Neurological	Seizures: clonic convulsions. Cerebrovascular accident: including brain haemorrhages, infarcts and ischaemic episodes. Neuropsychological changes: deficits in attention, concentration, memory and new learning skills. Movement disorders: e.g. tics, disturbed gait, stereotyped repetitive movements, choreiform movements.
Psychiatric	May mimic any psychiatric disorder. More commonly: • depression, with changes in mood and affect, sleep, activity • paranoia, ranging from hypervigilance to paranoid psychosis • anxiety and aggression, ranging from irritability and agitation to panic attacks or violence (more common in amphetamine and methamphetamine users) • delirium, with clouding of consciousness, disorientation, confusion • psychosis, characterised by paranoia and anxiety, impaired reality testing with loss of insight and delusions (e.g. ideas of reference, persecutory delusions) and perceptual disturbances (including misperceptions and visual, auditory or tactile (formication) hallucinations).
Respiratory	Smoking of cocaine and amphetamines can result in chronic lung damage (including pneumonia, pulmonary oedema, bronchitis).
Sexuality	Short-term stimulant use is often associated with increased sexual drive and performance. However, chronic use can lead to difficulties achieving orgasm, altered menstruation (oligomenorrhea, amenorrhoea) and galactorrhoea in women, and reduced libido, impotence and gynaecomastia in men.
Hyperpyrexia	Extremely elevated body temperature, which can contribute to seizures, cardiac arrhythmias and death. Rhabdomyolysis can also occur, resulting in acute renal and hepatic failure, disseminated intravascular coagulation and death.
Pregnancy	Stimulant use during pregnancy is associated with higher rates of obstetric complications (spontaneous abortion, miscarriage and placental abruption) and harm to the fetus.
Other	Weight loss (chronic loss of appetite and increased metabolism). Skin lesions and abscesses, due to adulterants, particularly in injectors.

Source: NSW Health (2008b). *Drug and alcohol withdrawal: Clinical practice guidelines: NSW*, p. 51. Sydney: NSW Health Reproduced by permission, NSW Ministry of Health. © 2015.

New psychoactive substances may be so new that little is known about potential withdrawal.

REHABILITATION FOR PEOPLE DEPENDENT ON ALCOHOL OR OTHER DRUGS

People who enter rehabilitation are not only learning to live without their drug or drugs of choice—they are learning a whole new way to live. For some, getting up at a set time, attending to personal hygiene and being at groups, classes or appointments on time is difficult. Many of the skills-based groups are confronting; living as part of a community can be difficult for those who have been homeless or who have become disconnected from family and friends. Over the period of the rehabilitation, people will have a chance to mend broken relationships, organise finances, improve physical health, have drug-related medical or psychiatric problems addressed, learn new skills to assist with future employment and personal life, settle outstanding legal matters and discover recreational opportunities not linked to drug use. The nurse may run the primary health clinic, assist with doctor's appointments, liaise with the pharmacy, conduct education sessions, run therapeutic groups or provide individual counselling. The nurse will also be responsible for first aid, triage and transfer to hospital in case of medical emergencies.

Each discipline has a different perspective on and understanding of dependence; this can enrich the whole rehabilitation experience for the person provided all staff are respectful of each other's views. Some rehabilitation centres adopt a particular philosophy; for example, some are based on the Twelve Step Model from Alcoholics Anonymous developed as the Minnesota Model (Anderson, McGovern & DuPont, 1999) or have a religious emphasis, while others focus on daily work patterns and may require committed input to the running of a farm or other business. Sometimes a drug rehabilitation centre is established based on a single person's successful recovery and personal leadership style; in these centres, there may not be a focus on evidence-based practice or any outcome measures done. Other centres are run as therapeutic communities. The cost of treatment in private clinics will preclude many from admission.

ACTIVITY

Rad (24) has just arrived at the rehabilitation centre where you are the RN in charge of the primary health clinic. Part of your role is to perform a health check on new patients. Rad has travelled for 12 hours in a train, and looks tired and stressed. He says to you: 'So I did the detox but I had to go a long way from home to get a place. Now I'm just wondering if it's all going to be worth it? They say it takes at least 2 weeks to come off ice [crystal methamphetamine] but the detox only keeps people for 5 days. I feel like I don't know who I am anymore, like I've lost myself somehow. I only want to hide. Maybe I should just go now?'

What would you say to Rad?

Psychosocial interventions in recovery

Psychosocial interventions in rehabilitation may include a range of different therapies. They aim to manage aspects of substance misuse based on both individual (internal) psychological attributes such as emotions, attitudes and behaviours, and social (external) factors such as family, community and culture. Interventions with the strongest evidence base are assessment and brief intervention, motivational interviewing (see Box 5.2), contingency management, cognitive behavioural therapy, psychodynamic therapy, dialectical behaviour therapy, self-help approaches (which now include internet-based assistance) and continuing care. Others are mindfulness-based stress reduction, acceptance and commitment therapy (ACT), couples or family therapy, and self-help groups such as Alcoholics Anonymous, Narcotics Anonymous, SMART Recovery and WHOS (We Help Our Selves) (NSW Ministry of Health, 2021). Behavioural approaches address capability, opportunity and motivation (West & Farrell, 2015). Relapse prevention skills are crucial, including identifying triggers and distinguishing a lapse from a relapse.

Active case management and efficient care coordination are important because people with a serious substance misuse problem are likely to require a range of other services as well as specific therapies for the alcohol or drug problem. A counselling style known as motivational interviewing (see Box 5.2) is helpful when working with this group. Although the principles

BOX 5.2 Principles of motivational interviewing

1. **Express empathy**
   Understanding the cycle of change can help the nurse to empathise, communicate a sense of respect and give direction to intervention strategies (Miller, 1995); an empathic therapeutic style is associated with greater long-term behaviour change.
2. **Develop discrepancy**
   Motivation for change occurs when people perceive a discrepancy between where they are and where they want to be. The object of this approach is to enhance and focus attention on such discrepancies with regard to alcohol and drug use (Miller, 1995); at this stage, the nurse may discuss concerns about the person's current level of use, what is positive about such use and what is causing problems (NSW Health, 2008a).
3. **Roll with resistance and avoid argumentation**
   New perspectives may be raised but not imposed: arguing is counterproductive and can create defensiveness. The simplest response to resistance is non-resistance; repeating the person's statement in a neutral form acknowledges and validates it, and can elicit an opposite reaction.
4. **Support self-efficacy**
   Self-efficacy is the belief that one can adopt a behaviour or accomplish a particular task; it is important because belief in the possibility of change is an effective motivator. The nurse facilitates informed choice of goal and method of treatment and communicates confidence and optimism (NCETA Consortium, 2004).

in the box are helpful for people wishing to gain an initial understanding of motivational interviewing, in the most recent text, the authors have modified these to engaging, focusing, evoking and planning (Miller & Rollnick, 2013). The mnemonic RULE is a helpful way to remember the principles: Resist the righting reflex, Understand the patient's own motivations, Listen with empathy, Empower the patient. The mnemonic OARS is a helpful way to remember the interviewing style: Open-ended questions, Affirmations, Reflections, Summarising (Hall, Gibbie & Lubman, 2012).

CONSIDERATION FOR PRACTICE

People are at highest risk of relapse within the first few months after stopping the misused substance. Vulnerability to triggers and intense cravings are a normal, although difficult, feature of the earlier stages of recovery. An acronym that can assist in recognising behaviours that lead to relapse is HALT: Hungry, Angry, Lonely and Tired. Nurses should emphasise the importance in preventing relapse of a balanced diet, adequate sleep, healthy recreation activities and a caring support system.

INTERPROFESSIONAL CARE

Working with people who have a substance misuse problem involves a range of disciplines, and for the care to be effective all these health professionals need to work as a team, whether the person is in acute withdrawal, undertaking a lengthy rehabilitation or being supported by an outreach service in the community. Teamwork and collaborative practice are essential in this setting (Levett-Jones et al., 2017). In the hospital setting, as well as nurses and doctors, the person with a substance misuse problem may need assistance from a social worker, a dietitian, any one of a number of specialist physicians, a mental health nurse, and a drug and alcohol nurse. In residential rehabilitation, a multidisciplinary team can include nurses, general practitioners, social workers, psychologists, counsellors, welfare workers, case managers, support workers and staff in recovery themselves. Educational programs and groups may be run by nurses, TAFE teachers, music teachers, art teachers, financial counsellors, nutritionists, yoga teachers, personal trainers, chefs, horticulturalists and tradespeople.

A person who elects to work with an outreach service may attend some of these groups and educational sessions and will also be supported by a key worker with regular appointments and phone calls. Among the staff the person encounters will be those who advocate complete abstinence, those who support the recovery model based on the 12-step model of Alcoholics Anonymous (which is dominant in the US) and those who adopt a harm minimisation approach (Recke, 2017).

National and international drug policy

The 'war on drugs' is a familiar phrase, but it has not reduced the international drug trade or the health consequences for people who use illicit drugs; it also suggests that a militarised response is appropriate, and in so doing shifts the focus away from providing healthcare and social support in a public health framework. People who use drugs can then be seen as collateral damage in this war, instead of as people who need to access quality healthcare because of some of their behaviours (Perlman & Jordan, 2017).

International drug policies vary widely and often reflect community values and expectations, as well as the vested interests of organisations and governments. Use of tobacco, alcohol and opioids were all generally accepted in the 19th century, but after World War 1, opioids and cocaine became subject to international controls, based partly on concerns about use of opium in the Far East, but also on US trade and strategic interests in that area (Berridge, 2010).

Options informing legal frameworks to govern supply and use include full prohibition (supply, possession and use are banned completely and are treated as criminal acts), depenalisation (use is a criminal act but the user may be diverted to treatment and health care), decriminalisation (possession and use attract civil penalties such as fines, although the drugs themselves are still illegal and supply is still a criminal offence) and legalisation (supply and use are legal). Portugal decriminalised use and possession of all illicit drugs in 2001 (Lee & Ritter, 2016).

Australian drug policies are based on the principle of harm minimisation. This encompasses three strategies:

1. Supply reduction to disrupt the production and supply of illegal drugs and to control and regulate legal substances.
2. Demand reduction to prevent people starting harmful drug use. This includes abstinence and treatment to reduce drug use. Priority substances are methamphetamines and other stimulants, alcohol, tobacco, cannabis, non-medical use of pharmaceuticals, opioids and new psychoactive substances (Commonwealth of Australia, 2019).
3. **Harm reduction** to reduce drug-related harms to both individuals and communities. Broad harm reduction strategies include demand reduction, supply reduction and environmental responses to help users in the safest way possible. These can be seen as 'the least worst option' (Hamilton & Rumbold, 2004, p. 136).

Health education, harm minimisation and health promotion

Health education is not the same thing as health promotion. Schools may provide some information about types of drugs and their effects as part of a personal development course, and there are many websites that also provide constantly updated information about drugs in common use (e.g. https://adf.org.au). Mass education campaigns in the form of television advertisements or large roadside hoardings capture the public's attention but may not have the desired effect. Education may be a first step in a move to change, but a systematic review of public education campaigns concluded that contrary to popular belief, some antidrug mass media campaigns may be damaging (Allara et al., 2015).

Harm minimisation is a component of current national drug policy and accepts that some people will continue to misuse substances in spite of the risk. This strategy therefore looks at providing ways to minimise the harms of this problematic use. A useful definition of harm minimisation is 'Approaches to drug policy that seek to minimise the harmful consequences of drug use to the individual, families and the community at large, and adopt a value-neutral position with regard to drug use per se' (Van Beek, 2013, p. 170). The value-neutral position is particularly important to nurses if they are going to view drug use as a health problem.

Harm minimisation is not intended to encourage or facilitate use, but rather to manage risks, although it can be misunderstood by some in the community. It decreases potential harms for people already using substances. Examples of harm minimisation strategies are:

- provision of needle and syringe exchange programs—AIVL (the Australian Injecting and Illicit Drug Users League) provides a state and territory listing of needle and syringe programs and a legal guide for users (www.aivl.org.au)
- information about safe injecting techniques
- education about what to do in case of overdose
- making Narcan (naloxone) readily available
- changing route of administration of drug
- establishing the Medically Supervised Injecting Centre in Sydney's Kings Cross in 2001
- NSW Health funding of *User's News* (https://nuaa.org.au)
- pill testing kits
- free water at large public events
- advising young people not to drive with somebody who is intoxicated with alcohol or drugs
- laws preventing service of alcohol to intoxicated people
- 'safe glass' containers in pubs to prevent injuries in brawls
- lock out times and earlier cessation of service where alcohol is available
- access to public transport after large events
- providing free transport home from hotels and clubs
- banning glass bottles at large open-air events.
- collapsible road signage and poles
- random breath testing that discourages people from driving when intoxicated or affected by drugs (see Figure 5.3)
- rules preventing smoking in public buildings
- asking people not to smoke near children
- distribution of condoms to prevent HIV and other STDs.

Sharma (2016) proposed a Multi Model Theory of health behaviour change, focusing on both starting the change and then continuing with the change. For the first, the person needs two-way communication with a health worker, then a belief in the ability to make the change in the future, then a physical environment that will support this; for the second, the person needs self-motivation and self-belief, with practice for change, and finally good social support.

Health promotion programs focus on prevention in a broad sense. They look ahead to potential future use. Strategies may be universal, selective or individual. Until science is able to predict accurately who will develop abuse or dependence, or even start using, universal strategies will continue to be important (Sloboda et al., 2009). Health education now refers to behaviour change, whereas the broad view today of health promotion is very similar to the new public health. The focus is on social justice, empowerment and the achievement of equity (Baum, 2008). To prevent a problem from happening, the focus should be on changing the factors that predict it (Catalano et al., 2011). Genetic vulnerability to addiction may be reduced by developing more effective social norms (Lamb et al., 2021). Becoming more involved in community activities was shown to be protective against a genetic risk for cannabis use (Thomas et al., 2021).

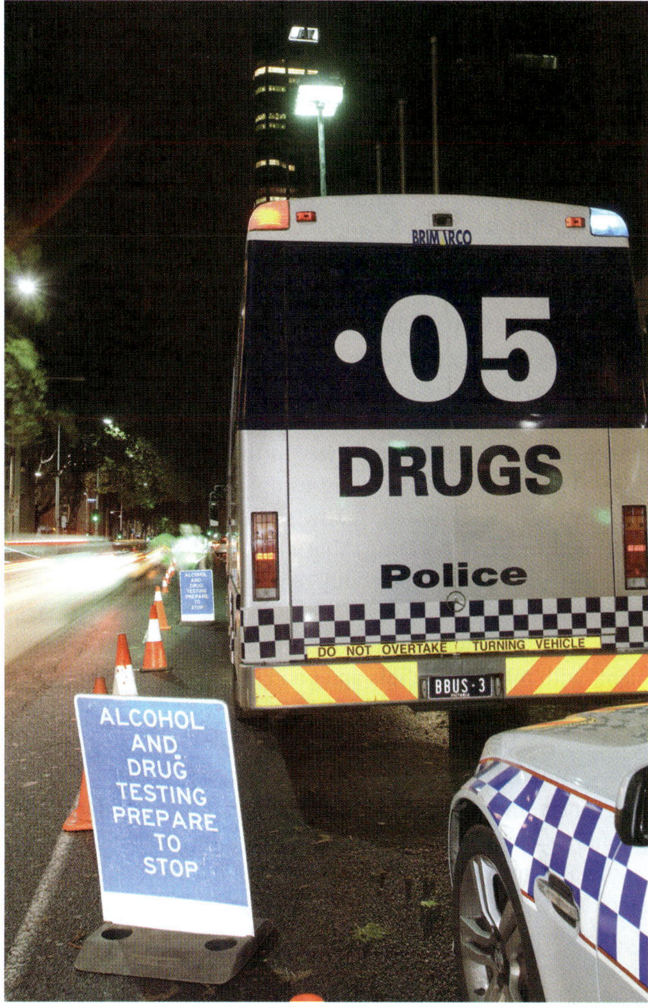

FIGURE 5.3 ***Alcohol and drug testing play an important role in reducing road trauma and help to prevent people from driving after drinking or taking drugs***

Source: Ashley Cooper/Alamy Stock Photo.

ACTIVITY

If you were elected to your local council, what strategies would you adopt and what changes might you make if planning a health promotion project to minimise harms from drug and alcohol use in your community, particularly to prevent young people from misusing substances? Which community groups and organisations (both public and private) would you involve in your project?

SPECIAL POPULATIONS

Adolescents

Adolescence is a period of great change—physical, social, emotional and intellectual—and the teenager can be vulnerable at this time. There is no single risk factor responsible for adolescent drug misuse; rather, multiple risk factors contribute (Rassool, 2010). However most young people at risk do not start using drugs; also, a risk factor for one person may not be a risk factor for another. Risk factors include early aggressive behaviour, lack of parental supervision, peer substance misuse, availability of drugs and poverty. Ineffective parenting, a chaotic home environment, and parents with criminal behaviours, mental illness or substance misuse problems contribute. Outside the home, aggression and impulsivity in the classroom, academic failure, poor social skills, drug-using peers and a belief that drug use is normal among fellow students are also significant (National Institute on Drug Abuse, 2003). A Malaysian study recorded similar findings with regard to peers, with school involvement as a protective factor (Razali & Kliewer, 2015), as did a Thai study with regard to peers and low school commitment, with religious beliefs and good social skills as protective factors (Wongtongkam et al., 2014).

Pregnant women

Pregnant women who go into acute withdrawal, particularly from alcohol or opioids, are at risk of miscarriage, premature labour, and fetal hypoxia and fetal distress. Risks from withdrawal from opioids are greater in the first and third trimester. Babies born to mothers who are using substances are likely to suffer neonatal abstinence syndrome (NAS). It is more common where the mother is opioid dependent and will be characterised by neurological excitability, gastrointestinal dysfunction and autonomic signs. The Finnegan scale is used to assess NAS. An opioid- dependent mother who is on the Opioid Substitution Treatment Program and prescribed methadone or buprenorphine will require the usual daily dose and extra pain relief during labour. For opioid-dependent women, opioid substitution is generally safer than opioid withdrawal. But vomiting of a methadone dose puts the mother and the fetus at risk of withdrawal. Parents should be advised of the association between maternal smoking during pregnancy, environmental tobacco smoke and sudden infant death syndrome. A baby born to a mother dependent on alcohol may have fetal alcohol syndrome (which is difficult to diagnose at birth but which has long-term implications as the child grows up) and/or physical and intellectual abnormalities (see www.fasdhub.org.au for more information). Pregnant women dependent on benzodiazepines should be transferred to a single, long-acting drug such as diazepam and slowly withdrawn (NSW Health, 2014).

Older people

The proportion of older people in the general population is increasing, and as it does, so does the proportion of those people who have substance misuse problems. Mental health issues including cognitive disorders, and complex combinations of substances, complicate the issues. Physical health problems and long-term use of prescribed medications such as hypnotics, anxiolytics and analgesics add to the difficulties, as do psychosocial factors such as bereavement, retirement, boredom, loneliness, depression and homelessness, which are associated with a higher rate of alcohol use (Royal College of Psychiatrists, 2011). Clues to alcohol misuse in older people include cognitive decline, falls, self-care deficits, missing appointments, hypertension, poor appetite, gastrointestinal problems, slurred speech, problems with vision or movement, incontinence, frequent presentations to the emergency department, delirium when hospitalised and seizures (DiBartolo & Jarosinski, 2017).

Alcohol misuse in older people (over age 65) is often not recognised, and if it is, is undertreated. However, if the long-term damage caused by alcohol misuse is becoming apparent, treatment may be offered. As people age, the liver enzymes that metabolise alcohol become less efficient and the CNS becomes more sensitive to drugs. Age-related decrease in lean body mass then increases the effective concentration of alcohol and other psychotropics in the body. Binge drinking is thought to pose higher risks for the older person in terms of morbidity and mortality, and mixing alcohol with opioids, benzodiazepines or sedatives can cause serious outcomes. Use of the AUDIT or of the geriatric version of the MAST can be helpful, as can brief interventions (Blow & Barry, 2016).

An older person in hospital for other reasons may undergo withdrawal from regular, long-term use of even low doses of benzodiazepines. The elderly are vulnerable to developing delirium. Usage even at low doses should not be stopped abruptly because of the risk, particularly for this group, of precipitating withdrawal.

PATIENT SAFETY COMPETENCY FRAMEWORK

3 Cultural competence 

The Patient Safety Competency Framework indicates that nursing students must demonstrate cultural competence by seeking to understand the person's cultural and spiritual values, needs, practices and perspectives, and avoid generalisations and stereotypes when discussing people from different cultural groups (Levett-Jones et al., 2017).

Aboriginal and Torres Strait Islander people

While Aboriginal and Torres Strait Islander people have been shown to be less likely than non-Indigenous people to consume alcohol, those who do are more likely to drink at high-risk levels, and are therefore more likely to experience the adverse physical and social effects of heavy alcohol consumption (AIHW, 2017b). Other commonly used substances for this population are cannabis and tobacco (NSW Health, 2014). Apart from ecstasy and cocaine, Indigenous people over age 14 use illicit drugs at a higher rate than the general population, although there were no significant changes in rate of use between 2013 and 2016

(AIHW, 2017b). The smoking rate fell from 46% in 2012–2013 to 43% in 2018–2019. In 2018–2019, 1 in 4 adults reported no use of alcohol in the preceding 12 months (AIHW, 2020a).

AOD staff caring for Indigenous people should be culturally competent and seek to understand the cultural needs of people from different communities by liaising with local Elders and key contacts. At times, the AOD worker may need to consider the substance misuse problem as a symptom of a broader community issue such as family violence, unemployment or financial stress (Lee et al., 2012).

The LGBTQIA+ community

Members of this community identified equity, inclusion and respect for diversity as key to effective mental healthcare (Rees, Crowe & Harris, 2021); these also apply when assistance with substance misuse is sought. Assumptions may be made by the nurse about choice of partner and family structure, and these can derail engagement and effective treatment. Ignorance, stigma and fear of rejection may compound these issues, but as there are higher rates of substance misuse in this community, what is needed is a non-judgmental approach combined with 'warmth and curiosity' (Sherer & Levousnis, 2020, p. 277).

Healthcare workers

Nurses and other healthcare workers have access to drugs and may sometimes misuse them as a way of coping with the demands of shift work and the workplace stress, and/or to attempt to manage pre-existing mental health issues. They may conceal their dependence because of concerns about loss of employment, legal sanctions, stigma and threats to career advancement. However, early intervention is key, and the new Nurse and Midwife Support website has been set up to assist nurses and midwives with these types of health concerns (see https://www.nmsupport.org.au). By law, registered health practitioners, employers and education providers are required to report 'notifiable conduct' by making a mandatory notification about a complaint or concern. 'Notifiable conduct' includes practising while intoxicated from alcohol or drugs (Australian Health Practitioner Regulation Agency, 2018).

CONCLUSION

Irrespective of their context of work, nurses will engage with people who have substance misuse problems. Current knowledge of common drugs used in the community, the ability to assess, offer a brief intervention and refer appropriately are critical and may help the person begin the journey towards recovery. This is more helpful than being judgmental and denying the person healthcare. Indeed, the International Council of Nurses (ICN) *Code of Ethics for Nurses* emphasises that attempting to 'target, capture, surveille or wage war' (Perlman & Jordan, 2017) will only drive the person away, with consequences, not only for that person, but for the wider community (ICN, 2012).

CHAPTER HIGHLIGHTS

- Substance misuse is the unsanctioned use of any chemical despite adverse effects on the individual's physical, psychological, interpersonal or social health.
- Substance dependence occurs when control over the chemical substance is lost and the individual must use increasing amounts to produce the desired effect (tolerance) and to avoid or relieve uncomfortable symptoms (withdrawal).
- Physical dependence can occur even with prescribed drugs such as opioids if the person takes them for a long period.
- Combinations of genetic, biological and psychosocial factors contribute to substance misuse or dependence.
- While alcohol is the most commonly used and misused substance, polysubstance misuse is frequent.
- Stress management, relapse prevention, social support and counselling are helpful strategies that should be often offered as part of an outreach or rehabilitation program, and sometimes following a managed withdrawal.

CONCEPT CHECK

1 In which stage of change are people not considering a change in their drinking or drug-taking behaviour and frequently described as being 'in denial'?
1 contemplation
2 pre-contemplation
3 preparation
4 action
5 relapse

2 Which of the following are the most appropriate questions to ask when interviewing a person who you suspect has been abusing alcohol?
1 'Typically, on how many days a week do you drink alcohol?'
2 'Have you been drinking lately?'
3 'You don't drink too much alcohol, do you?'
4 'I expect your drinking causes a lot of problems in your personal relationships?'

3 What is the rationale behind ordering thiamine (vitamin B_1) for a person with a history of chronic alcoholism?
1 to prevent acute pancreatitis
2 to prevent cirrhosis of the liver
3 to prevent hepatic encephalopathy
4 to prevent Wernicke's encephalopathy

4 Which of the following substances present the highest medical danger during withdrawal?
1 tobacco and methamphetamine
2 opioids and marijuana
3 alcohol and benzodiazepines
4 new psychoactive substances and hallucinogens

5 What is the rationale for prescribing disulfiram (Antabuse) for someone with alcohol abuse problems?
1 to decrease the discomfort of withdrawal symptoms
2 to decrease the pleasant, reinforcing effects of alcohol
3 to prevent the breakdown of alcohol, thereby inhibiting impulsive drinking through an adverse effect
4 to block the signs and symptoms of alcohol withdrawal

6 Harm minimisation aims to:
1 decrease the harms caused by substance misuse
2 assure people that drugs are safe if used recreationally
3 teach people to use only legal drugs
4 encourage adolescents to experiment with drugs

7 Which of the following statements is FALSE?
1 Smoking is the leading known cause of preventable death and disease among women.
2 Smoking rates for women have steadily declined since the 1950s.
3 Women who smoke during pregnancy have a higher risk of spontaneous abortions.
4 Women who smoke have an increased risk of stroke and heart disease.

8 Which statement illustrates an understanding of quality use of prescribed benzodiazepines?
1 'I can take as many as I need to feel better.'
2 'It's okay to give some to my daughter if she is stressing about exams.'
3 'My new pills must be safe because my GP prescribed them.'
4 'I know why my pills were prescribed, how they work, possible side-effects and how to take them correctly.'

9 Which of the following is a realistic goal for people with a substance misuse problem?
1 They will learn ways to deal with stressful situations instead of resorting to substance use.
2 They will refrain from using substances but only until craving for the substance has been eliminated.
3 They will focus exclusively on negative aspects of past behaviours and interpersonal relationships.
4 They will be able to use alcohol or drugs in moderation.

10 All of the following are TRUE except:
1 People may use or abuse alcohol and other drugs because of an underlying and undiagnosed mental health problem.
2 Many drugs both legal and illegal can cause symptoms which suggest mental illness.
3 People who have become dependent on substances cannot ever change their behaviour.
4 ASSIST, FRAMES, AUDIT, CAGE CIWA-Ar and COWS are all screening or assessment tools used in alcohol and other drug work.

BIBLIOGRAPHY

Agrawal, A. & Lynskey, M. (2008). Are there genetic influences on addiction: evidence from family, adoption and twin studies. *Addiction*, *103*, 1069–1081.

Ali, R., Gowing, L. & Harland, J. (2015). Screening and brief interventions. In P. Haber, C. Day & M. Farrell (eds), *Addiction medicine. Principles and practice* (pp. 126–142). Melbourne: IP Communications.

Allara, E., Ferri, M., Bo, A., Gasparrini, A. & Faggiano, F. (2015). Are mass-media campaigns effective in preventing drug use? A Cochrane systematic review and meta-analysis. *BMJ Open*, *5*, e007449.

American Psychiatric Association (APA) (2022). *Diagnostic and statistical manual of mental disorders DSM-5-TR*. (5th ed.). Washington, DC: American Psychiatric Association.

Anderson, D., McGovern, J. & DuPont, R. (1999). The origins of the Minnesota model of addiction treatment—A first person account. *Journal of Addictive Diseases*, *18*(1), 107–114.

Australian Commission on Safety and Quality in Health Care (ACSQHC) (2021). *National Safety and Quality Health Service Standards* (2nd ed.). Sydney: ACSQHC.

Australian Criminal Intelligence Commission (2021). *Illicit drug data report 2019–2020*. Canberra: Commonwealth of Australia.

Australian Health Practitioner Regulation Agency (2018). *Mandatory reporting*. Retrieved from https://www.ahpra.gov.au/

Australian Institute of Health and Welfare (AIHW) (2015). *National drug strategy household survey 2013*. Canberra: AIHW.

Australian Institute of Health and Welfare (AIHW) (2017a). *Non-medical use of pharmaceuticals. Trends, harms and treatment 2006–07 to 2015–16*. Canberra: AIHW.

Australian Institute of Health and Welfare (AIHW) (2017b). *National drug strategy household survey 2016. Detailed findings*. Drug Statistics series no. 31. Catalogue no. PHE 214. Canberra: AIHW.

Australian Institute of Health and Welfare (AIHW) (2020a). *National drug strategy household survey 2019*. Drug Statistics series no. 32. Catalogue no. PHE 270. Canberra: AIHW.

Australian Institute of Health and Welfare (AIHW) (2020b). *Australia's health 2020: In brief*. Australia's health series no. 17. Catalogue no. AUS 232. Canberra: AIHW.

Australian Institute of Health and Welfare (AIHW) (2022a). *Alcohol, tobacco and other drugs in Australia*. Web report. Canberra: AIHW.

Australian Institute of Health and Welfare (AIHW) (2022b). *Illicit drug use snapshot*. Canberra: AIHW.

Baum, F. (2008). *The new public health* (3rd ed.). South Melbourne: Oxford University Press.

Berridge, V. (2010). Why are some drugs legal and others not? *Of Substance*, *8*(1), 8–9.

Blow, F. & Barry, K. (2016). Drinking over the lifespan. Focus on older adults. *Alcohol Research: Current Reviews*, *38*(1), 115–120.

Brick, J. & Erickson, C. (2012). *Drugs, the brain, and behavior: The pharmacology of abuse and dependence*. Hoboken, NJ: Taylor & Francis.

Brighton, R. & Smith, K. (2018). Substance use disorders. In L. Moxham, M. Hazelton, E. Muir-Cochrane, T. Heffernan, C. Kneisl & E. Trigoboff (eds), *Contemporary psychiatric-mental health nursing. Partnerships in care*. Melbourne: Pearson.

Carlson, R., Kumar, N., Wong-Mckinstry, E., Ayyagari, S., Puri, N., Jackson, F. & Shashikumar, S. (2012). Alcohol withdrawal syndrome. *Critical Care Clinics*, *28*, 549–585. http://dx.doi.org/10.1016/j.ccc.2012.07.004

Catalano, R., Haggerty, K., Hawkins, J. & Elgin, J. (2011). Prevention of substance use and substance use disorders. Role of risk and protective factors. In Y. Kaminer & K. Winters (eds), *Clinical manual of adolescent substance abuse treatment* (Chapter 2). Washington DC: American Psychiatric Publishing.

Commonwealth of Australia (2019). *National alcohol strategy 2018–2026*. Canberra: Department of Health.

Commonwealth of Australia, Department of the Prime Minister and Cabinet (2015). *Final report of the National Ice Taskforce*. Canberra: Author.

Danielson, C., Amstadter, A., Dangelmaier, R., Resnick, H., Saunders, B. & Kilpatrick, D. (2009). Trauma-related risk factors for substance abuse among male versus female young adults. *Addictive Behaviors*, *34*, 395–399.

de Crespigny, C. & Talmet, J. (eds) (2012). *Alcohol, tobacco and other drugs: Clinical guidelines for nurses and midwives*. Version 3. Adelaide: The University of Adelaide School of Nursing/Drug and Alcohol Services South Australia.

Degenhardt, L., Chiu, W., Sampson, N. et al. (2008). Toward a global view of alcohol, tobacco, cannabis, and cocaine use: Findings from the WHO World Mental Health Surveys. *PLoS Medicine*, *5*, 1053–1067.

Department of Health (2014). *New psychoactive substances: What you need to know*. National Drug and Alcohol Research Centre Factsheet. Retrieved from https://www.comorbidity.edu.au

Department of Health and Ageing (2009). *Guidelines for the treatment of alcohol problems*. Canberra: Commonwealth of Australia.

DiBartolo, M. & Jarosinski, J. (2017). Alcohol use disorder in older adults: Challenges in assessment and treatment. *Issues in Mental Health Nursing*, *38*, 25–32.

DiClemente, C. (2005). Blueprint to build strong foundations for change. *Addiction Today*. Retrieved from https://www.addictiontoday.org/

Dziegielewski, S. (2015). *DSM-5 in action*. Hoboken, NJ: Wiley.

Foroud, T., Edenberg, H. & Crabbe, J. (2010). Who is at risk for alcoholism? *Alcohol Research and Health*, *33*(1 & 2), 64–75.

Ghodse, H. (2010). *Ghodse's drugs and addictive behaviour. A guide to treatment* (4th ed.). Cambridge: Cambridge University Press.

Griffiths, S., Murray, S. & Mond, J. (2016). The stigma of anabolic steroid use. *Journal of Drug Issues*, *46*(4), 446–456.

Guirguis, A. (2017). New psychoactive substances: A public health issue. *International Journal of Pharmacy Practice*, *25*, 323–325.

Hall, K. Gibbie, T. & Lubman, D. (2012). Motivational interviewing techniques. Facilitating behaviour change in the general practice setting. *Australian Family Physician*, *41*(9), 660–667.

Hamilton, M. & Rumbold, G. (2004). Addressing drug problems: The case for harm minimisation. In M. Hamilton, T. King & A. Ritter, *Drug use in Australia. Preventing harm*. South Melbourne: Oxford University Press.

Heather, N. (2017). Q: Is addiction a brain disease or a moral failing? A: Neither. *Neuroethics*, *10*, 115–124.

Hulse, G., White, J. & Cape, G. (2002). *Management of alcohol and drug problems*. South Melbourne: Oxford University Press.

International Council of Nurses (ICN) (2012). *The ICN Code of Ethics for Nurses*. Geneva: ICN.

Jellinek, E. (1946). *Phases in the drinking history of alcoholics*. New Haven, CT: Hillhouse Press.

Kanayama, G., Hudson, J. & Pope, H. (2008). Long-term psychiatric and medical consequences of anabolic-androgenic steroid abuse: A looming public health concern? *Drug and Alcohol Dependence*, *98*, 1–12.

Lamb, R., Stark, H. & Ginsburg, B. (2021). Implications of there being many paths to addiction and recovery. *Pharmacology, Biochemistry and Behavior*, *211*, 173299.

Lee, K., Freeburn, B., Ella, S., Miller, W., Perry, J. & Conigrave, K. (2012). *Handbook for Aboriginal alcohol and drug work*. Sydney: University of Sydney.

Lee, N., Johns, L., Jenkinson, R., Johnston, J., Connolly, K., Hall, K. & Cash, R. (2007). *Clinical treatment guidelines for alcohol and drug clinicians. No 14: Methamphetamine dependence and treatment*. Fitzroy, Vic.: Turning Point Alcohol and Drug Centre Inc.

Lee, N. & Ritter, A. (2016). Australia's recreational drug policies aren't working so what are the options for reform? *The Conversation*, 2 March. Retrieved from https://www.theconversation.com.au

Levett-Jones, T., Dwyer, T., Reid-Searl, K., Heaton, L., Flenady, T., Applegarth, J., Guinea, S. & Andersen, P. (2017). *Patient Safety Competency Framework (PSCF) for Nursing Students*. Sydney. Retrieved from http://psframework.wpengine.com/

Maldonado, J., Sher, Y., Ashouri, J., Hills-Evans, K., Swendsen, Lolak, S. & Miller, A. (2014). The 'Prediction of Alcohol Withdrawal Severity Scale' (PAWSS): Systematic literature review and pilot study of a new scale for the prediction of complicated alcohol withdrawal syndrome. *Alcohol*, *48*, 375–390. http://dx.doi.org/10.1016/alcohol.2014.01.004

Matthews, A., Sutherland, R., Peacock, A., Van Buskirk, J., Whittaker, E., Burns, L. & Bruno, R. (2017). I like the old stuff better than the new stuff? Subjective experiences of new psychoactive substances. *International Journal of Drug Policy*, *40*, 44–49.

Miller, W. B. (1995). *Motivational enhancement therapy with drug abusers*. The University of New Mexico. Retrieved from https://www.motivationalinterview.org

Miller, W. & Rollnick, S. (2013). *Motivational interviewing: Helping people change*. New York: Guilford Press.

Monds, L. & van Golde, C. (2017). Doctors and nurses can't always tell if someone's drunk or on drugs, and misdiagnosis can be dangerous. *The Conversation*, 5 July. Retrieved from https://www.theconversation.com.au

Moore, E., Mancusco, S., Slade, T., Galletly, C. & Castle, D. (2012). The impact of alcohol and illicit drugs on people with psychosis: The second Australian national survey of psychosis. *Australian and New Zealand Journal of Psychiatry*, *46*(9), 864–878.

Morley, K., Baillie, A., Leung, S., Sannibale, C., Teesson, M. & Haber, P. (2016). Is specialized integrated treatment for comorbid anxiety, depression and alcohol dependence better than treatment as usual in a public hospital setting? *Alcohol and Alcoholism*, *51*(4), 402–409.

National Centre for Education and Training on Addiction (NCETA) (2004). *Alcohol and other drugs: A handbook for health professionals*. Adelaide: Australian Government Department of Health and Ageing.

National Centre for Education and Training on Addiction (NCETA) Consortium (2004). *Resource kit for GP trainers on illicit drug issues*. Commonwealth of Australia. Retrieved from https://www.nceta.flinders.edu.au/

National Institute on Drug Abuse (2003). *Preventing drug use among children and adolescents. A research-based guide for parents, educators, and community leaders* (2nd ed.). Bethesda, MA: US Department of Health and Human Services.

NSW Health (2008a). *Drug and alcohol psychosocial interventions professional practice guidelines*. Sydney: NSW Health.

NSW Health (2008b). *Drug and alcohol withdrawal: Clinical practice guidelines: NSW*. Sydney: NSW Health.

NSW Health (2014). *Clinical guidelines for the management of substance use during pregnancy, birth and the postnatal period*. Sydney: NSW Health.

NSW Health (2015). *Managing nicotine dependence: A guide for NSW Health staff*. Sydney: NSW Health.

NSW Health (2018). *Fact sheet: Energy drinks and caffeine*. Sydney: NSW Health. Retrieved from https://www.health.nsw.gov.au/

NSW Ministry of Health (2021). *Handbook for nurses and midwives: Responding effectively to people who use alcohol and other drugs*. St Leonards: NSW Ministry of Health.

Nursing and Midwifery Board of Australia (NMBA) (2016). *Registered Nurse Standards for Practice*. Retrieved from https://www.nursingmidwiferyboard.gov.au/

Perlman, D. & Jordan, A. (2017). To neither target, capture, surveille, nor wage war: On-going need for attention to metaphor theory in care and prevention for people who use drugs. *Journal of Addictive Diseases*, *36*(1), 1–4.

Prochaska, J., Norcross, J. & DiClemente, C. (2013). Applying the stages of change. *Psychotherapy in Australia*, *19*(2), 10–15.

Quigley, A., Connolly, C., Palmer, B. & Helfgott, S. (2015). *A brief guide to the assessment and treatment of alcohol dependence* (2nd ed.). Perth: Drug and Alcohol Office.

Rassool, G. (2010). *Addiction for nurses*. Chichester, UK: Wiley-Blackwell.

Razali, M. & Kliewer, W. (2015). Risk and protective factors for recreational and hard drug use among Malaysian adolescents and young adults. *Addictive Behaviors*, *50*, 149–156.

Recke, L. (2017). Is it possible to recover from recovery? *Nordic Studies on Alcohol and Drugs*, *34*(2), 112–114.

Reddel, S., Bruno, R., Burns, L., Kirwan, A., Lokugi, K. & Dietze, P. (2013). Prevalence and associations of quetiapine fumarate misuse among an Australian national city sample of people who regularly inject drugs. *Addiction*, *109*, 295–302.

Rees, S., Crowe, M. & Harris, H. (2021). The lesbian, gay, bisexual and transgender communities' mental health care needs and experiences of mental health services: An integrative review of qualitative studies. *Journal of Psychiatric and Mental Health Nursing*, *28*, 578–589.

Rietschel, M. & Treutlein, J. (2013). The genetics of alcohol dependence. *Annals of the New York Academy of Sciences*, *1282*, 39–70.

Royal College of Psychiatrists (2011). *Our invisible addicts. First report of the older persons' substance misuse working group of the Royal College of Psychiatrists*. College Report CR165. London: Author.

Sansone, R. & Sansone, L. (2010). Is Seroquel developing an illicit reputation for misuse/abuse? *Psychiatry*, *7*(1), 13–16.

Schifano, F. (2014). Misuse of pregabalin and gabapentin: Cause for concern? *CNS Drugs*, *28*, 491–496.

Seear, K., Fraser, S., Moore, D. & Murphy, D. (2015). Understanding and responding to anabolic steroid injecting and hepatitis C risk in Australia: A research agenda. *Drugs Education Prevention and Policy*, *22*(5), 449–455.

Sharma, M. (2016). A new theory for health behaviour change: Implications for alcohol and drug education. *Journal of Alcohol and Drug Education*, *60*(1), 5–8.

Sherer, J. & Levousnis, P. (2020). LGBTQIA: Lesbian, gay, bisexual, transgender, queer or questioning, intersex, asexual or allied. In C. Marienfeld (ed.), *Absolute addiction psychiatry review* (pp. 277–287). New York: Springer. https://doi.org/10.1007/978-3-030-33404-8

Shield, K., Parry, C. & Rehm, J. (2013). Chronic diseases and conditions related to alcohol use. *Alcohol Research: Current Reviews*, *35*, 155–173. Retrieved from http://pubs.niaaa.nih.gov

Sloboda, Z., Cottler, L., Hawkins, J. & Pentz, M. (2009). Reflections on 40 years of drug abuse prevention research. *Journal of Drug Issues*, *39*(1), 179–196.

State Library of NSW (2018). *Drug Info factsheet: Steroids*. Retrieved from http://druginfo.sl.nsw.gov.au/

Sullivan, J., Sykora, K., Schneiderman, J., Naranjo, C. & Sellers, D. (1989). Assessment of alcohol withdrawal: The revised Clinical Institute Withdrawal Assessment for Alcohol Scale (CIWA-Ar). *British Journal of Addiction*, *84*(11), 1353–1357.

Sutherland, R., Karlsson, A., Price, O. et al. (2021). *Australian drug trends 2021: Key findings from the National Ecstasy and Related Drugs Reporting System (EDRS) interviews*. Sydney: National Drug and Alcohol Research Centre, UNSW.

Swan, A., Sciacchitano, L. & Berends, L. (2008). *Alcohol and other drug brief intervention in primary care*. Fitzroy, Vic.: Turning Point Alcohol and Drug Centre.

Teesson, M., Hall, W., Proudfoot, H. & Degenhardt, L. (2012). *Addictions* (2nd ed.). Hove East, Sussex/ New York, NY: Psychology Press.

Thomas, N., Salvatore, J., Gillespie, N., Aliev, F., Ksinan, A., Dick, D. & Spit for Science Working Group (2021). Cannabis use in college: Genetic predispositions, peers, and activity participation. *Drug and Alcohol Dependence, 219*, 108489.

Treloar, A., McMillan, M. & Stone, T. (2015). Authenticity: A critical element in the use of clinical anecdotes as stimulus material for undergraduates in mental health nursing. *Journal of Problem-Based Learning, 2*(1), 25–33.

van Amsterdam, J., Opperhuizen, A. & Hartgens, F. (2010). Adverse health effects of anabolic androgenic steroids. *Regulatory Toxicology and Pharmacology, 57*(1), 117–123.

Van Beek, I. (2013). Harm reduction: Reducing the harms from drug use. In A. Ritter, T. King & M. Hamilton, *Drug use in Australian society*. South Melbourne: Oxford University Press.

Volkow, N., Koob, G. & McLellan, T. (2016). Neurobiologic advances from the brain disease model of addiction. *The New England Journal of Medicine, 374*, 363–371.

Wesson, D. R. & Ling, W. (2003). The Clinical Opiate Withdrawal Scale (COWS). *Journal of Psychoactive Drugs, 35*(2), 253–259.

West, R. & Farrell, M. (2015). Behavioural science and addiction. In P. Haber, C. Day & M. Farrell (eds), *Addiction medicine. Principles and practice* (pp. 22–35). Melbourne: IP Communications.

Wongtongkam, N., Ward, P., Day, A. & Winefield, A. (2014). The influence of protective and risk factors in individual, peer and school domains on Thai adolescents' illicit drug use: A survey. *Addictive Behaviors, 39*, 1447–1451.

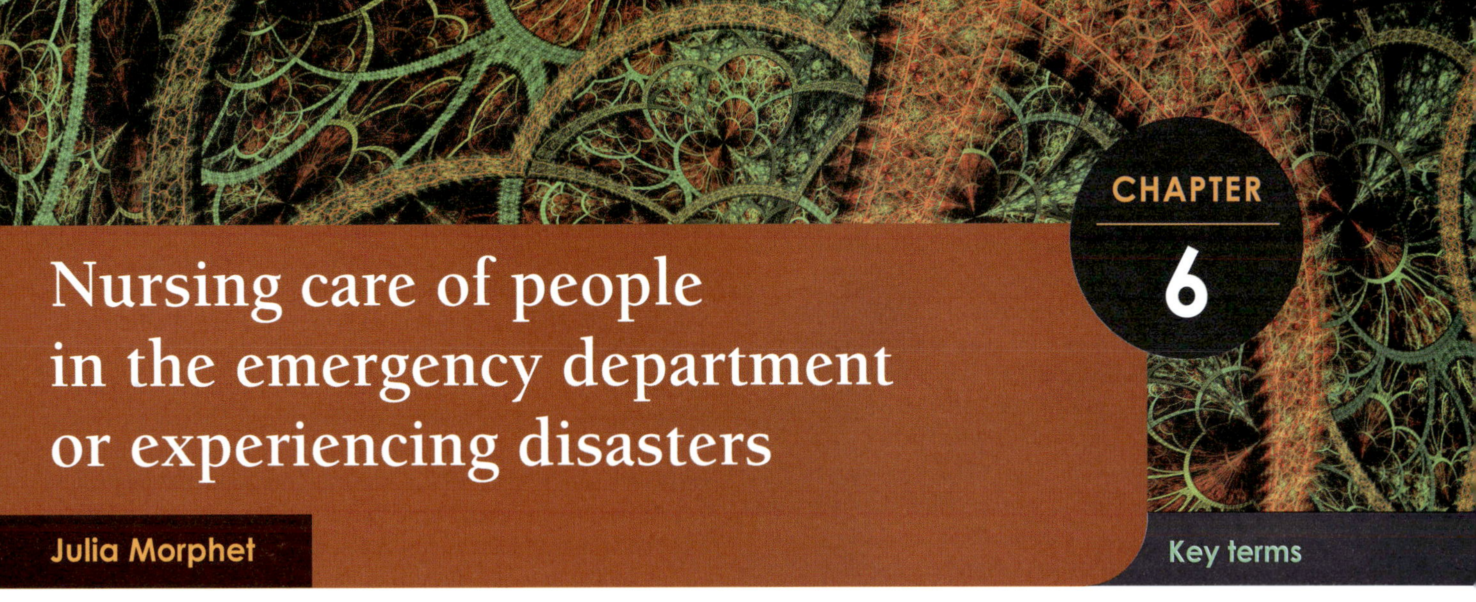

CHAPTER 6

Nursing care of people in the emergency department or experiencing disasters

Julia Morphet

Key terms

communication 108
disaster 113
epidemic 114
focused assessment 111
man-made disaster 113
mass casualty incident (MCI) 113
mitigation 116
natural disaster 113
pandemic 114
preparedness 116
primary survey 110
recovery 117
response 116
secondary survey 111
terrorism 114
triage 109

Learning outcomes

- Outline the role of the emergency department within the Australian healthcare system.
- Discuss the aims and purpose of the triage system.
- Outline the range of assessments conducted in the emergency department, including primary and secondary survey.
- Outline the processes of disaster planning, response and mitigation.
- Explain the scope of nursing practice in the emergency department.
- Define the meaning, types and classifications of disasters.
- Describe the common types of injuries or symptoms that are associated with a disaster.
- Identify ways that nurses are able to provide care to people with special considerations during a disaster.

Clinical competencies

- Demonstrate a structured approach to assessment using a primary/secondary survey.
- Assess health status of people who have experienced unexpected health breakdown.
- Use evidence-based research to plan and implement nursing care for people with injuries suffered as a result of a disaster.
- Using assessment skills, determine priority nursing diagnoses, and implement and evaluate individualised nursing interventions for people experiencing disasters.
- Provide skilled nursing care to treat disaster-related injuries.
- Integrate interprofessional care with an understanding of local, state and federal systems of disaster response.
- Evaluate and revise plan of care and interventions based on the person's condition, environmental factors and resources to promote, maintain or restore functional health status to people who have sustained injuries.

The emergency department (ED) is a common pathway for admission to hospital. Accidents, sudden illness and exacerbation of chronic conditions are just a few of the reasons people present to an ED. The ED is unique in the hospital setting as, in reality, there are no limits on the number of patient presentations, their ages or presenting complaints.

Although all nurses will be expected to care for victims of disasters, whether they work in acute care settings, ambulatory sites, long-term care facilities or in their communities, the ED is usually where people experiencing disasters receive initial care. It is often not possible to know where or when a disaster may strike. Because of this, nurses must be prepared to assist individuals, families, friends, healthcare workers, first responders and communities in their recovery from disastrous events.

There are a number of basic competencies that nurses should be cognisant of related to disaster preparedness and management of people in the ED. This chapter provides an introduction to the concepts important to understanding the role and function of emergency nurses, both within the ED setting and in the disaster setting.

EMERGENCY NURSING IN AUSTRALIA

The ED is a unique and unpredictable practice setting that provides a key access point for people who require urgent healthcare or admission to hospital (Australian Institute of Health and Welfare (AIHW), 2022). In Australia and New Zealand, all residents are entitled to present to public hospital EDs for free emergency healthcare, and approximately 30% of all hospital admissions come through the ED (AIHW, 2022).

The provision of quality emergency nursing care requires an extensive knowledge of body systems, disease processes, age groups, specialty populations, health promotion and education. The *Registered Nurse Standards for Practice* (Nursing and Midwifery Board of Australia (NMBA), 2016) emphasise the importance of comprehensive and systematic assessments, and emergency nurses must apply these skills to people with a diversity of undiagnosed illnesses and injuries. Emergency nurses must have the knowledge and skills to care for people of all ages and populations, in clinical areas ranging from minor injury clinics through to the resuscitation cubicles and triage (College of Emergency Nursing Australasia (CENA), 2020).

Emergency nurses must also be skilled at assessment, triage, emergency preparedness, resuscitation and crisis intervention (CENA, 2020). The busy and variable nature of the ED means that communication and teamwork are also essential emergency nursing skills.

Communication

Emergency nurses play a fundamental role in the assessment, management and disposition (transfer to a hospital ward or discharge home) of people within the ED (Cameron, Shaw & Parsons, 2020). Effective assessment and management of people in the ED is reliant on clear communication (Jones, Curtis & Shaban, 2021). **Communication** is the exchange of information between two or more people, groups or entities. It involves verbal and written exchanges, as well as body language, attitude and tone (Australian Commission on Safety and Quality in Health Care (ACSQHC), 2021). Emergency nurses need to communicate with people in the ED and their families, and the interprofessional healthcare team. Appropriate communication facilitates safe and timely interventions, and appropriate dispatch of people from the ED to hospital wards or the community.

Visits to the ED are usually episodic and often distressing. Emergency nurses use therapeutic communication to support people by providing them with information and explanations regarding processes, health conditions and plans of care specific to their needs. People accessing the ED have emphasised a desire to understand their condition and expected treatment and highlighted the importance of being 'listened to' to enable them to engage in their own care (Blackburn, Ousey & Goodwin, 2019). Clear communication also allows the emergency nurse to provide education for the person on health promotion, illness prevention and access to relevant community services. Communication must be clear, timely and understood by the recipient. Poor communication compromises care delivery, while good communication reduces errors and increases patient satisfaction (Lawrence et al., 2018). It has been reported that 20% of sentinel events in Australia were the result of communication failures (Victorian Quality Council, 2010). A strong emphasis on communication has seen this decline in recent years (Safer Care Victoria, 2022).

Communication between emergency nurses and other health professionals must be based on current, concise and timely information. The emergency nurse should be able to distinguish between urgent and non-urgent problems and convey this information clearly. Emergency nurses should ensure they have assessed the person and read their notes, and should have the person's health history available when communicating with other members of the healthcare team (Jones et al., 2021).

ISBAR (Identify, Situation, Background, Assessment, Request) is a tool that is used to help provide standardised structure to verbal communication both in the ED and in other clinical contexts to ensure timely, relevant and structured clinical handover.

Links to National Patient Safety Standards

NSQHS: Communicating for Safety Standard

This standard specifies that processes for structured clinical handover must be used to effectively communicate about the healthcare of patients.

Source: ACSQHC (2021). *National Safety and Quality Health Service Standards* (2nd ed.). Sydney: ACSQHC. © Australian Commission on Safety and Quality in Health Care.

TABLE 6.1 ISBAR

	SEQUENCE	INFORMATION TO BE COMMUNICATED
I	Identify	Identify yourself–name, position, location. Identify the person you are speaking about.
S	Situation	Explain WHY you are calling. Provide the person's age, gender, current status (stable, unstable).
B	Background	Give the relevant details such as presenting problems and clinical history. Include aspects of history, examination, investigations and management where relevant.
A	Assessment	Outline your assessment of the person. State what you think is going on. Give your interpretation of the situation. Don't leave the receiver to guess what you are thinking–tell them. Stating the obvious is helpful here.
R	Request	State what you want from them. Be clear about what you are requesting (e.g. review, transfer) and how urgently your request should be addressed.

Source: ACSQHC (2010). *OSSIE guide to clinical handover improvement*. Retrieved from https://www.safetyandquality.gov.au/publications-and-resources/resource-library/ossie-guide-clinical-handover-improvement.

ISBAR helps to prioritise information for both the transmitter (speaker) and the receiver. It decreases the chance of forgetting relevant information and helps to decrease assumptions by making the purpose of the communication obvious at the outset. Table 6.1 provides examples of information that should be communicated within each step of the tool.

TABLE 6.2 Australasian Triage Scale

ATS CATEGORY	TREATMENT ACUITY (MAXIMUM WAITING TIME)	PERFORMANCE INDICATOR THRESHOLD
ATS 1	Immediate	100%
ATS 2	10 minutes	80%
ATS 3	30 minutes	75%
ATS 4	60 minutes	70%
ATS 5	120 minutes	70%

Source: CENA (2015). *Triage and the Australasian Triage Scale*. Retrieved from https://acem.org.au/Content-Sources/Advancing-Emergency-Medicine/Better-Outcomes-for-Patients/Triage. © Australian College for Emergency Medicine (ACEM). Reproduced with permission.

The triage system in the emergency department

In 2020–2021, there were 8.8 million presentations to Australian public hospital EDs (AIHW, 2022). In New Zealand, there are almost 1 million presentations to EDs each year (New Zealand Ministry of Health, 2021). In light of the number and variety of people presenting to Australasian EDs, it is important that there are both appropriately skilled staff to care for people and a system in place to prioritise care and ensure the most effective utilisation of resources.

Triage is the process by which all people presenting to an ED for care are assessed and their care prioritised according to actual or potential severity of illness or injury; it is the first point of clinical contact for every person who presents to the ED in need of healthcare (Australasian College for Emergency Medicine (ACEM), 2016; CENA, 2015). Staff at triage must perform a rapid assessment on each person who presents to the ED and, commensurate with their findings, allocate each person a triage category based on the Australasian Triage Scale (ATS) (ACEM, 2016; CENA, 2015). The ATS is a five-level priority scale which determines the time and sequence in which people receive care (CENA, 2015). As illustrated in Table 6.2, each triage category equates to a maximum time a person can wait for emergency care (CENA, 2015). As such, the ATS categories indicate the level of clinical urgency for each person and ensure that resources are allocated according to need, resulting in the most critically ill people receiving the greatest resource allocation.

Triage is an autonomous role which should be undertaken by an experienced and appropriately prepared emergency nurse (CENA, 2015). The triage nurse has many responsibilities, including patient assessment and allocation of an ATS category, initiation of nursing interventions to improve patient outcomes (e.g. first aid), reassessment and management of people in the waiting room and provision of education to people in the ED and their family members (CENA, 2015).

To improve patient safety and facilitate early provision of care, many Australian EDs have introduced nurses who have a specialised role in the ED waiting room and are responsible for reassessing people who are waiting for care, communicating with them about their care and commencing interventions early. This role has been shown to improve person-centred care (Innes et al., 2021).

Triage decisions clearly affect a person's safety in determining the order in which people are seen. The Emergency Triage Education Kit (ETEK) was developed by the Australian Government to provide consistent education to triage nurses (Department of Health and Ageing, 2007), thereby supporting consistency in triage decision making. Consistency in triage decision making means that a person should receive the same triage category regardless of the ED to which they present or how busy the ED is when they arrive. Importantly, triage consistency ensures the appropriate utilisation of finite ED resources and optimal service delivery (CENA, 2015).

To improve delivery of emergency care, some EDs have introduced varied models of care. One example is streaming, in which, following triage, people are 'streamed' to the most appropriate care location and team. These models are designed to support department flow, but do not preclude the need for triage (ACEM, 2016).

Links to National Patient Safety Standards

NSQHS: Recognising and Responding to Acute Deterioration Standard

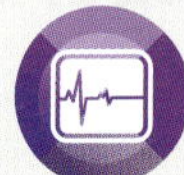

This standard highlights the need for organisational systems to support, promote recognise and response to patient deterioration.

Source: ACSQHC (2021). *National Safety and Quality Health Service Standards* (2nd ed.). Sydney: ACSQHC. © Australian Commission on Safety and Quality in Health Care.

Disaster triage

Civilian disasters also require a triage system to support the allocation of resources: however, this triage system is quite different from the ATS. While the ATS aims to ensure that the sickest people receive the most resources, disaster triage aims to achieve the greatest good for the greatest number of injured people. In disaster settings, decisions are made to first allocate resources to those who are likely to survive, rather than prioritise valuable resources such as blood products or a surgeon's time on those unlikely to survive. In disaster triage, the focus is not what is best for individuals, but what is best for the community.

As resources are often limited, in Australia, SMART triage tags are used to enable nationally consistent understanding of disaster triage (NSW Health Emergency Management Unit, 2017). SMART triage tags use colours to represent triage categories. They are waterproof and can be written on even when wet. Table 6.3 illustrates the disaster triage system used in Australasia. Box 6.1 shows key triage points to remember.

BOX 6.1 Key triage points to remember in mass casualty management

- Use a triage system that is easy to learn, easy to implement in stressful conditions and does not require advanced diagnostic skills, yet allows for basic interventions.
- Use the incident management system on every incident and wear personnel identification vests.
- Get accurate preliminary and final headcounts and relay this information to the incident commander.
- Do not fall into the trap of using your time by providing one-to-one care.
- Re-triage individuals frequently, at the incident, on arrival at the treatment area and periodically thereafter.
- Make certain the 'walking-wounded' are gathered and treated.
- Pre-plan for potential incidents that may occur.
- Be aware that emergency responders may be potential targets.
- Practise, practise, practise.

Source: Sasser et al. (2012). Guidelines for field triage of injured patients: Recommendations of the National Expert Panel on Field Triage, 2011. Centers for Disease Control and Prevention, *Morbidity & Mortality Weekly Report. Recommendations & Reports, 61*(RR-1), 1–20. Retrieved from https://www.cdc.gov/mmwr/preview/mmwrhtml/rr6101a1.htm.

Patient assessment in the emergency department

Primary survey

As people presenting to the ED are largely an undiagnosed population, assessment is focused on recognition of symptoms rather than disease processes. Assessment in emergency nursing is systematic and is guided by a *primary survey*, *secondary survey* and *focused assessment*. The Recognising and Responding to Acute Deterioration Standard of the NSQHS Standards identifies the importance of recognition and response to clinical deterioration (ACSQHC, 2021) and emphasises that deterioration should be recognised promptly, appropriate action must be taken, and that deterioration includes physiological changes as well as acute changes in cognition and mental state. Failure to identify that a person is deteriorating can have serious consequences, and this structured approach to assessment reduces the risk that signs or symptoms of illness are missed. The **primary survey** identifies life-threatening illnesses or

TABLE 6.3 Disaster triage system, by category

TRIAGE CATEGORY	LEVEL OF URGENCY	DESCRIPTION	COLOUR
1	Immediate priority	Casualties who require immediate life-saving procedures	Red
2	Urgent priority	Casualties who require surgical or medical intervention within 2-4 hours	Yellow
3	Delayed priority	Less serious cases whose treatment can safely be delayed beyond 4 hours	Green
4	Expectant priority	Casualties whose condition is so severe that they cannot survive despite the best available care and whose treatment would divert medical resources from salvageable people who may then be compromised	Blue
Deceased	N/A	Deceased casualties	Black

Source: Adapted from New South Wales Health Emergency Management Unit (2017). *Mass casualty triage—Smart triage packs*. Document number PD2017-037.

TABLE 6.4 Primary survey mnemonic

PRIMARY SURVEY MNEMONIC		EXAMPLES
D	Danger	Wet floor, trip hazards, violent visitors, infectious disease etc.
R	Response	Patient alert, responding to voice, pain, or unresponsive
S	Send for help	If patient unresponsive, send for help
A	Airway	Patent/stridor/drooling etc.
B	Breathing	Respiration rate, work of breathing, SpO_2
C	Circulation	Heart rate, strength and regularity, blood pressure, skin colour and temperature
D	Disability	Glasgow Coma Scale, temperature, blood glucose level, pain score
E	Exposure	Head to toe identifying abnormalities

conditions, and follows the DRSABCDE mnemonic (see Table 6.4) (Trauma Victoria, 2022). The DRSABCDE mnemonic is designed to aid the nurse in identifying actual or potential threats to airway, breathing, circulation, disability (i.e. neurological status) and exposure. Life-threatening illness or injury must be treated prior to continuing with the assessment (Trauma Victoria, 2022). For example, if the airway is not patent, the nurse should intervene to ensure airway patency before moving on to assess breathing. It is also important that these findings are reported to senior nursing and medical staff.

Danger to self has become more prominent since the COVID-19 pandemic, and it is important to consider risk of infection, as well as environmental risks, prior to proceeding further. If there is a risk of infection to staff, apply appropriate personal protective equipment (PPE) before progressing further. After ensuring the environment is safe to proceed, checking for a response and sending for help if needed, the emergency nurse should assess the person's airway for patency. Common causes of airway obstruction include foreign bodies, vomit or the person's tongue (Trauma Victoria, 2022). Signs of obstructed airway include audible stridor, gurgling, wheezing or snoring, a hoarse voice or drooling. If a person is talking, it can be concluded that their airway is patent. If a person has an obstructed airway, the nurse should call for help, then intervene by performing a head tilt/chin lift or jaw thrust (Australian and New Zealand Committee on Resuscitation (ANZCOR), 2021). The head tilt/chin lift can move the tongue from the pharynx, thus opening the airway (Trauma Victoria, 2022). If cervical injury is suspected, a jaw lift is preferred, as there is less risk of cervical spine movement (Trauma Victoria, 2022). The use of suction can also remove many obstructions if performed correctly (Trauma Victoria, 2022).

When the airway is patent, the nurse can assess breathing. This will include looking and feeling for rise and fall of the chest and listening for air entry. The emergency nurse will observe the work of breathing, including the use of accessory muscles during respiration, patient positioning, respiratory rate and chest symmetry. If the person is breathing, the emergency nurse should move on to assess circulation.

Assessing circulation entails feeling for rate, strength and regularity of pulse; checking blood pressure; and looking for sources of uncontrolled haemorrhage. If circulation is intact, the emergency nurse can assess for disability. This includes assessment of neurological status using the Glasgow Coma Scale (GCS) (see the chapter 'A person-centred approach to assessing the nervous system' for a description of the GCS), and assessment of pain. Pain can be assessed using a numerical rating scale (e.g. 0–10) or a visual analogue scale (horizontal or vertical lines on a continuum of increasing pain). Refer to the chapter 'Nursing care of people in pain' for more information about pain assessment.

In the person with a GCS less than 13 (or two points less than their normal), the emergency nurse may also measure the person's blood glucose level (BGL). Alterations to BGL can affect neurological status, with some people presenting unconscious or with signs similar to those of a stroke. The nurse can check for exposure by removing the person's clothing and performing a thorough examination. The primary survey is completed with an assessment of temperature and the initiation of treatments to minimise hypothermia.

Secondary survey

After the primary survey has been completed, and any life-threatening findings have been addressed, the secondary survey can commence. The **secondary survey** is a brief but thorough head-to-toe examination which aims to detect all signs and symptoms of illness or injury, with an emphasis on the need for continued reassessment of the person and evaluation of their response to interventions. The head-to-toe examination should include visual inspection, palpation and auscultation of the person's anterior and posterior body surfaces, looking for abnormalities (Trauma Victoria, 2022). Many actions occur simultaneously during the assessment and, while performing the head-to-toe physical assessment, the emergency nurse should also be gathering the person's health history.

Focused assessment

Following the primary and secondary survey, the emergency nurse should undertake a focused assessment of the body system or region of concern, as identified by the signs and symptoms or mechanism of injury (The Royal Children's Hospital Melbourne, 2017). The **focused assessment** should help to identify specific issues and guide treatment. For example, a person who presents with a painful wrist following a fall would be assessed for threats to ABCDE, have a secondary assessment, including collection of health history, followed by a focused assessment of the distal limb. A mental health assessment may be undertaken as part of the focused assessment if relevant (see the chapter 'Mental healthcare in the Australian context').

Once the person has been thoroughly assessed, any concerns—sometimes referred to as 'red flags' or 'early warnings'—must be identified, reported (using ISBAR) and documented. Abnormal vital signs, symptoms of a time-critical illness (e.g. acute myocardial infarction (AMI), stroke or envenomation) or a high-risk medical history (e.g. renal failure in a person with confusion) are all concerns which may be of threat to the person's life or limb.

HEALTH HISTORY The health history can be collected by asking questions of the person presenting to the ED and their carer/next of kin during the physical assessment. The health history should include the presenting problem and associated symptoms, the mechanism of injury (i.e. how the injury occurred) if relevant, current treatment for the presenting problem, relevant past medical and surgical history, medications, known allergies, immunisation status, family history and a social history.

INVESTIGATIONS Investigations assist in diagnosis of illness and injury, and subsequent development of a definitive plan of care for the person. Investigations can assist in the identification of people who are sick or have complex needs. It is important that emergency nurses understand the rationale for ordering specific investigations and the significance of each result, so that they understand the rationale for further management of the person. Many EDs in Australia and internationally (Burgess et al., 2021) have introduced protocols to allow emergency nurses to initiate investigations such as ordering pathology and distal limb x-rays. Nurse-initiated investigations have been shown to reduce length of stay in the ED (Burgess et al., 2021).

REASSESSMENT Following each intervention, an important responsibility of the emergency nurse is the reassessment of the person (CENA, 2020). The purpose of reassessment is twofold: (1) to ascertain if the intervention was effective, and (2) to establish if there are any undesired effects from the intervention. For example, a person who is hypotensive may be given a fluid bolus to improve blood pressure. Following the fluid bolus, the emergency nurse should reassess the person's heart rate and blood pressure to determine whether the intervention has achieved its purpose. The emergency nurse should also consider the undesired effect of a fluid bolus in some people (fluid overload), and assess for signs of this (i.e. assess work of breathing and listen to breath sounds).

DOCUMENTATION It is important in all areas of healthcare provision that each person's assessment findings and interventions are documented, and this is also true in the ED. Australasian EDs are moving towards a paperless environment, and for many emergency nurses, documentation from triage through to discharge is recorded in the electronic medical record. In the ED, nursing documentation will include the person's health history, nursing assessment and vital signs, interventions (including drugs and fluids administered), reassessment, and reporting of findings.

The scope of nursing practice in the emergency department

The scope of practice for Australasian emergency nurses is broad and highly specialised. Unlike nurses in most ward settings, emergency nurses care for people across the lifespan: delivering newborns; managing unwell children, adults and the elderly; and providing end-of-life care. The problems that people may present with also vary, from those with minor injuries to the critically ill. As a result, Australasian emergency nurses need to have excellent critical thinking and clinical reasoning skills, as well as an extensive clinical skill set. Emergency nurses need to consolidate the person's health history with assessment findings to determine appropriate nursing interventions and the degree of urgency with which interventions must occur.

Emergency nursing skills in Australasian EDs include the ability to provide simple first aid; insert IV cannulae and draw blood; select and apply appropriate wound dressings; apply plaster backslabs and splints to support injured limbs; close simple wounds using sutures; and provide appropriate oxygen delivery to people who are short of breath. As well as these clinical skills, emergency nurses have many advanced practice roles, including the collection and systematic interpretation of 12-lead electrocardiograms, haemodynamic monitoring and management of the intubated and mechanically ventilated adult or child.

As they are likely to care for people with a variety of illnesses, it is essential that emergency nurses possess considerable pharmacological knowledge. Pain is the most common presenting complaint in the ED, and many Australian EDs have introduced policies allowing emergency nurses to initiate oral analgesia (Varndell, Fry & Elliott, 2020), including Schedule 8 drugs, for people in pain.

Nurses have a central role in the timely discharge of people from the ED. Consistent triage decisions, nurse-initiated analgesia, timely assessment, nurse-initiated investigations, and recognition and reporting of abnormal findings all contribute to a rapid ED journey and achieving the national throughput targets. Communication of each person's requirements and plans of care facilitates the timely allocation of a hospital ward bed or the arrival of family to transport the person home.

Emergency Nurse Practitioners

Many Australian EDs also have Nurse Practitioners working in the ED team. Nurse Practitioners have completed formal education beyond that of the Registered Nurse, allowing them to work in an advanced practice role, making independent and collaborative decisions about people's healthcare needs. The scope of the Nurse Practitioner includes ordering investigations, diagnosis of illness, prescribing medications and referral of people to specialists as required (NMBA, 2021).

People with unique needs in the emergency department

EDs cater for a broad range of people, all with unique healthcare needs. However, some groups are recognised as collectively having specific needs that impact on clinical presentation, resource allocation, clinician experience and education requirements, and their equipment and environmental needs. These groups include those in the community who are more vulnerable, such as children, the elderly, people with aural or vision impairment, people with a mental illness and victims of violence. Other people with unique needs include obstetric patients, Aboriginal and Torres Strait Islander people, Māori people and people who are culturally and linguistically diverse. Emergency nurses are encouraged to provide person-centred care which considers the unique health needs of all people presenting to the ED and to address each person's needs in a culturally safe way.

PATIENT SAFETY COMPETENCY FRAMEWORK

1 Person-centred care 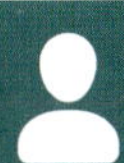

Person-centred care is central to safe and effective nursing care. The Patient Safety Competency Framework indicates that nursing students must demonstrate person-centred care by providing holistic care that takes into account the person's current situation, previous experiences and life history (Levett-Jones et al., 2017).

DISASTER NURSING

A disaster or mass casualty event has an impact on every nurse regardless of where they are working. Consequently, it is essential that every nurse is familiar with the disaster plans at federal, state, local government and institutional levels. Emergency and critical care nurses are on the front line during a disaster; however, nurses in all other areas must be prepared to receive victims and other new patients (there is often an increase in presentations of non-victim situations such as acute myocardial infarctions and asthma). Preparedness is the key to survival.

Definitions

A **disaster** is defined as:

1. *A serious disruption of the functioning of a community or a society involving widespread human, material, economic or environmental losses which exceeds the ability of the affected community or society to cope using its own resources.* (United Nations, 2009, p. 9)
2. *A situation or event, which overwhelms local capacity, necessitating a request to national or international level for external assistance; an unforeseen and often sudden event that causes great damage, destruction and human suffering.* (Center for Research on the Epidemiology of Disasters (CRED), 2009, p. 15)

For a disaster to be declared, CRED, EM-DAT (2018a) states that at least one of the following must be fulfilled:

- 10 or more people reported killed
- 100 or more people reported affected
- declaration of a state of emergency
- call for international assistance.

In contrast, a **mass casualty incident (MCI)** is defined as 'an event which generates more patients at one time than locally available resources can manage using routine procedures' (World Health Organization (WHO), 2007, p. 6). MCIs require 'exceptional emergency arrangements and additional or extraordinary assistance' (WHO, 2007, p. 6). Most people affected in an MCI *do not die*, and many deaths and long-term consequences for casualties are preventable with timely and appropriate intervention.

Worldwide, the number of disasters between 2017 and 2021 remained relatively constant at 550–610 disaster events per year (CRED, EM-DAT, 2022). The number of people affected by disasters follows a similar pattern—in the period above, the least number affected worldwide was 85,295,112 in 2018 and the greatest number affected was 108 million in 2019 and 2021 (CRED, EM-DAT, 2022).

Types of disasters

In the past, disasters were simply categorised as **natural** or **man-made** (technological), accidental or intentional. As there are more events than fit these definitions, the categories for disasters have been significantly expanded (see Table 6.5). Acts of terrorism are *not* contained within the new classification, and the WHO (2019) describes a sub-category within the man-made category to include civil unrest, war, terrorism and cyber security.

In recent years (2017–2021), Oceania has been affected by a number of significant natural disasters, resulting in 80 natural disaster events, 501 deaths and 1.88 million people affected, costing US$17,307,059. Of these, 22 natural disasters occurred in Australia, resulting in 81 deaths and 152,761 people affected, costing US$16,513,536 (CRED, EM-DAT, 2022).

TABLE 6.5 Classification of disasters

DISASTER GROUP	SUBGROUP	MAIN TYPE
Natural	Geophysical	Earthquake
		Mass movement
		Volcanic activity
		Tsunami
	Meteorological	Extreme temperature
		Fog
		Storms & cyclones
	Hydrological	Flood
		Landslide
		Wave action
	Climatological	Drought
		Glacial lake outburst
		Wildfire
	Biological	Airborne diseases
		Waterborne diseases
		Insect infestation
		Animal diseases
	Extraterrestrial	Impact (e.g. meteorite)
		Space weather
Human-induced	Technological	Industrial accident: chemical spill, structural collapse, gas leak, poisoning, radiation leak, other
		Transport accident: air, road, rail, water
		Explosion
		Fire
		Infrastructure disruption: power outage, cyber security
	Miscellaneous	Other

Sources: Adapted from WHO (2019). *Health emergency and disaster risk management framework*. Retrieved from https://apps.who.int/iris/handle/10665/326106; CRED, EM-DAT (2018b). *General classification of disasters*. Retrieved from http://www.emdat.be/classification.

Specifically, the Black Summer bushfires in NSW in 2019 (see Figure 6.1) and major flooding in New South Wales and Queensland in 2021 and 2022 (see Figure 6.2) resulted in significant losses. The Black Summer bushfires were unprecedented in their extent and intensity, with fire grounds covering 169,967 km^2 (7% of the state), resulting in 32 deaths and 1,959 people displaced. The NSW and Queensland floods in 2021 were reported to affect 54,000 people and resulted in 20 deaths (CRED, EM-DAT, 2022).

Disasters can also be unintentional, such as a campfire that has been left unattended which creates a massive bushfire. This is an example of an accidental man-made disaster. Inexplicably, many bush/grass fires are acts of arson—in 2013, in Western Australia alone 1,600 fires were deliberately lit (ABC News, 2019). Intentional disasters occur when harm and/or destruction is the primary aim of the perpetrators. Most disasters result in the destruction of property, loss of life and/or injury to person.

The potential for a disaster exists at any time when hazardous materials are involved as, by their nature, they pose a potential risk to life, health or property if they are released, due to their chemical, biological or physical nature. The hazard exists during any stage of use, from the production and storage of these substances to their transportation, use or disposal. A recent example was a fire in a Lebanon port which triggered the detonation of 2,750 tonnes of ammonium nitrate, killing 206 people, wounding 6,000 others and leaving 300,000 people homeless (CRED, EM-DAT, 2022). Hazardous materials are often involved in acts of terrorism.

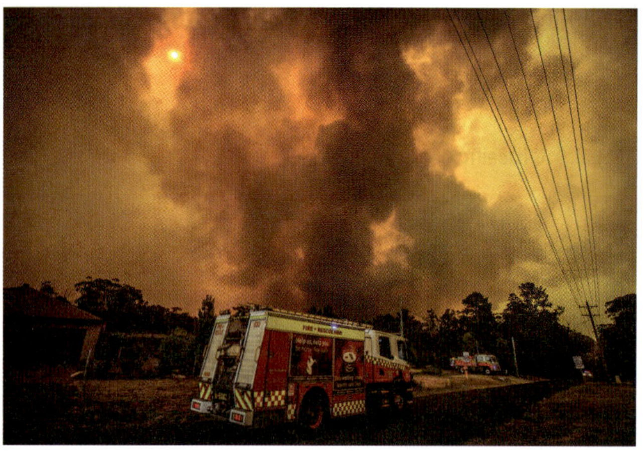

FIGURE 6.1 ***Black Summer bushfires, NSW, 2019***

Source: David Gray/Getty Images.

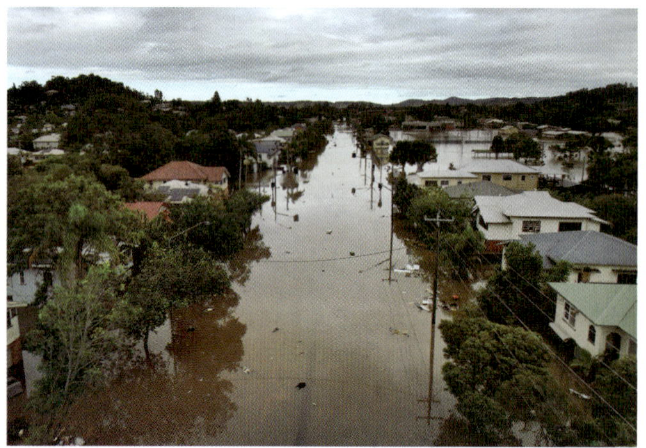

FIGURE 6.2 ***Flooding in New South Wales, 2022***

Source: Dan Peled/Getty Images.

An **epidemic** is defined as a widespread occurrence of an infectious disease (biological), localised to a particular community, region or population. Recent examples include the Ebola virus outbreak in the Democratic Republic of the Congo in 2020 and the dengue outbreak in Sudan in 2019 (WHO, 2022a).

However, as the global population travels more rapidly and easily, infectious diseases are spreading more readily, often before a traveller exhibits symptoms, and this can result in a **pandemic**—the worldwide spread of a disease (WHO, 2018)—as seen with COVID-19. The first cases of COVID-19 were reported in China in December 2019. By 10 January 2020, the WHO had released guidance on how to limit the spread (mitigation), and on 11 March 2020, the WHO declared the COVID-19 outbreak a global pandemic, which saw the entire globe initiating disaster response plans (preparedness and response). On 12 June 2022, more than 540 million people were reported to have had COVID-19 and more than 6 million people had died from the disease (Worldometer, 2022). The WHO estimates that between 80,000 and 180,000 healthcare workers died from COVID-19 between January 2020 and May 2021 (WHO, 2022b). This highlights the importance of access to appropriate PPE (preparedness). Coordinated containment measures included closure of borders to reduce travel and spread of disease, testing and contact tracing, stay at home measures including requirements to work and study from home where possible, cancellation of public events and gatherings, mandatory use of face masks and provision of income support (Our World in Data, 2022). Global focus on development of a vaccine and mandatory vaccination requirements in many countries also helped reduce the spread of this disease (WHO, 2022c).

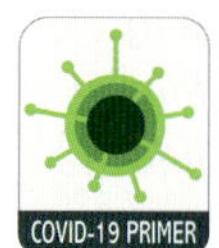

Terrorism

Terrorism is not a modern concept; the earliest recorded acts of terrorism are seen throughout the New Testament of the Holy Bible where the Zealots of Judea waged a campaign against the Romans to free Judea from foreign rule.

A terrorist act means an action or threat of action that meets both of the following criteria:

- *It intends to coerce or influence the public or any government by intimidation to advance a political, religious or ideological cause.*
- *It causes one or more of the following:*
  - *death, serious harm or danger to a person*
  - *serious damage to property*
  - *a serious risk to the health or safety of the public*

- *serious interference with, disruption to, or destruction of critical infrastructure such as a telecommunications or electricity network.* (Attorney-General's Department, 2022)

Terrorists use both conventional (e.g. bombs, guns) and non-conventional (e.g. chemical, biological and nuclear) means to achieve their end. A terrorist strike is not usually predictable. Government counter-terrorism efforts use surveillance with the aim of preventing or minimising danger to the public; however, there have been situations when surveillance information was not analysed correctly or not passed on to the relevant authorities. Surveillance relates to the collection and analysis of data to determine a change or significant trend in a group (Bradt et al., 2015). The goal of the surveillance system is to determine the status of the public's health and detect any sudden change in that status.

Healthcare providers have become a necessary component of terrorism surveillance, especially with biologically based agents. A disaster preparedness plan that outlines the protocol and procedures to be taken with a suspected bioterrorism attack, as well as the response to MCIs, should be established in every healthcare facility. Most countries have a central or federal disaster plan; for example, COMDISPLAN 2020 (Australian Government, 2020) and National Civil Defence Emergency Management Plan Order 2020 (New Zealand Government, 2020).

Common disaster-related injuries and related symptoms

Natural disasters

Tsunami can bring water waves travelling more than 800 km/h, and *cyclones* have winds of up to 200 km/h and flooding rains. Most deaths from tsunami and cyclones occur as a result of drowning, collapsed buildings or flying debris which becomes lethal in high winds (Queensland Disaster Management, 2018).

Thunderstorms bring the risk of a lightning strike. The short duration of a lightning strike results in a very short flow of current internally, despite the high voltage of lightning. However, the longer the duration of contact with high-voltage current, the greater the potential for tissue destruction. The greatest conductors of electrical current in the body are the nerves, muscles and blood vessels, which have a high electrolyte and water content. High resistors to electric current are bones, tendons and fat, due to their tendency to heat up and coagulate instead of transmitting current. Much of the energy current may be dissipated at the skin surface, resulting in significant surface burns (Blancher et al., 2018; Talley & O'Connor, 2017).

Thunderstorms can also trigger what is known as thunderstorm asthma, a reaction to the inhalation of very small grass pollens (Healthdirect, 2019). In November 2016, Melbourne experienced an unprecedented surge in asthma following a severe thunderstorm. Thousands of people suffered respiratory distress, EDs were overwhelmed and nine people died. The Victorian Government has developed an asthma risk forecasting system to minimise the risk of this disaster occurring again (Victorian Department of Health, 2021).

Floods, most commonly caused by heavy rainfall in Australia, can spread over thousands of square kilometres causing injury and destruction. Most flood-related deaths result when people attempt to drive, walk, swim or play in flood waters as the depth and current are easily misjudged.

Bushfires (or wildfires) are a common occurrence in Australia and, with a combination of high temperatures, high winds and dry but plentiful vegetation, can be lethal. Fire-related injuries include burns, smoke inhalation and toxic fume poisoning, the last being the most common.

Earthquakes have a high incidence of mortality and morbidity due to the multiple injury modalities, as seen in Christchurch in February 2011. The most common health effects experienced by victims of earthquakes include stress-related symptoms; wounds; bone, joint and muscle injuries; burns from explosions; clean-up injuries; gastrointestinal and respiratory problems; aggravation of chronic illnesses; obstetric complications; and death (Hall et al., 2017). Countries such as New Zealand and Japan are prone to earthquakes as they are situated on the boundaries of two constantly moving tectonic plates which cause frequent quakes. The incidence of earthquakes in Australia is lower because it is sitting on a single tectonic plate.

Technological injuries

Explosive or blast injuries are the result of explosive munitions, often involving car or package bombs. Care for people injured by blast injuries typically focuses on abdominal and lung injuries, penetrating wounds, traumatic amputations and burns. The level of injury depends on how close the victim was to the epicentre of the blast. More complex are injuries from dirty bombs, which contain a conventional explosive packed with radioactive waste by-products. When detonated, deadly radioactive particles are released into the environment, spreading in the wind like a dust cloud. In this way, dirty bombs reach far wider areas than the initial explosion (Centers for Disease Control and Prevention, 2018) and cause long-term effects as a result of radiation exposure changing cellular DNA. These changes can result in either cell/organ death or malignant changes within an organ.

Thermal burns are the most common mechanism resulting in injury and death associated with nuclear detonation. Thermal burn injuries can be severe and are treated like any other burn. Radiation suppresses the immune system, so special care must be taken to reduce the potential infection often associated with full-thickness burns (Cancio et al., 2017). More information on burn care can be found in the chapter 'Nursing care of people with burns'.

DISASTER PLANNING, RESPONSE AND MITIGATION

Disaster planning and risk reduction in Australia is informed by the United Nations Office for Disaster Risk Reduction (2015) Sendai Framework for Disaster Risk Reduction 2015–2030, the outcomes of which are stated as:

> *The substantial reduction of disaster risk and losses in lives, livelihoods and health and in the economic, physical, social, cultural and environmental assets of persons, businesses, communities and countries.* (United Nations Office for Disaster Risk Reduction, 2015, p. 12)

Disaster preparedness has been a priority issue for the Australian Government. There are federal and state disaster plans which involve defence forces, public health services, State Emergency Services, police, and fire and ambulance services. The main federal coordinating body is the National Emergency Management Agency (NEMA). There are disaster plans in each Australian state, and the Commonwealth Government Disaster Response Plan (COMDISPLAN) is the framework for states and territories to request Commonwealth assistance arising from any type of emergency.

Australia has introduced a warning system that is consistent across different types of disasters (see Table 6.6). The three levels of warning are: Advice (yellow), Watch and act (orange) and Emergency warning (red) (see Figure 6.3). The Australian Institute for Disaster Resilience (AIDR) delivers the Australian Disaster Resilience Handbook Collection on behalf of the Australian Government. Handbooks provide nationally consistent information about emergency management, such as *Health and Disaster Management* (AIDR, 2019), *Public Information and Warnings* (AIDR, 2021a) and *Emergency Planning* (AIDR, 2020).

Stages and phases of a disaster

Warfield (2015) outlines the *goals of disaster management* as follows:

1. Reduce, or avoid, losses from hazards.
2. Assure prompt assistance to victims.
3. Achieve rapid and effective recovery.

There are four disaster management phases to achieve these goals. The length of each phase greatly depends on the severity of the disaster.

1. *Mitigation:* reducing the effects of disaster
2. *Preparedness:* preparing and planning a response in advance
3. *Response:* putting the plans into action so that hazards are minimised and the needs of the victims met
4. *Recovery:* restoration of the community to a pre-disaster functional level.

Mitigation occurs when actions are taken that eliminate or reduce the chance of a disaster happening or reduce the effects of an unavoidable disaster. Information such as countermeasures and emergency risk are critical for mitigation to be successful. Appropriate building codes, road safety measures, vulnerability analyses, public education (e.g. early notification of extreme events, evacuation plans) and maintaining civil order all contribute to mitigation. A contemporary example is wearing a face mask to reduce the spread of COVID-19.

TABLE 6.6 Australian Warning System

WARNING LEVEL	DESCRIPTION
Advice	An incident has started. There is no immediate danger. Stay up to date in case the situation changes.
Watch and act	There is a heightened level of threat. Conditions are changing and you need to start taking action now to protect you and your family.
Emergency warning	An Emergency warning is the highest level of warning. You may be in danger and need to take action immediately. Any delay now puts your life at risk.

Source: AIDR (2021b). Australian Warning System. Retrieved from https://knowledge.aidr.org.au/resources/australian-warning-system/.

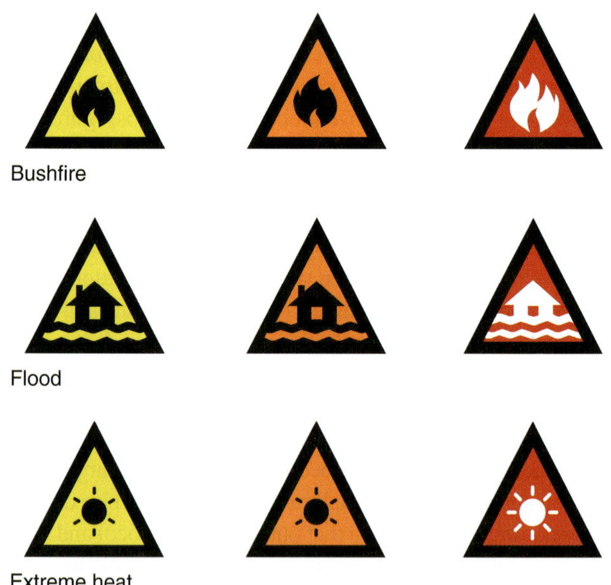

FIGURE 6.3 ***Examples of warning system***

Source: AIDR (2021b). Australian Warning System. Retrieved from https://knowledge.aidr.org.au/resources/australian-warning-system/.

Preparedness is having a comprehensive disaster plan in place that coordinates the efforts of public and private organisations such as the State Emergency Services, the military and all levels of government. Each organisation has specific roles and is able to mobilise quickly and effectively. This level of readiness enables a community to respond to any emergency situation.

The plan will be based on familiarity with possible disaster agents based on previous experiences, as well as experiences of others from various regions and countries. It is imperative that all people and agencies who may be involved in the disaster response be involved in the planning. In this way, information is shared and representatives from each agency explain and offer their respective resources and expertise and note deficiencies in the plan. Planning committees will exist on all levels—federal, regional, state, local and individual agency. Nurses participate in this facet of disaster planning by having a nurse representative on the planning committee at least at the agency level.

Response to disasters happens in the emergency stage and after the disaster event has occurred. The purpose of the emergency response is to act to maintain life, maintain health and evaluate and respond to the psychological needs of the affected community. The community has been rapidly assessed for damage, and the types and extent of injuries suffered, as well as the immediate needs of the community, have been determined. Hospital disaster planners must plan for the possibility that the next disaster may involve the hospital. The hospital's response may include the evacuation of people receiving care as well as relocating and operating from an independent facility. Surge capacity is the healthcare system's ability to rapidly expand beyond normal services to meet the increased demand for qualified personnel, medical care and public health in the event of a large-scale disaster. The aims of the Department of Health and Ageing's (2011) *National Health Emergency Response Arrangements* are to:

- outline the strategic authorities, responsibilities, arrangements and the mechanisms that enable a coordinated national health sector response to emergencies of national consequence
- inform and guide a coordinated Australian health sector response to, and recovery from, emergencies of national consequence
- provide a strategic planning framework for guidance to the future revisions of existing health sector emergency plans.

Recovery is the final phase and, as the word implies, it is the period when the emergency is under control and the community starts to rebuild. In this phase, the resources established in the disaster plan may be put into action. The recovery depends on the ability of the resources to meet the needs of the community affected. In many disasters, the available resources need to be supplemented by government and aid agencies. There is no distinct point at which immediate relief changes into recovery and then into long-term sustainable development. There is no set period for the recovery phase; this phase depends on the type of disaster. It can take years for a community to recover; some never return to their pre-disaster state.

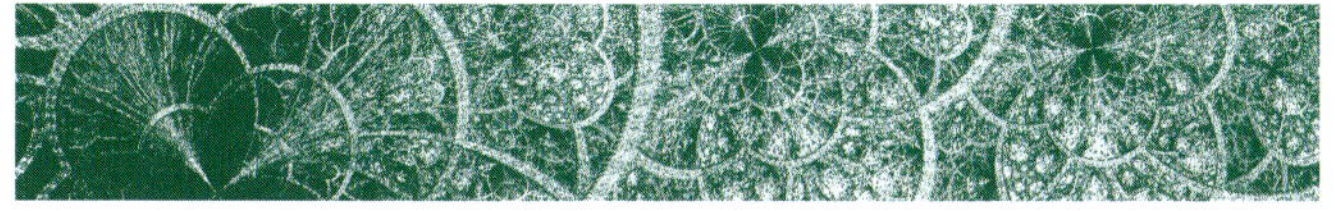

Nursing care

The role of the nurse in a disaster

Disaster nursing is a relatively new discipline internationally; however, it should be remembered that nurses have been on the front line of wars and disasters for over a century. The International Red Cross has deployed nurses to conflict zones since 1919. The World Association for Disaster and Emergency Medicine (WADEM), an international multidisciplinary organisation, established a nursing chapter in 2004. The role of nurses in a disaster situation in Australia is not clearly defined but depends greatly on a number of variables, including the nature of the disaster; the number of victims and severity of injuries; the location of the disaster and of the nurse; and the availability of supplies, rescue and command personnel, and other necessary resources. The nurse must be able to perform under stressful conditions but will not be expected to endanger self, other nurses or other rescuers. It is important to remember that during a disaster, access to normal services such as transport, communication, interpreters, food and water, and even medical care is going to be disrupted and at times not available. In addition, your colleagues may not react or respond to the disaster as you might expect.

The emergency nurse may be involved in first-line response (i.e. attending the disaster site) or be responsible for individuals attending the ED for stabilisation. All Australian hospitals have a disaster plan and increasingly these are put to the test.

Nurses may have to assume expanded roles in making decisions for the most appropriate treatment of casualties. Discussions should take place among doctors, nurses and policy makers regarding the necessity of nurses' expanded roles in crisis situations. Additionally, healthcare personnel should receive specialised training in order to be safe and competent practitioners of the expanded duties. This training must be practised and updated and those participating in the training must be tracked and notified of additional requirements as necessary. Nurses take on a variety of roles based on their expertise and the needs of the victims. Nurses will be expected to follow the emergency preparedness plans outlined in their communities and in their agencies of employment. It is critical that nurses work within their scope of practice, as victims of a disaster will present with a variety of individualised needs including anxiety, impaired verbal communication, ineffective or impaired coping, fear, post-trauma syndrome, powerlessness, injury and trauma.

Isolation and personal protective equipment (PPE)

People suspected of having a highly contagious disease, such as COVID-19 or H2N2 influenza, will need to be isolated to prevent spread of the disease to others. Airborne protection can be achieved with negative-pressure ventilation. All people entering the room should wear personal respiratory protective devices capable of filtering submicron particles.

Gas masks are used in a broad range of military, industrial and emergency situations to protect the user from hazardous dust, gas or other aerosols. Biological contaminants that are spread through aerosolised droplets create a threat to those not wearing PPE. A gas mask may be considered a high-performance respirator and is usually equipped with both eye protection and air supply protection or treatment. Protective clothing is made to guard against mild irritants and even serious lethal materials. Some protective suits are disposable, intended for one use only. Others are durable, multilayered fabrics that are completely impermeable and are reusable. State disaster plans include guidelines to inform healthcare workers and first responders about the correct level of PPE for various situations (Queensland Health, 2016).

The recommendations by the US Environmental Protection Agency (EPA) (2021) for personal protection clothing are listed in Box 6.2.

In addition to the isolation of individuals, special air handling systems are used in the isolation rooms to prevent the spread of the contaminated droplets into the general hospital air vents. Many hospitals have the capability to shut off airflow in contaminated areas to prevent the spread of contaminants to

BOX 6.2 EPA levels of protective clothing

Level A protection is required when the greatest potential for exposure to hazards exists and when the greatest level of skin, respiratory and eye protection is required. Examples of Level A clothing and equipment include:

- positive-pressure, full-face-piece self-contained breathing apparatus (SCBA) or positive-pressure supplied-air respirator with escape SCBA
- totally encapsulated chemical and vapour-protective suit
- inner and outer chemical-resistant gloves
- disposable protective suit, gloves and boots.

Level B protection is required under circumstances requiring the highest level of respiratory protection, with lesser level of skin protection. Examples of Level B protection include:

- positive-pressure, full-face-piece self-contained breathing apparatus (SCBA) or positive-pressure supplied-air respirator with escape SCBA
- inner and outer chemical-resistant gloves
- face shield
- hooded chemical-resistant clothing
- coveralls
- outer chemical-resistant boots.

Level C protection is required when the concentration and type of airborne substances is known and the criteria for using air-purifying respirators is met. Typical Level C equipment includes:

- full-face air-purifying respirators
- inner and outer chemical-resistant gloves
- hard hat
- escape mask
- disposable chemical-resistant outer boots.

Level D protection is the minimum protection required. Level D protection may be sufficient when no contaminants are present or work operations preclude splashes, immersion or the potential for unexpected inhalation or contact with hazardous levels of chemicals. Appropriate Level D protective equipment may include:

- gloves
- coveralls
- safety glasses
- face shield
- chemical-resistant, steel-toe boots or shoes.

Source: EPA (2021). *Personal protective equipment.* Retrieved from https://www.epa.gov/emergency-response/personal-protective-equipment.

other 'clean' areas of the hospital. The heating, ventilation, air conditioning and refrigeration (HVAC) systems are closely monitored and can be shut down in designated areas to avoid air intake from the outside as well, especially in cases of outdoor environmental contamination.

Recording victim data

Each health area has a trauma sheet to record data about victims of disasters. The categories on the data sheet include demographics, circumstances of the injury, injury conditions and disposition. The completion of this form will be initiated by the triage nurse and completed by the nurse who implements the treatment or transfers the injured person to another unit/department.

Psychosocial needs

The importance of mental health services for victims, the public, first responders and healthcare workers cannot be overstated in both emergency and disaster situations. People react to disasters in a variety of ways, both physically and behaviourally. Their reactions depend on the severity of their injuries, real and perceived threat and their proximity to the area of direct impact. The closer the person is to the area of impact and the longer the exposure, the greater the likelihood of a more severe reaction to the event.

THE THREE STAGES OF GENERAL ADAPTATION SYNDROME (GAS) General adaptation syndrome (GAS) is a psychological response to stressors. In a disaster or mass casualty event, it is the physiological responses aimed at survival.

Alarm reaction stage This is an autonomic nervous system (ANS) sympathetic branch 'fight or flight' response:

- The hypothalamus releases hormones called glucocorticoids.
- Glucocorticoids trigger the release of adrenaline and cortisol.
- Adrenaline increases heart rate and blood pressure rises.
- Blood sugar levels increase.

Resistance The body tries to counteract these physiological changes also controlled by the ANS parasympathetic branch.

- There is a reduction of the amount of cortisol produced. The heart rate and blood pressure begin to return to normal.
- This physical response can lead to a person struggling to concentrate and becoming irritable.

However, if the stressor remains, the body will stay in a state of alert and stress hormones continue to be produced.

Exhaustion stage After an extended period of stress, the body goes into the final stage of GAS. The body has depleted its energy resources by continually trying but failing to recover from the initial alarm reaction stage, and the person's body is no longer equipped to fight stress. The person experiences:

- tiredness
- depression
- anxiety
- feeling unable to cope.

If a person does not find ways to manage stress levels at this stage, they are at risk of developing stress-related health conditions (Legg, 2017).

Special considerations

Disasters are not selective in their victims—anyone in the target zone will be affected: young, old, impaired or healthy. As in most emergency situations, the very young and old are likely to be more vulnerable. Issues such as limited mobility and access to resources can impact on the younger and older person's ability to react to the crisis. The notion of community becomes important. Community knowledge, such as knowing where older people or young families live in your area, can help first responders to assist these victims and evacuate them to safety. When injured, the older person may have fewer physiological reserves due to the ageing process, and their chances of full recovery are reduced in accordance with the amount of time it takes to be rescued. The very young are dependent for all basic needs and have limited physiological reserves. If separated from their carer, they risk further harm. Therefore, restoring a carer's role is critical.

Each age group will have unique reactions to a disaster. Teenagers may take unnecessary risks such as crossing a flooding river—these behaviours result in an increase in the death and injury toll.

PEOPLE WITH MOBILITY AND SENSORY DEFICITS It is estimated that 1 in 4 Australians has some form of activity limitation due to a chronic condition (Department of Health, 2017). Many people require the use of assistive technology devices to accommodate mobility and other impairments. Careful planning must be in place in order to provide necessary support to this group during and after a disaster. Volunteers or staff can assist with relocation to a safe room or shelter when required; however, relocation can be problematic when access to this group of people is limited by the disaster. These individuals or their caregivers must provide input to service personnel to determine what kind of support services would be necessary in an emergency or disaster.

NON-ENGLISH-SPEAKING PEOPLE Providing information in a variety of languages is not unusual in Australian culture; however, information regarding actions to be taken during a disaster is often provided in English only. In addition, one cannot assume that people are literate in their own language. It is ideal to obtain the assistance of an interpreter who can translate information for those who do not speak English. Communication aids can be prepared in advance of disasters to be used during emergencies. The use of visual aids is very helpful.

IMMUNOCOMPROMISED PEOPLE The immunocompromised population is at greater risk of complications and death than the general population. Bottled water should be ready so the immunocompromised person can avoid drinking water of questionable purity. It is safest for this population of individuals to consume processed or tinned foods if they can be heated to the proper temperatures (Emmerich, 2016).

SPIRITUAL CONSIDERATIONS Religion tends to be a source of comfort for those who are experiencing the threat of loss of life, property or way of living. Churches, mosques, synagogues and religious leaders become active in supporting their congregations in times of disaster. Religious leaders should be actively involved in community planning for disaster preparedness, especially if certain religious considerations should be strictly followed where possible. In times of uncertainty, many individuals turn to their religion for answers and support. Access to normal spiritual activities and support may be interrupted and, in some cases, it falls to the nurse to provide spiritual care. The nurse does not need to believe in the same way the victim does; however, assisting them to carry out a religious ritual will assist in that person's recovery or journey to death.

Community-based care

Nurses are invaluable in disaster relief efforts, whether they are answering questions from their neighbours regarding the water supply in their communities or assisting in complex care using their advanced practice knowledge in a hospital.

Nurses have a responsibility to the public to maintain competence in nursing practice and to be cognisant of evolving threats to the public's health. Nurses must learn about anticipated and unexpected disasters, as well as their vital roles in emergency preparedness and response. Nurses will play a role in disaster response whether they work in acute care settings, long-term care, ambulatory care or in the community.

Teaching about disaster preparedness and appropriate actions is important in all communities. The Australian Government has become more active in educating the public at all stages of a disaster, as seen in the guides mentioned earlier. Disaster preparedness and response procedures should be practised on a regular basis prior to an emergency. A multitude of communication means are available through technological support systems, such as internal phones and handheld communication devices. Written and visual cue boards are often more useful because they are not reliant on power. Although these methods of communication have been challenged by disasters in Japan and the Black Saturday fires in Victoria, when services are limited, adaptation will occur.

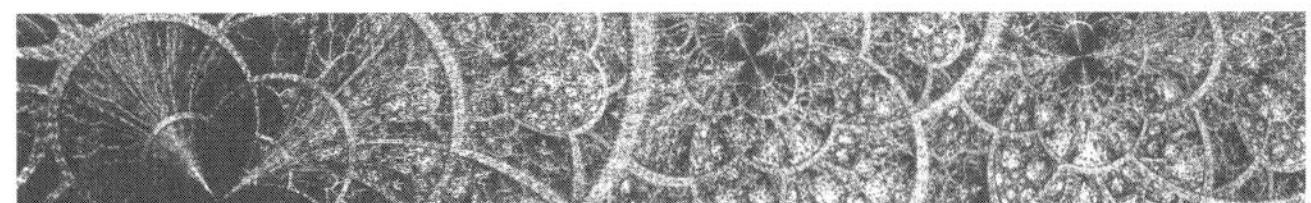

NURSING CARE PLAN A person with spinal injuries from being blown off a roof during a storm

Michael Vaughan, a 29-year-old carpenter, is married to Jacqui, 27; they have an 18-month-old daughter, Grace. The couple has just purchased an older house in the city that needs a great deal of work. Michael is fit and well and cannot remember the last time he needed to have medical assistance. During a heavy rainstorm with high winds, the roof started leaking. To protect his house, Michael climbed onto the roof to seal the leak. He did not secure himself on the roof and a gust of wind blew him to the ground, a fall of approximately 6 metres. He was transported to hospital by ambulance on a spine board with a cervical collar fitted. At the hospital's ED he was given a triage category of 2 because of the potential spinal injuries and height of his fall.

ASSESSMENT

Lisa Smith, RN, obtains a nursing assessment, as follows:

Primary survey

D(anger): Michael's cervical spine is secured and the spinal board is maintaining spinal alignment
R(esponse): Michael is alert and oriented to his surroundings
A(irway): Michael is able to talk articulately and without distress—airway patent, Cx collar in-place
B(reathing): Michael has equal air entry on both sides, chest rising is equal, R 26, SaO_2 96% on room air
C(irculation): Michael is pink and well perfused. HR 122, BP 100/60. All major pulses present, strong and equal. Right dorsalis pedis pulse is weak and thready. Capillary return is <2 secs except on the right leg below the knee.
D(isability): GCS 15. Numerical rating scale pain = 8/10

Secondary survey

Head: Conscious and alert, no lacerations on head.
Torso: Multiple bruises appearing on the right side, no tenderness over liver, spleen, kidneys, bowel sounds present and normal, no evidence of deformity to the chest cavity. Back examination by medical staff (log rolled) shows bruising on right side, no palpable deformity of spine or spinous processes.

Limbs: Arms normal in appearance and range of motion, no pain on palpation, no deformity seen. Bruising on right shoulder. Left leg and foot normal with no deformity or pain. Right leg is pale, cool, reduced sensation to touch, unable to move without severe pain.

Focused assessment (spine and right leg)

X-rays rule out any spinal injury or concerns about the cervical spine.

Examination of the right leg shows bruising on anterior surface. Slight deformity 10° laterally. Gentle palpation reveals disruption mid-shaft tibia and fibula.

A peripheral IV is initiated with continuous fluids. Michael is now fasting.

DIAGNOSES

- *Acute pain* related to right leg injury evidenced by pain score of 8.
- *Impaired circulation* to right leg related to displaced and separated fracture mid-shaft tibia and fibula evidenced by changes in colour, warmth, sensation and movement (CWSM).
- *Risk of hypovolaemia* due to internal haemorrhage related to leg fractures.

PLANNING

- Monitor Michael's GCS, respiratory rate, heart rate and rhythm, and blood pressure every half hour.
- Arrange orthopaedic review for management of fractured tibia and fibula.
- Assess Michael's signs and symptoms of pain and administer pain relief as required and prescribed.
- Observe for internal bleeding.
- Maintain hydration: monitor intake and output.
- Inspect posterior skin every 4 hours, document skin condition, report changes.
- Arrange education in regard to home safety.

Expected outcomes

- Pain relieved within 15 minutes with narcotic IVI.
- Return of circulation to right lower leg—surgical intervention required.
- Mobility restored—surgical intervention required.
- Remains normovolaemic.
- Skin remains intact.

IMPLEMENTATION

- Assess and record Michael's GCS, respiratory rate, heart rate and rhythm, and blood pressure every half hour.
- Administer IVI narcotics as per pain score and medication orders.
- Monitor and record pain scores every 30 minutes.
- Prepare Michael for surgery.
- Monitor CWSM every 15 minutes until surgery then 30/60 for 4 hours, 1/24 for 24 hours.
- Postoperative rehabilitation to restore pre-incident mobility.

EVALUATION

Michael was transferred to surgery for internal fixation of right tibia and fibula. He was admitted to the orthopaedic unit for 5 days then discharged home in a POP cast and non-weight-bearing on crutches.

CRITICAL THINKING IN THE NURSING PROCESS

1. Explain Michael's initial observations in relation to his pain and injury.
2. What post-surgical observations would indicate neurovascular compromise and what are the appropriate nursing interventions?
3. What are the major physiological considerations for Michael?
4. What could impede healing in Michael's situation?

REFLECTION ON THE NURSING PROCESS

1. Outline what you have learned from this case study.
2. How will you apply the systematic assessment process described in this case study in your future nursing practice?
3. What cues were important for the critical decision making?
4. How did you determine priority?

CHAPTER HIGHLIGHTS

- Triage in the ED is the process of sorting people using medical acuity as its basis.
- Emergency assessment consists of three stages: primary assessment, secondary assessment and a focused assessment.
- Emergency nursing interventions are focused on stabilisation and disposition.
- Clear communication is fundamental to safe, person-centred care in ED.
- Disasters require extraordinary efforts beyond those needed to respond to everyday emergencies.
- Nurses will be actively engaged in assessing the physical as well as the mental needs of victims, their families, first responders and other healthcare personnel.
- Nurses are actively involved in disaster mitigation, planning and response efforts by learning and practising their communities' and agencies' disaster preparedness systems.

CONCEPT CHECK

1 The primary aim of the Australasian Triage Scale is to:
1 ensure appropriate allocation of funding to the ED
2 ensure that ED care is delivered according to time of arrival to the ED
3 ensure that ED care is delivered according to clinical need
4 prevent ED overcrowding

2 The primary function of the emergency triage nurse is to:
1 provide first aid to people presenting to the ED
2 ensure that care is delivered according to time of arrival to the ED
3 assess and prioritise patient care
4 provide education and redirect people to appropriate community services

3 During the primary assessment of a collapsed victim, the nurse determines that the person has a patent airway. The next assessment the nurse makes includes:
1 the level of consciousness
2 observation for external bleeding
3 the status of the person's respiration
4 the rate and character of carotid or femoral pulses

4 A man is brought into the ED via ambulance following a high-speed motor vehicle accident. He is unconscious and bleeding profusely from the arm. In planning care for this man, the nurse gives the highest priority to the goal of:
1 maintaining the person's airway
2 assisting the person's breathing
3 controlling the bleeding
4 maintaining the person's fluid volume

5 The key difference between emergencies and disasters is that:
1 emergencies are controlled
2 disasters result from man-made errors
3 emergencies can typically be handled by available emergency services
4 disasters typically involve the local emergency services and no other agencies

6 The purpose of triage is to:
1 prioritise care according to actual or potential severity of illness or injury
2 test first responders on their triage classification categories
3 save those people who are in the most critical condition
4 do the greatest good for the greatest number with limited resources

7 Which of the following is true about personal protective equipment (PPE)?
1 PPE protects by creating a barrier against hazards.
2 Eye, face, head, foot and hand protection are addressed in PPE programs.
3 PPE should reduce the likelihood of occupational injury and/or illness.
4 Healthcare workers do not need to wear PPE if they follow strict handwashing protocol and universal precautions.

8 The goals of disaster management are:
1 preparedness, response and recovery
2 mitigation, response and recovery
3 reduce hazards, prompt assistance, effective recovery
4 mitigation, reduce hazards, prompt assistance, effective recovery

BIBLIOGRAPHY

ABC News (2019). *NSW bushfires that destroyed dozens of homes may have been deliberately lit, authorities say*. Retrieved from https://www.abc.net.au/

Attorney-General's Department (2022). *Australia's counter-terrorism laws*. Retrieved from https://www.ag.gov.au/. © Commonwealth of Australia 2022, Attorney-General's Department. Licensed under a Creative Commons Attribution 4.0 International licence, https://creativecommons.org/licenses/by/4.0/.

Australasian College for Emergency Medicine (ACEM) (2016). *Guidelines on the implementation of the Australasian Triage Scale in emergency departments*. Melbourne: ACEM.

Australian and New Zealand Committee on Resuscitation (ANZCOR) (2021). *ANZCOR guideline 4—Airway*. Melbourne: ANZCOR. Retrieved from https://resus.org.au/

Australian Commission on Safety and Quality in Health Care (ACSQHC) (2010). *OSSIE guide to clinical handover improvement*. Sydney: ACSQHC.

Australian Commission on Safety and Quality in Health Care (ACSQHC) (2021). *National Safety and Quality Health Service Standards* (2nd ed.). Sydney: ACSQHC.

Australian Government (2020). *COMDISPLAN 2020: Australian Government Disaster Response Plan*. Retrieved from https://www.homeaffairs.gov.au/

Australian Institute for Disaster Resilience (AIDR) (2019). *Health and disaster management*. Retrieved from https://www.aidr.org.au/

Australian Institute for Disaster Resilience (AIDR) (2020). *Emergency planning*. Retrieved from https://knowledge.aidr.org.au/

Australian Institute for Disaster Resilience (AIDR) (2021a). *Public information and warnings*. Retrieved from https://knowledge.aidr.org.au/

Australian Institute for Disaster Resilience (2021b). *Australian Warning System*. Retrieved from https://knowledge.aidr.org.au/

Australian Institute of Health and Welfare (AIHW) (2022). *Emergency department care activity*. Retrieved from https://www.aihw.gov.au/

Blackburn, J., Ousey, K. & Goodwin, E. (2019). Information and communication in the emergency department. *International Emergency Nursing*, *42*, 30–35.

Blancher, M., Albasini, F., Elsensohn, F. et al. (2018). Management of multi-casualty incidents in mountain rescue: Evidence-based guidelines of the International Commission for Mountain Emergency Medicine. *High Altitude Medicine & Biology*, *19*(2), 131–140.

Bradt, D. A., Bartley, B., Hibble, B. A & Varshney, K. (2015). Australasian disasters of national significance: An epidemiological analysis, 1900–2012. *Emergency Medicine Australasia*, *27*, 132–138.

Burgess, L., Kynoch, K., Theobald, K. & Keogh, S. (2021). The effectiveness of nurse-initiated interventions in the emergency department: A systematic review. *Australasian Emergency Care, 24*, 248–254.

Cameron, M., Shaw, V. & Parsons, M. (2020). Expanding the emergency nurse role to meet demand: Nurse and physician perspectives. *Emergency Nurse, 28*(6), 21–28.

Cancio, L. C., Sheridan, R. L., Dent, D. et al. (2017). Guidelines for burn care under austere conditions: Special etiologies: Blast, radiation, and chemical injuries. *Journal of Burn Care & Research, 38*(1), e482–e496.

Center for Research on the Epidemiology of Disasters (CRED) (2009). *Working paper: Disaster category classification and peril terminology for operational purposes*. Retrieved from http://www.emdat.be/

Center for Research on the Epidemiology of Disasters (CRED), EM-DAT (2018a). *Criteria for declaring a disaster*. Retrieved from http://www.emdat.be/

Center for Research on the Epidemiology of Disasters (CRED), EM-DAT (2018b). *General classification of disasters*. Retrieved from http://www.emdat.be/

Center for Research on the Epidemiology of Disasters (CRED), EM-DAT (2022). *Advanced search—World data*. Retrieved from https://www.emdat.be/data

Centers for Disease Control and Prevention (2018). *Frequently asked questions about dirty bombs*. Retrieved from https://www.cdc.gov/

College of Emergency Nursing Australasia (CENA) (2015). *Triage and the Australasian Triage Scale*. Melbourne: CENA.

College of Emergency Nursing Australasia (CENA) (2020). *Practice standards for the specialist emergency nurse* (4th ed.). Melbourne: CENA.

Department of Health (2017). *Chronic conditions*. Retrieved from http://www.health.gov.au/

Department of Health and Ageing (2007). *Emergency triage education kit*. Canberra: Australian Government.

Department of Health and Ageing (2011). *National health emergency response arrangements*. Retrieved from https://www.health.gov.au/

Emmerich, M. (2016) *Managing infection control in a disaster*. Retrieved from https://infectioncontrol.tips/

Hall, M. L., Lee, A. C. K., Cartwright, C., Marahatta, S., Karki, J. & Simkhada, P. (2017). The 2015 Nepal earthquake disaster: Lessons learned one year on. *Public Health, 145*, 39–44.

Healthdirect (2019). *Thunderstorm asthma*. Retrieved from https://www.healthdirect.gov.au/

Innes, K., Jackson, D., Plummer, V., Elliott, D. (2021). Exploration and model development for emergency department waiting room nurse role: Synthesis of a three-phase sequential mixed methods study. *International Emergency Nursing, 59*, 101075.

Jones, T., Curtis, K. & Shaban, R. (2021). Practice expectations for Australian graduate emergency nursing programs: A Delphi study. *Nurse Education Today, 99*, 104811.

Lawrence, P., Jarugula, R., Hazelwood, S., Fincher, G. & Hay, K. (2018). Wait times are not the problem! Detailed analysis of unsolicited patient complaints from a metropolitan Australian emergency department. *Emergency Medicine Australasia, 30*(5), 672–677.

Legg, T. J. (2017). *What to know about general adaptation syndrome*. Retrieved from https://www.medicalnewstoday.com/

Levett-Jones, T., Dwyer, T., Reid-Searl, K., Heaton, L., Flenady, T., Applegarth, J., Guinea, S. & Andersen, P. (2017). *Patient Safety Competency Framework (PSCF) for Nursing Students*. Sydney. Retrieved from http://psframework.wpengine.com/

New South Wales Health Emergency Management Unit (2017). *Mass casualty triage—Smart triage packs*. Retrieved from https://www1.health.nsw.gov.au/

New Zealand Government (2020). *National Civil Defence Emergency Management Plan Order 2015* (reprinted 2020). Retrieved from https://www.legislation.govt.nz/

New Zealand Ministry of Health (2021). *Emergency departments*. Retrieved from https://www.health.govt.nz/

Nursing and Midwifery Board of Australia (NMBA) (2016). *Registered Nurse Standards for Practice*. Retrieved from https://www.nursingmidwiferyboard.gov.au/

Nursing and Midwifery Board of Australia (NMBA) (2021). *Nurse Practitioner Standards for Practice*. Retrieved from https://www.nursingmidwiferyboard.gov.au/

Our World in Data (2022). *Policy responses to the coronavirus pandemic*. Retrieved from https://ourworldindata.org/

Queensland Disaster Management (2018). *Prevention, preparedness, response and recovery disaster management guideline transition*. Retrieved from http://www.disaster.qld.gov.au/

Queensland Health (2016). *Queensland Health mass casualty incident plan*. Retrieved from https://www.health.qld.gov.au/

Safer Care Victoria (2022). *Supporting patient safety: Learning from sentinel events. Annual report 2020–2021*. Retrieved from www.safercare.vic.gov.au/

Sasser, S. M., Hunt, R. C., Faul, M. et al. (2012). Guidelines for field triage of injured patients: Recommendations of the National Expert Panel on Field Triage, 2011. Centers for Disease Prevention and Control. *Morbidity & Mortality Weekly Report. Recommendations & Reports, 61*(RR-1), 1–20. Retrieved from https://www.cdc.gov/

Talley, N. J & O'Connor, S. (2017). *Clinical examination: A systematic guide to physical diagnosis* (8th ed.). Sydney: Churchill Livingston.

The Royal Children's Hospital Melbourne (2017). *Focused assessment*. Melbourne: RCH. Retrieved from https://www.rch.org.au/

Trauma Victoria (2022). *Primary survey*. Melbourne: Victorian Department of Health. Retrieved from http://trauma.reach.vic.gov.au/

United Nations (2009). *International strategy for disaster reduction: 2009 UNISDR terminology on disaster risk reduction*. Retrieved from https://www.unisdr.org/

United Nations Office for Disaster Risk Reduction (UNISDR) (2015). *Sendai framework for disaster risk reduction 2015–2030*. Retrieved from https://www.unisdr.org/

United States Environmental Protection Agency (EPA) (2021). *Personal protective equipment*. Retrieved from https://www.epa.gov/

Varndell, W., Fry, M. & Elliott, D. (2020). Pain assessment and interventions by nurses in the emergency department: A national survey. *Journal of Clinical Nursing, 29*(13–14), 2532–2362.

Victorian Department of Health (2021). *Epidemic thunderstorm asthma*. Retrieved from https://www.health.vic.gov.au/

Victorian Quality Council (2010). *Promoting effective communication among healthcare professionals to improve patient safety and quality of care*. Melbourne: Department of Health (Victoria).

Warfield, C. (2015). *The disaster management cycle*. Retrieved from https://www.gdrc.org/

World Health Organization (WHO) (2007). *Mass casualty management systems: Strategies and guidelines for building health sector capacity*. Retrieved from http://www.who.int/

World Health Organization (WHO) (2018). *Managing epidemics: Key facts about major deadly diseases*. Retrieved from http://www.who.int/

World Health Organization (WHO) (2019). *Health emergency and disaster risk management framework*. Geneva. Retrieved from http://www.who.int/

World Health Organization (WHO) (2022a). *Epidemic and pandemic-prone diseases: Outbreaks*. Retrieved from http://www.emro.who.int/

World Health Organization (WHO) (2022b). *Health and care worker deaths during COVID-19*. Retrieved from https://www.who.int/

World Health Organization (WHO) (2022c). *Timeline: WHO's COVID-19 response*. Retrieved from https://www.who.int/

Worldometer (2022). *COVID-19 coronavirus pandemic: Coronavirus cases*. Retrieved from https://www.worldometers.info/

UNIT 2 BUILDING CLINICAL COMPETENCE

Alterations in patterns of health

Clinical scenario

You have been assigned to care for the following four people for the 0700 shift in an emergency department (ED). Significant data obtained during report are as follows:

- Peter Black is a 46-year-old who was admitted to the ED 2 hours ago after being thrown 20 metres during a cyclone. When last taken, his vital signs were T 37.6°C, P 86, R 24 and BP 140/86. He had multiple abrasions and lacerations that were sutured in the emergency room. He is now complaining of numbness in both legs.
- Alice Jones is a 19-year-old woman with a history of asthma. She has not been using her preventer and came to the ED 3 hours ago complaining of shortness of breath. She has been having salbutamol nebulisers every 30 minutes. Her vital signs are T 37.2°C, P 90, R 26, BP 134/88, SpO_2 95% on room air.
- John Linner, aged 67, was brought in by his family 2.5 hours ago. He is in the terminal stages of colon cancer and the family are no longer able to care for him at home. Vital signs are T 36°C, P 54, R 10, BP 88/68. The family is requesting that a nurse check on Mr Linner because they feel that death is imminent.
- Paul Gregs, aged 47, was brought in by police after he was seen standing in the middle of the road directing traffic. He has a history of alcohol abuse, and on admission his alcohol level was 0.45. Current vital signs are T 36.7°C, P 110, R 30, BP 168/94. He is confused, agitated and diaphoretic.

Critical-thinking questions

1 In what order would you review these people after handover?
1.
2.
3.
4.

2 What top two priority nursing diagnoses would you choose for each of the people presented above? Can you explain, if asked, the rationale for your choices?

	Priority Nursing Diagnosis #1	Priority Nursing Diagnosis #2
Peter Black		
Alice Jones		
John Linner		
Paul Gregs		

3 After assessing Mr Black, which nursing intervention should the nurse perform first?
1. Call the doctor to report the numbness in his legs.
2. Have Mr Black perform active exercises to prevent thrombosis in his legs.
3. Ambulate Mr Black in the hall to promote circulation to his legs.
4. Medicate Mr Black for pain so he can move his legs better.

4 Outline the elements of the primary and secondary survey, and describe how you would apply them in relation to Peter Black.

5 What are the changes that occur in the airway with asthma?
1. oedema, bronchoconstriction, increased mucus production
2. oedema, bronchoconstriction, decreased mucus production
3. oedema, bronchodilation, decreased mucus production
4. oedema, bronchodilation, increased mucus production

6 Describe the focused respiratory assessment you would undertake on Alice Jones.

7 Prioritise four nursing interventions for Alice Jones.
1.
2.
3.
4.

8 With a history of alcoholism for 5 years, what is a priority nursing intervention in the plan of care for Mr Gregs?
1. Identify maladaptive behaviours that may contribute to the alcoholism.
2. Encourage participation in therapeutic group activities.
3. Teach the effects of alcohol on the body.
4. Use a respectful, non-judgmental approach to gain trust.

9 A prescription for naltrexone is given to Mr Gregs. He voices understanding of how to take the medication when he states:
1. 'I must avoid all forms of alcohol and narcotics while taking this medication.'
2. 'It is all right to take over-the-counter cold medications if I catch a cold.'
3. 'This medication will keep me from having withdrawal symptoms.'
4. 'I can get physically ill if I drink alcohol while taking this medication.'

10 When Mr Gregs was admitted to the ED, which laboratory studies would you expect to have taken? (Select all that apply.)
1. bilirubin
2. serum electrolytes
3. ALK
4. complete blood cell count
5. AST
6. WCC

11 To prepare the family for Mr Linner's death, the nurse institutes the following interventions:
1. Teach the stages of coping with the loss of their family member.
2. Explain the physical symptoms they may see as death approaches.
3. Discuss funeral and burial arrangements with the family.
4. Refer family to appropriate support groups to assist in dealing with death.

12 When preparing for the role the nurse will play in disaster relief, the nurse must first:
1. be able to apply basic first aid skills
2. be aware of decontamination procedures
3. serve on disaster preparedness committees
4. know how to take care of himself or herself

Case study

Mr Kim Lui is admitted to the emergency department with open left fractures of the tibia and fibula, left upper quadrant pain and reddened areas across the left shoulder, neck and chest. According to the paramedics, he was involved in a multiple-car crash on a freeway. On initial assessment he is found to be a non-English-speaking Korean, 28 years of age, is 1.8 m in height and weighs 54 kg. His vital signs are T 37°C, P 100, R 28 and shallow, BP 150/86. He indicates his pain scale level as 9 out of 10, even after being medicated with morphine in the ambulance.

After chest, abdominal and leg x-rays, Mr Lui is diagnosed with crushing injury and comminuted fractures of the left tibia and fibula, a haematoma on his spleen and bruising across the shoulder, neck and chest due to the seat belt. With the use of a translator, the doctor explains that he will have to have surgery to repair his fractures.

Blood is taken for the following pathology tests: full blood count (FBC) with differential, electrolytes, prothrombin time (PT), partial thromboplastin time (PTT) and blood gases. A urine specimen is sent to the laboratory for a urinalysis. Preoperative preparation is completed. The nurse tries to answer any questions Mr Lui has regarding the surgery and what will happen in the postoperative period. The nurse attempts to contact family members and a monk to see Mr Lui before he goes to surgery. At the ordered time, the nurse administers prescribed preoperative medication and Mr Lui is sent to the operating room.

Due to difficulty understanding the English language, pain and the need for surgery, Mr Lui is very anxious. The nursing diagnosis of *Anxiety* is appropriate for guiding preoperative nursing care. Anxiety is an uneasy feeling of not knowing what is going to happen. The pathophysiology of anxiety is anticipation of danger or a threat to health status that leads to a 'fight-or-flight' response from the sympathetic nervous system. Manifestations of anxiety are restlessness, tachycardia, rapid breathing, facial flushing, increased perspiration, weakness, tremors, and impaired attention and concentration. Complications of anxiety are nausea, vomiting, diarrhoea, loss of appetite, insomnia, immobility and powerlessness that can lead to panic or phobias.

Based on Mr Lui's medical diagnosis and treatment plan, anxiety is identified as the priority nursing diagnosis at this time.

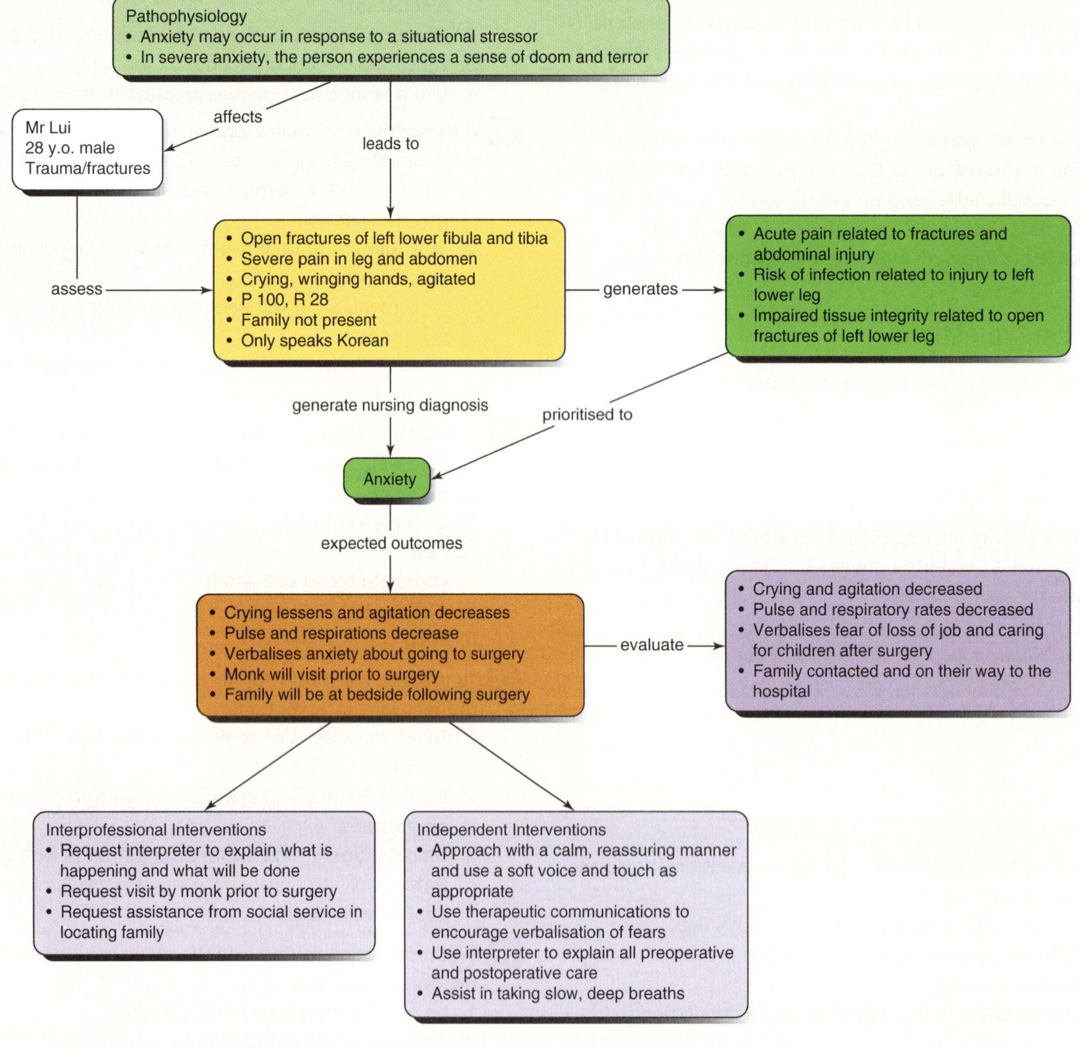

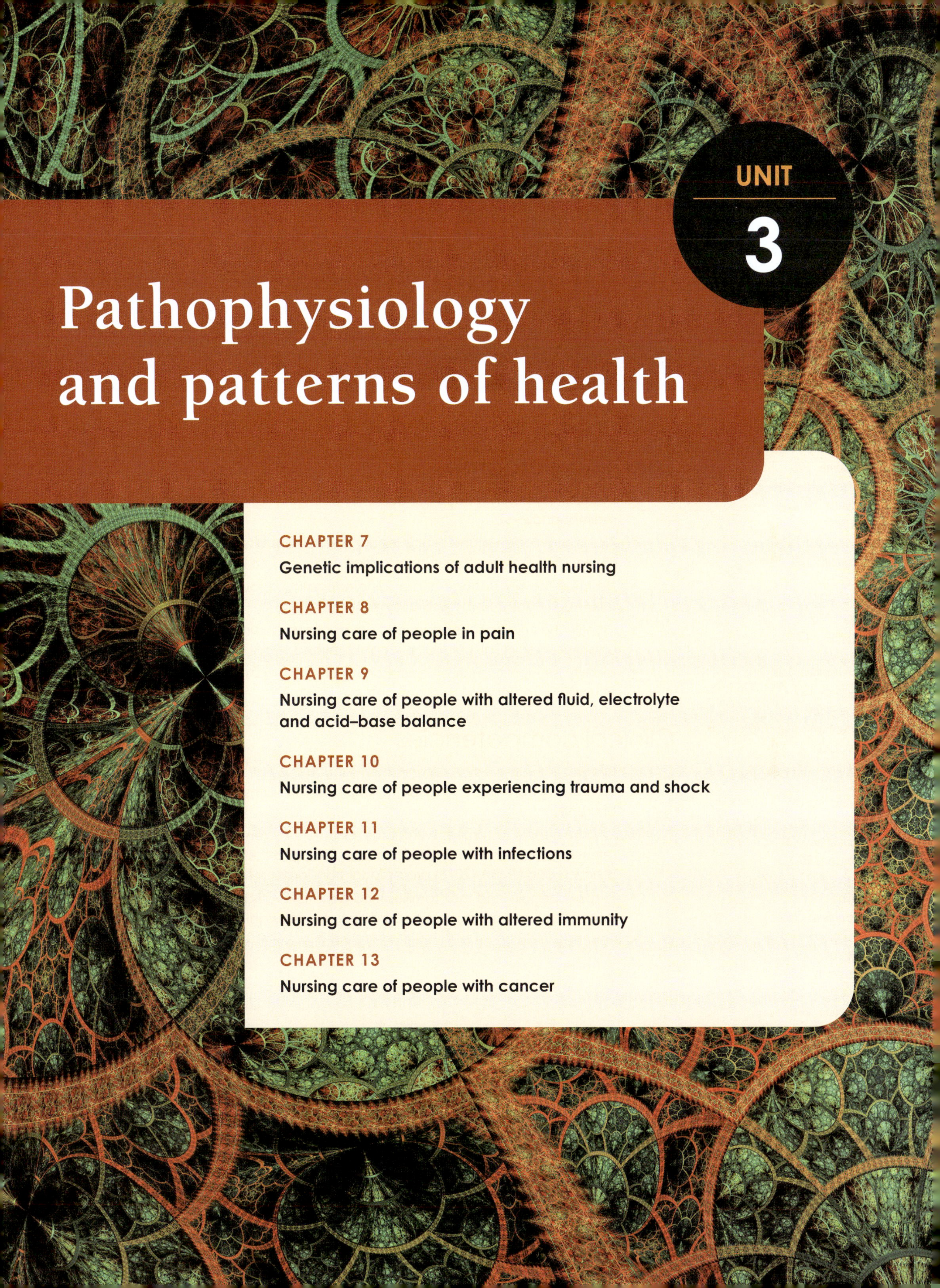

UNIT 3

Pathophysiology and patterns of health

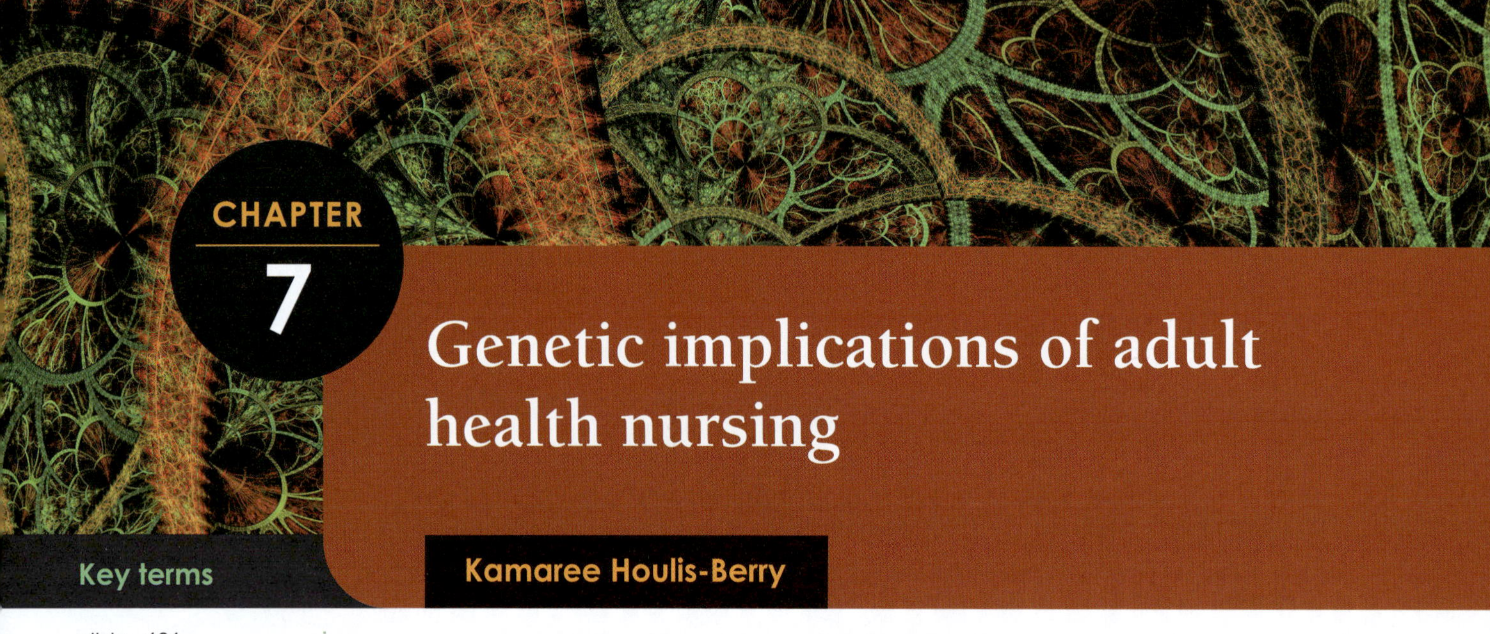

CHAPTER 7

Genetic implications of adult health nursing

Kamaree Houlis-Berry

Key terms

Learning outcomes

- Discuss the role of genetic concepts in health promotion and health maintenance.
- Apply knowledge of the principles of genetic transmission and risk factors for genetic disorders to nursing practice.
- Describe the significance of providing education about genetics and counselling follow-up in an ethically justifiable manner.
- Identify the implications of genetic advances for nursing practice with particular attention to spiritual, cultural, ethical, legal and social issues.
- Identify the significance of recent advances in human genetics in terms of healthcare delivery.

Clinical competencies

- Integrate genetic physical assessment and the use of a pedigree family history into nursing care according to the NMBA (2016) professional standards required of the RN.
- Identify people or families with actual or potential genetic problems and initiate referrals to appropriate professionals according to the relevant nurses' scope of practice and NMBA (2016) professional standards for the RN.
- Prepare people and their families for a genetic evaluation and facilitate the genetic counselling process according to the relevant nurses' scope of practice.
- Integrate genetic concepts into education for people and their families.

OVERVIEW OF GENETICS AND GENOMICS

Increasingly, nurses and midwives encounter people with conditions related to genetics, and thus they need the knowledge, skills and attitudes to effectively care for these people in culturally safe and ethically justifiable ways. The completion of the Human Genome Project (HGP) (see Box 7.1) has accelerated the incorporation of genetics into mainstream medical, midwifery and nursing practice. The HGP changed not only the way disease treatment is approached but, more importantly, how nurses and midwives look at health promotion and health maintenance. Thanks to the HGP, we now have a much better idea of the contribution of genetics to illness and wellness, targeted drug therapy (**pharmacogenetics**) and the development of genetic tests that identify those at risk of specific illnesses. We know now that most illnesses have a genetic component. We know that myocardial infarction, some forms of cancer, mental illness and diabetes, as well as addiction and Alzheimer's disease, are all caused by the interaction between at least one gene and complex environmental and social factors.

The explosion of knowledge about genetics and genomics brings significant nursing, medical, ethical and legal concerns, which all health professionals must consider. With the ability to predict the risk of developing many conditions comes a better understanding of how genetic and environmental and lifestyle factors interact to produce disease. In addition, we have the capacity to tailor treatments based on an understanding of the genetic basis of disease in the individual, and in all likelihood this will reduce the burden of these conditions on society and individuals. For example, population-based screening for colorectal cancer guidelines recommends that screening begin at age 50. It is now possible to adjust the guidelines to take into account genomic risk factors such as having a first-degree relative (parent, sibling or child) who developed cancer at a younger age, or people with multiple affected first-degree relatives, so that screening begins at an earlier age.

People and populations are increasingly offered predictive tests and carrier tests to determine if they are at risk of conditions such as Alzheimer's disease (AD), which is a major cause of disability in the older adult. Most AD cases are late in onset and are undoubtedly influenced by a combination of genetic and environmental factors. Inheritance plays a role in approximately 80% of cases (Cuyvers & Sleegers, 2016; Rao, Degnan & Levy, 2014) and has a risk association with the APOE 4 allele. The social and ethical implications of this knowledge are enormous. Would you want to know if you are at risk of Alzheimer's disease? Would you tell your life insurer? If you knew that you have a genetic risk of heart disease, would you be more likely to change your lifestyle? Should testing for Alzheimer's disease or Down syndrome be compulsory? If the tests are 'positive', should an affected fetus be aborted by state order because of the financial costs of lifelong care? These questions show the financial price we pay as individuals and members of society for information about our future health risks, as well as the social consequences, including unfair discrimination with regard to life insurance and employment.

DNA is at the centre of the state of our health (see Figure 7.1). We know that wellness and good health are associated with properly structured and functioning genes. If they are not functioning properly, ill health or an increased risk of disease can result. This includes not only the well-known genetic disorders and problems, but also complex conditions such as heart disease, stroke, diabetes and several kinds of cancer. The knowledge gained from human genome research has and will have a profound impact on the prevention, diagnosis, prediction and treatment of genetic disorders and complex diseases.

BOX 7.1 Human Genome Project

The Human Genome Project (HGP) is one of the great accomplishments in medical history. Funded in the United States by the National Institutes of Health and the Department of Energy in 1990, the mission of the now completed HGP was to map the complexities of chromosomes and the genes within them, and how they affect human health.

The ultimate goal was to sequence the human genome and identify all human genes. The completion of a high-quality reference sequence was announced in April 2003, marking 50 years since the publication in the journal *Nature* of the letter by James Watson and Francis Crick describing DNA's double-helix structure. Information obtained through the sequencing of the human genome has had a tremendous impact on finding the genes associated with human illness and health. Now that the HGP has been completed, research is being directed towards understanding the complex functions of cellular regulation, human variation and the interplay of genes and environment, and how all the cell organelles, genes and proteins work together in life's functions (USDOE Genome Programs, 2008).

INTEGRATING GENETICS AND GENOMICS INTO NURSING PRACTICE

Genetics generally focuses on one gene, whereas **genomics** involves multiple genes as well as interacting factors, such as environmental conditions and cultural and social influences, all of which affect the 'expression' or triggering of individual or groups of genes. Genetics and genomics have revolutionised how people perceive themselves, as well as their health status and their health potential. Therefore, nurses and midwives must integrate new genetic knowledge into practice. In 2016, the American Nurses Association (ANA) and International Society of Nurses in Genetics (ISONG) updated the 16 standards that measure the accountabilities for general, graduate-level prepared and advanced practice genetics/genomics nurses.

Kirk, Tonkin and Skirton (2014) published, for the National Genetics Education and Development Centre in the UK, a wide-ranging review and revised competence-based framework, including learning outcomes and practice indicators for nurses and specifically, midwives, in 2018. While the Australian

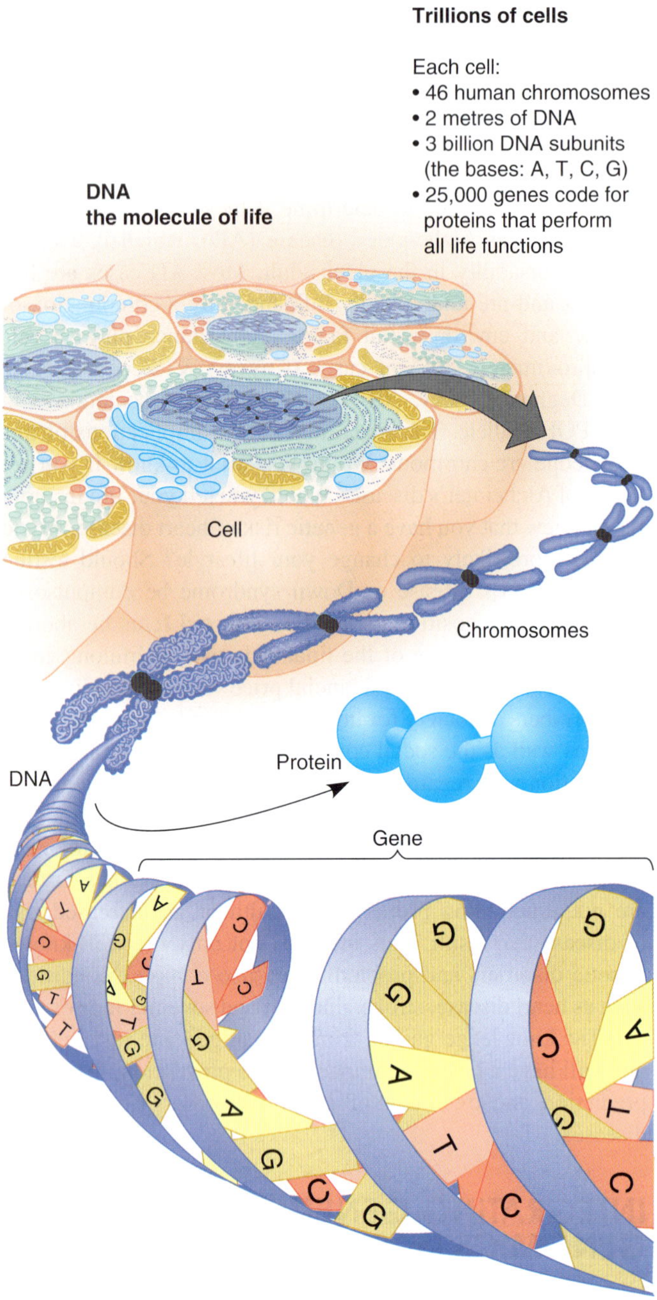

FIGURE 7.1 *Each cell nucleus throughout the body contains the genes, DNA and chromosomes that make up the majority of an individual's genome. The remaining portion of the human genome is in the mitochondria*

standards for the RN (Nursing and Midwifery Board of Australia (NMBA), 2016) do not specifically refer to genetics, Standard 4.3 states that the Registered Nurse, 'works in partnership to determine factors that affect the health and wellbeing of people and populations to determine priorities for action and/or referral' (p. 5), and Standard 4.4 assesses the resources available to inform planning, which would include a family history. Therefore, both the UK and US frameworks and competency standards have relevance for Australian nurses and midwives.

FOUNDATIONS OF GENETICS

Nurses need to have foundational knowledge of the cell, DNA, cell division, chromosomes and genes in order to deliver competent care and to enable people requiring assessment, support and referral to fully benefit from advances in genetics (see Box 7.2).

The cell is the basic unit of life and the working unit of all living systems. Life starts as a single cell, but the developed human body is made up of trillions of cells. These cells share common features, such as a nucleus that contains 46 chromosomes and organelles such as mitochondria. There are many different types of 'specialised' cells that function differently depending on their location. For example, pancreatic cells have a very different function from that of nerve cells.

All human cells, except mature red blood cells, contain a complete set of deoxyribonucleic acid (DNA) molecules. DNA molecules consist of long sequences of nucleotides or bases represented by the letters A, G, T and C. The order of these bases gives the exact instructions for the functioning of that particular cell. Writing the correct order of the bases using the above abbreviations represents the sequence of the bases in DNA. The entire DNA in a human cell is referred to as the **human genome**, or the complete set of inheritance for an individual. The human genome includes the DNA in the cell nucleus as well as the DNA found in the mitochondria, which will be discussed later in this section. Each person's genome is unique. Identical (monozygotic) twins are the exception because they develop from only one fertilised ovum and share identical DNA.

The cell nucleus contains about 183 cm of DNA that is tightly wound and packaged into 23 pairs of **chromosomes**, making a complete set of 46 chromosomes. The structure and number of chromosomes can be shown by a karyotype, or picture, of an individual's chromosomes (see Figure 7.2). There are two copies of each chromosome. One copy, or half of the complete set of these 46 chromosomes, is inherited from the mother and the other copy, or the other half of the 46 chromosomes, is inherited from the father. For example, an individual will have two of chromosome 1, one inherited from her mother and one inherited from her father. These two copies or pairs of

BOX 7.2 Using the people-first approach

Nurses must incorporate a 'people-first' philosophy and use genetic terminology that is sensitive to the maintenance of an individual's positive self-image. This can be accomplished by using terms such as 'unaltered' or 'wild-type' gene instead of 'normal' gene and 'altered gene'; 'altered, disease-producing gene' or 'gene alteration' instead of the terms 'mutated' or 'abnormal' gene when communicating genetic concerns.

wild-type = normal = expected = unaltered

versus

mutated = abnormal = defective = unexpected = altered

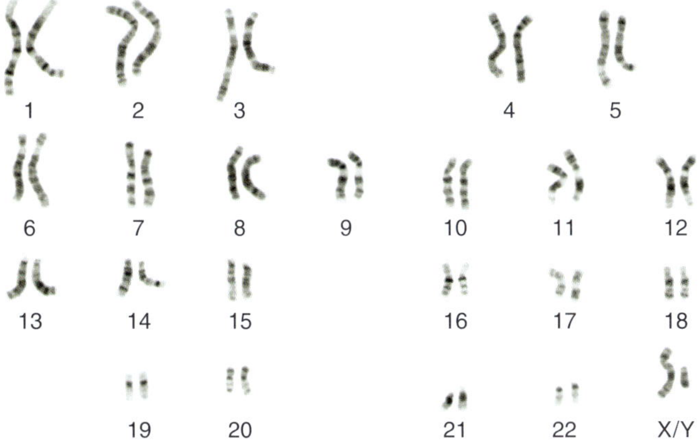

FIGURE 7.2 *A karyotype is a picture of an individual's chromosomes. It shows the chromosomal structure and number of the 22 pairs of autosomes and the sex chromosomes*

Source: Mediscan/Alamy Stock Photo.

inherited chromosomes are called **homologous chromosomes**. Chromosomes are numbered according to size, with chromosome 1 being the largest and chromosome 22 being the smallest. The first 22 pairs of chromosomes, known as **autosomes**, are alike in males and females. The 23rd pair, the **sex chromosomes**, determines an individual's gender. A female has two copies of the X chromosomes (one copy inherited from each parent), and a male has one X chromosome (inherited from his mother) and one Y chromosome (inherited from his father).

Cell division

Mitosis and meiosis are the two types of cell division in human cells. **Mitosis** is the process of making new cells and takes place in the **somatic**, or tissue, **cells** of the body. Cell division through mitosis heals wounds and replaces cells lost daily on skin surfaces and in the lining of gastrointestinal and respiratory tracts. In addition, mitosis is responsible for development. The mitotic activity of the zygote and its daughter cells is the foundation for a human's growth and development. The zygote undergoes mitosis to form a multicellular embryo, then fetus, then infant. Cell division through mitosis results in two cells, called *daughter cells,* that are genetically identical to the original cell, or *mother cell*, and each other.

Meiosis is also known as the reduction division of the cell. Meiosis occurs only in the sex cells of the testes and ovaries and results in the formation of the sperm and oocyte (gametes). Meiosis is very similar to mitosis in that it is a form of cell division; however, through a series of complex mechanisms, the amount of genetic material is reduced by half (23 chromosomes). This is very important because when the two sex cells combine during fertilisation, the total number of chromosomes (46) is present in the offspring's cells. The purpose of meiosis is to produce gametes, to reduce the number of chromosomes by half and to make new combinations of genetic material from crossing over and independent assortment processes, which allow diversity in the human population.

Chromosomal alterations

Alterations in chromosomes often occur during cell division (meiosis or mitosis) and are classified as either alterations in the number of chromosomes or structural alterations. They involve either part of or the whole chromosome. The clinical consequences of number and structural changes in the chromosomes in an individual vary depending on the amount and type of DNA affected by the alterations.

Alterations in chromosome number

An increase or decrease in chromosomal numbers can occur during meiosis or mitosis (see Box 7.3). Alterations often occur during meiosis because meiosis is a highly specific and complex process, and each new daughter cell must contain exactly one chromosome from each homologous pair of chromosomes. During meiosis, the paired chromosomes may fail to separate, resulting in daughter cells with either two copies or no copies of that chromosome. This is known as **nondisjunction**.

Nondisjunction creates an egg or sperm cell with either two copies or no copies of a particular chromosome. When these egg or sperm cells are fertilised by a normal gamete that contains 23 copies of all of the chromosomes, a zygote that is monosomic (one member of the chromosome pair is missing) or trisomic (having three chromosomes instead of the usual two) results. These circumstances produce such conditions as Turner's syndrome (**monosomy**) or Down syndrome (**trisomy** 21). As you have already read, normally each cell has 23 pairs of chromosomes, making a total of 46 chromosomes. One of these pairs, the sex chromosomes, determines the gender of the fetus (46XY for a boy and 46XX for a girl). In **Turner's syndrome** (affects about 1 in 2,500 girls), there will usually be only one X chromosome or portion of one missing in all or some of the cells. The reason for this total or partial loss of the chromosome usually cannot be found, but the loss occurs soon after conception. Sometimes there may be abnormalities in the X chromosome in only some cells in the body. This is referred to as mosaic Turner's syndrome; there may be few or no symptoms and fertility may not be affected. Parents need to be reassured that there was nothing either parent could have done to prevent this from happening; it is

BOX 7.3 Variations in chromosomal number

Aneuploidy—the condition when extra or missing chromosomes exist; if there is an addition or deletion of chromosome number and the individual lives, physical abnormalities and/or mental retardation are common.

Monosomy—the loss of a single chromosome from a pair; i.e. Turner's syndrome (45XO).

Trisomy—the gain of a single chromosome, making a total of three copies of a certain chromosome; i.e. trisomy 21 or Down syndrome.

Euploidy—the presence of the normal number of 46 chromosomes.

Polyploidy—the condition when more than two pairs of all the chromosomes are present.

a biological accident for which no one is responsible. Girls with Turner's syndrome are at risk of impairments in the cognitive, behavioural and social domains—learning disabilities, particularly with regard to spatial perception, visual–motor integration, mathematics, memory, the ability to formulate goals and plan action sequences to attain them, and attention span. To complicate matters, a female with 45XO Turner's syndrome may manifest an X-linked recessive disorder, such as haemophilia, because she has only one X chromosome.

The missing genes cause significant problems for the girl, but the main ones are:

- short stature (average height: 143 cm)
- lack of secondary sexual characteristics (failure to develop at puberty)
- infertility.

Klinefelter's syndrome, also known as the XXY condition, describes males who have an extra X chromosome in most of their cells. Klinefelter's syndrome is named after Dr Henry Klinefelter. Boys with Klinefelter's syndrome are born with at least one extra X chromosome (47 chromosomes in each cell, rather than the normal number of 46). Klinefelter's syndrome is also called 47XXY syndrome. It is thought to be caused by an error within the fertilised egg or the dividing cells as the baby develops. The presence of the Y chromosome ensures male sexual characteristics but, because the testicles are underdeveloped, there may not be enough testosterone production. This is why the penis and testicles are smaller than average, and why most men with Klinefelter's syndrome are infertile. Some researchers suspect that advanced maternal age may be a risk factor.

Down syndrome is named after Dr John Langdon Down who first identified the syndrome in 1866. Trisomy 21 (Down syndrome) is caused by an extra copy of chromosome 21. An obsolete term that should never be used to describe someone with Down syndrome is *mongolism*. The extra chromosome causes certain physical characteristics and affects intellectual development. In Australia, about 95% of all pregnant women consent to have a screening test to determine if the fetus is at risk of Down syndrome. About 1 in 20 (5%) women will be notified that the fetus is at increased risk. Only further testing will show which babies do have the problem. It is important to remember that even if the test shows that the baby is at low risk of Down syndrome the child may be born with other complications. Testing does NOT ensure the 'perfect baby'. Down syndrome occurs in all races and cultures. Approximately 1 in every 800 babies is born with Down syndrome. However, the actual rate is probably much higher than this because many women will choose to terminate their pregnancy.

Alterations in chromosome structure

Alterations in chromosome structure include inversions, deletions and duplications, and translocations. In a chromosomal inversion, a segment of a chromosome is reversed, changing the DNA sequence for that portion of the chromosome. It occurs when a chromosome breaks in two places and the piece between the breaks turns upside down and reattaches within the same chromosome. The clinical consequences of an inversion depend on how much chromosomal material is involved, where the inversion occurs and what type of inversion is present.

A chromosomal alteration that includes a missing (deletion) or additional (duplication) whole chromosome or segment of a chromosome is an unbalanced rearrangement. An unbalanced rearrangement can result in missing genes, confusing directions from the genes or too much gene product, which often results in a condition that is not compatible with life, or in altered physical and/or mental development. An example is cri du chat syndrome (intellectual disability, crying that sounds like a cat mewing and low-set ears). Cri du chat syndrome is an abnormality resulting in the deletion of a large part of the short arm of chromosome 5. **Translocation** (chromosomal reshuffling) occurs when a segment of a chromosome transfers or moves and attaches itself to another chromosome. An example is the reciprocal translocation that is found in 95% of people with chronic myelogenous leukaemia (CML). The contributing translocation occurs between chromosomes 9 and 22. The translocation results in a shortened chromosome 22, an observation first described by Nowell and Hungerford in 1960 and subsequently termed the Philadelphia (Ph^1) chromosome after the city where it was discovered. The translocation (two chromosomes break, then parts from each chromosome switch places) relocates an oncogene called Abl from the long arm of chromosome 9 to the long arm of chromosome 22. As a result, a new, abnormal gene called BCR produces Bcr-Abl tyrosine kinase, an abnormal protein that causes too many stem cells to develop into white blood cells (granulocytes or blasts). The exact cause of CML is unknown, though it is now known how the disease develops from genetic changes in myeloid cells.

Unlike the translocation responsible for Down syndrome, which occurs in the germ cells, the translocation responsible for CML occurs in somatic cells and therefore is not inheritable (Leukaemia Foundation, 2020; National Cancer Institute, 2022a; Nussbaum et al., 2015). Thus, environmental factors account for only a small number of CML cases and so family history does not appear to play a role in the development of CML.

Genes

Nurses must also have knowledge of genes—what they are and the role they play in homeostasis, as well as the consequences of gene alterations. How these gene alterations are inherited is also important for nursing and midwifery interventions and teaching the person who is at risk of, or who has, a known gene (DNA-based) condition. Knowledge of the function and inheritance of genes is implicit in health promotion as well as health maintenance of the person and their family.

A **gene** is a small portion (segment) of the nucleotide (base) sequence of a chromosome DNA molecule that can be identified as having a particular function or characteristic. These segments of DNA within each gene have specific directions for the functioning of the gene. This specific sequence of nucleotides (the genes and the variations therein) is referred to as the individual's **genotype**. Each chromosome contains numerous genes arranged in a linear order. Researchers currently believe there are about 20,000 to 30,000 genes in the human genome (Loscalzo et al., 2022; National Human Genome Research Institute, 2017). The number of genes present on each chromosome varies. Chromosome 1 is the largest chromosome and has the largest number of genes, with 2968. The Y chromosome has the smallest number of genes, with 231 (HGP, 2008).

All genes come in pairs because chromosomes come in pairs. The only exceptions to all genes being paired are the genes on the sex chromosomes (X and Y) present in males. All genes have a specific location on a specific chromosome. This is known as the **genetic locus**. For example, one of the many genes located on chromosome 19 is a gene for eye colour. There may be slight variations or different forms of a gene—for instance, green versus blue eye colour—and these different forms or versions of genes are called **alleles**. When an individual has two identical forms (alleles) of a gene, they are said to be **homozygous** (homo = same). If an individual has two different forms (alleles) of the gene, they are said to be **heterozygous** (hetero = different). Genes can be described as *altered* or *mutated*, when a change has taken place, or *expressed*, when the gene has an impact on the outward appearance of an individual and/or the functioning of cells. The observable, outward expression of an individual's entire physical, biochemical and physiological make-up, as determined by their genotype (alleles) and environmental factors, is referred to as **phenotype**. Phenotype may be expressed or observed as curly or straight hair or the presentation of signs and symptoms of a disease.

Function and distribution of genes

Although the function of more than 50% of the genes in the human genome is still unknown, we do know that about 2% of the genes give directions to parts of the cell for how to make proteins, what type of proteins to make and how much of a protein to make (HGP, 2008). These protein-directing genes are very important to life and functioning as a human being because proteins are very specialised and perform a variety of functions within the cell. These functions include transmitting messages between cells, fighting infection, directing genes to turn 'on' or 'off' and forming structures, as well as sensing light, taste and smell. Some gene activities change from moment to moment in response to tens of thousands of intra- and extracellular environmental signals (USDOE Genome Programs, 2008). An example of this is the feedback mechanism that stimulates a cell to produce insulin after eating lollies. After eating, a gene on chromosome 11 directs pancreatic cells to produce, modify and secrete insulin. Although the gene for producing insulin is present in all nucleated cells of the body, it is only functional in insulin-secreting pancreatic cells (Ikle & Gloyn, 2021).

Mitochondrial genes

Chromosomes in the cell nucleus are not the only site where genes reside. Several dozen that are involved in energy metabolism are located in the cell mitochondria (the 'powerhouse' of the cell). **Mitochondria** are concerned with energy production and metabolism. Some cells contain more mitochondria than others, but each mitochondrion contains its own copies of DNA, identified as mitochondrial DNA (mtDNA). Because ova have many mitochondria and sperm do not (most mitochondria are located in the tail of the sperm that detaches after fertilisation), mtDNA is primarily inherited from the mother. Therefore, mitochondrial genes and any diseases due to DNA alterations on those genes are transmitted through the mother in a matrilineal pattern. This pattern of inheritance is very different from the pattern of inheritance of genes found in the nucleus of the cell (Ikle & Gloyn, 2021). Thus, an affected female will pass the mtDNA mutation to all of her children; however, an affected male will not pass the mtDNA mutation to any of his children (Chen et al., 2020; Nussbaum et al., 2015). Signs and symptoms of conditions occurring as a result of mitochondrial gene alterations primarily involve high-energy tissues and organs such as skeletal muscles, liver, kidney, brain and nerve cells, ears, eyes, endocrine system and heart muscle. Symptoms develop over years as unhealthy or dying cells are not replaced. Hypertrophic cardiomyopathy, heart block, seizures and deafness are also associated with mtDNA gene alterations (Craven et al., 2017; Nussbaum et al., 2015). An Italian research team found that chronic kidney disease (CKD) is possibly linked to oxidative stress caused by dysregulation of the genes that control mitochondria (Singh Bhatti, Kaur Bhatti & Reddy, 2017).

Gene alterations and disease

A protein will malfunction and in many cases cause disease if any kind of alteration (mutation or change) is present in the order of the DNA sequence within a gene. These gene alterations can be inherited from one or either parent, or they can be acquired. *Mutations* inherited from a parent (hereditary mutations) are also known as *germline mutations* because the mutation exists in the reproductive sperm or ova of the parent. Consequently, the DNA in every cell of that offspring will have the gene alteration and also can be inherited from generation to generation.

The second kind of gene alteration is an *acquired mutation* or *somatic mutation*. These alterations occur in the DNA of cells of the individual throughout their life. They can result from errors during cell division (mitosis) or from environmental influences such as radiation or toxins (Centers for Disease Control and Prevention (CDC), 2020).

Today, we know that gene alterations are responsible for approximately 6,000 hereditary diseases. However, different gene alterations within a particular gene can result in a wide variety of signs and symptoms. Since it occurs in one of the first 22 pairs of chromosomes, the cystic fibrosis (CF) defect is autosomal. It is not sex-linked, so the disease can occur in either gender. For example, the CFTR gene for cystic fibrosis is a very large gene located on chromosome 7. More than 1,500 different mutations of this gene have been reported to cause cystic fibrosis (Ferraguti et al., 2011). The area of the CFTR gene that controls mucus production can have more than 300 different gene alterations, resulting in a variety of symptoms ranging from mild, to severe, or no symptoms at all (CDC, 2020). Gene alterations, not the genes themselves, cause genetic diseases and conditions. Since CF is a recessive trait, an affected individual must receive two defective genes in order to be born with CF. As with all chromosome pairs, one is inherited from the mother and one is inherited from the father. This means that both parents must carry the cystic fibrosis trait or have CF themselves in order to have a child with CF. People who are carriers have only one defective gene. They will not have CF and will not have any symptoms. On average, about 1 in 25 Australians and New Zealanders are genetic carriers for CF, but they are more likely to be a carrier if they are of Northern European descent (including the UK). If both parents are carriers, there is a 1 in 4 chance that each parent will pass on their defective gene, meaning their baby will also have CF. Interestingly, other factors probably influence the course of CF. For example, changes in genes other than CFTR might explain why some people with the disease are more severely affected than others. So far none of these factors have been identified.

All babies in Australia are screened for CF shortly after birth:

- Genetic testing may be available to determine if a person is a carrier of the faulty CFTR gene. The screening test may be offered pre-pregnancy and in pregnancy when there is a family history of CF or a blood relative is a genetic carrier for CF.
- Genetic screening may also be available as part of pre-pregnancy planning for those people with a high chance of being a genetic carrier for CF based on their family history. The screening will only pick up those who are carriers of one of the more common changes in the CFTR gene.

Other situations where gene alterations cause illness and disease are through gene interaction with the environment. These genes and conditions are referred to as multifactorial (Tromans & Barwell, 2022; Yang, 2019). Alterations in regulatory genes may also occur. Regulatory genes play a part in maintaining homeostasis or normal functioning. A regulatory gene mutation might lead to the loss of expression of a gene, to unexpected expression in a tissue in which it is usually silent or to a change in the time when a gene is usually expressed. An example of a regulatory gene mutation associated with disease includes the insulin gene region that increases the risk of type 1 diabetes (Ikle & Gloyn, 2021). Researchers have identified a gene, KIAA0350, that increases the risk of getting type 1 diabetes (insulin-dependent diabetes) (Grant, Wells & Rich, 2020). This finding does not mean that researchers know how to prevent diabetes in those who have these genetic mutations. Diabetes is a complex disorder and the risk of developing it is known to be affected by environmental factors and at least four other genes.

Gene alterations that decrease risk of disease

Although it is common to associate gene mutations with disease, it is important to remember that gene mutations can also be helpful and decrease the risk of disease. Gene alterations and genetic variations may also have a protective role in the expression of diseases. A common example is the protective value of the gene alteration that causes sickle cell disease. Those individuals with this gene alteration have protection against malaria. Another, less common example of a 'protective' gene alteration is the one on the receptor gene named CCR5. This mutation consists of a deletion within the DNA sequence. People who are homozygous for the CCR5 mutation (have two copies of the altered gene) are almost completely resistant to infection with HIV type I, and those who are heterozygous for the deletion (have one copy of the altered gene), progress much more slowly from the stage of HIV infection to AIDS (Lashley, Schneidereith & Kasper, 2015). As genomic research continues, more and more of these types of beneficial gene alterations will be identified.

Single nucleotide polymorphisms

Single nucleotide polymorphisms, or SNPs ('snips'), are one-letter (base pair) variations in the DNA sequence that occur in more than 1% of the population. In all people, 99.9% of the DNA is identical; SNPs are responsible for differences among individuals. **Polymorphisms** are DNA sequences that have many forms but give the genetic 'directions' for the same thing. Most of these differences have no effect on the individual. Some cause subtle differences in numerous characteristics in appearance such as widow's peak, tongue rolling and attached ear lobes. Other SNPs, however, affect an individual's risk of certain diseases and have a major impact on how the individual responds to environmental factors such as toxins, microbes and medications. Biological markers are important for the construction of chromosome maps and are easily tracked, stable segments of DNA. Scientists are mapping these areas of SNPs in order to move to the next step of identifying the multiple genes that are associated with diseases that are not caused by single-gene alterations—those complex diseases caused by multiple genes such as cancer, cardiovascular disease, some forms of mental illness and diabetes (Tromans & Barwell, 2022; Yang, 2019). More recently, an international collaboration has linked common SNPs on chromosome 5 to five different types of cancer, while at the same time conferring protection against melanoma. Of note, four of the five cancers have a strong environmental contribution to risk (smoking for lung and bladder cancer, UV light for skin cancer and HPV infection for cervical cancers) (Rafnar et al., 2009).

PRINCIPLES OF INHERITANCE

Knowledge of inheritance allows nurses and midwives not only to offer and reinforce genetic information to people and their families, but also to assist them in managing their care and in making reproductive decisions. The basic underlying principles of inheritance that health professionals can apply to inheritance risk assessment and teaching include: (1) all genes are paired, (2) only one gene of each pair is transmitted (passed on) to an offspring, and (3) one copy of each gene in the offspring comes from the mother and the other copy comes from the father. Understanding the Mendelian patterns of inheritance is made easier by relating these principles.

Mendelian patterns of inheritance

Conditions that are caused by a mutation or alteration of a single gene are known as *monogenic* or *single-gene disorders*. There are more than 6,000 known single-gene disorders occurring in about 1 in 200 births (HGP, 2008). The most common gene alterations that result in genetic disorders are categorised into Mendelian inheritance patterns because they are predictably passed on from generation to generation following Mendel's laws of inheritance. These single-gene mutations follow an autosomal dominant, autosomal recessive, **X-linked recessive** or **X-linked dominant** inheritance pattern. The first three of these patterns are the most common. Modes of transmission or inheritance for thousands of conditions resulting from monogenic alterations have been identified (McKusick/Nathans Institute of Genetic Medicine, 2022).

Recessive versus dominant disorders

The distinction between recessive and dominant phenotypes or disease presence (expression) lies in the amount of gene product (usually proteins) from the unaltered (**wild-type** or normal) **gene**. When the individual is heterozygous (has one unaltered gene and one altered gene), the altered gene as well as the disease is classified as recessive if half of the product produced from the unaltered gene is enough to maintain homeostasis and perform the expected function. Therefore, two altered genes must be present to cause a diseased state. If the altered gene causes disease even though the unaltered gene is producing the gene product, then the altered gene as well as the disease is classified as dominant (Nussbaum et al., 2015).

Autosomal dominant conditions

Autosomal dominant (AD) conditions are the result of an altered gene on any of the 22 autosomes or non-sex chromosomes (see Figure 7.3). More than half of the known Mendelian conditions are autosomal dominant. In AD conditions, disease occurs in spite of the fact that there exists one unaltered or normal gene. Also, homozygous dominant conditions are generally much more severe than heterozygous dominant conditions and are often lethal. Because homozygous dominant conditions are usually lethal and would result from *both parents being affected*, the nurse or midwife should consider an individual exhibiting an autosomal dominant condition as heterozygous. See Box 7.4 for characteristics of an AD pattern of inheritance.

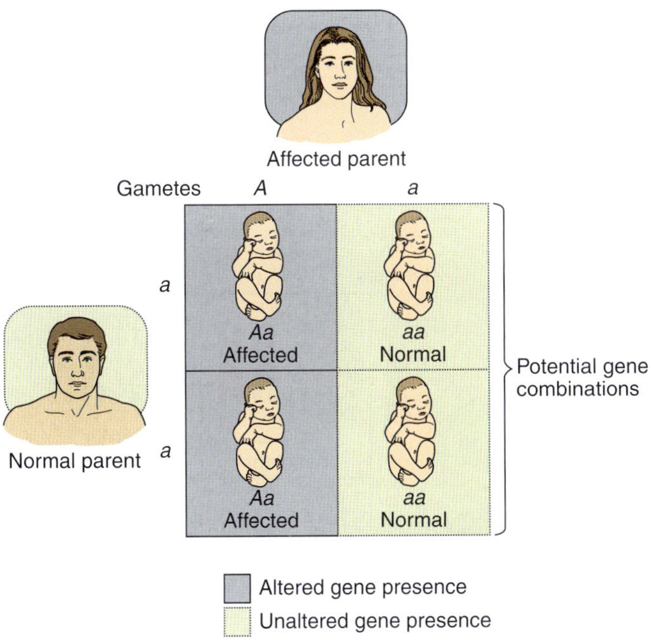

FIGURE 7.3 ***This Punnett square shows potential gene combinations (genotypes) and resulting phenotypes of children from parent genotypes with an autosomal dominant altered gene. Phenotypes are expressed (affected) when a male or female has one copy of the gene alteration***

BOX 7.4 Autosomal dominant Mendelian inheritance characteristics

(*Examples*: neurofibromatosis, breast and ovarian cancer, autosomal dominant polycystic kidney disease, Marfan's syndrome, Huntington's disease, familial hypercholesterolaemia.)

When the health professional gathers a family history, they should assess for any of the following characteristics of autosomal dominant inheritance:

1. Both males and females are affected.
2. Males and females are usually affected in equal numbers.
3. An affected child will have an affected parent and/or all generations will have an affected individual (appearing as a vertical pattern of affected individuals on the family pedigree).
4. Unaffected children of an affected parent will have unaffected offspring.
5. A significant proportion of isolated cases are due to a new mutation.

Autosomal recessive conditions

A gene or genetic condition is considered recessive when two copies of altered genes are needed to express the condition—for example, cystic fibrosis. Autosomal recessive (AR) conditions are the result of an altered gene on any of the 22 autosomes or non-sex chromosomes (see Figure 7.4). An individual with a recessive condition has inherited one altered gene from their mother and one from their father. In most cases, neither of the parents is affected and, therefore, each of the parents must have a single gene alteration on one chromosome of a pair and the normal, wild-type or unaltered form of the gene on the other chromosome. These parents would be known as **carriers** of the condition and they do not usually exhibit any signs and symptoms of the condition. Because the gene alteration occurs on a non-sex chromosome, both males and females have an equal chance of inheriting the altered gene from their parent. Generally, conditions that are autosomal recessive are more severe and have an earlier onset than conditions with other patterns of inheritance. Most inborn errors in metabolism or metabolic conditions are autosomal recessive. Many are enzyme defects and the functioning of the unaltered gene is sufficient to provide normal functioning in the person who is heterozygous or the carrier of one copy of the altered gene (Lashley et al., 2015). See Box 7.5 for characteristics of an AR pattern of inheritance.

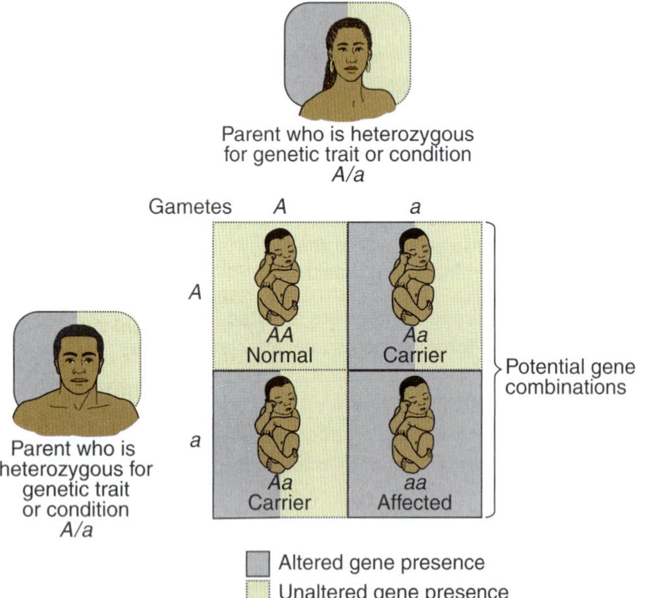

FIGURE 7.4 ***This Punnett square shows potential gene combinations (genotypes) and resulting phenotypes of children from parent genotypes with an autosomal recessive altered gene. Phenotypes are expressed (affected) when a male or female has two copies of the gene alteration***

BOX 7.5 Autosomal recessive Mendelian inheritance characteristics

(*Examples*: haemochromatosis type 1, cystic fibrosis, phenylketonuria, sickle cell anaemia.)

When the health professional gathers a family history, they should assess for any of the following characteristics of autosomal recessive inheritance:

1. **Both males and females are affected.**
2. **Males and females are usually affected in equal numbers.**
3. **An affected child will have an unaffected parent but may have affected siblings (appearing as a horizontal pattern of affected individuals on the family pedigree).**
4. **The condition may appear to skip a generation.**
5. **The parents of the affected child may be consanguineous (close blood relatives).**
6. **The family may be descendants of a certain ethnic group that is known to have a more frequent occurrence of a certain genetic condition.**

X-linked recessive conditions

X-linked conditions are the result of an altered gene on the X chromosome. Unlike the autosomes, the sex chromosome, X, is unevenly distributed to males and females. The female has two X chromosomes and the male has only one. Thus, the family history and pattern of inheritance has a characteristic distribution pattern among the males and females in the family (see Figure 7.5). Because the male has only one copy of any

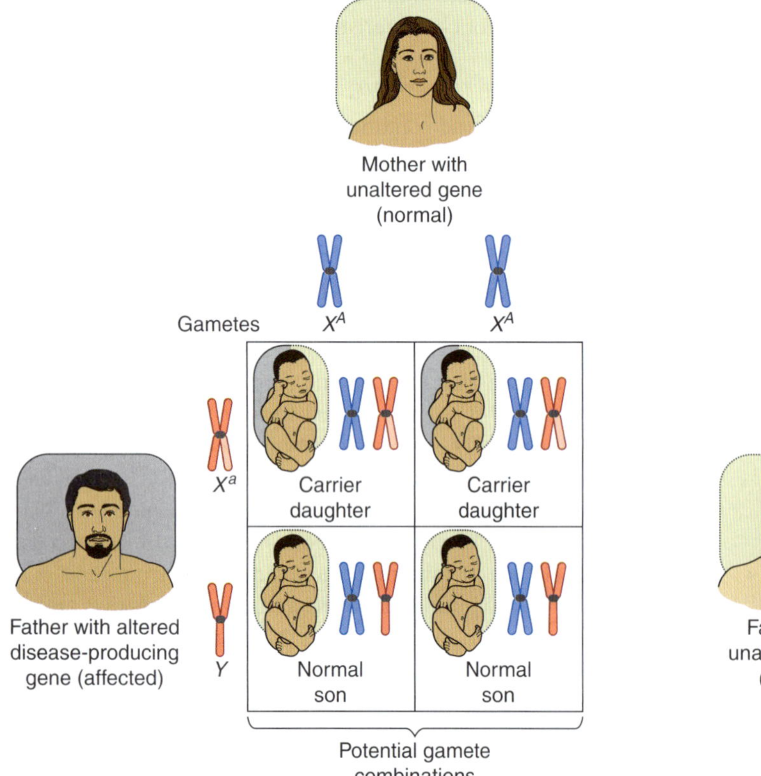

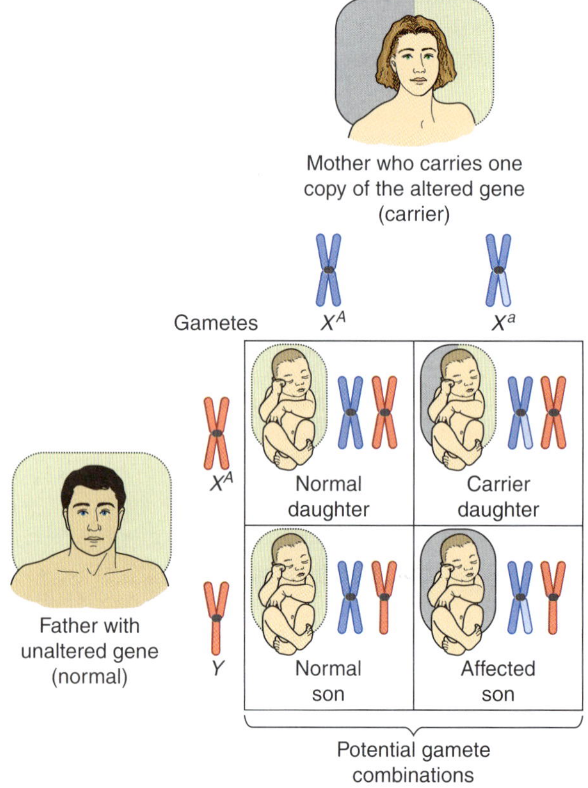

FIGURE 7.5 ***These Punnett squares show potential gene combinations (genotypes) and resulting phenotypes of children from different parent genotypes with an X-linked recessive altered gene. Phenotypes are expressed (affected) in a male with only one copy of the gene alteration and in a female with two copies of the altered gene***

gene on the X chromosome, it becomes the only copy available to give direction for those particular functions of these genes regardless of whether it is considered dominant or recessive in the female. Thus, if any of these genes are altered, an unaltered counterpart is not present to 'override' the altered functioning gene.

The consequences of the altered gene on an X chromosome will be expressed in all males. Females, on the other hand, will have two copies and the unaltered gene generally compensates for the altered gene, making the female a carrier. The male receives his X chromosome from his mother and his Y chromosome from his father. The female offspring receives an X chromosome from each of her parents. Thus, all affected males will pass on the altered X chromosome to all of his daughters who will be carriers of the altered gene. A male can never transmit an altered gene on the X chromosome to his sons because the male will transmit only the Y chromosome to his sons. Because of these transmission patterns, the most commonly occurring transmission of an X-linked condition is through a female who is a carrier of an altered gene. See Box 7.6 for characteristics of an X-linked recessive pattern of inheritance.

X-linked dominant conditions

X-linked dominant conditions also exist but are very rare. The inheritance pattern for X-linked inheritance differs from autosomal inheritance only because the X chromosome has no homologous chromosome in the male; the male has an X and a Y chromosome. For an X-linked dominant disorder, if the father carries the abnormal X gene, all of his daughters will inherit the disease but no sons will have the disease. If the mother carries the abnormal X gene, 50% of all her children (daughters and sons) will inherit the disease tendency. The other children inherit the normal copy of the chromosome. If a male is affected, the condition is severe and often lethal. A family history of multiple male miscarriages may be a sign of an X-linked dominant condition. X-linked dominant diseases are very uncommon, but some inherited forms of rickets are transmitted in this manner. Very few genes have been discovered on the Y chromosome.

BOX 7.6 X-linked recessive Mendelian inheritance characteristics

(*Examples*: haemophilia A; Duchenne muscular dystrophy.) When gathering a family history, the health professional should assess for any of the following characteristics of X-linked recessive inheritance:

1. More males will be affected than females; rarely seen in females.
2. An affected male will have all carrier daughters.
3. There is no male-to-male inheritance.
4. Affected males are related by carrier females.
5. Females may report varying milder symptoms of the condition.
6. A new sporadic case could be due to a new mutation.

Variability in classic Mendelian patterns of inheritance

Along with understanding the classic Mendelian inheritance patterns, several other concepts are also important for families to understand when health professionals are assisting people with, or at risk of inheriting, a genetic disorder. These include the following exceptions or variations to the traditional Mendelian patterns of inheritance.

Penetrance

Penetrance is the probability that a gene will be expressed phenotypically. It is an 'all or none' concept, in that either the gene will be expressed (even if mildly expressed) or it will not be expressed at all. Penetrance can be measured in the following way. In a certain group of individuals with the same genotype, what percentage of them will exhibit at least some signs and/or symptoms of the condition? If the number is less than 100%, then that condition is said to show reduced penetrance. For example, the gene alterations that cause achondroplasia exhibit 100% penetrance and all individuals with one copy of the gene alteration will exhibit signs and symptoms of the disease (Daly et al., 2021; Nussbaum et al., 2015).

New mutation

When there is no previous history of a condition, including even subtle signs and symptoms of the disease in any other immediate or distant family member, the disease may be caused by a spontaneous new mutation. This case is usually called *de novo* mutation. New mutations of a gene are most frequently seen in autosomal dominant conditions because one copy of an altered gene is all that is necessary to elicit a state of altered health. Autosomal dominant diseases known to have high mutation rates include neurofibromatosis, achondroplasia (dwarfism) and Marfan's syndrome. New mutations are also possible in autosomal recessive diseases, although rarely expressed because two altered genes are necessary for signs and symptoms to appear. Finally, new mutations are often seen in X-linked recessive disorders, such as haemophilia A, since a male with just one altered gene will demonstrate the disease.

Anticipation

Anticipation is said to occur when successive generations of a family exhibit more severe signs and symptoms of certain diseases and the disease often has an earlier onset. An example is myotonic dystrophy type 1, an autosomal dominant condition characterised by a range of signs and symptoms including myotonia, muscle weakness, cataracts and cardiac arrhythmias. The congenital form is severe, causing intellectual disability, and may be life threatening. Most children with this congenital form of myotonic dystrophy have a mildly affected mother who may not even be aware she has the disease (Nussbaum et al., 2015). The severity of the condition, as well as the age of onset, is determined by the number of trinucleotide repeats. Trinucleotide repeats are short DNA sequences such as the CTG base sequence of the gene DMPK that are repeated to more than 2,000 times, resulting in alterations in the protein products produced by the gene and varying signs and symptoms.

Variable expressivity

Expressivity is used to describe the severity of the **gene expression** of the phenotype. When people with the same genetic make-up (genotype) exhibit signs and/or symptoms with varying degrees of severity, the phenotype is described as *achondroplasia* exhibit 100% penetrance (Nussbaum et al., 2015).

Neurofibromatosis type 1 (NF1) is a common autosomal dominant disorder which displays considerable inter- and intra-familial variability in phenotypic expression. Although neurofibromatosis has 100% penetrance, variable expressivity can occur within family members with each family member exhibiting a variety of signs and/or symptoms.

Multifactorial (polygenic or complex) disorders

Many birth defects such as cleft lip and palate, as well as many adult-onset conditions such as cancer, mental illnesses, asthma, diabetes, obesity, heart disease and Alzheimer's disease, have a multifactorial cause. **Multifactorial** conditions occur as a result of several gene (polygenic) variations, lifestyle and environmental influences that work together. The polygenic concept is illustrated with the multiple genes involved in an individual's susceptibility for breast cancer. These genes have been identified on chromosomes 6, 11, 13, 14, 15, 17 and 22. Exactly which genes interrelate and how many environmental influences are enough to cause the presentation of many of the common complex diseases or conditions is not known. It is now known that the birth defect spina bifida is caused by the action of several genes, but its prevalence also depends on the amount of folate in the diet. Hypertension is influenced by a number of genes, but also by obesity. The precise causes of multiple sclerosis (MS) are largely unknown. MS is most likely a multifactorial condition involving interaction between genetic, lifestyle and environmental factors. It is well documented that MS also runs in some families. There are probably a number of genes that cause susceptibility to MS as well as affecting the severity and progression of the disease. The major contributing genes for many common complex conditions have now been identified.

Multifactorial conditions accumulate in families, but these conditions do not follow the characteristic Mendelian pattern of inheritance seen with single-gene conditions. Inheritable recurrence risks vary in multifactorial conditions. With information gathered from a family history, basic occurrence risks can be assessed for an individual. For instance, premature death in a first-degree relative, two affected first-degree relatives, and two second-degree maternal or paternal relatives with at least one individual having premature onset of the disease are all considered high inheritance risks. Moderate risks include an individual having a first-degree relative with late or unknown disease onset or two second-degree relatives from the same lineage with late or unknown disease onset. An individual having no affected relatives or a negative family history, or only one affected second-degree relative from one or both sides of the pedigree, is considered average or general population risk (American College of Obstetricians and Gynecologists, 2020; National Cancer Institute, 2022b).

Recurrence risks refer to whether or not a condition will occur again in subsequent pregnancies. Because a Mendelian pattern is not present, statistical percentages can be used to represent the chance that parents have a condition that will occur in another child. The risk of recurrence is higher when more than one family member is affected. The recurrence risk after the first affected child is 4%, whereas the recurrence risk after a second affected child increases to 10%. It is also known that the recurrence risk increases with an increase in severity of the defect.

INTERPROFESSIONAL CARE

Many health professionals work together in the screening, diagnosis, identification, prediction and treatment of genetic disorders. The goals of collaborative care are early diagnosis through testing and assessment, prediction and development of an effective treatment plan, psychosocial support to enhance decision making and coping, and referral to a genetic specialist as needed.

Genetic testing

Genetic testing may be used for a person's clinical management, for making personal decisions or for assisting in reproductive choices. A genetic test is very different from other types of clinical tests. Genetic tests involve the analysis of DNA, RNA, chromosomes and serum levels of specific enzymes or metabolites. Enzymes and metabolites are part of the protein products that genes produce. DNA, RNA and/or chromosomes are unique for each individual and the results have personal, social, financial and legal implications. Some genetic tests are diagnostic, while others are predictive or inform the individual of an increased risk of acquiring a disease or condition. A 'positive' genetic test may indicate that an asymptomatic individual will develop a genetic condition, but a prediction of the onset or severity of the condition cannot be made.

Complications also arise in a person's understanding because a negative test result cannot guarantee that the disease or condition might not develop in the future, often because environmental influences cannot be measured or controlled. Also, the genetic test may have only been able to detect the most common gene mutations and not all of the disease-producing gene alterations are known or available for inclusion in clinical testing. People may learn that they will develop a genetic condition such as Huntington's disease, for which there is no treatment. People may find out through genetic testing that they are a carrier and they have unknowingly passed the altered disease-producing gene on to their children.

Finally, the implications of genetic test results are far reaching. While confidentiality and autonomy for the individuals are always foremost for the nurse, the implications for the person's children, grandchildren, siblings and other extended family members who share a percentage of the same genes can be life altering. This information may be very confusing and very different from how they have perceived healthcare in the past and how they perceived the implications of a simple 'blood test'.

TYPES OF GENETIC TESTS Nurses and midwives should understand that genetic tests can be classified into two categories: screening and diagnostic. A positive screening genetic test result notifies the person of an increased risk or probability but must always be confirmed by diagnostic testing. Screening genetic tests are most commonly completed in prenatal, newborn and carrier circumstances. In contrast, a diagnostic test can definitively validate or eliminate a genetic disorder in the symptomatic person and then direct clinical management. Box 7.7 lists some of the positive and negative aspects of genetic testing.

Several categories of genetic tests included as subcategories of screening and diagnostic genetic tests follow:

- *Newborn screening*. In Australia, the Guthrie test is offered to mothers of all newborn infants and provides a means to identify children who have an increased risk of developing more than 30 genetic diseases such as phenylketonuria, CF and hypothyroidism. Some researchers are lobbying for newborns to be tested for fragile X syndrome, which is the most common cause of inherited intellectual disability, even though in Australia it affects only about 1 in 3,600 males and between 1 in 4,000 and 1 in 6,000 females. The syndrome is caused by a genetic abnormality on the X chromosome, where a single sequence of three DNA base pairs is repeated many times, with devastating consequences.
- *Carrier testing* is completed on asymptomatic individuals who may be carriers of one copy of a gene alteration that can be transmitted to future children in an autosomal recessive or X-linked pattern of inheritance. This may be part of a couple's premarriage or preconception planning if they belong to a particular ethnic group with known risks of developing genetic disorders such as sickle cell anaemia and haemophilia. It may be necessary to determine the exact gene mutation from an affected family member prior to carrier testing. This is often completed through lineage analysis. In Australia, the haemoglobinopathies are the only group of conditions for which population screening is widely offered and which is government funded. The thalassaemias are the most common single gene disorders in the world's population and are a common cause of hereditary anaemia. Recent immigration to Australia, especially from South-East Asia, has introduced large numbers of people from areas where alpha-thalassaemia is common. Screening programs, particularly antenatal testing, are used to detect the carrier state for alpha-thalassaemia as well as the Hb variants in the homozygous form, or in combination with alpha-thalassaemia, which may cause severe disease. In some Australian states there are also population screening programs for cystic fibrosis and autosomal recessive conditions more common in Ashkenazi (Eastern European) Jewish individuals; this screening is generally offered on a user-pays basis.
- *Preimplantation genetic diagnosis (PGD)*. Parents with a family history of a serious or fatal genetic condition now have the option of combining IVF and genetic testing, in a technique known as preimplantation genetic diagnosis (PGD). Couples using PGD first need to use IVF procedures to generate embryos. A single cell can then be removed from the early embryo without damaging it. This cell can be tested to see if it carries the genetic defect that causes the condition. Only embryos that do not carry the defective gene are implanted in the mother. Some couples have used PGD on embryos to determine if they can provide a bone marrow transplant for a sick sibling. The bone marrow cells for the sick sibling are taken from the umbilical cord blood of the new baby. Using this process of tissue typing, these babies are sometimes called 'saviour siblings', as they have the potential to save their brother or sister's life.
- Regulations regarding this use of PGD testing vary from country to country. In Australia, some states have PGD regulations and others do not.
- *Predictive genetic testing* is usually made available to the asymptomatic individual and includes both predispositional and presymptomatic testing. A positive predispositional testing result will indicate there is an increased risk that the individual might eventually develop the disease. Common examples include breast cancer and hereditary non-polyposis colorectal cancer. A presymptomatic test is performed when development of the disease is certain if the gene alteration is present. The Australian Breast Cancer Network (2018) *position statement* explains that an extensive family history of breast cancer is a known predictive risk factor for the disease. A strong family history can indicate an inherited predisposition through the presence of a germline mutation in genes associated with breast cancer. A germline mutation is a mutation that occurs in the genetic material of the egg or sperm

BOX 7.7 Positive and negative outcomes related to genetic testing

Benefits of genetic testing

Provides for:

- Early screening and preventive measures
- Future planning and life preparation
- Lifestyle adaptations
- Decreased confusion and anxiety
- Psychological stress relief
- Reproductive choices
- Informed extended family members
- Early medical and/or surgical intervention
- Cost of medical follow-up reduced (if negative result).

Possible negative outcomes of genetic testing

- Survivor guilt
- Loss of identity
- No treatment may exist
- Employability and insurability affected
- Confusion about accessing healthcare and resources
- Risk of invasion of confidentiality and privacy
- Social stigmatisation.

Source: Data from Secretary's Advisory Committee on Genetic Testing (SACGT), National Institutes of Health, 2000. *Enhancing the oversight of genetic tests: Recommendations of the SACGT*. Retrieved from https://www4.od.nih.gov/.

and can be passed on at conception. Inherited gene mutations account for 5% to 10% of all breast cancer. Some research suggests that BRCA1 and BRCA2 are tumour suppressor genes; that is, genes whose loss of function can lead to neoplastic growth. However, other studies point to the role of BRCA1 and BRCA2 in DNA repair, where inadequate repair may cause additional mutations and ultimately cancer.

- The estimated frequency of BRCA1 or BRCA2 gene mutation carriers in the general population is 1 per 1,000 people. The frequency in specific population groups has also been estimated: for those of Ashkenazi Jewish descent, the rate of BRCA1 or BRCA2 gene mutation carriers is 1 per 50 to 100 people.
- Women with inherited mutations in genes such as BRCA1 and BRCA2 have a potentially high risk of developing breast cancer and for developing the disease at an earlier age. Those carrying mutations are also at increased risk of cancers of the ovary and fallopian tube (and perhaps other cancers). It is important to note that the risk of developing breast cancer never reaches 100%, which means that those with inherited gene mutations have a genetic predisposition to the disease but are not certain to develop it.
- Predictive genetic testing is medically indicated when the seriousness and mortality of the disease can be reduced with knowledge of the gene alteration. Life planning and lifestyle choices can be influenced by predictive testing. In Australia, premiums for private health insurance are not based on risk assessment according to the individual's present or past health or their family history. Premiums for life insurance products, which include cover for life, disability and trauma, and business and bank loans, are calculated according to the present and past health of the applicant and any genetic information, including their family history or any genetic test result (underwritten). The Investment and Financial Services Association Ltd (IFSA) has a policy on genetic testing and life insurance which states that no applicant will be required to undergo a predictive genetic test. Under Australian law, an application for a life insurance product is required to disclose any health or genetic information known to the applicant (Newson et al., 2017; Tiller, Otlowski & Lacaze, 2017). Other uses of genetic testing include organ transplantation tissue typing and pharmacogenetic testing, which involves predicting or studying the person's response to particular medications (American Society of Human Genetics (ASHG), 2019; National Health and Medical Research Council (NHMRC), 2011). Predictive tests and carrier tests are now being offered to determine if people are at risk of conditions such as Alzheimer's disease (AD). The precise causation of AD is not fully understood. However, some cases of early-onset AD are caused by a number of genetic mutations on chromosomes 21, 14 and 1. Scientists have recently discovered that the mutations seen in early-onset AD are not involved in this form of disease. The three genes linked to familial Alzheimer's disease are presenilin 1 (PSEN1), presenilin 2 (PSEN2) and the amyloid precursor protein (APP); these and the mutations that cause Alzheimer's disease cause abnormal proteins to be formed (Dementia Australia, 2022a, 2022b). Dozens of studies have confirmed that the APOE-D4 allele increases the risk of developing AD. In September 2009, researchers identified three genes (CLU, PICALM and CR1) that significantly increase the risk of someone developing AD. Three of the genes have roles in protecting the brain from damage. Changes in the genes may remove this protection or may even turn them into 'killers'. Ongoing research to better understand dementia and AD continue today (Dementia Australia, 2022a, 2022b).

DIAGNOSING CHROMOSOMAL ALTERATIONS Microscopic examination of chromosomes through a karyotype can reveal chromosomal alterations such as chromosomal additions, deletions, gross breaks, and rearrangements or rejoinings (translocations) (USDOE Genome Programs, 2008). Among other things, these chromosomal alterations are responsible for many forms of cancer and, more importantly, particular tumour types. Chromosomal diagnostic examination can be accomplished with a simple blood sample and skin or buccal cell sampling. A karyotype is completed in a cytogenetics laboratory. Chromosomes can be identified by their size and unique light and dark banding patterns. The pairs of autosomal chromosomes are arranged from 1 to 22 according to each chromosome's size, unique banding patterns and centromere position. The sex chromosomes complete the picture, with the X chromosome(s) first, then the Y chromosome (if present). The karyotype shows all of the chromosome pairs lined up and positioned on a piece of paper, allowing for visual chromosomal analysis. (See Figure 7.2 earlier in this chapter.) The final report contains numerical data that includes the total number of chromosomes present. If there is an additional or deleted chromosome, it is identified with a plus (+) or minus (−) symbol. For example, the male individual with 47, XY, +18 has 47 chromosomes (instead of the expected number of 46) that include an additional chromosome 18. Guidelines for writing results of karyotyping are determined by the International System of Human Cytogenetic Nomenclature (ISCN). These guidelines allow for use of a standardised universal language by cytogenetic laboratories and in medical publications.

DIAGNOSING GENE ALTERATIONS With the rapidly expanding advances in technology and the identification of genes in the human genome, the availability of genetic, DNA (gene)-based tests has grown tremendously. Currently, more than 1,000 genetic tests are available with more becoming available each day (USDOE Genome Programs, 2008). **DNA-based tests** involve new, sophisticated technology that permits the examination of the DNA itself. Genetic testing that is DNA-based can be obtained from blood, bone marrow, amniotic fluid, fibroblast cells of the skin, or buccal cells from the mouth. Genetic testing includes different types of DNA-based tests. The appropriate genetic tests may be testing for a specific mutation. This would be used if a family member was known to have a genetic condition and could therefore be tested for that particular gene alteration. Another way to examine DNA is by running a panel of mutations. This is done when there are a specific number of identified genes that the majority of individuals with a genetic condition have—for instance, a panel of the three mutations on the BRCA1 gene that are common in the Ashkenazi Jewish population. A third type of DNA-based test is a complete gene sequence (ASHG, 2019; NHMRC, 2011).

Quality and accuracy of genetic tests

Genetic nurses have expressed concerns that genetic tests are becoming available too quickly, with no regulation of the companies that are offering genetic tests. The quality, accuracy and reliability of genetic test results are not measured against any common standard. Individuals often make hard and irrevocable life-altering decisions after receiving test results, so accuracy and reliability are essential. Also, in most cases, minimal or no education is provided for the individual who is undergoing testing; nor is there any quality counselling or follow-up after the results are given to the individual. Genetic tests are often offered by laboratories before the tests have been proven safe, effective and practical. Because the majority of genetic conditions are rare, there is often only one laboratory offering the genetic test that is needed. Recently, concerns have been voiced about 'direct-to-consumer' genetic testing. Genetic tests are being offered at 'walk-in' locations and also via the internet. Individuals can receive results of genetic tests in private without a physician's order and fear of discrimination, but also without education or knowledge of the implications of the test results.

Concerns also exist related to test validity, test sensitivity and specificity, the quality of the laboratory performing the test, and the competence of the person's healthcare provider to interpret the test results. **Test sensitivity** refers to how specifically the test identifies (positive test result) individuals who are affected and/or who have the disease phenotype. A test with a high degree of sensitivity has very few false negatives and many true positives. **Test specificity** refers to how specifically the test does not identify (negative test result) individuals who are unaffected or do not have the disease phenotype. A test with a high degree of specificity has very few false positives (SACGT, 2000). The laboratory selected for the genetic test should have a CLIA88 (Clinical Laboratories Improvement Amendments of 1988) certification (CDC, 2022).

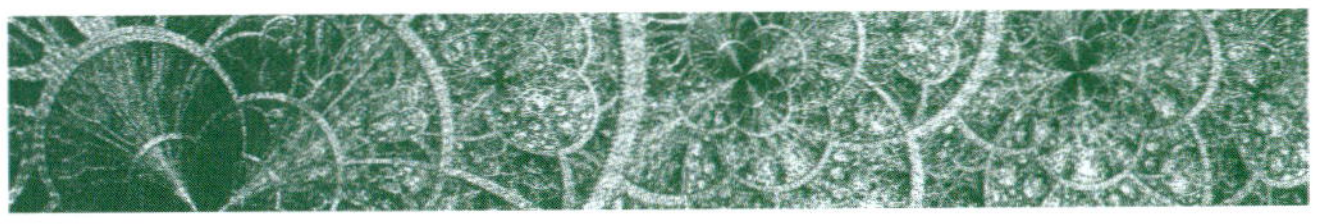

Nursing care

The role of the nurse in genetic testing

With knowledge of available genetic tests and the many implications related to genetic testing, the nurse can assist people as they weigh choices regarding genetic testing. As consumers of multimedia, people often have unreliable sources for information related to genetic testing. They may form many misconceptions about the types of genetic tests available and what information these different types of genetic tests are able and not able to provide. Nurses involved in education about genetic testing must include education for the individual and the family. Communication with the person about genetic testing should include an assessment of the positive and negative outcomes of the test. Are there existing treatments for the condition being tested? Psychological issues should also be emphasised. Who will be affected by the test results? Will the test results be shared with extended family members?

The nurse is responsible for alerting people to their right to make an informed decision prior to any genetic testing, with consideration of the special circumstances arising from the family, culture and community life. All genetic testing should be voluntary and it is the nurse's responsibility to ensure that the consent process includes discussion of the risks and benefits of the test, including any physical harm as well as potential psychological and societal injury by stigmatisation, discrimination and emotional stress (Bunnik, Janssens & Schemer, 2014; ISONG, 2018; NHMRC, 2011).

Above all, nurses have a responsibility to fully educate people about the multiple issues related to genetic testing. People should engage in genetic testing with full knowledge and confidentiality, and autonomously. Informed consent may be given verbally, although some laboratories require written consent. Prior to the testing, the people should have an idea of the probability of a positive or negative result, if one can be determined by the person's or family history (ASHG, 2019; NHMRC, 2011). To deliver the expected standard of care, it is imperative that the nurse includes these issues when developing an educational plan for the person anticipating the use of genetic testing and as part of the informed consent process.

Ensuring confidentiality and privacy for genetic testing

Although confidentiality and privacy are integral parts of delivery of care for all nurses, this issue is of even more concern as it relates to genetic information. Results of genetic tests can be far reaching and can affect employment and insurance options. Will the results affect the person's ability to obtain and/or maintain insurance coverage? Can an employer refuse to hire or promote an individual because of genetic testing results? Can genetic information be released to the courts, the armed forces, schools or adoption agencies? Would a person with a known gene alteration for Huntington's disease be offered a scholarship to the best university? There is debate over whether genetic privacy is different from medical privacy. Nurses should inform people of their rights and responsibilities regarding who will have access to the genetic test results. Those providing the genetic tests must provide the person with assurance that the results will be handled confidentially and that there will be no access to the genetic information by a third party without written permission of the individual being tested.

Results of genetic tests should only be communicated directly to the individual who gave the consent. No outside governmental, employment or insurance organisations should ever have access to genetic test results without the written permission of individuals. People should confirm how they will receive the test results. They should ask who will have access to the test results and what will happen to the DNA sample after the test is completed. In the majority of cases, results of genetic tests should not be shared with extended family members without written permission. Healthcare providers are legally liable to maintain that confidence. Exceptions to the individual's privacy may be made only when the individual refuses to inform extended family members when there is a very high probability of irreversible harm for an extended family member and informing the family member can prevent the harm (Grace & Milliken, 2022; Johnson et al., 2020). Every effort should be made to educate the individual about the benefits of informing extended family members if applicable. Genetic testing should ideally be accompanied by pre-test and post-test counselling by genetic specialists or by another knowledgeable healthcare provider.

Psychosocial issues

Although family and individual anxiety may be decreased with a negative test result, potential problems do exist and the nurse or midwife must be prepared to address them. Concerns about carrier status may interfere with development of intimacy and interpersonal relationships. Non-paternity may be revealed through genetic testing. For example, the parents of a child born with an autosomal recessive condition will be considered carriers of the altered gene the majority of the time. To counsel the parents about future pregnancies, the parents would be tested to confirm their genotype and non-paternity may become an issue. A positive test result may lead to feelings of unworthiness, confusion, anger, depression and self-image disturbance. Survivor guilt may affect adults with negative results if their siblings are positive. The individual carrying a gene alteration for a late-onset disease may have an increased tendency for risky behaviours and may choose not to be a positive member of society. Relatives of an individual affected with a genetic disorder may be very frightened when they realise what their own future might be (SACGT, 2000). The individual who has inherited an altered disease-producing gene may foster deep resentment towards the parent who carries the altered gene. Parents and older generations may feel tremendous guilt for passing the altered gene to their children and grandchildren (Bilkey et al., 2019).

Economic issues

The nurse should consider the cost of genetic tests, which can range from hundreds to thousands of dollars, depending on the size of the gene being tested. In Australia, many of the tests are sent to overseas organisations for analysis.

Genetic tests differ from routine medical tests in many ways. The risks and benefits of genetic testing are numerous and complicated. Nurses have an obligation to maintain their knowledge regarding genetic testing, to advocate for the person, and to maintain ethical standards of care. Above all, nurses and midwives must be able to recognise the limits of their expertise and know how to refer a person to genetic specialists and additional resources.

Assessment

Health promotion and health maintenance

Health promotion and health maintenance of the person are viewed as the foundations of all nursing and midwifery care. However, most individuals do not know their complete genetic make-up. Some know they carry an altered gene that causes a specific disease, but the majority of individuals do not know with certainty what their future health status will be. With no sure knowledge of genetic make-up or whether a certain alteration in health status will occur (e.g. heart disease), healthy lifestyles are not always a priority. Imagine, then, if people knew their statistical risks for developing or inheriting disease by having complete access to the types of genes in their cells? Health promotion and health maintenance teaching and nursing interventions would be based on specific genes. The nurse could provide important, life-saving nutritional information to people based on their specific risks, and each individual then might be more inclined to maintain a proper diet, give up their sedentary lifestyle, increase exercise and decrease fast-food intake. Personal lifestyle choices would become more personal and monitoring health might take on a new meaning.

With knowledge of genetic conditions, the nurse can ensure health teaching and early detection of complications from genetic conditions with emphasis on primary and secondary care interventions. For example:

- A woman with a strong family history and/or mutations in the BRCA1 and BRCA2 tumour suppressor genes should begin monthly self breast exams and have screening clinical breast exams and mammographies at an earlier age than the general population.
- A man with a strong family history and/or mutations in the BRCA1 and BRCA2 tumour suppressor genes should report any mass, tenderness or swelling in the breast tissue and maintain early screening for prostate cancer.
- Aggressive colonoscopy screening every 1 to 2 years beginning at age 25 is important for the individual with a positive family history and/or mutations in the MLH1/MSH2 gene, which increases the risk of hereditary nonpolyposis colorectal cancer.

People receiving early intervention and health-promotion-focused care can live longer and with a much better quality of life than those who do not. The nurse must be able to identify both community-based and genetic-based resources that are available to assist the person with strategies to support both health promotion and health maintenance activities.

By simply integrating into practice the genetic aspects of assessment, observation and history gathering, the nurse can improve the standard of care delivered and have a very positive impact on the person. The nurse does not need to be a genetic expert, but with heightened awareness, appropriate inquiries and referrals to genetic specialists can be completed.

Health history

Nurses can improve the standard of nursing care and have a positive impact on people by integrating genetic concepts into their existing practice of inspection, observation and history gathering. Nurses should be able to recognise genetic features of physical assessment, basic patterns of inheritance and predisposition to development of disease. As health professionals integrate genetic concepts into their delivery of care, appropriate inquiries and referrals to genetic specialists can be completed.

Although family history has long been a part of nursing assessments, the relative importance of this assessment piece has recently increased as our knowledge of the interaction of genes and the environment has expanded. In phenotypically 'healthy' individuals, an accurate and complete family history can identify a single-gene (Mendelian) disorder or a mitochondrial, multifactorial or chromosomal inheritance pattern as well as guide the prevention, diagnosis and treatment of common complex diseases such as cardiovascular disease and cancer. A family history illustrates the interaction of genes and the environment for an individual and consequently provides a basis for individualised disease prevention. Although an individual's inheritance risks from their own genotype are non-modifiable, knowledge of an individual's increased risk of chronic disease can influence lifestyle choices, clinical management, and sometimes risk reduction and prevention of the disease. Knowledge of a family history can also guide diagnostic workups and clinical treatment (Ikle & Gloyn, 2021).

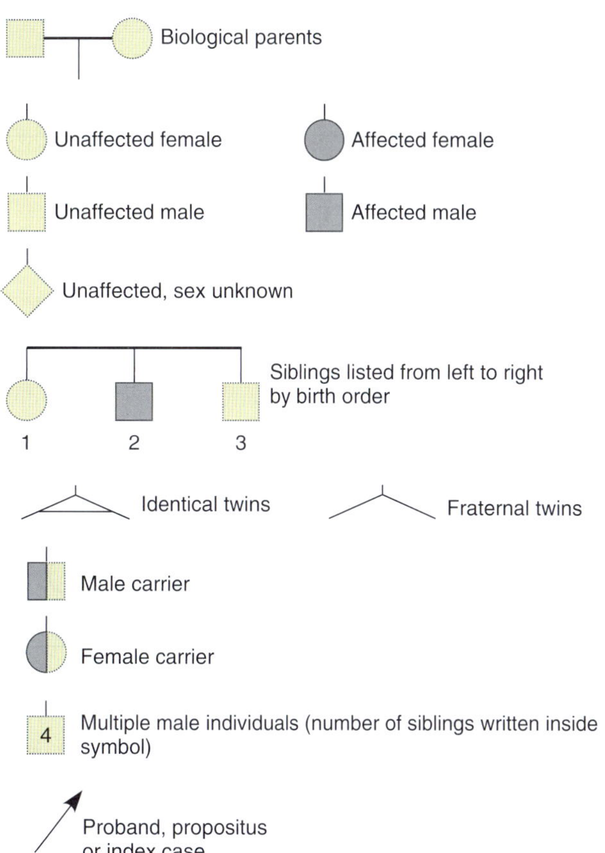

FIGURE 7.6 ***Selected standardised symbols for use in drawing a pedigree***

Pedigrees

A nurse should know how to take a family history, record the history in a pedigree and think 'genetically'. A pedigree is a pictorial representation or diagram of the medical history of a family. Multiple symbols are utilised to present this picture (see Figure 7.6), and the finished pedigree presents a family's medical data and biological relationship information at a glance (see Figure 7.7). A pedigree provides the nurse, genetic counsellor or geneticist with a clear, visual representation of relationships of affected individuals to the immediate and extended family. It can identify other individuals in the family who might benefit from a genetic consultation. It can also identify a single-gene alteration pattern of inheritance or a cluster of multifactorial conditions, and a referral and/or reproductive risk teaching for the individual and family can result. A family's learning can be enhanced by the visual teaching contribution a pedigree can provide and which may also clarify any inheritance misunderstandings or misconceptions. Box 7.8 lists steps for creating a family pedigree. If correctly and fully completed, a pedigree allows all healthcare professionals working with the individual or family to quickly see what history and background information has been collected (see Box 7.9).

It is important to gather a three-generation family pedigree even if the nurse believes this is a first occasion of the condition within a family (see Figure 7.7). A condition without any identifiable inheritance pattern on the pedigree may be due to a new mutation or variable expressivity. Throughout the process of gathering family history assessment data, the nurse must remember family confidentiality at all times: all information related to a pedigree is confidential information. The history may reveal sensitive details that include infertility problems, elective termination of pregnancies or non-paternity. This information may not even be known by a current partner or immediate and extended family members. Other sensitive issues include pregnancies conceived by technology, a history of suicides, drug or alcohol abuse, and same-sex relationships. Box 7.10 lists ethical implications of genetic information.

Challenges inherent in recalling the family history include the person's inability to remember any conditions that may have been surgically repaired and then forgotten, or reporting conditions that may have been attributed incorrectly to other causes. Also, the family history may contain information previously unknown to extended family members. Reproductive decisions may have been made that were against the family's religious or cultural beliefs. Both

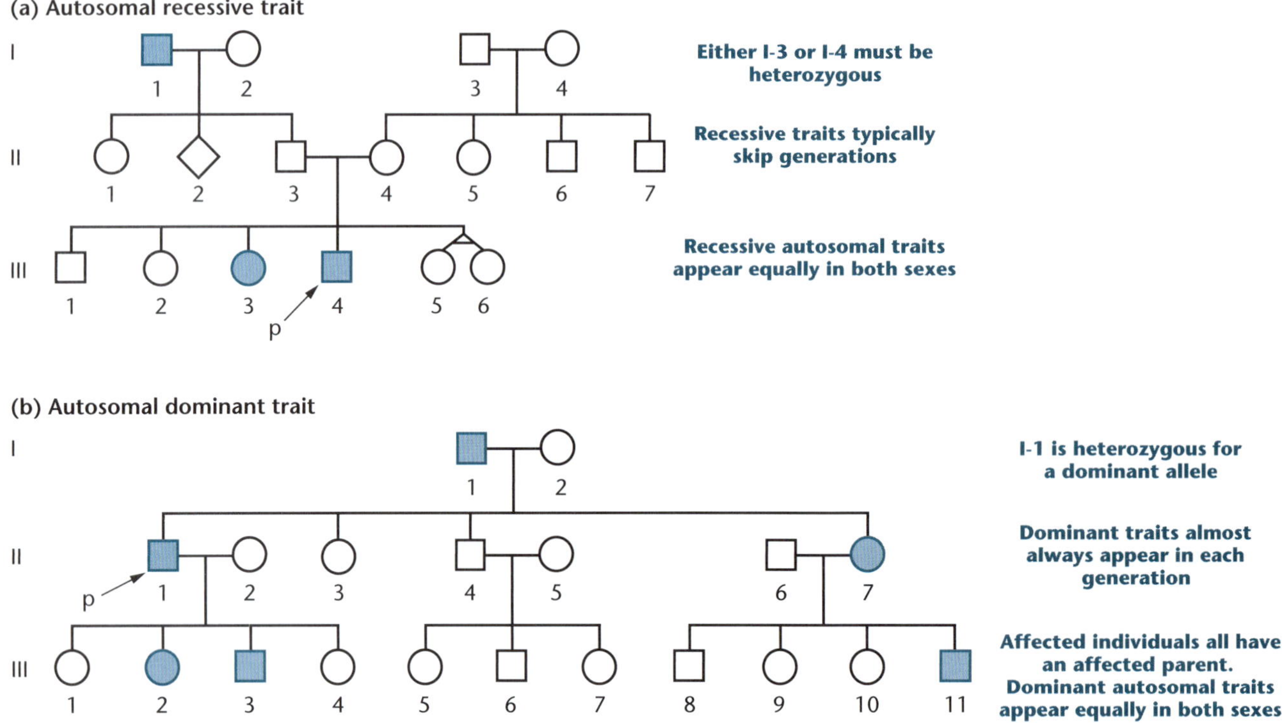

FIGURE 7.7 *Sample three-generation pedigree. A, A representative pedigree for a single character or genetic condition through three generations. B, The most probable genotypes of each individual in the pedigree for an autosomal recessive condition, represented by AA, Aa or aa*

Source: Klug et al. (2019). *Concepts of genetics* (12th ed.), p. 60, Figure 3.13. © 2019. Reprinted by permission of Pearson Education, Inc., Upper Saddle River, New Jersey.

immediate and extended family members may be unaware of these 'family skeletons' and the person may be very reluctant to reveal this information (Beery, Workman & Eggert, 2018; Bennett, 2010).

Genetic physical assessment

An assessment of newborns and children with a genetics focus on minor and major anomalies is essential. A minor anomaly or malformation is an unusual or morphological feature that in itself is of no serious medical or cosmetic concern to the individual or family. A major anomaly is a serious structural defect at birth that may interfere with normal functioning of body systems and may lead to a lifelong disability or even an early death (Healthdirect, 2022; Watson & Ban, 2021).

Some children grow into adults whose physical features may or may not have been recognised as potential links to genetic conditions. Anomalies that exist after a person is beyond expected developmental and cognitive milestones may go unnoticed, but they may still be important. The nurse can pick up cues to genetic problems by inspecting the person and other family members. If practical, nurses should ask to look at family photographs and examine them for common dysmorphic features and family traits. Subjective assessment data can also be valuable. A person's complaints of fatigue and joint pain may indicate the onset of hereditary haemochromatosis. A physical assessment that includes a genetics focus is important for nurses when caring for people of any age. An undiagnosed genetic condition may also have implications for reproductive decisions the person makes. However, genetic assessments and genetic referrals are important throughout the lifespan.

Nursing diagnosis and interventions

Nurses are responsible for comprehensively delivering the correct standard of care to people, but at the same time being aware of the limitations of their own knowledge and expertise. In addition to the continuous integration of genetic aspects into nurses' assessments of family history and physical assessment, nurses and midwives are also responsible for carrying out interventions that include initiating referrals to genetic specialists and delivering care to the individual or family in any of the following ways. Nursing diagnoses to consider include:

- *Anticipatory grieving*
- *Anxiety*
- *Disturbed body image*
- *Ineffective coping*
- *Decisional conflict*
- *Interrupted family processes*
- *Ineffective health maintenance*
- *Deficient knowledge*
- *Powerlessness*
- *Spiritual distress.*

BOX 7.8 Steps in drawing a pedigree

I. How to:
1. Work in pencil.
   a. Family historians often remember additional relatives and details only after questioning is almost completed.

II. Organisation:
1. Begin recording data in the middle of the sheet of paper.
   a. Allow enough room for both the maternal and paternal sides of the family.
2. Use only standard pedigree symbols.
   a. For example, males are represented by squares and females by a circle.
3. The male individual in a couple is placed on the left of the relationship line and the paternal side of the family also goes on the left-hand side of the paper.

III. Determining family relationships:
1. The clinician should determine the relationships within the family by asking questions such as:
   - Do you have a partner or are you married?
   - How many biological brothers and sisters do you have?
   - How many children do you have?
   - Do all the children have the same biological father?
   - Do all the children share the same mother and father?
2. Referral to 'the baby's father or mother' can be helpful until a relationship or marriage is established between the parents.
3. Referral to a 'union' if marriage does not exist can also help communication.
4. Determine if each individual is married, has children, signs and symptoms, etc., before continuing on to the next individual.
5. Always ask if there is any chance the mother could be related to the father or if any other parents in the family are blood relatives.
   - To determine consanguinity.

IV. Who should or should not be included:
1. To ensure accuracy, the pedigree should include the parents, offspring, siblings, aunts, uncles, grandparents and first cousins of the individual seeking counselling.
2. Detailed information about the spouses of the proband's family can be omitted unless there is a history of some kind of disorder or condition. The proband is the first clinically affected family member diagnosed with a genetic disorder. For example, a baby born with Down syndrome may be the proband.
3. Eliminating people or any information that do not contribute any valuable information can help keep the pedigree small and more manageable.

V. Recording the family history:
1. Determine the approximate size of the family.
2. Record the family's ethnic background at the top of the page.
3. The initial drawing should begin with the proband, or the person who is affected with the genetic condition.
   a. This is usually the reason someone is seeking a genetic referral.
4. The proband is marked with an arrow on the pedigree.
5. Draw and mark the symbols for the brothers and sisters of the proband. Draw the relationship line, the line of descent, marriage or union line, and symbols for the parents of the proband.
   a. Repeat this step for any children of the proband or children of the proband's brothers and sisters.
6. Children resulting from a mating (siblings) should be recorded in descending order of their birth, with the oldest sibling on the left.
7. Continue with symbols for all immediate relatives drawn previously and then draw and mark symbols for paternal grandparents and indicated relatives followed by the same for the maternal grandparents and relatives.
8. A legend key should contain all of the correct symbols for each indicated disease.
9. Record the age of onset of common and complex diseases and/or conditions such as coronary heart disease; diabetes mellitus; hypertension; colon, breast, ovarian or endometrial cancer; and stroke.
10. The pedigree should include at least three generations.
    a. Generations are symbolised by Roman numerals along the left-hand side of the paper with the first generation marker, I, at the top.
    b. Each person in the generation should follow an imaginary horizontal line from left to right.
11. The names of each individual (maiden names in case of married women) and their dates of birth should be included along with half-siblings, pregnancy losses, stillbirths, previous marriages and adopted children.

VI. Other:
1. Consanguinity may be suspected if the historian repeatedly gives the same last name on both sides of the family.
   a. Consanguinity can be confirmed by asking if any relatives in the family have ever had a child together.

VII. Completing the pedigree:
1. When completed, the pedigree should be dated and signed with the name, credentials and position of the person drawing it.

Source: Data from Bennett (2010). *The practical guide to the genetic family history* (2nd ed.). New York: Wiley-Liss.

BOX 7.9 Specific facts and health information to include in a pedigree

- Age/birth date or year of birth
- Age of death (year, if known)
- Cause of death
- Age at diagnosis
- Full siblings versus half- or step-siblings
- Pregnancy with gestational age (last menstrual period (LMP)) or estimated date of delivery (EDD)
- Infertility versus no children by choice
- Pregnancy complications with gestational ages noted (e.g. 6 wks, 32 wks)
- Miscarriage (spontaneous abortion (SAB))
- Stillbirth (SB)
- Pregnancy termination (TOP)
- Relevant health information (e.g. height and weight)
- Affected/unaffected status—define shading of symbols in a legend key
- Ethnic background
- Consanguinity
- Date pedigree taken or updated
- Name of person who took pedigree and credentials
- Key or legend

BOX 7.10 Ethical implications of genetic information

Clinicians must consider the enormity of the ethical issues facing all families who have knowledge of their genetic make-up. The ethical issues a nurse may have to discuss with the person are numerous. A few of the issues are listed below.

Access to information

- Who should have access to personal genetic information and how will it be used?
- Do insurers, employers, courts, police force, schools, universities, adoption agencies and the armed forces have a right to access this information?

Self-perception

- How does personal genetic information affect an individual's perception of self?
- How does personal genetic information affect society's perceptions of that individual?
- How does personal genetic information affect an individual's cultural identity?
- How is self-identity and self-worth affected by a confirmed genetic risk or condition?

Family roles and relationships

- Should an individual be tested for an autosomal dominant condition if the siblings and/or parents are opposed to knowing if they, themselves, have the altered gene?
- Should potential mates have genetic information?
- Should two people with increased genetic risk be prohibited from having children?
- Should a child be tested?
- Should the father be told if genetic testing and/or genetic counselling reveals non-paternity?
- Should adoption records contain a complete genetic history of the biological parents?
- Is there an obligation to tell other family members if an altered gene that demands a change in lifestyle (nutrition, exercise, smoking, etc.) is diagnosed?
- Is there an obligation to tell other family members if an altered gene that causes early debilitation and/or death is diagnosed?

Informed consent

- Are all individuals receiving true informed consent and do they understand all of the consequences of agreeing to even a simple blood test in the doctor's office that may reveal a diagnosis or increased risk of a genetic condition?

Health and life insurance

- Should insurance companies have access to genetic test results?
- Should medical insurance costs be higher for people with a known gene disease-producing alteration?
- Should medical insurance costs be higher for people with a known increased risk of disease because of any gene alteration?
- Should medical insurance costs be higher for people with known increased risk of disease because of any gene alteration if they make unhealthy lifestyle choices and do nothing to lower their risk?
- Should the individual be covered by medical insurance at all?
- Should individuals pay higher costs if they have children?
- Should individuals be required to have a large life insurance policy to financially protect their families?

Financial

- Should the child be eligible for government grants or any scholarship money?
- Should society be expected to financially support children through government programs or private insurance?
- What is the motivation to save money for the future?

Employment

- Should an employer have access to an individual's genetic profile?
- Should a young adult be hired even though they will burden the company with multiple sick days, higher insurance financial support, etc.?
- Should the individual receive promotional opportunities and increased job responsibilities if the employer knows there will be a large number of lost work days?
- Will the individual's productivity be affected by the genetic condition?

Genetic referrals and counselling

After gathering assessment data that incorporates genetic concepts, the nurse and/or midwife is able to initiate a referral to genetic specialists if there are indicators for a genetic referral (see Box 7.11). The nurse and/or midwife should provide the person with information about the advantages of a referral to genetic specialists and the disadvantages of not following through with the referral. The nurse should inform the person that a genetic referral can provide information and answer many questions they may have concerning genetic health. Questions regarding the conditions, inheritance, availability of treatment, as well as economic, insurance and future implications, can be addressed.

People who are concerned about genetic disease may benefit from a genetic consultation whether or not genetic testing is available for that condition. Many people seek information and coping strategies as much as they do test results. Referral of a person with a suspected genetic problem to a geneticist or genetic clinic is an expected nursing responsibility in the same way as are referrals to a dietitian or a social worker. When in doubt, the nurse should contact a genetic counsellor or geneticist to discuss concerns.

PREPARATION FOR GENETIC REFERRALS AND GENETIC COUNSELLING Not knowing what to expect from a genetic referral is common, and fear of the unknown may cause anxiety for the person. To facilitate the referral to a genetic specialist, the clinical nurse should educate the person so that they know what to expect during as well as after a genetic evaluation.

Usually, before the first genetic evaluation visit the person will be contacted to provide a detailed medical and family history and to make an appointment for genetic consultation. The person should be prepared to give as exact a family history as possible so that a detailed three-generation pedigree can be constructed. The person should be informed that a genetic consultation usually lasts several hours. During the appointment, a genetic clinical nurse, genetic counsellor and/or physician will perform an initial interview, and a geneticist will examine the person in order to establish an accurate diagnosis. Tests may be ordered. These may include chromosome (cytogenetic) analysis, DNA-based testing, x-rays, biopsy, biochemical tests and linkage studies (Lashley et al., 2015). After the exam and the completion of any applicable testing, the geneticist and/or genetic counsellor will discuss the findings with the person and make recommendations. The discussion will include the natural history of the condition, the inheritance patterns, the current preventive or treatment options, and the risks to the person and/or family. The visit will also include opportunities for questions and answers, as well as the assessment and evaluation of the person's understanding. It is typical for the information retention of a person facing a new genetic diagnosis to be very low. This makes it imperative for the clinician to take advantage of opportunities to reinforce genetic concepts at a later time when the person is ready.

As the visit concludes, the person can expect appropriate referrals to be made, discussion of available services or research studies, and possible scheduling of a follow-up visit. A summary of the information is usually sent to the person, and their healthcare provider will receive a report if requested by the person.

BOX 7.11 Adult indicators for a referral to a genetic specialist

Adult history assessment data

- Several closely related individuals affected with the same or related conditions:
  - Breast and ovarian cancer
  - Colon and endometrial cancer
  - Diabetes
  - Hypertension
  - Coronary heart disease
  - Thyroid cancer
  - Colon polyps
- A common disorder with earlier age of onset than typical (increase concern if it occurs in more than one family member):
  - Breast cancer: < 45–50 years of age or premenopausal
  - Colon cancer: < 45–50 years of age
  - Prostate cancer: < 45–60 years of age
  - Vision loss: < 55 years of age
  - Hearing loss: < 50–60 years of age
  - Dementia: < 60 years of age
  - Heart disease: < 40–60 years of age
  - Stroke: < 60 years of age
- A sudden or unexpected death in someone who 'seemed' healthy:
  - Renal disease
  - Asthma
  - Suicides

An individual with:

- Two or more conditions
- A medical condition and dysmorphic features
- Developmental delay with dysmorphic features and/or physical birth anomalies
- Learning disabilities
- Behavioural problems
- Unexplained:
  - Movement disorders
  - Seizures
  - Hypotonia
  - Ataxia
  - Infertility
- Disproportionate tall or short stature
- Proportionate short stature with dysmorphic features
- Atypical sexual development
- Premature ovarian failure

Source: American Medical Association (2004). *Family medical history in disease prevention.* Retrieved from https://www.ama-assn.org/resources/doc/genetics/family_history02.pdf. Used with permission of the American Medical Association.

Genetic healthcare providers present the person with information to promote informed decisions. They are also sensitive to the importance of protecting the individual's autonomy. A challenge during any visit to a genetic specialist is providing non-directive counselling. People should be permitted to make decisions that are not influenced by any biases or values from the nurse, counsellor or geneticist. Many people are accustomed to practitioners and nurses providing direction and guidance in their decision making so they may be very uncomfortable with the non-directional approach of the nurse. They may believe that the nurse or healthcare provider is withholding very bad news. The nurse should discuss the positives and negatives of each decision and present as many options as possible through the use of therapeutic listening and communication skills (Beery et al., 2018).

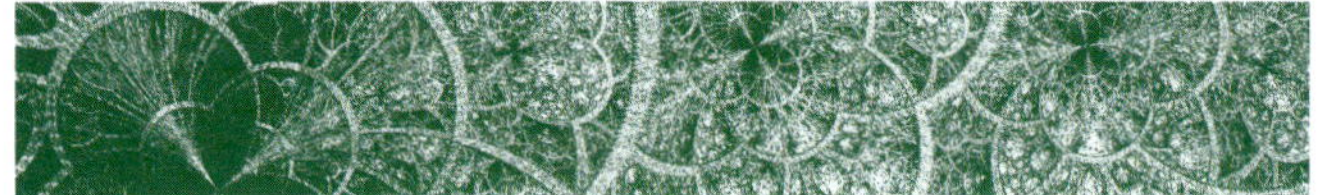

EDUCATION

The nurse and/or midwife must be aware of available genetic resources and participate in educating the person on genetic disorders as well as health promotion and prevention. Informing people of what to expect from a genetic referral, as well as clarifying and/or reinforcing information obtained during a genetic referral or from genetic test results, is also important.

Prior to teaching, the clinician assesses the person's cultural and religious beliefs. Are the gene alterations viewed as uncontrollable and believed to be occurring secondary to cultural belief, such as a stranger looking at the person? Or, are the gene alterations considered a 'punishment'? A person's readiness to learn can be influenced by cultural or religious beliefs and values. Obtaining educational materials in the person's native language will also help facilitate the teaching–learning experience.

The clinician must be aware of common inheritance misconceptions such as a person's belief that, with a 25% recurrence risk, after one child is affected, the next three children will be unaffected, or with a 50% recurrence risk, every other child will be affected. The recurrence risk *for each pregnancy* should be continually stressed by the nurse. People often believe that a family member has inherited the genetic condition because they look like or 'take after' a relative with a genetic condition. When new gene alterations or mutations are discussed, people will often exhibit surprise because no one else in the family has the condition, so they perceive that the trait or condition cannot possibly be inherited (Bennett, 2010). Helping people to understand these genetic concepts is fundamental to delivering the required standard of genetic nursing care.

Psychosocial care

To meet the person's psychosocial needs, the nurse should identify the person's expectations and needs, as well as their cultural and spiritual values and belief system. From where does the person receive strength? Denial of the genetic diagnosis is common and nurses must be aware of the person's state of acceptance. Individuals often will not believe that a chronic genetic condition exists. Nurses must also provide care to help alleviate any anxiety and/or guilt in the person. Anxiety about the unknown is common when awaiting diagnosis or test results, but individuals also experience anxiety from not understanding the future implications of a confirmed genetic disease. Guilt may be associated with knowledge of the existence of a genetic condition in a family. The nurse must support people as they contemplate telling extended family members, friends and neighbours about a confirmed diagnosis. People often do not want to tell extended family members until they are ready. The nurse should encourage open discussion and the expression of fears and concerns. Feelings of guilt and shame are very common as a person deals with the loss of the expectation and dream of a healthy, productive life. Reinforce that genetic alterations are caused by changes within a gene and not by superstitions related to sin or other cultural beliefs. However, it is important to remember that everyone has superstitions or beliefs and the nurse must remain non-judgmental. As mothers, fathers, siblings and extended family members provide continuous care for the person with a genetic condition, depression can result. Depression also can occur in the individual with the chronic condition. The clinician must maintain awareness of the possibility of depression and be proactive in obtaining support for the individual or family.

The nurse also is responsible for assessing the person's coping mechanisms as well as available family, spiritual, cultural and community support systems. Genetic conditions can cause a permanent strain on family dynamics and relationships. The counsellor may need to help the person reaffirm their own self-worth and value (Lashley et al., 2015). If seen in an academic setting, people may feel they are part of a 'production line' even though they are present for a very private problem (Beery et al., 2018). It is important to be sensitive to these perceptions, provide open communication and encourage discussion of feelings. Growth and development, and meeting adult developmental milestones, can be altered by actual or potential genetic disorders. Especially unique is the potential or actual inheritance of a late-onset condition such as Huntington's disease. The person with this altered gene may not meet any of the developmental tasks in moving through adulthood. Should the person get married, attend university, save money or worry about the future? The nurse must identify the impact of genetic knowledge on activities of daily living but also on movement through developmental milestones. Both individual and family strengths need to be identified.

Working in collaboration with the other members of the healthcare team, nurses can refer the person to a support group. However, it is important to have the person's permission if the nurse is providing their name and contact information to a support group.

Another key role for the team is to help people with the often difficult task of communicating genetic information such as inheritance patterns to extended family members. Cultural values of autonomy and privacy are affected when a person must consider whether to communicate genetic information to extended family members who may also carry the altered gene. The history of a genetic alteration that may or may not cause disease can be extensive within a family, affecting multiple family members. Family members often have difficulty understanding that some genetic conditions have variable expressivity. Members of the extended family often are shocked and feel a profound sense of guilt that they are the one who has carried the gene alteration that caused their loved one to have a genetic condition.

Careful self-assessment of feelings is essential for every member of the team. Nurses play an important role in advocating for people and support their decisions even if the decisions contradict their own ideals and morals. Coping with genetic revelations and making genetic-related treatment decisions are difficult activities for everyone. Team members must remember that people will need resources and support and also help in gathering information about reproductive options.

Evaluation

Expected outcomes of delivering healthcare with a genetic focus include:

- The person will make informed and voluntary decisions related to genetic health issues.
- The person will accurately identify:
  - basic genetic concepts and simple inheritance risk probabilities
  - what to expect from a genetic referral
  - the influence of genetic factors in health promotion and health maintenance
  - differences between medical and genetic tests
  - social, legal and ethical issues related to genetic testing.

VISIONS FOR THE FUTURE

Nurses are often the primary caregivers to whom people turn for information, guidance and clarification of ideas. Their role is essential not only in providing direct nursing care but as a member of the community. As more information about the genetic revolution becomes available to consumers—in areas such as pharmacogenomics, gene transfer, ethics, genetic engineering and stem cell research—the role of nurses not only remains vital but will also grow enormously. Clinicians should remain educated, informed, knowledgeable and ready to discuss trends and changes with individuals and their families.

PATIENT SAFETY COMPETENCY FRAMEWORK

5 Clinical reasoning

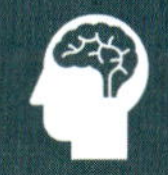

The Patient Safety Competency Framework indicates that nursing students must demonstrate clinical reasoning through the ability to accurately assess, interpret and respond to individual patient data in a systematic and timely way (Levett-Jones et al., 2017).

CHAPTER HIGHLIGHTS

- Nurses and midwives are responsible for basic genetic knowledge and for delivering the expected standard of genetic nursing care.
- When cell division does not occur as expected, chromosomal alterations on the autosomes or sex chromosomes can result.
- Chromosomal alterations can be seen in a human karyotype.
- Protein-directing genes are very important to life and functioning as a human being because proteins are very specialised and perform a variety of functions within the cell.
- Different forms of genes are alleles.
- A person may be identified as heterozygous or homozygous for a single gene.
- Some gene alterations cause disease and some are protective from disease.
- Mitochondrial gene alterations are inherited from the mother and primarily involve high-energy organs such as skeletal muscles, brain and heart muscle.
- Multifactorial inheritance does not follow Mendelian inheritance patterns.
- Genetic healthcare providers present the person and their family with information to promote informed decisions.
- Many types of genetic tests are available and they differ from routine medical tests.
- All genetic tests have special considerations related to social, financial, ethical and legal implications.
- Basic genetic nursing care involves family risk assessment through a detailed family history, drawing a three-generation pedigree and integrating genetic concepts into a physical assessment.
- Care should be taken in initiating a referral to a genetic specialist.
- Knowledge of the principles of inheritance allows the clinician not only to offer and reinforce genetic information to individuals and their families, but also to assist them in managing their care and in making reproductive decisions.
- Genetic concepts can be applied to health promotion and health maintenance.
- The nurse must be aware of the social, ethical, cultural and spiritual issues related to the delivery of healthcare.

CONCEPT CHECK

1 A person you are caring for is discussing the inheritance of an autosomal dominant trait. He has the condition and his wife does not. They have one child without the condition. The nurse would be correct in explaining to the person that he is most likely which genotype?

1 FF
2 Ff
3 ff
4 X_fY

2 A male diagnosed with Fabry disease is admitted to the unit. Which statement made by the person would indicate to the nurse that he understands Mendelian inheritance concepts? 'I have the disease because ...' (Select all that apply.)

1 'my mother had Fabry disease and my father did not'
2 'my father's mother had Fabry disease'
3 'my grandmother's brother had Fabry disease'
4 'my father has Fabry disease'

3 The nurse is providing information regarding genetic testing to a couple who believe they are carriers of an autosomal recessive gene alteration. Which statement is appropriate?

1 'If both of you are carriers, all of your sons will be affected and all of your daughters will be carriers.'
2 'Chromosomal studies will reveal if you are actually a carrier.'
3 'Newborn screening will reveal if your child is affected.'
4 'During the genetic evaluation, you will be asked to provide at least a three-generation family history.'

4 The nurse knows that which assessment data obtained during a family history may suggest a genetic condition or inherited susceptibility to a common disease? (Select all that apply.)

1 breast cancer at age 33
2 a sibling who died unexpectedly while playing basketball at age 66
3 colon polyps in four third-degree relatives
4 a brother's unexplained infertility

5 When analysing a family pedigree, the nurse/midwife notes the pedigree demonstrates that successive generations contain affected individuals, both males and females are affected, and there is no father-to-offspring inheritance. What is the most likely pattern of inheritance?

1 autosomal dominant
2 autosomal recessive
3 X-linked recessive
4 multifactorial
5 mitochondrial

6 When developing a teaching plan, which statement/s is/are a correct rationale regarding the health promotion and health maintenance benefits from an assessment of family history? (Select all that apply.)

1 Clinical treatment options can be more focused.
2 Prophylactic treatments can be started early.
3 Specific diet, exercise regimen and genotype can be determined.
4 Single-gene alteration can be diagnosed.

7 The nurse is recording a family pedigree. Which would be correct to include in drawing the pedigree?

1 Detailed information is important for all people recorded on the pedigree.
2 The maternal side of the family should be placed on the left of the page.
3 The proband is marked with an arrow and a 'P'.
4 Two generations should be recorded and labelled with Roman numerals.

8 The clinician would consider which assessment finding(s) as minor anomalies? (Select all that apply.)

1 café au lait spots
2 ear pits
3 atrial septal defect (ASD)
4 hypertelorism

9 Which are appropriate concepts for the clinician to include when developing a teaching plan for the individual prior to genetic testing? (Select all that apply.)

1 Predispositional genetic tests are medically indicated when the seriousness and mortality of the disease can be reduced with knowledge of the gene alteration.
2 To meet quality assurance, laboratories should hold a CLIA88 certification.
3 A mutation panel contains the most common gene alterations, but may not include all of the disease-causing mutations.
4 Family members affected by genetic test results have a legal right to the test results.

10 The person asks the nurse if a genetic referral is necessary. Which information would be appropriate for the nurse to provide? Most likely genetic specialists will: (Select all that apply.)

1 provide direction for important decision making
2 complete chromosomal studies
3 ask to see photographs of relatives
4 provide information about the natural history of the condition

BIBLIOGRAPHY

American College of Obstetricians and Gynecologists (ACOG) (2020). *Committee on Genetics—Opinion: Family history as a risk assessment tool.* Retrieved from https://www.acog.org

American Medical Association (2004). *Family medical history in disease prevention.* Retrieved from https://www.ama-assn.org/

American Nurses Association and International Society of Nurses in Genetics, Inc. (ANA/ISONG) (2016). *Genetics/Genomics nursing: Scope and standards of practice* (2nd ed.). Washington, DC: American Nurses Publishing.

American Society of Human Genetics (ASHG) (2019). *Genetic testing, privacy and healthcare.* Retrieved from https://www.ashg.org/

Australian Breast Cancer Network (2018). *Position statement: Family history and hereditary breast cancer.* Retrieved from https://www.bcna.org.au/

Beery, T. A., Workman, M. L. & Eggert, J. A. (2018). *Genetics and genomics in nursing and healthcare* (2nd ed.). Philadelphia: FA Davis Company.

Bennett, R. L. (2010). *The practical guide to the genetic family history* (2nd ed.). New York: Wiley-Liss.

Bilkey, G. A., Burns, B. I., Coles, E. P. et al. (2019). Genomic testing for human health and disease across the life cycle: Applications and ethical, legal, and social challenges. *Frontiers in Public Health*, 7. https://doi.org/10.3389/fpubh.2019.00040. Retrieved from https://www.frontiersin.org

Bunnik, E. M., Janssens, A. C. W. & Schemer, M. H. N. (2014). Informed consent in direct-to-consumer personal genome testing: The outline of a model between specific and genetic consent. *Bioethics, 28*(7), 343–381.

Centers for Disease Control and Prevention (CDC) (2020). *Genomics & precision health: Genetic testing.* Retrieved https://www.cdc.gov

Centers for Disease Control and Prevention (CDC) (2022). *Clinical Laboratory Improvement Amendments (CLIA).* Retrieved from https://www.cdc.gov

Chen, Z., Wang, Z. H., Zhang, G. et al (2020). Mitochondrial DNA segregation and replication restrict the transmission of detrimental mutation. *Journal Cell Biology, 219*(7). https://doi.org/10.1083/jcb.201905160

Craven, L., Tang, M.-X., Gorman, G. S. et al. (2017). Novel reproductive technologies to prevent mitochondrial disease. *Human Reproduction Update, 23*(5), 501–519.

Cuyvers, E. & Sleegers, K. (2016). Genetic variations underlying Alzheimer's disease: Evidence from genome-wide association studies and beyond. *The Lancet Neurology, 15*(8), 857–868.

Daly, M. B., Pal, T., Berry, M. P. et al. (2021). NCCN clinical practice guidelines in oncology: Genetic/familial high-risk assessment: breast, ovarian, and pancreatic (Version 2.2021). *Journal of the National Comprehensive Cancer Network, 19*(1), 77–102. doi: 10.6004/jnccn.2021.0001

Dementia Australia (2022a). *Causes of dementia*. Retrieved from https://www.dementia.org.au/

Dementia Australia (2022b). *Genetics of dementia*. Retrieved from https://www.dementia.org.au/

Ferraguti, G., Pierandrei, S., Bruno, S. M., Ceci, F., Strom, R. & Lucarelli, M. (2011). A template for mutational data analysis of the CFTR gene. *Clinical Chemistry and Laboratory Medicine, 49*(9), 1447.

Grace, P. & Milliken, A. (eds) (2022). *Clinical ethics handbook for nurses: Emphasizing context, communication and collaboration.* New York: Springer.

Grant, S. F. A., Wells, A. D. & Rich, S. S. (2020). Next steps in the identification of gene targets for type 1 diabetes. *Diabetologia, 63*, 2260–2269. https://doi.org/10.1007/s00125-020-05248-8

Healthdirect (2022). *Body dysmorphic disorder*. Retrieved from https://www.healthdirect.gov.au/

Human Genome Project (HGP) (2008). *From genome to the proteome*. Retrieved from https://www.ornl.gov/

Ikle, J. M. & Gloyn, A. L. (2021). A brief history of diabetes genetics: Insights for pancreatic beta-cell development and function. *Journal of Endocrinology, 250*(3), R23–R35. Retrieved from https://joe.bioscientifica.com/

International Society of Nurses in Genetics (ISONG) (2018). *Position statement: Informed decision-making and consent related to genetic testing (clinical and research): The role of the nurse*. Retrieved from https://www.isong.org/

Johnson, S. B., Slade, I., Giubilini, A. & Graham, M. (2020). Rethinking the ethical principles of genomic medicine services. *European Journal of Human Genetics, 28*, 147–154. https://doi.org/10.1038/s41431-019-0507-1

Kirk, M., Tonkin, E. & Skirton, H. (2014). An iterative consensus-building approach to revising a genetics/genomics competency framework for nurse education in the UK. *Journal of Advanced Nursing, 70*(2), 405–420.

Klug, W. S., Cummings, M. R., Spencer, C. A., Palladino, M. A. & Killian, D. (2019). *Concepts of genetics* (12th ed.). Upper Saddle River: Pearson Education Limited.

Lashley, F. R., Schneidereith, T. A. & Kasper, E. C. (2015). *Lashley's essential clinical genetics in nursing practice* (2nd ed.). New York: Springer.

Leukaemia Foundation (2020). *Chronic myeloid leukaemia (CML)*. Retrieved from https://www.leukaemia.org.au/

Levett-Jones, T., Dwyer, T., Reid-Searl, K., Heaton, L., Flenady, T., Applegarth, J., Guinea, S. & Andersen, P. (2017). *Patient Safety Competency Framework (PSCF) for Nursing Students*. Sydney. Retrieved from http://psframework.wpengine.com/

Loscalzo, J., Fauci, A. S., Kasper, D. L., Hauser, S. L. & Longo, D. (2022). *Harrison's principles of internal medicine* (21st ed.). New York: McGraw Hill Medical.

McKusick/Nathans Institute for Genetic Medicine (eds) (2022). *Online Mendelian Inheritance in Man*. Retrieved from https://omim.org

National Cancer Institute (2022a). *Chronic myelogenous leukemia*. Retrieved from https://www.cancer.gov/

National Cancer Institute (2022b). *Cancer genetics risk assessment and counselling: Health professional version*. Retrieved from https://www.cancer.gov/

National Health and Medical Research Council (NHMRC) (2011). *DNA genetic testing in the Australian context*. Retrieved from https://www.nhmrc.gov.au/

National Human Genome Research Institute (2017). *Universal genomics instructor handbook and toolkit*. Retrieved from https://www.genome.gov/

Newson, A. J., Tiller, J., Keogh, L. A., Otlowski, M. & Lacaze, P. (2017). Genetics and insurance in Australia: Concerns around self-regulated industry. *Public Health Genomics, 20*(4), 247–256.

Nowell, P. C. & Hungerford, D. A. (1960). A minute chromosome in human chronic granulocytic leukemia. *Science, 142*, 1497.

Nursing and Midwifery Board of Australia (NMBA) (2016). *Registered Nurse Standards for Practice*. Retrieved from https://www.nursingmidwiferyboard.gov.au/

Nussbaum, R. L., McInnes, R. R., Willard, H. F. & Boerkoel, C. F. (2015). *Thompson & Thompson genetics in medicine* (8th ed.). Sydney: Elsevier Australia.

Rafnar, T., Sulem, P., Stacey, S. N. et al. (2009). Sequence variants at the TERT-CLPTM1L locus associate with many cancer types. *Nature Genetics*, February, *41*(2), 221–227.

Rao, A. T., Degnan, A. J. & Levy, L. M. (2014). Genetics of Alzheimer disease. *American Journal of Neuroradiology, 35*(3), 418–423.

Secretary's Advisory Committee on Genetic Testing (SACGT), National Institutes of Health (2000). *Enhancing the oversight of genetic tests: Recommendations of the SACGT*. Retrieved from https://www.od.nih.gov/

Singh Bhatti, J., Kaur Bhatti, G. & Reddy, P. H. (2017). Mitochondrial dysfunction and oxidative stress in metabolic disorders: A step towards mitochondria based therapeutic strategies. *Biochimica et Biophysica Acta—Molecular Basis of Disease, 1863*(2017), 1066–1077. http://dx.doi.org/10.1016/j.bbadis.2016.11.010 0925-4439

Tiller, J., Otlowski, M. & Lacaze, J. (2017). Should Australia ban the use of genetic test results in life insurance? *Frontiers in Public Health, 5*. Retrieved from https://www.ncbi.nlm.nih.gov/

Tromans, E. & Barwell, J. (2022). Clinical genetics: Past, present and future. *European Journal of Human Genetics, 30*, 991–992. Retrieved from https://www.nature.com/

US Department of Energy (USDOE) Genome Programs (2008). *Genomics and its impact on science and society: The Human Genome Project and beyond*. Retrieved from https://permanent.fdlp.gov/

Watson, C. & Ban, S. (2021). Body dysmorphic disorder in children and young people. *British Journal of Nursing, 30*(3), 160–164. doi: 10.12968/bjon.2021.30.3.160

Yang, Y. B. (2019). The role of genetics in medicine: A future of precision medicine. *British Columbia Medical Journal (BCMJ), 61*(10), 388–389.

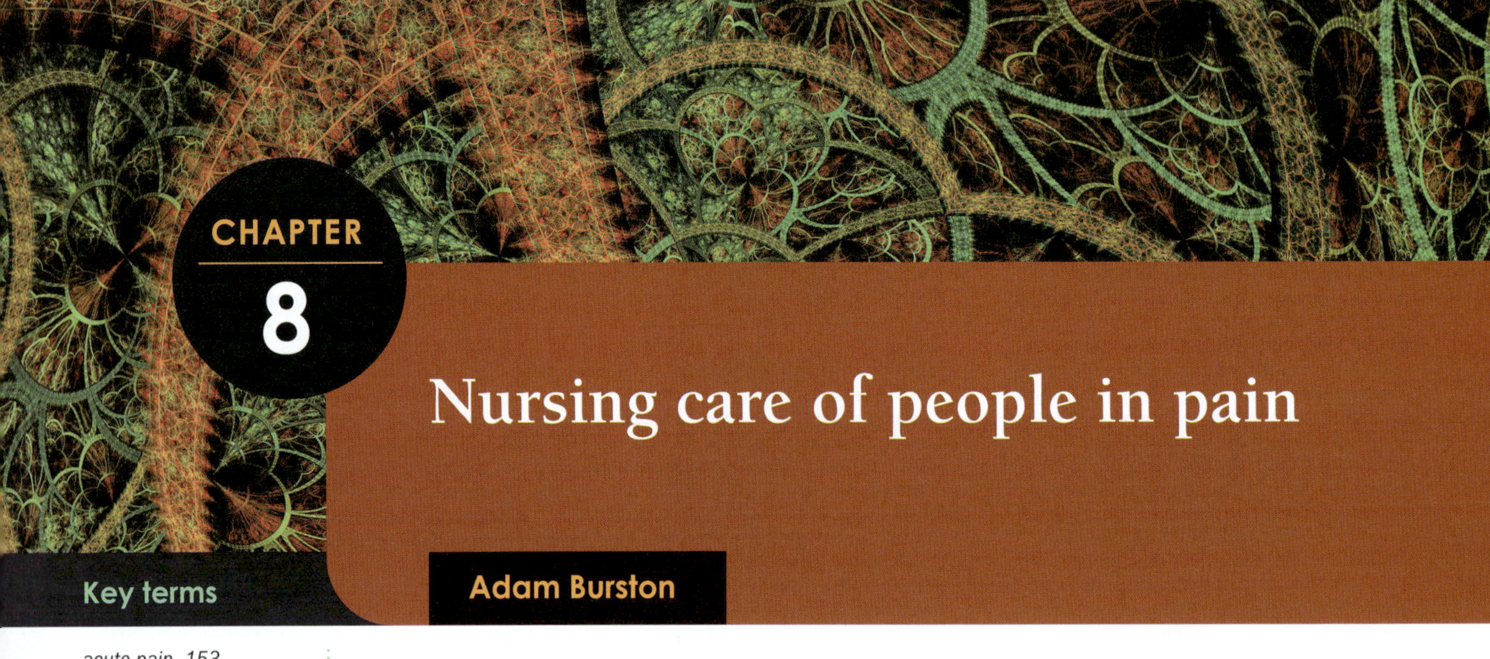

CHAPTER 8

Nursing care of people in pain

Adam Burston

Key terms

acute pain 153
addiction 161
analgesic 160
breakthrough pain 154
cancer pain 155
central pain 155
neuropathic pain 155
nociception 151
nociceptors 151
pain tolerance 155
persistent (chronic) pain 154
phantom pain 155
procedural pain 154
titrate 165
transdermal 165

Learning outcomes

- Describe the neurophysiology and theories of pain.
- Compare and contrast definitions and characteristics of acute and chronic pain.
- Discuss factors affecting individualised responses to pain.
- Clarify myths and misconceptions about pain.
- Introduce interprofessional care for the person in pain and discuss pharmacological and non-pharmacological treatment alternatives.
- Describe a framework for providing individualised nursing care for the person experiencing pain.

Clinical competencies

- Conduct comprehensive pain assessment.
- Assess the effect of pain on physical, psychological and social function.
- Support autonomy for the person with pharmacological and non-pharmacological management strategies.
- Administer medications and monitor effects knowledgeably and safely.
- Promote autonomy in pain management through collaboration with the person, their family and significant others to assess pain and plan effective pain management.
- Evaluate effectiveness of pain management strategies and use this to revise plans of care.

The International Association for the Study of Pain (IASP) defines pain as 'an unpleasant sensory and emotional experience associated with actual or potential tissue damage, or described in terms of such damage' (IASP, 2020). Pain is a subjective response, not always measureable or observable, to both physical and psychological stressors which all people experience at some point during their lives. Although pain is usually experienced as uncomfortable and unwelcome, it also serves a protective role; pain may also warn of potential health-threatening conditions. For this reason, pain needs to be assessed and considered as an essential vital sign.

Each individual pain event is a distinct personal experience. It is influenced by physiological, cognitive, psychological, sociocultural and spiritual factors.

NEUROPHYSIOLOGY AND THEORIES OF PAIN

Neurophysiology

The peripheral nervous system is composed of two types of neurons: sensory and motor. Pain is perceived through the sensory neurons and responded to through the motor neurons. Connections or synapses occur within the spinal cord and again within the central nervous system (CNS), where cognitive analysis of the painful stimulus leads to a response.

Nerve receptors of pain are called **nociceptors** (see Figure 8.1). These are the nerve receptors that are sensitive to pain (noxious stimuli) and give an immediate response when stimulated. They are located at the ends of small afferent neurons and are woven throughout all tissues of the body, except the brain. Nociceptors are especially numerous in the skin and muscles. Pain occurs when biological, mechanical, thermal, electrical or chemical factors stimulate nociceptor activity to the spinal cord. The intensity and duration of the stimuli determines the sensation.

Reactions are caused either by persistent mechanical, chemical or thermal stimuli that create a cascade of chemical mediators which can act directly on the cell or via a messenger system to activate **nociception**. Bradykinin, a polypeptide element of the kinin protein system, is a pain-producing chemical; other biochemical sources of pain include prostaglandins, substance P, histamine, leukotriene B, hydrogen ions and serotonin (ANZCA 2020; Crisp et al., 2020). These biochemicals are thought to bind to nociceptors in response to noxious stimuli, causing the nociceptors to initiate pain impulses.

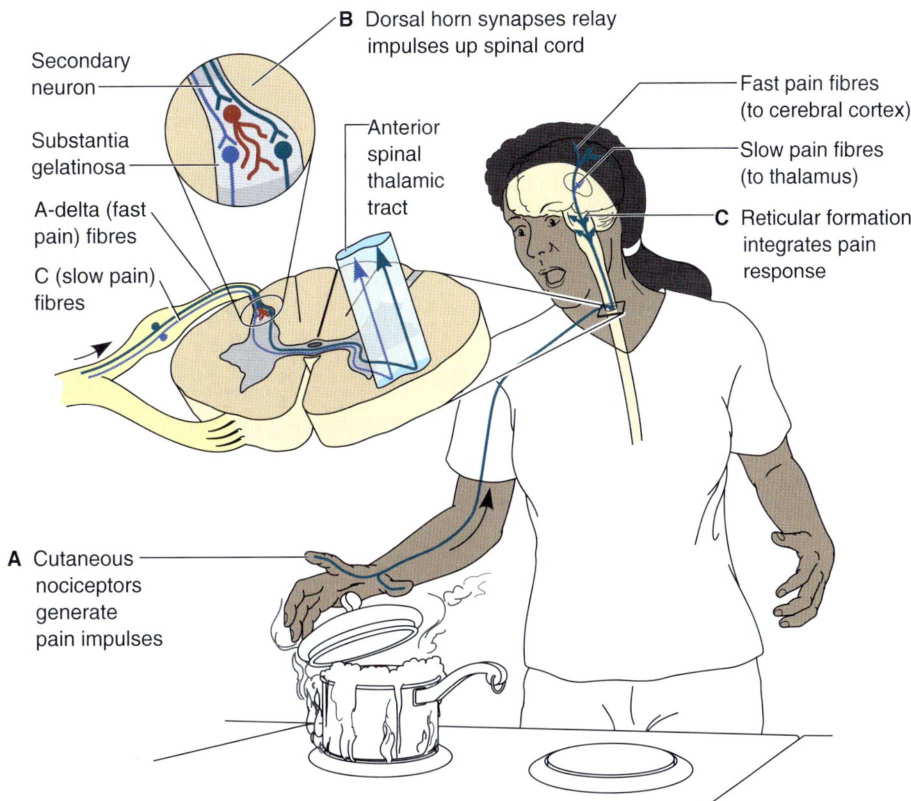

FIGURE 8.1 *A, Cutaneous nociceptors generate pain impulses that travel via A-delta and C fibres to the spinal cord's dorsal horn. B, Secondary neurons in the dorsal horn pass impulses across the spinal cord to the anterior spinothalamic tract. C, Slow pain impulses ascend to the thalamus, while fast pain impulses ascend to the cerebral cortex. The reticular formation in the brainstem integrates the emotional, cognitive and autonomic responses to pain*

Ascending pain pathways

The ascending pathways of pain are illustrated in Figure 8.1 and are summarised as follows:

1. Pain is perceived by the nociceptors in the periphery of the body—for example, in the skin or viscera. Cutaneous pain is transmitted through two types of nerve fibres that transmit signals:
   - A-delta fibres are medium-diameter, myelinated and respond primarily to high-intensity mechanical or heat stimuli, causing sharp, stabbing-like pain.
   - Smaller C nerve fibres are small-diameter, unmyelinated and respond to lower-intensity thermal, chemical or mechanical cold stimuli, resulting in a dull and aching type of pain. The pain from deep body structures (such as muscles and viscera) is primarily transmitted by C fibres and is commonly associated with persistent pain.

   Both A-delta and C fibres are involved in most injuries. For example, if a person bangs their elbow, A-delta fibres transmit this pain stimulus within 0.1 second. The person feels this pain as a sharp, localised, smarting sensation. One or more seconds after the blow, the person experiences a duller, aching, diffuse sensation of pain impulses carried by the C fibres.
2. Second-order sensory neurons transmit the impulses from the afferent neurons (A-delta fibres and C fibres) through the dorsal horn of the spinal cord, where they synapse in the substantia gelatinosa. This first synapse is important for modulation input in the CNS. The impulses then cross over to the anterior and lateral spinothalamic tracts.
3. The impulses of the second-order neurons ascend via the anterior and lateral spinothalamic tracts and pass through the medulla and midbrain to the thalamus.
4. In the thalamus and cerebral cortex, the pain impulses are perceived, described, localised and interpreted, and a response is formulated. A noxious impulse becomes pain when the sensation reaches conscious levels and is perceived and evaluated by the person experiencing the sensation.

Some pain impulses ascend along the paleospinothalamic tract in the medial section of the spinal cord. These impulses enter the reticular formation and the limbic systems, which integrate emotional and cognitive responses to pain. Interconnections in the autonomic nervous system may also cause an autonomic response to the pain. In addition, deep nociceptors often converge on the same spinal neuron, resulting in pain that is experienced in a part of the body other than its origin.

Inhibitory mechanisms

Efferent fibres run from the reticular formation and midbrain to the substantia gelatinosa in the dorsal horns of the spinal cord. Along these fibres, pain may be inhibited or modulated. The analgesia system is a group of midbrain neurons that transmits impulses to the pons and medulla, which in turn stimulate a pain inhibitory centre in the dorsal horns of the spinal cord. The exact nature of this inhibitory mechanism is unknown.

The most clearly defined chemical inhibitory mechanism is fuelled by endorphins (endogenous morphines) which are naturally occurring opioid peptides present in neurons in the brain, spinal cord and gastrointestinal tract. Endorphins in the brain are released in response to afferent noxious stimuli, whereas endorphins in the spinal cord are released in response to efferent impulses. Endorphins work by binding with opiate receptors on the neurons to inhibit pain impulse transmission (see Figure 8.2).

Pain theories

Several theories attempt to explain the response to pain and the diversity of human experiences with pain. Specificity and pattern theories describe nerve impulses of varying intensity terminating in pain centres in the forebrain. These theories provide explanations of the neurophysiological basis of pain.

The gate-control theory

In 1965, Melzack and Wall postulated the gate-control theory (Bryant et al., 2019). A gating mechanism exists at the spinal cord level where nerve transmission may be blocked by competing impulses. This explains the ability of even low-intensity stimulation such as light brushing of the skin to successfully block the experience of pain. Pain perception results from the interaction of two systems: the substantia gelatinosa in the dorsal horns of the spinal cord

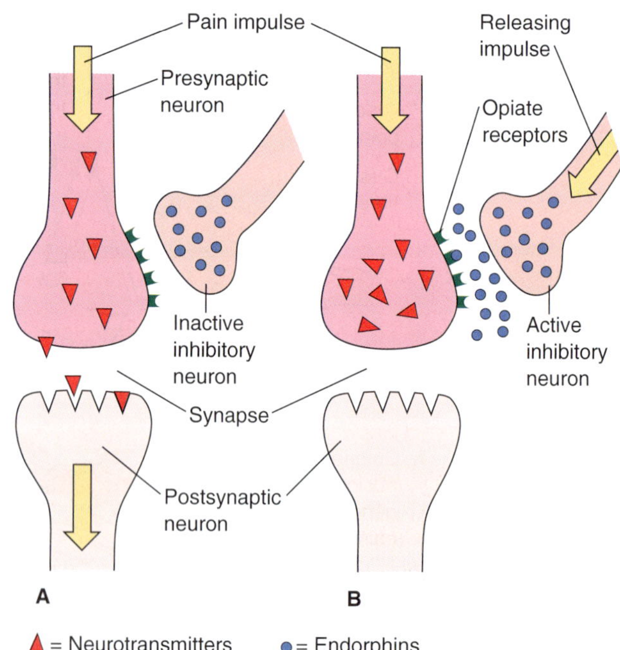

FIGURE 8.2 *A, Pain impulse causes presynaptic neuron to release burst of neurotransmitters across synapse. These bind to postsynaptic neuron and propagate impulse. B, Inhibitory neuron releases endorphins, which bind to presynaptic opiate receptors. Neurotransmitter release is inhibited and pain impulse is interrupted*

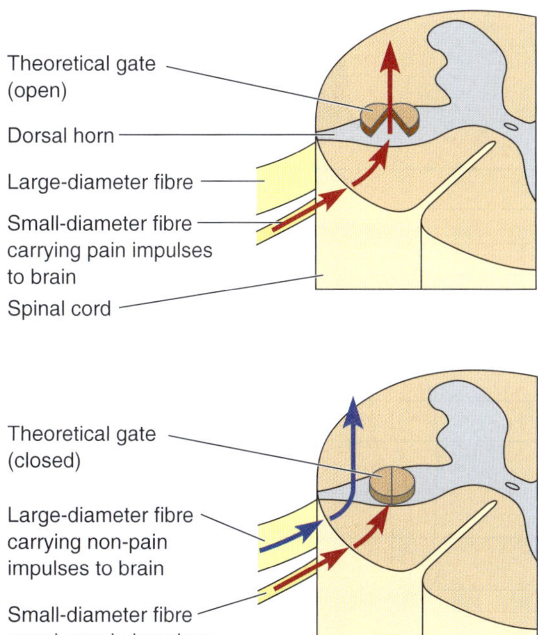

FIGURE 8.3 *The spinal cord component of the gate-control theory. Pain transmission by small-diameter fibres is blocked when large-diameter fibres carrying touch impulses dominate, closing the gate in the substantia gelatinosa*

(see Figure 8.3), which regulates impulses entering or leaving the spinal cord; and an inhibitory system within the brainstem.

A-delta and C fibres in the spinal cord carry fast and slow pain impulses, while large-diameter A-beta fibres carry impulses for tactile stimulation from the skin. In the substantia gelatinosa, these impulses encounter a 'gate' thought to be opened and closed by the domination of either the large-diameter or the small-diameter fibres. If impulses along the small-diameter pain fibres outnumber impulses along the large-diameter touch fibres, the gate is open, and pain impulses travel unimpeded to the brain. If impulses from the touch fibres predominate, they will close the gate, and the pain impulses will be 'turned away' at the gate. This explains why light stimulation such as massaging a stubbed toe can reduce the intensity and duration of the pain.

The second system described by gate-control theory is the inhibitory system located in the brainstem. It is believed that cells in the midbrain, activated by a variety of stimuli such as opiates, psychological factors, or even simply the presence of pain itself, signal receptors in the medulla which in turn stimulate nerve fibres in the spinal cord to block the transmission of impulses from pain fibres. Ongoing research demonstrates that the control and modulation of pain is much more complex than the description supplied by gate-control theory, which served as a basis for further research about pain-modulating systems. Ongoing theory development of the neuromatrix integrates cultural, genetic, attention, expectation, personality and stress factors with basic neurophysiological function. This neuromatrix is particularly useful to understand chronic pain and phantom limb pain, considering there is no defined relationship between tissue injury and the pain experience.

Central sensitisation

Another pain theory that is quite significant in clinical terms describes the effect of sensitising the central and peripheral nervous system to painful stimuli. Central sensitisation manifests as pain hypersensitivity. This theory suggests painful signals create a cascade of changes in the nervous system, which in turn increase the responsiveness of the peripheral and central neurons. These changes, in turn, amplify light touch and pressure, causing enhanced after sensations, increased temporal summation and response to future signals (Nijs et al., 2021). Studies of infants undergoing painful procedures show that those who received analgesia experienced reduced sensitivity to future painful events, while those who did not receive analgesia experienced greater sensitivity (The Royal Children's Hospital Melbourne, 2021). Sensitisation occurs from nociceptive barrage as well as inflammation following an injury or incision. In adults this theory indicates the value of preventing sensitisation as well as treating perceived pain with multimodal pain therapy.

DEFINITIONS AND CHARACTERISTICS OF PAIN

Acute pain

Acute pain has a sudden onset, is usually temporary, is localised and is the common, everyday pain that most people know. Pain that lasts for less than 3 months and has an identified cause is classified as acute pain (Balasubramanian, 2021). The onset is usually immediate, most often resulting from tissue injury from trauma, surgery or inflammation. The pain is often sharp and localised, although it may radiate. Acute pain warns of actual or potential injury to tissues. As a stressor, it initiates the fight-or-flight autonomic stress response. Characteristic physical responses include tachycardia, rapid and shallow respirations, increased blood pressure, dilated pupils, sweating, pallor and alterations to blood sugar levels. The three major types of acute pain are as follows:

1. *Somatic pain* arises from nerve receptors originating in the skin or close to the surface of the body. Somatic pain may be either sharp and localised, or dull and diffuse. It is often accompanied by nausea and vomiting.
2. *Visceral pain* arises from body organs and is dull and poorly localised because of the low number of nociceptors. The viscera are sensitive to stretching, inflammation and ischaemia, but relatively insensitive to cutting and temperature extremes. Visceral pain is associated with nausea and vomiting, hypotension and restlessness. It often radiates or is referred; that is, perceived at a location other than that of the painful stimulus. It may be described as cramping, intermittent pain or colicky pain.
3. *Referred pain* is perceived in an area distant from the site of the stimuli and commonly occurs with visceral pain. Visceral fibres synapse at the level of the spinal cord, close to fibres innervating other subcutaneous tissue areas of the body (see Figure 8.4). Pain in a spinal nerve

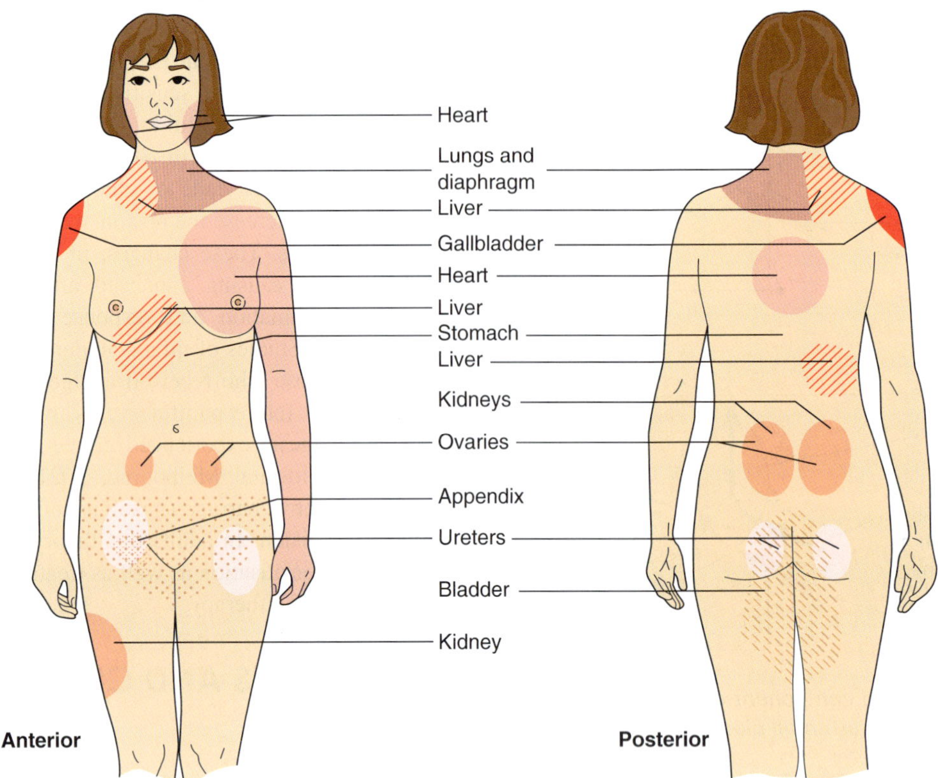

FIGURE 8.4 *Referred pain is the result of the convergence of sensory nerves from certain areas of the body before they enter the brain for interpretation. For example, a toothache may be felt in the ear, pain from inflammation of the diaphragm may be felt in the shoulder and pain from ischaemia of the heart muscle (angina) may be felt in the left arm*

may be felt over the skin in any body area innervated by sensory neurons that share that same spinal nerve route. Body areas defined by spinal nerve routes are called dermatomes (see the chapter 'A person-centred approach to assessing the nervous system').

Persistent (chronic) pain

Persistent (chronic) pain is ongoing and prolonged pain. It may be associated with a known cause, such as malignancy. It may arise also from acute situations such as post trauma, herpes zoster, acute back pain and postoperative surgical pain. It is defined as 'pain in one or more anatomical regions, persisting or recurring for longer than 3 months, associated with significant emotional distress, when symptoms are not better accounted for by another diagnosis' (Balasubramanian, 2021, pp. 2–3).

Predictive factors for chronic post-surgical pain include preoperative, intraoperative and postoperative factors:

- Preoperative considerations include moderate to severe pain lasting for more than one month, repeat surgery, psychological vulnerability (e.g. catastrophising), preoperative anxiety.
- Intraoperative considerations include a surgical approach with risk of nerve damage.
- Postoperative factors include pain (acute, moderate to severe), radiation to the area, depression and anxiety (adapted from ANZCA, 2020).

Neurological changes that can occur with persistent pain are changes in perception. Physical changes that result are loss of muscle mass, deconditioning, postural changes, alterations in appetite and weight, constipation and sleep disturbances. Persistent pain is complex and is poorly understood.

The 'persistent (chronic) pain syndrome' refers to the unspecific behaviours that can occur with persistent pain. Often a cycle of persistent pain and disability causes physical deconditioning, drug tolerance, reduced activity, passive treatments, distorted beliefs and social stresses such as financial pressures, altered gender roles and the destruction of intimate relationships. From a psychological perspective, the person with persistent pain experiences anxiety, stress, depression and sleep disturbance (Hruschak et al., 2021). Although persistent pain may range from mild to severe, its unrelenting presence often results in the pain itself becoming a pathological process requiring intervention.

Breakthrough pain

Breakthrough and incident, or 'procedural', pain relates to how pain progresses through time. **Breakthrough pain** occurs between doses of analgesia; it can be prevented by giving breakthrough analgesia more frequently, increasing the dose of the analgesia, or increasing the slow (continuous) release medication. **Procedural pain** occurs when procedures, dressings or activity increase the pain experience. Procedural pain can often be predicted, and analgesia should be available and given prior to the activity commencing.

Neuropathic pain

Neuropathic pain may be acute or chronic resulting from injury or disease that affects the peripheral or central nervous systems. Acute neuropathic pain may result from lesions or entrapment of nerves (Brown et al., 2020). Neuropathic pain can be caused by numerous factors such as trauma, surgery, inflammation, toxicity, and immunological and vascular changes affecting either the central nervous or the peripheral nervous systems of the body. Examples of neuropathic pain arising from the CNS are post-stroke pain and spinal cord injury. Peripheral causes of neuropathic pain are diabetic neuropathy, HIV-related neuropathies and tumours invading the nerve area and surgery.

Common surgical procedures associated with a higher incidence postoperatively of persistent neuropathic pain are amputation (phantom limb pain), thoracotomy, mastectomy, hernia repair and cholecystectomy (ANZCA, 2020). The person with neuropathic pain will often state their pain is burning, shooting or electric; they might comment on numbness in and around the area or the sensation of pins and needles. Diagnosis is usually made with a detailed history, personal description and pain assessment.

- *Complex regional pain syndrome (CRPS)* is neuropathic pain that commonly results from nerve damage related to minor trauma (Haight et al., 2021). CRPS is recognised as a persistent pain condition in which functional restoration and integrated rehabilitation focused upon functional restoration and quality-of-life improvement is necessary (Hudson et al., 2021). Common features of CRPS are continuous, severe pain (usually burning or electric), trophic changes (hair and nails alter in growth), vasospasm changes (vasodilation causing the limb to become hot, red and swollen, followed by vasoconstriction) and limb immobility causing muscle wasting. During the recovery phase, patients report CRPS-related pain, generalised pain, movement restriction, reliance on medication and stiffness (Llewelyn et al., 2018) as the primary challenges to overcome.
- *Neuralgias* are painful conditions that result from damage to a peripheral nerve caused by infection or disease. Post-herpetic neuralgia (following shingles) is an example occurring in 50% of those who are over 50 years and 75% of those who are over 75 years. Trigeminal neuralgia can occur as an acute exacerbation of neuropathic pain. Most causes are idiopathic and the main treatment is with topiramate or carbamazapine (ANZCA, 2020).

Phantom pain

Phantom pain is a common condition among amputees. Phantom pain commonly resembles pre-injury pain (if it was present) and is exacerbated by stump problems, ill-fitting prostheses and back pain. Phantom pain also occurs in other parts of the body after surgical removal (e.g. mastectomy, tongue). Phantom pain is *not* phantom sensation, which resolves over time as the sensation retreats into the stump and is a contributory mechanism to phantom pain development (ANZCA, 2020).

Central pain

Central pain is related to a lesion in the brain or spinal cord that may spontaneously produce a high-frequency burst of impulses from the ascending spinothalamocortical pathways; their relays or end stations in the brain or spinal cord create a sensation of pain. A vascular lesion, tumour, trauma or inflammation may also cause central pain. Thalamic pain is most common, severe, spontaneous and often continuous. Hyperaesthesia (an abnormal sensitivity to touch, pain or other sensory stimuli) may occur on the side of the body opposite the lesion in the thalamus. The perception of body position and movement may also be lost.

Cancer pain

Cancer pain is a common condition of those with advanced cancer. Cancer pain is often persistent, arising from a number of factors (e.g. the disease process, the prescribed treatment, resultant disability and subsequent comorbidity problems). Cancer pain can be very challenging to manage and is often a mixture of nociceptive and neuropathic, with acute and persistent features creating problems of breakthrough and procedural pain.

FACTORS AFFECTING RESPONSES TO PAIN

Physical response to pain involves specific and often predictable neurological changes. In fact, everyone has the same pain *threshold* and perceives pain stimuli at the same stimulus intensity. For example, heat is perceived as painful at 44°C to 46°C, the range at which it begins to damage tissue. What varies is *tolerance*, which is based on perception of, and reaction to, pain. When a person is described as highly sensitive to pain, this is a reference to their **pain tolerance**, which is the amount of pain a person can endure before outwardly responding to it. The ability to tolerate pain may be decreased by repeated episodes of pain, fatigue, anger, anxiety and sleep deprivation. The use of such practices as heat/cold, position, relaxation, distraction, hypnosis, spiritual practices, medications and alcohol may increase pain tolerance. The individualised response to pain is

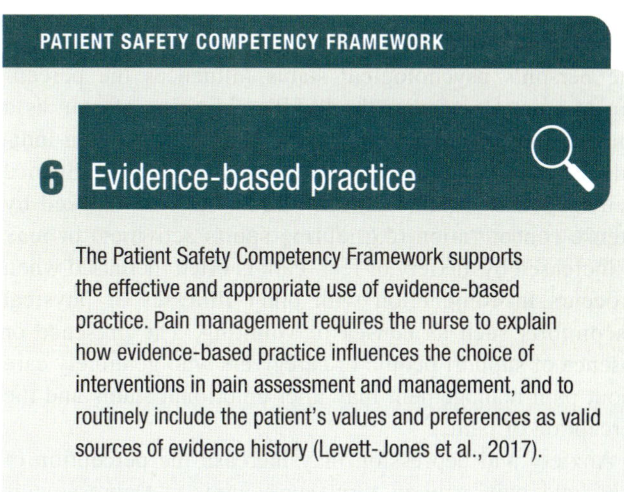
PATIENT SAFETY COMPETENCY FRAMEWORK

6 Evidence-based practice

The Patient Safety Competency Framework supports the effective and appropriate use of evidence-based practice. Pain management requires the nurse to explain how evidence-based practice influences the choice of interventions in pain assessment and management, and to routinely include the patient's values and preferences as valid sources of evidence history (Levett-Jones et al., 2017).

shaped by multiple and interacting factors, including sociocultural influences, emotional status, past experiences with pain, the source and meaning of the pain, the person's knowledge base and their age.

Sociocultural influences

A person's response to pain is strongly influenced by family, community and culture. Sociocultural influences affect the way in which a person tolerates pain, interprets the meaning of pain, and reacts verbally and non-verbally to the pain. For example, if a person comes from a social background where normative behaviour is that males should not cry and must tolerate pain stoically, rather than expressing his discomfort a male person may appear withdrawn and refuse pain medication. On the other hand, when open and intense emotional expression is accepted as the social norm, a person may demonstrate their discomfort clearly and be comfortable requesting pain medication.

Cultural norms also influence an individual's experience of pain, including how much pain to tolerate, what types of pain to report, who to report the pain to and what kind of treatment to seek. For example, some cultural norms place value on 'being a good patient', which may cause the person to avoid 'complaining' about their pain, whereas a person from another sociocultural background may value seeking information about pain, which may lead them to discuss their pain often and in detail. However, behaviours vary greatly within cultural and social groups, and from generation to generation. The nurse should approach each person as an individual, observing them carefully, taking the time to ask questions and avoiding making assumptions.

The nurse also brings with them a set of personal sociocultural values, beliefs and experiences about pain. If these values, beliefs and experiences differ from those of the person, the assessment and management of pain may be based on the values of the nurse rather than on the needs of the person. It is not uncommon to hear staff compare their own personal experiences of pain with the person receiving care (e.g. 'When I had my appendix removed, I had two paracetamol and I was fine; this person doesn't need a PCA [patient-controlled analgesia] machine.').

Psychological status

The person's psychological status influences the perception of pain. Remember the IASP's definition of pain as a *sensory and emotional experience*; therefore, how an individual feels psychologically and emotionally will influence their response to pain. Pain sensations may be blocked by intense concentration (e.g. during sports activities) or may be increased by anxiety or fear. Pain is often increased when it occurs in conjunction with other illnesses or physical discomforts such as nausea or vomiting. The presence or absence of support people or caregivers who genuinely care about pain management may alter emotional status and the perception of pain.

Anxiety and depression may increase the perception of pain, and pain may in turn cause anxiety. Depression is clearly linked to pain and is generally associated with higher pain intensity (ANZCA, 2020). In addition, the muscle tension commonly found with anxiety can create its own source of pain. This association explains why non-pharmacological interventions such as relaxation or guided imagery are helpful in relieving or decreasing pain. Fatigue, lack of sleep and depression also are related to pain experiences. Pain interferes with a person's ability to fall asleep and stay asleep, and thus induces fatigue. In turn, fatigue can lower pain tolerance.

Past experiences with pain

Previous experiences with pain are likely to influence the person's response to a current pain episode. If supportive adults responded to childhood experiences with pain appropriately, the adult usually will have a healthy attitude to pain. If, however, the person's pain was responded to with exaggerated emotions or neglectful indifference, that person's future responses to pain may be exaggerated or denied.

The responses of healthcare providers to the person in pain can influence their response during the next pain episode. If providers respond to pain with effective strategies and a caring attitude, the person will remain more comfortable during any subsequent pain episode, and anxiety will be avoided. If, however, the pain is not adequately relieved, or if the person feels that empathetic care was not given, anxiety about the next pain episode sets up the person for a more complex and therefore more painful event.

Source and meaning

The meaning associated with the pain influences the experience of pain. For example, the pain of labour to deliver a baby is experienced differently from the pain following removal of a major organ for cancer. Because pain is the major signal for health problems, it is strongly linked to all associated meanings of health problems, such as disability, loss of role and death. For this reason, it is important to explain the aetiology and prognosis of pain to the person receiving care.

Knowledge

A lack of understanding of the source, outcome and meaning of pain can contribute negatively to the pain experience. The nurse needs to assess the person's readiness to learn, use methods of teaching that are effective for the person and family, and evaluate learning carefully. Teaching must include the process of the pain, its predictable course (if possible) and the proposed plan of care. In addition, nurses should discuss strategies for managing pain and encourage the person to communicate preferences for pain relief. Involving the person's significant others regarding the presence of pain and how they can help promote effective relief will assist in achieving a holistic approach to pain management.

Age

Age influences a person's perception and expression of pain and the physical changes that will influence drug requirements (see Table 8.1). Dangerous misconceptions exist regarding the management of pain in older adults.

TABLE 8.1 Physical changes related to ageing and their influence on drug requirements

PHYSICAL CHANGE	EFFECT	OUTCOME
Cardiac output	Drug concentrations after bolus	Require smaller bolus dose
Muscle mass	Change in drug distribution	Potential for unwanted side effects
Liver function	Influences drug elimination	Drug accumulation
Renal function	Influences drug excretion	Drug accumulation
Cerebral blood flow	Alters response to analgesia	Unwanted and unexpected side effects can occur

Sources: ANZCA (2020). *Acute pain management: Scientific evidence* (5th ed.). Melbourne: Australian and New Zealand College of Anaesthetists; Fitzgerald, Tripp & Halksworth-Smith (2017). Assessment and management of acute pain in older people: Barriers and facilitators to nursing practice. *Australian Journal of Advanced Nursing, 35*(1), 48–57.

Misconceptions regarding ageing

1. *Pain is expected in the older adult.* While the occurrence of pain is common in the older adult, it is often not recognised or is undertreated (Eliopoulos, 2021; Vafeas & Slatyer, 2021); however, it is still an indicator of an underlying clinical issue. Often believing that pain is a part of growing older, the person may ignore pain or self-medicate with over-the-counter medications. Individuals in this age group may fail to acknowledge pain, believing that it is inevitable or fearing dependency if they alarm their loved ones (Eliopoulos, 2021; Vafeas & Slatyer, 2021).
2. *Pain perception decreases with age.* Age does not change the perception of acute pain. It is essential to apply specific methods to assessing pain in the older adult as well as emphasising the education of healthcare staff in using appropriate pain assessment tools (ANZCA, 2020; Schofield, 2018).
3. *When older adults report pain, they are attention seeking.* This is highly unlikely. Do not forget that some older people suffer mute myocardial infarction and experience painless peritonitis, pancreatitis and cholecystitis (Eliopoulos, 2021; Vafeas & Slatyer, 2021). The elderly are at a greater risk of mortality and morbidity if pain is not relieved.
4. *Opiates are dangerous in older adults.* When opiates are prescribed, the factors identified in Table 8.1 need to be considered.
5. *Opiate use causes addiction in older adults.* Older adults may hesitate to ask for pain medicine because they fear addiction and loss of independence (Brown et al., 2020).

Pain assessment in older adults may be difficult when the person is experiencing cognitive impairment and has difficulty communicating descriptions of pain. When discussing pain with the older person, it can be better to use terms they use when self-reporting pain, such as 'aching' or 'soreness'. Some adults with a cognitive impairment can describe current, usual or worse pain when a standardised pain scale is used, such as the verbal descriptor of 'mild, moderate or severe'. However, many older people with moderate to severe dementia cannot complete self-report instruments, so informal caregivers are commonly the pain assessment information source (ANZCA, 2020; Bullock et al., 2019).

Dementia is most common in older people and is a substantial barrier to accurate pain management (Dementia Australia, 2022). Recommended methods for pain assessment include: (1) behavioural observations, (2) documenting baseline behaviours and activity patterns and monitoring changes that might indicate the need for further pain assessment, and (3) effective communication with informal caregivers/family.

FAST FACTS

- Older people have the highest rate of illness and surgical procedures associated with pain; they also have the highest rate of complications associated with surgical interventions.
- Persistent pain is common in older adults. For those over 70 years of age, 50% of those living in the community and 80% of those in residential care suffer persistent pain.
- Musculoskeletal pain affecting major joints and back, or neuropathic pain from diabetic neuropathy and post-herpetic neuralgia have an increased prevalence in the ageing population.
- Concurrent illnesses are common in the elderly, making clinical presentation complex and sometimes difficult.
- Cognitive impairment enhances the risk of poor pain control, negatively influencing the individual's quality of life.

Sources: ANZCA (2020). *Acute pain management: Scientific evidence* (5th ed.). Melbourne: Australian and New Zealand College of Anaesthetists; Youngcharoen (2022). A cross-sectional study of factors associated with nurses' postoperative pain management practices for older patients. *Nursing Open*. https://doi.org/10.1002/nop2.1281

Pain in the paediatric population

Historically, infants and young children were assumed to have a lack of pain sensation; however, it is now understood that due to a more robust inflammatory response and lack of central inhibitory influence, their response to pain may be even greater than that of adults. The nurse plays a central role in the assessment and management of pain in this context. Selecting the most appropriate pain assessment tool for the child's developmental stage and facilitating communication with parents and the healthcare team are central. Without a strategic and consistent approach, nurses may fail to recognise, treat or prevent pain (Martin et al., 2019).

It is recommended that health professionals should anticipate painful experiences, monitor the condition of the child and provide adequate information about what to expect and appropriate measures to reduce the distress to children and parents (Foote, 2019). Involving the child (if age appropriate) in pain assessment is more effective than relying on parental observations alone (Gorito et al., 2022).

Optimal pain control can be achieved using a variety of techniques. These may range from deep sedation or anaesthesia to cognitive behavioural strategies such as imagery and relaxation. Whatever strategy is used, a quiet environment with calm parents and clear and confident instruction will assist the paediatric person experiencing pain (Truba & Hoyle, 2014).

Pain and cultural diversity

Substantial diversity exists in the expression of pain and acceptable ways in which pain is managed. To provide culturally safe care, the nurse must endeavour to be as familiar as possible with this nuanced diversity. Not only does diversity exist across cultural groups, but also within cultural groups. Communication, based upon forming therapeutic relationships, is central to this. Interpreter support may be required to bridge communication barriers. Ineffective communication about pain, be it pain assessment, intervention or evaluation, hinders the delivery of culturally congruent care (Lor, Rabago & Backonja, 2021).

Within the pain management context, patient-controlled analgesia may be used to provide efficient and effective analgesia (ANZCA, 2020). Pain is subjective and nurses may underestimate the pain of those from a different cultural background. For example, in one American study, Asian patients received 24% lower doses of analgesics postoperatively than Caucasian people; however, both groups used similar amounts of opioid analgesia when using a PCA (Brown et al., 2020).

Pain and Indigenous Australians

Aboriginal and Torres Strait Islander peoples are considered to be particularly vulnerable in relation to healthcare. In 2015–2017, life expectancy at birth for Aboriginal and Torres Strait Islander males was 71.6 years and for females 75.6 years, which remain noticeably lower than for non-Indigenous Australians (Australian Institute of Health and Welfare (AIHW), 2022). Significant burden from mental health illness, substance use disorders, injuries, cardiovascular disease, cancer and musculoskeletal conditions persists (AIHW, 2022). Pain is a common symptom associated with these conditions.

Arthur and Rolan (2019) identified specific challenges such as misunderstanding due to levels of health literacy, patient dissatisfaction with healthcare providers from misaligned expectations, experiencing negative stereotypes, disconnection between patient and nurses regarding culturally appropriate ways of expressing and managing pain and how it should be treated, and an expectation to adopt pain behaviours from the nurse's culture.

A culturally safe assessment of the person is required, with sensitivity to pain tolerance, language barriers and tendencies to display a stoic attitude to pain demonstrated. Where possible, nurses should use interpreters, Indigenous health workers or liaison officers. As with other high-risk patient groups, Indigenous Australians often have multiple comorbidities, which may influence the types of analgesics prescribed.

MYTHS AND MISCONCEPTIONS ABOUT PAIN

Myths and misconceptions about pain and its management are common in both healthcare providers and the general population. Some of the most common misconceptions are:

- *Pain is a result, not a cause.* According to the traditional view of pain, it is only a symptom of a condition. However, it is now recognised that unrelieved or poorly relieved pain sets up further responses such as central sensitisation, amplifying pain sensations and delaying rehabilitation.
- *Persistent pain is really a masked form of depression.* Serotonin plays a chemical role in pain transmission and is also the major modulator of depression. Therefore, pain and depression are chemically related, not mutually exclusive. It is common to find them coexisting.
- *Opioid medication is too risky to be used to treat persistent pain.* This common misconception often deprives the person experiencing pain of the most effective source of pain relief. It is true that other methods should be tried first; however, if they prove ineffective, opioids should be considered as an appropriate alternative.
- *It is best to wait until the person has pain before giving medication.* It is now widely accepted that anticipating pain has a noticeable effect on the amount of pain a person experiences. Offering pain relief before a pain event is well on its way can lessen the pain. Remember that agony is harder to manage.
- *Many people lie about the existence or severity of their pain.* The most reliable source of pain severity is the person's score, as they will rarely lie about their pain.
- *Postoperative pain is best treated with intramuscular injections.* The most commonly used postoperative pain relief for many years was morphine or pethidine given intramuscularly. However, both have adverse effects, such as late-onset respiratory depression, they are painful to give and they can irritate the tissues (causing tissue abscess). Pethidine is short acting and also produces norpethidine, a CNS stimulant that can cause seizures. Most experts now do not recommend pethidine to manage postoperative pain (Pandharipande & McGrane, 2017).
- *Pain relief interferes with diagnosis.* Pain is the single most common reason that people present to an emergency department (ED).
- A common misconception is that analgesia given prior to medical assessment will mask the pathology and therefore diagnosis. In the case of abdominal pain, research shows that pain relief will not interfere with the diagnostic process in adults and children (ANZCA, 2020). Despite a prevailing attitude that pain management is an essential part of quality medical care, pain management in the ED is difficult because of the short-term associations

with the person, increased vigilance against drug abuse and the myth that diagnosis is impaired by pain relief. Nevertheless, 60% of people presenting to Australian EDs with abdominal pain are satisfied with their analgesia on discharge (ANZCA, 2020).

INTERPROFESSIONAL CARE AND PHARMACOLOGICAL/ NON-PHARMACOLOGICAL TREATMENT ALTERNATIVES

Effective analgesia relief results from collaboration among healthcare providers, particularly nurses, as it is the nursing staff that most closely cares for the person 24 hours a day, especially in an acute situation. For those with more persistent pain problems, there are pain clinics staffed by teams of healthcare professionals who use a multidisciplinary approach to manage persistent pain. Therapies may include traditional pharmacological agents as well as psychotherapy, biofeedback, hypnosis, acupuncture, massage and other treatments. Hospices for palliation provide a multifaceted approach to pain management (see the chapter 'Nursing care of people experiencing loss, grief and death').

Non-pharmacological strategies to manage pain

KNOWLEDGE AND INFORMATION Knowledge and information will assist the person in managing their pain. Give direct, clear, concise information that the person understands, but do not make them more anxious and distressed. A clear, concise plan of action that has been discussed with the person will assist in effective pain management.

RELAXATION Relaxation involves learning activities that deeply relax the body and mind. Relaxation distracts the person, lessens the effects of stress from pain, increases pain tolerance, increases the effectiveness of other analgesic measures, and increases perception of pain control. In addition, by teaching the person relaxation techniques, the nurse acknowledges the person's pain and provides reassurance that the person will receive help in managing the pain (Lok, Ibrahim & Sidani, 2020). Examples of relaxation activities include:

- *Diaphragmatic breathing* can relax muscles, improve oxygen levels and provide a feeling of release from tension. The technique for diaphragmatic breathing is described and illustrated in the chapter 'Nursing care of people having surgery'.
- *Progressive muscle relaxation* may be used alone or in conjunction with deep breathing to help manage pain. The person should be taught to tighten one group of muscles (such as those of the face), hold the tension for a few seconds and then relax the muscle group completely. The person should repeat these actions for all parts of the body.
- *Guided imagery*, also called *creative visualisation*, is the use of the imaginative power of the mind to create a scene or sensory experience that relaxes the muscles and moves the attention of the mind away from the pain experience. To use guided imagery, the person must be able to concentrate, use their imagination and follow directions. The nurse can facilitate this technique by asking the person for some descriptions of what they find most relaxing. The nurse then speaks to the person in a calming, soothing voice about those places or situations. Audio recordings are available to assist with guided imagery.
- *Meditation and mindfulness* is a process whereby the person empties the mind of all sensory data and, typically, concentrates on a single object, word or idea. This activity produces a deeply relaxed state in which oxygen consumption decreases, muscles relax and endorphins are produced. At its deepest level, the meditative state may resemble a trance.

DISTRACTION Distraction involves the redirection of the person's attention away from the pain and on to something that the person finds more pleasant. Examples of distracting activities are practising focused breathing and listening to or doing some form of rhythmic activity to music.

Distraction may also involve the individual participating in an activity that promotes pleasure and stimulates laughter, as laughing for 20 minutes or more is known to produce an increase in endorphins that may continue to give pain relief even after the person stops laughing.

BIOFEEDBACK Biofeedback is an electronic method of measuring physiological responses, such as brain waves, muscle contraction and skin temperature, and then 'feeding' this information back to the person. Most biofeedback units consist of electrodes placed on the skin and an amplification unit that transforms data into visual cues, such as coloured lights. The person thus learns to recognise stress-related responses and to replace them with relaxation responses. Eventually, the person learns to repeat independently those actions that produce the desired brain wave effect.

Relaxation helps alleviate the anxiety that often accompanies and complicates pain (Vagnoli et al., 2019). Additionally, biofeedback gives the person a measure of control over the response to pain.

HYPNOSIS Hypnosis is a trance state in which the mind becomes extremely suggestible. To achieve hypnosis, the person sits or lies down in a dimly lit, quiet room. The therapist suggests that the person relax and fix attention on an object. The therapist then repeats, in a calming, soothing voice, simple phrases such as instructions to relax and listen to the therapist's voice. Eventually the person hears only the therapist's voice; during this state, the therapist may then make suggestions to encourage pain relief.

COGNITIVE BEHAVIOURAL THERAPY Cognitive behavioural therapy (CBT) is a proven psychosocial intervention in chronic pain and is effective across the lifespan. CBT assists the patient in exploring pain beliefs and associated pain behaviours, and has proven beneficial in addressing depression, anxiety, stress and functional status (Hadley & Novitch, 2021).

Manual therapies

PHYSIOTHERAPY Physiotherapy can offer a range of pain management strategies—for example, graded reactivation programs, therapeutic ultrasound and exercises to increase strength and flexibility to promote pre-injury functional status.

MASSAGE Massage has been shown to assist in post-surgical abdominal pain and thoracic surgery. Pain scores are not necessarily lowered, but there is a reduction in the unpleasantness of pain (ANZCA, 2020).

HEAT AND COLD THERAPY Heat and cold therapy are commonly used as strategies to relieve pain; however, evidence regarding their effectiveness is inconsistent.

ACUPUNCTURE Acupuncture is an ancient Chinese system involving the stimulation of certain specific points on the body to enhance the flow of vital energy (chi) along pathways called meridians. Acupuncture points can be stimulated by the insertion and withdrawing of needles, the application of heat, massage, laser, electrical stimulation or a combination of these methods. Only care providers with special training can use this method.

TRANSCUTANEOUS ELECTRICAL NERVE STIMULATION A transcutaneous electrical nerve stimulation (TENS) unit consists of a low-voltage transmitter connected by wires to electrodes placed by the person as directed by the physical therapist (see Figure 8.5). The person experiences a gentle tapping or vibrating sensation over the electrodes. The person can adjust the voltage to achieve maximum pain relief. It is believed that TENS electrodes stimulate the large-diameter A-delta fibres, activating inhibitory networks in the dorsal horn, which reduces the nociceptive transmission of the C fibres.

A TENS unit is most commonly used to relieve persistent benign pain. Thorough education is essential, including an explanation of the manufacturer's directions, instructions on where to place the electrodes and the importance of placing the electrodes on clean, unbroken skin. The clinical use of TENS has been extensively studied (Johnson et al., 2022). TENS offers several advantages: avoidance of drug side effects, person control and good interaction with other therapies. Disadvantages are its cost and the need for initial expert training. When choosing a TENS machine, make sure it is portable, has adjustable amplitude, can be managed by the user and has built-in output short-circuit protection. TENS should not be used by people with cardiac pacemakers and implanted defibrillators.

HYPERBARIC OXYGEN THERAPY This therapy is defined as the intermittent inhalation of 100% oxygen in a hyperbaric chamber at a pressure higher than 1 absolute atmosphere (1 ATA = 760 mmHg, the normal atmospheric pressure at sea level) (Sutherland et al., 2015).

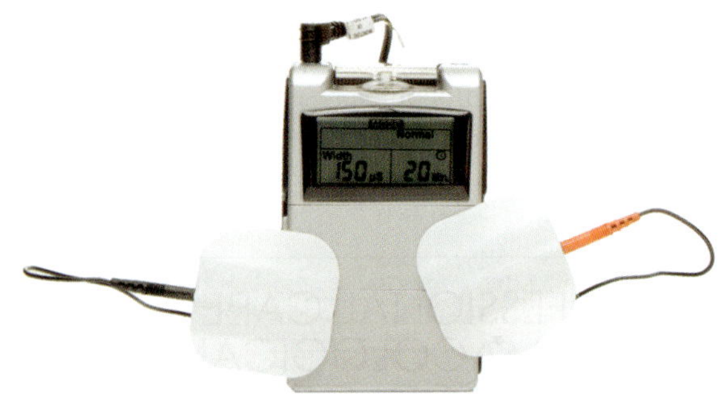

FIGURE 8.5 ***The TENS unit is believed to assist in pain management in the ways described in the gate-control theory. Electrodes that deliver low-voltage electrical stimuli are placed directly on the person over painful areas***

Source: © Rob Byron/Shutterstock.com.

Hyperbaric therapy is increasingly being tried and researched to manage neuropathic pain as well as headaches, cancer pain and postoperative pain, and has demonstrated some effectiveness (Pejic & Frey, 2018).

Pharmacological strategies for managing pain

MEDICATION Medications are the most common approach to pain management. A variety of drugs with many kinds of delivery systems are available. These drugs include simple analgesics, non-steroidal anti-inflammatory drugs (NSAIDs), opioids, antidepressants and local anaesthetic agents. In addition to administering the prescribed medications, the nurse may act independently in choosing the dosage and timing. The nurse is also responsible for assessing the side effects of the medications, evaluating their effectiveness and providing education. The nurse's roles in pain relief are those of advocate, educator and direct caregiver.

The World Health Organization (WHO) 'ladder of analgesia' effectively guides the use of medications (Anekar & Cascella, 2022) (see Figure 8.6). Analgesics are used progressively until pain is reduced or relieved, reflecting the interactive nature of these types of medications. Initially a simple analgesic (e.g. paracetamol) is used. A person will then progress to NSAIDs and then to opioid medications. Box 8.1 describes terms associated with pain medication.

Simple analgesics Simple **analgesics** such as paracetamol produce analgesia and reduce fever. The exact mechanism of action is uncertain, but it is used to treat mild to moderate pain. It is absorbed rapidly in the small intestine after oral administration, having an effect in approximately 30 minutes. Paracetamol can be given rectally, though absorption is erratic; there is also an intravenous preparation giving analgesia in approximately 10 minutes. Paracetamol should be given with caution to children and those who are underweight or have liver or renal dysfunction.

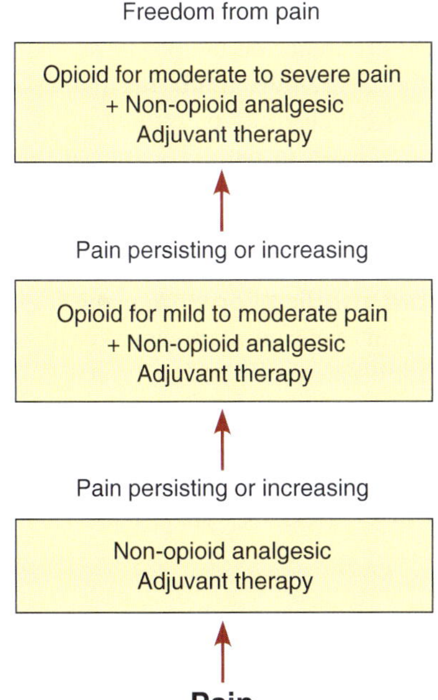

FIGURE 8.6 ***The WHO analgesic ladder illustrates the process for selection of analgesic medications for pain management***

Source: Reprinted from WHO (2018). *WHO guidelines for the pharmacological and radiotherapeutic management of cancer pain in adults and adolescents*, p. 70. Retrieved from https://www.who.int/. Copyright (2018). World Health Organization.

NSAIDs NSAIDs (non-steroidal anti-inflammatory drugs) act on peripheral nerve endings and minimise pain by interfering with prostaglandin synthesis. These medications provide analgesic effects by reducing inflammation and by perhaps blocking the generation of noxious impulses. Examples include aspirin, diclofenac and ibuprofen. The NSAIDs have prostaglandin synthesis. These medications anti-inflammatory, analgesic and antipyretic actions. NSAIDs are useful (providing renal function is adequate) for mild to moderate pain and continue to be effective when combined with opioids for moderate to severe pain. The cyclooxygenase-2 (COX-2) selective NSAIDs (celecoxib, parecoxib) are newer formulations; although less harmful to gastric mucosa, their usage has been questioned because of cardiac-associated adverse reactions and care must always be taken when prescribing regarding the person's renal function.

NSAIDs have minimal side effects if used on a short-term basis, but side effects can and do occur when used over a long period for persistent pain problems.

BOX 8.1 Terms associated with pain medications (usually opioids)

- **Addiction**: a disease characterised by aberrant drug-seeking behaviour that includes compulsive use of a substance, cravings and loss of control despite the negative biopsychosocial consequences.
- *Substance abuse disorder*: the use of any chemical substance for other than a medical purpose that causes a disintegration of the person and their life commitments.
- *Physical drug dependence*: a physiological need for a substance that results in physical withdrawal symptoms if it is not supplied or the amount is reduced suddenly. Common withdrawal symptoms include agitation, insomnia, yawning, tachycardia, sneezing and diarrhoea.
- *Psychological drug dependence*: a psychological need for a substance. If the substance is not supplied, psychological withdrawal symptoms occur, including anxiety and irritability.
- *Drug tolerance*: the process by which the body requires a progressively greater amount of a drug to achieve the same results.
- *Equianalgesic*: having the same analgesic effect when administered to the same individual. Drug dosages are equianalgesic if they have the same effect as morphine sulfate 10 mg administered parenterally.
- *Pseudoaddiction*: behaviours resembling drug seeking; often as a result of receiving inadequate analgesia.

Links to National Patient Safety Standards

NSQHS: Medication Safety Standard

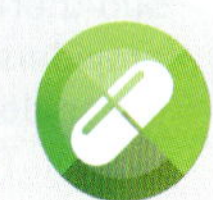

The intention of this standard is to 'ensure clinicians are competent to safely prescribe, dispense and administer appropriate medicines and to monitor medicine use' and that 'consumers are informed about medicines and understand their individual medicine needs and risks' (Australian Commission on Safety and Quality in Health Care (ACSQHC), 2021, p. 36).

Medication safety is supported by a range of initiatives across interprofessional teams, including the implementation of a National Inpatient Medication Chart (NIMC), safe labelling practice, quality education and training, and accurate reconciliation and administration of medications (ACSQHC, 2021). Nurses play an integral role in the safe administration of medicines to an informed consumer.

Source: ACSQHC (2021). *National Safety and Quality Health Service Standards* (2nd ed.). Sydney: ACSQHC. © Australian Commission on Safety and Quality in Health Care.

Tramadol Tramadol is a centrally acting synthetic analgesic that is used for moderate to severe pain. Tramadol has a three-way action, having some opioid activity and also inhibiting the re-uptake of noradrenaline and serotonin. Because it is not completely an opioid, tramadol has been classed as a Schedule 4 medication. Its analgesic effect is comparable to that of codeine. It can be used for moderate to severe pain, though it is not as powerful as morphine. Tramadol is contraindicated in those with epilepsy, as seizures have been reported, but it causes less respiratory depression, gastric stasis and constipation than the opioids (Martinez, Guichard & Fletcher, 2015). Tramadol is available in oral (immediate and slow release) and intravenous preparations.

Opioids Opioids are derivatives of the opium plant. ('Opioid' is the preferred term as 'narcotic' has negative connotations.) These medications (and their synthetic forms) are the pharmacological treatment of choice for moderate to severe pain. Examples are morphine, codeine and fentanyl. Opioid analgesics produce analgesia by binding to opioid receptors both within and outside the CNS (Cooney & Quinlan-Colwell, 2020). A common myth among healthcare professionals is that using opioids for analgesia poses a real threat of addiction. When opioids are used as recommended, there is little to no risk of addiction (see Box 8.2). Nursing implications for opioids are found in the 'Medication administration' box.

A summary of the common opioids, their preparations and the brand names available in Australia is shown in Table 8.2, and general adverse effects of opioids are listed in Box 8.3.

ADJUVANTS There are a number of drugs that are often used in pain management that assist with analgesia or control specific symptoms. These drugs are often referred to as the adjuvants or co-analgesics.

Antidepressants Tricyclic antidepressants within the tricyclic chemical group act on the production and retention of serotonin in the CNS, thus inhibiting pain sensation. They also promote normal sleeping patterns, further alleviating the suffering of the person in pain. They are useful with neuropathic pain. Common drugs used in this class are amitriptyline, nortriptyline and doxepin.

Anticonvulsant medications Anticonvulsant medications such as gabapentin (Neurontin), pregabalin (Lyrica) and carbamazepine (Tegretol) are useful with neuropathic pain, including phantom limb pain, shingles (herpes zoster), migraine headaches and diabetic neuropathic pain. These drugs reduce pain and sleep disruption. Although these drugs are primarily used to treat epilepsy (seizures), they are also used to treat nerve pain conditions.

Ketamine Ketamine is a dissociative anaesthetic and has the action of being an NMDA (N-methyl-D-asparate) antagonist. Tissue damage that causes continual nociception or neuropathic pain activates NMDA, which subsequently produces sensitisation of the central nervous system. Low-dose ketamine calms down this NMDA reaction and is used clinically for the person with persistent pain, opioid tolerance, substance abuse issues or a neuropathic pain state.

Nitrous oxide Nitrous oxide is useful for women in labour and for some dressings and procedures that are painful. Despite its analgesic and sedative effects, it has minimal cardiovascular or respiratory depressive effects. Neurological and bone marrow problems can develop with regular use, so relevant assessment should occur at regular intervals. To help prevent neurological problems, methionine, folic or folinic acid and vitamin B_{12} should be prescribed (ANZCA, 2020).

BOX 8.2 Pain management and substance use history

The person with a substance use disorder often experiences sub-therapeutic dosing of opioid medications for pain. When providers suspect or learn of substance use, they tend to order lower doses than they would for a person of similar age and weight. Despite significant data showing very little addiction as the result of treating pain with adequate pain relief, prescribers still tend to under-treat pain in the person with a substance use disorder. When the person with a substance use disorder has an acute injury, they usually need greater doses of pain medication because of the tolerance they have developed from repeated exposure to opioids and other drugs. The person with chronic cancer or non-cancer pain can display opioid tolerance due to perioperative opioid administration, particularly opioids of high potency (ANZCA, 2020).

During the acute stress of injury or infection, withholding pain medication is an added stressor. Nurses attempting to advocate for the comfort needs of a person experiencing addiction may encounter resistance around this issue. This creates a potential ethical as well as a professional dilemma. Therefore, where possible, use a pain service to assist in a person's analgesic management.

Providing analgesics for a person with pain who has a history of, or ongoing, substance use can be challenging. It is important to clearly communicate all information about medications and accessibility to the providers. Giving appropriate analgesic relief will help prevent the person sourcing medications illegally. Dose escalation may be monitored with careful assessment and random urine screens if requested by medical staff.

If diversion of the drug or inappropriate use of the prescribed medication is suspected, then opioids can be prescribed with restrictions (e.g. collecting limited amounts at one time, or only after review by a medical practitioner). Detoxification is a matter for the person to determine when they are over their crisis.

MEDICATION ADMINISTRATION Opioid analgesics

Opioid analgesics are used to treat severe pain. Drugs in this category include morphine, codeine, opium derivatives and synthetic substances. Morphine and codeine are pure chemical substances isolated from opium. They decrease the awareness of the sensation of pain by binding to opiate receptors in the brain and spinal cord. It is also believed they diminish the transmission of pain impulses by altering cell membrane permeability to sodium and by affecting the release of neurotransmitters for efferent nerves sensitive to noxious stimuli. People can develop a tolerance to opioids and psychological and physical dependence. For the person who has had an acute painful assault and is now requiring slow-release preparations in the short term, ensure that there is an overall strategy to decrease their opioid consumption. For example, the person is given a written reduction plan to follow, a written reduction regimen is sent to their general practitioner, or the person is sent to a specialised pain medicine clinic to assist with opioid reduction.

NURSING RESPONSIBILITIES

- Assess allergies or adverse effects from any opioids previously experienced by the person.
- Assess for any respiratory disease, such as asthma or sleep apnoea, that might increase the risk of respiratory depression.
- Assess the characteristics of the pain and the effectiveness of medications that have been previously used to treat pain.
- Measure and record baseline vital signs before administering the medication.
- Administer the medication following established guidelines.
- Opioids are regulated by individual state laws; the nurse and witness must record the date, time, person's name, type and amount of the drug used and sign the entry in the Schedule 8 book (commonly known as the DD—dangerous drugs—book). A witness must check the medication is given to the correct person. If the medication is disposed of after it is signed out, this must be recorded and witnessed in the Schedule 8 book.
- Keep an opioid antagonist, such as naloxone, immediately available to treat respiratory depression.
- Monitor vital signs, level of consciousness, papillary response, nausea, bowel function, urinary function and analgesic effectiveness.
- Use non-invasive methods of pain management and multimodal analgesics in conjunction with opioid medications.

HEALTH EDUCATION FOR THE PERSON WITH PAIN, THEIR FAMILY AND SIGNIFICANT OTHERS

- The use of opioids to treat severe pain is unlikely to cause addiction.
- Do not drink alcohol.
- Do not take over-the-counter medications unless approved by the healthcare provider.
- Increase intake of fluids and fibre in the diet to prevent constipation.
- The drugs often cause dizziness, drowsiness and impaired thinking; use caution when driving or making critical decisions.

TABLE 8.2 Common opioids available in Australia

OPIOID	PREPARATION	BRAND NAME
Morphine	Oral syrup (immediate release)	Ordine
	Oral tablet (immediate release)	Anamorph/Severdol
	Oral tablet/capsule (sustained release)	MSContin/Kapanol
	Injection (immediate release)	Morphine sulfate/Tartrate
Oxycodone	Oral tablet/capsule/elixir	Endone, Oxycodone, OxyNorm
	(immediate release)	Oxycontin
	Oral tablet (sustained release)	Prolodone
	Suppository (absorption uncertain)	Oxycodone
	Injection (immediate release)	
Fentanyl	Lozenge (immediate release)	Atiq
	Transdermal patch (sustained release)	Durogesic
	Injection (immediate release)	Sublimaze
Hydromorphone	Oral liquid/tablet/injection (immediate release)	Dilaudid
	Oral (sustained release)	Junista
Methadone (absorption independently variable)	Oral syrup	Physeptone syrup/Biodone Forte
	Oral tablets	Physeptone
	Injection	Physeptone
Codeine	Oral tablet/linctus (immediate release)	Codeine phosphate
Pethidine	Injection (immediate release)	Pethidine

BOX 8.3 General adverse effects of opioids

Neurological symptoms are often dose-dependent and may include sedation, dysphoria, confusion, dizziness, mental cloudiness, euphoria, miosis, muscle rigidity and seizures. It is usually advised that people do not drive, work heavy machinery or make critical decisions when initially taking these medications.

Respiratory symptoms are often dose-related and may include cough suppression, respiratory depression, bronchospasm and asthma.

Cardiovascular symptoms may include bradycardia, hypotension and vasodilation.

Gastrointestinal symptoms may include nausea, vomiting, constipation, loss of appetite and biliary colic.

Dermatological symptoms may include itch, sweating, flushing and rash.

Urinary symptoms may include urinary retention and changes in bladder and sphincter tone.

Neuroendocrine symptoms tend to develop after long-term use. They include a reduction in some hypothalamic-releasing hormones, which affects the gonads, adrenal cortex and endorphins.

Opioid rotation is common, especially for persistent pain as different opioids act on different receptors. Therefore, often a specialist will rotate the person on to a different opioid in the hope of producing more effective pain relief at a reduced dose. Sometimes equianalgesic tables are used to aid this rotation process, but these must be used with caution as each individual has different tolerances and preferences.

Local anaesthetics Local anaesthetics block the initiation and transmission of nerve impulses in a local area, thus also blocking pain sensations. Common examples of these drugs are lignocaine, bupivacaine and ropivacaine.

Local anaesthetics can be delivered by a variety of methods—for example, a single-dose nerve injection, as wound infiltration, or via topical application. All have been shown to aid analgesia. Delivery can also be made directly to the sheath of a nerve through a peripheral nerve catheter offering a continuous nerve blockade when the catheter is connected to an ongoing local anaesthetic infusion. When this latter method is used, nurses must be competent in the delivery system and the hospital should have standard protocols and policies to manage this technique. Side effects can occur from receiving local anaesthetics, such as trauma to the anaesthetised area and local anaesthetic toxicity from accidental intravascular injection.

Bisphosphonates Bisphosphonates are medications that target malignant tumours growing in bone. Referred to as osseous metastases, these expanding, painful tumours impair function. Bisphosphonates stabilise bone, slowing or preventing the development of tumours, and have a pain-relieving benefit which exceeds that of steroids and NSAIDs. Disodium pamidronate (Aredia) is effective with breast cancer metastases and multiple myeloma. A newer generation bisphosphonate, zoledronic acid (Aclasta), is useful with bony metastases secondary to lung, prostate, renal cell and other solid tumours (Mathew & Brufsky, 2015).

Radiopharmaceuticals Radiopharmaceuticals are unsealed substances produced in a nuclear reactor that emit a beta particle or an electron. The radioactivity is particularly damaging to malignant cells and is a safe and effective treatment for bony metastases. Radiopharmaceuticals are particularly useful in the management of those with prostate cancer and painful osteoblastic metastases confirmed on bone scan. Negative effects may include severe renal dysfunction or severe bone marrow depression.

Treatments may be given intravenously or orally. Care of the person treated with radiopharmaceuticals must follow radiation precautions, disposing of all body fluids quickly and thoroughly. Urine excretion is essentially completed in the first 6 hours.

Duration of action

Each pharmacological agent has a unique absorption and duration of action. Remember that no drug will have a totally predictable course of action because each person absorbs, metabolises and excretes medications at different dosage levels. The only way to obtain reliable data about the effectiveness of the medication for the individual person is to assess how that person responds. Therefore, the best choice is to individualise the dosing schedule.

There are two major descriptors of dosing schedules. The first type is for medications prescribed 'on a regular basis', such as paracetamol, NSAIDs and slow-release opioid preparations. These medications are usually given regularly if the person experiences constant pain predictably during a 24-hour period. The second type of dosing schedule is 'on an as-needed basis' (prn)—meaning *pro re nata* (Latin for 'as circumstances may require')—whereby immediate-release opioid medications are commonly used. Note that prn medication should be administered:

- as soon as the pain begins or prior to onset
- when increased pain is anticipated, such as when an activity or procedure is planned (e.g. a dressing) or when the regular prescribed medication does not cover all the pain. This is often the case in treating cancer pain as breakthrough medications may be required.

Giving analgesics before the pain occurs or increases gives the person confidence in the certainty of pain relief and thereby avoids some of the untoward effects of pain. The benefits of a preventive approach can be summarised as follows:

- The person may spend less time in pain.
- Frequent analgesic administration may allow for smaller doses and less analgesic administration.
- Smaller doses will in turn mean fewer side effects.

- The person's fear and anxiety about the return of pain will decrease.
- The person will probably be more physically active and avoid the difficulties caused by immobility.
- The swift and effective management of acute pain can prevent persistent pain states occurring.

The side effects of a medication can become difficult to manage if the dosage is too high, and the person may suffer unnecessary pain because of reluctance to endure side effects. The best formula for adequate dosage is a balance between effective analgesia and minimal side effects. Within prescribed limits, the nurse can choose the most appropriate dose according to the person's response. It is also the role of the nurse to inform the doctor and request a review of their analgesics if the prescribed dosage does not meet the person's needs.

Routes of administration

ORAL ROUTE The oral route is the simplest route for both person and nurse. Special nursing care is still required, because some medications must be given with food, some are irritating to the gastrointestinal system and some people may have trouble swallowing pills. Liquids, elixirs, capsules, soluble preparations and slow-release formulations are available for special applications.

RECTAL ROUTE The rectal route is helpful for those who are unable to swallow; however, absorption is unpredictable. The rectal route is contraindicated in those with diarrhoea, those with neutropenia and those who have had rectal surgery.

TRANSDERMAL MEDICATION The **transdermal** or 'patch' form of medication is increasingly being used because it is simple, painless and delivers a continuous level of medication (see Figure 8.7). Transdermal medications are easy to store and apply. Reapplication depends on the type of patch used (every 72 hours for fentanyl patches or 7 days for buprenorphine). Additional short-acting medication is often needed for breakthrough pain. Over-dosage can occur; therefore, it is important to start with a low-dose patch and **titrate** (which means to increase or decrease the dose in small increments) to the effective level. Again, these patches are good for those who are not eating or drinking; however, for those who sweat profusely or have a fever or inflammation of the skin, expect an increased absorption rate. Exercise and use of electric blankets or heating pads may also accelerate absorption of the medication and cause respiratory depression.

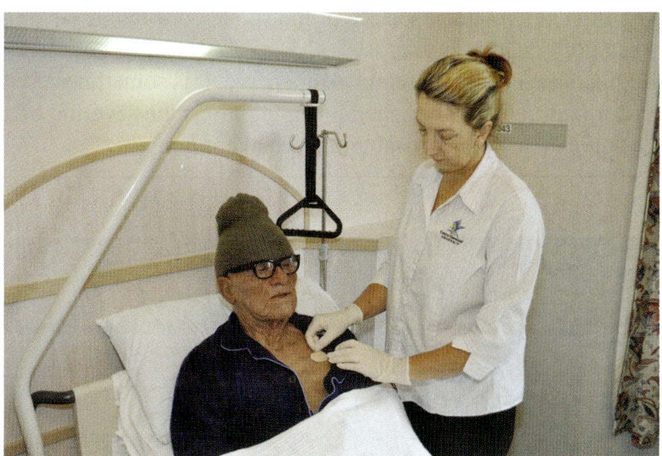

FIGURE 8.7 ***The transdermal patch administers medication in predictable doses***

Source: Courtesy of Tracy Levett-Jones.

To apply a medication transdermally, apply to a hairless area of skin that is not irritated or broken. The area of skin needs to be cleaned and then the patch applied. Apply the patch immediately upon opening the package and ensure that the contact is complete, especially around the edges. The effectiveness of a patch is dependent on its absorption, and the next patch should always be applied to a different site. When first applying a transdermal medication, expect 12 to 24 hours (for fentanyl) and up to 3 days (for buprenorphine) until a therapeutic level is absorbed; also, when discontinuing expect a similar decline in level because of the medication reservoir in the skin. If the person complains of severe light-headedness, is pale, sweaty and weak, the medical officer needs to be informed immediately and the patch removed.

INTRAMUSCULAR INJECTION Intramuscular injection was once the most popular route for pain medication administration. Its disadvantages include uneven absorption from the muscle (resulting in delayed respiratory depression), discomfort on administration, and the time needed to prepare and administer the medication. It is also recognised that the quality of analgesia is inferior to that of intravenous patient-controlled analgesia.

INTRAVENOUS ROUTE The intravenous (IV) route provides the most rapid onset, usually ranging from 1 to 15 minutes. Medication can be given by drip, bolus or person-controlled analgesia (PCA)—a pump with a control mechanism that affords the person self-management of pain. The advantages of PCA are dose precision, timeliness and convenience. The person does not have to wait for a nurse to assess the need for pain medication, then procure and deliver the analgesia (Cooney & Quinlan-Colwell, 2020). Respiratory depression and sedation are minimised when plasma levels of opioids are steady (Burchum & Rosenthal, 2021). Several drugs are available for this route. The disadvantages are the nursing care needed for any intravenous line, the potential for infection, the cost of disposable supplies and ensuring that only the actual patient presses the PCA button. For this reason, the PCA method of administration requires careful education coupled with close and attentive monitoring.

SUBCUTANEOUS ROUTE The subcutaneous (SC) route is accepted; its disadvantages are similar to those of the intramuscular route.

EPIDURAL ROUTE The epidural route is invasive and requires more extensive nursing care but it may provide better analgesia and postoperative recovery than intravenous delivery. When opioids are inserted into the epidural space they are usually combined with local anaesthetics. This mixture can be given as an infusion or as a 'top-up'. When this combination of drugs is used the person experiences better analgesia, earlier bowel recovery, earlier mobility and a shorter length of hospital stay than with the intravenous route (ANZCA, 2020). Nursing implications for the person receiving PCA are discussed later in this chapter.

INTRATHECAL ROUTE The intrathecal route involves the placement of drugs (usually opioids, local anaesthetics or both) into the cerebrospinal fluid. When medication is inserted into the intrathecal space, it is usually as a single injection, and much smaller doses are required compared to the epidural route.

REGIONAL ANALGESIA Regional analgesia is commonly known as 'a nerve block'. Nerve blocks use local anaesthetics (sometimes in combination with a steroidal drug, depending on the situation) injected into or near a nerve, usually in an area between the nociceptor and the dorsal root. In the post-operative situation, nerve blocks can be either a single-shot injection or run as a continuous peripheral nerve block infusion (CPNB). When a CPNB is ordered, strict protocols, procedures and standards must be adhered to so as to ensure safety.

In the persistent-pain setting the procedure may be performed to determine the precise location of the source of the pain: pain relief indicates that the injection site is the source of the pain. Temporary nerve blocks may give the person enough relief to:

- develop a more hopeful attitude that pain relief is possible
- allow local procedures to be performed without causing discomfort
- exercise and move the affected part.

If the nerve block is successful, a permanent neurolytic agent can be used to give long-term analgesia.

SURGERY As an analgesic measure, surgery is usually performed only after all other methods have failed. Those who need this measure should understand possible risks such as reduced motor function or incontinences. Surgical procedures used to relieve pain are shown in Figure 8.8 and include the following:

- A *rhizotomy* is destruction of the dorsal spinal roots. It is most often performed to relieve back/neck pain. A rhizotomy can be performed by a spinal or neurosurgeon: the nerve fibres are surgically severed. Rhizotomies may also be performed by a pain specialist who injects a chemical, or uses a radiofrequency current or cryotherapy, to selectively destroy painful fibres. These types of rhizotomy are called percutaneous and usually offer temporary pain relief.
- A *sympathectomy* involves blocking the ganglia of sympathetic nerves, usually in the lumbar region, often with local anaesthetic or surgery. The sympathetic nerves play an important role in producing and transmitting the sensation of pain.
- A *cordotomy* is an incision into the anterolateral tracts of the spinal cord to interrupt the transmission of pain. Because it is difficult to isolate the nerves responsible for upper body pain, this surgery is most often performed for pain in the abdominal region and legs, including severe pain from terminal cancer. A percutaneous cordotomy produces lesions of the anterolateral surface of the spinal cord by means of a radiofrequency current.
- A *neurectomy* is the removal of a nerve. It is sometimes used for pain relief. A peripheral neurectomy is the severing of a nerve at any point distal to the spinal cord.

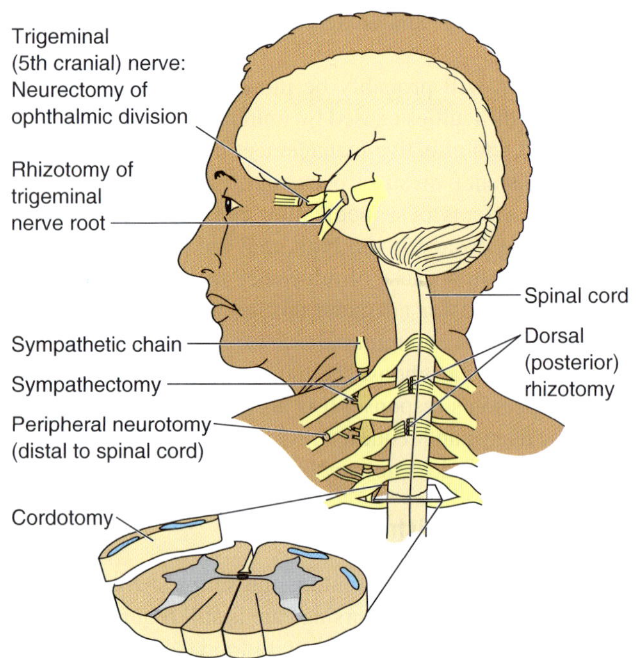

FIGURE 8.8 ***Surgical procedures are used to treat severe pain that does not respond to other types of management. They include cordotomy, neurectomy, sympathectomy and rhizotomy***

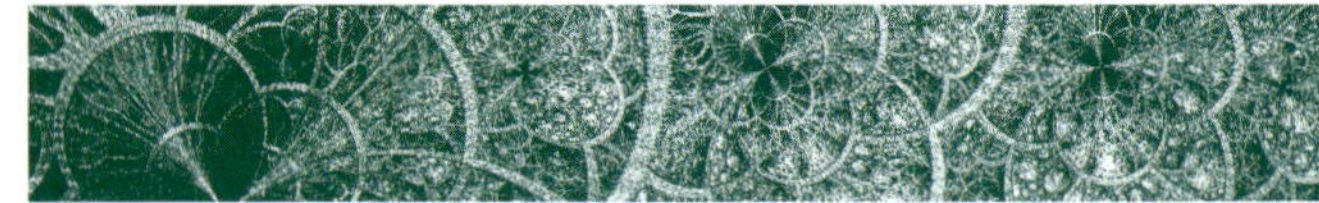

Nursing care

Assessment

Nursing assessment of the person with pain presents perhaps more of a challenge than almost any other type of illness or injury because of the subjectivity of pain and the effects it has on the individual.

A comprehensive approach to pain assessment is essential to ensure adequate and appropriate interventions. The five assessment areas are: (1) health history, (2) physiological response, (3) examination, (4) behavioural response, and (5) response to treatment.

1. Health history

Before commencing an in-depth assessment, discuss:

- The definition of the word 'pain' to ensure that the person and the nurse are communicating on the same level. It is often helpful to use the person's own words when describing the pain. For example, the person may talk about discomfort as opposed to pain.
- Explain that the report of pain is important for promoting recovery, not just for achieving temporary comfort.
- Ask the person to establish a comfort-function goal. This is a level of pain that does not interfere with or prevent the performance of essential activities of recovery or living. The person's history of the pain can be assessed by using the PQRST technique (Jarvis, Jarvis & Botti, 2021):
  P = What precipitated (triggered, stimulated) the pain? Has anything relieved the pain? What is the pattern of the pain (constant, episodic)?
  Q = What are the qualities of the pain? How would you describe the pain (sharp, stabbing, aching, burning, stinging, deep, crushing, vice-like, gnawing)?
  R = What is the region (location) of the pain? Can you put your finger on where the pain is? Does the pain radiate to other areas of the body?
  S = What is the severity or intensity of the pain?
  T = What is the timing of the pain? When does it begin, how long does it last and how is it related to other events in the person's life?
- What precipitated (triggered, stimulated, makes it worse) the pain? What palliates (what makes it better, has anything relieved) the pain? What is the pattern of the pain?
- What are the quality and quantity of the pain? Is it sharp, stabbing, aching, burning, stinging, deep, crushing, vice-like, gnawing? A reliable indicator of the presence and degree of pain is the person's own statement about the pain. The McGill Pain Questionnaire is a useful tool in assessing the person's subjective experience of the pain. It asks the person to locate the pain, to describe the quality of the pain, to indicate how the pain changes with time and to rate the intensity of the pain. (see Table 8.3).
- What is the region (location) of the pain? Does the pain radiate to other areas of the body?
- What is the timing of the pain? When does it begin, how long does it last (continuous or intermittent) and how is it related to other events in the person's life?
- What is the severity of the pain? The most common method to assess the severity of pain is a pain rating scale. Several scales are illustrated in Figure 8.9.

If you are caring for the person with an established persistent pain condition in an acute care setting, remember to ask what their normal pain score is when they are managing their life in the community. It is not unusual for those with a persistent pain condition to give higher pain scores.

- For the person who does not understand English or numerals, a scale using colours (e.g. light blue no pain through to bright red worst possible pain) or pain faces may be helpful. Often pain assessment is made while a person is sedentary. In this state the person may experience less pain than when active and falsely estimate tolerable pain ratings. Provide guidelines for setting goals.

The following nursing interventions will help the nurse assess for pain using a pain rating scale:

- Ensure consistent communication. Explain the specific pain rating scale used. If a word descriptor scale is used, verify that the person can read the language being used. If a numerical scale is used, be sure the person can count to 10. If the person is not able to report pain because of communication difficulties, intubation, emotional disturbances or cognitive impairments, monitor the manifestations of pain by taking vital signs, assessing skin temperature and moisture, observing pupils, observing facial expressions, position in bed, guarding of body parts and restlessness. Autonomic responses to pain may result in increased blood pressure, tachycardia, rapid respirations and perspiration and dilated pupils. Other responses to pain include grimacing, clenching the hands, muscle rigidity, guarding, restlessness and nausea. The person with chronic pain may have a blunted affect.
- Be sure the person is able to report pain. Cognitive impairment challenges this ability and bespoke assessment strategies are needed (Cascella et al., 2019).

The following nursing interventions will help the nurse assess for pain using other measures:

- Look for indicators of pain, such as grimacing, restlessness, rubbing, stillness, verbal or non-verbal vocalisations and holding on to an object tightly.

TABLE 8.3 Pain questionnaires in common use

PAIN QUESTIONNAIRE	FOCUS OF ASSESSMENT
McGill Pain Questionnaire (Melzack, 1975)	Subjective descriptors of pain
Revised Oswestry Disability Questionnaire (RODQ) (Page et al., 2001)	Assessment specific to back pain
Leeds Assessment of Neuropathic Symptoms and Signs (LANSS) (Bennett, 2001)	For use in patients with chronic persisting pain; allows for sensory descriptions of pain
Brief Pain Inventory (BPI) (Atkinson et al., 2011)	Focuses on patient outcomes related to pain intensity and pain interference

**Note*: all pain questionnaires identified in the table are in current use and are commonly used across a variety of settings. Other pain questionnaires exist.

NURSING CARE PLAN A person receiving patient-controlled analgesia

Patient-controlled analgesia (PCA) is used to manage moderate to severe pain. Specialised lockable infusion pumps are used to control the delivery of intravenous analgesia, most commonly opioid medications such as morphine or fentanyl. A push button device is attached to the infusion pump that, when pressed by the patient, administers a prescribed bolus of medication. Alternatively, PCA pumps can be set to provide a continuous background infusion, with the bolus dose used (by the patient) as additional breakthrough analgesia.

PCA is frequently used in the management of acute and acute postoperative pain but has also been used for short-term management of chronic pain. The use of this delivery method improves patient autonomy by giving the patient an element of control over the administration of analgesia, reducing waiting times for pain relief, but also, in many instances, reducing the ultimate amount of analgesia used by the patient. A lockout timing mechanism is built into PCA protocols to reduce risk of harm, most specifically from over-use of the medications. This mechanism prevents the patient from receiving another dose of medication within a specified timeframe from the last dose administered. As opioids are usually used, the medication order includes guidelines for the implementation of clinical review, or a rapid response review in the instance of an acute change in the patient's condition. Additionally, a standing order for the administration of naloxone (to reverse opioid overdose) is commonly prescribed.

NURSING CARE

- Familiarise yourself with the appropriate facility policies, guidelines and documentation. This may include a requirement to complete formal competency assessment before you are permitted to provide nursing care related to PCA.
- Assess the capacity of the patient to use PCA appropriately and effectively. Ensure the patient has:
  - the cognitive capacity to understand the correct use of PCA
  - the physical capacity to use PCA effectively
  - consented to use of PCA as a pain management approach.
- Ensure the medication order is correct, legible and includes all of the necessary details.
- Ensure the patient has patent and secure intravenous access.
- Provide appropriate supplemental oxygen therapy.
- Obtain and prepare medication (syringe or pre-mixed bag) as per facility policy.
- Provide patient education:
  - Explain the correct use of the PCA pump and familiarise the patient with the equipment.
  - Explain the in-built lockout period (and how this reduces the risk of accidental overdose), bolus dose mechanism and background infusion (if prescribed).
  - Clearly explain that only the patient is to press the PCA button (to reduce risk of accidental opioid overdose).
  - Discuss potential adverse effects of the medication/s, and signs and symptoms the patient must be aware of.
  - Discuss general safety considerations associated with attachment to an intravenous pump for example, restricted mobilisation.
  - Explain the ongoing monitoring nursing staff will conduct.
- Conduct monitoring of the patient and the PCA infusion as per facility policy. This will commonly include hourly monitoring of respiratory status, pain score, sedation score, supplemental oxygen therapy rate, bolus doses attempted and delivered, background infusion (if applicable) and total amount of medication administered.
- Liaise with the multidisciplinary team for discontinuation of PCA when appropriate.

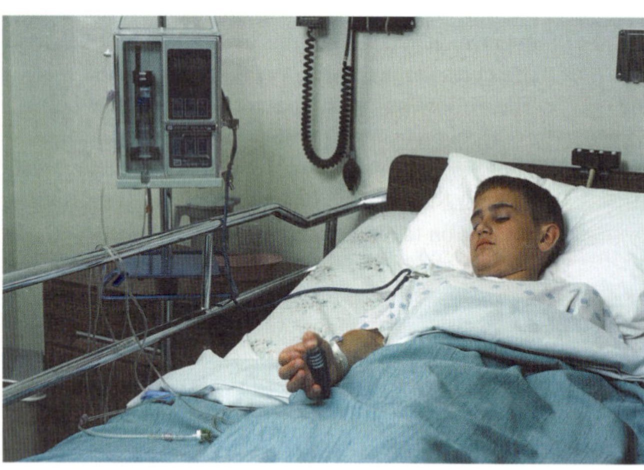

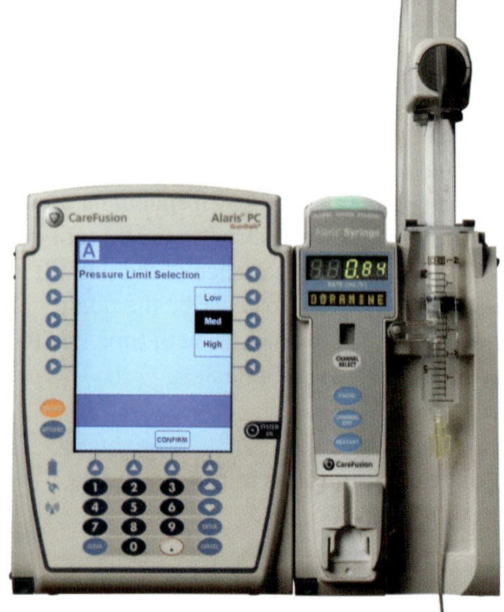

PCA units allow the person to self-manage severe pain. The units may be portable or mounted on intravenous poles

Source: *Left*, © Roy Ramsey/Pearson Education; *right*, courtesy and © Becton, Dickinson and Company.

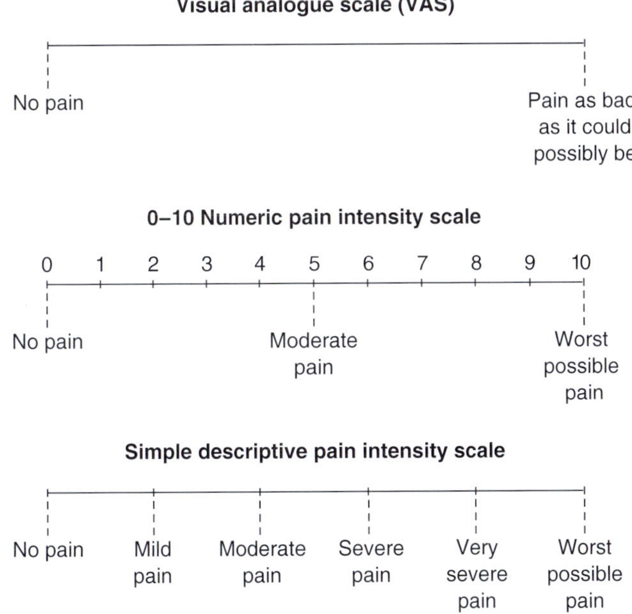

FIGURE 8.9 ***Examples of commonly used pain scales***

- Pain has been shown to increase adverse behaviours such as wandering, carer resistance, socially inappropriate behaviours and delusional thoughts. Ensure pain is considered as part of the assessment of all aged care residents (Tosato et al., 2012).
- Ask a family member or caregiver, if they suspect the person has pain, to serve as a proxy pain rating.

2. Physiological response

When the body experiences acute pain, the stress response is initiated. This metabolic response releases neuroendocrine hormones systemically and a local release of cytokines at the injury site. Surgical stimuli that cause pain can influence the sympathetic efferent nerves, causing an increase in myocardial oxygen demand, influencing heart rate and blood pressure. Gastric motility is often reduced, so the potential for a paralytic ileus can develop. Injury/surgery to the upper abdominal or the thoracic area can cause difficulty in coughing, which can result in reduced functional residual capacity. If this persists, then ventilation perfusion problems can occur.

For those suffering with persistent pain, loss of muscle mass and physical deconditioning can occur. As these symptoms continue, movement restrictions develop, and insomnia, fatigue and a change in appetite may occur.

3. Examination

Examination of the person should include observation, auscultation, palpation and percussion of the sensitive areas. The doctor will also undertake a physical assessment that does not cause any undue pain. Discuss the person's normal ability to perform activities of daily living and how this acute or chronic condition has affected this. Observe for pain behaviours and non-verbal clues such as facial expression and body language.

Assess the effect the pain has on the person's sleep pattern. Note any pre-existing medical or pain conditions that could influence the person's current condition. Investigations ordered by the medical staff should assist in confirming clinical impressions.

4. Behavioural response

It is essential to assess the person's response to any treatment given for pain. If you give a medication for pain relief, go back and *assess* its effectiveness, especially with respect to functional abilities. The person's satisfaction must also be noted in response to their pain treatments, whether a treatment helped, had no effect on, or increased their pain. Meticulous documentation is critical as future pain regimens may be based on this.

5. Responses to treatment

Some behaviours are so typical of people in pain that the behaviours are referred to as pain behaviours. They include bracing or guarding the painful part, taking medication, crying, moaning, grimacing, withdrawing from activity and socialisation, becoming immobile, talking about pain, holding the painful area, breathing with increased effort, exhibiting a sad facial expression and being restless.

Behavioural responses to pain may or may not coincide with the person's report of pain and are not reliable cues to the pain experience. For example, one person may rate pain at an 8 on a 0–10 scale (where 0 = no pain and 10 = worst imaginable) while laughing or walking down the hall, while another may deny pain completely but be reluctant to move and grimace or moan. Denial of pain may be for a variety of reasons, including fear of injections, fear of drug addiction, misinterpretation of terms (the person may not think that aching, soreness or discomfort qualify as pain) or the belief that healthcare providers alone decide when a person is experiencing pain. Some may deny pain as part of an attempt to deny that there is something wrong with them. Others, by contrast, may think that 'as-needed' medications will be given only if their pain rating is high. Discrepancies between the person's report of pain and behavioural responses may be influenced by certain factors—for example, sociocultural factors, emotional state, knowledge, past experiences and age, and relaxation or distraction techniques.

SELF-MANAGEMENT OF PAIN The person's attempts to manage pain are useful additions to the assessment database. This information is individualised and specific to each person; it includes many factors such as culture, age and knowledge. Obtain detailed descriptions of actions the person or significant others used, and when and how these measures were applied and how well they worked.

CONSIDERATION FOR PRACTICE

Do not assume that the older person or the person with a cognitive impairment is not experiencing pain or is unable to identify its intensity.

Nursing diagnoses and interventions

Acute or persistent pain

Assess the characteristics of the pain by asking the person to:

- Point to the pain location or mark the pain location on a figure drawing. *Pain location provides information about the aetiology of the pain and the type of pain being experienced.*
- Rate the intensity of the pain at rest and during movement by using a pain scale (1 to 10, with 10 being the worst pain ever experienced), a visual analogue scale (a scale on which pain is marked on a continuum from no pain to severe pain), or with word descriptors (such as the McGill Pain Questionnaire, and mild, moderate or severe). Use the same scale with each assessment. *The intensity of pain is a subjective experience. The perception of the intensity of pain is affected by the person's degree of concentration or distraction, state of consciousness and expectations.*
- Describe the quality of the pain. For example, say to the person: 'Describe what your pain feels like.' If necessary, provide word descriptors for the person to select from. *Descriptive terms provide insight into the nature and perception of the pain. In addition, the location and type of pain (e.g. acute versus persistent) affect the quality.*
- Describe the pattern of the pain, including time of onset, duration, persistence and times without pain. It is also important to ask whether the pain is worse at regular times of the day and whether it has any relationship to activity. *The pattern of pain provides clues about cause and location.*
- Describe any precipitating or relieving factors. *Precipitating factors include sleep deficits, anxiety, temperature extremes, excessive noise, anxiety, fear, depression and activity.*
- Describe the meaning of the pain, including its effects on lifestyle, self-concept, roles and relationships. *The person with acute pain may believe the pain is a normal response to injury, or that it signals serious illness and death. Pain is a stressor that may affect the person's ability to cope effectively. The person with persistent pain may have concerns about addiction to pain medication, cost, social interactions, sexual activity and relationships with significant others.*
- Monitor manifestations of pain by assessing skin temperature and moisture; observing pupils; observing facial expressions, position in bed and guarding of body parts; and noting restlessness. *Autonomic responses to pain may result in increased blood pressure, tachycardia, rapid respirations, perspiration and dilated pupils. Other responses to pain include grimacing, clenching the hands, muscle rigidity, guarding, restlessness and nausea. The person with persistent pain may have a blunted, flat affect with a tired facial appearance. (Remember, if the person has persistent pain, vital signs may not be increased.)*
- Acknowledge the person's pain by verbally recognising the presence of the pain, listen carefully to the description of pain, and act to help the person manage the pain. *Because pain is a personal, subjective experience, the nurse must convey belief in the person's pain. By doing so, the nurse reduces the person's anxiety and thereby lessens their pain.* See the 'Translation to practice' box.
- Provide optimal pain relief with prescribed analgesics, determining the preferred route of administration. Provide pain-relieving measures for severe pain on a regular around-the-clock basis or by self-administration (such as with a PCA pump). *The person is part of the decision-making process and can exert some control over the situation by choosing the administration route. Analgesics are usually most effective when they are administered before pain occurs or becomes severe. Around-the-clock administration has been proven to provide better pain management for both acute and persistent pain. Do not crush or break, or allow the person to chew, controlled-release oral preparations; a dose meant to be slowly absorbed that is absorbed rapidly may lead to a toxic overdose and death.*
- Evaluate and monitor the effects of analgesics and other pain-relieving measures and teach family members or significant others to be alert for adverse reactions to pain medications. Sedation, constipation, nausea and dizziness are common side effects. *Excessive sedation can progress to significant respiratory depression. Oxygen saturation should be checked regularly. Protocols will vary within your institution. Prevent falls that may result from sedation or dizziness. If the person has symptoms of excessive opioid dosage, antidotes are available. Naloxone is used for opioid overdose. Titrate naloxone slowly. Never push an entire dose all at once. Administer only enough naloxone to eliminate adverse effects such as respiratory depression or excessive sedation. If excessive naloxone is administered, the person may experience acute withdrawal and will have no pain relief. It may take considerable time to re-establish a therapeutic comfort level.*
- Determine the level of sedation the person will tolerate. *For those with persistent pain or cancer pain who need high doses of opioids, sedation may interfere with quality of life and neither the person nor the family want them to be sedated.* Several classes of drugs can be used to counteract sedation. They are usually given in the morning so that they will not interfere with night sleep. Amphetamines, especially methylphenidate (Ritalin), is the most commonly used; modafinil (Modavigil) has been used for several years; and donepezil (Aricept), which is used for the symptoms of Alzheimer's disease, reduces sedation and fatigue (MIMS, 2022).

TRANSLATION TO PRACTICE Barriers and facilitators to effective pain management

Pain, pain assessment and pain management have been investigated extensively. Pharmacological and non-pharmacological interventions, the importance of patient autonomy in pain management, validation of pain assessment tools and the subjectiveness of pain experiences have been explored in depth. Yet, in practice, pain management interventions still demonstrate inconsistent effectiveness. Translating research evidence to practice is difficult and requires careful consideration of the barriers and facilitators to implementation.

Two recently published systematic reviews (one of the highest levels of research evidence) identified common barriers and facilitators to effective pain management. Mala, Forster and Kain (2021) explored nurse and midwife competence in providing pain management for neonatal patients. Likewise, Rababa, Al-Sabbah and Hayajneh (2021) investigated pain assessment and management, but with critical care patients.

Similarities were evident in both studies, including:

- lack of knowledge about, or underuse of, pain assessment tools (barrier)
- absence of, or limitations in, standardised guidelines/protocols (barrier)
- adequate and ongoing training in pain assessment/management (facilitator)
- parent/patient involvement in pain assessment (facilitator)
- team approaches, collaboration and effective team communication (facilitator).

Additionally, Mala et al. (2021) identified clear evidence-based guidelines and appropriate use of pain assessment tools as facilitators and the level of personal and professional experience with pain management as a barrier. For Rababa et al. (2021), the critical care patients' inability to communicate was highlighted as a barrier.

The studies highlight two key points for the novice practitioner. First, commonality in pain management exists regardless of the clinical context. Therefore, ongoing education, effective communication within teams that includes the patient/family, the appropriate use of recognised pain assessment tools and clear, robust guidelines on pain management can improve clinical practice regardless of the clinical context. Second, there are always contextual differences across the diverse clinical landscape that must be accounted for. Therefore, the ability of the nurse to tailor pain assessment and management skills to suit their unique practice context is a critical skill to develop.

CRITICAL THINKING IN PERSON-CENTRED CARE

1 Reflect on your own experiences with pain. Evaluate how these experiences help or hinder your assessments and interventions for a person in pain.
2 You are caring for a young man who has multiple injuries from a motorcycle accident. He tells you his pain is so bad that he just wants to die. Describe and explain how you would respond, and why.
3 You are caring for an 80-year-old man with diabetes who has had his left foot amputated for gangrene. He is restless and moaning. Another nurse tells you to give only one-half of the ordered dose of opioids because 'he is old and there is a danger of respiratory depression'. Assess this nurse's suggested intervention and explain how you would handle this situation.
4 Nurses tend to underestimate and under-medicate pain.' Discuss this statement using recent published research.

- Teach the person and family non-pharmacological methods of pain management, such as relaxation, distraction and cutaneous stimulation. *These techniques are especially useful when used in conjunction with pain medications and may also be useful in managing persistent pain.*
- Provide comfort measures, such as changing position, massage, oral care, skin care and changing bed linen. *Basic comfort measures for personal cleanliness, skin care and mobility promote physical and psychosocial wellbeing, lessening the perception of pain.*

NURSING CARE PLAN A person with persistent pain

Susan Akers, aged 37, is currently being seen at an outpatient clinic for persistent non-malignant pain. She works at a local paper factory. She has a 3-year history of neck and shoulder pain that usually is accompanied by headaches. She believes the pain is related to lifting objects at work, but it is now precipitated by activities of daily living. Susan is absent from work approximately three times a month and states that the absences are due to her pain and headaches. She has been seeking care in the local emergency department on an average of twice monthly for injections for pain. She takes Panadeine Forte and Valium as needed (usually 3 or 4 times a day). Susan is divorced and has two teenage children. She states that she has several friends in the area, but her parents and siblings live interstate.

ASSESSMENT

During the nursing history, Susan rates her pain during an acute episode as a 7 on a 1 to 10 scale. She states that lifting objects and moving her hands and arms above shoulder level causes sharp pain. The pain never really goes away, but it does decrease with upper extremity rest. She says that when she lifts a lot at work, she has difficulty sleeping that night. She takes two Panadeine Forte tablets every 4 hours when the pain is severe, but does not get complete relief. The medical officer diagnoses muscular pain.

(continued)

NURSING CARE PLAN A person with persistent pain (continued)

DIAGNOSIS

- *Persistent pain* related to muscle inflammation resulting from repetitive movement and lifting of heavy objects manifested by pain on movement that lessens at rest and in response to analgesia.

PLANNING

After negotiating expected outcomes and intervention techniques, opioid analgesia and distraction techniques are to be used during the acute phase of management. Non-opioid analgesia is to be used after the acute phase and review of the work environment is to be undertaken.

Expected outcomes

- Return for follow-up visits with a journal of activities and pain experiences.
- After 3 to 5 days on regularly scheduled doses of pain medication, report a decrease in the level of pain from 7 to 3 or 4 on a 1 to 10 scale.
- Decreased number of absences from work.
- Modify activities at work and at home, especially when pain is intense.

IMPLEMENTATION

- Encourage discussion of pain and acknowledge belief in Susan's report of pain.
- Consult with a doctor for a non-opioid analgesic with a minimum of side effects and instruct in maintaining regular dosing schedules.
- For episodes of acute pain, take opioid analgesics as soon as the pain begins and every 4 hours, while continuing the dosage of non-opioid analgesic.
- Teach one relaxation technique that is personally useful.
- Explore distraction techniques such as listening to music, watching comedies or reading.
- Provide contact phone number and instruct to call if pain is unrelieved with narcotic and non-opioid analgesics.

EVALUATION

Susan returns for scheduled follow-up visits with a completed journal of her activities and associated pain. She reports that taking oral opioid analgesics has relieved her pain and that within 3 weeks non-opioid analgesics have brought her pain under control. She also reports that her supervisor has reassigned her to a position that requires no lifting. She now rates her pain at 2 or 3 on a 1 to 10 scale. She has missed only 1 day of work in the last 3 months and reports that her children and friends have helped with her household tasks when she has requested they do so.

CRITICAL THINKING IN THE NURSING PROCESS

1. Describe three factors that support the statement 'Pain is a personal experience.'
2. Susan asks you how often she should take her pain medications. Do you tell her to (a) take them on a regular basis, or (b) wait until she experiences pain? Which action would you choose, and why?
3. Susan is at risk of constipation. Why, and what information would you provide?

REFLECTION ON THE NURSING PROCESS

1. What have you learned from the case study that you will apply to your clinical practice?
2. If someone is non-adherent with the negotiated care plan and returns to the pain clinic with continued discomfort, consider some of the reasons this non-adherence may have occurred.

- Provide person and family education, and make referrals if necessary to assist with coping, such as financial support services and home care. *The person (and family) with pain requires information about medications, non-invasive techniques for pain management and sources of assistance with home-based care. The person with acute pain requires information about the expected course of pain resolution.*

Community-based care

Educate the person, family and significant others regarding:

- specific medications to be taken, including the frequency, potential side effects, possible interactions and any special precautions to be taken (such as taking with food or avoiding alcohol)
- how to take or administer the medication (see Table 8.4)

TABLE 8.4 Providing long-term analgesia at home

ROUTE	DRUG	NURSING IMPLICATIONS
Oral	Oxycodone	Available in a slow-release formulation for 12-hour dosing (Oxycontin) and as fast-acting formulations (Endone or Endone elixir) for breakthrough pain.
Oral	Morphine	Formulated as slow-release particles in a capsule (Kapanol). If the person cannot swallow the capsule, it may be sprinkled over food or given by gastric tube. Morphine can also be given as a slow-release tablet (MsContin) or as immediate-release preparations either as a tablet (Anamorph) or capsule (Sevredol) or an elixir (Ordine).
Transdermal	Fentanyl	A patch absorbed slowly through the skin (Durogesic, Fenpatch, Denpax); allows 72-hour dose schedule. Takes up to 12 hours to achieve therapeutic level; when discontinued, therapeutic effect will decay slowly. A lozenge formulation fentanyl citrate (Actiq, Abstral) absorbed through the buccal cavity can be used to treat breakthrough cancer pain in opioid-tolerant people.

- the importance of taking analgesics before the pain becomes severe
- an explanation that the risk of addiction to analgesics is very small when they are used appropriately for pain relief
- the importance of scheduling periods of rest and sleep.

In addition, suggest the following resources:

- pain clinics
- community support groups
- International Association for the Study of Pain (IASP)
- Australian Pain Society (APS)
- Cancer Council Australia.

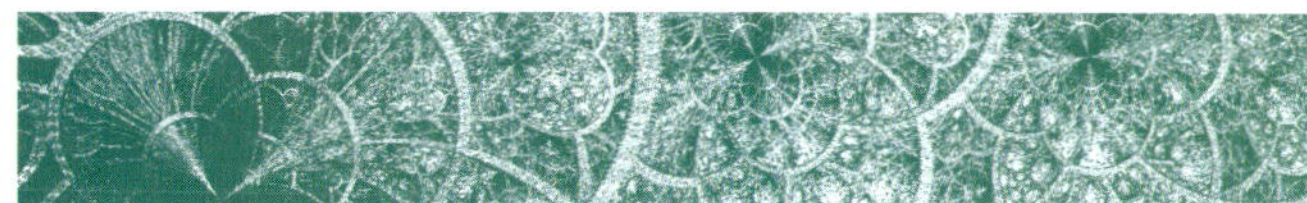

CHAPTER HIGHLIGHTS

- Pain is perceived in the central nervous system. Opioids, and other analgesics, block the perception of pain; NSAIDs and most non-pharmacological interventions block or decrease the transmission of pain from the periphery to the CNS. Measures to block the sensitisation of pain-transmitting fibres can be used prior to painful procedures.
- There are many types of pain, and treatment varies according to the type and combination of types. Acute pain usually decreases as healing progresses; persistent pain has acute exacerbations and compounds acute pain. Breakthrough pain is recognised as an increase in pain intensity that occurs when the peak and duration of medications are reached. Procedural pain occurs in relation to a change or increase in activity. Central pain results from CNS lesions. Phantom pain occurs after amputation, seeming to originate in the missing body part.
- Myths and misconceptions exist about pain and its management. The person's perceived cause of pain and the best self-care method to relieve pain provide pertinent assessment information.
- People's response to pain is influenced by their emotional state, past experiences with pain and the meaning they attribute to the experience of pain. The person with a diagnosis of malignancy or a poor prognosis may have an interpretation of pain that is significantly different from the person experiencing temporary states such as curative surgery or labour and childbirth.
- Older adults perceive pain as intensely as younger adults. The dosages of opioids they may need is variable, as older adults may have difficulty metabolising or eliminating medications.
- Assertively assess pain in the older person. Older adults may hesitate to report pain for fear of losing independence or being considered a nuisance. Cognitive impairment makes self-report of pain less available. Behavioural scales for assessing pain are useful when the person cannot give a self-report.
- Addiction is believed to be a neurophysiological disease, heavily influenced by social determinants of health. The person with addiction to opioids may need greater doses of opioids to control pain because of the tolerance they may have developed through usage.
- Pain management includes assessment, planning, intervention and evaluation. It is important to verify that interventions have been effective. If not, interventions must be identified that bring pain down to a level of intensity with which the person feels satisfied.

CONCEPT CHECK

1 Which of the following statements suggests a misconception of pain?

1 It is best to wait until a person has pain before giving medication.
2 Anxiety can cause pain and pain can cause anxiety.
3 Pethidine is no longer recommended for postoperative pain.
4 The rationale for use of a TENS unit is supported by the gate-control theory.

2 You are taking a health history for a person who has taken a NSAID for several years. What would be an appropriate question to ask?

1 'Do you understand what this drug could do to you?'
2 'Have you ever vomited blood or had very dark stools?'
3 'Do you know that you may become addicted to this drug?'
4 'Have you noticed any problems with your breathing?'

3 You are replacing a transdermal analgesic patch. Where on the body would you place it?

1 on one side of the buttocks
2 below the navel, midline on the abdomen
3 on the anterior thigh
4 on the upper torso

4 Which of the following statements would be most useful in determining the quality of a person's pain?

1 'Tell me where you hurt.'
2 'Rate your pain on a scale of 0 to 10.'
3 'Describe what your pain feels like.'
4 'Tell me how this pain affects your sleep.'

5 The person has orders for intravenous patient-controlled analgesia (PCA). The following principles are true, except:

1 basal doses are continuous
2 overdose cannot occur
3 a 10-minute lockout each hour allows six bolus doses
4 unused bolus doses cannot accumulate

6 The most common side effects of opioid analgesics are:

1 anuria, diplopia and cough
2 constipation, nausea and sedation
3 pruritus, constipation and hallucinations
4 dysphagia, fever and gastritis

7 The preferred route of opioid administration for persistent pain is:

1 transdermal
2 oral
3 intravenous
4 rectal

8 The equivalent dose of an oral drug compared to the intravenous preparation of the same drug:
1 is equal dosage
2 is twice the intravenous dose
3 varies according to the medication
4 is one-half the intravenous dose

9 People treated for persistent pain may need additional pain management strategies for:
1 breakthrough pain
2 acute pain
3 end-of-dose pain
4 all of the above

BIBLIOGRAPHY

Anekar, A. A. & Cascella, M. (2022). *WHO analgesic ladder*. Retrieved from https://www.ncbi.nlm.nih.gov/

Arthur, L. & Rolan, P. (2019). A systematic review of western medicine's understanding of pain experience, expression, assessment, and management for Australian Aboriginal and Torres Strait Islander Peoples. *Pain Reports*, *4*(6), e764–e764. https://doi.org/10.1097/PR9.0000000000000764

Atkinson, T. M., Rosenfeld, B. D., Sit, L. et al. (2011). Using confirmatory factor analysis to evaluate construct validity of the Brief Pain Inventory (BPI). *Journal of Pain and Symptom Management*, *41*(3), 558–565.

Australian and New Zealand College of Anaesthetists and Faculty of Pain Medicine (ANZCA) (2020). *Acute pain management: Scientific evidence* (5th ed.). Melbourne: Australian and New Zealand College of Anaesthetists.

Australian Commission on Safety and Quality in Health Care (ACSQHC) (2021). *National Safety and Quality Health Standards* (2nd ed.). Sydney: ACSQHC.

Australian Institute of Health and Welfare (AIHW) (2022). *Australia's health 2022*. Retrieved from https://www.aihw.gov.au/

Balasubramanian, S. (2021). Pain—Definition and classification. In T. Vasu, S. Balasubramanian, M. Kodivalasa & P. M. Ingle, *Chronic pain management*. TFM Publishing. ISBN 9781910079928.

Bennett, M. (2001). The LANSS Pain Scale: The Leeds Assessment of Neuropathic Symptoms and Signs. *Pain*, *92*(1–2), 147–157.

Brown, D., Edwards, H., Seaton, L. & Buckley, T. (2020). *Lewis's medical–surgical nursing: Assessment and management of clinical problems* (5th ANZ ed.). Chatswood, NSW: Mosby Elsevier Australia.

Bryant, B., Knights, K., Darroch, S. & Rowland, A. (2019). *Pharmacology for health professionals* (5th ed.). Chatswood, NSW: Elsevier Australia.

Bullock, L., Bedson, J., Jordan, J. L., Bartlam, B., Chew-Graham, C. A. & Campbell, P. (2019). Pain assessment and pain treatment for community-dwelling people with dementia: A systematic review and narrative synthesis. *International Journal of Geriatric Psychiatry*, *34*(6), 807–821. https://doi.org/10.1002/gps.5078

Burchum, J. & Rosenthal, L. D. (2021). *Lehne's pharmacology for nursing care* (11th ed.). Elsevier US Evolve.

Cascella, M., Bimonte, S., Saettini, F. & Muzio, M. R. (2019). The challenge of pain assessment in children with cognitive disabilities: Features and clinical applicability of different observational tools. *Journal of Paediatrics and Child Health*, *55*(2), 129–135. https://doi.org/10.1111/jpc.14230

Cooney, M. F. & Quinlan-Colwell, A. (2020). *Assessment and multimodal management of pain: An integrative approach*. Philadelphia: Elsevier.

Crisp, J., Douglas, C., Rebeiro, G. & Waters, D. (2020). *Potter and Perry's fundamentals of nursing* (6th ANZ ed.). Chatswood, NSW: Mosby Elsevier Australia.

Dementia Australia (2022). *What is good care?* Retrieved from https://www.dementia.org.au/

Eliopoulos, E. (2021). *Gerontological nursing* (10th ed.). Philadelphia: Wolters Kluwer/Lippincott Williams & Wilkins.

Fitzgerald, S., Tripp, H. & Halksworth-Smith, G. (2017). Assessment and management of acute pain in older people: Barriers and facilitators to nursing practice. *Australian Journal of Advanced Nursing*, *35*(1), 48–57.

Foote, J. M. (2019). Communication, physical, and developmental assessment of the child and family. In M. J. Hockenberry, D. Wilson & C. C. Rodgers (eds), *Wong's nursing care of infants and children* (11th ed.). St Louis, MO: Elsevier.

Gorito, V., Monjardino, T., Azevedo, I. & Lucas, R. (2022). Potentially unrecognised pain in children: Population-based birth cohort study at 7 years of age. *Journal of Paediatrics and Child Health*, *58*(3), 474–480. https://doi.org/10.1111/jpc.15749

Hadley, G. & Novitch, M. B. (2021). CBT and CFT for chronic pain. *Current Pain and Headache Reports*, *25*(5), 35. https://doi.org/10.1007/s11916-021-00948-1

Haight, E. S., Huck, N. A., Jordan, C. E. & Tawfik, V. L. (2021). Complex regional pain syndrome: An introduction. In E. F. Lawson & J. P. Castellanos (eds), *Complex regional pain syndrome*. Cham: Springer. https://doi.org/10.1007/978-3-030-75373-3_1

Hruschak, V., Flowers, K. M., Azizoddin, D. R., Jamison, R. N., Edwards, R. R. & Schreiber, K. L. (2021). Cross-sectional study of psychosocial and pain-related variables among patients with chronic pain during a time of social distancing imposed by the coronavirus disease 2019 pandemic. *Pain*, *162*(2), 619–629. https://doi.org/10.1097/j.pain.0000000000002128

Hudson, J., Lake, E., Soruit, E. et al. (2021). Comprehensive rehabilitation of patients with complex regional pain syndrome. In E. F. Lawson & J. P. Castellanos (eds), *Complex regional pain syndrome*. Cham: Springer. https://doi.org/10.1007/978-3-030-75373-3_7

International Association for the Study of Pain (IASP) (2020). *Revised definition of pain*. Retrieved from https://www.iasp-pain.org/

Jarvis, C., Jarvis, S. & Botti, A. (2021). Pain assessment. In C. Jarvis, A. Eckhardt, E. Watt & H. Forbes (eds), *Jarvis's health assessment & physical examination* (3rd ANZ ed.). Chatswood, NSW: Elsevier Australia.

Johnson, M. I., Paley, C. A., Jones, G., Mulvey, M. R. & Wittkopf, P. G. (2022). Efficacy and safety of transcutaneous electrical nerve stimulation (TENS) for acute and chronic pain in adults: A systematic review and meta-analysis of 381 studies (the meta-TENS study). *BMJ Open*, *12*(2), e051073–e051073. https://doi.org/10.1136/bmjopen-2021-051073

Levett-Jones, T., Dwyer, T., Reid-Searl, K., Heaton, L., Flenady, T., Applegarth, J., Guinea, S. & Andersen, P. (2017). *Patient Safety Competency Framework (PSCF) for Nursing Students*. Sydney. Retrieved from http://psframework.wpengine.com/

Llewellyn, A., McCabe, C. S., Hibberd, Y. et al. (2018). Are you better? A multi-centre study of patient-defined recovery from Complex Regional Pain Syndrome. *European Journal of Pain*, *22*(3), 551–564. https://doi.org/10.1002/ejp.1138

Lok, J., Ibrahim, S. & Sidani, S. (2020). Registered Nurses' awareness, acceptability and use of music for the management of pain and anxiety in clinical practice. *Complimentary Therapies in Clinical Practice*, *40*. https://doi.org/10.1016/j.ctcp.2020.101203

Lor, M., Rabago, D. & Backonja, M. (2021). 'There are so many nuances ...': Health care providers' perspectives of pain communication with patients in primary care settings. *Journal of Transcultural Nursing*, *32*(5), 575–582. https://doi.org/10.1177/1043659620959437

Mala, O., Forster, E. M. & Kain, V. (2021). Neonatal nurse and midwife competence regarding pain management in neonates: A systematic review. *Advances in Neonatal Care*, *22*(2), E34–E42. https://doi.org/10.1097/ANC.0000000000000911

Martin, S. D., Maxtin, M., Smalling, K. & Park, S. (2019). Pain assessment and management in children. In M. J. Hockenberry, D. Wilson & C. C. Rodgers (eds), *Wong's nursing care of infants and children* (11th ed.). St Louis, MO: Elsevier.

Martinez, V., Guichard, L. & Fletcher, D. (2015). Effect of combining tramadol and morphine in adult surgical patients: A systematic review and meta-analysis of randomized trials. *British Journal of Anaesthesia*, *114*(3), 384–395.

Mathew, A. & Brufsky, A. (2015). Bisphosphonates in breast cancer. *International Journal of Cancer*, *137*(4), 753–764.

Melzack, R. (1975). The McGill Pain Questionnaire: Major properties and scoring methods. *Pain*, *1*(3), 277–299.

MIMS (2022). *Donepezil*. Retrieved from https://www.mims.co.uk/

Nijs, J., George, S. Z., Clauw, D. J. et al. (2021). Central sensitisation in chronic pain conditions: Latest discoveries and their potential for precision medicine. *The Lancet: Rheumatology*, 3(5), e383–e392. https://doi.org/10.1016/S2665-9913(21)00032-1

Page, S. J., Shawaryn, M. A., Cernich, A. N. & Linacre, J. M. (2001). Scaling of the revised Oswestry low back pain questionnaire. *Archives of Physical Medicine and Rehabilitation*, *83*(11), 1579–1584.

Pandharipande, P. & McGrane, S. (2017). Pain control in the critically ill patient. *UpToDate*. Retrieved from https://www.uptodate.com/

Pejic, W. & Frey, N. (2018). *Hyperbaric oxygen therapy for the treatment of chronic pain: A review of clinical effectiveness and cost-effectiveness*. Ottawa: Canadian Agency for Drugs and Technologies in Health.

Rababa, M., Al-Sabbah, S. & Hayajneh, A. A. (2021). Nurses' perceived barriers to and facilitators of pain assessment and management in critical care patients: A systematic review. *Journal of Pain Research*, *14*, 3475–3491. https://doi.org/10.2147/JPR.S332423

Schofield, P. (2018). The assessment of pain in older people: UK national guidelines. *Age and Ageing, 47*(suppl. 1), i1–i22.

Sutherland, A. M., Clarke, H. A., Katz, J. & Katznelson, R. (2015). Hyperbaric oxygen therapy: A new treatment for chronic pain? *PAIN Practice, 16*(5), 620–628.

The Royal Children's Hospital Melbourne (2021). *Clinical guideline nursing: Sucrose (oral) for procedural pain management in infants*. Retrieved from https://www.rch.org.au/

Tosato, M., Lukas, A., van der Roest, H. G., Danese, P., Antocicco, M., Finne-Soveri, H., Nikolaus, F. Landi, F. & Bernabei, R. (2012). Association of pain with behavioural and psychiatric symptoms among nursing home residents with cognitive impairment. Results from the SHELTER study. *Pain, 153*, 305–310.

Truba, N. & Hoyle, J. D. (2014). Pediatric pain. *Journal of Pain Management, 7*(3), 235.

Vafeas, C. & Slatyer, S. (2021). *Gerontological nursing: A holistic approach to the care of older people*. Chatswood, NSW: Elsevier.

Vagnoli, L., Bettini, A., Amore, E., De Masi, S. & Messeri, A. (2019). Relaxation-guided imagery reduces perioperative anxiety and pain in children: A randomized study. *European Journal of Pediatrics, 178*(6), 913–921. https://doi.org/10.1007/s00431-019-03376-x

World Health Organization (WHO) (2018). *WHO guidelines for the pharmacological and radiotherapeutic management of cancer pain in adults and adolescents*. Retrieved from https://www.who.int/

Youngcharoen, P. (2022). A cross-sectional study of factors associated with nurses' postoperative pain management practices for older patients. *Nursing Open*. https://doi.org/10.1002/nop2.1281

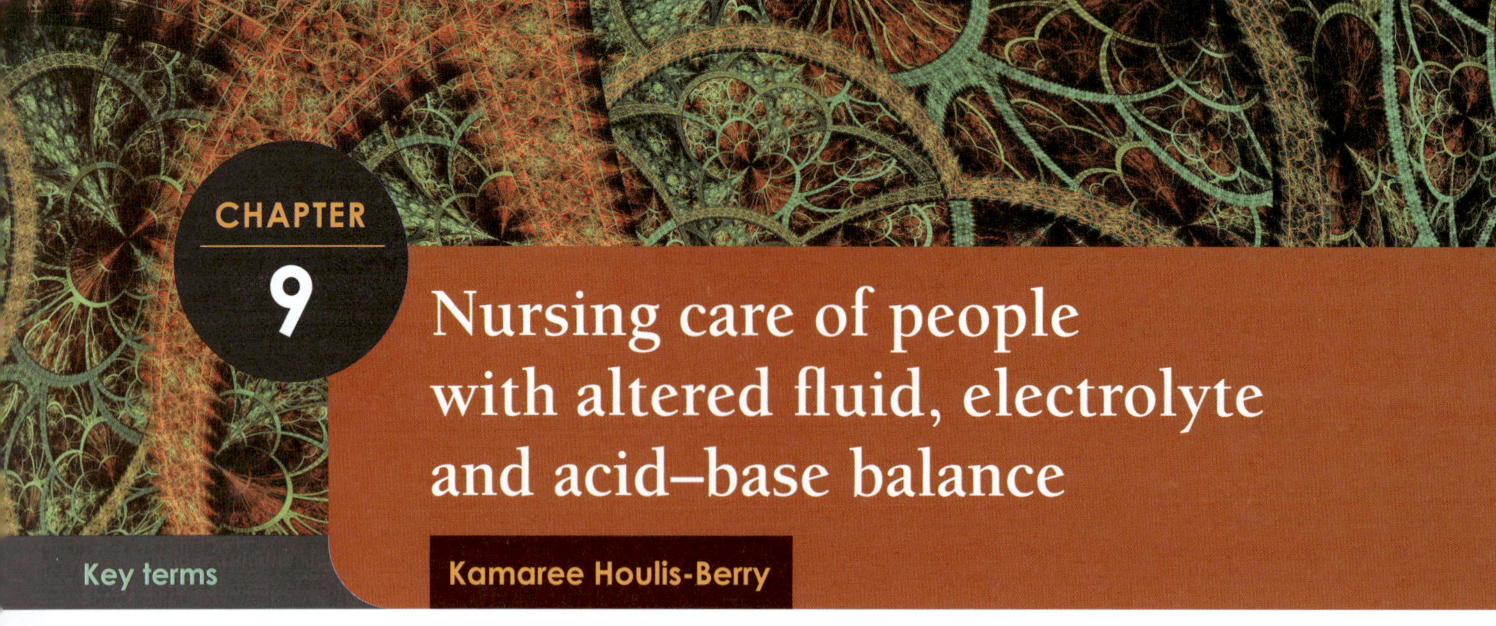

CHAPTER 9

Nursing care of people with altered fluid, electrolyte and acid–base balance

Kamaree Houlis-Berry

Key terms

Learning outcomes

- Describe the functions and regulatory mechanisms that maintain water and electrolyte balance in the body.
- Compare and contrast the causes, effects and care of the person with fluid volume or electrolyte imbalance.
- Explain the pathophysiology and manifestations of imbalances of sodium, potassium, calcium, magnesium and phosphorus.
- Describe the causes and effects of acid–base imbalances.

Clinical competencies

- Assess and monitor the person's fluid, electrolyte and acid–base balance.
- Administer fluids and medications knowledgeably and safely.
- Determine priority nursing diagnoses, based on assessment data, to select and implement individualised nursing interventions.
- Deliver pertinent information to the person and their family about diet and medications used to restore, promote and maintain fluid, electrolyte and acid–base balance.
- Integrate interprofessional care into care of a person with altered fluid, electrolyte and acid–base balance.

Changes in the normal distribution and composition of body fluids often occur in response to illness and trauma. These changes affect fluid balance of the intracellular and extracellular compartments of the body, the concentration of electrolytes within fluid compartments and the body's hydrogen ion concentration (pH). Normal physiological processes depend on a relatively stable state in the internal environment of the body. The fluid volume, electrolyte composition and pH of both intracellular and extracellular spaces must remain constant within a relatively narrow range to maintain health and life.

Homeostasis is the body's tendency to maintain a state of physiological balance in the presence of constantly changing conditions. Homeostasis is necessary if the body is to function optimally at a cellular level and as a total organism. Homeostasis depends on multiple factors in both the external and internal environments, such as available oxygen in the air and nutrients in food, as well as normal body temperature, respiration and digestive processes. The normal volume, composition, distribution and pH of body fluids reflect a state of homeostasis.

Changes in the normal volume of fluids, their composition, distribution, and relative acidity or alkalinity have the potential to disrupt most functional health patterns. Imbalances of fluids, electrolytes and pH affect the ability to maintain activities of daily living (the activity–exercise pattern), think clearly (the cognitive–perceptual pattern) and engage in self-care (the health perception–health management pattern). Conversely, alterations in a number of health patterns affect the ability to maintain homeostasis. Alterations in the nutritional–metabolic pattern affect the ability to consume adequate food and fluids. Disruptions of the elimination pattern may lead to retention or loss of excess amounts of fluids and electrolytes. Disrupted heart or respiratory function, which falls within the activity–exercise pattern, has the potential to affect fluid, electrolyte and acid–base balance.

The goal in managing fluid, electrolyte and acid–base imbalances is to re-establish and maintain a normal balance. Nursing care includes identifying and assessing a person who is likely to develop imbalances, monitoring the person for early manifestations, and implementing collaborative and nursing interventions to prevent or correct imbalances. Effective nursing interventions require an understanding of both multiple processes that maintain fluid, electrolyte and acid–base balance, and of the causes and treatment of imbalances that occur (Marieb & Hoehn, 2018).

Mechanisms that maintain normal fluid and electrolyte balance are discussed first, followed by sections on fluid imbalances and electrolyte imbalances. Discussion of normal acid–base balance precedes discussion of acid–base imbalances. Case studies related to selected fluid, electrolyte and acid–base disorders are found throughout the chapter.

OVERVIEW OF NORMAL FLUID AND ELECTROLYTE BALANCE

Fluid and electrolyte balance in the body involves regulatory mechanisms that maintain the composition, distribution and movement of fluids and electrolytes. This section provides an overview of fluid and electrolyte balance in the body. It is followed by discussion of fluid volume and electrolyte balance disorders.

Body fluid composition

Body fluid is composed of water and various dissolved substances (solutes).

Water

Water is the primary component of body fluids. It functions in several ways to maintain normal cellular function. Water provides a medium for the transport and exchange of nutrients and other substances such as oxygen, carbon dioxide and metabolic wastes to and from cells; provides a medium for metabolic reactions within cells; assists in regulating body temperature through the evaporation of perspiration; provides form for body structure and acts as a shock absorber; provides insulation and acts as a lubricant.

Total body water constitutes about 60% of total body weight, but this amount varies with age, gender and the amount of body fat. Total body water decreases with ageing; in the older adult, body water may decrease to 45% to 50% of total body weight (Marieb & Hoehn, 2018). Adipose tissue contains comparatively little water. In the person who is obese, the proportion of water to total body weight is less than in the person of average weight; in a person who is very thin, the proportion of water to total body weight is greater than in the person of average weight. Adult females have a greater ratio of fat to lean tissue mass than adult males; therefore, they have a lower percentage of body water content.

To maintain normal fluid balance, body water intake and output should be approximately equal. The average fluid intake and output usually is about 2,500 mL over a 24-hour period. Food and fluids consumed provide the majority of water gain; carbohydrate metabolism and other metabolic processes produce an additional small amount.

Urine production and excretion account for most water loss. The average daily urine output is 1,200 to 1,500 mL in adults. At least 400 mL of highly concentrated urine per day is required to excrete metabolic wastes produced by the body (Marieb & Hoehn, 2018). *Insensible* water loss (which normally cannot be measured) occurs through the skin, lungs and faeces. These losses, while normally small, can increase significantly during exercise, when environmental temperatures are high, and during illness that increases the respiratory rate, perspiration or gastrointestinal (GI) losses (particularly diarrhoea). Table 9.1 shows the sources of fluid gain and loss.

Electrolytes

Body fluids contain both water molecules and chemical compounds. These chemical compounds can either remain intact in solution or separate (dissociate) into discrete particles. **Electrolytes** are substances that dissociate in solution to form charged particles called ions. *Cations* are positively charged electrolytes; *anions* are negatively charged electrolytes. For example, sodium chloride (NaCl) in solution dissociates into

TABLE 9.1 Balanced fluid gain and loss for an adult

	SOURCE	AMOUNT (mL)
Gain	Fluids taken orally	1,200
	Water in food	1,000
	Water as by-product of food metabolism	300
		↓
	Total	**2,500**
		↑
Loss	Urine	1,500
	Faeces	200
	Perspiration	300
	Respiration	500

a sodium ion, a cation carrying a positive charge (Na^+), and a chloride ion, an anion carrying a negative charge (Cl^-). Electrolytes may be *univalent*, with only one unit of electrical charge, such as sodium (Na^+) and chloride (Cl^-); or they may be *divalent*, carrying two units of electrical charge, such as magnesium (Mg^{2+}) and phosphate (HPO_4^{2-}).

Electrolytes have many functions, including assisting in regulating water balance, regulating and maintaining acid–base balance, and contributing to enzyme reactions essential for neuromuscular activity.

The concentration of electrolytes in body fluids generally is measured in milliequivalents per litre of water (mEq/L). A *milliequivalent* is a measure of the chemical combining power of the ion. For example, 100 mEq of sodium (Na^+) can combine with 100 mEq of chloride (Cl^-) to form sodium chloride (NaCl). Sodium, potassium and chloride usually are measured in milliequivalents. In some cases, the amount of an electrolyte in body fluid may be measured by weight in milligrams per 100 mL (1 decilitre, dL) of water (mg/dL). Calcium, magnesium and phosphorus often are measured by weight in milligrams per decilitre. Other laboratories use the International System of Measurements, or SI units.

Body fluid distribution

Body fluid is classified by its location inside or outside cells. *Intracellular fluid* (ICF) is found within cells. It accounts for approximately 40% of total body weight (see Figure 9.1) and is essential for normal cell function, providing a medium for metabolic processes. *Extracellular fluid* (ECF) is located outside cells and accounts for approximately 20% of total body weight. ECF is classified by location: interstitial fluid is located in the spaces between most of the cells of the body. It accounts for approximately 15% of total body weight.

- Intravascular fluid, called *plasma*, is contained within the arteries, veins and capillaries. It accounts for approximately 5% of total body weight.
- Transcellular fluid includes urine, digestive secretions and perspiration, as well as cerebrospinal, pleural, synovial, intraocular, gonadal and pericardial fluids.

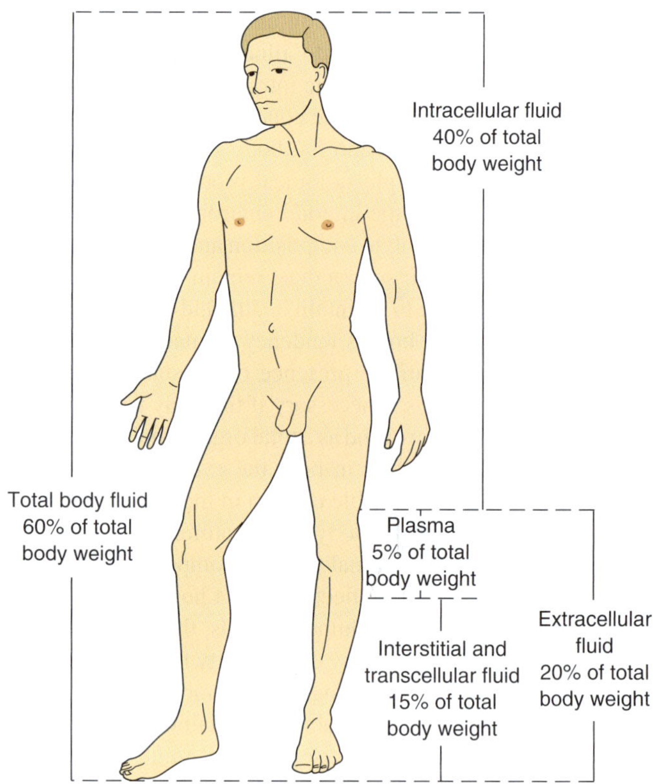

FIGURE 9.1 *The major fluid compartments of the body*

A trace amount of water is found in bone, cartilage and other dense connective tissues; this water is not exchangeable with other body fluids.

ECF is the transport medium that carries oxygen and nutrients to, and waste products from, the cells. For example, plasma transports oxygen from the lungs and glucose from the digestive system to the tissues. These solutes diffuse through the capillary wall into the interstitial space and from there across the cell membrane into the cells. Waste products of metabolism (e.g. carbon dioxide and hydrogen ions) diffuse from the intracellular space into the interstitial space and from there into plasma via the capillary walls. Plasma then transports these waste products to the lungs and kidneys for elimination (Marieb & Hoehn, 2018).

Although the overall concentration of solutes in ICF and ECF is nearly identical, the concentration of specific electrolytes differs significantly between these compartments, as shown in Figure 9.2. ICF contains high concentrations of potassium (K^+), magnesium (Mg^{2+}) and phosphate (PO_4^{2-}), as well as other solutes such as glucose and oxygen. Sodium (Na^+), chloride (Cl^-) and bicarbonate (HCO_3^-) are the principal extracellular electrolytes. The high sodium concentration in ECF is essential to regulating body fluid volume. The concentration of potassium in ECF is low. There is a minimal difference in electrolyte concentration between plasma and interstitial fluid. Normal values for electrolytes in plasma are shown in Table 9.2.

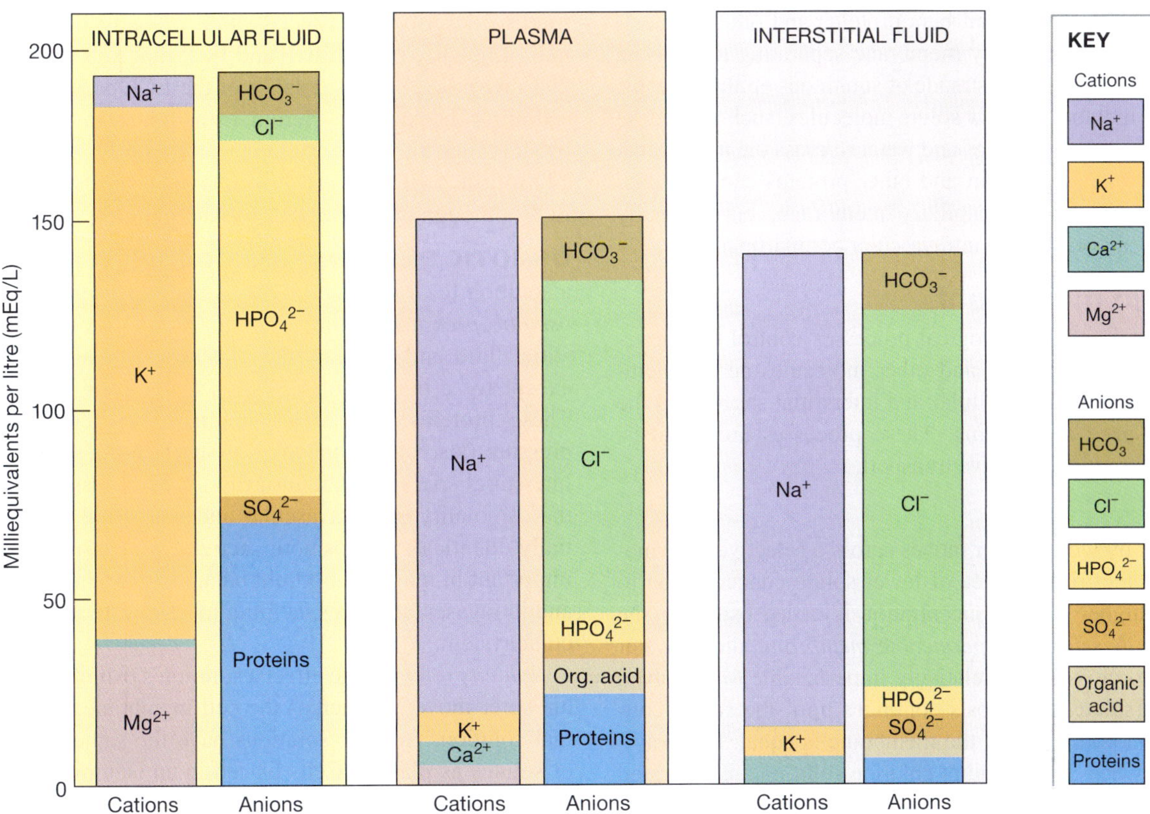

FIGURE 9.2 *Electrolyte composition (cations and anions) of body fluid compartments*

Source: Martini, Nath & Bartholomew (2018). *Fundamentals of anatomy and physiology* (11th ed.). © 2018 Reprinted by permission of Pearson Education, Inc.

The body fluid compartments are separated by several types of membranes:

- Cell membranes separate interstitial fluid from intracellular fluid.
- Capillary membranes separate plasma from interstitial fluid.
- Epithelial membranes separate transcellular fluid from interstitial fluid and plasma. These membranes include the mucosa of the stomach, intestines and gallbladder; the pleural, peritoneal and synovial membranes; and the tubules of the kidney.

A cell membrane consists of layers of lipid and protein molecules. The layering of these molecules controls the passage of fluid and solutes between the cell and interstitial fluid. The cell membrane is selectively permeable; that is, it allows the passage of water, oxygen, carbon dioxide and small

TABLE 9.2 Normal values for electrolytes and serum osmolality

SERUM COMPONENT	VALUES	
ELECTROLYTES	CONVENTIONAL UNITS	SI UNITS
Sodium (Na^+)	135-145 mEq/L	135-145 mmol/L
Chloride (Cl^-)	95-105 mEq/L	95-105 mmol/L
Bicarbonate (HCO_3^-)	22-30 mEq/L	22-30 mmol/L
Calcium (Ca^{2+}) (total)	9-11 mg/dL	2.3-2.8 mmol/L
Potassium (K^+)	3.5-5.3 mEq/L	3.5-5.0 mmol/L
Phosphate/inorganic phosphorus (PO_4^{2-})	1.7-2.6 mEq/L (2.5-4.5 mg/dL)	0.8-1.5 mmol/L
Magnesium (Mg^{2+})	1.5-2.5 mg/dL (1.8-3.0 mEq/L)	0.8-1.3 mmol/L
Serum osmolality	280-300 mOsm/kg	275-295 mmol/kg

water-soluble molecules, but bars proteins and other intracellular colloids. The capillary membrane separating the plasma from the interstitial space is made of squamous epithelial cells. Pores in the membrane allow solute molecules (such as glucose and sodium), dissolved gases and water to cross the membrane. Minute amounts of albumin and other proteins can also pass through the pores of a capillary membrane, but normally plasma proteins stay in the intravascular compartment.

Body fluid movement

Four chemical and physiological processes control the movement of fluid, electrolytes and other molecules across membranes between the intracellular and interstitial spaces and the interstitial space and plasma. These processes are osmosis, diffusion, filtration and active transport.

Osmosis

The process by which water moves across a selectively permeable membrane from an area of lower solute concentration to an area of higher solute concentration is called **osmosis** (see Figure 9.3). A *selectively permeable membrane* allows water molecules to cross but is relatively impermeable to dissolved substances (solutes). Osmosis continues until the solute concentration on both sides of the membrane is equal. For example, if pure water and a sodium chloride solution are separated by a selectively permeable membrane, then water molecules will move across the membrane to the sodium chloride solution. Osmosis is the primary process that controls body fluid movement between the ICF and ECF compartments.

OSMOLARITY AND OSMOLALITY The concentration of a solution may be expressed as the osmolarity or osmolality of the solution. *Osmolarity* refers to the quantity of solutes per litre of solution (by volume); it is reported in milliosmoles per litre (mOsm/L) in a solution. *Osmolality* refers to the quantity of solutes per kilogram of water (by weight); it is reported in milliosmoles per kilogram (mOsm/kg). Because osmotic activity in the body is regulated by the number of active particles (solutes) per kilogram of water, osmolality is used to describe the concentration of body fluids. The normal osmolality of both ICF and ECF ranges between 275 and 295 mOsm/kg. The osmolality of the ECF depends chiefly on sodium concentration. Serum osmolality may be estimated by doubling the serum sodium concentration (approximately 142 mEq/L). Glucose and urea contribute to the osmolality of ECF, although to a lesser extent than sodium.

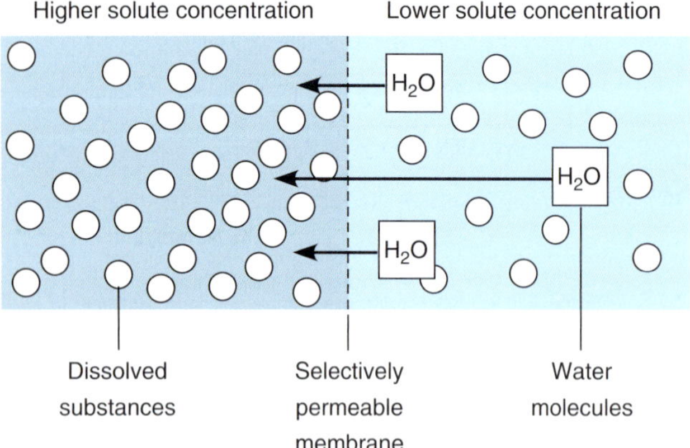

FIGURE 9.3 ***Osmosis. Water molecules move through a selectively permeable membrane from an area of low solute concentration to an area of high solute concentration***

OSMOTIC PRESSURE AND TONICITY The power of a solution to draw water across a membrane is known as the *osmotic pressure* of the solution. The composition of interstitial fluid and intravascular plasma is essentially the same except for a higher concentration of proteins in the plasma. These proteins (especially albumin) exert colloid osmotic pressure (also called oncotic pressure), pulling fluid from the interstitial space into the intravascular compartment. Because the osmolality of intravascular and interstitial fluid is essentially identical, the osmotic activity of plasma proteins is important in maintaining fluid balance between the interstitial and intravascular spaces, helping to hold water within the vascular system.

Tonicity refers to the effect a solution's osmotic pressure has on water movement across the cell membrane of cells within that solution. *Isotonic* solutions have the same concentration of solutes as plasma. Cells placed in an isotonic solution will neither shrink nor swell because there is no net gain or loss of water within the cell and no change in cell volume (see Figure 9.4A). Normal saline (0.9% sodium chloride solution) is an example of an isotonic solution.

Hypertonic solutions have a greater concentration of solutes than plasma. In their presence, water is drawn out of a cell, causing it to shrink (see Figure 9.4B). A 3% sodium chloride solution is hypertonic. *Hypotonic* solutions (such as 0.45% sodium chloride) have a lower solute concentration than plasma (see Figure 9.4C). When red blood cells are placed in a hypotonic solution, water moves into the cells, causing them to swell and rupture (*haemolyse*).

The concepts of osmotic draw and tonicity are important in understanding the pathophysiological changes that occur with fluid and electrolyte imbalances, as well as treatment measures. For example, an increased sodium concentration of extracellular fluid pulls water from the ICF compartment into the ECF compartment, causing cells to shrink. In this case, administering a hypotonic intravenous solution to reduce the sodium concentration and osmolality of ECF will facilitate water movement back into the cells.

Diffusion

The process by which solute molecules move from an area of high solute concentration to an area of low solute concentration to become evenly distributed is called **diffusion** (see Figure 9.5). The two types of diffusion are simple and facilitated diffusion. *Simple diffusion* occurs by the random movement of particles through a solution. Water, carbon dioxide, oxygen and solutes move between plasma and the interstitial space by simple diffusion through the capillary membrane. Water and solutes move into the cell by passing through protein channels or by dissolving in the lipid cell membrane.

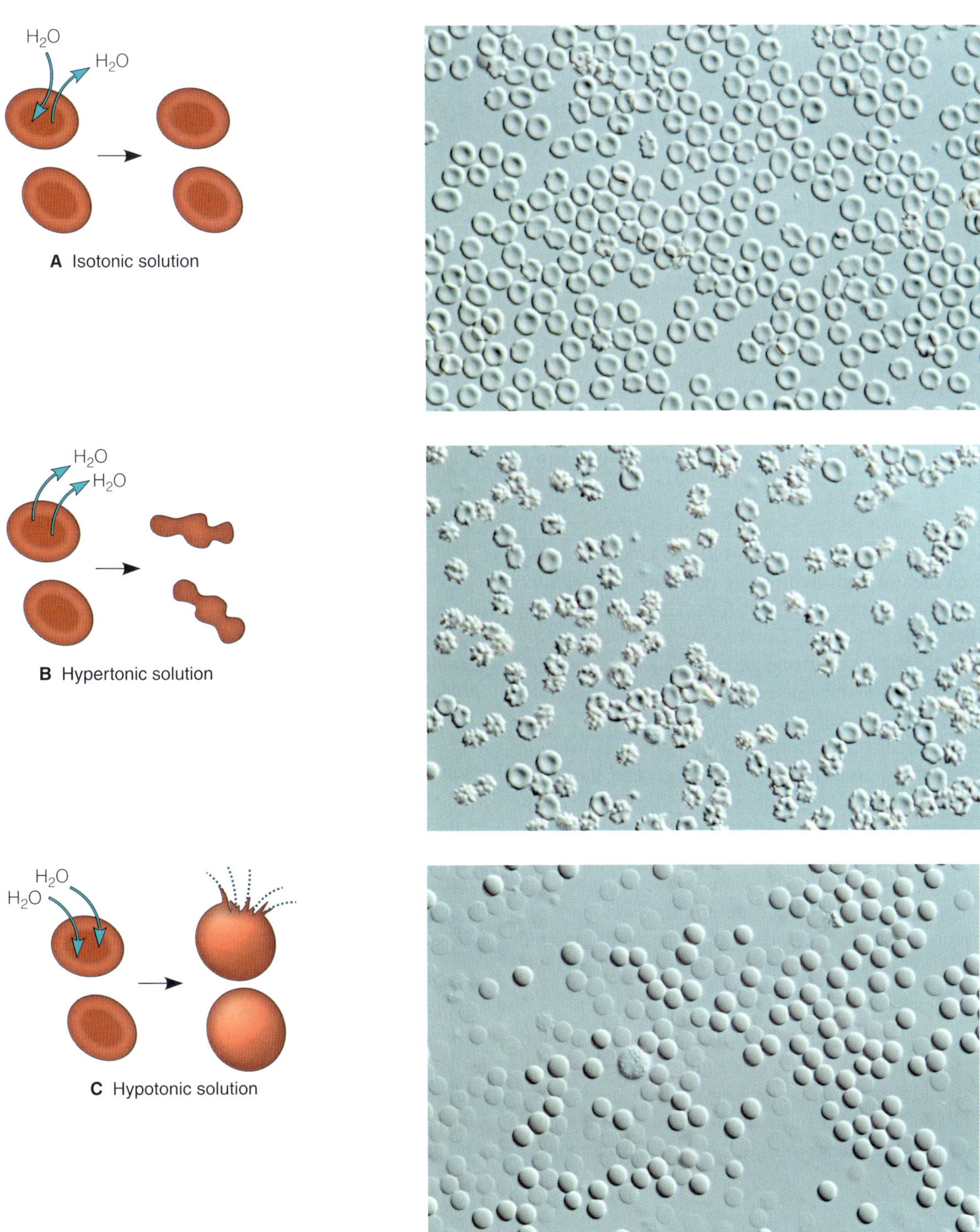

FIGURE 9.4 ***The effect of tonicity on red blood cells. A, In an isotonic solution, red blood cells neither gain nor lose water, retaining their normal biconcave shape. B, In a hypertonic solution, cells lose water and shrink in size. C, In a hypotonic solution, cells absorb water and may burst (haemolysis)***

Source: Photos © Herve Conge, ISM/Science Photo Library.

Facilitated diffusion, also called carrier-mediated diffusion, allows large water-soluble molecules, such as glucose and amino acids, to diffuse across cell membranes. Proteins embedded in the cell membrane function as *carriers*, helping large molecules cross the membrane.

The rate of diffusion is influenced by a number of factors, such as the concentration of solute and the availability of carrier proteins in the cell membrane. The effect of both simple and facilitated diffusion is to establish equal concentrations of the molecules on both sides of a membrane.

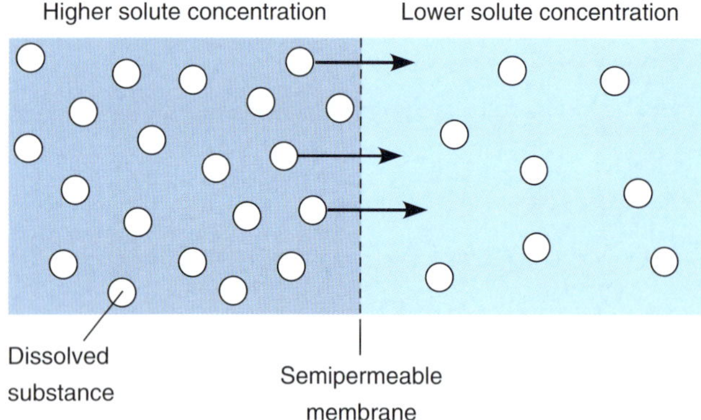

FIGURE 9.5 ***Diffusion. Solute molecules move through a semipermeable membrane from an area of high solute concentration to an area of low solute concentration***

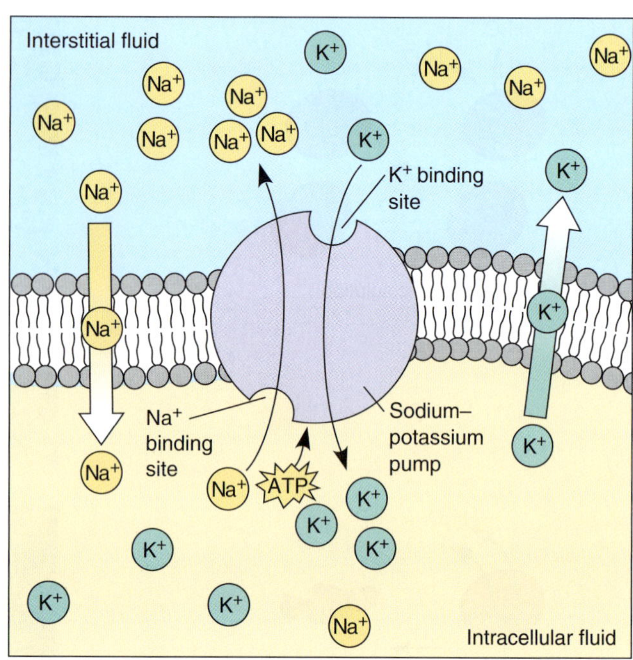

FIGURE 9.7 ***The sodium–potassium pump. Sodium and potassium ions are moved across the cell membranes against their concentration gradients. This active transport process is fuelled by energy from ATP***

Filtration

The process by which water and dissolved substances (solutes) move from an area of high hydrostatic pressure to an area of low hydrostatic pressure is called **filtration**. This usually occurs across capillary membranes. *Hydrostatic pressure* is created by the pumping action of the heart and gravity against the capillary wall. Filtration occurs in the glomerulus of the kidneys, as well as at the arterial end of capillaries.

A balance of hydrostatic (filtration) pressure and osmotic pressure regulates the movement of water between the intravascular and interstitial spaces in the capillary beds of the body. Hydrostatic pressure within the arterial end of the capillary pushes water into the interstitial space. Hydrostatic pressure within the interstitial space opposes this movement to some degree. At the venous end of the capillary, the osmotic force of plasma proteins draws fluid back into the capillary (see Figure 9.6).

Active transport

Active transport allows molecules to move across cell membranes and epithelial membranes against a concentration gradient. This movement requires energy (adenosine triphosphate, or ATP) and a carrier mechanism to maintain a higher concentration of a substance on one side of the membrane than on the other. The sodium–potassium pump is an important example of active transport (see Figure 9.7). High concentrations of potassium in intracellular fluids and of sodium in extracellular fluids are maintained because cells actively transport potassium from interstitial fluid (where the concentration of potassium is about 5 mEq/L) into intracellular fluid (where the potassium concentration is about 150 mEq/L).

Body fluid regulation

Homeostasis requires several regulatory mechanisms and processes to maintain the balance between fluid intake and excretion. These include thirst, the kidneys, the renin–angiotensin–aldosterone mechanism, antidiuretic hormone and atrial natriuretic peptide. These mechanisms affect the volume, distribution and composition of body fluids.

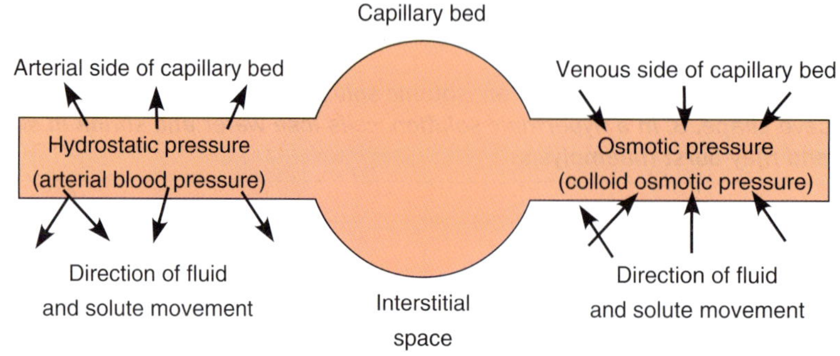

FIGURE 9.6 ***Fluid balance between the intravascular and interstitial spaces is maintained in the capillary beds by a balance of filtration at the arterial end and osmotic draw at the venous end***

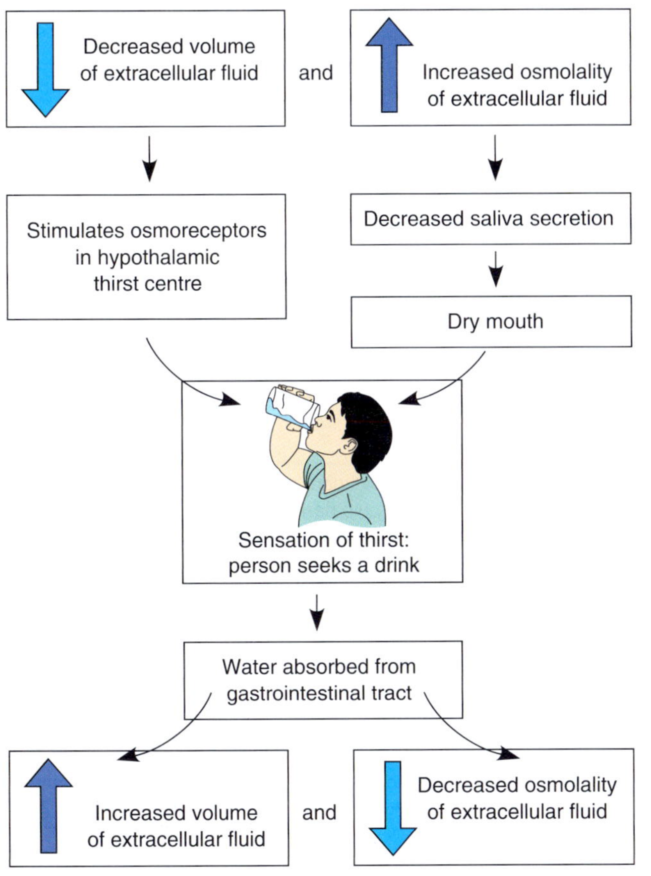

FIGURE 9.8 ***Factors stimulating water intake through the thirst mechanism***

Thirst

Thirst is the primary regulator of water intake. Thirst plays an important role in maintaining fluid balance and preventing dehydration. The thirst centre, located in the brain, is stimulated when the blood volume drops because of water losses or when serum osmolality (solute concentration) increases (see Figure 9.8).

The thirst mechanism is highly effective in regulating extracellular sodium levels. Increased sodium in ECF increases serum osmolality, stimulating the thirst centre. Fluid intake in turn reduces the sodium concentration of ECF and lowers serum osmolality. Conversely, a drop in serum sodium and low serum osmolality inhibit the thirst centre.

> **CONSIDERATION FOR PRACTICE**
>
> **The thirst mechanism declines with ageing, making older adults more vulnerable to dehydration and hyperosmolality (high serum osmolality). People with an altered level of consciousness or who are unable to respond to thirst are also at risk.**

Kidneys

The kidneys are primarily responsible for regulating fluid volume and electrolyte balance in the body. They regulate the volume and osmolality of body fluids by controlling the excretion of water and electrolytes. In adults, about 170 L of plasma are filtered through the glomeruli every day. By selectively reabsorbing water and electrolytes, the kidneys maintain the volume and osmolality of body fluids. About 99% of the glomerular filtrate is reabsorbed, and only about 1,500 mL of urine is produced over a 24-hour period.

Renin–angiotensin–aldosterone system

The renin–angiotensin–aldosterone system works to maintain intravascular fluid balance and blood pressure. A decrease in blood flow or blood pressure to the kidneys stimulates specialised receptors in the juxtaglomerular cells of the nephrons to produce renin, an enzyme. Renin converts angiotensinogen (a plasma protein) in the circulating blood into angiotensin I. Angiotensin I travels through the bloodstream to the lungs, where it is converted to angiotensin II by angiotensin-converting enzyme (ACE). Angiotensin II is a potent vasoconstrictor; it raises the blood pressure. It also stimulates the thirst mechanism to promote fluid intake and acts directly on the kidneys, causing them to retain sodium and water. Angiotensin II stimulates the adrenal cortex to release aldosterone. Aldosterone promotes sodium and water retention in the distal nephron of the kidney, restoring blood volume (see Figure 9.9).

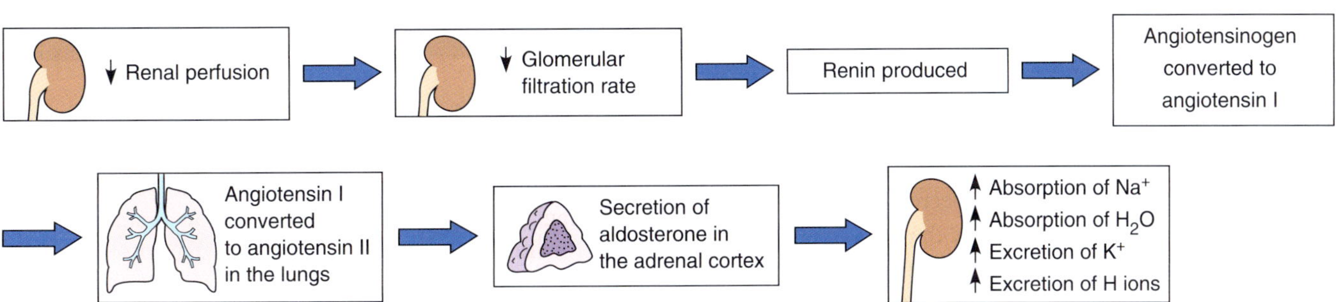

FIGURE 9.9 ***The renin–angiotensin–aldosterone system. Decreased blood volume and renal perfusion set off a chain of reactions, leading to release of aldosterone from the adrenal cortex. Increased levels of aldosterone regulate serum K^+ and Na^+, blood pressure and water balance through effects on the kidney tubules***

Antidiuretic hormone

Antidiuretic hormone (ADH), released by the posterior pituitary gland, regulates water excretion from the kidneys. Osmoreceptors in the hypothalamus respond to increases in serum osmolality and decreases in blood volume, stimulating ADH production and release. ADH acts on the distal tubules of the kidney, making them more permeable to water and thus increasing water reabsorption. With increased water reabsorption, urine output falls, blood volume is restored and serum osmolality drops as the water dilutes body fluids (see Figure 9.10).

In addition to decreased blood volume and increased serum osmolality, increased amounts of ADH are released in response to stress, pain, surgery and anaesthesia, some medications such as morphine and barbiturates, and mechanical ventilation. Its release is inhibited by ethanol, medications such as phenytoin, as well as increased circulating blood volume and decreased serum osmolality.

Two disorders of ADH production illustrate the effect of ADH on water balance and urine output. First, diabetes insipidus is a condition characterised by deficient ADH production. The lack of ADH causes the distal tubules and collecting ducts of the kidney to be impermeable to water, so little water is reabsorbed into the bloodstream. As a result, copious, very dilute urine is excreted. Water loss leads to increased concentration of the plasma or increased serum osmolality. ADH is not released in response to the serum hyperosmolality, but the thirst mechanism is stimulated and the person drinks additional fluids, maintaining high urine output. In the other condition, the syndrome of inappropriate ADH secretion (SIADH), excess ADH is released. Increased water reabsorption causes increased fluid volume and scant, concentrated urine output. These diseases of the pituitary gland are discussed in the chapter 'Nursing care of people with endocrine disorders'.

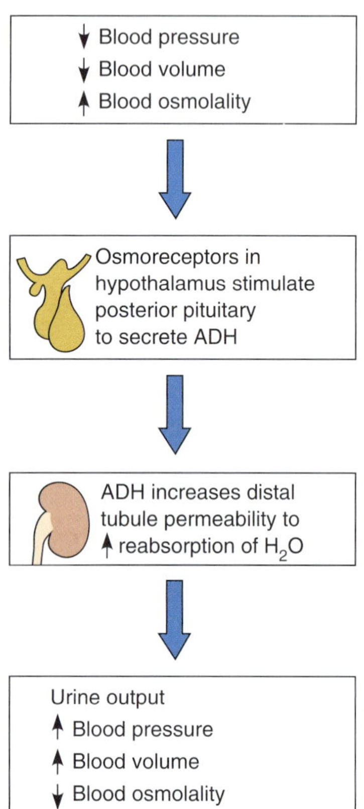

FIGURE 9.10 ***Antidiuretic hormone (ADH) release and effect. Increased serum osmolality or a fall in blood volume stimulates the release of ADH from the posterior pituitary. ADH increases the permeability of distal tubules, promoting water reabsorption***

Atrial natriuretic peptide

Atrial natriuretic peptide (ANP) is a hormone released by atrial muscle cells in response to distension from fluid overload. ANP affects several body systems, including the cardiovascular, renal, neural, gastrointestinal and endocrine systems, but it primarily affects the renin–angiotensin–aldosterone system. ANP opposes this system by inhibiting renin secretion and blocking the secretion and sodium-retaining effects of aldosterone. As a result, ANP promotes sodium wasting and diuresis (increased urine output) and causes vasodilation.

Fluid and electrolyte imbalances

THE PERSON WITH FLUID VOLUME DEFICIT

Fluid volume deficit (FVD) is a decrease in intravascular, interstitial and/or intracellular fluid in the body. FVDs may be due to excessive fluid losses, insufficient fluid intake or failure of regulatory mechanisms and fluid shifts within the body. FVD is a relatively common problem that may exist alone or in combination with other electrolyte or acid–base imbalances. The term **dehydration** refers to loss of water alone, even though it often is used interchangeably with fluid volume deficit.

Pathophysiology

The most common cause of FVD is excessive loss of gastrointestinal fluids from vomiting, diarrhoea, gastrointestinal suctioning, intestinal fistulas and intestinal drainage. Other causes of fluid losses include excessive renal losses of water and sodium from diuretic therapy, renal disorders or endocrine disorders, inability to swallow fluids, oral trauma, water and sodium losses during sweating from excessive exercise or increased environmental temperature, haemorrhage and chronic abuse of laxatives and/or enemas. Older adults in particular are at risk of FVD (see the 'Nursing care of the older adult' box).

NURSING CARE OF THE OLDER ADULT Fluid volume deficit

Changes in the normal ageing process affect homeostasis in several ways. In older adults, the percentage of total body water is about 10% lower than in younger or middle-aged adults, and thus they have less body reserve. Lean muscle mass is lower in older adults, and the percentage of body fat is higher; as a result, water accounts for about 50% of the total body weight (TBW) of an older man and about 45% of the TBW of an older woman. Sodium and water regulation become less efficient with ageing. Renal blood flow and glomerular filtration decline with ageing; the kidneys are less able to effectively concentrate the urine and conserve sodium and water. The perception of thirst decreases, interfering with the thirst mechanism. Consequently, the older adult may become dehydrated without being aware of the need to increase fluid intake.

Undetected fever in older adults can increase the total body need for water with every degree of temperature. Dehydration can cause a fever and further compound dehydration in the older adult. Older adults who have self-care deficits or who are confused, depressed, tube fed, on bed rest or taking medications (such as sedatives, tranquillisers, diuretics and laxatives) are at greatest risk for fluid volume imbalance. Older adults without air-conditioning are at risk during extremely hot weather. In addition, functional changes and illnesses can affect fluid balance. For example, fear of incontinence can lead to self-limiting of fluid intake; physical disabilities associated with age-related illnesses, such as arthritis or stroke, may limit access to fluids; and cognitive impairments can interfere with recognition of thirst and the ability to respond to it.

Manifestations of FVD may be more difficult to recognise in the older adult. A change in mental status, memory or attention may be an early manifestation. Skin turgor is less reliable as an indicator of dehydration, although assessing turgor over the sternum or on the inner aspect of the thigh may be more effective. Dry oral mucous membranes, increased tongue furrows, subnormal temperature, tachycardia and a pinched facial expression are also indicative of dehydration. Orthostatic vital signs may not demonstrate typical changes in the dehydrated older adult.

FVD can develop slowly or rapidly, depending on the type of fluid loss. Loss of extracellular fluid volume can lead to *hypovolaemia*, decreased circulating blood volume. Electrolytes often are lost along with fluid, resulting in an *isotonic FVE.* When both water and electrolytes are lost, the serum sodium level remains normal, although levels of other electrolytes such as potassium may fall. Fluid is drawn into the vascular compartment from the interstitial spaces as the body attempts to maintain tissue perfusion. This eventually depletes fluid in the intracellular compartment as well (McCance & Huether, 2018).

Hypovolaemia stimulates regulatory mechanisms to maintain circulation. The sympathetic nervous system is stimulated, as is the thirst mechanism. ADH and aldosterone are released, prompting sodium and water retention by the kidneys. Severe fluid loss can lead to cardiovascular collapse.

Two other types of FVD—hypovolaemic FVD and hypertonic FVD—are discussed as effects of sodium imbalance in that section of this chapter.

Third spacing

Third spacing is a shift of fluid from the vascular space into an area where it is not available to support normal physiological processes. Fluid may be sequestered in the abdomen or bowel, or in such other actual or potential body spaces as the pleural or peritoneal spaces. Fluid may also become trapped within soft tissues following trauma or burns. The trapped fluid is unavailable to support cardiovascular or renal function; therefore, it represents a volume loss.

Increased vascular permeability or decreased protein levels can trigger third spacing (Loscalzo et al., 2022). Stress hormones released in response to tissue trauma or sepsis (catecholamines in particular) promote redistribution of blood to vital organs (heart and brain). Renal blood flow falls, stimulating the renin–angiotensin–aldosterone system. This promotes sodium and water retention to maintain intravascular volume. The blood vessel and tissue damage caused by surgery stimulates the release of inflammatory mediators such as histamine and prostaglandins. These substances lead to local vasodilation and increased capillary permeability, allowing fluid to accumulate in interstitial tissues.

Assessing the extent of FVD resulting from third spacing is difficult. It may not be reflected by changes in weight or intake-and-output records and it may not become apparent until after organ malfunction occurs (Giddens, 2021; Metheny, 2012). Delays in recognition and treatment can lead to irreversible shock and multi-organ system failure (Burns & Delgado, 2018; Perrin & MacLeod, 2017).

Manifestations

With a rapid fluid loss (such as with haemorrhage or uncontrolled vomiting), manifestations of hypovolaemia develop rapidly. When the loss of fluid occurs more gradually, the person's fluid volume may be very low before symptoms develop. See 'Multisystem effects of FVD'.

Rapid weight loss is a good indicator of FVD. Each litre of body fluid weighs about 1 kg. The severity of the FVD can be estimated by the percentage of rapid weight loss: a loss of 2–5% of total body weight represents a mild FVD; 6–9% moderate FVD; and 10% or greater, severe FVD (Giddens, 2021; Metheny, 2012).

Loss of interstitial fluid causes skin turgor to diminish. When pinched, the skin of a person with FVD remains elevated. Loss of skin elasticity with ageing makes this assessment finding less accurate in older adults. Tongue turgor is not generally affected by age; therefore, assessing the size, dryness and longitudinal furrows of the tongue may be a more accurate indicator of FVD.

Postural or orthostatic hypotension is a sign of hypovolaemia. A drop of more than 15 mmHg in systolic blood pressure when changing from a lying to a standing position often indicates loss of intravascular volume. Venous pressure falls as well, causing flat neck veins, even when the person is recumbent. Loss of intravascular fluid causes the haematocrit to increase.

Multisystem effects of fluid volume deficit (FVD)

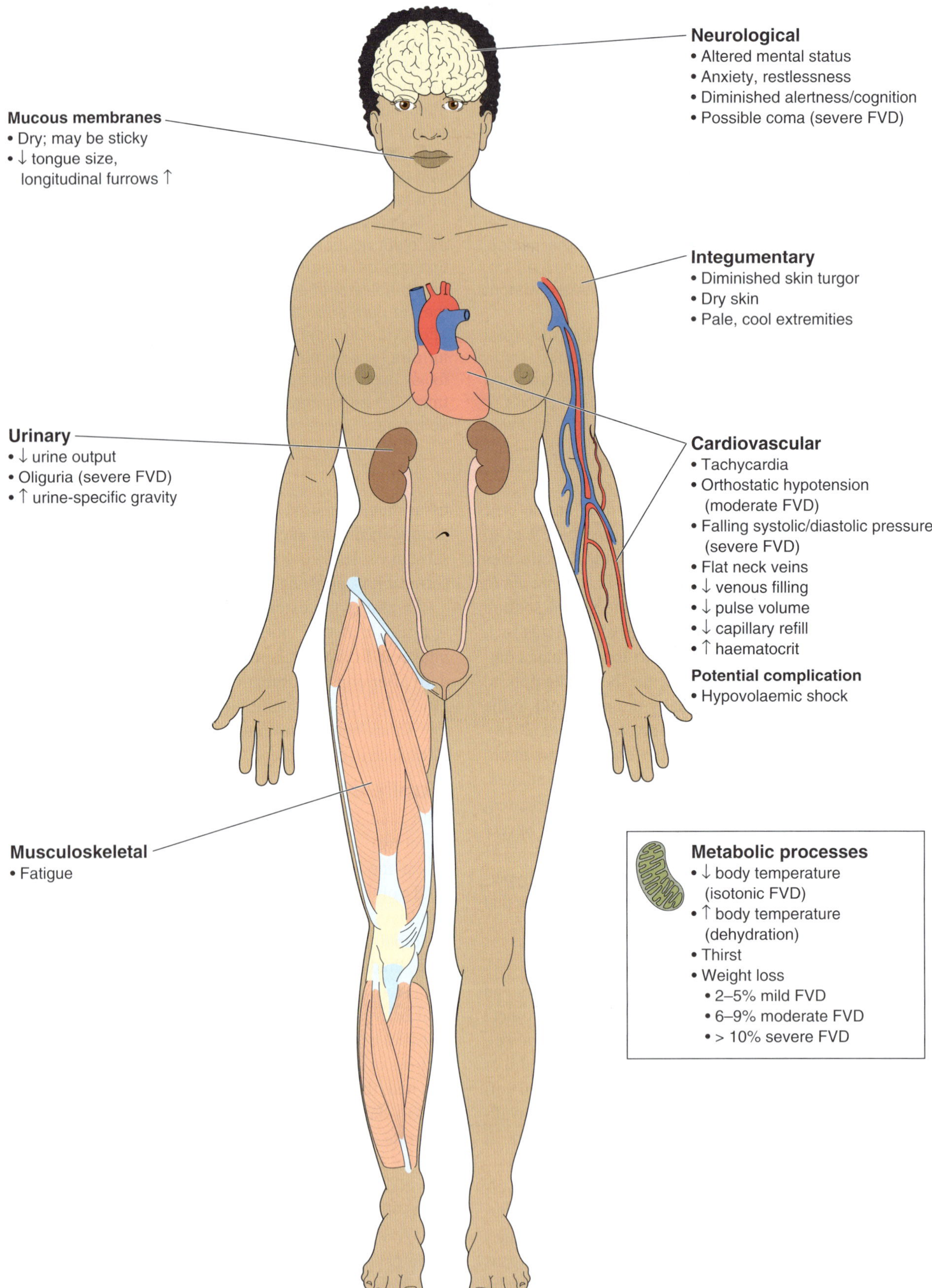

TABLE 9.3 Comparison of assessment findings in a person with fluid imbalance

ASSESSMENT	FLUID DEFICIT	FLUID EXCESS
Blood pressure	Decreased systolic Postural hypotension	Increased
Heart rate	Increased	Increased
Pulse amplitude	Decreased	Increased
Respirations	Normal	Moist crackles Wheezes
Jugular vein	Flat	Distended
Oedema	Rare	Dependent
Skin turgor	Loose, poor turgor	Taut
Output	Low, concentrated	May be low or normal
Urine-specific gravity	High	Low
Weight	Loss	Gain

Compensatory mechanisms to conserve water and sodium and maintain circulation account for many of the manifestations of FVD, such as tachycardia; pale, cool skin (vasoconstriction); and decreased urine output. The specific gravity of urine increases as water is reabsorbed in the tubules. Table 9.3 compares assessment findings for fluid deficit and fluid excess.

INTERPROFESSIONAL CARE

The primary goals of care related to FVD are to prevent deficits in people at risk and to correct deficits and their underlying causes. Depending on the acuity of the imbalance, treatment may include replacement of fluids and electrolytes by the intravenous, oral or enteral routes. When possible, the oral or enteral route is preferred for administering fluids. In acute situations, however, intravenous fluid administration is necessary.

Diagnosis

Laboratory and diagnostic tests may be ordered when FVD is suspected. Such tests measure:

- *Serum electrolytes.* In an isotonic fluid deficit, sodium levels are within normal limits; when the loss is water only, sodium levels are high. Decreases in potassium are common.
- *Serum osmolality.* Measurement of serum osmolality helps to differentiate isotonic fluid loss from water loss. With water loss, osmolality is high; it may be within normal limits with an isotonic fluid loss.
- *Haemoglobin and haematocrit.* The haematocrit often is elevated due to loss of intravascular volume and haemoconcentration.
- *Urine-specific gravity and osmolality.* As the kidneys conserve water, both the specific gravity and osmolality of urine increase.
- *Haemodynamic pressures.* The mean arterial pressure (MAP), *central venous pressure* (CVP), right atrial pressure (RAP) and pulmonary artery wedge pressure (PAWP) are decreased in severe FVD (Burns & Delgado, 2018; Perrin & MacLeod, 2017). The technique for measuring CVP is outlined in Box 9.1.

Fluid management

Oral rehydration is the safest and most effective treatment for FVD in alert people who are able to take oral fluids. Adults require a minimum of 1,500 mL of fluid per day or approximately 30 mL per kg of body weight (ideal body weight is used to calculate fluid requirements for the person who is obese) for maintenance. Fluids are replaced gradually, particularly in older adults, to prevent rapid rehydration of the cells. In general, fluid deficits are replaced at a rate of approximately 30% to 50% of the deficit per 24 hours.

For mild fluid deficits in which the loss of electrolytes has been minimal (e.g. moderate exercise in warm weather), water alone may be used for fluid replacement. When the fluid deficit is more severe and when electrolytes have also been lost (e.g. FVD due to vomiting and/or diarrhoea, strenuous exercise for longer than an hour or two), a carbohydrate/electrolyte solution such as a sports drink, ginger ale or a rehydrating solution is more appropriate. These solutions provide sodium, potassium, chloride and kilojoules to help meet metabolic needs.

INTRAVENOUS THERAPY When the fluid deficit is severe or the person is unable to ingest fluids, the intravenous route is used to administer replacement fluids. Table 9.4 describes the types, tonicity and uses of commonly administered intravenous fluids. Isotonic electrolyte solutions (0.9% NaCl or Ringer's solution) are used to expand plasma volume in a hypotensive person or to replace abnormal losses, which are usually isotonic in nature. Normal saline (0.9% NaCl) tends to remain in the vascular compartment, increasing blood volume. When administered rapidly, however, this solution can precipitate acid–base imbalances, so balanced electrolyte solutions such as lactated Ringer's solution are preferred to expand plasma volume.

Five per cent dextrose in water (D5W) or 0.45% NaCl (one-half normal saline or 1/2 NS) is given to provide water to treat total body water deficits. D5W is isotonic (similar in tonicity to the plasma) when administered and thus does not provoke haemolysis of red blood cells. The dextrose is metabolised to carbon dioxide and water, leaving free water available for tissue needs. Hypotonic saline solution

BOX 9.1 Measuring central venous pressure with a manometer

CVP is a haemodynamic monitoring method for evaluating fluid volume status. It measures mean right atrial pressure by means of a catheter. The CVP catheter is inserted by a doctor, most often at the person's bedside, into the antecubital, internal jugular or subclavian vein. Either a haemodynamic monitoring system (see the chapter 'Nursing care of people with coronary heart disease') or a manual system may be used to measure the CVP. Nursing responsibilities in measuring CVP are as follows:

1. Explain to the person and their family what is being done.
2. Prior to the first measurement, take baseline vital signs and measure the level of the right atrium on the person's thorax. This is usually at the fourth intercostal space on the lateral chest wall, midway between the anterior and posterior chest. This site, called the *phlebostatic axis*, is marked and used as the reference point for all measurements.
3. If possible, place the bed in the same position for each reading, usually with the person supine and the head of the bed flat. Elevating the head of the bed to as much as 60 degrees usually does not affect the accuracy of the CVP reading in a person who is haemodynamically stable (Urden, Stacy & Lough, 2021).
4. Use a carpenter's level to check the level of the measuring device to make sure the transducer or the 0 on the manometer is level with the phlebostatic axis (see figure).
5. Remove any air bubbles in the line.
6. If using a manometer, turn the stopcock so that fluid flows into the manometer, filling it a few centimetres above the expected reading. Then turn the stopcock to open the line between the manometer and the person. The fluid level will fall and then reach a point at which it fluctuates with the person's respirations. This point is recorded as the CVP.
7. After the measurement is taken, turn the stopcock so that the fluid can again flow from the fluid source to the person.

Normal values

When CVP is measured using a manometer, normal values range from 2 to 8 cm water. With a haemodynamic monitoring system, the normal CVP range is 2 to 5 mmHg. A low CVP indicates inadequate venous return from fluid deficit and hypovolaemia or due to peripheral vasodilation. A high CVP indicates fluid overload, cardiac problems that decrease cardiac contractility or pulmonary disorders that increase pulmonary vascular resistance.

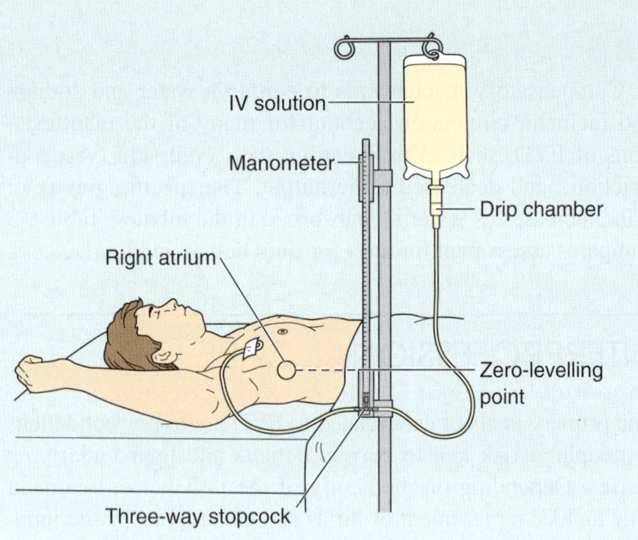

(0.45% NaCl with or without added electrolytes) or 5% dextrose in 0.45% sodium chloride (D5 1/2 NS) are used as maintenance solutions (Giddens, 2021; Metheny, 2012). These solutions provide additional electrolytes such as potassium, a buffer (lactate or acetate) as needed and water. When dextrose is added, they also provide a minimal number of kilojoules.

FLUID CHALLENGE A fluid challenge, the rapid administration of a designated amount of intravenous fluid, may be performed to evaluate fluid volume when urine output is low and cardiac or renal function is questionable. A fluid challenge helps prevent fluid volume overload resulting from intravenous fluid therapy when cardiac or renal function is compromised. Nursing responsibilities for a fluid challenge are as follows:

- Obtain and document baseline vital signs, breath sounds, urine output and mental status.
- Administer (by IV infusion) an initial fluid volume of 200 to 300 mL over 5 to 10 minutes.
- Re-evaluate baseline data at the end of the 5 or 10-minute infusion period.
- Administer additional fluid until a specified volume is infused or the desired haemodynamic parameters are achieved.

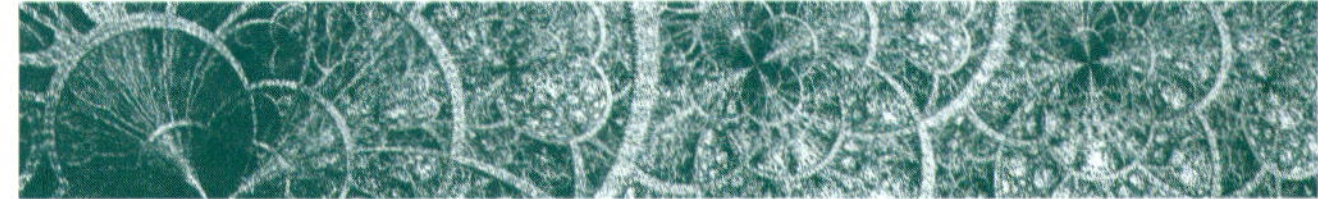

Nursing care

Nurses are responsible for identifying if a person is at risk of FVD, initiating and carrying out measures to prevent and treat FVD, and monitoring the effects of therapy.

Health promotion

Health promotion activities focus on teaching people to prevent FVD. Discuss the importance of maintaining adequate fluid intake, particularly when exercising and during hot weather. Advise people to use commercial sports drinks to replace both water and electrolytes when exercising during warm weather. Instruct people to maintain fluid intake when ill, particularly during periods of fever or when diarrhoea is a problem.

Discuss the increased risk of FVD with older adults and provide information about prevention. Teach older adults (and their caregivers) that thirst decreases with ageing and urge them to maintain a regular fluid intake of about 1,500 mL per day, regardless of perception of thirst.

TABLE 9.4 Commonly administered intravenous fluids

	FLUID AND TONICITY	USES
Dextrose in water solutions	5% dextrose in water (D_5W) Isotonic	Replaces water losses Provides free water necessary for cellular rehydration Lowers serum sodium in hypernatraemia
	10% dextrose in water ($D_{10}W$) Hypertonic	Provides free water Provides nutrition (supplies 340 kcal/L)
	20% dextrose in water ($D_{20}W$) Hypertonic	Supplies 680 kcal/L May cause diuresis
	50% dextrose in water ($D_{50}W$) Hypertonic	Supplies 1,700 kcal/L Used to correct hypoglycaemia
Saline solutions	0.45% sodium chloride Hypotonic	Provides free water to replace hypotonic fluid losses Maintains levels of plasma sodium and chloride
	0.9% sodium chloride Isotonic	Expands intravascular volume Replaces water lost from extracellular fluid Used with blood transfusions Replaces large sodium losses (as from burns)
	3% sodium chloride Hypertonic	Corrects serious sodium depletion
Combined dextrose and saline solution	5% dextrose and 0.45% sodium chloride Isotonic	Provides free water Provides sodium chloride Maintenance fluid of choice if there are no electrolyte imbalances
Multiple electrolyte solutions	Hartmann's solution Isotonic (electrolyte concentrations of sodium, potassium, chloride and calcium are similar to plasma levels)	Expands the intracellular fluid Replaces extracellular fluid losses
	Lactated Ringer's solution Isotonic (similar in composition of electrolytes to plasma but does not contain magnesium)	Replaces fluid losses from burns and the lower gastrointestinal tract Fluid of choice for acute blood loss

Carefully monitor a person at risk of abnormal fluid losses through routes such as vomiting, diarrhoea, nasogastric suction, increased urine output, fever or wounds. Monitor fluid intake in a person with a decreased level of consciousness, disorientation, nausea and anorexia, and physical limitations.

Assessment

Collect assessment data through the health history interview and physical examination.

- *Health history*: risk factors such as medications, acute or chronic renal or endocrine disease; precipitating factors such as hot weather, extensive exercise, lack of access to fluids, recent illness (especially if accompanied by fever, vomiting and/or diarrhoea); onset and duration of symptoms.
- *Physical assessment*: weight; vital signs including orthostatic blood pressure and pulse; peripheral pulses and capillary refill; jugular neck vein distension; skin colour, temperature, turgor; level of consciousness and mentation; urine output. See Box 9.2 for physical assessment changes in the older adult.
- *Diagnostic tests*: serum osmolality and electrolytes, haemoglobin and haematocrit (expect values to fall with rehydration), urine-specific gravity and osmolality, central venous pressure readings.

BOX 9.2 Assessing older adults: fluid volume deficit

With ageing, the elasticity of skin decreases. As a result, turgor diminishes, even in the well-hydrated older adult. This makes skin turgor less reliable when assessing for FVD. In addition, some older adults experience postural hypotension, even when well hydrated. Allow the older adult to stand quietly for a full minute before rechecking blood pressure and pulse when measuring orthostatic vital signs.

Nursing diagnoses and interventions

The focus for nursing diagnoses and interventions for the person with *Fluid volume deficit* is on managing the effects of the deficit and preventing complications.

Deficient fluid volume

A person with a FVD due to abnormal losses, inadequate intake or impaired fluid regulation requires close monitoring as well as immediate and ongoing fluid replacement.

- Assess intake and output accurately, monitoring fluid balance. In acute situations, hourly intake and output may be indicated. *Urine output should be 30 to 60 mL per hour (unless renal failure is present). Urine output of less than 30 mL per hour indicates inadequate renal perfusion and an increased risk of acute renal failure and inadequate tissue perfusion (Perrin & MacLeod, 2017).*

CONSIDERATION FOR PRACTICE

Report a urine output of less than 30 mL per hour to the attending doctor.

- Assess vital signs, CVP and peripheral pulse volume at least every 4 hours. *Hypotension, tachycardia, low CVP and weak, easily obliterated peripheral pulses indicate hypovolaemia.*
- Weigh daily under standard conditions (time of day, clothing and scale). *In most instances (except third spacing), changes in weight accurately reflect fluid balance.* (See the 'Translation to practice' box.)
- Administer and monitor the intake of oral fluids as prescribed. Identify beverage preferences and provide these on a schedule. *Oral fluid replacement is preferred when the person is able to drink and retain fluids.*
- Administer IV as prescribed using an electronic infusion pump. Monitor for indicators of fluid overload if rapid fluid replacement is ordered: dyspnoea, tachypnoea, tachycardia, increased CVP, jugular vein distension and oedema. *Rapid fluid replacement may lead to hypervolaemia, resulting in pulmonary oedema and cardiac failure, particularly in the person with compromised cardiac and renal function.*
- Monitor laboratory values: electrolytes, serum osmolality and haematocrit. *Rehydration may lead to changes in serum electrolytes, osmolality and haematocrit. In some cases, electrolyte replacement may be necessary during rehydration.*

Ineffective tissue perfusion

A fluid volume deficit can lead to decreased perfusion of renal, cerebral and peripheral tissues. Inadequate renal perfusion can lead to acute renal failure. Decreased cerebral perfusion leads to changes in mental status and cognitive function, causing restlessness, anxiety, agitation, excitability, confusion, vertigo, fainting and weakness.

- Monitor for changes in level of consciousness and mental status. *Restlessness, anxiety, confusion and agitation may indicate inadequate cerebral blood flow and circulatory collapse.*
- Monitor serum urea and creatinine and cardiac enzymes, reporting elevated levels to the doctor. *Elevated levels may indicate impaired renal function or cardiac perfusion related to circulatory failure.*
- Turn at least every 2 hours. Provide good skin care and monitor for evidence of skin or tissue breakdown. *Impaired circulation to peripheral tissues increases the risk of skin breakdown. Turn frequently to relieve pressure over bony prominences. Keep skin clean, dry and moisturised to help maintain integrity.*

Risk of injury

The person with FVD is at risk of injury because of dizziness and loss of balance resulting from decreased cerebral perfusion secondary to hypovolaemia.

- Institute safety precautions, including keeping the bed in a low position, using side rails as needed, and slowly raising the person from supine to sitting or sitting to standing position. *Using safety precautions and allowing time for the blood pressure to adjust to position changes will reduce the risk of injury.*

TRANSLATION TO PRACTICE Evidence-based practice for determining fluid needs for the person in long-term care

Residents of long-term care facilities are at significant risk of developing FVD. Most are elderly, many have some degree of dementia, and a significant number are dependent on caregivers to provide fluids. Dehydration, when it occurs, can be a sentinel health event leading to serious and potentially life-threatening secondary problems (Gaspar, 2011; Woodward, 2013).

Various standards for determining the amount of fluid a resident requires have been developed. These standards vary in complexity from a simple 30 mL fluid per kilogram of body weight to a formula that uses body surface area to determine fluid needs. A retrospective study by Gaspar (2011) compared four different formulas, ultimately recommending a formula based on the height and weight of the resident to determine fluid intake.

IMPLICATIONS FOR NURSING

As noted at the beginning of this chapter, the percentage of total body water varies with age and the amount of lean body tissue to adipose tissue. Likewise, fluid requirements of residents in long-term care facilities vary, necessitating attention to the needs of the individual. Furthermore, caregivers are more likely to attend to an individualised plan for a resident's fluid intake than to a generalised recommendation to 'push fluids'. This plan should include not only the target amount of daily fluid intake but also residents' preferences for the type, temperature and timing of fluid intake.

CRITICAL THINKING IN PERSON-CENTRED CARE

1. Why are older adults more vulnerable to dehydration and FVD than younger adults?
2. Identify factors in long-term care settings that increase the risk for FVD. Consider the setting, residents and caregivers.
3. Develop a teaching plan about resident fluid intake for caregivers in a long-term care facility.

- Teach the person and their family members how to reduce orthostatic hypotension:
  a. Move from one position to another in stages; for example, raise the head of the bed before sitting up, and sit for a few minutes before standing.
  b. Avoid prolonged standing.
  c. Rest in a recliner rather than in bed during the day.
  d. Use assistive devices to pick up objects from the floor, rather than stooping.

  Teaching measures to reduce orthostatic hypotension reduces the person's risk of injury. Prolonged bed rest increases skeletal muscle weakness and decreases venous tone, contributing to postural hypotension. Prolonged standing allows blood to pool in the legs, reducing venous return and cardiac output.

Community-based care

Depending on the severity of the fluid volume deficit, the person may be managed in the home or residential facility or may be admitted to an acute care facility. Assess the person's understanding of the cause of the deficit and the fluids necessary for providing replacement. Address the following topics when preparing the person and their family for home care:

- The importance of maintaining adequate fluid intake (at least 1,500 mL per day; more if extra fluid is being lost through perspiration, fever or diarrhoea).
- Manifestations of fluid imbalance and how to monitor fluid balance.
- How to prevent fluid deficit:
  - Avoid exercising during extreme heat.
  - Increase fluid intake during hot weather.
  - If vomiting, take small frequent amounts of ice chips or clear liquids, such as weak tea, flat cola or ginger ale.
  - Reduce intake of coffee, tea and alcohol, which increase urine output and can cause fluid loss.
- Replacement of fluids lost through diarrhoea with fruit juices or bouillon, rather than large amounts of tap water.
- Alternative sources of fluid (such as gelatine, frozen juices or ice-cream) for effective replacement of lost fluids.

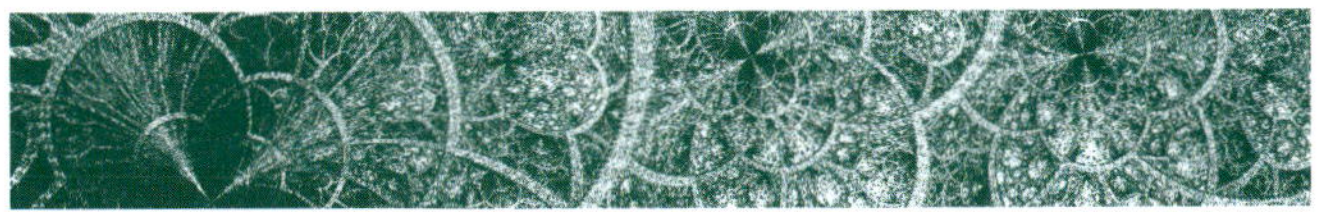

PATIENT SAFETY COMPETENCY FRAMEWORK

5 Clinical reasoning

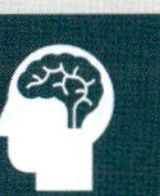

The Patient Safety Competency Framework indicates that nursing students must demonstrate clinical reasoning through the ability to accurately assess, interpret and respond to individual patient data in a systematic and timely way (Levett-Jones et al., 2017).

FLUID VOLUME EXCESS

Fluid volume excess (FVE) results when both water and sodium are retained in the body. FVE may be caused by fluid overload (excess water and sodium intake) or by impairment of the mechanisms that maintain homeostasis. The excess fluid can lead to excess intravascular fluid (hypervolaemia) and excess interstitial fluid (**oedema**).

Pathophysiology

FVE usually results from conditions that cause retention of both sodium and water. These conditions include heart failure, cirrhosis of the liver, renal failure, adrenal gland disorders, corticosteroid administration and stress conditions causing the release of ADH and aldosterone. Other causes include an excessive intake of sodium-containing foods, drugs that cause sodium retention and the administration of excess amounts of sodium-containing intravenous fluids (such as 0.9% NaCl or Ringer's solution). This *iatrogenic* (induced by the effects of treatment) cause of FVE primarily affects a person with impaired regulatory mechanisms.

In FVE, both water and sodium are gained in about the same proportions as normally exists in extracellular fluid. The total body sodium content is increased, which in turn causes an increase in total body water. Because the increase in sodium and water is isotonic, the serum sodium and osmolality remain normal and the excess fluid remains in the extracellular space.

Stress responses activated before, during and immediately after surgery commonly lead to increased ADH and aldosterone levels, leading to sodium and water retention. In the immediate postoperative period, however, this additional fluid tends to be sequestered in interstitial tissues and is unavailable to support cardiovascular and renal function (see the 'Third spacing' section earlier in this chapter). This sequestered fluid is reabsorbed into the circulation within about 48 to 72 hours after surgery. Although it is then normally eliminated through a process of diuresis, a person with heart or kidney failure is at risk of developing fluid overload (McCance & Huether, 2018).

Manifestations and complications

Excess extracellular fluid leads to hypervolaemia and circulatory overload. Excess fluid in the interstitial space causes peripheral or generalised oedema. Manifestations of FVE with related pathophysiology are described in Table 9.5.

Heart failure is not only a potential cause of FVE, but also a potential complication of the condition if the heart is unable to increase its workload to handle the excess blood volume. Severe fluid overload and heart failure can lead to pulmonary oedema, a medical emergency. See the chapter 'Nursing care of people with cardiac disorders' for more information about heart failure and pulmonary oedema.

INTERPROFESSIONAL CARE

Managing FVE focuses on prevention in a person at risk, treating its manifestations and correcting the underlying cause. Management includes limiting sodium and water intake and administering diuretics.

TABLE 9.5 Manifestations of fluid volume excess

MANIFESTATIONS	RELATED PATHOPHYSIOLOGY
Peripheral oedema, or if severe, **anasarca** (severe, generalised oedema)	Excess fluid in the interstitial spaces, usually resulting from conditions that cause retention of both sodium and water (e.g. heart failure, renal failure and stress responses causing the release of ADH and aldosterone, such as surgery)
Full bounding pulse, distended neck and peripheral veins, increased central venous and right atrial pressures, cough, **dyspnoea** (laboured or difficult breathing), **orthopnoea** (difficult breathing when supine)	Circulatory overload from increased water and sodium retention
Dyspnoea at rest	Mobilisation (reabsorption) of fluid from peripheral tissues increases circulatory fluid volume
Tachycardia and hypertension	Increased circulatory fluid volume
Reduced oxygen saturation	As fluid increases in the interstitial spaces and alveoli, gas exchange is impaired, leading to hypoxia and hypercapnia
Moist crackles on auscultation of the lungs, pulmonary oedema	Excess fluid in pulmonary interstitial spaces and alveoli
Increased urine output (**polyuria**)	Increased circulatory volume and increased perfusion of the renal arteries increases amount of filtrate produced in glomerulus
Ascites (excess fluid in the peritoneal cavity)	Increased filtration pressure due to hypervolaemia
Decreased haematocrit and BUN	Dilutional effect of increased circulatory volume
Altered mental status and anxiety	Pressure on the cerebral cortex from cerebral hypertension and oedema causes decreased oxygenation (hypoxia) of neurons
Pulmonary oedema	Elevation of left-sided filling pressures from increased circulatory volume and heart failure increase pressures in pulmonary vascular system

Diagnosis

The following laboratory tests may be ordered.

- *Serum electrolytes* and *serum osmolality* are measured. Serum sodium and osmolality usually remain within normal limits.
- *Serum haematocrit* and *haemoglobin* often are decreased due to plasma dilution from excess extracellular fluid.
- Additional tests of *renal* and *liver function* (such as serum urea and creatinine and liver enzymes) may be ordered to help determine the cause of FVE if it is unclear.

Medications

Diuretics are commonly used to treat FVE. They inhibit sodium and water reabsorption, increasing urine output. The three major classes of diuretics, each of which acts on a different part of the kidney tubule, are as follows:

1. Loop diuretics act in the ascending loop of Henle.
2. Thiazide-type diuretics act on the distal convoluted tubule.
3. Potassium-sparing diuretics affect the distal nephron.

The nursing implications for diuretics are outlined in the 'Medication administration' box.

BOX 9.3 Fluid restriction guidelines

- **Subtract requisite fluids (e.g. ordered IV fluids, fluid used to dilute IV medications) from total daily allowance.**
- **Divide remaining fluid allowance:**
  - **day shift: 50% of total**
  - **evening shift: 25% to 33% of total**
  - **night shift: remainder.**
- **Explain the fluid restriction to the person and family members.**
- **Identify preferred fluids and intake pattern.**
- **Place allowed amounts of fluid in small glasses (gives perception of a full glass).**
- **Offer ice chips (when melted, ice chips are approximately half the frozen volume).**
- **Provide frequent mouth care.**
- **Provide sugarless chewing gum (if allowed) to reduce thirst sensation.**

Treatments

FLUID MANAGEMENT Fluid intake may be restricted in a person who has FVE. The amount of fluid allowed per day is prescribed by the primary attending doctor. All fluid intake must be calculated, including meals and that used to administer medications orally or intravenously. Box 9.3 provides guidelines for a person with a fluid restriction.

DIETARY MANAGEMENT Because sodium retention is a primary cause of FVE, a sodium-restricted diet is often prescribed. This is particularly important for people with a history of heart or renal failure (McCance & Huether, 2018; Metheny, 2012; Stevenson et al., 2018). Australian adults typically consume 2.5 to 3 g of sodium every day; recommended sodium intake is 500 to 2,000 mg per day, or 1 teaspoon (Food Standards Australia New Zealand, 2015; National Health and Medical Research Council, 2013). The primary dietary sources of sodium are the salt shaker, processed foods and foods themselves (see Box 9.4).

A mild sodium restriction can be achieved by instructing the person and primary food preparer in the household to reduce the amount of salt in recipes by half, avoid using the salt shaker during meals and avoid foods that contain high levels of sodium (either naturally or because of processing). In moderate and severely sodium-restricted diets, salt is avoided altogether, as are all foods containing significant amounts of sodium.

MEDICATION ADMINISTRATION **Diuretics for fluid volume excess**

Diuretics increase urinary excretion of water and sodium. They are categorised into three major groups: loop diuretics, thiazide and thiazide-like diuretics, and potassium-sparing diuretics. Diuretics are used to enhance renal function and to treat vascular fluid overload and oedema. Common side effects include orthostatic hypotension, dehydration, electrolyte imbalance and possible hyperglycaemia. Diuretics should be used with caution in the older adult. Examples of each major type follow.

LOOP DIURETICS

Frusemide (Lasix)
Ethacrynic acid
Bumetanide

Loop diuretics inhibit sodium and chloride reabsorption in the ascending loop of Henle. (See the chapter 'Nursing care of people with kidney disorders' for the anatomy of the kidneys.) As a result, loop diuretics promote the excretion of sodium, chloride, potassium and water.

THIAZIDE AND THIAZIDE-LIKE DIURETICS

Bendroflumethiazide
Chlorothiazide
Hydrochlorothiazide
Chlorthalidone
Indapamide

Thiazide and thiazide-like diuretics promote the excretion of sodium, chloride, potassium and water by decreasing absorption in the distal tubule.

POTASSIUM-SPARING DIURETICS

Spironolactone (Aldactone)
Amiloride HCl (Midamor)

Potassium-sparing diuretics promote excretion of sodium and water by inhibiting sodium–potassium exchange in the distal tubule.

HEALTH EDUCATION FOR THE PERSON AND THEIR FAMILY

- The drugs will increase the amount and frequency of urination.
- The drugs must be taken even when you feel well.
- Take the drugs in the morning and afternoon to avoid having to get up at night to urinate.
- Change position slowly to avoid dizziness.
- Report the following to your attending doctor: dizziness; trouble breathing; or swelling of face, hands or feet.
- Weigh yourself every day and report sudden gains or losses.
- Avoid using the salt shaker when eating.
- If the drug increases potassium loss, consume drinks and foods high in potassium, such as orange juice and bananas.
- Do not use salt substitutes if you are taking a potassium-sparing diuretic.

BOX 9.4 Foods high in sodium

Processed meat and fish
- Bacon
- Sausage
- Luncheon meat and other cold cuts
- Smoked fish

Selected dairy products
- Buttermilk
- Cottage cheese
- Cheeses
- Ice-cream

Processed grains
- Cracker biscuits
- Most dry cereals

Most canned goods
- Meats
- Vegetables
- Soups

Snack foods
- Salted popcorn
- Nuts
- Potato chips/pretzels
- Gelatine desserts

Condiments and food additives
- Barbecue sauce
- Saccharin
- Pickles
- Chilli sauce
- Soy sauce
- Meat tenderisers
- Salted margarine
- Worcestershire sauce
- Salad dressings

Naturally high in sodium
- Brains
- Oysters
- Kidneys
- Prawns
- Dried fruit
- Crab
- Spinach
- Lobster
- Carrots

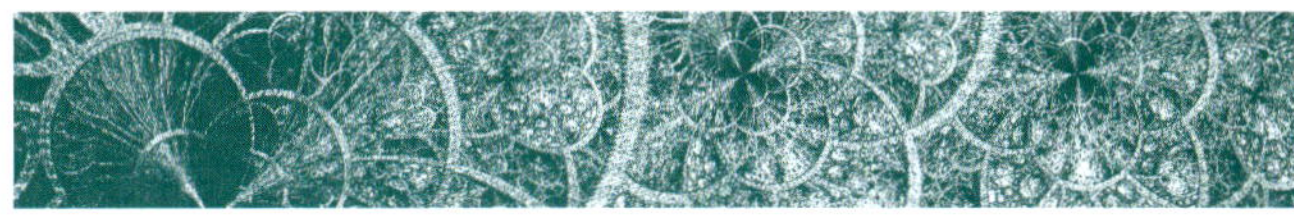

Nursing care

Nursing care focuses on preventing FVE in a person at risk and on managing problems resulting from its effects. See 'Nursing care plan: a person with fluid volume excess'.

Health promotion

Health promotion related to FVE focuses on teaching preventive measures to a person who is at risk (e.g. people who have heart or kidney failure). Discuss the relationship between sodium intake and water retention. Provide guidelines for a low-sodium diet and teach the person to carefully read food labels to identify 'hidden' sodium, particularly in processed foods. Instruct the person at risk to weigh themself on a regular basis, using the same scales, and to notify their primary attending doctor if they gain more than 2 kg in a week or less. Carefully monitor the person receiving intravenous fluids for signs of hypervolaemia. Reduce the flow rate and promptly report manifestations of fluid overload to the doctor.

NURSING CARE PLAN A person with fluid volume excess

Dorothy Smith is a 45-year-old Indigenous woman hospitalised with acute renal failure that developed as a result of acute glomerulonephritis. She is expected to recover, but she has very little urine output. Ms Smith is a single mother of two teenage sons. Until her illness, she was active in caring for her family, her career as a primary school teacher's aide and community activities.

ASSESSMENT

Mike Penning, Ms Smith's nurse, notes that she is in the oliguric phase of acute renal failure and that her urine output for the previous 24 hours is 250 mL; this low output has been constant for the past 8 days. She gained 0.45 kg in the past 24 hours. Laboratory test results from that morning are sodium, 155 mEq/L (normal 135 to 145 mEq/L); potassium, 5.3 mEq/L (normal 3.5 to 5.0 mEq/L); calcium, 7.6 mg/dL (normal 8.0 to 10.5 mg/dL) and urine-specific gravity 1.008 (normal 1.010 to 1.030). Ms Smith's serum creatinine and urea are high; however, her ABGs are within normal limits.

In his assessment of Ms Smith, Mike notes the following:

- BP 160/92; P 102, with obvious neck vein distension; R 28, with crackles and wheezes; head of bed elevated 30 degrees; T 37.0°C.
- Periorbital and sacral oedema present; 3+ pitting bilateral pedal oedema; skin cool, pale and shiny.
- Alert, oriented; responds appropriately to questions.
- States she is thirsty, slightly nauseated and extremely tired.

Ms Smith is receiving intravenous frusemide and is on a 24-hour fluid restriction of 500 mL plus the previous day's urine output to manage her FVE.

DIAGNOSES

- *Excess fluid volume* related to acute renal failure
- *Risk of impaired skin integrity* related to fluid retention and oedema
- *Risk of impaired gas exchange* related to pulmonary congestion
- *Activity intolerance* related to FVE, fatigue and weakness

PLANNING

- Advise Ms Smith that she needs to be weighed twice daily, at 0600 and 1800 hours to monitor fluid balance daily.
- Explain to Ms Smith that the nurses will be monitoring vital signs and SaO_2 every 4 hours and the reasons for monitoring vital signs.
- Explain the purpose for Ms Smith being placed on restricted fluids and suggested ways to maintain the fluid restriction.
- Explain to Ms Smith that all fluids consumed and all urine output will need to be measured and documented on a fluid balance chart.
- Instruct and educate Ms Smith on the importance of oral hygiene and the effectiveness of moistened oral applicators to prevent mouth dryness.
- Advise Ms Smith of the importance of sitting out of bed on a chair three times a day and of the necessity to call for assistance when ambulating or if dyspnoea is increasing.
- Explain the importance of keeping the head of the bed elevated 30 to 40 degrees and the importance of not staying in one position for a prolonged period of time.
- Attend to pressure area care as required to maintain skin integrity.

Expected outcomes

- Regain fluid balance, as evidenced by weight loss, decreasing oedema and normal vital signs.
- Experience decreased dyspnoea.
- Maintain intact skin and mucous membranes.
- Increase activity levels as prescribed.

IMPLEMENTATION

- Weigh Ms Smith at 0600 and 1800 daily and record the findings.
- Document and review the vital signs, fluid balance chart 4 hourly.
- Obtain, measure and document urine-specific gravity every 8 hours.
- Discuss and consult with Ms Smith about her compliance with the prescribed fluid restriction.
- Consult with Ms Smith about her ability to move and inspect her skin for any signs of pressure areas.
- Consult with Ms Smith and identify her ability to maintain oral hygiene. Provide extra assistance if required to maintain oral care every 2 to 4 hours.
- Consult with Ms Smith and identify if the elevation of the head of bed is reducing the dyspnoea.
- Observe and monitor Ms Smith's ability to sit out of bed and ambulate safely without increasing shortness of breath and fatigue.

EVALUATION

At the end of the shift, Mike evaluates the effectiveness of the plan of care and continues all diagnoses and interventions. Ms Smith has gained no weight and her urinary output during this shift is 170 mL. Her urine-specific gravity remains at 1.008. Her vital signs are unchanged, but her crackles and wheezes have decreased slightly. Her skin and mucous membranes are intact. Ms Smith tolerated the bedside chair without dyspnoea or fatigue.

CRITICAL THINKING IN THE NURSING PROCESS

1. What is the pathophysiological basis for Ms Smith's increased respiratory rate, blood pressure and pulse?
2. Explain how elevating the head of the bed 30 to 40 degrees facilitates respirations.
3. Suppose Ms Smith says, 'I would really like to have all my fluids at once instead of spreading them out.' How would you reply and why?
4. Outline a plan for teaching Ms Smith about diuretics.

REFLECTION ON THE NURSING PROCESS

1. As the Registered Nurse, how do you know if the education pertaining to fluid restriction has been effective?
2. Outline what you have learned from this case study that you will apply to your future practice.

Assessment

Collect assessment data through the health history interview and physical examination.

- *Health history*: risk factors such as medications, heart failure, acute or chronic renal or endocrine disease; precipitating factors such as a recent illness, change in diet or change in medications; recent weight gain; complaints of persistent cough, shortness of breath, swelling of feet and ankles, or difficulty sleeping when lying down.
- *Physical assessment*: weight; vital signs; peripheral pulses and capillary refill; jugular neck vein distension; oedema; lung sounds (crackles or wheezes), dyspnoea, cough and sputum; urine output; mental status.
- *Diagnostic tests*: monitor serum electrolytes and osmolality, haemoglobin and haematocrit, urine-specific gravity.

Nursing diagnoses and interventions

Nursing diagnoses and interventions for the person with FVE focus on the multisystem effects of the fluid overload.

Excess fluid volume

Nursing care for the person with excess fluid volume includes collaborative interventions such as administering diuretics and maintaining a fluid restriction, as well as monitoring the status and effects of the excess fluid volume. This is particularly critical in older adults because of the age-related decline in cardiac and renal compensatory responses.

- Assess vital signs, heart sounds, CVP and volume of peripheral arteries. *Hypervolaemia can cause hypertension, bounding peripheral pulses, a third heart sound (S_3) due to the volume of blood flow through the heart and high CVP readings.*
- Assess for the presence and extent of oedema, particularly in the lower extremities, the back, and sacral and periorbital areas. *Initially, oedema affects the dependent portions of the body—the lower extremities of the ambulatory person and the sacrum of the bedridden person. Periorbital oedema indicates more generalised oedema.*

> **CONSIDERATION FOR PRACTICE**
>
> **Assess urine output hourly. Maintain accurate intake and output records. Note urine output of less than 30 mL per hour or a positive fluid balance on 24-hour total intake and output calculations. Heart failure and inadequate renal perfusion may result in decreased urine output and fluid retention.**

- Obtain daily weights at the same time of day, using approximately the same clothing and balanced scales. *Daily weights are one of the most important gauges of fluid balance. Acute weight gain or loss represents fluid gain or loss. Weight gain of 2 kg is equivalent to 2 L of fluid gain.*
- Administer oral fluids cautiously, adhering to any prescribed fluid restriction. Discuss the restriction with the person and significant others, including the total volume allowed, the rationale, and the importance of reporting all fluid taken. *All sources of fluid intake, including ice chips, are recorded to avoid excess fluid intake.*
- Provide oral hygiene at least every 2 hours. *Oral hygiene contributes to the comfort of the person and keeps mucous membranes intact; it also helps to relieve thirst if fluids are restricted.*
- Teach the person and significant others about the sodium-restricted diet and emphasise the importance of checking before bringing foods to the person on this diet. *Excess sodium promotes water retention; a sodium-restricted diet is ordered to reduce water gain.*
- Administer prescribed diuretics as ordered, monitoring the person's response to therapy. *Loop or high-ceiling diuretics such as frusemide can lead to rapid fluid loss and signs of hypovolaemia and electrolyte imbalance.*
- Promptly report significant changes in serum electrolytes or osmolality or abnormal results of tests done to determine contributing factors to the FVE. *Gradual correction of serum electrolytes and osmolality is expected; however, aggressive diuretic therapy can lead to over-correction.*

Risk of impaired skin integrity

Tissue oedema decreases oxygen and nutrient delivery to the skin and subcutaneous tissues, increasing the risk of injury.

- Frequently assess skin, particularly in pressure areas and over bony prominences. *Skin breakdown can progress rapidly when circulation is impaired.*
- Reposition the person at least every 2 hours. Provide skin care with each position change. *Frequent position changes minimise tissue pressure and promote blood flow to tissues.*
- Provide an egg-crate mattress or alternating pressure mattress, foot cradle, heel protectors and other devices to reduce pressure on tissues. *These devices, which distribute pressure away from bony prominences, reduce the risk of skin breakdown.*

Risk of impaired gas exchange

With FVE, gas exchange may be impaired by oedema of pulmonary interstitial tissues. Acute pulmonary oedema is a serious and potentially life-threatening complication of pulmonary congestion.

- Auscultate lungs for presence or worsening of crackles and wheezes; auscultate heart for extra heart sounds. *Crackles and wheezes indicate pulmonary congestion and oedema. A gallop rhythm (S_3) may indicate diastolic overloading of the ventricles secondary to FVE.*
- Place in Fowler's position if dyspnoea or orthopnoea is present. *Fowler's position improves lung expansion by decreasing the pressure of abdominal contents on the diaphragm.*
- Monitor oxygen saturation levels and **arterial blood gases (ABGs)** for evidence of impaired gas exchange (SaO_2 < 92% to 95%; PaO_2 < 80 mmHg). Administer oxygen as indicated. *Oedema of interstitial lung tissues can interfere with gas exchange and delivery to body tissues. Supplemental oxygen promotes gas exchange across the alveolar–capillary membrane, improving tissue oxygenation.*

Community-based care

Teaching for home care focuses on managing the underlying cause of FVE and preventing future episodes of excess fluid volume. Address the following topics when preparing the person and the family for home care:

- Signs and symptoms of excess fluid and when to contact the attending doctor.
- Prescribed medications: when and how to take, intended and adverse effects, what to report to attending doctor.
- Recommended or prescribed diet; ways to reduce sodium intake; how to read food labels for salt and sodium content; use of salt substitutes, if allowed.
- If restricted, the amount and type of fluids to take each day; how to balance intake over 24 hours.
- Monitoring weight; changes reported to attending doctor.
- Ways to decrease dependent oedema:
  a. Change position frequently.
  b. Avoid restrictive clothing.
  c. Avoid crossing the legs when sitting.
  d. Wear support stockings or hose.
  e. Elevate feet and legs when sitting.
- How to protect oedematous skin from injury:
  a. Do not walk barefoot.
  b. Buy good-fitting shoes; shop in the afternoon when feet are more likely to be swollen.
- Using additional pillows or a recliner to sleep, to relieve orthopnoea.

BOX 9.5 Teaching people to reduce sodium intake

- Reducing sodium intake will help the body excrete excess sodium and water.
- The body needs less than one-tenth of a teaspoon of salt per day.
- Approximately one-third of sodium intake comes from salt added to foods during cooking and at the table; one-quarter to one-third comes from processed foods; and the rest comes from food and water naturally high in sodium.
- Sodium compounds are used in foods as preservatives, leavening agents and flavour enhancers.
- Many non-prescription drugs (such as analgesics, cough medicine, laxatives and antacids), as well as toothpastes and mouthwashes, contain high amounts of sodium.
- Low-sodium salt substitutes are not really sodium-free and may contain half as much sodium as regular salt.
- Use salt substitutes sparingly; larger amounts often taste bitter instead of salty.
- The preference for salt will eventually diminish.
- Salt, monosodium glutamate, baking soda and baking powder contain substantial amounts of sodium.
- Read labels.
- In place of salt or salt substitutes, use herbs, spices, lemon juice, vinegar and wine as flavouring when cooking.

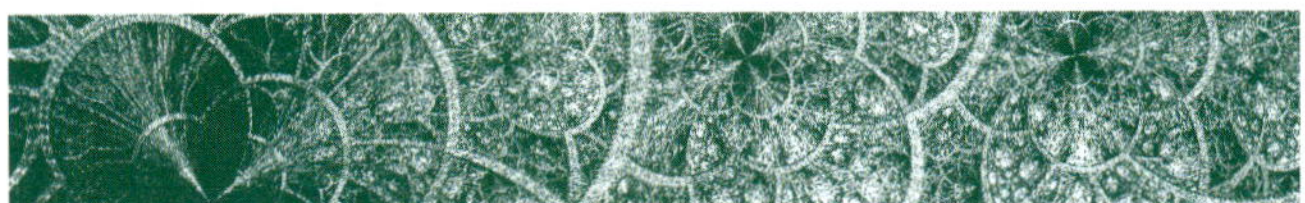

SODIUM IMBALANCE

Sodium is the most plentiful electrolyte in ECF, with normal serum sodium levels ranging from 135 to 145 mEq/L. Sodium is the primary regulator of the volume, osmolality and distribution of ECF. It is also important for maintaining neuromuscular activity. Because of the close interrelationship between sodium and water balance, disorders of fluid volume and sodium balance often occur together. Sodium imbalances affect the osmolality of ECF and water distribution between the fluid compartments. When sodium levels are low (hyponatraemia), water is drawn into the cells of the body, causing them to swell. In contrast, high levels of sodium in ECF (hypernatraemia) draw water out of body cells, causing them to shrink. See Box 9.5 for information on teaching the person to help reduce sodium intake.

Overview of normal sodium balance

Most of the body's sodium comes from dietary intake. Other sources of sodium include prescription drugs and certain self-prescribed remedies. Sodium is primarily excreted by the kidneys. A small amount is excreted through the skin and the gastrointestinal (GI) tract.

The kidney is the primary regulator of sodium balance in the body. The kidney excretes or conserves sodium in response to changes in vascular volume. A fall in blood volume prompts several mechanisms that lead to sodium and water retention:

- The renin–angiotensin–aldosterone system (see Figure 9.9) is stimulated. Angiotensin II prompts the renal tubules to reabsorb sodium. It also causes vasoconstriction, slowing blood flow through the kidney and reducing glomerular filtration. This further reduces the amount of sodium excreted. Angiotensin II promotes the release of aldosterone from the adrenal cortex. In the presence of aldosterone, more sodium is reabsorbed in the cortical collecting tubules of the kidney and more potassium is eliminated in the urine.
- ADH is released from the posterior pituitary (see Figure 9.10). ADH promotes sodium and water reabsorption in the distal tubules of the kidney, reducing urine output and expanding blood volume.

  By contrast, when blood volume expands, sodium and water elimination by the kidneys increases.
- The **glomerular filtration rate** (the rate at which plasma is filtered through the glomeruli of the kidney) increases, allowing more water and sodium to be filtered and excreted.
- ANP is released by cells in the atria of the heart. ANP increases sodium excretion by the kidneys.
- ADH release from the pituitary gland is inhibited. In the absence of ADH, the distal tubule is relatively impermeable to water and sodium, allowing more to be excreted in the urine. Table 9.6 summarises the causes and effects of sodium imbalances.

The person with hyponatraemia

Hyponatraemia is a serum sodium level of less than 135 mEq/L. Hyponatraemia usually results from a loss of sodium from the body, but it may also be caused by water gains that dilute ECF.

TABLE 9.6 Causes and manifestations of sodium imbalances

IMBALANCE	POSSIBLE CAUSES	MANIFESTATIONS
Hyponatraemia Serum sodium < 135 mEq/L Critical value < 120 mEq/L *Other lab values* Serum osmolality < 280 mOsm/kg Critical value < 250 mOsm/kg	• Excess sodium loss through kidneys, GI tract or skin • Water gains related to renal disease, heart failure or cirrhosis of the liver • SIADH • Excessive hypotonic IV fluids	• Anorexia, nausea, vomiting, abdominal cramping and diarrhoea • Headache • Altered mental status • Muscle cramps, weakness and tremors • Seizures and coma
Hypernatraemia Serum sodium > 145 mEq/L Critical value > 160 mEq/L *Other lab values* Serum osmolality > 295 mOsm/kg Critical value > 325 mOsm/kg	• Altered thirst • Inability to respond to thirst sensation or obtain water • Profuse sweating • Diarrhoea • Diabetes insipidus • Oral electrolyte solutions or hyperosmolar tube-feeding formulas • Excess IV fluids such as normal saline, 3% or 5% sodium chloride or sodium bicarbonate	• Thirst • Increased temperature • Dry, sticky mucous membranes • Restlessness • Weakness • Altered mental status • Decreasing level of consciousness • Muscle twitching • Seizures

Pathophysiology

Excess sodium loss can occur through the kidneys, GI tract or skin. Diuretic medications, kidney diseases or adrenal insufficiency with impaired aldosterone and cortisol production can lead to excessive sodium excretion in urine. Vomiting, diarrhoea and gastrointestinal suction are common causes of excess sodium loss through the GI tract. Neurological conditions such as stroke, cerebral haemorrhage, trauma or surgery can cause cerebral salt wasting. Sodium may also be lost when gastrointestinal tubes are irrigated with water instead of saline or when repeated tap-water enemas are administered (Norris, 2018). Excessive sweating or loss of skin surface (as with an extensive burn) can also cause excessive sodium loss.

Water gains that can lead to hyponatraemia may occur with:

- systemic diseases such as heart failure, renal failure or cirrhosis of the liver
- syndrome of inappropriate secretion of antidiuretic hormone (SIADH), in which water excretion is impaired
- excessive administration of hypotonic intravenous fluids.

Hyponatraemia causes a drop in serum osmolality. Water shifts from ECF into the intracellular space, causing cells to swell and reducing the osmolality of intracellular fluid. Many of the manifestations of hyponatraemia can be attributed to cellular oedema and hypo-osmolality (McCance & Huether, 2018; Tran, Tantsis & Ging, 2017).

Manifestations

The manifestations of hyponatraemia depend on the rapidity of onset, the severity and the cause of the imbalance. If the condition develops slowly, manifestations are usually not experienced until the serum sodium levels reach 125 mEq/L. In addition, the manifestations of hyponatraemia vary depending on extracellular fluid volume. Early manifestations of hyponatraemia include muscle cramps, weakness and fatigue from its effects on muscle cells. Gastrointestinal function is affected, causing anorexia, nausea and vomiting, abdominal cramping and diarrhoea.

As sodium levels continue to decrease, the brain and nervous system are affected by cellular oedema. Neurological manifestations progress rapidly when the serum sodium level falls below 120 mEq/L and include headache, depression, dulled sensorium, personality changes, irritability, lethargy, hyperreflexia, muscle twitching and tremors. If serum sodium falls to very low levels, convulsions and coma are likely to occur. When hyponatraemia is associated with decreased ECF volume, the manifestations are those of hypovolaemia (*hypotonic dehydration*). In hyponatraemia associated with FVE, manifestations include those of hypervolaemia.

INTERPROFESSIONAL CARE

Interprofessional management of hyponatraemia focuses on restoring normal blood volume and serum sodium levels.

Diagnosis

The following laboratory tests may be ordered:

- *Serum sodium* and *osmolality* are decreased in hyponatraemia (serum sodium < 135 mEq/L; serum osmolality < 275 mOsm/kg).
- A *24-hour urine specimen* is obtained to evaluate sodium excretion. In conditions associated with normal or increased extracellular volume (such as SIADH), urinary sodium is increased; in conditions resulting from losses of isotonic fluids (e.g. sweating, diarrhoea, vomiting and third-space fluid accumulation), by contrast, urinary sodium is decreased.

Medications

When both sodium and water have been lost (hyponatraemia with hypovolaemia), sodium-containing fluids are given to replace both water and sodium. These fluids may be given by mouth, nasogastric tube or intravenously. Isotonic Ringer's solution or isotonic saline (0.9% NaCl) solution may be administered. Cautious administration of intravenous 3% or 5% NaCl solution may be necessary in a person who has very low plasma sodium levels (110 to 115 mEq/L).

Loop diuretics are administered to a person who has hyponatraemia with normal or excess ECF volume. Loop diuretics promote an isotonic diuresis and fluid volume loss without hyponatraemia. Thiazide diuretics are avoided because they cause a relatively greater sodium loss in relation to water loss.

In addition, drugs to treat the underlying cause of hyponatraemia may be administered.

Fluid and dietary management

If hyponatraemia is mild, increasing the intake of foods high in sodium may restore normal sodium balance. Fluids often are restricted to help reduce ECF volume and correct hyponatraemia.

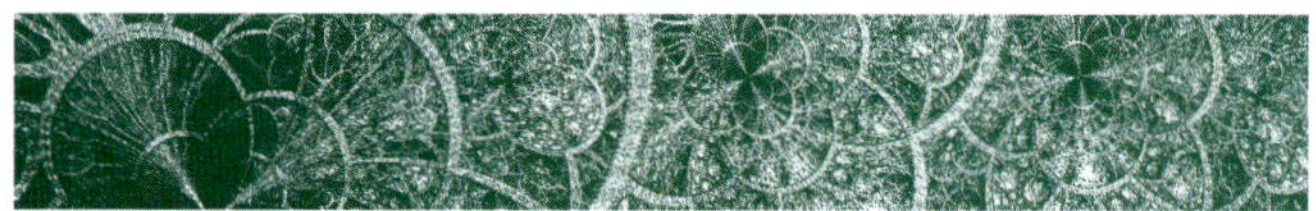

Nursing care

Nursing care of the person with hyponatraemia focuses on identifying the person at risk and managing problems resulting from the systemic effects of the disorder.

Health promotion

People at risk of mild hyponatraemia include those who participate in activities that increase fluid loss through excessive perspiration (diaphoresis) and then replace those losses by drinking large amounts of water. This includes athletes, people who do heavy labour in high environmental temperatures and older adults living in non-air-conditioned settings during hot weather. Teach the following to people who are at risk:

- manifestations of mild hyponatraemia, including nausea, abdominal cramps and muscle weakness
- the importance of drinking liquids containing sodium and other electrolytes at frequent intervals when perspiring heavily, when environmental temperatures are high and/or if watery diarrhoea persists for several days.

Assessment

Assessment data related to hyponatraemia include the following:

- *Health history*: current manifestations, including nausea and vomiting, abdominal discomfort, muscle weakness, headache and other symptoms; duration of symptoms and any precipitating factors such as heavy perspiration, vomiting or diarrhoea; chronic diseases such as heart or renal failure, cirrhosis of the liver or endocrine disorders; current medications.
- *Physical assessment*: mental status and level of consciousness; vital signs, including orthostatic vitals and peripheral pulses; presence of oedema or weight gain.
- *Diagnostic tests*: serum sodium and osmolality; serum potassium.

Nursing diagnoses and interventions

Risk of imbalanced fluid volume

Because of its role in maintaining fluid balance, sodium imbalances often are accompanied by water imbalances. In addition, treatment of hyponatraemia can affect the person's fluid balance.

> **CONSIDERATION FOR PRACTICE**
>
> **Carefully monitor the person receiving sodium-containing intravenous solutions for signs of hypervolaemia (increased blood pressure and CVP, tachypnoea, tachycardia, gallop rhythm S_3 and/or S_4 heart sounds, shortness of breath, crackles). Hypertonic saline solutions can lead to hypervolaemia, particularly in the person with cardiovascular or renal disease.**

- Monitor intake and output, weigh daily and calculate 24-hour fluid balance. *Fluid excess or deficit may occur with hyponatraemia.*
- Use an intravenous flow control device to administer hypertonic saline (3% and 5% NaCl) solutions; carefully monitor flow rate and response. *Hypertonic solutions can increase the risk of pulmonary and cerebral oedema due to water retention. Careful monitoring is vital to prevent these complications and possible permanent damage.*
- If fluids are restricted, explain the reason for the restriction, the amount of fluid allowed and how to calculate fluid intake. *Teaching increases the person's sense of control and compliance.*

For additional nursing interventions that may apply to the person with hyponatraemia, review the discussions of FVD and FVE.

Risk of ineffective cerebral tissue perfusion

The person with severe hyponatraemia experiences fluid shifts that cause an increase in intracellular fluid volume. This can cause brain cells to swell, increasing pressure within the cranial vault.

- Monitor serum electrolytes and serum osmolality and report abnormal results. *As serum sodium levels fall, the manifestations and neurological effects of hyponatraemia become increasingly severe.*
- Assess for neurological changes, such as lethargy, altered level of consciousness, confusion and convulsions. Monitor mental status and orientation. Compare baseline data with continuing assessments. *Serum sodium levels of 115 to 120 mEq/L can cause headache, lethargy and decreased responsiveness; sodium levels less than 110 to 115 mEq/L may cause seizures and coma.*
- Assess muscle strength and tone and deep tendon reflexes. *Increasing muscle weakness and decreased deep tendon reflexes are manifestations of increasing hyponatraemia.*

> **CONSIDERATION FOR PRACTICE**
>
> **Maintain a quiet environment and institute seizure precautions in the person with severe hyponatraemia. Severe hyponatraemia can lead to seizures and it is evidenced that a quiet environment reduces neurological stimulation. It is pertinent to maintain the person's safety and reduce the risk of injury from seizures by using precautions, such as ensuring that side rails are up, lowering the height of the bed and having airway equipment readily available.**

Community-based care

Teaching for home care focuses on the underlying cause of the sodium deficit and often on prevention. Teach the person who has experienced hyponatraemia and those who are at risk of developing hyponatraemia about the following:

- manifestations of mild and more severe hyponatraemia to report to the primary attending doctor
- the importance of regular serum electrolyte monitoring if taking a potent diuretic or on a low-sodium diet
- types of foods and fluids to replace sodium orally if dietary sodium is not restricted
- older adults' increased risk for hyponatraemia from the effects of medications and potential fluid imbalances.

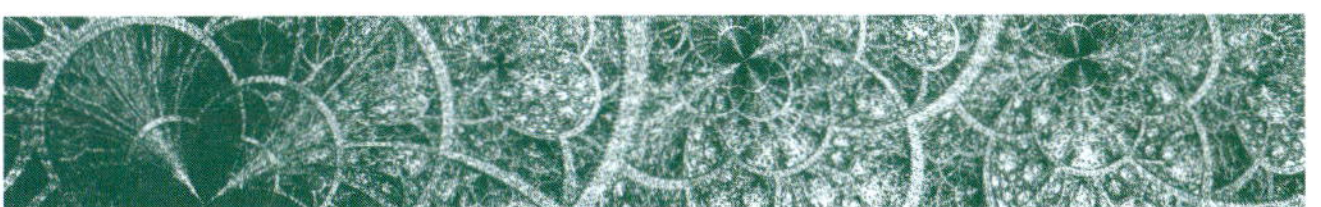

The person with hypernatraemia

Hypernatraemia is a serum sodium level greater than 145 mEq/L. It may develop when sodium is gained in excess of water or when water is lost in excess of sodium. Either FVD or FVE often accompanies hypernatraemia. Older adults with diminished thirst or who have limited access to water are at particular risk for hypernatraemia (Loscalzo et al., 2022).

Pathophysiology

Two regulatory mechanisms protect the body from hypernatraemia: (1) excess sodium in ECF stimulates the release of ADH so more water is retained by the kidneys, and (2) the thirst mechanism is stimulated to increase the intake of water (Giddens, 2021; Metheny, 2012). These two factors increase extracellular water, diluting the excess sodium and restoring normal levels. Because of the effectiveness of these mechanisms, hypernatraemia almost never occurs in the person who has an intact thirst mechanism and access to water.

Water deprivation is a cause of hypernatraemia in the person who is unable to respond to thirst due to altered mental status or physical disability. Excess water loss may occur with watery diarrhoea or increased insensible losses (due to fever, hyperventilation, excessive perspiration or massive burns). Unless water is adequately replaced, the person with diabetes insipidus (see the chapter 'Nursing care of people with endocrine disorders') also may develop hypernatraemia. Excess sodium intake can result from ingestion of excess salt or hypertonic intravenous solutions. People who experience near-drowning in seawater are at risk of hypernatraemia, as are people with heat stroke.

Manifestations

Hypernatraemia (also known as *hypertonic dehydration*) causes hyperosmolality of ECF. As a result, water is drawn out of cells, leading to cellular dehydration. The most serious effects of cellular dehydration are seen in the brain. As brain cells contract, neurological manifestations develop. The brain itself shrinks, causing mechanical traction on cerebral vessels. These vessels may tear and bleed. Although the brain rapidly adapts to hyperosmolality to minimise the water loss, acute hypernatraemia can cause widespread cerebral vascular bleeding (Metheny, 2012; Norris, 2018).

Thirst is the first manifestation of hypernatraemia. If thirst is not relieved, the primary manifestations relate to altered neurological function (see Table 9.6). Initial lethargy, weakness and irritability can progress to seizures, coma and death in severe hypernatraemia. Both the severity of the sodium excess and the rapidity of its onset affect the manifestations of hypernatraemia.

INTERPROFESSIONAL CARE

Treatment of hypernatraemia depends on its cause. Hypernatraemia is corrected slowly (over a 48-hour period) to avoid development of cerebral oedema secondary to a shift of water into the brain cells.

Diagnosis

The following laboratory and diagnostic tests may be ordered:

- *Serum sodium levels* are greater than 145 mEq/L in hypernatraemia.
- *Serum osmolality* is greater than 295 mOsm/kg in hypernatraemia.
- The *water deprivation test* may be conducted to identify diabetes insipidus. Water and all other fluids are withheld for a specified period of time. During this time, urine specimens are obtained for osmolality and specific gravity. No change in these values supports the diagnosis of diabetes insipidus.

Medications

The principal treatment for hypernatraemia is oral or intravenous water replacement. Hypotonic intravenous fluids such as 0.45% NaCl solution or 5% dextrose in water (which is isotonic when administered but provides pure water when the glucose is metabolised) may be administered to correct the water deficit. Diuretics may also be given to increase sodium excretion (Lukitsch, 2021; Mestrom et al., 2021).

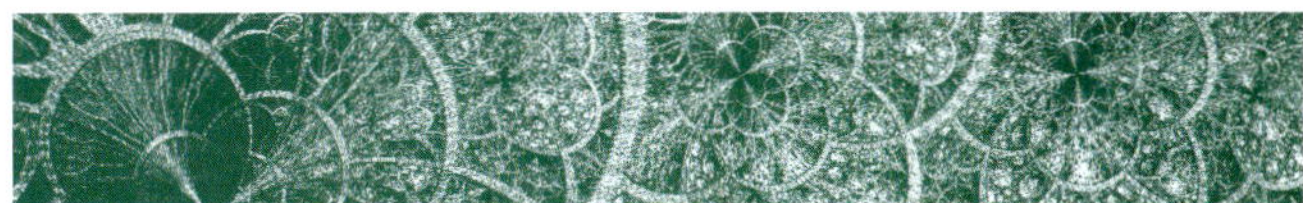

Nursing care

The primary focus of nursing care related to hypernatraemia is prevention. Measures to prevent hypernatraemia include identifying risk factors, teaching the person and caregivers, monitoring laboratory test results and working with the interprofessional team to reduce the potential for hypernatraemia.

Health promotion

Education pertaining to hypernatremia is required for the person at risk of hypernatraemia, as well as their attending doctors, and is essential to prevent this electrolyte disorder. Instruct caregivers of debilitated people who are unable to perceive or respond to thirst to offer fluids at regular intervals. If the person is unable to maintain adequate fluid intake, contact the medical staff about an alternative route for fluid intake (e.g. a feeding tube). Teach attending doctors the importance of providing adequate water for the person receiving tube feedings (many of which are hypertonic).

Assessment

Assessment data related to hypernatraemia include the following:

- *Health history*: duration of symptoms and any precipitating factors such as water deprivation, increased water loss due to heavy perspiration, temperature or rapid breathing, diarrhoea, excess salt intake or diabetes insipidus; current medications; perception of thirst.

- *Physical assessment*: vital signs including temperature; mucous membranes; altered mental status or level of consciousness; manifestations of FVE or FVD.
- *Diagnostic tests*: monitor serum sodium and osmolality, serum potassium.

Nursing diagnoses and interventions

Risk of injury

Mental status and brain function may be affected by hypernatraemia itself or by rapid correction of the condition that leads to cerebral oedema. In either case, closely monitor the person and take precautions to reduce risk of injury.

- Monitor and maintain fluid replacement to within the prescribed limits. Monitor serum sodium levels and osmolality; report rapid changes to the attending doctor. *Rapid water replacement or rapid changes in serum sodium or osmolality can cause fluid shifts within the brain, increasing the risk of bleeding or cerebral oedema.*
- Monitor neurological function, including mental status, level of consciousness and other manifestations such as headache, nausea, vomiting, elevated blood pressure and decreased pulse rate. *Both hypernatraemia and rapid correction of hypernatraemia affect the brain and brain function. Careful monitoring is vital to detect changes in mental status that may indicate cerebral bleeding or oedema.*
- Institute safety precautions as necessary: keep the bed in its lowest position, side rails up and padded, and an airway at the bedside. *The person with a sodium disorder is at risk of injury due to seizure activity and changes in mental status.*
- Keep clocks, calendars and familiar objects at the bedside. Orient to time, place and circumstances as needed. Allow significant others to remain with the person as much as possible. *An unfamiliar environment and altered thought processes can further increase the person's risk of injury. Significant others provide a sense of security and reduce the person's anxiety.*

Community-based care

When preparing the person who has experienced hypernatraemia for home care, discuss the following topics:

- the importance of responding to thirst and consuming adequate fluids (if the person is dependent on a caregiver, stress to the caregiver the importance of regularly offering fluids)
- if prescribed, guidelines for following a low-sodium diet (see Box 9.5)
- use and effects (intended and unintended) of any prescribed diuretic or other medication
- the importance of following a schedule for regular monitoring of serum electrolyte levels and reporting manifestations of imbalance to the attending doctor.

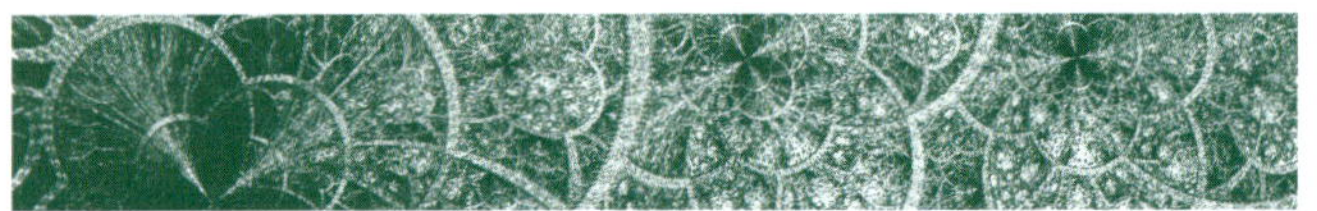

POTASSIUM IMBALANCE

Potassium, the primary intracellular cation, plays a vital role in cell metabolism and cardiac and neuromuscular function. The normal serum (ECF) potassium level is 3.5 to 5.0 mEq/L.

Overview of normal potassium balance

Most potassium in the body is found within the cells (ICF), which have a concentration of 140 to 150 mEq/L. This significant difference in the potassium concentrations of ICF and ECF helps maintain the resting membrane potential of nerve and muscle cells; either a deficit or an excess of potassium can adversely affect neuromuscular and cardiac function. The higher intracellular potassium concentration is maintained by the sodium–potassium pump.

To maintain its balance, potassium must be replaced daily. Normally, potassium is supplied in food. Virtually all foods contain potassium, although some foods and fluids are richer sources of this element than others (see Box 9.6).

The kidneys eliminate potassium very efficiently; even when potassium intake is stopped, the kidneys continue to excrete it. Because the kidneys do not conserve potassium well, significant amounts may be lost through this route. However, because the kidneys are the principal organs involved in the elimination of potassium, renal failure can lead to potentially serious elevations of serum potassium.

Aldosterone helps regulate potassium elimination by the kidneys. An increased potassium concentration in ECF stimulates aldosterone production by the adrenal gland. The kidneys respond to aldosterone by increasing potassium excretion. Changes in aldosterone secretion can profoundly affect the serum potassium level.

Normally only small amounts of potassium are lost in the faeces, but substantial amounts may be lost from the gastrointestinal tract with diarrhoea or through drainage from an ileostomy (a permanent opening into the small bowel).

Potassium constantly shifts into and out of the cells. This movement between ICF and ECF can significantly affect the serum potassium level. For example, potassium shifts into or out of the cells in response to changes in hydrogen ion

BOX 9.6 Foods high in potassium

Fruits
- Apricots
- Avocados
- Bananas
- Dates
- Oranges
- Raisins

Vegetables and vegetable juices
- Carrots
- Cauliflower
- Mushrooms
- Peas
- Potatoes
- Spinach
- Tomatoes

Meats and fish
- Beef
- Chicken
- Kidney
- Liver
- Lobster
- Pork
- Salmon
- Tuna
- Turkey

Milk products
- Buttermilk
- Chocolate milk
- Evaporated milk
- Low-fat yoghurt
- Milk

TABLE 9.7 Causes and manifestations of potassium imbalances

IMBALANCE	CAUSES	MANIFESTATIONS
Hypokalaemia Serum potassium < 3.5 mEq/L Critical value < 2.5 mEq/L	• Excess GI losses: vomiting, diarrhoea, ileostomy drainage • Renal losses: diuretics, hyperaldosteronism • Inadequate intake • Shift into cells: alkalosis, rapid tissue repair	Cardiovascular • Arrhythmias • ECG changes Gastrointestinal • Nausea and vomiting • Anorexia • Decreased bowel sounds • Ileus Musculoskeletal • Muscle weakness • Leg cramps
Hyperkalaemia Serum potassium > 5.0 mEq/L Critical value > 6.5 mEq/L	• Renal failure • Potassium-sparing diuretics • Adrenal insufficiency • Excess potassium intake (e.g. excess potassium replacement) • Aged blood • Shift out of cells: cell and tissue damage, acidosis	Cardiovascular • Tall, peaked T waves, widened QRS • Arrhythmias • Cardiac arrest Gastrointestinal • Nausea and vomiting • Abdominal cramping • Diarrhoea Neuromuscular • Muscle weakness • Paraesthesias • Flaccid paralysis

concentration (pH, discussed later in this chapter) as the body strives to maintain a stable acid–base balance.

The significant difference between intracellular and extracellular potassium concentrations is vital to the resting membrane potential of cells. Resting membrane potential, in turn, is necessary for transmitting nerve impulses. Potassium imbalances affect transmission and conduction of nerve impulses, maintenance of normal cardiac rhythms and contraction of skeletal and smooth muscle (McCance & Huether, 2018).

As the primary intracellular cation, potassium plays a major role in regulating the osmolality of ICF and is involved in metabolic processes. Potassium is necessary for the storage of glycogen in skeletal muscle cells. Table 9.7 summarises the causes and manifestations of potassium imbalances.

The person with hypokalaemia

Hypokalaemia is an abnormally low serum potassium (less than 3.5 mEq/L). It usually results from excess potassium loss, although the hospitalised person may be at risk of hypokalaemia because of inadequate potassium intake.

Pathophysiology

Excess potassium may be lost through the kidneys or the GI tract. These losses deplete total potassium stores in the body.

- Excess potassium loss through the kidneys often is secondary to drugs such as potassium-wasting diuretics, corticosteroids, amphotericin B and large doses of some antibiotics. Hyperaldosteronism, a condition in which the adrenal glands secrete excess aldosterone, also causes excess elimination of potassium through the kidneys. Glucosuria and osmotic diuresis (e.g. associated with diabetes mellitus) also cause potassium wasting through the kidneys (Giddens, 2021; Metheny, 2012).
- Gastrointestinal losses of potassium result from severe vomiting, gastric suction, or loss of intestinal fluids through diarrhoea or ileostomy drainage.

Potassium intake may be inadequate in the person who is unable or unwilling to eat for prolonged periods. The person who is hospitalised is at risk, especially when on extended parenteral fluid therapy with solutions that do not contain potassium. The person with anorexia nervosa or alcoholism may develop hypokalaemia due to both inadequate intake and loss of potassium through vomiting, diarrhoea, or laxative or diuretic use.

A *relative* loss of potassium occurs when potassium shifts from ECF into the cells. This usually is due to loss of hydrogen ions and alkalosis, although it also may occur during periods of rapid tissue repair (e.g. following a burn or trauma), in the presence of excess insulin (insulin promotes potassium entry into skeletal muscle and liver cells), during acute stress or because of hypothermia. In these instances, the total body stores of potassium remain adequate.

Manifestations

Hypokalaemia affects the transmission of nerve impulses, interfering with the contractility of smooth, skeletal and cardiac muscle, as well as the regulation and transmission of cardiac impulses.

- Characteristic electrocardiogram (ECG) changes of hypokalaemia include flattened or inverted T waves, the development of U waves and a depressed ST segment (see Figure 9.11). The most serious cardiac effect is an increased risk of atrial and ventricular arrhythmias (abnormal rhythms). Hypokalaemia increases the risk of digitalis toxicity in the person receiving this drug used to treat heart failure (see the chapter 'Nursing care of people with cardiac disorders').

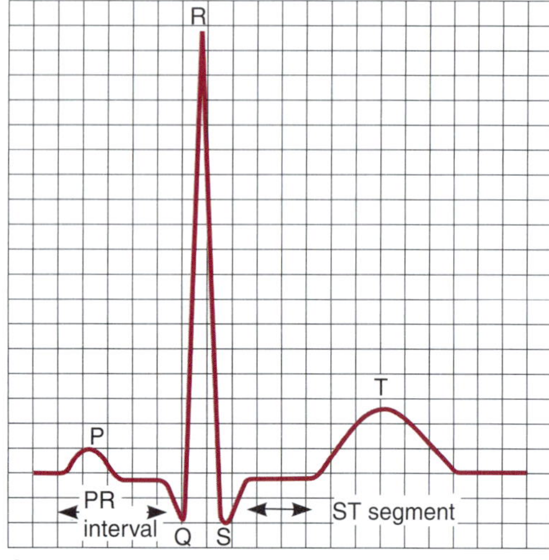

A

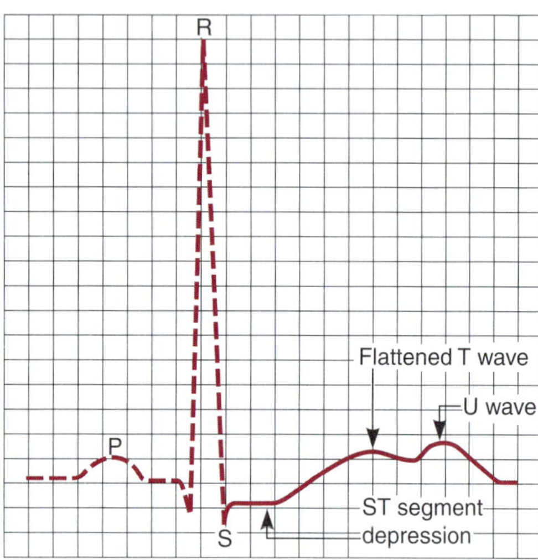

B

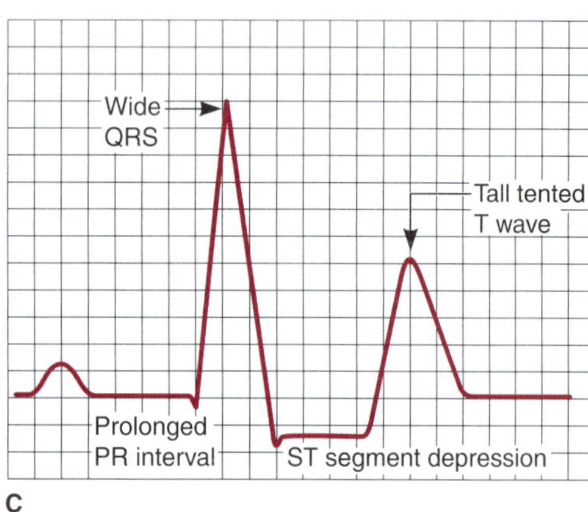

C

FIGURE 9.11 ***The effects of changes in potassium levels on the electrocardiogram (ECG). A, Normal ECG; B, ECG in hypokalaemia; C, ECG in hyperkalaemia***

- Hypokalaemia affects both the resting membrane potential and intracellular enzymes in skeletal and smooth muscle cells. This causes skeletal muscle weakness and slowed peristalsis of the GI tract. Muscles of the lower extremities are affected first, then the trunk and upper extremities. This effect of hypokalaemia is magnified when serum calcium levels are above normal.
- Carbohydrate metabolism is affected by hypokalaemia. Insulin secretion is suppressed, as is the synthesis of glycogen in skeletal muscle and the liver.

Hypokalaemia also can affect kidney function, particularly the ability to concentrate urine. Severe hypokalaemia can lead to rhabdomyolysis, a condition in which muscle fibres disintegrate, releasing myoglobin to be excreted in the urine.

Manifestations of hypokalaemia are more pronounced when potassium losses occur acutely. When hypokalaemia develops gradually, potassium shifts out of the cells, helping maintain the ratio of intracellular to extracellular potassium. As a result, the neuromuscular manifestations of hypokalaemia are less severe. See 'Multisystem effects of hypokalaemia'.

INTERPROFESSIONAL CARE

The management of hypokalaemia focuses on prevention and treatment of a deficiency.

Diagnosis

The following laboratory and diagnostic tests may be ordered:

- *Serum potassium* (K^+) is used to monitor potassium levels in the person who is at risk of, or who is being treated for, hypokalaemia. A serum K^+ of 3.0 to 3.5 mEq/L is considered mild hypokalaemia. Moderate hypokalaemia is defined as a serum K^+ of 2.5 to 3.0 mEq/L and severe hypokalaemia as a serum K^+ of less than 2.5 mEq/L (Giddens, 2021; Metheny, 2012).
- *Arterial blood gases (ABGs)* are measured to determine acid–base status. An increased pH (alkalosis) often is associated with hypokalaemia. (See Table 9.11 later in this chapter for normal ABG values.)
- *Renal function studies*, such as *serum urea and creatinine,* may be ordered to evaluate for potential causes or effects of hypokalaemia.
- *ECG recordings* are obtained to evaluate the effects of hypokalaemia on the cardiac conduction system.

Medications

Oral and/or parenteral potassium supplements are given to prevent and, as needed, treat hypokalaemia. To prevent hypokalaemia in the person taking nothing by mouth, potassium chloride is added to IV fluids. The dose used to treat hypokalaemia includes the daily maintenance requirement, replacement of ongoing losses (e.g. gastric suction) and additional potassium to correct the existing deficit. Several days of therapy may be required. Commonly prescribed potassium supplements, their actions and nursing implications are described in the 'Medication administration' box.

Nutrition

A diet high in potassium-rich foods is recommended for the person at risk of developing hypokalaemia or to supplement drug therapy (see Box 9.6).

Multisystem effects of hypokalaemia

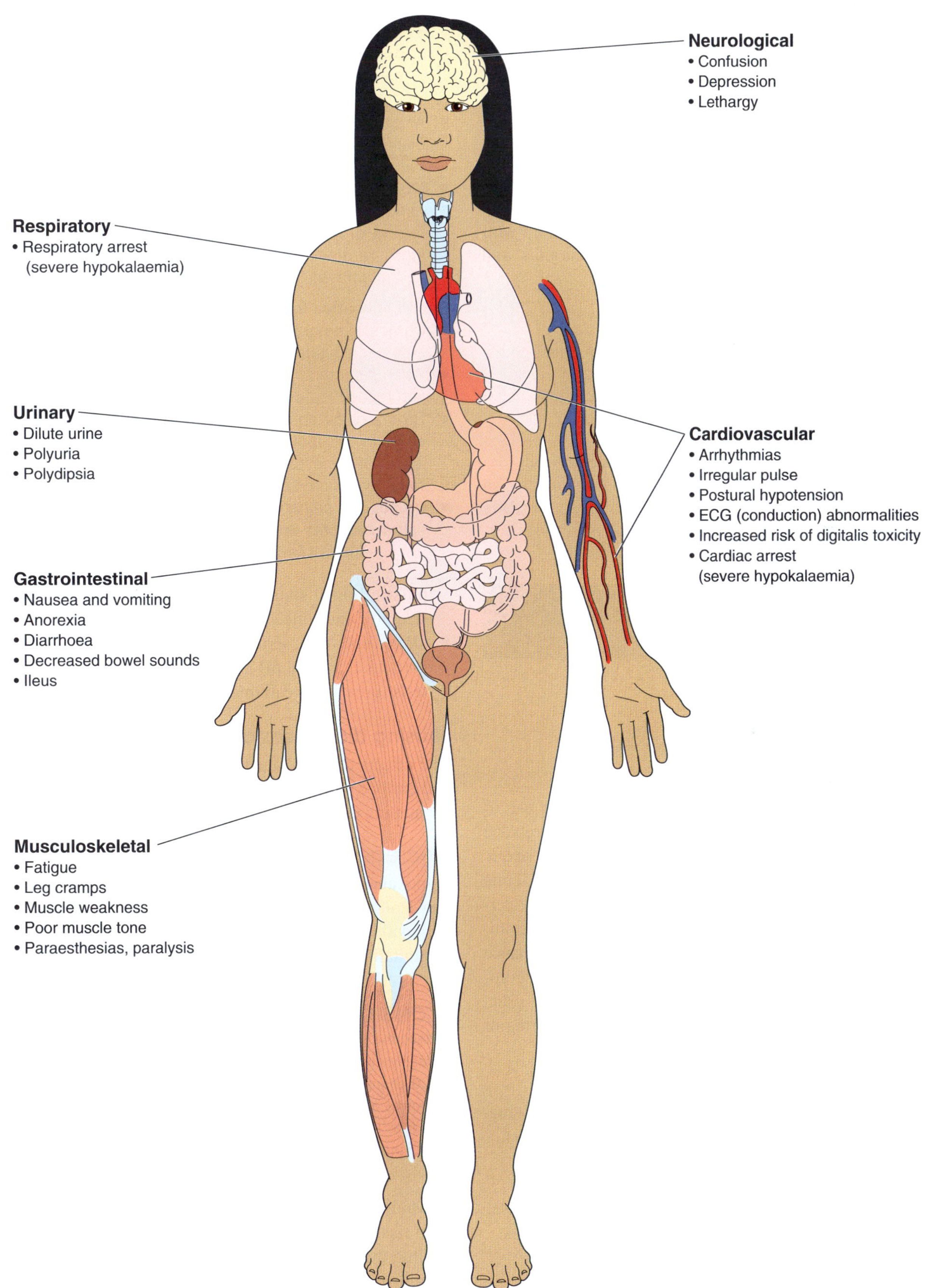

MEDICATION ADMINISTRATION Hypokalaemia

POTASSIUM SOURCES
Potassium acetate
Potassium bicarbonate
Potassium citrate
Potassium chloride
Potassium gluconate

Potassium is rapidly absorbed from the gastrointestinal tract; potassium chloride is the agent of choice, because low chloride often accompanies low potassium. Potassium is used to prevent and/or treat hypokalaemia (e.g. with parenteral nutrition and potassium-wasting diuretics and prophylactically after major surgery).

Nursing responsibilities

- When giving oral forms of potassium:
  a. Dilute or dissolve effervescent, soluble or liquid potassium in fruit or vegetable juice or cold water.
  b. Chill to increase palatability.
  c. Give with food to minimise GI effects.
- When giving parenteral forms of potassium:
  a. Check correct infusion rate and administer slowly.
  b. Check appropriate administration mode and use as an additive (usually NOT administered IV push and NOT added to fluids already hanging).
  c. Do *not* administer undiluted.
  d. Assess injection site frequently for signs of pain and inflammation.
  e. Use an infusion control device.
- Assess for abdominal pain, distension, gastrointestinal bleeding; if present, do not administer medication. Notify the attending doctor.
- Monitor fluid intake and output.
- Assess for manifestations of hyperkalaemia: weakness, feeling of heaviness in legs, mental confusion, hypotension, cardiac arrhythmias, changes in ECG, increased serum potassium levels.

Health education for the person and their family

- Do not take potassium supplements if you are also taking a potassium-sparing diuretic.
- When parenteral potassium is discontinued, eat potassium-rich foods.
- Do not chew enteric-coated tablets or allow them to dissolve in the mouth, as this may affect the potency and action of the medications.
- Take potassium supplements with meals.
- Do not use salt substitutes when taking potassium (most salt substitutes are potassium-based).

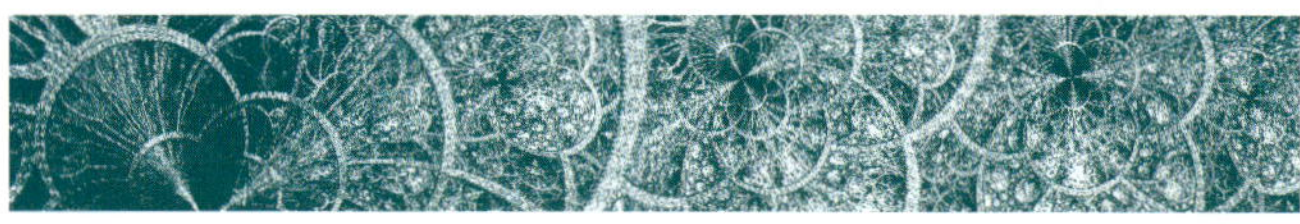

Nursing care

See 'Nursing care plan: a person with hypokalaemia'.

Health promotion

When providing general health education, discuss the use of balanced electrolyte solutions (e.g. sports drinks) to replace abnormal fluid losses (excess perspiration, vomiting or severe diarrhoea). Discuss the necessity of preventing hypokalaemia with the at-risk person. Provide diet teaching and refer the person with anorexia nervosa for counselling. Stress the potassium-losing effects of taking diuretics and using laxatives to enhance weight loss. Discuss the potassium-wasting effects of most diuretics with the person taking these drugs and encourage a diet rich in high-potassium foods, as well as regular monitoring of serum potassium levels.

Assessment

Assessment data related to hypokalaemia include the following:

- *Health history*: current manifestations, including anorexia, nausea and vomiting, abdominal discomfort, muscle weakness or cramping, and other symptoms; duration of symptoms and any precipitating factors such as diuretic use, prolonged vomiting or diarrhoea; chronic diseases such as diabetes, hyperaldosteronism or Cushing's syndrome; current medications.
- *Physical assessment*: mental status; vital signs, including orthostatic vitals, apical and peripheral pulses; bowel sounds, abdominal distension; muscle strength and tone.
- *Diagnostic tests*: serum electrolytes, K^+, Na^+ and Ca^{2+} in particular, arterial pH and other ABG results, renal function tests (urea and creatinine), ECG changes.

Nursing diagnoses and interventions

The effects of hypokalaemia on cardiac impulse transmission and cardiac and skeletal muscle function are the highest priority nursing care focus.

Decreased cardiac output

Hypokalaemia affects the strength of cardiac contractions and can lead to arrhythmias that further impair cardiac output. Hypokalaemia also alters the response to cardiac drugs, such as digitalis and the anti-arrhythmics.

CONSIDERATION FOR PRACTICE

Place the person with severe hypokalaemia on a cardiac monitor. Closely monitor cardiac rhythm and observe for characteristic ECG changes of hypokalaemia (ST segment depression, flattened T waves and U waves). Report rhythm changes immediately and treat as indicated. Severe hypokalaemia can cause life-threatening arrhythmias.

- Monitor serum potassium levels, particularly in the person at risk of hypokalaemia (those with excess losses due to drug therapy, gastrointestinal losses or who are unable to consume a normal diet). Report abnormal levels to the attending doctor. *Potassium must be replaced daily, because the body is unable to conserve it. Either lack of*

NURSING CARE PLAN A person with hypokalaemia

Rose Ortiz is a 72-year-old widow who lives alone, although close to her daughter's home. Ms Ortiz has mild heart failure and is being treated with digoxin (Lanoxin) 0.125 mg, frusemide (Lasix) 40 mg PO daily and a mildly restricted sodium diet (2 g daily). For the last several weeks, Ms Ortiz has complained that she feels weak and sometimes faint, light-headed and dizzy. Serum electrolyte tests ordered by her doctor reveal a potassium level of 2.4 mEq/L. Potassium chloride solution (K Ciel 20 mEq/15 mL) PO twice daily is prescribed and Ms Ortiz is referred to Nancy Walters, RN, for follow-up care.

ASSESSMENT

Ms Ortiz's health history reveals that she has rigidly adhered to her sodium-restricted diet and has been compliant in taking her prescribed medications, with the exception of occasionally taking an additional 'water pill' when her ankles swell. She takes a laxative every evening to ensure a daily bowel movement. Ms Ortiz states that she is reluctant to take the potassium chloride the doctor has ordered because her neighbour complains that his potassium supplement upsets his stomach. Physical assessment findings include T 36.8°C, P 70, R 20 and BP 138/84. Muscle strength in her upper extremities is normal and equal; lower extremity strength is weak but equal. No sensory deficits are apparent.

DIAGNOSES

- *Risk of injury* related to muscle weakness.
- *Risk of ineffective health maintenance* related to lack of knowledge about how diuretic therapy and laxative use affect potassium levels.

PLANNING

- Advise Ms Ortiz about the potential hazards of negotiating stairs.
- Highlight awareness of potential medication side effects and adverse effects and explain how taking additional tablets may have contributed to hypokalaemia.
- Consider alternative measures to prevent constipation without using laxatives on a regular basis (e.g. high-fibre diet, adequate fluid intake).
- Explain purpose of the prescribed potassium and its role in reversing muscle weakness.
- Instruct and educate Ms Ortiz on the importance of taking the medication (potassium supplement) after breakfast and supper. Advise to call if gastric irritation occurs.
- Discuss dietary sources of potassium and provide a list of potassium-rich foods.

EXPECTED OUTCOMES

- Maintain potassium level within normal limits (3.5 to 5.0 mEq/L).
- Regain normal muscle strength.
- Remain free of injury.
- Verbalise understanding of the effects of diuretic therapy and laxatives on potassium levels.
- Identify measures to avoid gastrointestinal irritation when taking oral potassium.
- Identify potassium-rich foods.

IMPLEMENTATION

- To observe and monitor Ms Ortiz's ability to safely ambulate up and down stairs.
- Discuss and consult with Ms Ortiz if there have been any heart palpations, dizziness which could be a result of side effects of frusemide.
- Discuss and consult with Ms Ortiz about her dietary intake with a focus on high fibre and fluids.
- Discuss with Ms Ortiz her compliance with medication administration after food, advising report of any gastric irritation.
- Review Ms Ortiz's dietary intake, identifying that she is eating potassium-rich food sources.

EVALUATION

On a follow-up visit 1 week later, Ms Ortiz states that her muscle weakness, dizziness and other symptoms have resolved. She is taking the prescribed drugs as directed and is using laxatives only 2 or 3 times a week. Ms Ortiz reports that she has increased her intake of both potassium-rich foods and fluids and high-fibre foods. Her potassium level is within normal limits.

CRITICAL THINKING IN THE NURSING PROCESS

1. What is the pathophysiological basis for Ms Ortiz's muscle weakness and dizziness?
2. How might the chronic overuse of laxatives contribute to hypokalaemia?
3. Describe the interaction of digitalis, diuretics and potassium.
4. Develop a plan of care for Ms Ortiz for the nursing diagnosis of *Perceived constipation*.

REFLECTION ON THE NURSING PROCESS

1. As the Registered Nurse, how do you know that education pertaining to medication compliance has been effective?
2. What communication and education strategies could you use when providing care for a person with hypokalaemia?

intake or abnormal losses of potassium in the urine or gastric fluids can lead to hypokalaemia.

- Monitor vital signs, including orthostatic vitals and peripheral pulses. *As cardiac output falls, the pulse becomes weak and thready. Orthostatic hypotension may be noted with decreased cardiac output.*
- Monitor the person taking digitalis for toxicity. Monitor response to anti-arrhythmic drugs. *Hypokalaemia potentiates digitalis effects and increases resistance to certain anti-arrhythmics.*
- Dilute intravenous potassium and administer using an electronic infusion device. In general, potassium is given no faster than 10 to 20 mEq/hour. Closely monitor intravenous flow rate and response to potassium replacement. *Rapid potassium administration is dangerous and can lead to hyperkalaemia and cardiac arrest.*

CONSIDERATION FOR PRACTICE

Never administer undiluted potassium directly into the vein.

Activity intolerance

Muscle cramping and weakness are common early manifestations of hypokalaemia. The lower extremities are usually affected initially. This muscle weakness can cause the person to fatigue easily, particularly with activity.

- Monitor skeletal muscle strength and tone, which are affected by moderate hypokalaemia. *Increasing weakness, paraesthesias or paralysis of muscles or progression of affected muscles to include the upper extremities or trunk can indicate a further drop in serum potassium levels.*
- Monitor respiratory rate, depth and effort; heart rate and rhythm; and blood pressure at rest and following activity. *Tachypnoea, dyspnoea, tachycardia and/or a change in blood pressure may indicate decreasing ability to tolerate activities. Report changes to the attending doctor.*
- Assist with self-care activities as needed. *Increasing muscle weakness can lead to fatigue and affect the ability to meet self-care needs.*

Risk of imbalanced fluid volume

- Maintain accurate intake and output records. *Gastrointestinal fluid losses can lead to significant potassium losses.*
- Monitor bowel sounds and abdominal distension. *Hypokalaemia affects smooth muscle function and can lead to slowed peristalsis and paralytic ileus.*

Acute pain

Discomfort is common when intravenous potassium chloride at a concentration of more than 40 mEq/L is given into a peripheral vein.

- When possible, administer intravenous KCl through a central line. *The rapid blood flow through central veins dilutes the KCl solution, decreasing discomfort.*
- Spread the total daily dose of KCl over 24 hours to minimise the concentration of intravenous solutions. *High concentrations of KCl are irritating to vein walls, particularly if inflammation is present.*
- Discuss with the doctor the use of a small amount of lidocaine prior to or with the infusion. *Both a lidocaine bolus given at the infusion site and a small amount of lidocaine in the intravenous infusion have been shown to at least partially relieve discomfort associated with concentrated potassium solutions (Giddens, 2021; Metheny, 2012).*

Community-based care

The focus in preparing the person with or at risk of hypokalaemia is prevention. Discharge planning focuses on teaching self-care practices. Include the following topics when preparing the person and family for home care:

- recommended diet, including a list of potassium-rich foods
- prescribed medications and potassium supplements, their use, and desired and unintended effects
- using salt substitutes (if recommended) to increase potassium intake; avoiding substitutes if taking a potassium supplement or potassium-sparing diuretic
- manifestations of potassium imbalance (hypokalaemia or hyperkalaemia) to report to the attending doctor
- recommendations for monitoring serum potassium levels
- if taking digitalis, manifestations of digitalis toxicity to report to the attending doctor
- managing gastrointestinal disorders that cause potassium loss (vomiting, diarrhoea, ileostomy drainage) to prevent hypokalaemia.

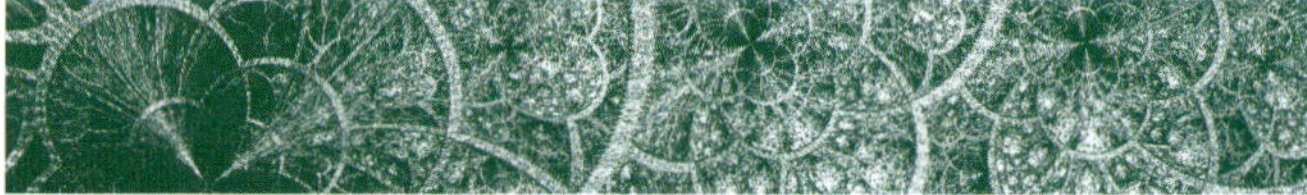

The person with hyperkalaemia

Hyperkalaemia is an abnormally high serum potassium level (greater than 5 mEq/L). Hyperkalaemia can result from inadequate excretion of potassium, excessively high intake of potassium, or a shift of potassium from the intracellular to the extracellular space. *Pseudohyperkalaemia* (an erroneously high serum potassium reading) can occur if the blood sample haemolyses, releasing potassium from blood cells, before it is analysed. Hyperkalaemia affects neuromuscular and cardiac function.

Pathophysiology

Impaired renal excretion of potassium is a primary cause of hyperkalaemia. Untreated renal failure, adrenal insufficiency (e.g. Addison's disease or inadequate aldosterone production) and medications (such as potassium-sparing diuretics, the antimicrobial drug trimethoprim and some NSAIDs) impair potassium excretion by the kidneys.

In the person with a normal renal excretion of potassium, excess oral potassium (e.g. by supplement or use of salt substitutes) rarely leads to hyperkalaemia. Rapid intravenous administration of potassium or transfusion of aged blood can lead to hyperkalaemia. A shift of potassium ions from the intracellular space can occur in acidosis, with severe tissue trauma, during chemotherapy and due to starvation. In acidosis, excess hydrogen ions enter the cells, displacing potassium and causing it to shift into the extracellular space. The extent of this shift is greater with metabolic acidosis than with respiratory acidosis (see 'Acid–base disorders' later in this chapter).

Hyperkalaemia alters the cell membrane potential, affecting the heart, skeletal muscle function and the GI tract. The most harmful consequence of hyperkalaemia is its effect on cardiac function. The cardiac conduction system is affected first, with slowing of the heart rate, possible heart blocks and prolonged depolarisation. ECG changes include peaked T waves, a prolonged PR interval and widening of the QRS complex (see Figure 9.11). Ventricular arrhythmias develop and cardiac arrest may occur. Severe hyperkalaemia decreases the strength of myocardial contractions (McCance & Huether, 2018).

Skeletal muscles become weak and paralysis may occur with very high serum potassium levels. Hyperkalaemia causes smooth muscle hyperactivity, leading to gastrointestinal disturbances.

The seriousness of hyperkalaemia is based on the serum potassium (K^+) level and ECG changes.

- *Mild hyperkalaemia:* serum K^+ between 5 and 6.5 mEq/L; ECG changes limited to peaked T wave.
- *Moderate hyperkalaemia:* serum K^+ between 6.5 and 8 mEq/L; ECG changes limited to peaked T wave.
- *Severe hyperkalaemia:* serum K^+ greater than 8 mEq/L; ECG shows absent P waves and widened QRS pattern.

Manifestations

The manifestations of hyperkalaemia result from its effects on the heart, skeletal and smooth muscles. Early manifestations include diarrhoea, colic (abdominal cramping), anxiety, paraesthesias, irritability, and muscle tremors and twitching. As serum potassium levels increase, muscle weakness develops, progressing to flaccid paralysis. The lower extremities are affected first, progressing to the trunk and upper extremities. The heart rate may be slow (bradycardia) and irregular. The ECG shows T-wave changes and, at high serum potassium levels, widening of the QRS complex and absence of P waves.

INTERPROFESSIONAL CARE

The management of hyperkalaemia focuses on returning the serum potassium level to normal by treating the underlying cause and avoiding additional potassium intake. The choice of therapy for existing hyperkalaemia is based on the severity of the hyperkalaemia.

Diagnosis

The following laboratory and diagnostic tests may be ordered:

- *Serum electrolytes* show a serum potassium level greater than 5.0 mEq/L. Low calcium and sodium levels may increase the effects of hyperkalaemia; therefore, these electrolytes are usually measured as well.
- *ABGs* are measured to determine if acidosis is present.
- An *ECG* is obtained and *continuous ECG monitoring* is instituted to evaluate the effects of hyperkalaemia on cardiac conduction and rhythm.

Medications

Medications are administered to lower the serum potassium and to stabilise the conduction system of the heart. For moderate to severe hyperkalaemia, calcium gluconate is given intravenously to counter the effects of hyperkalaemia on the cardiac conduction system. While the effect of calcium gluconate lasts only for 1 hour, it allows time to initiate measures to lower serum potassium levels. To rapidly lower these levels, regular insulin and 50 g of glucose are administered. Insulin and glucose promote potassium uptake by the cells, shifting potassium out of ECF. In some cases, a β_2-agonist such as salbutamol may be given by nebuliser to temporarily push potassium into the cells. Sodium bicarbonate may be given to treat acidosis. As the pH returns towards normal, hydrogen ions are released from the cells and potassium returns into the cells.

To remove potassium from the body, sodium polystyrene sulfonate, a resin that binds potassium in the GI tract, may be administered orally or rectally. If renal function is normal, diuretics such as frusemide are given to promote potassium excretion. Commonly prescribed drugs, their actions and nursing implications are listed in the 'Medication administration' box.

Dialysis

When renal function is severely limited, either peritoneal dialysis or haemodialysis may be implemented to remove excess potassium. These measures are invasive and are typically used only when other measures are ineffective. See the chapter 'Nursing care of people with kidney disorders' for more information about dialysis.

PATIENT SAFETY COMPETENCY FRAMEWORK

9 Medication safety

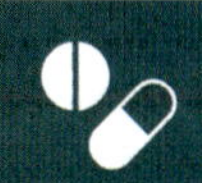

The Patient Safety Competency Framework indicates that nursing students must show medication safety by demonstrating the ability to administer and monitor the therapeutic use of medications, and responding appropriately to medication errors and adverse drug effects (Levett-Jones et al., 2017).

Links to National Patient Safety Standards

NSQHS: Medication Safety Standard

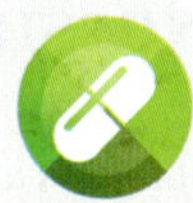

Intention of this standard is to 'ensure clinicians are competent to safely prescribe, dispense and administer appropriate medicines and to monitor medicine use' and that 'consumers are informed about medicines and understand their individual medicine needs and risks' (Australian Commission on Safety and Quality in Healthcare (ACSQHC), 2021, p. 36).

Medication safety is supported by a range of initiatives across interprofessional teams, including the implementation of a National Inpatient Medication Chart (NIMC), safe labelling practice, quality education and training, and accurate reconciliation and administration of medications (ACSQHC, 2021). Nurses play an integral role in the safe administration of medicines to an informed consumer.

Source: ACSQHC (2021). *National Safety and Quality Health Service Standards* (2nd ed.). Sydney: ACSQHC. © Australian Commission on Safety and Quality in Health Care.

MEDICATION ADMINISTRATION Hyperkalaemia

DIURETICS

Potassium-wasting diuretics, such as frusemide (Lasix), may be used to enhance renal excretion of potassium.

Nursing responsibilities

- Monitor serum electrolytes.
- Monitor and record weight at regular intervals under standard conditions (same time of day, balanced scale, same clothing).
- Monitor intake and output.

INSULIN, HYPERTONIC DEXTROSE AND SODIUM BICARBONATE

Insulin, hypertonic dextrose (10% to 50%) and sodium bicarbonate are used in the emergency treatment of moderate to severe hyperkalaemia. Insulin promotes the movement of potassium into the cell and glucose prevents hypoglycaemia. The onset of action of insulin and hypertonic dextrose occurs within 30 minutes and is effective for approximately 4 to 6 hours.

Sodium bicarbonate elevates the serum pH; potassium is moved into the cell in exchange for hydrogen ion. Sodium bicarbonate is particularly useful in the person with metabolic acidosis. Onset of effects occurs within 15 to 30 minutes and is effective for approximately 2 hours.

Nursing responsibilities

- Administer intravenous insulin and dextrose over prescribed interval of time using an infusion pump.
- Administer sodium bicarbonate as prescribed. It may be administered as an intravenous bolus or added to a dextrose-in-water solution and given by infusion.
- In the person receiving sodium bicarbonate, monitor for sodium overload, particularly in the person with hypernatraemia, heart failure and renal failure.
- Monitor the ECG pattern closely.
- Monitor serum electrolytes (K^+, Na^+, Ca^{2+}, Mg^{2+}) frequently during treatment.

CALCIUM GLUCONATE AND CALCIUM CHLORIDE

Intravenous calcium gluconate or calcium chloride is used as a temporary emergency measure to counteract the toxic effects of potassium on myocardial conduction and function.

Nursing responsibilities

- Closely monitor the ECG of the person receiving intravenous calcium, particularly for bradycardia.
- Calcium should be used cautiously in the person receiving digitalis, because calcium increases the cardiotonic effects of digitalis and may precipitate digitalis toxicity, leading to arrhythmias.

SODIUM POLYSTYRENE SULFONATE AND SORBITOL

Sodium polystyrene sulfonate is used to treat moderate or severe hyperkalaemia. Categorised as a cation exchange resin, sodium polystyrene sulfonate exchanges sodium or calcium for potassium in the large intestine. Sorbitol is given with sodium polystyrene sulfonate to promote bowel elimination. Sodium polystyrene sulfonate and sorbitol may be administered orally, through a nasogastric tube or rectally as a retention enema. The usual dosage is 20 g three or four times a day with 20 mL of 70% sorbitol solution.

Nursing responsibilities

- Because sodium polystyrene sulfonate contains sodium, monitor the person with heart failure and oedema closely for water retention.
- Monitor serum electrolytes (K^+, Na^+, Ca^{2+}, Mg^{2+}) frequently during therapy.
- Restrict sodium intake in the person who is unable to tolerate increased sodium load (e.g. those with CHF or hypertension).
- Sodium polystyrene sulfonate should not be given to people at risk of intestinal necrosis, including postoperative patient, those who have a history of bowel obstruction, ischaemic bowel disease or those who have had a renal transplant.

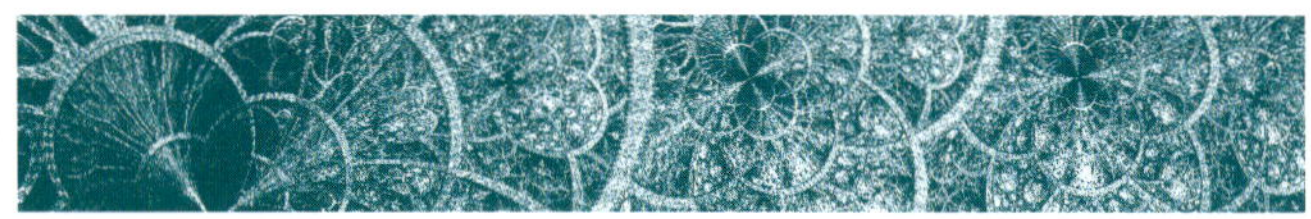

Nursing care

Nursing care focuses related to hyperkalaemia include identifying the at-risk person, preventing hyperkalaemia and addressing problems resulting from the systemic effects of hyperkalaemia. See 'Nursing care plan: a person with hyperkalaemia'.

Health promotion

Those at the greatest risk of developing hyperkalaemia include people taking potassium supplements (prescribed or over-the-counter), using potassium-sparing diuretics or salt substitutes, and experiencing renal failure. Athletes participating in competition sports such as body building and using anabolic steroids, muscle-building compounds or 'energy drinks' also may be at risk of hyperkalaemia.

Teach all people to read food and dietary supplement labels carefully. Discuss the importance of taking prescribed potassium supplements as ordered and not increasing the dose unless prescribed by the attending doctor. Advise the person taking a potassium supplement or potassium-sparing diuretic to avoid salt substitutes, which usually contain potassium. Discuss the importance of maintaining an adequate fluid intake (unless a fluid restriction has been prescribed) to maintain renal function and eliminate potassium from the body.

Assessment

Assessment data related to hyperkalaemia include the following:

- *Health history*: current manifestations, including numbness and tingling, nausea and vomiting, abdominal cramping, muscle weakness, palpitations; duration of symptoms and

NURSING CARE PLAN A person with hyperkalaemia

Monty Longacre, a 51-year-old male, has end-stage renal failure. He arrives at the emergency clinic complaining of shortness of breath on exertion and extreme weakness.

ASSESSMENT

Mr Longacre tells the nurse, Janet Allen, RN, that he normally receives dialysis 3 times a week. He missed his last treatment, however, to attend his father's funeral. During the past several days, he has eaten a number of fresh oranges he received as a gift. Physical assessment findings include T 37.3°C, P 100, R 28, BP 168/96, 2^+ pretibial oedema and a 3.6-kg weight gain since his last haemodialysis treatment 4 days ago. Laboratory and diagnostic tests show the following abnormal results:

- K^+ 6.5 mEq/L (normal 3.5 to 5 mEq/L)
- urea 118 mg/dL (normal 7 to 18 mg/dL)
- creatinine 14 mg/dL (normal 0.7 to 1.3 mg/dL)
- HCO_3^- 17 mEq/L (normal 22 to 26 mEq/L)
- peaked T wave noted on ECG.

Mr Longacre is placed on continuous ECG monitoring and the physician prescribes haemodialysis. As an interim measure to lower the serum potassium, the medical officer prescribes $D_{50}W$ (25 g of dextrose), one ampule, to be administered intravenously with 10 units of regular insulin over 30 minutes.

DIAGNOSES

- *Activity intolerance* related to skeletal muscle weakness.
- *Risk of decreased cardiac output* related to hyperkalaemia.
- *Risk of ineffective health maintenance* related to inadequate knowledge of recommended diet.
- *Excess fluid volume* related to renal failure.

PLANNING

- Advise Mr Longacre that the nurses will be monitoring and documenting in the case notes all fluid intake and urine output.
- Explain the purpose of follow up treatments of venepuncture and electrocardiographs (ECGs).
- Educate Mr Longacre about the causes of hyperkalaemia.
- Explain the importance of the medically prescribed requirement of haemodialysis.
- Discuss dietary sources and provide a list of foods to prevent hyperkalaemia.

Expected outcomes

- Gradually resume usual physical activities.
- Maintain serum potassium level within normal range.
- Verbalise causes of hyperkalaemia, the importance of haemodialysis treatments as scheduled and the role of diet in preventing hyperkalaemia.

IMPLEMENTATION

- To observe, monitor and document fluid intake and fluid output.
- To follow up on the collection of serum potassium and review serum potassium results and report abnormalities to the medical officer. Attend to ECGs as ordered by the medical officer or as required and report findings to the medical officer.
- Review Mr Longacre's knowledge pertaining to causes of hyperkalaemia and the relationship between haemodialysis and hyperkalaemia.
- Discuss and consult with Mr Longacre about the importance of avoiding foods high in potassium to prevent or control hyperkalaemia.

EVALUATION

Following emergency treatment and haemodialysis, Mr Longacre's ECG and serum potassium level have returned to normal. His muscle strength has returned to near normal and he verbalises an understanding of his prescribed haemodialysis regimen. Janet Allen provides verbal and written information about hyperkalaemia, and the importance of complying with the haemodialysis regimen and of limiting intake of dietary sources of potassium in renal failure. She also furnishes a list of foods high in potassium and cautions against using potassium-containing salt substitutes and non-prescription drugs.

CRITICAL THINKING IN THE NURSING PROCESS

1. What information given by Mr Longacre indicated that he might be experiencing hyperkalaemia?
2. Why was continuous ECG monitoring instituted as an emergency measure?
3. What additional emergency measures might have been instituted if Mr Longacre's serum potassium level had been 8.5 mEq/L and his ECG had shown changes in impulse conduction?
4. Develop a care plan for Mr Longacre for the nursing diagnosis of *Anxiety*.

REFLECTION ON THE NURSING PROCESSM

1. Identify and outline what you have learned from this case study and how will you apply it to your future nursing practice.
2. What communication and education strategies could you use when caring for a person with a nursing diagnosis of *Anxiety*?

any precipitating factors such as use of salt substitutes, potassium supplements or reduced urine output; chronic diseases such as renal failure or endocrine disorders; current medications.

- *Physical assessment*: apical and peripheral pulses; bowel sounds; muscle strength in upper and lower extremities; ECG pattern.
- *Diagnostic tests*: serum electrolytes, potassium, sodium and calcium in particular; ABGs; digitalis levels; ECG.

Nursing diagnoses and interventions

The effects of excess potassium on the electrical conduction and contractility of the heart are the highest priority for nursing care, particularly when the serum potassium level is 6.5 mEq/L or higher.

Risk of decreased cardiac output

Hyperkalaemia affects depolarisation of the atria and ventricles of the heart. Severe hyperkalaemia can cause arrhythmias with ventricular fibrillation and cardiac arrest. The cardiac effects of hyperkalaemia are more pronounced when the serum potassium level rises rapidly. Low serum sodium and calcium levels, high serum magnesium levels and acidosis contribute to the adverse effects of hyperkalaemia on the heart muscle.

- Closely monitor the response to intravenous calcium gluconate, particularly in people taking digitalis. *Calcium increases the risk of digitalis toxicity.*

> **CONSIDERATION FOR PRACTICE**
> **Monitor the ECG pattern for development of peaked, narrow T waves, prolongation of the PR interval, depression of the ST segment, widened QRS interval and loss of the P wave. Notify the doctor of changes. Progressive ECG changes from a peaked T wave to loss of the P wave and widening of the QRS complex indicate an increasing risk of arrhythmias and cardiac arrest.**

Risk of activity intolerance

Both hypokalaemia (low serum potassium levels) and hyperkalaemia (high serum potassium levels) affect neuromuscular activity and the function of cardiac, smooth and skeletal muscles. Hyperkalaemia can cause muscle weakness and even paralysis.

- Monitor skeletal muscle strength and tone. *Increasing weakness, muscle paralysis or progression of affected muscles to affect the upper extremities or trunk can indicate increasing serum potassium levels.*
- Monitor respiratory rate and depth. Regularly assess lung sounds. *Muscle weakness due to hyperkalaemia can impair ventilation. In addition, medications such as sodium bicarbonate or sodium polystyrene sulfonate can cause fluid retention and pulmonary oedema in the person with pre-existing cardiovascular disease.*
- Assist with self-care activities as needed. *Increasing muscle weakness can lead to fatigue and affect the ability to meet self-care needs.*

Risk of imbalanced fluid volume

Renal failure is a major cause of hyperkalaemia. The person with renal failure also is at risk of fluid retention and other electrolyte imbalances.

- Closely monitor serum potassium, serum urea and creatinine. Notify the doctor if serum potassium level is greater than 5 mEq/L or if serum urea and creatinine levels are increasing. *Serum urea and creatinine are the primary indicators of renal function. Levels of these substances rise rapidly in acute renal failure, more slowly in chronic renal failure* (see the chapter 'Nursing care of people with kidney disorders').
- Maintain accurate intake and output records. Report an imbalance of 24-hour totals and/or urine output less than 30 mL/hour. *Oliguria (scant urine) or anuria (no urine output) may indicate renal failure and an increased risk of hyperkalaemia and FVE.*
- Monitor the person receiving sodium bicarbonate for FVE. *Increased sodium from injection of a hypertonic sodium bicarbonate solution can cause a shift of water into the extracellular space.*
- Monitor the person receiving cation exchange resins and sorbitol for FVE. *The resin exchanges potassium for sodium or calcium in the bowel. Excessive sodium and water retention may occur.*

Community-based care

Preventing future episodes of hyperkalaemia is the focus when preparing the person for home care. Include the family, a significant other or a caregiver when teaching the following topics:

- recommended diet and any restrictions, including salt substitutes and foods high in potassium
- medications to be avoided, including over-the-counter and fitness supplements
- follow-up appointments for lab work and evaluation.

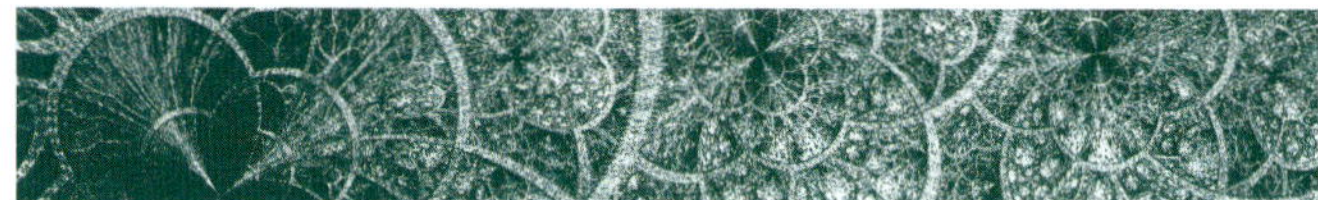

CALCIUM IMBALANCE

Calcium is one of the most abundant ions in the body. The normal adult total serum calcium concentration is 8.5 to 10.0 mg/dL.

Overview of normal calcium balance

Calcium is obtained from dietary sources, although only about 20% of the calcium ingested is absorbed into the blood. The remainder is excreted in faeces. Extracellular calcium is excreted by the kidneys. Approximately 99% of the total calcium in the body is bound to phosphorus to form the minerals in bones and teeth. The remaining 1% is in extracellular fluid. About half of this extracellular calcium is ionised (free); it is this ionised calcium that is physiologically active. The remaining extracellular calcium is bound to protein or other ions. Ionised calcium is essential to a number of processes: stabilising cell membranes; regulating muscle contraction and relaxation; and maintaining cardiac function and blood clotting.

Serum calcium levels are regulated by the interaction of three hormones: parathyroid hormone (PTH), calcitonin and calcitriol (a metabolite of vitamin D). When serum calcium levels fall, the parathyroid glands secrete PTH, which mobilises skeletal calcium stores, increases calcium absorption in the intestines and promotes calcium reabsorption by the kidneys (see Figure 9.12).

Calcitriol facilitates this process by stimulating calcium release from the bones, absorption in the intestines and reabsorption by the kidneys. Calcitonin is secreted by the thyroid gland in response to high serum calcium levels. Its effect on serum calcium levels is the opposite of PTH: it inhibits the movement of calcium out of bone, reduces intestinal absorption of calcium, and promotes calcium excretion by the kidneys.

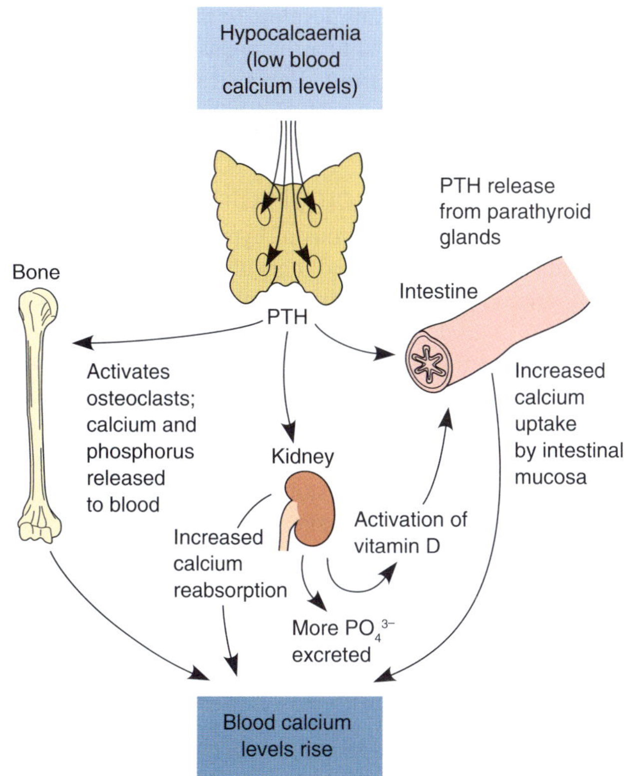

FIGURE 9.12 ***Low calcium levels (hypocalcaemia) trigger the release of parathyroid hormone (PTH), increasing calcium ion levels through stimulation of bones, kidneys and intestines***

Serum calcium levels are also affected by acid–base balance. When hydrogen ion concentration falls and the pH rises (alkalosis), more calcium is bound to protein. While the total serum calcium remains unchanged, less calcium is available in the ionised, active form. Conversely, when hydrogen ion concentration increases and the pH falls (acidosis), calcium is released from protein, making more ionised calcium available.

Finally, the total amount of calcium in blood plasma fluctuates with plasma protein levels, particularly the albumin level. As the albumin level falls, the total amount of plasma calcium declines. Table 9.8 summarises the causes and manifestations of calcium imbalances.

TABLE 9.8 Causes and manifestations of calcium imbalances

IMBALANCE	CAUSES	MANIFESTATIONS
Hypocalcaemia Serum calcium < 8.5 mg/dL or 4.3 mEq/L Critical value < 6.0 mg/dL	• Parathyroidectomy or neck surgery • Acute pancreatitis • Inadequate dietary intake • Lack of sun exposure • Lack of weight-bearing exercise • Drugs: loop diuretics, calcitonin • Hypomagnesaemia, alcohol abuse • Acute renal failure with hyperphosphataemia	Neuromuscular • Tetany • Paraesthesias • Muscle spasms • Positive Chvostek's sign • Positive Trousseau's sign • Laryngospasm • Seizures • Anxiety, confusion, psychoses Cardiovascular • Decreased cardiac output • Hypotension • Arrhythmias Gastrointestinal • Abdominal cramping • Diarrhoea
Hypercalcaemia Serum calcium > 10 mg/dL or 5.3 mEq/L Critical value > 13.0 mg/dL	• Hyperparathyroidism • Some cancers • Prolonged immobilisation • Paget's disease • Excess milk or antacid intake • Chronic renal failure with associated hyperparathyroidism	Neuromuscular • Muscle weakness, fatigue • Decreased deep tendon reflexes Behavioural • Personality changes • Altered mental status • Decreasing level of consciousness Gastrointestinal • Abdominal pain • Constipation • Anorexia, nausea, vomiting Cardiovascular • Arrhythmias • Hypertension Renal • Polyuria, thirst

The person with hypocalcaemia

Hypocalcaemia is a total serum calcium level of less than 8.5 mg/dL. Hypocalcaemia can result from decreased total body calcium stores or low levels of extracellular calcium with normal amounts of calcium stored in bone. The systemic effects of hypocalcaemia are caused by decreased levels of ionised calcium in extracellular fluid.

Risk factors

Certain populations of people are at greater risk of hypocalcaemia: people who have had a parathyroidectomy (removal of the parathyroid glands), older adults (especially women), people with lactose intolerance and those with alcoholism. People who have undergone bariatric surgery for weight loss are at risk due to decreased food intake and malabsorption (Chakhtoura et al., 2016; Dewey & Heuberger, 2011). Older adults often consume less milk and milk products (good sources of calcium) and may have less exposure to the sun (a source of vitamin D). Older adults also may be less active, promoting calcium loss from bones. They are more likely to be taking drugs that interfere with calcium absorption or promote calcium excretion (e.g. frusemide). Older women are at particular risk after menopause because of reduced oestrogen levels. Intolerance to lactose (found in milk and milk products) causes diarrhoea and often limits the intake of milk and milk products, leading to possible calcium deficiency. Ethanol, or drinking alcohol, has a direct effect on calcium balance, reduces its intestinal absorption and interferes with other processes involved in regulating serum calcium levels.

Pathophysiology

Common causes of hypocalcaemia are hypoparathyroidism (see the chapter 'Nursing care of people with endocrine disorders') resulting from surgery (parathyroidectomy, thyroidectomy, radical neck dissection) and acute pancreatitis. In the person who has undergone surgery, symptoms of hypocalcaemia usually occur within the first 24 to 48 hours but they may be delayed.

CONSIDERATION FOR PRACTICE

Carefully monitor the person who has undergone neck surgery for manifestations of hypocalcaemia. Check serum calcium levels and report changes.

Additional causes of hypocalcaemia include other electrolyte imbalances (such as hypomagnesaemia or hyperphosphataemia), alkalosis, malabsorption disorders that interfere with calcium absorption in the bowel and inadequate vitamin D (due to lack of sun exposure or malabsorption). Hyperphosphataemia often occurs in acute renal failure, with reciprocal hypocalcaemia. Massive transfusion of banked blood also can lead to hypocalcaemia. Citrate is added to blood to prevent clotting and as a preservative. When blood is administered faster than the liver can metabolise the citrate, it can bind with calcium, temporarily removing ionised calcium from circulation. Many drugs increase the risk of hypocalcaemia, including loop diuretics (such as frusemide), anticonvulsants (such as phenytoin and phenobarbital), phosphates (including phosphate enemas) and drugs that lower serum magnesium levels (such as cisplatin and gentamicin) (Giddens, 2021; Metheny, 2012).

Extracellular calcium acts to stabilise neuromuscular cell membranes. This effect is reduced in hypocalcaemia, increasing neuromuscular irritability. The threshold of excitation of sensory nerve fibres is lowered as well, leading to paraesthesias (altered sensation). The nervous system becomes more excitable and muscle spasms develop. In the heart, this change in cell membranes can lead to arrhythmias such as ventricular tachycardia and cardiac arrest. Hypocalcaemia decreases the contractility of cardiac muscle fibres, leading to decreased cardiac output.

Manifestations and complications

The most serious manifestations of hypocalcaemia are **tetany** (tonic muscular spasms) and convulsions. Numbness and tingling around the mouth (circumoral) and in the hands and feet develop. Muscle spasms of the face and extremities occur and deep tendon reflexes become hyperactive. Chvostek's sign, contraction of the facial muscles produced by tapping the facial nerve in front of the ear (see Figure 9.13A), and Trousseau's sign, carpal spasm induced by inflating a blood pressure cuff on the upper arm to above systolic blood pressure for 2 to 5 minutes (see Figure 9.13B), indicate increased neuromuscular excitability in the person without obvious symptoms.

Tetany can cause bronchial muscle spasms, simulating an asthma attack and visceral muscle spasms, producing acute abdominal pain. Cardiovascular manifestations include hypotension, possible bradycardia (slow heart rate) and ventricular arrhythmias.

Serious complications of hypocalcaemia include airway obstruction and possible respiratory arrest from laryngospasm, ventricular arrhythmias and cardiac arrest, heart failure and convulsions.

INTERPROFESSIONAL CARE

Management of hypocalcaemia is directed towards restoring normal calcium balance and correcting the underlying cause.

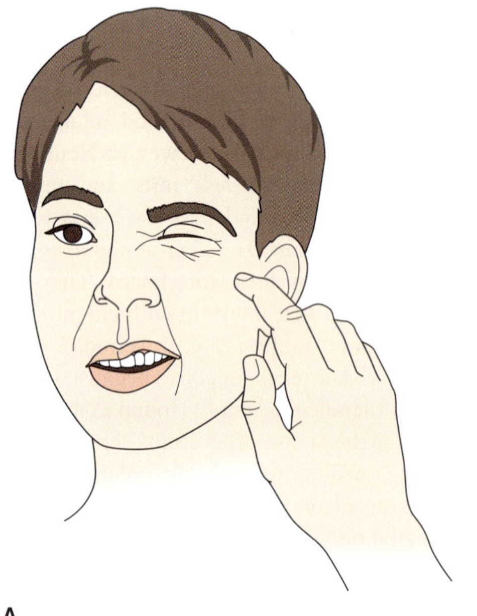

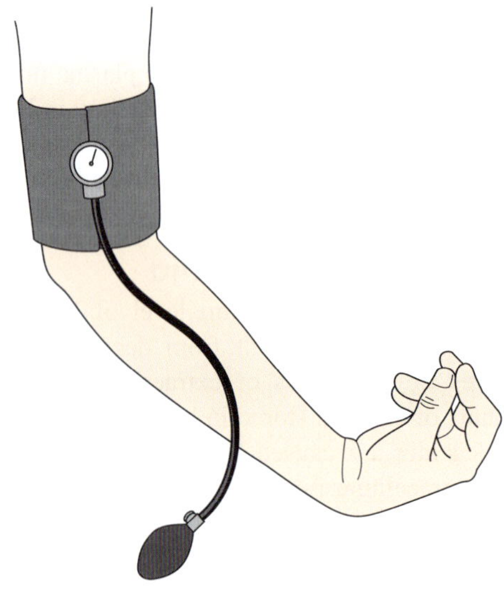

FIGURE 9.13 *A, Positive Chvostek's sign. B, Positive Trousseau's sign*

Diagnosis

The following laboratory and diagnostic tests may be ordered when hypocalcaemia is known or suspected.

- *Total serum calcium*, the amount of ionised (active) calcium available, is usually estimated. In the person who is critically ill, however, *ionised calcium* may be directly measured using ion selective electrodes. Direct measurement of ionised calcium requires special handling of the blood specimen, including placing the specimen on ice and analysing it immediately.
- *Serum albumin*, because the albumin level affects serum calcium results. When the albumin level is low (hypoalbuminaemia), the amount of ionised calcium may remain normal even though the total calcium level is low.
- *Serum magnesium*, because hypocalcaemia is often associated with hypomagnesaemia (serum magnesium < 1.6 mg/dL). In this case, normal magnesium levels must be restored to correct the hypocalcaemia.
- *Serum phosphate*; hyperphosphataemia (serum phosphate > 4.5 mg/dL) can lead to hypocalcaemia because of the inverse relationship between phosphorus and calcium. (As phosphate levels rise, calcium levels fall.)
- *Parathyroid hormone (PTH)*, to identify the possible diagnoses of hyperparathyroidism.
- An *ECG*, to evaluate the effects of hypocalcaemia on the heart, such as a prolonged ST segment.

Medications

Hypocalcaemia is treated with oral or intravenous calcium. The person with severe hypocalcaemia is treated with intravenous calcium to prevent life-threatening problems such as airway obstruction. The most common intravenous calcium preparations include calcium chloride and calcium gluconate. Although calcium chloride contains more elemental calcium than calcium gluconate, it also is more irritating to the veins and may cause venous sclerosis (hardening of the vein walls) if given into a peripheral vein. Intravenous calcium preparations can cause necrosis and sloughing of tissue if they extravasate into subcutaneous tissue. Rapid drug administration can lead to bradycardia and possible cardiac arrest due to overcorrection of hypocalcaemia with resulting hypercalcaemia. See the 'Medication administration' box for further information on calcium administration.

Oral calcium preparations (calcium carbonate, calcium gluconate or calcium lactate) are used to treat chronic, asymptomatic hypocalcaemia. Calcium supplements may be combined with vitamin D, or vitamin D may be given alone to increase gastrointestinal absorption of calcium.

Nutrition

A diet high in calcium-rich foods may be recommended for the person with chronic hypocalcaemia or with low total body stores of calcium. Box 9.7 lists foods that are high in calcium.

BOX 9.7 Foods high in calcium

- Cottage cheese
- Canned sardines and salmon
- Cheese
- Rhubarb
- Milk
- Broccoli
- Cream
- Yoghurt
- Ice-cream
- Spinach
- Tofu

MEDICATION ADMINISTRATION Calcium salts

CALCIUM SALTS
Calcium carbonate
Calcium chloride
Calcium citrate
Calcium gluconate
Calcium lactate

Calcium salts are given to increase calcium levels when there is a deficit (a total body deficit or inadequate levels of extracellular calcium). Calcium is necessary to maintain bone structure and for multiple physiological processes, including neuromuscular and cardiac function as well as blood coagulation. In the presence of vitamin D, calcium is well absorbed from the gastrointestinal tract. Severe hypocalcaemia is treated with intravenous calcium preparations.

Nursing responsibilities

Oral calcium salts:

- Administer 1 to 1.5 hours after meals and at bedtime.
- Give calcium tablets with a full glass of water.

Intravenous calcium salts:

- Assess IV site for patency. Do not administer calcium if there is a risk of leakage into the tissues.
- May be given by slow IV push (dilute with sterile normal saline for injection prior to administering) or added to compatible parenteral fluids such as NS, lactated Ringer's solution or D5W.
- Administer into the largest available vein; use a central line if available.
- Do not administer with bicarbonate or phosphate because a precipitate (insoluble salt) will form (Metheny, 2012).
- Continuously monitor ECG when administering IV calcium to the person taking digitalis, due to increased risk of digitalis toxicity.
- Frequently monitor serum calcium levels and response to therapy.

Health education for the person and their family

- Take calcium tablets with a full glass of water 1 to 2 hours after meals. Do not take with food or milk. If possible, do not take within 1 to 2 hours of other medications.
- Maintain adequate vitamin D intake through diet or exposure to the sun to promote calcium absorption.
- Calcium carbonate can cause constipation. Eat a high-fibre diet and maintain a generous fluid intake to prevent constipation.

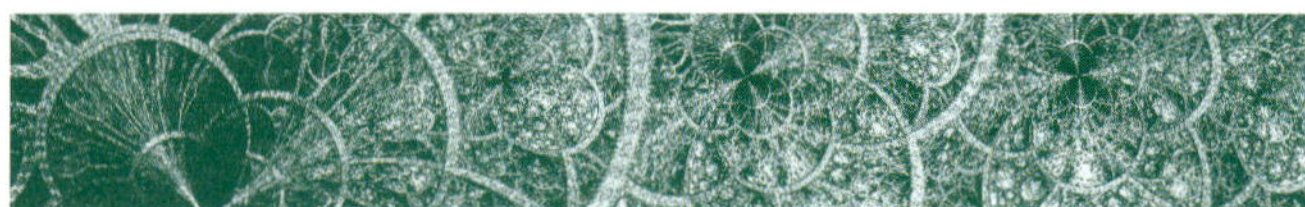

Nursing care

Health promotion

Because of the large stores of calcium in bones, most healthy adults have a very low risk of developing hypocalcaemia. However, a deficit of total body calcium is often associated with ageing, increasing the risk of osteoporosis, fractures and disability. Women have a higher risk of developing osteoporosis than men, due to lower bone density and hormonal influences. Educate women of all ages about the importance of maintaining adequate calcium intake through diet and, as needed, calcium supplements. Stress the relationship between weight-bearing exercise and bone density and encourage women to engage in a regular aerobic and weight-training exercise regimen. Discuss hormone replacement therapy and its potential benefits during and after menopause. See the chapter 'Nursing care of people with musculoskeletal disorders' for more information about osteoporosis.

Assessment

Assessment data related to hypocalcaemia include the following:

- *Health history*: current manifestations, including numbness and tingling around the mouth and of hands and feet, abdominal pain, shortness of breath; acute or chronic diseases such as pancreatitis, liver or kidney disease; current medications.
- *Physical assessment*: muscle spasms; deep tendon reflexes; Chvostek's sign and Trousseau's sign; respiratory rate and depth; vital signs and apical pulse; heart rate and rhythm; presence of convulsions.
- *Diagnostic tests*: serum electrolytes (calcium, magnesium, phosphate and potassium, in particular), serum albumin, thyroid and parathyroid hormone levels; ECG.

Nursing diagnoses and interventions

The effect of hypocalcaemia on neuromuscular irritability, with the risk of muscle spasm and convulsions, is the highest priority for nursing care of the person.

Risk of injury

The person with hypocalcaemia is at risk of injury from possible laryngospasm, cardiac arrhythmias or convulsions. In addition, too rapid administration of intravenous calcium or extravasation of the medication into subcutaneous tissues can lead to injury.

CONSIDERATION FOR PRACTICE

Laryngeal spasm is a respiratory emergency, requiring immediate intervention to maintain ventilation and gas exchange.

- Frequently monitor airway and respiratory status. Report changes such as respiratory **stridor** (a high-pitched, harsh inspiratory sound indicative of upper airway obstruction), or increased respiratory rate or effort, to the doctor. *These changes may indicate laryngeal spasm due to tetany.*
- Monitor cardiovascular status, including heart rate and rhythm, blood pressure and peripheral pulses. *Hypocalcaemia decreases myocardial contractility, causing reduced cardiac output and hypotension. It also can cause bradycardia or ventricular arrhythmias. Cardiac arrest may occur in severe hypocalcaemia.*
- Continuously monitor ECG in the person receiving intravenous calcium preparations, especially if the person also is taking digitalis. *Rapid administration of calcium salts can lead to hypercalcaemia and cardiac arrhythmias. Calcium administration increases the risk of digitalis toxicity and resultant arrhythmias.*
- Provide a quiet environment. Institute seizure precautions such as raising the side rails and keeping an airway at the bedside. *A quiet environment reduces central nervous system stimuli and the risk of convulsions in the person with tetany.*

Community-based care

In preparing the person with hypocalcaemia for discharge and home care, consider the circumstances leading to low serum calcium levels. Discuss risk factors for hypocalcaemia specific to the person and provide information about managing these risk factors to avoid future episodes of hypocalcaemia. Educate about prescribed medications, including calcium supplements. Provide a list of foods high in calcium, as well as sources of vitamin D if recommended. Discuss symptoms to report to the attending doctor and stress the importance of follow-up care as scheduled.

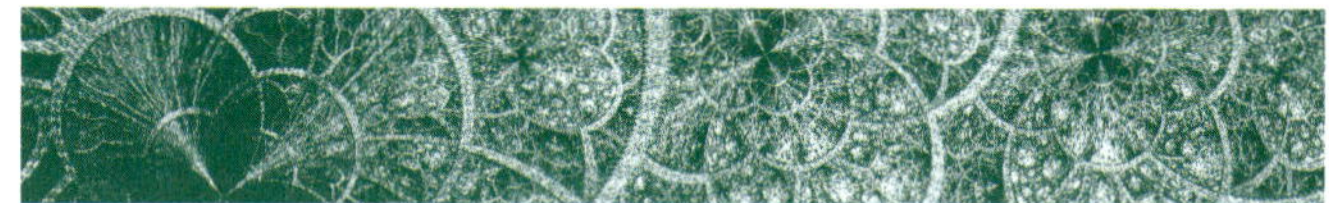

The person with hypercalcaemia

Hypercalcaemia is a serum calcium value greater than 10.0 mg/dL. Excess ionised calcium in ECF can have serious widespread effects.

Pathophysiology

Hypercalcaemia usually results from increased resorption of calcium from the bones. The two most common causes of bone resorption are hyperparathyroidism and malignancies. In hyperparathyroidism, excess PTH is produced. This causes calcium to be released from bones, as well as increased calcium absorption in the intestines and retention of calcium by the kidneys. Hypercalcaemia is a common complication of malignancies. It may develop as a result of bone destruction by the tumour or due to hormone-like substances produced by the tumour itself. Prolonged immobility and lack of weight-bearing activity also causes increased resorption of bone with calcium release into extracellular fluids. Self-limiting hypercalcaemia also may follow successful kidney transplant. Levels of parathyroid hormone may be altered in chronic renal failure, leading to increased serum calcium levels.

Increased intestinal absorption of calcium also can lead to hypercalcaemia. This may result from excess vitamin D, overuse of calcium-containing antacids or excessive milk ingestion. Renal failure and some drugs such as thiazide diuretics and lithium can interfere with elimination of calcium by the kidneys, causing high serum calcium levels.

The effects of hypercalcaemia largely depend on the degree of serum calcium elevation and the length of time over which it develops. In general, higher serum calcium levels are associated with more serious effects. Calcium has a stabilising effect on the neuromuscular junction; hypercalcaemia decreases neuromuscular excitability, leading to muscle weakness and depressed deep tendon reflexes. Gastrointestinal motility is reduced as well. In the heart, calcium exerts an effect similar to digitalis (see the chapter 'Nursing care of people with cardiac disorders'), strengthening contractions and reducing the heart rate. Hypercalcaemia affects the conduction system of the heart, leading to bradycardia and heart blocks. The ability of the kidneys to concentrate urine is impaired by hypercalcaemia, causing excess sodium and water loss and increased thirst (McCance & Huether, 2018).

Extremely high serum calcium levels affect mental status. This is thought to be due to increased calcium in cerebrospinal fluid. Behavioural effects range from personality changes to confusion, impaired memory and acute psychoses.

Manifestations and complications

Manifestations of hypercalcaemia relate to its effects on neuromuscular activity, the central nervous system (CNS), the cardiovascular system and the kidneys. Decreased neuromuscular excitability causes muscle weakness and fatigue, as well as gastrointestinal manifestations such as anorexia, nausea, vomiting and constipation. CNS effects may include confusion, lethargy, behaviour or personality changes, and coma. Cardiovascular effects include arrhythmias, ECG changes and possible hypertension. Hypercalcaemia causes polyuria and, as a result, increased thirst.

Complications of hypercalcaemia can affect several different organ systems. Peptic ulcer disease may develop due to increased gastric acid secretion. Pancreatitis can occur as a result of calcium deposits in pancreatic ducts. Excess calcium can precipitate out of urine to form kidney stones. Hypercalcaemic crisis, an acute increase in the serum calcium level, can lead to cardiac arrest.

INTERPROFESSIONAL CARE

The management of hypercalcaemia focuses on correcting the underlying cause and reducing the serum calcium level. Treatment is particularly important in the person who has one or more of the following: serum calcium levels greater than 12 mg/dL, overt symptoms of hypercalcaemia, compromised renal function and inability to maintain an adequate fluid intake.

Diagnosis

The laboratory and diagnostic tests that may be ordered and the resultant findings are as follows:

- *Serum electrolytes* show a total serum calcium greater than 10.0 mg/dL.
- *Serum PTH* levels are measured to identify or rule out hyperparathyroidism as the cause of hypercalcaemia.
- *ECG* changes in hypercalcaemia include a shortened QT interval, shortened and depressed ST segment and widened T wave. Bradycardia or heart block may be identified on the ECG.
- *Bone density* scans may be done to monitor bone resorption and the effects of treatment measures on mineralisation of bone.

Medications

Measures to promote calcium elimination by the kidneys and reduce calcium resorption from bone are used to treat hypercalcaemia. In acute hypercalcaemia, intravenous fluids are given (see the 'Fluid management' section that follows) with a loop diuretic such as frusemide to promote elimination of excess calcium. Calcitonin, which promotes the uptake of calcium into bones, also may be used to rapidly lower serum calcium levels.

A number of drugs that inhibit bone resorption are available. The bisphosphonates (pamidronate and etidronate) are commonly used to treat hypercalcaemia associated with malignancies. These drugs also are used to prevent and treat osteoporosis. Nursing implications for calcitonin and bisphosphonate drugs are presented in the 'Medication administration' boxes in the chapter 'Nursing care of people with musculoskeletal disorders'. When a bisphosphonate drug is ineffective in correcting hypercalcaemia, mithramycin (a chemotherapeutic agent) may be used.

Rapid reversal of hypercalcaemia in emergency situations may be accomplished by intravenous administration of sodium phosphate or potassium phosphate. Calcium binds to phosphate, thus decreasing serum calcium levels. Paradoxically, complications of this therapy can include fatal hypocalcaemia resulting from binding of the ionised calcium and soft tissue calcifications.

Other drug therapies include the use of intravenous plicamycin to inhibit bone resorption. Glucocorticoids (cortisone), which compete with vitamin D, and a low-calcium diet may be prescribed to decrease gastrointestinal absorption of calcium, inhibit bone resorption and increase urinary calcium excretion. Also, calcitonin may be prescribed to decrease skeletal mobilisation of calcium and phosphorus, and to increase renal output of calcium and phosphorus. See the chapter 'Nursing care of people with endocrine disorders' for more information about and nursing implications of glucocorticoid therapy.

Fluid management

Intravenous fluids, usually isotonic saline, are administered to the person with severe hypercalcaemia to restore vascular volume and promote renal excretion of calcium. Isotonic saline is used because sodium excretion is accompanied by calcium excretion. Careful assessment of cardiovascular and renal function is done prior to fluid therapy; the person is carefully monitored for evidence of fluid overload during treatment.

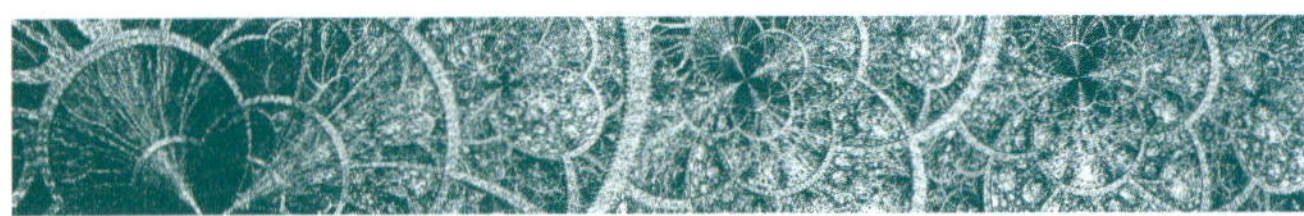

Nursing care

Health promotion

Identify and monitor the person at risk of hypercalcaemia. Promote mobility in the person when possible. Assist the hospitalised person to ambulate as soon as possible. In the home setting, discuss the benefits of regular weight-bearing activity with the person, families and caregivers. Encourage a generous fluid intake of up to 3 to 4 L per day. Encourage the person at risk to limit their intake of milk and milk products, as well as calcium-containing antacids and supplements. In addition, the person with prolonged immobility or hypercalcaemia is encouraged to consume fluids that increase the acidity of urine (which inhibits calcium stone formation), such as cranberry or prune juice.

Assessment

Assessment data related to hypercalcaemia include the following:

- *Health history*: current manifestations, including weakness or fatigue, abdominal discomfort, nausea or vomiting, increased urination and thirst; changes in memory or thinking; duration of symptoms and any risk factors such as excess intake of milk or calcium products, prolonged immobility, malignancy, renal failure or endocrine disorders; current medications.
- *Physical assessment*: mental status and level of consciousness; vital signs, including apical pulse; bowel sounds; muscle strength of upper and lower extremities; deep tendon reflexes.
- *Diagnostic tests*: serum electrolytes, urinary calcium, ECG and cardiac rhythm monitoring.

> **CONSIDERATION FOR PRACTICE**
>
> **Remember, calcium has a stabilising or sedative effect on neuromuscular transmission. Therefore:**
>
> - **Hypocalcaemia → increased neuromuscular excitability, muscle twitching, spasms and possible tetany**
> - **Hypercalcaemia → decreased neuromuscular excitability, muscle weakness and fatigue.**

Nursing diagnoses and interventions

Risk of injury

The person with hypercalcaemia is at risk of injury due to changes in mental status, the effects of hypercalcaemia on muscle strength and loss of calcium from bones.

> **CONSIDERATION FOR PRACTICE**
>
> **Monitor cardiac rate and rhythm, treating and/or reporting arrhythmias as indicated. Prepare for possible cardiac arrest; keep emergency resuscitation equipment readily available. Hypercalcaemia can cause bradycardia, various heart blocks and cardiac arrest. Immediate treatment may be necessary to preserve life.**

- Institute safety precautions if confusion or other changes in mental status are noted. *Changes in mental status may impair judgment and the person's ability to maintain own safety.*
- Observe for manifestations of digitalis toxicity, including vision changes, anorexia, and changes in heart rate and rhythm. Monitor serum digitalis levels. *Hypercalcaemia increases the risk of digitalis toxicity.*
- Promote fluid intake (oral and/or intravenous) to keep the person well hydrated and maintain dilute urine. Encourage fluids such as prune or cranberry juice to help maintain acidic urine. *Acidic, dilute urine reduces the risk of calcium salts precipitating out to form kidney stones.*
- If excess bone resorption has occurred, use caution when turning, positioning, transferring or ambulating. *Bones that have lost excess calcium may fracture with minimal stress or trauma (pathological fractures).*

Risk of excess fluid volume

Large amounts of isotonic intravenous fluid often are administered to help correct acute hypercalcaemia, leading to a risk of hypervolaemia. The person with pre-existing cardiac or renal disease is at particular risk.

- Closely monitor intake and output. *A loop diuretic such as frusemide may be necessary if urinary output does not keep up with fluid administration.*
- Frequently assess vital signs, respiratory status and heart sounds. *Increasing pulse rate, dyspnoea, adventitious lung sounds and an S_3 on auscultation of the heart may indicate excess fluid volume and potential heart failure.*
- Place in semi-Fowler's to Fowler's position. *Elevating the head of the bed improves lung expansion and reduces the work of breathing.*
- Administer diuretics as ordered, monitoring response. *Loop diuretics may be ordered to help eliminate excess fluid and calcium.*

Community-based care

Discuss the following topics when preparing the person for discharge:

- Avoid excess intake of calcium-rich foods and antacids.
- Use prescribed drugs to prevent excess calcium resorption. Discuss their dose, use, and desired and possible adverse effects.
- Increase fluid intake to 3 to 4 L per day; increase the intake of acid ash foods (meats, fish, poultry, eggs, cranberries, plums, prunes); increase dietary fibre and fluid intake to prevent constipation.
- Maintain weight-bearing physical activity to prevent hypercalcaemia.
- Report early manifestations of hypercalcaemia.
- Follow recommended schedule for monitoring serum electrolyte levels.

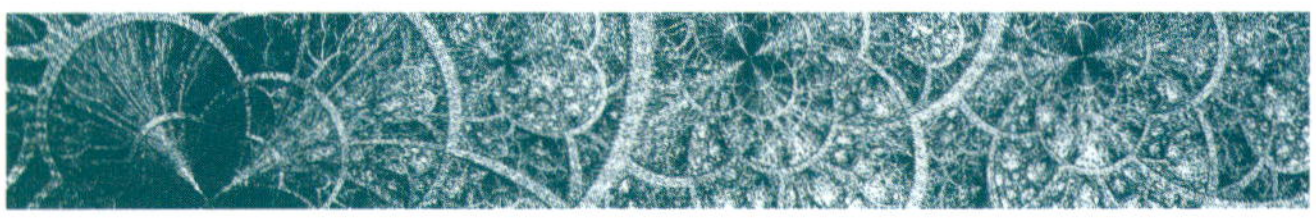

MAGNESIUM IMBALANCE

Only about 1% of the magnesium in the human body is in extracellular fluid; the rest is found within the cells and in bone. The normal serum concentration of magnesium ranges from 1.8 to 2.6 mg/dL (1.5 to 2.5 mEq/L).

Overview of normal magnesium balance

Magnesium is obtained through the diet (it is plentiful in green vegetables, grains, nuts, meats and seafood) and is excreted by the kidneys. Magnesium is vital to many intracellular processes, including enzyme reactions and synthesis of proteins and nucleic acids. Magnesium exerts a sedative effect on the neuromuscular junction, decreasing acetylcholine release. It is an essential ion for neuromuscular transmission and cardiovascular function. The physiological effects of magnesium are affected by both potassium and calcium levels. Approximately 65% of extracellular magnesium is ionised; the remainder is bound to protein. Table 9.9 summarises common causes and manifestations of magnesium imbalances.

The person with hypomagnesaemia

Hypomagnesaemia is a magnesium level of less than 1.6 mg/dL. It is a common problem, particularly in the critically ill person. Hypomagnesaemia may be caused by deficient magnesium intake, excessive losses, or a shift between the intracellular and extracellular compartments.

Risk factors

Loss of gastrointestinal fluids, particularly from diarrhoea, an ileostomy or intestinal fistula, is a major risk factor for hypomagnesaemia. Disruption of nutrient absorption in the small intestine also increases the risk. Chronic alcoholism is a common cause of deficient magnesium levels. Multiple factors associated with alcoholism contribute to hypomagnesaemia: deficient nutrient intake, increased gastrointestinal losses, impaired absorption and increased renal excretion. Other risk factors for hypomagnesaemia include:

- protein–kilojoule malnutrition or starvation
- endocrine disorders, including diabetic ketoacidosis
- drugs such as loop or thiazide diuretics, aminoglycoside antibiotics, amphotericin B and cyclosporin
- rapid administration of citrated blood (banked blood)
- kidney disease.

Pathophysiology

Magnesium deficiency usually occurs along with low serum potassium and calcium levels. The effects of hypomagnesaemia relate not only to the magnesium deficiency but also to hypokalaemia and hypocalcaemia.

Hypomagnesaemia causes increased neuromuscular excitability, with muscle weakness and tremors. The accompanying hypocalcaemia contributes to this effect. In the CNS, this increased neural excitability can lead to seizures and changes in mental status. Deficient intracellular magnesium in the myocardium increases the risk of cardiac arrhythmias and sudden death. Hypokalaemia increases this risk. Hypomagnesaemia also increases the risk of digitalis toxicity. Chronic hypomagnesaemia may contribute to hypertension, probably due to increased vasoconstriction.

TABLE 9.9 Causes and manifestations of magnesium imbalances

IMBALANCE	CAUSES	MANIFESTATIONS
Hypomagnesaemia Serum magnesium < 1.6 mg/dL Critical value < 1 mg/dL	• Chronic alcoholism • GI losses: intestinal suction, diarrhoea, ileostomy • Impaired absorption • Inadequate replacement • Increased excretion: drugs, renal disease, osmotic diuresis	Neuromuscular • Muscle weakness, tremors • Tetany, seizures Gastrointestinal • Dysphagia • Anorexia, nausea, vomiting, diarrhoea Cardiovascular • Tachycardia • Arrhythmias • Hypertension CNS • Mood and personality changes • Paraesthesias
Hypermagnesaemia Serum magnesium > 2.6 mg/dL or 2.1 mEq/L Critical value > 4.7 mg/dL	• Renal insufficiency or failure • Excess intake of antacids, laxatives • Excess magnesium administration	Neuromuscular • Muscle weakness • Depressed deep tendon reflexes Gastrointestinal • Nausea and vomiting Cardiovascular • Hypotension • Bradycardia • Cardiac arrest CNS • Respiratory depression • Coma

Manifestations and complications

Neuromuscular manifestations of hypomagnesaemia include tremors, hyper-reactive reflexes, positive Chvostek's and Trousseau's signs (see Figure 9.13), tetany, paraesthesias and seizures. CNS effects include confusion, mood changes (apathy, depression, agitation), hallucinations and possible psychoses. An increased heart rate and ventricular arrhythmias are common, especially when hypokalaemia is present or the person is taking digitalis. Cardiac arrest and sudden death may occur. Gastrointestinal manifestations include nausea, vomiting, anorexia, diarrhoea and abdominal distension.

INTERPROFESSIONAL CARE

Hypomagnesaemia is diagnosed by measuring serum electrolyte levels. The ECG shows a prolonged PR interval, widened QRS complex and depression of the ST segment with T-wave inversion. Treatment is directed towards prevention and identification of an existing deficiency. Magnesium is added to intravenous total parenteral nutrition solutions to prevent hypomagnesaemia.

In the person able to eat, a mild deficiency may be corrected by increasing the intake of foods rich in magnesium (see Box 9.8) or with oral magnesium supplements. Oral magnesium supplements may cause diarrhoea, however, limiting their use.

The person with manifestations of hypomagnesaemia is treated with parenteral magnesium sulfate. Treatment is continued for several days to restore intracellular magnesium levels. Magnesium may be given intravenously or by deep intramuscular injection. Renal function is evaluated prior to administration, and serum magnesium levels are monitored during treatment. The intravenous route is used for severe magnesium deficiency or if neurological changes or cardiac arrhythmias are present. See the 'Medication administration' box for the nursing implications of parenteral magnesium sulfate.

BOX 9.8 Foods high in magnesium

- Green, leafy vegetables
- Oranges
- Seafood
- Grapefruit
- Meat
- Chocolate
- Wheat bran
- Milk
- Coconut
- Legumes
- Refined sugar
- Bananas

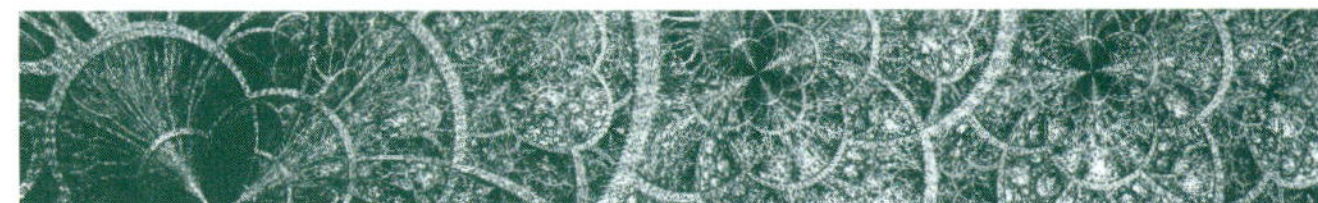

Nursing care

Health promotion

Discuss the importance of maintaining adequate magnesium intake through a well-balanced diet, particularly with those at risk (people with alcoholism, malabsorption or bowel surgery). Many hospitalised people are at risk of hypomagnesaemia due to protein–kilojoule malnutrition and other disorders. Monitor serum magnesium levels, reporting changes to the healthcare provider.

Assessment

In addition to asking questions related to risk factors for hypomagnesaemia, use the guidelines for assessing the person with hypokalaemia and hypocalcaemia for subjective and objective assessment data. Monitor diagnostic studies such as serum electrolytes, serum albumin levels and the ECG. Monitor GI function, including bowel sounds and abdominal distension.

MEDICATION ADMINISTRATION Magnesium sulfate

Magnesium sulfate is used to prevent or treat hypomagnesaemia. It is also used as an anticonvulsant in severe eclampsia or pre-eclampsia. It may be given intravenously or by intramuscular injection.

NURSING RESPONSIBILITIES

- Assess serum magnesium levels and renal function tests (serum urea and creatinine) prior to administering. Notify the attending doctor if magnesium levels are above normal limits or renal function is impaired.
- Frequently monitor neurological status and deep tendon reflexes during therapy. Withhold magnesium and notify the attending doctor if deep tendon reflexes are hypoactive or absent.
- Monitor intake and output.
- Administer IM doses deep into the ventral or dorsal gluteal sites.
- Intravenous magnesium sulfate may be given slowly by IV or by continuous infusion.

HEALTH EDUCATION FOR THE PERSON AND FAMILY

Explain purpose and duration of treatment. Discuss reason for frequent neurological and reflex assessments.

Nursing diagnoses and interventions

Nursing care for the person with hypomagnesaemia focuses on careful monitoring of manifestations and responses to treatment, promoting safety, the person and family education, and administering prescribed medications.

Risk of injury

- Monitor serum electrolytes, including magnesium, potassium and calcium. *Magnesium deficiency often is accompanied by deficiencies of potassium and calcium.*
- Monitor gastrointestinal function, including bowel sounds and abdominal distension. *Hypomagnesaemia reduces gastrointestinal motility.*
- Initiate cardiac monitoring, reporting and treating (as indicated) ECG changes and arrhythmias. In the person receiving digitalis, monitor for digitalis toxicity. *Low magnesium levels can precipitate ventricular arrhythmias, including lethal arrhythmias such as ventricular fibrillation.*
- Assess deep tendon reflexes frequently during intravenous magnesium infusions and prior to each intramuscular dose. *Depressed tendon reflexes indicate a high serum magnesium level.*
- Maintain a quiet, darkened environment. Institute seizure precautions. *Increased neuromuscular and CNS irritability can lead to seizures. A quiet, dark environment reduces stimuli.*

Community-based care

Prior to discharge, instruct the person to increase dietary intake of foods high in magnesium and provide information about magnesium supplements. In addition, if alcohol abuse has precipitated a magnesium deficit, discuss alcohol treatment options, including inpatient treatment and support groups such as Alcoholics Anonymous, Al-Anon and/or Al Teen.

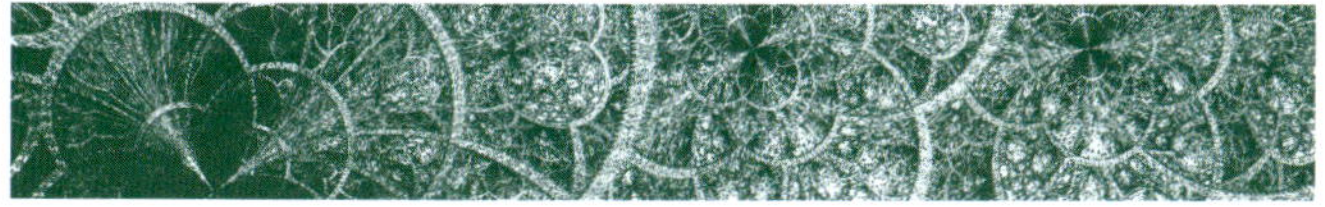

The person with hypermagnesaemia

Hypermagnesaemia is a serum magnesium level greater than 2.6 mg/dL. It is much less common than hypomagnesaemia. Hypermagnesaemia can develop in renal failure, particularly if magnesium is administered parenterally or orally (e.g. magnesium-containing antacids or laxatives). Older adults are at risk of hypermagnesaemia, as renal function declines with ageing and they are more likely to use over-the-counter laxatives and other preparations that contain magnesium.

Pathophysiology and manifestations

Elevated serum magnesium levels interfere with neuromuscular transmission and depress the central nervous system. Hypermagnesaemia also affects the cardiovascular system, potentially causing hypotension, flushing, sweating and bradyarrhythmias.

Predictable manifestations occur with increasing serum magnesium levels. With lower levels, nausea and vomiting, hypotension, facial flushing, sweating and a feeling of warmth occur. As levels increase, signs of CNS depression appear (weakness, lethargy, drowsiness, weak or absent deep tendon reflexes). Marked elevations cause respiratory depression, coma and compromised cardiac function (ECG changes, bradycardia, heart block and cardiac arrest).

INTERPROFESSIONAL CARE

The management of hypermagnesaemia focuses on identifying and treating the underlying cause. All medications or compounds containing magnesium (such as antacids, intravenous solutions or enemas) are withheld. In the person with renal failure, haemodialysis or peritoneal dialysis is instituted to remove the excess magnesium.

Calcium gluconate is administered intravenously to reverse the neuromuscular and cardiac effects of hypermagnesaemia. The person may require mechanical ventilation to support respiratory function and a pacemaker to maintain adequate cardiac output.

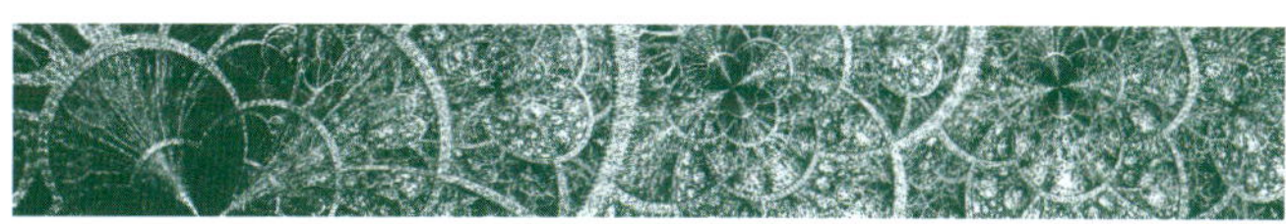

Nursing care

Nursing care includes instituting measures to prevent and identify hypermagnesaemia in the person at risk, monitoring for critical effects of hypermagnesaemia and providing measures to ensure the person's safety. Consider the following nursing diagnoses for the person with hypermagnesaemia:

- *Decreased cardiac output* related to altered myocardial conduction.
- *Risk of ineffective breathing pattern* related to respiratory depression.
- *Risk of injury* related to muscle weakness and altered level of consciousness.
- *Risk of ineffective health maintenance* related to lack of knowledge about use of magnesium-containing supplements, antacids, laxatives and enemas.

Community-based care

Discharge teaching and planning focus on instructions to avoid magnesium-containing medications, including antacids, mineral supplements, cathartics and enemas (see Box 9.9).

BOX 9.9 Medications containing magnesium

Antacids
- Gelusil
- Milk of magnesia
- Mylanta
- Gaviscon

Laxatives
- Milk of magnesia
- Magnesium oxide
- Magnesium citrate
- Epsom salts

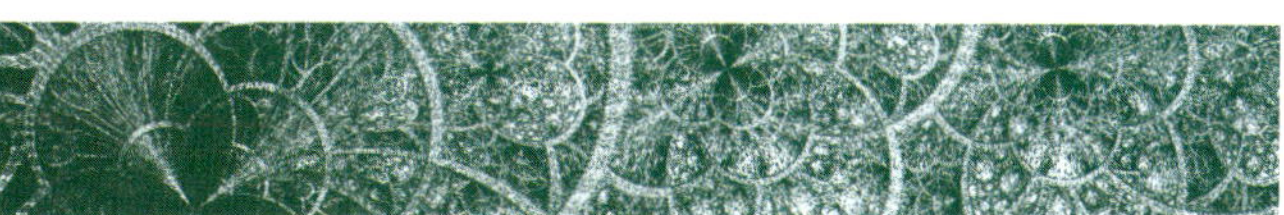

PHOSPHATE IMBALANCE

Although most phosphate (85%) is found in bones, it is the primary intracellular anion. About 14% is in intracellular fluid and the remainder (1%) is in extracellular fluid. The normal serum phosphate (or phosphorus) level in adults is 2.5 to 4.5 mg/dL. Phosphorus levels vary with age, gender and diet.

Overview of normal phosphate balance

Phosphate is essential to intracellular processes such as the production of ATP, the fuel that supports muscle contraction, nerve cell transmission and electrolyte transport. Phosphate is vital for red blood cell function and oxygen delivery to tissues; nervous system and muscle function; and the metabolism of fats, carbohydrates and protein. It also assists in maintaining acid–base balance.

Phosphorus is ingested in the diet, absorbed in the jejunum and primarily excreted by the kidneys. When phosphate intake is low, the kidneys conserve phosphorus, excreting less. An inverse relationship exists between phosphate and calcium levels: when one increases, the other decreases. Regulatory mechanisms for calcium levels (parathyroid hormone, calcitonin and vitamin D) also influence phosphate levels. The causes and manifestations of phosphate imbalances are summarised in Table 9.10.

The person with hypophosphataemia

Hypophosphataemia is a serum phosphorus of less than 2.5 mg/dL. Low serum phosphate levels may indicate a total body deficit of phosphate or a shift of phosphate into the intracellular space, the most common cause of hypophosphataemia. Decreased gastrointestinal absorption of phosphate or increased renal excretion of phosphate also can cause low phosphate levels. Hypophosphataemia often is *iatrogenic*—that is, related to treatment. Selected causes of hypophosphataemia include the following:

- *Refeeding syndrome* can develop when the malnourished person is started on enteral or total parenteral nutrition. Glucose in the formula or solution stimulates insulin release, which promotes the entry of glucose and phosphate into the cells, depleting extracellular phosphate levels.
- Medications frequently contribute to hypophosphataemia, including intravenous glucose solutions, antacids (aluminium or magnesium-based antacids bind with phosphate), anabolic steroids and diuretics.
- Alcoholism affects both the intake and absorption of phosphate.
- Hyperventilation and respiratory alkalosis cause phosphate to shift out of extracellular fluids into the intracellular space.
- Other causes include diabetic ketoacidosis with excess phosphate loss in the urine, stress responses and extensive burns.

Pathophysiology and manifestations

Most effects of hypophosphataemia result from depletion of ATP and impaired oxygen delivery to the cells due to a deficiency of the red blood cell enzyme 2,3-DPG. Severe hypophosphataemia affects virtually every major organ system:

- *Central nervous system*: reduced oxygen and ATP synthesis in the brain causes neurological manifestations such as irritability, apprehension, weakness, paraesthesias, lack of coordination, confusion, seizures and coma.
- *Haematological*: oxygen delivery to the cells is reduced. Haemolytic anaemia (excessive red blood cell destruction) may develop due to lack of ATP in red blood cells.
- *Musculoskeletal*: decreased ATP causes muscle weakness and release of creatinine phosphokinase (CPK, a muscle enzyme); acute rhabdomyolysis (muscle cell breakdown) can develop. Muscle cell destruction, in turn, can lead to acute renal failure as myoglobin, a muscle cell protein, exerts a toxic effect on the kidney tubule.
- *Respiratory*: chest muscle weakness can interfere with effective ventilation, leading to respiratory failure.

TABLE 9.10 Causes and manifestations of phosphate imbalances

IMBALANCE	CAUSES	MANIFESTATIONS
Hypophosphataemia Serum phosphorus < 2.5 mg/dL Critical value < 1 mg/dL	• Shift of phosphorus into cells • IV glucose administration • Total parenteral nutrition without phosphorus • Aluminium- or magnesium-based antacids • Diuretic therapy • Alcoholism	• Paraesthesias • Muscle weakness • Muscle pain and tenderness • Confusion, decreasing level of consciousness • Seizures • Bone pain, osteomalacia • Anorexia, dysphagia • Decreased bowel sounds • Possible acute respiratory failure
Hyperphosphataemia Serum phosphate > 4.5 mg/dL Critical value > 90 mg/dL	• Renal failure • Chemotherapy • Muscle tissue trauma • Sepsis • Severe hypothermia • Heat stroke	• Circumoral and peripheral paraesthesias • Muscle spasms • Tetany • Soft tissue calcification

- *Cardiovascular*: hypophosphataemia decreases myocardial contractility; decreased oxygenation of the heart muscle can cause chest pain and arrhythmias.
- *Gastrointestinal*: anorexia can occur, as well as dysphagia (difficulty swallowing), nausea and vomiting, decreased bowel sounds and possible ileus due to reduced gastrointestinal motility.

INTERPROFESSIONAL CARE

Treatment for hypophosphataemia is directed at prevention, treating the underlying cause of the disorder and replacing phosphate. An improved diet and oral phosphate supplement may restore normal phosphate levels in the person with a mild to moderate deficiency. Intravenous phosphate (sodium phosphate or potassium phosphate) is given when serum phosphate levels are less than 1 mg/dL. Oral phosphate supplements are then continued for up to 1 week to restore intracellular phosphate levels (Metheny, 2012).

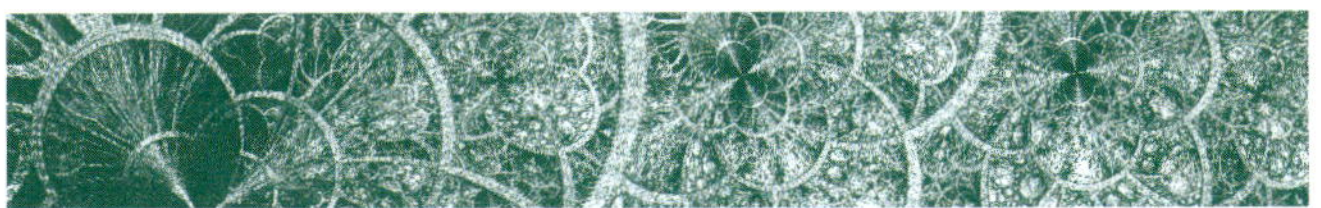

Nursing care

Nurses can be instrumental in identifying the person at risk of phosphate deficiency and preventing it from developing. Nurses should closely monitor serum electrolyte values in the person at risk, including those who are malnourished, receiving intravenous glucose solutions or total parenteral nutrition, or being treated with diuretic therapy or antacids that bind with phosphate. Nursing diagnoses that may be appropriate for the person with hypophosphataemia include:

- *impaired physical mobility* related to muscle weakness and poor coordination
- *ineffective breathing pattern* related to weakened muscles of respiration
- *decreased cardiac output* related to reduced myocardial contractility
- *risk of injury* related to muscle weakness and altered mental status.

Community-based care

In preparing for discharge, educate the person and family about the causes and manifestations of hypophosphataemia. Discuss the importance of avoiding phosphorus-binding antacids, unless prescribed. Stress the need for a well-balanced diet to maintain an adequate intake of phosphate.

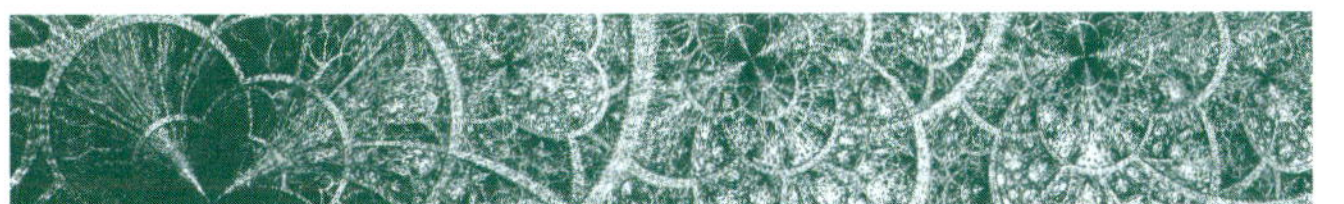

The person with hyperphosphataemia

Hyperphosphataemia is a serum phosphate level greater than 4.5 mg/dL. As with other electrolyte imbalances, it may be the result of impaired phosphate excretion, excess intake or a shift of phosphate from the intracellular space into extracellular fluids.

- Acute or chronic renal failure is the primary cause of impaired phosphate excretion.
- Rapid administration of phosphate-containing solutions can increase serum phosphate levels. This can include phosphate enemas. In addition, excess vitamin D increases phosphate absorption and can lead to hyperphosphataemia in the person with impaired renal function.
- A shift of phosphate from the intracellular to the extracellular space can occur during chemotherapy, due to sepsis or hypothermia, or because of extensive trauma or heat stroke.
- Because phosphate levels are affected by serum calcium concentrations, disruption of the mechanisms that regulate calcium levels (e.g. hypoparathyroidism, hyperthyroidism or vitamin D intoxication) can lead to hyperphosphataemia.

Pathophysiology and manifestations

Excessive serum phosphate levels cause few specific symptoms. The effects of high serum phosphate levels on nerves and muscles (muscle cramps and pain, paraesthesias, tingling around the mouth, muscle spasms, tetany) are more the result of hypocalcaemia that develops secondary to an elevated serum phosphorus level. The phosphate in the serum combines with ionised calcium and the ionised serum calcium level falls.

Calcification of soft tissues can occur with high phosphate levels. Phosphates bind with calcium to precipitate in soft tissues such as the kidneys and other organs. Soft tissue calcification can impair the function of affected organs.

INTERPROFESSIONAL CARE

Treatment of the underlying disorder often corrects hyperphosphataemia. When this is not feasible, phosphate-containing drugs are eliminated and intake of phosphate-rich foods such as organ meats and milk and milk products is restricted. Agents that bind with phosphate in the GI tract (such as calcium-containing antacids) may be prescribed. If renal function is adequate, intravenous normal saline may be given to promote renal excretion of phosphate. Dialysis may be necessary to reduce phosphate levels in the person with renal failure.

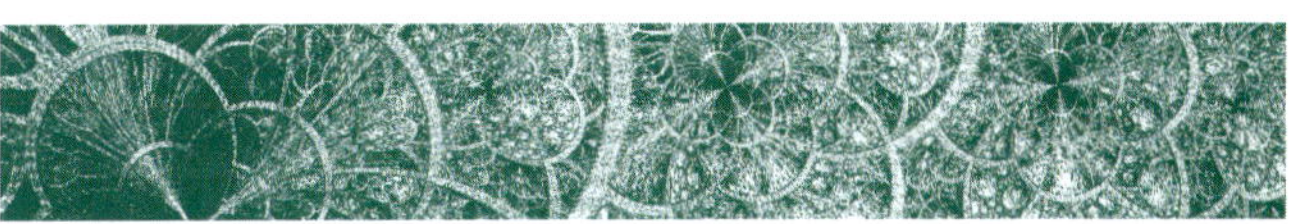

Nursing care

When providing nursing care for the person with hyperphosphataemia, monitor the person for laboratory data revealing an excess of phosphorus and a deficit of calcium, as well as the signs of hypocalcaemia.

Community-based care

Discuss the risk of hyperphosphataemia related to using phosphate preparations as laxatives or enemas, particularly with the person who has other risk factors for the disorder. When preparing the person for discharge, teach about the use of phosphate-binding preparations as ordered and dietary phosphate restrictions.

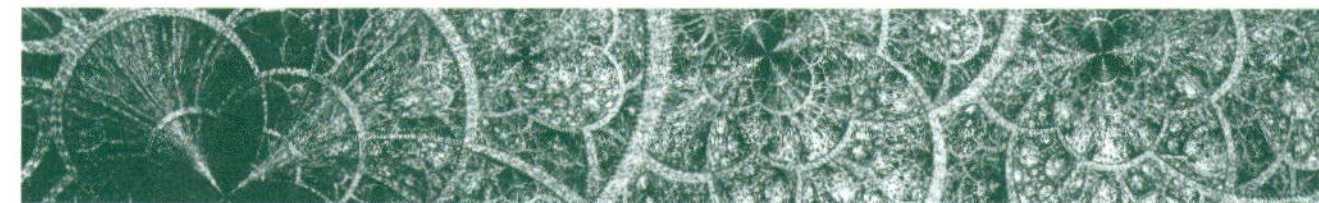

Acid–base disorders

Homeostasis and optimal cellular function require maintenance of the hydrogen ion (H^+) concentration of body fluids within a relatively narrow range. Hydrogen ions determine the relative acidity of body fluids. **Acids** release hydrogen ions in solution; **bases** (or **alkalis**) accept hydrogen ions in solution. The hydrogen ion concentration of a solution is measured as its pH. The relationship between hydrogen ion concentration and pH is inverse; that is, as hydrogen ion concentration increases, the pH falls and the solution becomes more acidic. As hydrogen ion concentration falls, the pH rises and the solution becomes more alkaline or basic. The pH of body fluids is slightly basic, with the normal pH ranging from 7.35 to 7.45. (A pH of 7 is neutral.)

REGULATION OF ACID–BASE BALANCE

A number of mechanisms work together to maintain the pH of the body within this normal range. Metabolic processes in the body continuously produce acids, which fall into two categories: volatile acids and non-volatile acids. **Volatile acids** can be eliminated from the body as a gas. Carbonic acid (H_2CO_3) is the only volatile acid produced in the body. It dissociates (separates) into carbon dioxide (CO_2) and water (H_2O); the carbon dioxide is then eliminated from the body through the lungs. All other acids produced in the body are *non-volatile acids* that must be metabolised or excreted from the body in fluid. Lactic acid, hydrochloric acid, phosphoric acid and sulfuric acid are examples of non-volatile acids. Most acids and bases in the body are weak; that is, they neither release nor accept a significant amount of hydrogen ions.

Three systems work together in the body to maintain the pH despite continuous acid production: buffers, the respiratory system and the renal system.

Buffer systems

Buffers are substances that prevent major changes in pH by removing or releasing hydrogen ions. When excess acid is present in body fluid, buffers bind with hydrogen ions to minimise the change in pH. If body fluids become too basic or alkaline, buffers release hydrogen ions, restoring the pH. Although buffers act within a fraction of a second, their capacity to maintain pH is limited. The major buffer systems of the body are the bicarbonate–carbonic acid buffer system, the phosphate buffer system and protein buffers.

The bicarbonate–carbonic acid buffer system can be illustrated by the following equation:

$$CO_2 + H_2O \leftrightarrow H_2CO_3 \leftrightarrow H^+ + HCO_3^-$$

Bicarbonate (HCO_3^-) is a weak base; when an acid is added to the system, the hydrogen ion in the acid combines with bicarbonate and the pH changes only slightly. Carbonic acid (H_2CO_3) is a weak acid produced when carbon dioxide dissolves in water. If a base is added to the system, it combines with carbonic acid and the pH remains within the normal range. Although the amounts of bicarbonate and carbonic acid in the body vary to a certain extent, as long as a ratio of 20 parts bicarbonate (HCO_3^-) to 1 part carbonic acid (H_2CO_3) is maintained, the pH remains within the 7.35 to 7.45 range (see Figure 9.14).

The normal serum bicarbonate level is 24 mEq/L and that of carbonic acid is 1.2 mEq/L. Thus, the ratio of bicarbonate to carbonic acid is 20:1. It is this ratio that maintains the pH within the normal range. Adding a strong acid to extracellular fluid depletes bicarbonate, changing the 20:1 ratio and causing the pH to drop below 7.35. This is known as **acidosis**. Addition of a strong base depletes carbonic acid as it combines with the

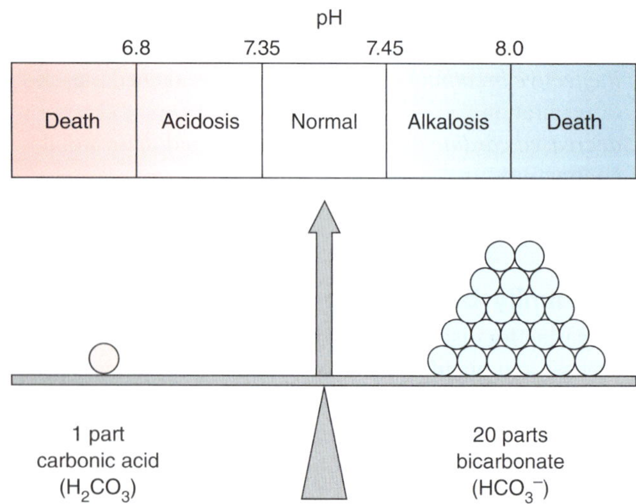

FIGURE 9.14 ***The normal ratio of bicarbonate to carbonic acid is 20:1. As long as this ratio is maintained, the pH remains within the normal range of 7.35 to 7.45***

base. The 20:1 ratio again is disrupted and the pH rises above 7.45, a condition known as **alkalosis**.

Intracellular and plasma proteins also serve as buffers. Plasma proteins contribute to buffering of extracellular fluids. Proteins in intracellular fluid provide extensive buffering for organic acids produced by cellular metabolism. In red blood cells, haemoglobin acts as a buffer for hydrogen ions when carbonic acid dissociates. Inorganic phosphates also serve as extracellular buffers, although their roles are not as important as the bicarbonate–carbonic acid buffer system. Phosphates are, however, important intracellular buffers, helping to maintain a stable pH within cells.

Respiratory system

The respiratory system (and the respiratory centre of the brain) regulates carbonic acid in the body by eliminating or retaining carbon dioxide. Carbon dioxide is a potential acid; when combined with water, it forms carbonic acid (see previous equation), a volatile acid. Acute increases in either carbon dioxide or hydrogen ions in the blood stimulate the respiratory centre in the brain. As a result, both the rate and depth of respiration increase. The increased rate and depth of lung ventilation eliminate carbon dioxide from the body and carbonic acid levels fall, bringing the pH to a more normal range. Although this compensation for increased hydrogen ion concentration occurs within minutes, it becomes less effective over time. The person with chronic lung disease may have consistently high carbon dioxide levels in their blood.

Alkalosis, by contrast, depresses the respiratory centre. Both the rate and depth of respiration decrease and carbon dioxide is retained. The retained carbon dioxide then combines with water to restore carbonic acid levels and bring the pH back within the normal range.

Renal system

The renal system is responsible for the long-term regulation of acid–base balance in the body. Excess non-volatile acids produced during metabolism normally are eliminated by the kidneys. The kidneys also regulate bicarbonate levels in extracellular fluid by regenerating bicarbonate ions as well as reabsorbing them in the renal tubules. Although the kidneys respond more slowly to changes in pH (over hours to days), they can generate bicarbonate and selectively excrete or retain hydrogen ions as needed. In acidosis, when excess hydrogen ion is present and the pH falls, the kidneys excrete hydrogen ions and retain bicarbonate. In alkalosis, the kidneys retain hydrogen ions and excrete bicarbonate to restore acid–base balance.

Assessment of acid–base balance

Acid–base balance is evaluated primarily by measuring arterial blood gases (ABGs).

Arterial blood is used because it reflects acid–base balance throughout the entire body better than venous blood. Arterial blood also provides information about the effectiveness of the lungs in oxygenating blood. The elements measured are pH, $PaCO_2$, PaO_2 and bicarbonate level.

CONSIDERATION FOR PRACTICE

Arteries are high-pressure vessels, in contrast to veins. Obtaining an arterial blood sample requires specialised training. It may be done by a doctor, a Registered Nurse, a respiratory therapist or a laboratory technician who has been trained in drawing ABGs. Apply firm pressure to the puncture site for 2 to 5 minutes after the needle is withdrawn to prevent bleeding into the surrounding tissues.

The **$PaCO_2$** measures the pressure exerted by dissolved carbon dioxide in the blood and reflects the respiratory component of acid–base regulation and balance. The $PaCO_2$ is regulated by the lungs. The normal value is 35 to 45 mmHg. A $PaCO_2$ of less than 35 mmHg is known as *hypocapnia*; a $PaCO_2$ greater than 45 mmHg is *hypercapnia*.

The **PaO_2** is a measure of the pressure exerted by oxygen that is dissolved in the plasma. Only about 3% of oxygen in the blood is transported in solution; most is combined with haemoglobin. However, it is the dissolved oxygen that is available to the cells for metabolism. As dissolved oxygen diffuses out of plasma into the tissues, more is released from haemoglobin. The normal value for PaO_2 is 80 to 100 mmHg. A PaO_2 of less than 80 mmHg is indicative of *hypoxaemia*. The PaO_2 is valuable for evaluating respiratory function, but is not used as a primary measurement in determining acid–base status.

CONSIDERATION FOR PRACTICE

You will see the abbreviations $PaCO_2$ and PaO_2 used interchangeably with PCO_2 and PO_2. The 'P' stands for partial pressure: the pressure exerted by the gas dissolved in the blood. The 'a' indicates that the sample is arterial blood. Because these measurements rarely are done on venous blood, the 'a' is often omitted from the abbreviation.

The **serum bicarbonate** (HCO_3^-) reflects the renal regulation of acid–base balance. It is often called the metabolic component of ABGs. The normal HCO_3^- value is 22 to 26 mEq/L.

The **base excess (BE)** is a calculated value also known as *buffer base capacity*. The base excess measures substances that can accept or combine with hydrogen ions. It reflects the degree of acid–base imbalance by indicating the status of the body's total buffering capacity. It represents the amount of acid or base that must be added to a blood sample to achieve a pH of 7.4. This is essentially a measure of increased or decreased bicarbonate. The normal value for base excess for arterial blood is −3.0 to +3.0. Normal ABG values are summarised in Table 9.11.

ABGs are analysed to identify acid–base disorders and their probable cause, to determine the extent of the imbalance and to monitor treatment. When analysing ABG results, it is important to use a systematic approach. First evaluate each individual measurement, then look at the interrelationships to determine the person's acid–base status (see Box 9.10).

TABLE 9.11 Normal arterial blood gas values

VALUE	NORMAL RANGE	SIGNIFICANCE
pH	7.35 to 7.45	Reflects hydrogen ion (H^+) concentration • < 7.35 = acidosis • > 7.45 = alkalosis
$PaCO_2$	35 to 45 mmHg	Partial pressure of carbon dioxide (CO_2) in arterial blood • < 35 mmHg = hypocapnia • > 45 mmHg = hypercapnia
PaO_2	80 to 100 mmHg	Partial pressure of oxygen (O_2) in arterial blood • < 80 mmHg = hypoxaemia
HCO_3^-	22 to 26 mEq/L	Bicarbonate concentration in plasma
BE	-3 to $+3$	Base excess; a measure of buffering capacity

ACID–BASE IMBALANCE

Acid–base imbalances fall into two major categories: acidosis and alkalosis. Acidosis occurs when the hydrogen ion concentration increases above normal (pH below 7.35). Alkalosis occurs when the hydrogen ion concentration falls below normal (pH above 7.45).

Acid–base imbalances are further classified as *metabolic* or *respiratory* disorders. In metabolic disorders, the primary change is in the concentration of bicarbonate. In metabolic acidosis, the amount of bicarbonate is decreased in relation to the amount of acid in the body (see Figure 9.15A). It can develop as a result of abnormal bicarbonate losses or because of excess non-volatile acids in the body. The pH falls below 7.35 and the bicarbonate concentration is less than 22 mEq/L. Metabolic alkalosis, by contrast, occurs when there is an excess of bicarbonate in relation to the amount of hydrogen ion (see Figure 9.15B). The pH is above 7.45 and the bicarbonate concentration is greater than 26 mEq/L.

In respiratory disorders, the primary change is in the concentration of carbonic acid. Respiratory acidosis occurs when carbon dioxide is retained, increasing the amount of carbonic acid in the body (see Figure 9.16A). As a result, the pH falls to less than 7.35 and the $PaCO_2$ is greater than 45 mmHg. When too much carbon dioxide is 'blown off', carbonic acid levels fall and respiratory alkalosis develops (see Figure 9.16B). The pH rises to above 7.45 and the $PaCO_2$ is less than 35 mmHg.

Acid–base disorders are further defined as primary (simple) and mixed. Primary disorders usually are due to one cause. For example, respiratory failure often causes respiratory acidosis due to retained carbon dioxide; renal failure usually causes metabolic acidosis due to retained hydrogen ion and impaired bicarbonate production. Table 9.12 summarises primary acid–base imbalances with common causes of each. Mixed disorders occur from combinations of respiratory and metabolic disturbances. For example, a person in cardiac arrest develops a mixed respiratory and metabolic acidosis due to lack of ventilation (and retained CO_2) and hypoxia of body tissues that leads to anaerobic metabolism and acid by-products (excess non-volatile acids).

BOX 9.10 Interpreting arterial blood gases

1. Look at the pH.
   - pH < 7.35 = acidosis
   - pH > 7.45 = alkalosis
2. Look at the $PaCO_2$.
   - $PaCO_2 < 35$ mmHg = hypocapnia; more carbon dioxide is being exhaled than normal
   - $PaCO_2 > 45$ mmHg = hypercapnia; carbon dioxide is being retained
3. Evaluate the pH–$PaCO_2$ relationship for a possible respiratory problem.
   - If the pH is < 7.35 (acidosis) and the $PaCO_2$ is > 45 mmHg (hypercapnia), retained carbon dioxide is causing increased H^+ concentration and respiratory acidosis.
   - If the pH is > 7.45 (alkalosis) and the $PaCO_2$ is < 35 mmHg (hypocapnia), low carbon dioxide levels and decreased H^+ concentration are causing respiratory alkalosis.
4. Look at the bicarbonate.
   - If the HCO_3^- is < 22 mEq/L, bicarbonate levels are lower than normal.
   - If the HCO_3^- is > 26 mEq/L, bicarbonate levels are higher than normal.
5. Evaluate the pH, HCO_3^- and BE for a possible metabolic problem.
   - If the pH is < 7.35 (acidosis), the HCO_3^- is < 22 mEq/L and the BE is < -3 mEq/L, then low bicarbonate levels and high H^+ concentrations are causing metabolic acidosis.
   - If the pH is > 7.45 (alkalosis), the HCO_3^- is > 26 mEq/L and the BE is $> +3$ mEq/L, then high bicarbonate levels are causing metabolic alkalosis.
6. Look for compensation.

   Renal compensation:
   - In respiratory acidosis (pH < 7.35, $PaCO_2$ 45 mmHg), the kidneys retain HCO_3^- to buffer the excess acid, so the HCO_3^- is > 26 mEq/L.
   - In respiratory alkalosis (pH > 7.45, $PaCO_2$ < 35 mmHg), the kidneys excrete HCO_3^- to minimise the alkalosis, so the HCO_3^- is < 22 mEq/L.

   Respiratory compensation:
   - In metabolic acidosis (pH < 7.35, $HCO_3^- < 22$ mEq/L), the rate and depth of respirations increase, increasing carbon dioxide elimination, so the $PaCO_2$ is < 35 mmHg.
   - In metabolic alkalosis (pH 7.45, $HCO_3^- > 26$ mEq/L), respirations slow, carbon dioxide is retained, so the $PaCO_2$ is > 45 mmHg.
7. Evaluate oxygenation.
   - $PaO_2 < 80$ mmHg = hypoxaemia; possible hypoventilation
   - $PaO_2 > 100$ mmHg = hyperventilation

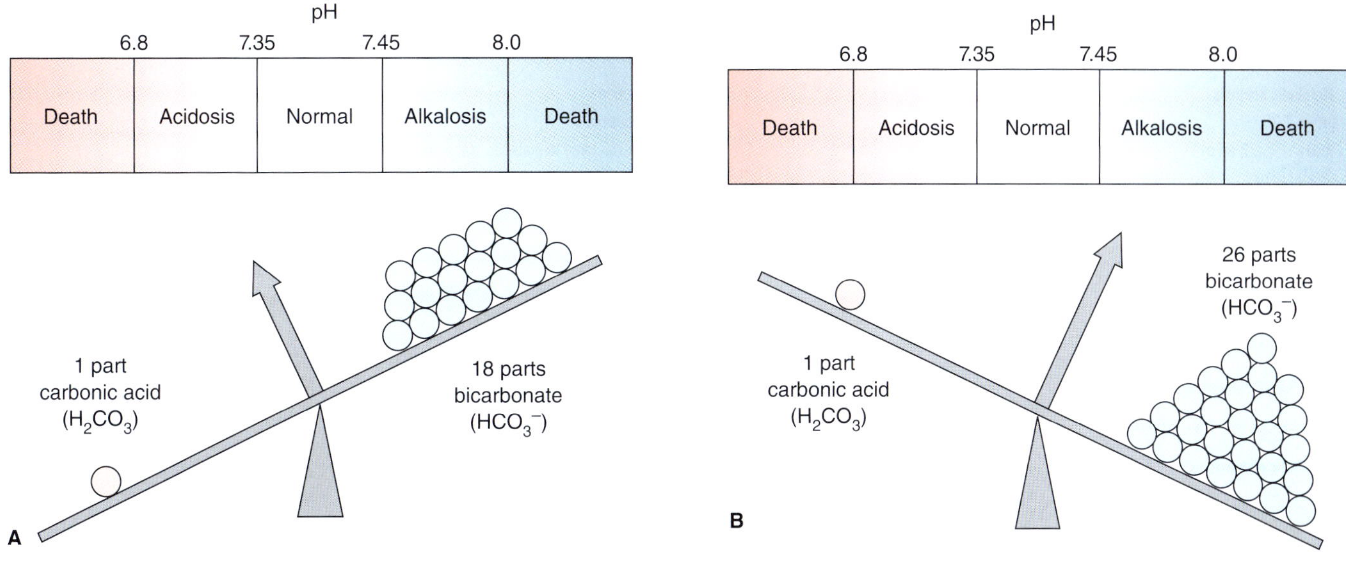

FIGURE 9.15 ***Metabolic acid–base imbalances. A, Metabolic acidosis. B, Metabolic alkalosis***

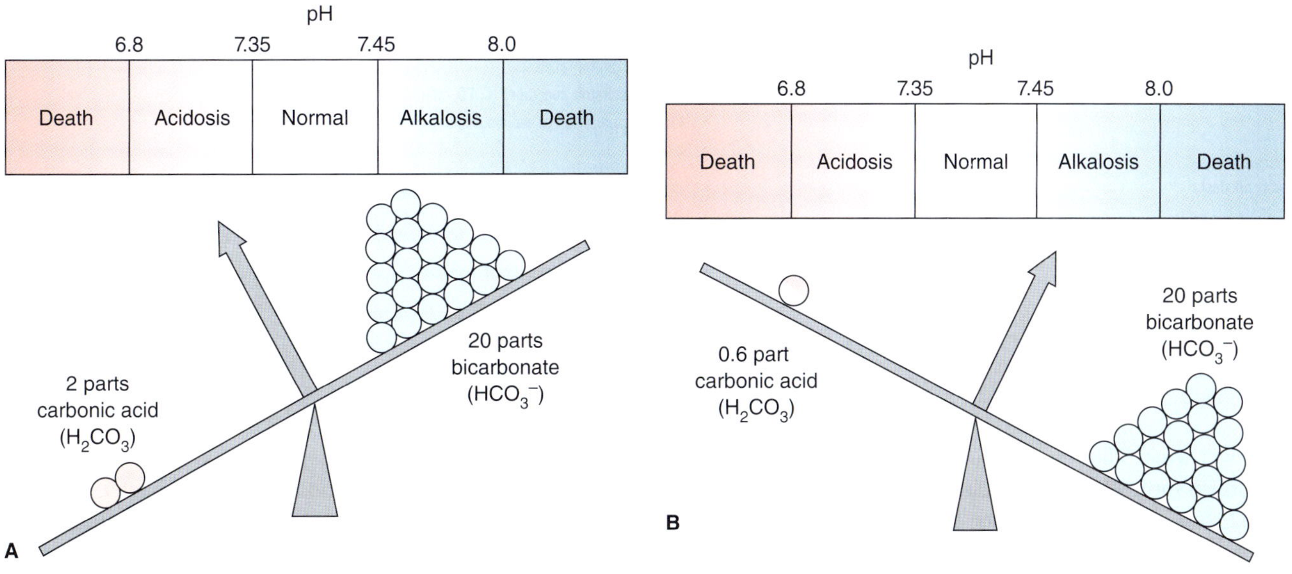

FIGURE 9.16 ***Respiratory acid–base imbalances. A, Respiratory acidosis. B, Respiratory alkalosis***

FAST FACTS

- Simple acid–base imbalances are more commonly seen than mixed imbalances. Common causes of simple acid–base imbalances include:
  - diabetic ketoacidosis (metabolic acidosis)
  - chronic obstructive lung disease (respiratory acidosis)
  - anxiety-related (psychogenic) hyperventilation (respiratory alkalosis).
- The critically ill person is at higher risk of mixed acid–base imbalances.

Compensation

With primary acid–base disorders, compensatory changes in the other part of the regulatory system occur to restore a normal pH and homeostasis. In metabolic acid–base disorders, the change in pH affects the rate and depth of respirations. Therefore, this affects carbon dioxide elimination and the $PaCO_2$, helping restore the carbonic acid to bicarbonate ratio. The kidneys compensate for simple respiratory imbalances. The change in pH affects both bicarbonate conservation and hydrogen ion elimination (see Table 9.12).

Compensatory changes in respirations occur within minutes of a change in pH. These changes, however, become less

TABLE 9.12 Common causes of primary acid–base imbalances

IMBALANCE	COMMON CAUSES
Metabolic acidosis pH < 7.35 HCO_3^- < 22 mEq/L *Critical values* pH < 7.20 HCO_3^- < 10 mEq/L	↑ Acid production • Lactic acidosis • Ketoacidosis related to diabetes, starvation or alcoholism • Salicylate toxicity ↓ Acid excretion • Renal failure ↑ Bicarbonate loss • Diarrhoea, ileostomy drainage, intestinal fistula • Biliary or pancreatic fistulas ↑ Chloride • Sodium chloride IV solutions • Renal tubular acidosis • Carbonic anhydrase inhibitors
Metabolic alkalosis pH > 7.45 HCO_3^- > 26 mEq/L *Critical values* pH > 7.60 HCO_3^- > 40 mEq/L	↑ Acid loss or excretion • Vomiting, gastric suction • Hypokalaemia ↑ Bicarbonate • Alkali ingestion (bicarbonate of soda) • Excess bicarbonate administration
Respiratory acidosis pH < 7.35 $PaCO_2$ > 45 mmHg *Critical values* pH < 7.2 $PaCO_2$ > 77 mmHg	• Acute respiratory acidosis • Acute respiratory conditions (pulmonary oedema, pneumonia, acute asthma) • Opiate overdose • Foreign body aspiration • Chest trauma • Chronic respiratory acidosis • Chronic respiratory conditions (COPD, cystic fibrosis) • Multiple sclerosis, other neuromuscular diseases • Stroke
Respiratory alkalosis pH > 7.45 $PaCO_2$ > 35 mmHg *Critical values* pH > 7.60 $PaCO_2$ < 20 mmHg	• Anxiety-induced hyperventilation (e.g. anxiety) • Fever • Early salicylate intoxication • Hyperventilation with mechanical ventilator

effective over time. The renal response takes longer to restore the pH but is a more effective long-term mechanism. If the pH is restored to within normal limits, the disorder is said to be *fully compensated*. When these changes are reflected in ABG values but the pH remains outside normal limits, the disorder is said to be *partially compensated*.

The person with metabolic acidosis

Metabolic acidosis (bicarbonate deficit) is characterised by a low pH (< 7.35) and a low bicarbonate (< 22 mEq/L). It may be caused by excess acid in the body or loss of bicarbonate from the body. When metabolic acidosis develops, the respiratory system attempts to return the pH to normal by increasing the rate and depth of respirations. Carbon dioxide elimination increases and the $PaCO_2$ falls (< 35 mmHg).

Risk factors

Metabolic acidosis rarely is a primary disorder; it usually develops during the course of another disease:

- *Acute lactic acidosis* usually results from tissue hypoxia due to shock or cardiac arrest.
- A person with type 1 diabetes mellitus is at risk of developing *diabetic ketoacidosis*. (See the chapter 'Nursing care of people with diabetes mellitus' for more information about diabetes and its complications.)
- *Acute* or *chronic renal failure* impairs the excretion of metabolic acids.
- Diarrhoea, intestinal suction or abdominal fistulas increase the *risk of excess bicarbonate loss*.

Other common causes of metabolic acidosis are listed in Table 9.12.

Pathophysiology

Three basic mechanisms that can cause metabolic acidosis are:

- accumulation of metabolic acids
- excess loss of bicarbonate
- an increase in chloride levels.

An accumulation of metabolic acids can result from excess acid production or impaired elimination of metabolic acids by the kidney. Lactic acidosis develops due to tissue hypoxia

BOX 9.11 Unravelling the anion gap

Calculation of the anion gap can help identify the underlying mechanism in metabolic acidosis if it is unclear.

The number of cations (positively charged ions) and anions (negatively charged ions) in ECF normally is equal (see Figure 9.2). Not all of these ions, however, are measured in laboratory testing (e.g. organic acids and proteins). The anion gap is calculated by subtracting the sum of two measured anions, chloride and bicarbonate, from the concentration of the major cation, sodium (see figure). The normal anion gap is 8 to 12 mEq/L.

Excess acids in ECF are buffered by bicarbonate, reducing serum bicarbonate levels and the total measured concentration of anions. This increases the anion gap (B in figure). When bicarbonate is lost from the body or chloride levels increase, however, the anion gap remains within normal limits (C in figure). This occurs because an increase or decrease in one of these negatively charged ions causes a corresponding change in the other to maintain balance (e.g. ↓HCO_3^- ↔↑Cl^-) and there is no change in the amount of unmeasured anions.

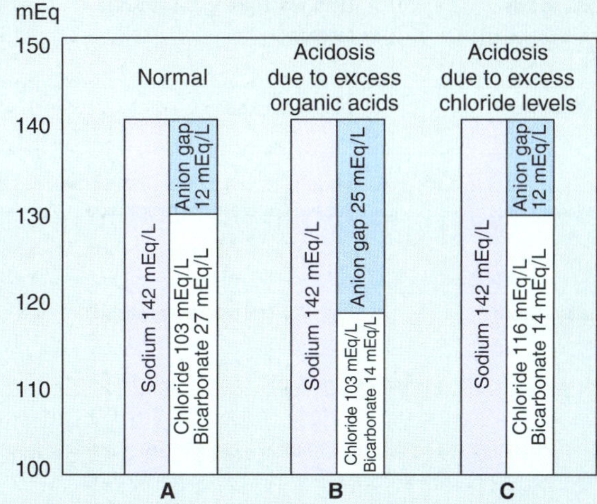

Illustration of the anion gap in metabolic acidosis. A, Normal anion gap. B, High anion gap caused by excess acids. C, Normal anion gap with hyperchloremia

and a shift to anaerobic metabolism by the cells. Lactate and hydrogen ions are produced, forming lactic acid. Both oxygen and glucose are necessary for normal cell metabolism. When intracellular glucose is inadequate due to starvation or a lack of insulin to move it into cells, the body breaks down fatty tissue to meet its metabolic needs. In this process, fatty acids are released, which are converted to ketones; ketoacidosis develops. Aspirin (acetylsalicylic acid) breaks down into salicylic acid in the body. Substances such as aspirin, methanol (wood alcohol) and ethylene (contained in antifreeze and solvents) cause a toxic increase in body acids by either breaking down into acid products (salicylic acid) or stimulating metabolic acid production (Norris, 2018). Renal failure impairs the body's ability to excrete excess hydrogen ions and form bicarbonate.

Excess metabolic acids increase the hydrogen ion concentration of body fluids. The excess acid is buffered by bicarbonate, leading to what is known as a high **anion gap** acidosis (see Box 9.11).

The pancreas secretes bicarbonate-rich fluid into the small intestine. Intestinal suction, severe diarrhoea, ileostomy drainage or fistulas can lead to excess loss of bicarbonate. Hyperchloraemic acidosis can develop when excess chloride solutions (such as NaCl or ammonium chloride) are infused, causing a rise in chloride concentrations. It may be related to renal disease or administration of carbonic anhydrate inhibitor diuretics. The anion gap remains normal in metabolic acidosis due to bicarbonate loss or excess chloride.

Acidosis depresses cell membrane excitability, affecting neuromuscular function. It also increases the amount of free calcium in ECF by interfering with protein binding. Severe acidosis (pH of 7.0 or less) depresses myocardial contractility, leading to a fall in cardiac output. If kidney function is normal, acid excretion and ammonia production increase to eliminate excess hydrogen ions.

Acid–base imbalances also affect electrolyte balance (see Table 9.13). In acidosis, potassium is retained as the kidney excretes excess hydrogen ions. Excess hydrogen ions also enter the cells, displacing potassium from the intracellular space to maintain the balance of cations and anions within the cells. The effect of both processes is to increase serum potassium levels. Also in acidosis, calcium is released from its bonds with plasma proteins, increasing the amount of ionised (free) calcium in the blood. Magnesium levels may fall in acidosis. See Box 9.11 for information on anion gap acidosis.

Manifestations

Metabolic acidosis affects the function of many body systems. Its general manifestations include weakness and fatigue, headache and general malaise. Gastrointestinal function is affected, causing anorexia, nausea, vomiting and abdominal pain. The level of consciousness declines, leading to stupor and coma. Cardiac arrhythmias develop and cardiac arrest may occur. The skin is often warm and flushed. Skeletal problems may develop in chronic acidosis, as calcium and phosphate are released from the bones. Manifestations of compensatory mechanisms are seen. The respirations are

TABLE 9.13 Compensation for simple acid–base imbalances

PRIMARY DISORDER	CAUSE	COMPENSATION	EFFECT ON ABGS
Metabolic acidosis	Excess non-volatile acids; bicarbonate deficiency	Rate and depth of respirations increase, eliminating additional CO_2	↓ pH ↓ HCO_3^- ↓ $PaCO_2$
Metabolic alkalosis	Bicarbonate excess	Rate and depth of respirations decrease, retaining CO_2	↑ pH ↑ HCO_3^- ↑ $PaCO_2$
Respiratory acidosis	Retained CO_2 and excess carbonic acid	Kidneys conserve bicarbonate to restore carbonic acid: bicarbonate ratio of 1:20	↓ pH ↑ $PaCO_2$ ↑ HCO_3^-
Respiratory alkalosis	Loss of CO_2 and deficient carbonic acid	Kidneys excrete bicarbonate and conserve H^+ to restore carbonic acid: bicarbonate ratio	↑ pH ↓ $PaCO_2$ ↓ HCO_3^-

deep and rapid, known as Kussmaul's respirations. The person may complain of shortness of breath or dyspnoea. (See the 'Manifestations' box.)

MANIFESTATIONS Metabolic acidosis

- Anorexia
- Nausea and vomiting
- Abdominal pain
- Weakness
- Fatigue
- General malaise
- Decreasing levels of consciousness
- Arrhythmias
- Bradycardia
- Warm, flushed skin
- Hyperventilation (Kussmaul's respirations)

INTERPROFESSIONAL CARE

Management of metabolic acidosis focuses on treating the underlying cause of the disorder and correcting the acid–base imbalance.

Diagnosis

The following laboratory and diagnostic tests may be ordered:

- *ABGs* generally show a pH of less than 7.35 and a bicarbonate level of less than 22 mEq/L. A compensatory decrease in $PaCO_2$ to less than 35 mmHg is usually present.
- *Serum electrolytes* demonstrate elevated serum potassium levels and possible low magnesium levels. The total calcium may remain unchanged, although more physiologically active ionised calcium is available. Sodium, chloride and bicarbonate levels are used to calculate the anion gap.
- The *ECG* may show changes that reflect both the acidosis (particularly when severe) and the accompanying hyperkalaemia.
- Other diagnostic studies such as the blood glucose and renal function studies may be ordered to identify the underlying cause of metabolic acidosis.

Medications

An alkalinising solution such as bicarbonate may be given if the pH is less than 7.1 to reduce the effects of the acidosis on cardiac function. Sodium bicarbonate is the most commonly used alkalinising solution; others include lactate, citrate and acetate solutions (which are metabolised to bicarbonate). Alkalinising solutions are given intravenously for severe acute metabolic acidosis. In chronic metabolic acidosis, the oral route is used.

The person treated with bicarbonate must be carefully monitored. Rapid correction of the acidosis may lead to metabolic alkalosis and hypokalaemia. Hypernatraemia and hyperosmolality may develop as well, leading to water retention and fluid overload.

Treatment for diabetic ketoacidosis includes intravenous insulin and fluid replacement. (See the chapter 'Nursing care of people with diabetes mellitus' for the treatment of diabetic ketoacidosis.) Alcoholic ketoacidosis is treated with saline solutions and glucose. Treatment for lactic acidosis from decreased tissue perfusion (e.g. shock or cardiac arrest) focuses on correcting the underlying problem and improving tissue perfusion. The person with chronic renal failure and mild or moderate metabolic acidosis may or may not require treatment, depending on the pH and bicarbonate levels. When metabolic acidosis is due to diarrhoea, treatment includes correcting the underlying cause and providing fluid and electrolyte replacement.

CONSIDERATION FOR PRACTICE

As metabolic acidosis is corrected, potassium shifts back into the intracellular space. This can lead to hypokalaemia and cardiac arrhythmias. Carefully monitor serum potassium levels during treatment.

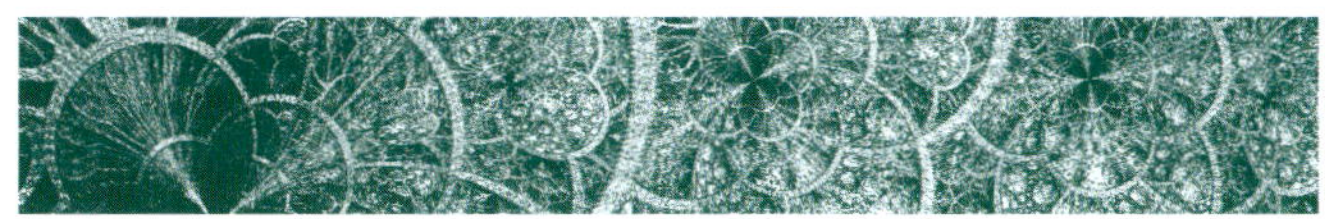

Nursing care

Nurses frequently provide care for people diagnosed with metabolic acidosis, although the focus of care often is the disorder underlying the acidosis (e.g. diabetes mellitus, renal failure) rather than the acidosis itself. For this reason, it is vital for the nurse to be aware of the effects of the acidosis and its implications for nursing care.

Health promotion

To promote health in the person at risk of metabolic acidosis, it is important for the nurse to discuss the management of the underlying disease process (e.g. type 1 diabetes or renal failure), especially preventing complications such as diabetic ketoacidosis and metabolic acidosis. Because early manifestations of metabolic acidosis (e.g. fatigue, general malaise, anorexia, nausea, abdominal pain) resemble those of common viral disorders such as 'the flu', stress the importance of promptly seeking treatment if these symptoms develop.

Assessment

Assessment data related to metabolic acidosis include the following:

- *Health history*: current manifestations, including anorexia, nausea, vomiting, abdominal discomfort, fatigue, lethargy, other symptoms; duration of symptoms and any precipitating factors such as diarrhoea, ingestion of a toxin such as aspirin, methanol or ethylene; chronic diseases such as diabetes or renal failure, cirrhosis of the liver or endocrine disorders; current medications.
- *Physical assessment*: mental status and level of consciousness; vital signs including respiratory rate and depth; apical and peripheral pulses; skin colour and temperature; abdominal contour and distension; bowel sounds; urine output.
- *Diagnostic tests*: ABGs, serum electrolytes, tests for underlying disorders.

Nursing diagnoses and interventions

Nursing management of a person with metabolic acidosis often focuses on the primary disorder (e.g. diabetic ketoacidosis or renal failure); however, the acidosis itself has effects that must be attended to when providing care.

Decreased cardiac output

Metabolic acidosis affects cardiac output by decreasing myocardial contractility, slowing the heart rate and increasing the risk of arrhythmias. The accompanying hyperkalaemia increases the risk of decreased cardiac output as well (see the earlier discussion about hyperkalaemia).

- Monitor vital signs, including peripheral pulses and capillary refill. *Hypotension, diminished pulse strength and slowed capillary refill may indicate decreased cardiac output and impaired tissue perfusion. Poor tissue perfusion can increase the risk of lactic acidosis.*
- Monitor the ECG pattern for arrhythmias and changes characteristic of hyperkalaemia. Notify the doctor of changes. *Progressive ECG changes such as widening of the QRS complex indicate an increasing risk of arrhythmias and cardiac arrest. Arrhythmias further decrease cardiac output, possibly intensifying the degree of acidosis.*
- Monitor laboratory values, including ABGs, serum electrolytes and renal function studies (serum urea and creatinine). *Frequent monitoring of laboratory values allows evaluation of the effectiveness of treatment as well as early identification of potential problems.*

Risk of excess fluid volume

Administering bicarbonate to correct acidosis increases the risk of hypernatraemia, hyperosmolality and FVE.

- Monitor and maintain fluid replacement as ordered. Monitor serum sodium levels and osmolality. *Bicarbonate administration can cause hypernatraemia and hyperosmolality, leading to water retention.*
- Monitor heart and lung sounds, CVP and respiratory status. *Increasing dyspnoea, adventitious lung sounds, a third heart sound (S_3) due to the volume of blood flow through the heart, and high CVP readings are indicative of hypervolaemia and should be reported to the attending doctor.*
- Assess for oedema, particularly in the back, sacral and periorbital areas. *Initially, oedema affects dependent tissues—the back and sacrum in the person who is bedridden. Periorbital oedema indicates more generalised oedema.*
- Assess urine output hourly. Maintain accurate intake and output records. Note urine output less than 30 mL/hour or a positive fluid balance on 24-hour total intake and output calculations. *Heart failure and inadequate renal perfusion may lead to decreased urine output.*
- Obtain daily weights using consistent conditions. *Daily weights are an accurate indicator of fluid balance.*
- Administer prescribed diuretics as ordered, monitoring the person's response to therapy. *Loop or high-ceiling diuretics such as frusemide can lead to further electrolyte imbalances, especially hypokalaemia. This is a significant risk like that seen during correction of metabolic acidosis.*

Risk of injury

Mental status and brain function are affected by acidosis, increasing the risk of injury.

- Monitor neurological function, including mental status, level of consciousness and muscle strength. *As the pH falls, mental functioning declines, leading to confusion, stupor and a decreasing level of consciousness.*
- Institute safety precautions as necessary: keep the bed in its lowest position, side rails raised. *These measures help protect the person from injury resulting from confusion or disorientation.*
- Keep clocks, calendars and familiar objects at the bedside. Orient to time, place and circumstances as needed. Allow significant others to remain with the person as much as

possible. *An unfamiliar environment and altered thought processes can further increase the risk of injury. Significant others provide a sense of security and reduce anxiety.*

Nursing care also includes measures to treat the underlying disorder, such as diabetic ketoacidosis. Refer to the chapters on diabetes ('Nursing care of people with diabetes mellitus') and renal failure ('Nursing care of people with kidney disorders') for specific interventions.

Community-based care

Discharge planning and teaching focus on the underlying cause of the imbalance. The person who has developed ketoacidosis as a result of diabetes mellitus, starvation or alcoholism needs interventions and teaching to prevent future episodes of acidosis. Diet, medication management and alcohol dependency treatment are vital teaching areas. When metabolic acidosis is related to renal failure, the person should be referred for management of the renal failure itself. The person who has experienced diarrhoea or excess ileostomy drainage leading to bicarbonate loss requires information about appropriate diarrhoea treatment strategies and when to call their healthcare provider.

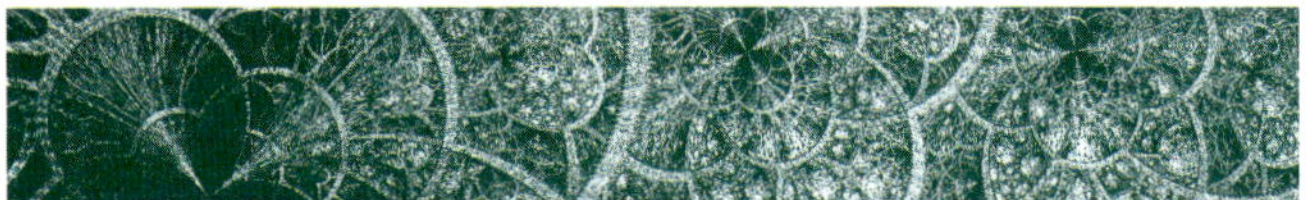

The person with metabolic alkalosis

Metabolic alkalosis (bicarbonate excess) is characterised by a high pH (> 7.45) and high bicarbonate (> 26 mEq/L). It may be caused by loss of acid or excess bicarbonate in the body. When metabolic alkalosis develops, the respiratory system attempts to return the pH to normal by slowing the respiratory rate. Carbon dioxide is retained and the $PaCO_2$ increases (> 45 mmHg).

Risk factors

As is the case with other acid–base imbalances, metabolic alkalosis rarely occurs as a primary disorder. Risk factors include hospitalisation, hypokalaemia and treatment with alkalinising solutions (e.g. bicarbonate).

Pathophysiology

Hydrogen ions may be lost via gastric secretions, through the kidneys or because of a shift of H^+ into the cells. Metabolic alkalosis due to loss of hydrogen ions usually occurs because of vomiting or gastric suction. Gastric secretions are highly acidic (pH 1 to 3). When these are lost through vomiting or gastric suction, the alkalinity of body fluids increases. This increased alkalinity results from both the loss of acid and selective retention of bicarbonate by the kidneys as chloride is depleted. (Chloride is the major anion in ECF; when it is lost, bicarbonate is retained as a replacement anion.)

Increased renal excretion of hydrogen ions can be prompted by hypokalaemia as the kidneys try to conserve potassium, excreting hydrogen ions instead. Hypokalaemia contributes to metabolic alkalosis in another way as well. When potassium shifts out of cells to maintain extracellular potassium levels, hydrogen ions shift into the cells to maintain the balance between cations and anions within the cell.

Excess bicarbonate usually occurs as a result of ingesting antacids that contain bicarbonate or overzealous administration of bicarbonate to treat metabolic acidosis. Common causes of metabolic alkalosis are summarised in Table 9.12.

In alkalosis, more calcium combines with serum proteins, reducing the amount of ionised (physiologically active) calcium in the blood. This accounts for many of the common manifestations of metabolic alkalosis. Alkalosis also affects potassium balance: hypokalaemia not only can cause metabolic alkalosis (discussed earlier), but it also can result from metabolic alkalosis. Hydrogen ions shift out of the intracellular space to help restore the pH, prompting more potassium to enter the cells and depleting ECF potassium. The high pH depresses the respiratory system as the body retains carbon dioxide to restore the carbonic acid to bicarbonate ratio.

Manifestations and complications

Manifestations of metabolic alkalosis (see the 'Manifestations' box) occur as a result of decreased calcium ionisation and are similar to those of hypocalcaemia, including numbness and tingling around the mouth, fingers and toes; dizziness; Trousseau's sign; and muscle spasm. As the respiratory system compensates for metabolic alkalosis, respirations are depressed, and respiratory failure with hypoxaemia and respiratory acidosis may develop.

MANIFESTATIONS Metabolic alkalosis

- Confusion
- Decreasing level of consciousness
- Hyperreflexia
- Tetany
- Arrhythmias
- Hypotension
- Seizures
- Respiratory failure

INTERPROFESSIONAL CARE

Interprofessional management of metabolic alkalosis focuses on diagnosing and correcting the underlying cause.

Diagnosis

The following laboratory and diagnostic tests may be ordered:

- *ABGs* show a pH greater than 7.45 and bicarbonate level greater than 26 mEq/L. With compensatory hypoventilation, carbon dioxide is retained and the $PaCO_2$ is greater than 45 mmHg.
- *Serum electrolytes* often demonstrate decreased serum potassium (< 3.5 mEq/L) and decreased chloride (< 95 mEq/L) levels. The serum bicarbonate level is high. Although the total serum calcium may be normal, the ionised fraction of calcium is low.
- *Urine pH* may be low (pH 1 to 3) if metabolic acidosis is caused by hypokalaemia. The kidneys selectively retain

potassium and excrete hydrogen ions to restore ECF potassium levels. Urinary chloride levels may be normal or greater than 250 mEq/24 hours.

- The *ECG pattern* shows changes similar to those seen with hypokalaemia. These changes may be due to hypokalaemia or to the alkalosis.

Medications

Treatment of metabolic alkalosis includes restoring normal fluid volume and administering potassium chloride and sodium chloride solution. The potassium restores serum and intracellular potassium levels, allowing the kidneys to more effectively conserve hydrogen ions. Chloride promotes renal excretion of bicarbonate. Sodium chloride solutions restore FVDs that can contribute to metabolic alkalosis. In severe alkalosis, an acidifying solution such as dilute hydrochloric acid or ammonium chloride may be administered. In addition, drugs may be used to treat the underlying cause of the alkalosis.

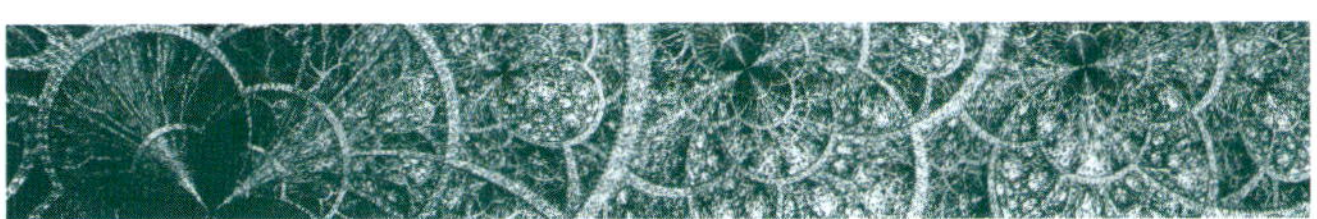

Nursing care

Health promotion

Health promotion activities focus on teaching a person the risks of using sodium bicarbonate as an antacid to relieve heartburn or gastric distress. Stress the availability of other effective antacid preparations and the need to seek medical evaluation for persistent gastric symptoms. In the hospital setting, carefully monitor laboratory values for the person at risk of developing metabolic alkalosis, particularly people undergoing continuous gastric suction.

Assessment

Focused assessment data related to metabolic alkalosis include the following:

- *Health history*: current manifestations, such as numbness and tingling, muscle spasms, dizziness, other symptoms; duration of symptoms and any precipitating factors such as bicarbonate ingestion, vomiting, diuretic therapy or endocrine disorders; current medications.
- *Physical assessment*: vital signs, including apical pulse and rate and depth of respirations; muscle strength; deep tendon reflexes.
- *Diagnostic tests*: ABGs, serum electrolytes.

Nursing diagnoses and interventions

As with metabolic acidosis, nursing care of the person with metabolic alkalosis often focuses on intervening for responses to the primary problem, rather than the alkalosis itself. However, the risk of impaired gas exchange is a priority problem, especially with severe metabolic alkalosis.

Risk of impaired gas exchange

Respiratory compensation for metabolic alkalosis depresses the respiratory rate and reduces the depth of breathing to promote carbon dioxide retention. As a result, the person is at risk of impaired gas exchange, especially in the presence of underlying lung disease.

- Monitor respiratory rate, depth and effort. Monitor oxygen saturation continuously, reporting an oxygen saturation level of less than 95% (or as ordered). *The depressed respiratory drive associated with metabolic alkalosis can lead to hypoxaemia and impaired oxygenation of tissues. Oxygen saturation levels of less than 90% indicate significant oxygenation problems.*
- Assess skin colour; note and report cyanosis around the mouth. *Central cyanosis, seen around the mouth and oral mucous membranes, indicates significant hypoxia.*
- Monitor mental status and level of consciousness (LOC). Report decreasing LOC or behaviour changes such as restlessness, agitation or confusion. *Changes in mental status or behaviour may be early signs of hypoxia.*
- Place in semi-Fowler's or Fowler's position as tolerated. *Elevating the head of the bed facilitates alveolar ventilation and gas exchange.*
- Schedule nursing care activities to allow rest periods. *The person who is hypoxaemic has limited energy reserves, necessitating frequent rest and limited activities.*
- Administer oxygen as ordered or necessary to maintain oxygen saturation levels. *Supplemental oxygen can help maintain blood and tissue oxygenation despite depressed respirations.*

Deficient fluid volume

A person with metabolic alkalosis often has an accompanying FVD.

- Assess vital signs, CVP and peripheral pulse volume at least every 4 hours. *Hypotension, tachycardia, low CVP and weak, easily obliterated peripheral pulses indicate hypovolaemia.*
- Weigh daily under standard conditions (time of day, clothing and scale). *Rapid weight changes accurately reflect fluid balance.*
- Administer intravenous fluids as prescribed using an electronic infusion pump. Monitor for indicators of fluid overload if rapid fluid replacement is ordered: dyspnoea, tachypnoea, tachycardia, increased CVP, jugular vein distension and oedema. *Rapid fluid replacement may lead to hypervolaemia, resulting in pulmonary oedema and cardiac failure, particularly in a person with compromised cardiac and renal function.*

CONSIDERATION FOR PRACTICE

Assess intake and output accurately, monitoring fluid balance. In acute situations, hourly intake and output may be indicated. Urine output of less than 30 mL/hour indicates inadequate tissue perfusion, inadequate renal perfusion and an increased risk of acute renal failure.

- Monitor serum electrolytes, osmolality and ABG values. *Rehydration and administration of potassium chloride will affect both acid–base and fluid and electrolyte balance. Careful monitoring is important to identify changes.*

Community-based care

When preparing the person with metabolic alkalosis for discharge, consider the cause of the alkalosis and any underlying factors. For example, provide teaching about the following:

- using appropriate antacids for heartburn and gastric distress
- using potassium supplements as ordered or eating high-potassium foods to avoid hypokalaemia if taking a potassium-wasting diuretic or if aldosterone production is impaired
- contact the primary attending doctor if uncontrolled or extended vomiting develops.

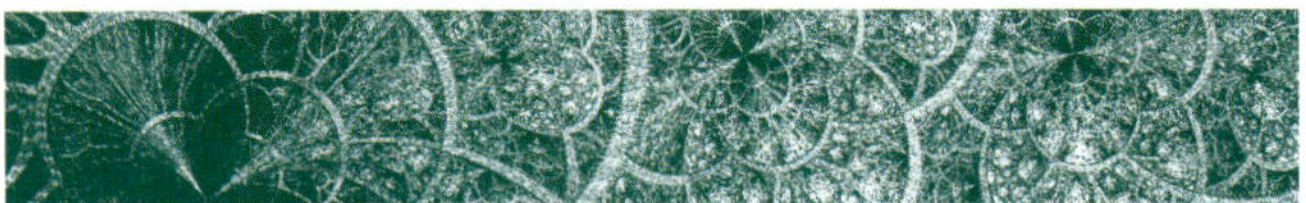

The person with respiratory acidosis

Respiratory acidosis is caused by an excess of dissolved carbon dioxide or carbonic acid. It is characterised by a pH less than 7.35 and a $PaCO_2$ greater than 45 mmHg. Respiratory acidosis may be either acute or chronic. In chronic respiratory acidosis, the bicarbonate is higher than 26 mEq/L as the kidneys compensate by retaining bicarbonate.

Risk factors

Acute or chronic lung disease (e.g. pneumonia or chronic obstructive pulmonary disease (COPD)) is the primary risk factor for respiratory acidosis. Other conditions that depress or interfere with ventilation, such as excess narcotic analgesics, airway obstruction or neuromuscular disease, also are risk factors for respiratory acidosis. Selected causes of respiratory acidosis are listed in Table 9.12.

Pathophysiology

Both acute and chronic respiratory acidosis results from carbon dioxide retention caused by alveolar hypoventilation. Hypoxaemia (low oxygen in the arterial blood) frequently accompanies respiratory acidosis.

ACUTE RESPIRATORY ACIDOSIS Acute respiratory acidosis occurs due to a sudden failure of ventilation. Chest trauma, aspiration of a foreign body, acute pneumonia and overdoses of narcotic or sedative medications can lead to this condition. Because acute respiratory acidosis occurs with the sudden onset of hypoventilation—for example, with cardiac arrest—the $PaCO_2$ rises rapidly and the pH falls markedly. A pH of 7 or lower can occur within minutes (Metheny, 2012). The serum bicarbonate level initially is unchanged because the compensatory response of the kidneys occurs over hours to days.

Hypercapnia (increased carbon dioxide levels) affects neurological function and the cardiovascular system. Carbon dioxide rapidly crosses the blood–brain barrier. Cerebral blood vessels dilate and, if the condition continues, intracranial pressure increases and *papilloedema* (swelling and inflammation of the optic nerve where it enters the retina) develops. Peripheral vasodilation also occurs and the pulse rate increases to maintain cardiac output.

CHRONIC RESPIRATORY ACIDOSIS Chronic respiratory acidosis is associated with chronic respiratory or neuromuscular conditions such as COPD, asthma, cystic fibrosis or multiple sclerosis. These conditions affect alveolar ventilation because of airway obstruction, structural changes in the lung or limited chest wall expansion. Most people with chronic respiratory acidosis have COPD with chronic bronchitis and emphysema. (See the chapter 'Nursing care of people with gas exchange disorders' for more information about COPD.)

In chronic respiratory acidosis, the $PaCO_2$ increases over time and remains elevated. The kidneys retain bicarbonate, increasing bicarbonate levels, and the pH often remains close to the normal range.

The acute effects of hypercapnia may not develop because carbon dioxide levels rise gradually, allowing compensatory changes to occur. When carbon dioxide levels are chronically elevated, the respiratory centre becomes less sensitive to the gas as a stimulant of the respiratory drive. The PaO_2 provides the primary stimulus for respirations. A person with chronic respiratory acidosis is at risk of developing *carbon dioxide narcosis*, with manifestations of acute respiratory acidosis, if the respiratory centre is suppressed by administering excess supplemental oxygen.

> **CONSIDERATION FOR PRACTICE**
>
> **Carefully monitor neurological and respiratory status in the person with chronic respiratory acidosis who is receiving oxygen therapy. Immediately report a decreasing LOC or depressed respirations.**

Manifestations

The manifestations of acute and chronic respiratory acidosis differ. In acute respiratory acidosis, the rapid rise in $PaCO_2$ levels causes manifestations of hypercapnia. Cerebral vasodilation causes manifestations such as headache, blurred vision, irritability and mental cloudiness. If the condition continues, the level of consciousness progressively decreases. Rapid and dramatic changes in ABGs can lead to unconsciousness and ventricular fibrillation, a potentially lethal cardiac arrhythmia. The skin of the person with acute respiratory acidosis may be warm and flushed and the pulse rate is elevated.

The manifestations of chronic respiratory acidosis include weakness and a dull headache. Sleep disturbances, daytime

MANIFESTATIONS **Respiratory acidosis**

ACUTE RESPIRATORY ACIDOSIS
- Headache
- Warm, flushed skin
- Blurred vision
- Irritability, altered mental status
- Decreasing level of consciousness
- Cardiac arrest

CHRONIC RESPIRATORY ACIDOSIS
- Weakness
- Dull headache
- Sleep disturbances with daytime sleepiness
- Impaired memory
- Personality changes

sleepiness, impaired memory and personality changes also may be manifestations of chronic respiratory acidosis (see the 'Manifestations' box).

INTERPROFESSIONAL CARE

A person with acute respiratory failure usually requires treatment in the emergency department or intensive care unit. The focus is on restoring adequate ventilation and gas exchange. Hypoxaemia often accompanies acute respiratory acidosis, so oxygen is administered as well. Supplemental oxygen is administered with caution to the person with chronic respiratory acidosis.

Diagnosis

The following laboratory and diagnostic tests may be ordered:

- *ABGs* show a pH of less than 7.35 and a $PaCO_2$ of more than 45 mmHg. In acute respiratory acidosis, the bicarbonate level is initially within normal range but increases to greater than 26 mEq/L if the condition persists. In chronic respiratory acidosis, both the $PaCO_2$ and the HCO_3^- may be significantly elevated.
- *Serum electrolytes* may show hypochloraemia (chloride level < 98 mEq/L) in chronic respiratory acidosis.
- *Pulmonary function tests* may be done to determine if chronic lung disease is the cause of the respiratory acidosis. However, these studies would not be done during the acute period.
- Additional diagnostic tests may be done to identify the underlying cause of the respiratory acidosis. *Chest x-ray* and *sputum studies* (cytology and culture) may be ordered to identify an acute or chronic lung disorder. If drug overdose is suspected, *serum levels* of the drug may be obtained.

Medications

Bronchodilator drugs may be administered to open the airways and antibiotics prescribed to treat respiratory infections. If excess narcotics or anaesthetic has caused acute respiratory acidosis, drugs to reverse their effects (such as naloxone) may be given.

Respiratory support

Treatment of respiratory acidosis, either acute or chronic, focuses on improving alveolar ventilation and gas exchange. The person with severe respiratory acidosis and hypoxaemia may require intubation and mechanical ventilation. (See the chapter 'Nursing care of people with gas exchange disorders' for more information about these procedures.) The $PaCO_2$ level is lowered slowly to avoid complications such as cardiac arrhythmias and decreased cerebral perfusion. In a person with chronic respiratory acidosis, oxygen is administered cautiously to avoid carbon dioxide narcosis.

Pulmonary hygiene measures, such as breathing treatments or percussion and drainage, may be instituted. Adequate hydration is important to promote removal of respiratory secretions.

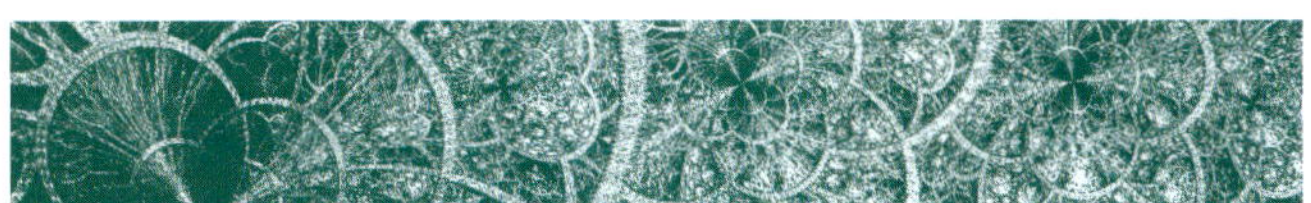

Nursing care

See 'Nursing care plan: a person with acute respiratory acidosis'.

Health promotion

Health promotion activities related to respiratory acidosis focus on identifying, monitoring and teaching the person at risk. Carefully monitor the person receiving anaesthesia, narcotic analgesics or sedatives for signs of respiratory depression. Monitor the response of a person with a history of chronic lung disease to oxygen therapy. Educate the person who has an identified risk of respiratory acidosis (such as people using narcotic analgesia for cancer pain and those with chronic lung disease) and their families about early manifestations of respiratory depression and acidosis, and instruct them to contact their attending doctor immediately if manifestations develop.

Assessment

Assessment data related to respiratory acidosis include the following:

- *Health history*: current manifestations, including headache, irritability or lethargy, difficulty thinking, blurred vision and other symptoms; duration of symptoms and any precipitating factors such as drug use or respiratory infection; chronic diseases such as cystic fibrosis or COPD; current medications.
- *Physical assessment*: mental status and level of consciousness; vital signs; skin colour and temperature; rate and depth of respirations, pulmonary excursion, lung sounds; examination of optic fundus for possible papilloedema.
- *Diagnostic tests*: ABGs, serum electrolytes; white blood cell count (indicator of infection), sputum culture results, serum drug and toxicology results.

NURSING CARE PLAN A person with acute respiratory acidosis

Marlene Hurd, age 76, is eating lunch with her friends when she suddenly begins to choke and is unable to breathe. After several minutes of trying, an attendant at the senior centre successfully dislodges some meat caught in Ms Hurd's throat using the Heimlich manoeuvre. Ms Hurd is taken by ambulance to the emergency department for follow-up because she was apnoeic for 3 to 4 minutes, her respirations are shallow and she is disoriented.

ASSESSMENT

Ms Hurd is placed in an observation room. Oxygen is started at 4 L/min per nasal cannula. David Love, the nurse admitting Ms Hurd, makes the following assessments: T 37.6°C, P 102, R 36 and shallow, BP 146/92. Skin is warm and dry. Alert but restless and not oriented to time or place; she responds slowly to questions. Stat ABGs are drawn, a chest x-ray is done and D_5 1/2 NS is started intravenously at 50 mL/h.

The chest x-ray shows no abnormality. ABG results are pH 7.38 (normal: 7.35 to 7.45), $PaCO_2$ 48 mmHg (normal: 35 to 45 mmHg), PaO_2 92 mmHg (normal: 80 to 100 mmHg) and HCO_3^- 24 mEq/L (normal: 22 to 26 mEq/L).

DIAGNOSES

- *Impaired gas exchange* related to temporary airway obstruction.
- *Anxiety* related to emergency hospital admission.
- *Risk of injury* related to confusion.

PLANNING

- Explain the need to monitor vital signs and the need for oxygen therapy to Ms Hurd and significant others.
- Explain the purpose for follow-up treatments of ABGs and continuous monitoring.
- Maintain a calm, quiet environment.
- Provide reorientation and explain all activities.
- Explain the importance of keeping the side rails in place and call bell within reach.

EXPECTED OUTCOMES

- Regain normal gas exchange and ABG values.
- Be oriented to time, place and person.
- Regain baseline mental status.
- Remain free of injury.

IMPLEMENTATION

- Monitor ABGs as per medical officer orders and collect ABG every 2 hours and report findings to the medical officer.
- Review ABG collection site pre and post collection of bloods.
- Monitor vital signs and respiratory status (including oxygen saturation) every 15 minutes for the first hour then every hour.
- Assess colour of skin, nail beds and oral mucous membranes every hour.
- Provide mouth hygiene hourly while O_2 is being administered.
- Assess mental status and orientation every hour.
- Monitor anxiety level as evidenced by restlessness and agitation.

EVALUATION

Ms Hurd remains in the emergency department for 6 hours. Her ABGs are still abnormal and David Love now notes the presence of respiratory crackles and wheezes. She is less anxious and responds appropriately when asked about her name, time and place. Because she has not regained normal gas exchange, Ms Hurd is admitted to the hospital for continued observation and treatment.

CRITICAL THINKING IN THE NURSING PROCESS

1. Describe the pathophysiological process that led to acute respiratory acidosis in Ms Hurd.
2. Describe the effect of acidosis on mental function.
3. What teaching would you provide to Ms Hurd to prevent future episodes of choking?

REFLECTION ON THE NURSING PROCESS

1. Identify and outline what you have learned from this case study and how you will apply it to your future nursing practice.
2. As the Registered Nurse, what communication and education strategies can you use to ensure Ms Hurd is able to prevent further episodes of choking?

Nursing diagnoses and interventions

Restoring effective alveolar ventilation and gas exchange is the priority of interprofessional and nursing care for the person with respiratory acidosis.

Impaired gas exchange

- Frequently assess respiratory status, including rate, depth, effort and oxygen saturation levels. *Decreasing respiratory rate and effort along with decreasing oxygen saturation levels may signal worsening respiratory failure and respiratory acidosis.*
- Promptly evaluate and report ABG results to the doctor and respiratory therapist. *Rapid changes in carbon dioxide or oxygen levels may necessitate modification of the treatment plan to prevent complications of overcorrection of respiratory acidosis.*
- Place in semi-Fowler's to Fowler's position as tolerated. *Elevating the head of the bed promotes lung expansion and gas exchange.*
- Administer oxygen as ordered. Carefully monitor response. Reduce the oxygen flow rate or percentage and immediately report increasing somnolence. *Supplemental oxygen can suppress the respiratory drive in the person with chronic respiratory acidosis.*

CONSIDERATION FOR PRACTICE

Frequently assess level of consciousness. A decline in LOC may indicate increasing hypercapnia and the need for increasing ventilatory support (such as intubation and mechanical ventilation).

Ineffective airway clearance

- Frequently auscultate breath sounds (whether on or off a mechanical ventilator). *Increasing adventitious sounds or decreasing breath sounds (faint or absent) may indicate worsening airway clearance due to obstruction or fatigue.*
- Encourage the person with chronic respiratory acidosis to use pursed-lip breathing. *Pursed-lip breathing helps maintain open airways throughout exhalation, promoting carbon dioxide elimination.*
- Frequently reposition and encourage ambulation as tolerated. *Repositioning, sitting at the bedside and ambulation promote airway clearance and lung expansion.*
- Encourage fluid intake of up to 3,000 mL per day as tolerated or allowed. *Fluids help liquefy secretions and hydrate respiratory mucous membranes, promoting airway clearance.*
- Administer medications such as inhaled bronchodilators as ordered. *Inhaled bronchodilators help to relieve bronchial spasm, dilating airways.*
- Provide percussion, vibration and postural drainage as ordered. *Pulmonary hygiene measures such as these help to loosen respiratory secretions so they can be coughed out of airways.*

Community-based care

Planning and educating for home care focuses on the problem that caused the person to develop respiratory acidosis. The person who developed acute respiratory acidosis as a result of acute pneumonia or chest trauma may only require education to prevent future problems. If acute respiratory acidosis occurred secondary to a narcotic overdose, determine if the drug was prescribed for pain or if it was an illicit street drug. Provide education to the person who requires narcotic medication on a continuing basis. Refer the person using illicit drugs to a substance abuse counsellor or treatment centre as appropriate.

For a person with chronic lung disease, discuss ways to avoid future episodes of acute respiratory failure. Encourage the person to be immunised against pneumococcal pneumonia and influenza. Discuss ways to avoid acute respiratory infections and measures to take when respiratory status is further compromised.

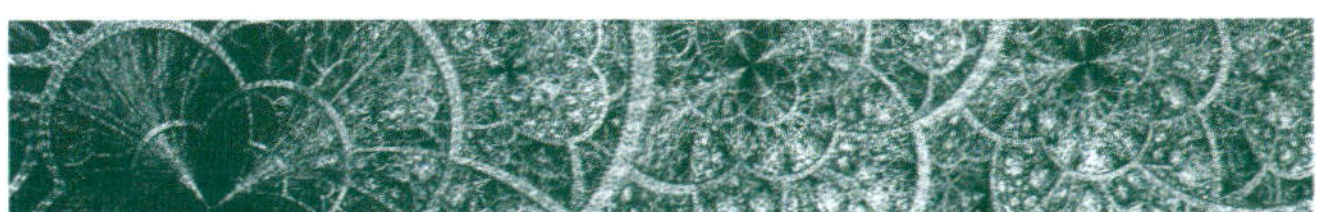

The person with respiratory alkalosis

Respiratory alkalosis is characterised by a pH greater than 7.45 and a $PaCO_2$ of less than 35 mmHg. It is always caused by hyperventilation leading to a carbon dioxide deficit.

Risk factors

Anxiety with hyperventilation is the most common cause of respiratory alkalosis; therefore, anxiety disorders increase the risk of this acid–base imbalance. In the person who is critically ill, mechanical ventilation is a risk factor for respiratory alkalosis.

Pathophysiology

In acute respiratory alkalosis, the pH rises rapidly as the $PaCO_2$ falls. Because the kidneys are unable to rapidly adapt to the change in pH, the bicarbonate level remains within normal limits. Anxiety-based hyperventilation is the most common cause of acute respiratory alkalosis. Other physiological causes of hyperventilation include high fever, hypoxia, Gram-negative bacteraemia and thyrotoxicosis. Early salicylate intoxication (aspirin overdose), encephalitis and high progesterone levels in pregnancy directly stimulate the respiratory centre, potentially leading to hyperventilation and respiratory alkalosis. Hyperventilation also can occur during anaesthesia or mechanical ventilation if the rate and tidal volume (depth) of ventilations are excessive.

If hyperventilation continues, the kidneys compensate by eliminating bicarbonate to restore the bicarbonate to carbonic acid ratio. The bicarbonate level is lower than normal in chronic respiratory alkalosis and the pH may be close to the normal range.

Alkalosis increases binding of extracellular calcium to albumin, reducing ionised calcium levels. As a result, neuromuscular excitability increases and manifestations similar to hypocalcaemia develop. Low carbon dioxide levels in the blood cause vasoconstriction of cerebral vessels, increasing the neurological manifestations of the disorder.

Manifestations

The manifestations of respiratory alkalosis include light-headedness, a feeling of panic and difficulty concentrating, circumoral and distal extremity paraesthesias, tremors and positive Chvostek's and Trousseau's signs. The person also may experience tinnitus, a sensation of chest tightness and palpitations (cardiac arrhythmias). Seizures and loss of consciousness may occur. (See the 'Manifestations' box.)

MANIFESTATIONS Respiratory alkalosis

- Dizziness
- Numbness and tingling around mouth, hands and feet
- Palpitations
- Dyspnoea
- Chest tightness
- Anxiety/panic
- Tremors
- Tetany
- Seizures, loss of consciousness

INTERPROFESSIONAL CARE

Management of respiratory alkalosis focuses on correcting the imbalance and treating the underlying cause.

Diagnosis

ABGs generally show a pH greater than 7.45 and a $PaCO_2$ of less than 35 mmHg. In chronic hyperventilation, there is a compensatory decrease in serum bicarbonate to less than 22 mEq/L and the pH may be near normal.

Medications

A sedative or anti-anxiety agent may be necessary to relieve anxiety and restore a normal breathing pattern. Additional drugs to correct any underlying problems other than anxiety-induced hyperventilation may be ordered.

Respiratory therapy

The usual treatment for anxiety-related respiratory alkalosis involves instructing the person to breathe more slowly and having the person breathe into a paper bag or rebreather mask. This allows rebreathing of exhaled carbon dioxide, increasing $PaCO_2$ levels and reducing the pH. If excessive ventilation by a mechanical ventilator is the cause of respiratory alkalosis, ventilator settings are adjusted to reduce the respiratory rate and tidal volume as indicated. When hypoxia is the underlying cause of hyperventilation, oxygen is administered.

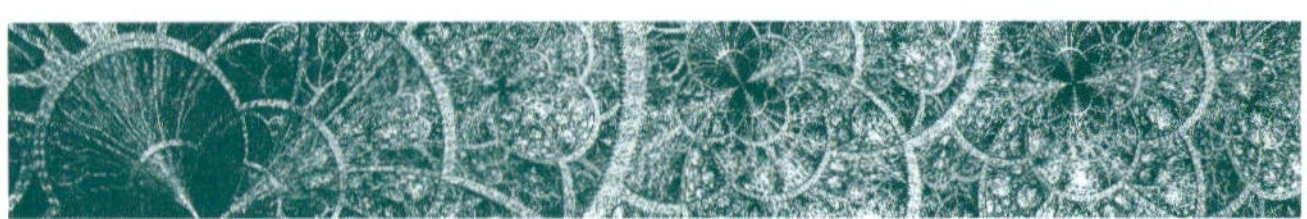

Nursing care

Health promotion

Identify the person at risk in the hospital (e.g. a person on mechanical ventilation or who has a fever or infection) and monitor assessment data and ABGs to identify early manifestations of hyperventilation and respiratory alkalosis.

Assessment, diagnoses and interventions

Ineffective breathing pattern

The usual cause of hyperventilation and respiratory alkalosis is psychological, although physiological disorders also can lead to hyperventilation. It is important not only to address the hyperventilation but also to identify the underlying cause.

- Assess respiratory rate, depth and ease. Monitor vital signs (including temperature) and skin colour. *Assessment data can help identify the underlying cause, such as a fever or hypoxia.*
- Obtain subjective assessment data such as the circumstances leading up to the current situation, current health and recent illnesses, or medication use and current manifestations. *Subjective data provide cues to the cause and circumstances of the hyperventilation response.*
- Reassure the person that they are not experiencing a heart attack and that symptoms will resolve when breathing returns to normal. *Manifestations of hyperventilation and respiratory alkalosis such as dyspnoea, chest tightness, or pain and palpitations can mimic those of a heart attack.*
- Instruct the person to maintain eye contact and breathe with you to slow the respiratory rate. *These measures help to make the person aware of respirations and provide a sense of support and control (Flynn Makic & Martinez-Kratz, 2022).*
- Have the person breathe into a paper bag. *This allows the person to rebreathe exhaled carbon dioxide, increasing the $PaCO_2$ and decreasing the pH.*
- Protect the person from injury. *If hyperventilation continues to the point at which the person loses consciousness, respirations will return to normal, as will acid–base balance.*
- If the person has experienced repeated episodes of hyperventilation or has a chronic anxiety disorder, refer for counselling. *Counselling can help the person develop alternative strategies for dealing with anxiety.*

Community-based care

Planning and teaching for home care are directed towards the underlying cause of hyperventilation. If anxiety precipitated the episode, discuss anxiety management strategies with the person. Refer the person and family to a counsellor if appropriate. Teach the person to identify a hyperventilation reaction and how to breathe into a paper bag to manage it at home.

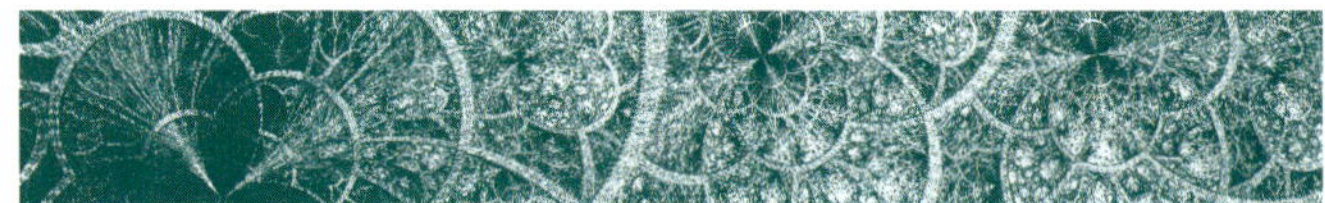

CHAPTER HIGHLIGHTS

- **The volume and composition of body fluid are normally maintained by a balance of fluid and electrolyte intake; elimination of water, electrolytes and acids by the kidneys; and hormonal influences. Change in any of these factors can lead to a fluid, electrolyte or acid–base imbalance that adversely impacts on health.**
- **Fluid, electrolyte and acid–base imbalances can affect all body systems, especially the cardiovascular system, the central nervous system and the transmission of nerve impulses. Conversely, primary disorders of the respiratory, renal, cardiovascular, endocrine or other body systems can lead to an imbalance of fluids, electrolytes or acid–base status.**
- **Fluid and sodium imbalances commonly are related; both affect serum osmolality.**
- **Potassium imbalances are commonly seen in the person with acute or chronic illnesses. Both hypokalaemia and hyperkalaemia affect cardiac conduction and function. Carefully monitor cardiac rhythm and status in the person with very low or very high potassium levels.**
- **Calcium imbalances primarily affect neuromuscular transmission: hypocalcaemia increases neuromuscular irritability; hypercalcaemia depresses neuromuscular transmission. Magnesium imbalances have a similar effect.**
- **Acid–base imbalances may be caused by either metabolic or respiratory problems. Simple acid–base imbalances (respiratory or metabolic acidosis or alkalosis) are more commonly seen than mixed imbalances.**

- Buffers, lungs and kidneys work together to maintain acid-base balance in the body. Buffers respond to changes almost immediately; the lungs respond within minutes; the kidneys, however, require hours to days to restore normal acid-base balance.
- The lungs compensate for metabolic acid-base imbalances by excreting or retaining carbon dioxide. This is accomplished by increasing or decreasing the rate and depth of respirations.
- The kidneys compensate for respiratory acid-base imbalances by producing and retaining or excreting bicarbonate and by retaining or excreting hydrogen ions.
- Careful monitoring of respiratory and cardiovascular status, mental status, neuromuscular function and laboratory values is an important nursing responsibility for the person with fluid, electrolyte or acid-base imbalances.

CONCEPT CHECK

1 A person is admitted to the emergency department with hypovolaemia. Which intravenous solution would the nurse anticipate administering?
1 Ringer's solution
2 10% dextrose in water
3 3% sodium chloride
4 0.45% sodium chloride

2 When assessing a person with FVD, the nurse would expect to find:
1 increased pulse rate and blood pressure
2 dyspnoea and respiratory crackles
3 headache and muscle cramps
4 orthostatic hypotension and flat neck veins

3 The nurse caring for a person with acute hypernatraemia includes which of the following in the plan of care? (Select all that apply.)
1 Conduct frequent neurological checks.
2 Restrict fluids to 1,500 mL per day.
3 Orient to time, place and person frequently.
4 Maintain intravenous access.
5 Limit length of visits.

4 Laboratory results for a person show a serum potassium level of 2.2 mEq/L. Which of the following nursing actions is of highest priority for this person?
1 Keep the person on bed rest.
2 Initiate cardiac monitoring.
3 Start oxygen at 2 L/min.
4 Initiate seizure precautions.

5 The nurse evaluates teaching about calcium supplement therapy as effective when the person states that she will take her calcium tablets:
1 all at one time in the morning
2 with meals
3 as needed for tremulousness
4 with a full glass of water

6 A person who is known to be an alcoholic presents with confusion, hallucinations and a positive Chvostek's sign. Which medication(s) should the nurse anticipate administering?
1 magnesium sulfate
2 calcium chloride
3 insulin and glucose
4 sodium bicarbonate

7 Arterial blood gas results for a person show pH 7.21, PaO_2 98 mmHg, $PaCO_2$ 32 mmHg and HCO_3^- 17 mEq/L. The nurse correctly interprets these values as indicative of which of the following acid-base imbalances?
1 metabolic acidosis
2 metabolic alkalosis
3 respiratory acidosis
4 respiratory alkalosis

8 A person is admitted with a suspected heroin overdose and a respiratory rate of 5 to 6 breaths per minute. Which of the following assessment data would the nurse anticipate? (Select all that apply.)
1 pH 7.29
2 alert and oriented
3 $PaCO_2$ 54 mmHg
4 HCO_3^- 32 mEq/L
5 skin warm and flushed

9 The nurse caring for a person undergoing several days of gastric decompression recognises that the person is at risk of which of the following acid-base imbalances?
1 metabolic acidosis
2 metabolic alkalosis
3 respiratory acidosis
4 respiratory alkalosis

10 A person undergoing mechanical ventilation following a severe chest wall injury and flail chest complains of chest tightness, anxiety and feeling as though she cannot get enough air. She is afraid she is having a heart attack. The nurse should first:
1 administer prescribed analgesic
2 contact respiratory therapy to evaluate ventilator settings
3 obtain arterial blood gases
4 notify the doctor

BIBLIOGRAPHY

Australian Commission on Safety and Quality in Health Care (ACSQHC) (2021). *National Safety and Quality Health Service Standards* (2nd ed.). Sydney: ACSQHC.

Burns, S. M. & Delgado, S. A. (2018). *AACN essentials of critical care nursing* (4th ed.). New York: McGraw Hill Medical.

Chakhtoura, M., Nakhouls, N., Akl, E. A., Mantzoros, C. S. & El Hajj Fuleihan, G. A. (2016). Guidelines on vitamin D replacement in bariatric surgery: Identification and systematic appraisal. *Metabolism: Clinical and Experimental*, *65*(4), 586–597. https://doi.org/10.1016/j.metabol.2015.12.013

Dewey, M. & Heuberger, R. (2011). Vitamin D and calcium status and appropriate recommendations in bariatric surgery patients. *Gastroenterology Nursing*, *34*(5), 367–374.

Flynn Makic, M. B. & Martinez-Kratz, M. R. (eds) (2022). *Ackley and Ladwig's nursing diagnosis handbook: An evidence based guide to planning care* (13th ed.). St Louis, MO: Elsevier.

Food Standards Australia New Zealand (2015). *Sodium and salt*. Retrieved from https://www.foodstandards.gov.au

Gaspar, P. (2011). Comparison of four standards for determining adequate water intake of nursing home residents. *Research and Theory for Nursing Practice*, *25*(1), 11–22.

Giddens, J. F. (2021). *Concepts of nursing practice* (3rd ed.). St Louis, MO: Elsevier.

Levett-Jones, T., Dwyer, T., Reid-Searl, K., Heaton, L., Flenady, T., Applegarth, J., Guinea, S. & Andersen, P. (2017). *Patient Safety Competency Framework (PSCF) for Nursing Students*. Sydney. Retrieved from http://psframework.wpengine.com/

Loscalzo, J., Fauci, A. S., Kasper, D. L., Hauser, S. L. & Longo, D. (2022). *Harrison's principles of internal medicine* (21st ed.). New York: McGraw Hill Medical.

Lukitsch, I. (2021). *Hypernatremia medication*. Retrieved from http://emedicine.medscape.com/

Marieb, E. & Hoehn, K. (2018). *Human anatomy and physiology* (11th ed.). Upper Saddle River, NJ: Pearson Education Limited.

Martini, F., Nath, J. & Bartholomew, E. (2018). *Fundamentals of anatomy and physiology* (11th ed.). Upper Saddle River, NJ: Pearson Education Limited.

McCance, K. L. & Huether, S. E. (2018). *Pathophysiology: The biologic basis for disease in adults and children* (8th ed.). St Louis, MO: Elsevier.

Mestrom, E. H. J. van der stam, J. A., te Pas, E. E. et al. (2021). Increased sodium intake and decreased sodium excretion in ICU-acquired hypernatremia: A prospective cohort study. *Journal of Critical Care*, *63*, 68–75. https://doi.org/10.1016/j.jcrc.2021.02.002

Metheny, N. M. (2012). *Fluid and electrolyte balance: Nursing considerations* (5th ed.). Sudbury: Jones & Bartlett Learning.

National Health and Medical Research Council (NHMRC). (2013). *Australian dietary guidelines*. Canberra: Australian Government.

Norris, T. L. (2018). *Porth's pathophysiology: Concepts of altered health states* (10th ed.). Philadelphia: Lippincott Williams & Wilkins.

Perrin, K. O. & MacLeod, C. E. (2017). *Understanding the essentials of critical care nursing* (3rd ed.). Upper Saddle River, NJ: Pearson Prentice Hall.

Stevenson, J., Tong, A., Campbell, K. L., Craig, J. C. & Lee, V. W. (2018). Perspectives of healthcare providers on the nutritional management of patients on haemodialysis in Australia: An interview study. *BMJ Open*, *8* doi: 10.1136/bmjopen-2017-020023

Tran, M. M. A., Tantsis, E. M. & Ging, J. (2017). In children requiring intravenous fluid for hydration maintenance, which out of hypotonic saline and isotonic saline is less likely to result in the development of hyponatremia? *Journal of Paediatrics and Child Health*, *53*(3), 309–313.

Urden, L. D., Stacy, K. M. & Lough, M. E. (2021). *Critical care nursing: Diagnosis and management* (9th ed.). St Louis, MO: Elsevier.

Woodward, M. (2013). *Guidelines to effective hydration in aged care facilities*. Heidelberg West, Vic.: Heidelberg Repatriation Hospital.

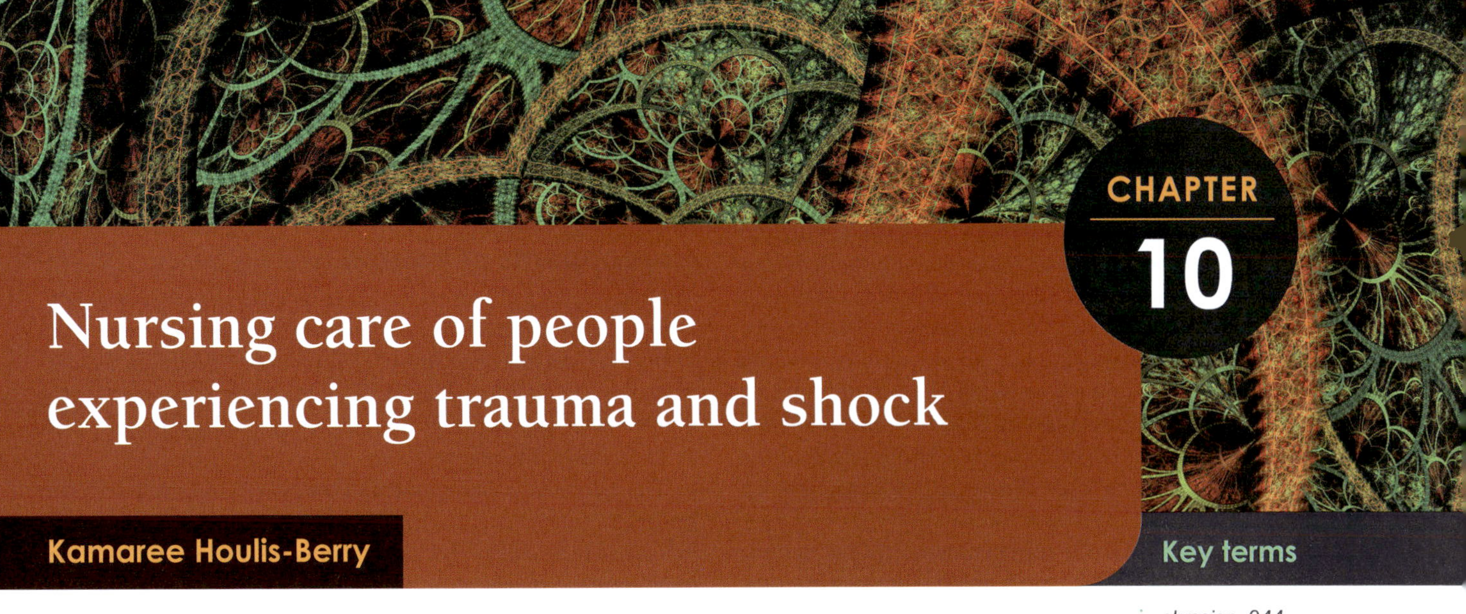

CHAPTER 10

Nursing care of people experiencing trauma and shock

Kamaree Houlis-Berry

Learning outcomes

- Describe the components and types of trauma including causes, effects to diagnose and management of life-threatening injuries.
- Discuss diagnostic tests, medications, blood transfusion and intravenous fluids used in assessing people experiencing trauma and shock.
- Explain organ donation and forensic implications of traumatic injury or death.
- Discuss the risk factors, aetiologies and pathophysiologies of hypovolaemic shock, cardiogenic shock, obstructive shock and distributive shock.
- Describe the role of the nurse in trauma prevention education and evaluate a plan of care to restore the functional health status of people experiencing trauma.

Clinical competencies

- Obtain initial data about the person experiencing trauma to include history taking, assessment, review of medical history and communication with pre-hospital and other healthcare providers and family members.
- Communicate and document significant data and changes in the condition of a person who has sustained trauma.
- Evaluate responses to medical and surgical interventions for people sustaining multiple trauma and shock.
- Formulate nursing diagnoses based on manifestations recognised during the nursing assessment.
- Develop a plan of care for the person experiencing trauma based on scientific knowledge and individual diversity.
- Describe the role of the nurse in trauma prevention education and evaluate a plan of care to restore the functional health status of people experiencing trauma.
- Advocate for people's rights as indicated by documents that address end-of-life issues.

Key terms

THE PERSON EXPERIENCING TRAUMA

Trauma is defined as injury to human tissues and organs resulting from the transfer of energy from the environment. In the past the term 'trauma' has been associated with the word 'accident'. *Accident* means that the injury occurred without intent, a result of random chance. We now know that a considerable number of injuries are preventable and not of random chance. Intentional and non-intentional trauma encompass a variety of injuries resulting from motor vehicle crashes, pedestrian injuries, gunshot wounds, falls, violence towards others or self-inflicted violence. The injuries, disabilities and deaths resulting from these acts constitute a major healthcare challenge.

Injury is a leading cause of morbidity, mortality and permanent disability in Australia, with the number of hospitalisations steadily increasing each year over the past decade, and now exceeding 544,000 people.

- The three major causes of hospitalised injuries are falls, contact with objects or transport accidents.
- Injuries account for 8.4% of the burden of disease (impact of living with illness and injury and dying prematurely), costing $8.9 billion in health expenditure.
- Males account for 55% of hospitalised injuries and 62% of injury deaths.
- Indigenous Australians are twice as likely as non-Indigenous Australians to be seriously injured, and twice as likely to die of an injury.
- Each year, 13,800 lives are lost as a result of injury (Australian Institute of Health and Welfare (AIHW), 2022).

Trauma usually occurs suddenly, leaving the person and family with little time to prepare for its consequences. Nurses provide a vital link in both the physical and psychosocial care for the injured person and family. In caring for the person who has experienced trauma, nurses must consider not only the initial physical injury but also its long-term consequences, including rehabilitation. Trauma may alter the person's previous way of life, potentially affecting independence, mobility, cognitive thinking and appearance.

Components of trauma

Trauma results from an abnormal exchange of energy between a host and a mechanism in a predisposing environment. The *host* is the person or group at risk of injury. Multiple factors influence the host's potential for injury: age, sex, race, economic status, pre-existing illnesses and use of substances such as street drugs and alcohol.

The *mechanism* is the source of the energy transmitted to the host. The energy exchanged can be mechanical, gravitational, thermal, electrical, physical or chemical. Table 10.1 lists the most common mechanisms for each type of energy. Mechanical energy is the most common type of energy transferred to a host in trauma. The most common mechanical source of injury in all adult age groups is the motor vehicle.

When describing a traumatic injury, *intention* is included as a component. Most gunshot and stab wounds are examples of intentional injuries. It is important to remember, however, that some gunshot wounds are unintentional, such as those that occur when children play with guns. Other common unintentional injuries result from motor vehicle crashes, falls, drowning and fires.

The final component of trauma is the *environment*. For example, a road that has become slippery after a storm is a physical environment that may contribute to an injury. Occupation is an important environmental factor to consider. Those in certain occupations face a high risk of trauma; examples include police officers, firefighters, professional athletes, race car drivers and taxi drivers. One's social environment also influences risk of injury; see the 'Meeting individualised needs' box for one example—domestic violence.

TABLE 10.1 Common mechanisms of injury by energy source

ENERGY SOURCE	COMMON MECHANISMS OF INJURY
Mechanical	Motor vehicles Firearms Machines
Gravitational	Falls
Thermal	Heating appliances Fire Freezing temperatures
Electrical	Wires, sockets and other electrical objects Lightning
Physical	Fists, feet and other body parts (as in physical assault) Sharp objects, such as knives Ultraviolet radiation Ionising radiation Water (drowning) Other submersion agents (e.g. grain) Explosions
Chemical	Drugs Poisons Industrial chemicals

MEETING INDIVIDUALISED NEEDS **Assessing older adult abuse and domestic violence**

INTIMATE PARTNER VIOLENCE (IPV)

Most incidents of domestic violence are not reported; therefore, it is believed that the available data greatly underestimate the true magnitude of the problem. From the findings of the *Family, Domestic and Sexual Violence in Australia* report (AIHW, 2021), it is noted that 1 in 6 women and 1 in 16 men, since the age of 15, have been subjected to physical and/or sexual violence by a current or previous cohabitating partner, with more than half (54%) of the women experiencing more than one violent incident. Family and domestic violence is a leading cause of homelessness for women with children and occurs at higher rates for Indigenous Australians. Intimate partner violence contributes to more burden of disease (illness impact, premature death and disability) than any other risk factor for Australian women aged 25–44. Domestic violence is a widespread problem that occurs regardless of age, sex, race, socioeconomic status or education.

VIOLENCE AND THE OLDER ADULT

Elder abuse is any act, in a relationship where there is an implication of trust that results in harm to an older person, over 65 years of age. This can range from physical or emotional assault to intimidation, neglect or financial exploitation. Wilful deprivation of food or medical care is also included (Australian Human Rights Commission, 2021; Kaspiew et al., 2019). Data indicates that between 2% and 5% of older Australians have experienced abuse, up to 80% of perpetrators are family members of the victims (the large majority being their children), financial and psychological abuse are the most common forms of abuse and women are twice as likely as men to be victims of abuse (Attorney General's Department, 2022; Australian Human Rights Commission, 2021; Kaspiew et al., 2019).

DIAGNOSIS OF ABUSE

The general approach to diagnosis in abuse situations is challenging as the abuse is often hidden. With spousal, older adult or child abuse, the task of identification is complex. The following are clues to identify violence-related injuries:

- injuries that do not correlate with the history
- injuries that suggest a defensive posture
- injuries during pregnancy
- pattern injuries
- pattern burns
- sexual abuse/rape
- unusual or unexplained fractures
- signs of confinement
- unusual interaction between the person and the caregiver
- lack of medical attention; immunisations not up to date; poor dental health
- unexplained dehydration or malnutrition.

Types of trauma

Minor trauma causes injury to a single part or system of the body and is usually treated in a general practitioner's clinic or in the hospital emergency department. A fracture of the clavicle, a small second-degree burn and a laceration requiring sutures are examples of minor trauma. **Major**, or **multiple**, **trauma** involves serious single-system injury (such as the traumatic amputation of a leg) or multiple-system injuries. Multiple trauma is most often the result of a motor vehicle crash.

Trauma is further classified as either blunt or penetrating. **Blunt trauma** occurs when there is no communication between the damaged tissues and the outside environment. It is caused by various forces including *deceleration* (a decrease in the speed of a moving object), *acceleration* (an increase in the speed of a moving object), *shearing* (forces occurring across a plane, with structures slipping across each other), *compression* and *crushing*. Blunt forces often cause multiple injuries that can affect the head, spinal cord, bones, thorax and abdomen. Blunt trauma is frequently caused by motor vehicle crashes, falls, assaults and sports activities.

Penetrating trauma occurs when a foreign object enters the body, causing damage to body structures. Structures commonly affected include the brain, lungs, heart, liver, spleen, the intestines and the vascular system. Examples of penetrating trauma are gunshot or stab wounds and impalement.

Other types of trauma include inhalation injuries from gases, smoke or steam; burn or freezing injuries; and blast injuries from explosions. Blast injuries result from the temperature and velocity of air movement and the force of projectiles from the explosion. Blast injuries are more severe in water than in air because blast waves travel further and faster in water. Trauma from blast injuries includes pulmonary oedema and haemorrhage, damage to abdominal organs, burns, penetrating injuries and ruptured tympanic membranes.

Outcome studies show a correlation between survival rates of multiple trauma victims and rapid response times by pre-hospital providers, coupled with appropriate decision making with regard to transporting the victim to a facility capable of treating their injuries (American College of Emergency Physicians, 2022; Australian College for Emergency Medicine, 2021). As a result, a system was devised to assist pre-hospital providers to make the appropriate decisions. People experiencing trauma are classified as class 1, 2 or 3 based on factors including mechanism of injury, vehicle speed, height of falls and location of penetrating injuries. Class 3 trauma is the least severe. An example would be a same-level fall without loss of consciousness or significant injury. Class 1 trauma involves life-threatening injuries likely to require medical specialists or immediate surgical intervention. While any hospital emergency department should be capable of caring for class 3 trauma people, people meeting class 1 or 2 criteria should be transported to a designated trauma centre when possible. Facilities designated as trauma centres have medical specialists and surgical coverage available or on call 24 hours a day.

Effects of traumatic injury

Death is a common result of serious traumatic injury, and falls into one of three categories related to the time span between injury and death: immediate, early or late. Immediate death happens within minutes at the scene from such injuries as a torn thoracic aorta or decapitation. Early death occurs within several hours of the injury from shock or delay in recognising injuries—causes may be major abdominal or thoracic injuries, or progression of intracranial haemorrhage. Late death generally occurs one or more days after the injury and results from multiple organ failure, sepsis and coagulopathies.

Because of the serious consequences of trauma, it is important to rapidly identify the person's injuries and institute appropriate interventions quickly. Following are common results of trauma and interventions necessary for good outcomes.

Airway obstruction

Maintenance of the airway and cervical spine are the highest priority in the trauma patient. Other distracting injuries may take the inexperienced practitioner away from the airway, but if the airway is not patent (open) and the person is unable to deliver oxygen to vital organs all other interventions are futile.

Assessment includes determining airway patency. If the person is unresponsive, manual opening of the airway using a jaw-thrust or chin-lift manoeuvre is necessary. The jaw thrust is the recommended manoeuvre for people having suspected cervical spine injury. Once the airway is opened, the practitioner must identify any potential obstruction from the tongue, loose teeth, foreign bodies, bleeding, secretions, vomitus or oedema. If the person is responsive and can vocalise, that is a good indication that the airway is clear.

Any time the nurse performs an intervention it is important to reassess the effectiveness of the intervention. For example, if the nurse suctions the airway to remove vomitus, they would reassess the airway after suctioning to determine if that intervention was successful or if the airway needs to be suctioned a second time.

All trauma victims should receive high-flow oxygen until stabilised. Assessment of breathing effectiveness is paramount. Assessment should include whether the person has spontaneous breathing, good rise and fall of the chest, determination of skin colour, general rate and depth of respirations, use of abdominal or accessory muscles, position of the trachea, observation of chest wall integrity and presence of jugular vein distension, bilateral breath sounds and any surface trauma. Consider pulse oximetry and cardiac monitoring as well.

In addition to suctioning, other available airway adjuncts include oral or nasal pharyngeal airways, oxygen delivery devices, laryngeal mask airways, Combitubes and endotracheal intubation (see Figure 10.1). Intubation is the preferred method of airway management if the person is unable to maintain oxygenation or an open airway.

People experiencing trauma may exhibit several aspects of airway management that are unique and require special preparation and precautions, as discussed next.

CLOSED HEAD INJURY Changes in haemodynamics, oxygenation and ventilation should be minimised in order to maintain adequate cerebral perfusion pressure. Anaesthetic agents should allow rapid control of the airway while minimising increase in intracranial pressure and supporting haemodynamic stability.

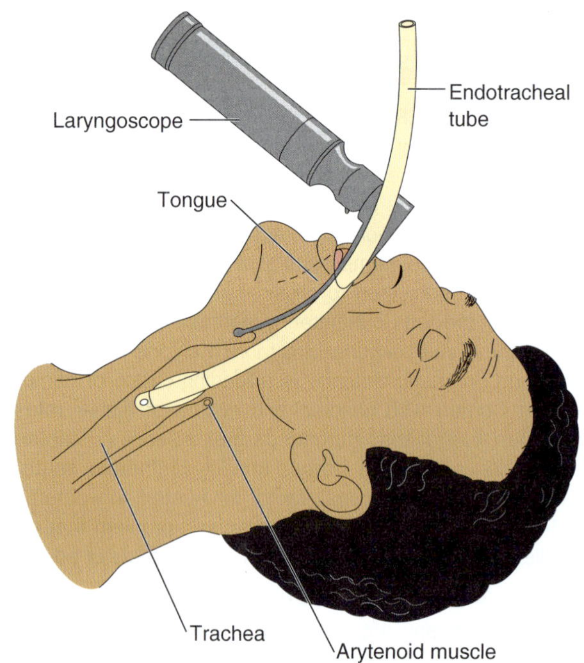

FIGURE 10.1 ***Placement of an oral endotracheal tube (ETT) for intubation. When the ETT is in place, air or oxygen can be blown into the external opening of the tube and enter the trachea***

The goal is to maintain a $PaCO_2$ of 35 to 40 mmHg. Lignocaine administered 3 to 5 minutes prior to intubation can blunt an increase in ICP that is secondary to laryngeal stimulation. In a normotensive person, beta-blockers may be given 2 to 3 minutes prior to intubation to attenuate the sympathetic response. Effective induction agents that may be used are etomidate, rocuronium or thiopental (Curtis et al., 2019; Kochanek et al., 2019).

MAXILLOFACIAL TRAUMA Significant distortion of normal anatomy occurs in facial trauma and respiratory compromise is not uncommon. Even in victims who present with mild respiratory compromise, rapid deterioration from oedema or haemorrhage can occur. A surgical airway may be the only alternative.

DIRECT AIRWAY TRAUMA Penetrating trauma to the neck is associated with a high degree of morbidity and mortality. Airway involvement includes dyspnoea, cyanosis, subcutaneous emphysema, hoarseness or air bubbling from the wound. Orotracheal intubation with rapid-sequence intubation is the technique of choice. The key is early identification of the need for intubation before the person has no airway at all. Tracheobronchial injury occurs in approximately 10% to 20% of people with penetrating neck injuries.

CERVICAL SPINE INJURY In the presence of a presumed cervical spine injury, precautions for securing an airway are consistently applied. Approximately 1.5% to 3% of major trauma victims have clinically significant cervical spine injuries (Rabinstein, 2019). Oral intubation with manual in-line axial head and neck stabilisation is a safe method.

The probability of cervical spine injury is decreased if the following criteria are met:

- absence of midline cervical spine tenderness
- normal alertness
- absence of intoxication
- absence of a painful distracting injury
- no focal neurological defects.

BURNS Burn victims with airway compromise require aggressive management. Upper airway oedema associated with inhalation or enclosed-space fires can progress during the post-burn phase. Securing an airway sooner rather than later is the goal. See the chapter 'Nursing care of people with burns' for nursing care of the person with burns.

Thoracic effects

TENSION PNEUMOTHORAX A **pneumothorax** results when air enters the potential space between the parietal and visceral pleura. The thorax is completely filled by the lungs, and surface tension between the pleural surfaces holds the lungs to the chest wall. Air present in the pleural space will eventually collapse the lungs. A **tension pneumothorax** is a life-threatening condition and requires immediate intervention. On inspiration, air enters the pleural space but cannot escape on expiration; this then increases intrapleural pressure. This pressure collapses the lung and causes a shift in the mediastinal contents, resulting in compression of the heart, great vessels, trachea and, eventually, the unaffected lung. In turn, this causes the following signs and symptoms:

- severe respiratory distress
- hypotension
- jugular vein distension
- tracheal deviation towards the uninjured side
- cyanosis.

The immediate short-term lifesaving intervention is a needle thoracotomy, in which a large-bore needle is inserted into the second intercostal space at the midclavicular line (see Figure 10.2).

FLAIL CHEST Flail chest is the fracture of two or more ribs in two or more separate locations, leading to an unstable thoracic wall segment. Paradoxical movement of the chest wall is seen, with the area sinking into the chest cavity with inspiration and protruding with expiration. The area must be supported quickly to re-establish effective respiration and subsequent ventilation.

THORACIC CONTUSION AND RUPTURE Bruising of thoracic tissue is referred to as contusion. Pulmonary contusion is the most common traumatic chest injury, mostly from motor vehicle accidents. As a shock wave force travels through the parenchyma, diffuse haemorrhage and alveolar oedema develop, impairing gas exchange. Diaphragmatic rupture is a rare traumatic injury but can result in herniation of abdominal contents into the thoracic cavity, causing respiratory compromise.

Myocardial contusion results in extravasation of red blood cells into the myocardial fibres. As myocardial cells are injured, it is believed that cardiac output diminishes due to reduction in contractile strength. Myocardial rupture is an acute traumatic tear of any structures of the heart, and although rare it is fatal.

Cardiac tamponade occurs when blood or fluid collects in the pericardial sac. Resulting in myocardial compression, this condition is potentially life threatening and should be addressed immediately with pericardiocentesis (see the chapter 'Nursing care of people with cardiac disorders').

Aortic rupture (transection) can result from acceleration–deceleration injury or blunt chest trauma. This injury is commonly fatal due to profuse bleeding.

Haemorrhage

When the person has suffered an injury that causes external haemorrhage, such as severing of an artery, the bleeding must be controlled immediately. This may be done by applying direct pressure over the wound and applying pressure over arterial pressure points (see Figure 10.3).

Internal haemorrhage may result from either blunt or penetrating traumatic injury. Discovering the cause and location of the injury, as well as the extent of related blood loss, are the

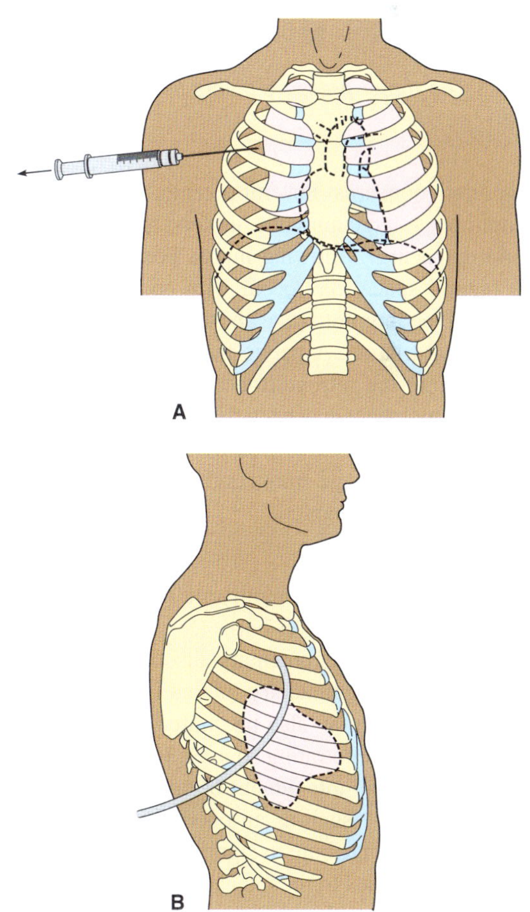

FIGURE 10.2 *A needle thoracotomy may be used in the emergency treatment of a tension pneumothorax. A, A large-gauge needle is introduced and air and fluid are aspirated. B, Alternatively, a chest tube may be inserted and connected to a chest drainage system*

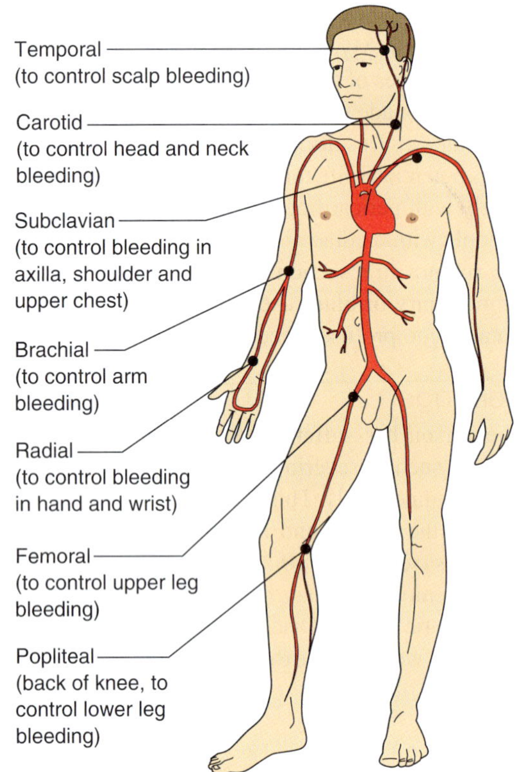

FIGURE 10.3 *The major pressure points used for the control of bleeding*

most important concerns. Several potential spaces in the body can accommodate large amounts of blood that may accumulate (called third spacing) following injury. For example, bleeding into the pleural space may occur with chest trauma (haemothorax) and bleeding into the abdominal cavity may occur with abdominal trauma. A pelvic fracture may cause massive haemorrhage into the retroperitoneal region. Once the source of internal haemorrhage has been recognised, interventions are initiated, including operative control of bleeding and continual assessment. Haemorrhage may result in hypovolaemic shock (discussed later in the chapter).

Integumentary effects

Injuries to the integument generally are not as serious as other injuries, with the exception of burns (see the chapter 'Nursing care of people with integumentary disorders'). The primary organ involved in integumentary trauma is the skin; however, underlying structures may also be injured. Injuries may result from either blunt or penetrating sources. It is important to evaluate all injuries to the integument because they may indicate a more serious injury such as an open fracture. Additionally, large wounds may contribute to significant blood loss.

Five specific injuries to the integument are contusions, abrasions, puncture wounds, lacerations and full-thickness avulsion injuries (see Figure 10.4). **Contusions**, or superficial tissue injuries, result from blunt trauma that causes the breakage of small blood vessels and bleeding into the surrounding tissue. **Abrasions** or partial-thickness denudations of an area of integument generally result from falls or scrapes. **Puncture wounds** occur when a sharp or blunt object penetrates the integument.

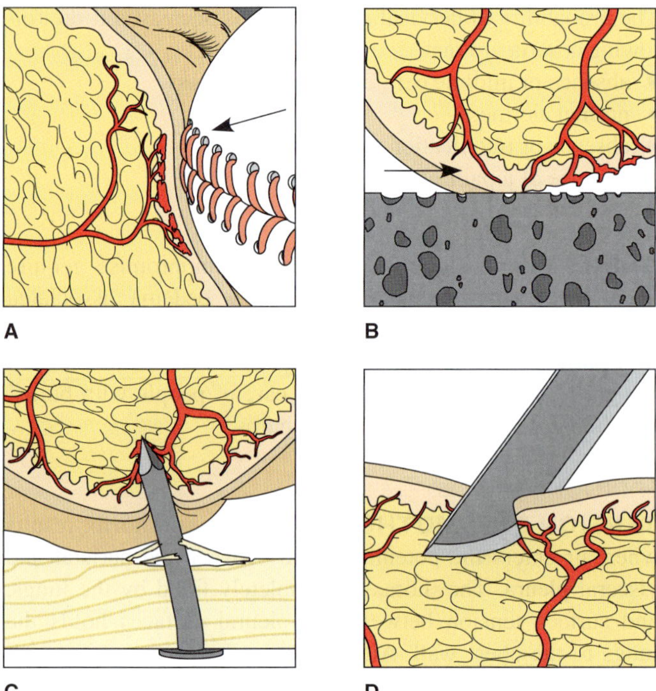

FIGURE 10.4 *Traumatic injuries to the skin include A, contusion; B, abrasion; C, puncture wound; D, laceration*

Lacerations are open wounds that result from sharp cutting or tearing. Injuries to the integument are at risk of contamination from dirt, debris or foreign objects. Infection may cause further physical stress to the person with multiple injuries. **Full-thickness avulsion injuries** are injuries that result in loss of all of the layers of the skin, causing fat and muscle to be exposed. The size of the wound impacts on both the length of time necessary for healing to take place and the risk of infection. These types of injuries are treated by allowing new skin to grow from the edges, suturing the wound together, reattaching avulsed skin or by skin grafting.

Abdominal effects

The abdomen contains both solid organs (liver, spleen and pancreas) and hollow organs (stomach and intestines). Direct trauma to the abdomen can lacerate and compress the solid organs and cause burst injuries to the hollow organs. Blood vessels may be torn and organs may be displaced from their blood supply, producing life-threatening haemorrhage. Damage to the mesenteric vessels supplying the bowel can result in bowel ischaemia and infarction. Injury to the stomach, pancreas and small bowel may allow digestive enzymes to leak into the abdominal cavity. Rupture of the large bowel results in escape of faeces, which causes peritonitis. Blunt or penetrating trauma to the abdomen may also cause rupture of the diaphragm with herniation of the abdominal organs into the thoracic cavity. The immediate threat following abdominal trauma is haemorrhage and the later threat is peritonitis.

Musculoskeletal effects

Musculoskeletal injuries may occur alone or with multiple injuries as the result of blunt or penetrating trauma. Musculoskeletal injuries usually are not considered a high priority in the care of the person with multiple injuries. Exceptions are the life or limb-threatening musculoskeletal injury, such as a dislocated hip, pulseless extremity or significant blood loss such as from a femur or pelvic fracture. Musculoskeletal injuries may provide clues to the presence of other serious injuries; for example, a fractured clavicle may indicate an associated thoracic injury. Care of the person who has suffered a musculoskeletal injury is discussed in the chapter 'Nursing care of people with musculoskeletal disorders'.

Neurological effects

Head injuries are a common type of injury sustained as the result of trauma. Injuries to the spinal cord resulting in loss of neurological function are devastating outcomes of trauma, but they are much less common than head injuries. Most head and spinal cord injuries result from blunt trauma and are sustained in motor vehicle crashes. Falls, sports injuries and assault are other sources of neurological injury. Care of the person with a neurological injury is discussed in the chapters 'Nursing care of people with intracranial disorders' and 'Nursing care of people with neurological disorders'.

Multiple organ dysfunction syndrome

Multiple organ dysfunction syndrome (MODS) is a common complication of severe injury and a frequent cause of death in intensive care units. MODS is a progressive impairment of two or more organ systems. This is the result of an uncontrolled inflammatory response to severe injury or illness.

People at risk of MODS are those with a disturbance in homeostasis resulting from one or a combination of the following conditions:

- infection
- injury
- inflammation
- ischaemia
- immune response
- intoxication of substances
- iatrogenic factors.

The primary organ systems involved in MODS are the respiratory, renal, hepatic, haematological, cardiovascular, gastrointestinal and neurological systems. Supportive therapy depends on the identification of correctable causes and this may be one or a combination of several therapies. Surgical intervention, antibiotic administration, corticosteroid administration and correction coagulopathies are some of the therapies used for this condition. The occurrence of MODS following traumatic injuries causes more than half of the late mortality following trauma.

Effects on the family

Trauma usually occurs suddenly and with little warning. It may result in death or cause injury serious enough to alter both the person's and the family's lives. The suddenness and seriousness of the event are precipitating factors in the development of a psychological crisis. During the past decade, some emergency departments have instituted care plans that allow families to be present during resuscitation. This policy is not without controversy, but it should be considered when appropriate in conjunction with institution work practices.

INTERPROFESSIONAL CARE

Interprofessional care of the trauma victim depends on a team approach. Providing trauma care with a team focus helps each team member know their role. Prompt delegation of tasks and responsibilities improves the person's chances of survival and decreases the morbidity that may result from traumatic injuries.

Pre-hospital care

The major functions of pre-hospital care include injury identification, critical interventions and rapid transport.

INJURY IDENTIFICATION Emergency care of the person experiencing trauma is based on rapid assessment to identify injuries and begin appropriate interventions. Injuries that indicate the need for trauma centre care include:

- penetrating injuries to the abdomen, pelvis, chest, neck or head
- spinal cord injuries with deficit
- crushing injuries to the abdomen, chest or head
- major burns
- injuries leading to airway compromise or obstruction.

Many methods help healthcare providers determine the seriousness of the person's injuries and the potential for survival. Scoring systems such as the Champion Revised Trauma Scoring System can be helpful (see Table 10.2). Furthermore, additional research suggests that routine measurements including oxygen saturation (SpO_2) and temperature have emerged as

TABLE 10.2 Champion Revised Trauma Scoring System

TEST	SCORE	CODED VALUE
Glasgow Coma Scale*	13 to 15	4
	9 to 12	3
	6 to 8	2
	4 to 5	1
	3	0
Systolic blood pressure (mmHg)	> 89	4
	76 to 89	3
	50 to 75	2
	1 to 49	1
	0	0
Respiratory rate (breaths/min)	10 to 29	4
	> 29	3
	6 to 9	2
	1 to 5	1
	0	0
	Total score:	______

The highest possible total score is 12. The lowest possible score is 0. The higher the total score, the greater the chance of survival.

*See the chapter 'A person-centred approach to assessing the nervous system' for instructions for using the Glasgow Coma Scale.

Source: Based on Centers for Disease Control and Prevention (2012). Guidelines for field triage of injured patients. *Morbidity and Mortality Weekly Report, 61*(RR-1). Retrieved from https://www.cdc.gov.

strong predictors (de Alencar Domingues et al., 2018; Filipescu et al., 2020; Jeong et al., 2017). A primary trauma assessment must be rapid and comprehensive. As a prompt, using an alphabetical mnemonic can be helpful:

- **A** is airway assessment (with cervical spine immobilisation) to determine if the airway is patent, maintainable or non-maintainable.
- **B** is breathing evaluation for spontaneous respirations or ventilator impedance—such as by rib fractures or a collapsed lung.
- **C** is circulatory assessment by palpating peripheral and central pulses; assessing capillary refill, skin colour and temperature; and identifying any external sources of bleeding.
- **D** is disability and refers to neurological status. Assessment includes level of consciousness and pupillary function assessment, response to verbal or painful stimuli, and assessment of blood glucose level.
- **E** is exposure/environment where a whole-body assessment for any obvious injuries is completed while ensuring that hypothermia does not occur (i.e. use of heated blankets, warmed intravenous fluids).

PATIENT SAFETY COMPETENCY FRAMEWORK

5 Clinical reasoning

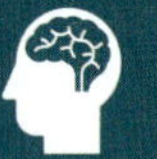

The Patient Safety Competency Framework indicates that nursing students must demonstrate clinical reasoning through the ability to accurately assess, interpret and respond to individual patient data in a systematic and timely way (Levett-Jones et al., 2017).

Secondary assessment usually begins while the primary assessment is underway. This assessment extends the alphabetical mnemonic.

- **F** is a full set of vital signs. It may also stand for having family members present during treatment.
- **G** is giving comfort measures, both physical and emotional, to the person and family.
- **H** is head-to-toe assessment and medical history that includes visual and manual assessment as well as auscultation.
- **I** is inspection of posterior surfaces for any injuries.

The Glasgow Coma Scale is another scoring system that is used to quantify the level of consciousness following traumatic brain injury (see the chapter 'A person-centred approach to assessing the nervous system').

CRITICAL INTERVENTIONS As life-threatening problems are identified during the primary assessment, appropriate on-the-scene interventions must be performed immediately. These include providing life support, immobilising the cervical spine, managing the airway and treating haemorrhage and shock.

Immobilisation of the person's cervical spine is a primary intervention. The person is placed on a spine board and a cervical collar and head immobiliser are applied (see Figure 10.5). The cervical spine may also be immobilised by log rolling the person onto a board, placing towel rolls or a head immobiliser along the sides of their head, and securing them to the board. If the person was wearing a helmet at the time of injury, the helmet should remain on until they arrive at the hospital, unless their airway is at risk. If necessary, healthcare personnel at the scene will remove the helmet by manipulating it over the person's nose and ears while holding their head and neck immobile; safe removal requires at least two people. Improper removal risks injury or additional injury to the spinal cord.

If the person's airway is patent, oxygen is administered. Ventilations may be assisted with a bag-valve-mask resuscitator

Links to National Patient Safety Standards

NSQHS: Recognising and Responding to Acute Deterioration Standard

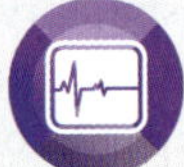

The intention of this standard is to ensure that a person's acute deterioration is recognised promptly and appropriate action is taken (Australian Commission on Safety and Quality in Health Care (ACSQHC), 2021). This includes the person's physical, mental and cognitive condition.

Implementing this standard is achieved by the establishment and maintenance of sytems for recognising and responding to clinical deterioration early. These systems include processes that recognise clinical deterioration and escalating care to ensure appropriate action is taken in people whose condition is deteriorating.

Effective communication should exist across all individuals involved in a person's care (including the person themself and their significant others).

Caring for individuals experiencing trauma and shock requires the need to observe, recognise and monitor physiological changes that could signal a person's deterioration.

Efficient and appropriate systems are imperative to ensure the safety of not only the person receiving appropriate care, but also any other individual involved in their care.

Source: ACSQHC (2021). *National Safety and Quality Health Service Standards* (2nd ed.). Sydney: ACSQHC.

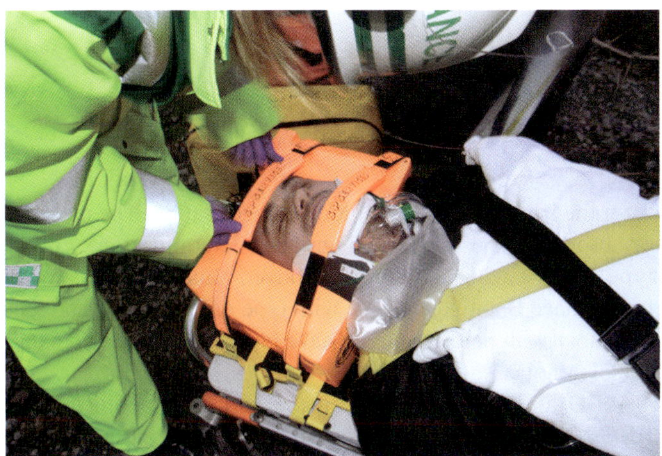

FIGURE 10.5 ***Immobilisation of the cervical spine at the scene of the accident is essential to prevent further injury to the spinal cord. The combined use of a hard cervical collar, head blocks and tape best restricts flexion, extension, rotation and lateral bending of the neck***

Source: Michael Donne/Science Photo Library/Alamy Stock Photo.

until airway management is achieved. Active external bleeding is controlled by direct pressure. Measures to reverse shock (discussed later in the chapter) are initiated.

RAPID TRANSPORT People who have multiple injuries must be transported as soon as possible to a regional trauma centre. The most common modes of rapid transport are ground ambulance and air ambulance, which includes helicopters specially staffed and equipped to care for trauma victims. Figure 10.6 shows a flight nurse assessing a person. Stable people within access of a ground ambulance are best transported by ground. Unstable people and those injured in the wilderness or other areas in which ground access is difficult may best be transported by air. When these transport systems are unavailable, the person is transported by any possible means.

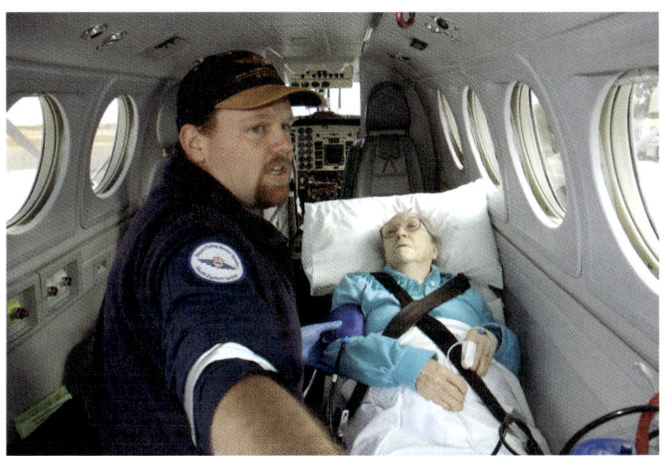

FIGURE 10.6 ***Flight nurses provide initial assessment, stabilisation and support for people with trauma***

Source: Royal Flying Doctor Service.

Emergency department care

ON ARRIVAL Multidisciplinary care and teamwork are required to ensure assessment and resuscitation strategies are implemented in a timely manner. Initial assessment and evaluation follow the process of primary survey, resuscitation, secondary survey, diagnosis, then definitive treatment or transfer to an appropriate healthcare facility that can provide this treatment.

DIAGNOSIS The diagnostic tests ordered once the person reaches the hospital depend on the type of injury they have sustained. Tests that may be ordered for victims of trauma include the following:

- *Blood type and crossmatch* involves typing the person's blood for ABO antigens and Rhesus (Rh) factor, screening the blood for antibodies and crossmatching the person's serum and donor red blood cells.
- *Arterial blood gases* evaluates oxygenation, acid–base balance and the presence of metabolic or respiratory compensatory mechanisms.
- *Full blood examination, electrolytes and coagulation* may be ordered after stabilisation and resuscitation.
- *Blood glucose level* to identify correctable cause of decreased level of consciousness; also early hypoglycaemia has been linked to increase risk of infection and mortality post trauma.
- *Blood alcohol level* measures the amount of alcohol in a person's blood. Studies have found that between 20% and 50% of people who are injured may be intoxicated. Alcohol alters the person's level of consciousness and response to pain.
- *Urinalysis*—perform dipstick to exclude occult haematuria. *Urine drug screen* may also be ordered. Like alcohol, drugs such as cocaine alter the person's level of consciousness and overall response to the primary survey.
- *Radiography*—anterior posterior chest x-ray to aid in diagnosis and confirmation of endotracheal or invasive central line placement; pelvic film for identification of pelvic fractures.
- *Focused abdominal sonography in trauma (FAST)* exam is a portable ultrasound examination used to identify the presence of free fluid in body cavities where it is not supposed to be. Primary focus is on the peritoneum, but the technician can also look at the pleura and pericardium.
- *Diagnostic peritoneal lavage* determines the presence of blood in the peritoneal cavity, which may indicate abdominal injury. This test is generally done in the emergency department. A local anaesthetic (such as lignocaine) is injected subcutaneously and a small incision is made in the lower abdomen. A catheter is placed into the peritoneal cavity and any free blood is aspirated. If free blood is found, the person is taken to the operating room for exploratory surgery. If no free blood is aspirated, 1 L of a warm isotonic crystalloid solution (such as normal saline) is rapidly infused into the peritoneal cavity and then allowed to drain by gravity. If the solution returns pink and is found to have the presence of red blood cells, white blood cells, bile, food or

faeces, the test is considered positive and the person is taken to the operating room for exploratory surgery. This procedure has been used less since the inception of the FAST exam.

- *Pregnancy test* for any woman of childbearing age rules out the potential for pregnancy and fetal injury.
- *Computed tomography (CT) scans* can discover injuries to the brain, skull, spine, spinal cord, chest and abdomen.
- *Magnetic resonance imaging (MRI) scans* can discover injuries to the brain and spinal cord.

MEDICATIONS Medications used to treat the person who has experienced trauma depend on the type and severity of the injuries, as well as the degree of traumatic shock that is present. The following general categories of medications may be used. (Fluid administration and the drugs listed are covered later in the chapter in discussion of the collaborative care of the person in shock.)

- Blood components and crystalloids are administered intravenously in the initial treatment of traumatic shock to replace intravascular volume.
- Inotropic drugs (drugs that increase myocardial contractility) are given to increase cardiac output and improve tissue perfusion. These drugs, administered only after fluid volume restoration, include dopamine hydrochloride, dobutamine hydrochloride and isoprenaline hydrochloride (Isuprel).
- Vasopressors may be administered in conjunction with fluid replacement to treat neurogenic, septic or anaphylactic shock. Examples of vasopressors include dopamine, adrenaline and noradrenaline.
- Opioids administered by bolus or continuous infusion are used to treat pain as soon as possible. However, the effects of the pain medications may alter the person's responses and mask potential injuries. If pain medications are administered, they must be carefully regulated and the person must be closely monitored.
- Immunisation: if the person has penetrating and open wounds, tetanus immunisation status must be determined. If they are unable to remember when the last tetanus immunisation was given or are unable to answer, tetanus prophylaxis is given.

BLOOD TRANSFUSIONS Blood and blood components are initially produced in the body and then donated for use by another person through a **transfusion** (an infusion of blood or blood components). A person may be given whole blood, packed red blood cells (RBCs), platelets, plasma, albumin, clotting factors, prothrombin or cryoprecipitate (see Table 10.3). Blood and blood components increase the amount of haemoglobin available to carry oxygen to the cells, improve haemoglobin and haematocrit levels during active bleeding, increase intravascular volume and replace deficient substances such as platelets and clotting factors.

Each person has one of four blood types: A, B, AB or O. The blood group antigens A and B, present on RBC membranes, form the basis for the ABO blood categorisation. The presence or absence of these inherited antigens determines one's blood type. People with blood type A have A antigens, those with type B have B antigens, those with type AB have both antigens and those with neither antigen have blood type O (called a universal donor).

> **FAST FACTS**
>
> - Type AB blood is the 'universal recipient'.
> - Type O blood is the 'universal donor'.

ABO antibodies develop in the serum of people whose RBCs lack the corresponding antigen; these antibodies are called anti-A and anti-B. The person with blood type B has A antibodies, the person with type A has B antibodies, the person with type O has both types of antibodies and the person with blood type AB has no antibodies (called a universal recipient).

A third antigen on the RBC membrane is D. People who are Rh positive (RH^+) have the D antigen, whereas people who are Rh negative (RH^-) do not. These antigens and antibodies may cause ABO and Rh incompatibilities.

A transfusion of incompatible blood causes haemolysis (breakdown) of the RBCs and agglutination of erythrocytes. (*Agglutination* is the clumping of cells which results from their interaction with specific antibodies.) The ABO blood group names and compatibilities are listed in Table 10.4.

Before RBCs or whole blood can be administered, a series of procedures determine donor and recipient ABO types and Rh groups. These procedures—called a *type and crossmatch*—are performed by mixing the donor cells with the recipient's serum and watching for agglutination. If none occurs, the blood is considered compatible.

Despite meticulous procedures for matching blood types and antigens, blood transfusion reactions may still occur. The most common is a *febrile reaction*. Antibodies within the person receiving the blood are directed against the donor's white blood cells, causing fever and chills. Febrile reactions typically begin during the first 15 minutes of the transfusion. The use of leucocyte-reduced blood will avoid future febrile reactions.

Hypersensitivity reactions result when antibodies in the person's blood react against proteins, such as immunoglobulin A, in the donor blood. Hypersensitivity reactions may appear during or after the transfusion. The manifestations of hypersensitivity reaction include *urticaria* (the appearance of reddened wheals of various sizes on the skin) and itching.

Haemolytic reactions, the most dangerous transfusion reactions, usually result from an ABO incompatibility. Clumping RBCs block capillaries, decreasing blood flow to vital organs. In addition, macrophages engulf the clumped RBCs, releasing free haemoglobin into the circulating blood; the haemoglobin is then filtered by the kidneys and may block the renal tubules causing renal failure. Haemolytic reactions usually begin after infusion of 100 to 200 mL of the incompatible blood.

TABLE 10.3 Volume resuscitation therapies

COMPONENT	INDICATIONS	ADVANTAGES	DISADVANTAGES
Compound sodium lactate (or Hartmann's solution)	Restoration of circulating volume Replacement of electrolyte deficits	Good availability Safe to use Low cost Aids in buffering acidosis	Rapid movement from the intravascular to the extravascular space, leading to three or more times requirement for replacement
Normal saline	Restoration of circulating volume Vehicle compatible with administration of blood	Good availability Low cost Safe to use	Hyperchloraemic acidosis associated with prolonged use of sodium solutions
Whole blood	Replaces blood volume and oxygen-carrying capacity in haemorrhage and shock	Contains RBCs, plasma proteins, clotting factors and plasma	Contains few platelets or granulocytes; deficient in clotting factors V and VII Greatest risks are for incompatibility or circulatory overload Risk of transmitting blood-borne pathogens
Packed RBCs	Restoration of intravascular volume Replacement of oxygen-carrying capacity	One unit of RBCs should increase the haemoglobin of a 70 kg adult by approximately 1 g/L in the absence of volume overload or continuing blood loss	Red cells require compatibility testing Risk of transmitting blood-borne pathogens Should be warmed to prevent hypothermia Contains little or no clotting factors
Platelets	Significant thrombocytopenia (platelet count less than 50×10^9/L) Continued haemorrhage	Compatibility testing is not required Typical platelet transfusion should raise the platelets of a 70 kg adult approximately $20 - 40 \times 10^9$/L	Post-exposure prophylaxis with anti-Rh immune globulin should be considered following Rh^+ platelet transfusion to an Rh^- woman Risk of transmitting blood-borne pathogens
Albumin	Expends blood volume in shock and trauma	Good availability	Is not a substitute for whole blood Hypersensitivity reactions can occur Risk of transmitting blood-borne pathogens
Fresh frozen plasma (FFP)	Documented coagulopathy Restoration of clotting factors Supplies plasma proteins	Crossmatching and Rh compatibility not required	Thawed by transfusion service provider–takes approx. 30 mins Should be ABO compatible Risk of transmitting blood-borne pathogens
Cryoprecipitate	Coagulopathy with low fibrinogen Restoration of fibrinogen	Rh type not important	Risk of transmitting blood-borne pathogens Contains haemagglutinins Should be ABO compatible, as intravascular haemolysis can occur if a large volume of ABO-incompatible cryoprecipitate is administered

Manifestations of a haemolytic reaction include flushing of the face, a burning sensation along the vein, headache, urticaria, chills, fever, lumbar pain, abdominal pain, chest pain, nausea and vomiting, tachycardia, hypotension and dyspnoea. If any of these manifestations appear, the blood transfusion must be immediately discontinued.

Other risks to people receiving blood include circulatory overload, electrolyte imbalances and infectious diseases such as hepatitis or cytomegalovirus.

People who have experienced trauma of any severity have had substantial blood loss and are usually in hypovolaemic shock. Blood replacement is the treatment of choice to restore oxygen-carrying capacity. People in severe shock with active bleeding are given universal type O red blood cells immediately. Those with less severe injuries or bleeding may be stabilised with other types of fluids until type-specific or crossmatched blood is available.

Some emergency departments and trauma centres use autotransfusion to provide blood for transfusions for the person with multiple injuries and/or severe shock. Autotransfusion is a method of blood administration in which special equipment collects and returns the person's own blood. The chest cavity is the typical source of blood to be autotransfused.

TABLE 10.4 Blood group types and compatibilities

BLOOD GROUP	RBC AGGLUTINOGENS	SERUM AGGLUTINOGENS	COMPATIBLE DONOR BLOOD GROUPS	INCOMPATIBLE DONOR BLOOD GROUPS
A	A	Anti-B	A, O	B, AB
B	B	Anti-A	B, O	A, AB
AB	A, B	None	A, B, AB, O	None
O	None	Anti-A, anti-B	O	A, B, AB

Note: Group O is often called the universal donor, and group AB is called the universal recipient.

Links to National Patient Safety Standards

NSQHS: Blood Management Standard

The intention of this standard is to ensure that a patient's own blood is safely and appropriately managed, and that any blood and blood products patients receive are safe and appropriate (ACSQHC, 2021).

Implementing this standard is achieved by the establishment of systems to optimise and conserve patient's blood and to ensure safe, appropriate prescription and administration of blood and blood products. These systems include processes facilitating accurate documentation, storage, transport, use and disposal. Effective communication regarding risks, benefits and use should exist across all individuals involved in a person's care (including the person themself and their significant others).

Caring for individuals experiencing haematological conditions will often result in the need to administer blood or blood products in order to manage the person's condition. As with any biological material, various risks are involved in all facets of this treatment. Efficient and appropriate systems are imperative to ensure the safety of not only the person receiving the product, but also any other individual involved in their care.

Source: ACSQHC (2021). *National Safety and Quality Health Service Standards* (2nd ed.). Sydney: ACSQHC. © Australian Commission on Safety and Quality in Health Care.

PATIENT SAFETY COMPETENCY FRAMEWORK

7 Preventing, minimising and responding to adverse events

The Patient Safety Competency Framework indicates that nursing students must prevent, minimise and respond to adverse events by anticipating and responding to human and systems factors that have the potential to jeopardise patient safety, and take appropriate actions to prevent reoccurrence of errors and near misses (Levett-Jones et al., 2017).

Nursing considerations for blood transfusion therapy are described in the 'Medication administration' box.

Emergency surgery

Immediate surgical intervention is indicated when the person remains in shock despite resuscitation and there is no obvious external sign of blood loss. Abdominal and chest x-ray, ultrasound studies, diagnostic peritoneal lavage or CT scan may be performed to help identify the potential source of the blood loss. It is important for the emergency or trauma nurse to speak with the family as soon as possible and keep them informed about what is happening to their family member. Unfortunately, the need for emergency surgery may not allow time for family members or significant others to see their loved one before transfer to the operating room.

Organ donation

The *Australian Organ and Tissue Donation and Transplantation Authority Act 2008* saw the establishment of the Australian Transplant Authority in January 2009. The focus of the Act was to implement the national reform package on organ and tissue donation by working with states and territories, clinicians, consumers and the community sector to build a world-leading organ and tissue donation and transplantation system for Australia. Under this Act, the Australian Organ Donor Registry (AODR) is the register of legal consent and is the only official national register for organ and tissue donation in Australia. The AODR ensures that consent (or objection) to donating organs and tissue for transplantation can be verified 24 hours a day, 7 days a week by authorised medical personnel, anywhere in Australia.

Consent for organ donation may be given not only by the donor but also by a spouse, adult children, parents, adult siblings, guardian or any adult authorised to do so. The Act also encourages people to carry donor cards. It is rare for a donation to proceed without the agreement of family or next-of-kin with their loved one's decision.

The increased success of organ transplant has made it a more common and valuable method of prolonging and improving life; however, many people are still waiting for organs and many people who may be suitable organ donors die each year from trauma. Organs and tissues that may be transplanted include bones, eyes, liver, lungs, skin, muscles and tendons, pancreas, intestines, kidneys, heart and heart valves.

The organ donation process begins with identification of the potential organ donor, which includes most people.

Certain factors are considered when determining if a person is an appropriate organ donor. They include:

- the circumstances of how, where and when a person dies
- any medical history
- age is considered, but it is more important to assess how the organs are working/functioning.

The family needs to be made aware of the person's prognosis and presented with the option of donating their organs. Both the family's and the person's feelings about organ donation must be explored. Even if the person carries an organ

MEDICATION ADMINISTRATION Blood transfusion

The risk of and seriousness of blood transfusion reactions require that extreme caution be taken when blood is administered. Most fatal transfusion reactions are the result of human error. Although general guidelines are provided here, each institution has specific policies and procedures that must be followed. Prior to beginning the transfusion, the nurse must determine that typed and crossmatched blood is available and collect the needed equipment: a blood administration set, a large-bore intravenous catheter (usually 18- or 19-gauge) and normal saline solution. Only normal saline is used with a blood transfusion as dextrose causes clumping of RBC and distilled water causes haemolysis.

NURSING RESPONSIBILITIES

- Obtain the person's consent.
- Assess for any previous reactions to blood.
- Explain the procedure to the person and answer any questions.
- Using aseptic non-touch technique, prepare the intravenous equipment. Prime the administration set with the saline.
- If venous access is not already in place, organise insertion of the intravenous needle (following body substance precautions) and begin administering the saline.
- Using institutional procedure, obtain the blood from the blood bank or laboratory. Administer the blood immediately; if this is not possible, return it to the blood bank or laboratory.
- Check and document that the donor and recipient blood have been tested and are compatible. This usually involves two nurses, each verifying that:
  a. An order for blood has been written.
  b. Type and crossmatch have been done.
  c. The name of the person and the name on the blood bag are identical.
  d. The number assigned to the unit of blood is identical to the one on the requisition for the blood.
  e. Blood type and Rh factor are compatible.
  f. The blood has not exceeded its expiration date.
  g. The unit of blood is intact and has no bubbles or discolouration.
- Identify the person by reading the armband identification and, if conscious, asking the person to tell you their name. Check the armband identification against the unit of blood labelling.
- Gently invert the blood bag several times to mix the plasma and RBCs.
- Take and record vital signs as a baseline.
- Attach the unit of blood to the administration set and begin the transfusion at a slow rate of about 2 mL per minute. (Some trauma victims may have blood infused at a rapid rate. If blood is infused rapidly, it may need to be warmed through an appropriate warming device during administration to prevent hypothermia.) Stay with the person for at least the first 15 minutes of the transfusion, monitoring for manifestations of a reaction and taking their vital signs.
- Continue to monitor the person during the transfusion, assessing for manifestations of hypersensitivity or haemolytic reactions, and taking and recording vital signs as directed by institutional policy.
- After the first 15 minutes the rate of infusion is increased. If there is no danger of fluid volume overload, most people can tolerate an infusion of a unit of blood (ranging from 250 to 500 mL depending on the blood component administered) in 2 hours. The unit of blood must be administered within 3 to 4 hours; after this time it has warmed and begins to deteriorate.
- Take the following actions if manifestations of a reaction occur:
  a. Stop the infusion of blood immediately and notify the physician. Continue to infuse the saline.
  b. Take vital signs and assess manifestations.
  c. Compare the blood slip with the unit of blood to ensure that an identification error was not made.
  d. Save the blood bag and any remaining blood for return to the laboratory for further tests to determine the cause of the reaction.
  e. Follow institutional policy for collecting urine and venous blood samples.
  f. Continue to monitor the person and provide prescribed interventions to treat hypersensitivity or haemolytic manifestations.

HEALTH EDUCATION FOR THE PERSON AND FAMILY

- In terms of viral safety, Australia has one of the safest blood supplies in the world. The possible risks of blood transfusions include transmission of infectious diseases and acquired immune deficiency syndrome (AIDS). However, with careful handling and storage of blood, bacterial contamination is rare. Although hepatitis may be transmitted by contaminated blood, new tests for hepatitis antibodies in donor blood are reducing this risk. Many people are afraid of contracting AIDS from blood even though donor screening and HIV-antibody testing of donor blood have virtually eliminated the transmission of HIV by blood transfusion.
- During the transfusion, immediately report any warm feelings, chills, itching, feelings of weakness or fainting, or difficulty breathing.
- Report any signs of a delayed transfusion reaction: chills, fever, cough, difficulty breathing, hives, itching or changes in circulation, and seek medical care immediately.
- Discuss any religious or cultural considerations related to blood transfusion.

donation card, many institutions will not remove any organs without a signature from a family member or other authorised person. The nurse must always respect the family's concerns and feelings during this process. Some members of certain cultural groups may have religious constraints or issues of mistrust that may interfere with the donation process. Donation coordinators facilitate the process and are responsible for contacting family and discussing options.

BOX 10.1 Brain death criteria

Clinical signs

- Irreversible condition
- No motor response in the cranial nerve distribution to noxious stimulation of the face, trunk and four limbs, AND no response in the trunk or limbs to noxious stimulation within the cranial nerve distribution
- Apnoea with a $PaCO_2$ greater than 60 mmHg
- No pupillary responses to light
- No gag, cough or corneal reflex
- No vestibulo-ocular reflexes on ice-cold caloric testing
- Absence of toxic, electrolyte, metabolic or endocrine disorders
- Hypothermia is not present and blood pressure is adequate

Confirmatory tests

- Cerebral blood flow study
- Electroencephalogram

Box 10.1 lists **brain death criteria**. Irreversible loss of all brain function is to be clinically confirmed. Along with the person being examined by two experienced medical practitioners, in some cases ancillary testing such as angiography or radionucleotide imaging will be used to provide additional evidence. Once brain death has been confirmed, the family must also understand the diagnosis and be allowed time to accept the person's death.

When caring for an adult person who is an organ donor, the nurse ensures the following are maintained:

- mean arterial blood pressure of greater that 60 mmHg to keep the person's organs perfused until removal
- urine output at greater than 0.5 mL/kg/hr. This is usually accomplished by administering fluids and/or inotropic agents such as dopamine
- oxygen saturation at 90% or greater.

Forensic considerations

Injuries often happen under circumstances that require legal investigation. Many injuries, particularly penetrating trauma, may involve criminal activity. Therefore, the nurse must recognise the need to identify, store and properly transfer potential evidence for medico-legal investigations.

Each item of clothing removed from the person must be placed in a breathable container, such as a paper bag, and documented appropriately. Bullets or knives should be labelled, with their source specified, and given to the proper authorities. Holes found in clothing should not be disturbed. When it is necessary to cut off clothing, these areas should be avoided and never cut through if at all possible.

The person's hands may yield important evidence, such as powder burns or residue on the skin, or tissue or hair samples beneath the fingernails. In the case of death, it is recommended that paper bags be placed over the person's hands if the presence of evidence is suspected; otherwise, the evidence should be collected from nail clippings.

Identify all wounds and document these findings with pictures, diagrams or written descriptions. Once the evidence has been collected, identified and properly stored, ensure that it is given to the appropriate authorities. A chain of custody needs to be maintained throughout the entire process. All evidence must be identified and labelled, and documentation procedures must chronicle where and in whose possession the evidence has been. For the chain of custody to remain intact, the evidence must remain in the continuous possession of identified people and be marked and sealed in tamper-proof containers.

PATIENT SAFETY COMPETENCY FRAMEWORK

2 Therapeutic communication

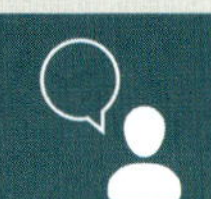

The Patient Safety Competency Framework indicates that nursing students must demonstrate therapeutic communication by using verbal and non-verbal communication skills to convey respect and empathy, and to encourage the person to express their feelings and needs, while at the same time maintaining professional boundaries (Levett-Jones et al., 2017).

Links to National Patient Safety Standards

NSQHS: Communicating for Safety Standard

The intention of this standard is to 'ensure timely, purpose-driven and effective communication and documentation that support continuous, coordinated and safe care for patients' (ACSQHC, 2021, p. 48).

Implementing this standard is achieved by the establishment and maintenance of systems and processes that support effective communication and documentation at high-risk times, including clinical governance and quality improvement, correct identification and procedure matching, communication at clinical handover and of critical information and documentation.

Source: ACSQHC (2021). *National Safety and Quality Health Service Standards* (2nd ed.). Sydney: ACSQHC. © Australian Commission on Safety and Quality in Health Care.

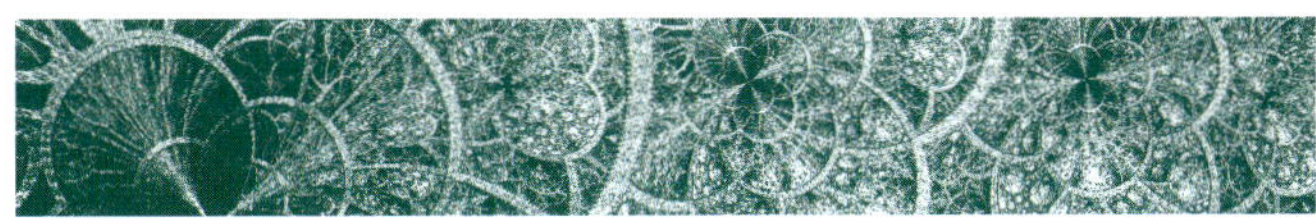

Nursing care

Nursing care of the person who has been injured begins with a primary assessment and the initiation of collaborative interventions for any life-threatening injuries. Nursing care is directed towards the person's specific responses to trauma.

Health promotion

Prevention efforts can reduce the incidence and severity of trauma. Areas of health promotion and trauma prevention interventions for individuals and communities include the following:

- *Motor vehicle safety*: seat belts, air bags, helmets, driving under the influence of alcohol or drugs, reckless driving, visual or cognitive deficits in the older adult, mobile phone use, driver fatigue.
- *Home safety*: electrical wiring, falls, burns, drowning, snow and ice removal.
- *Farm safety*: operating heavy equipment, safe storage of chemicals such as fertilisers.
- *Work safety*: operating work equipment, wearing safety equipment, removal of jewellery.
- *Relationships*: domestic violence, child abuse, older adult abuse or neglect.
- *Communities*: condition of streets, neighbourhood safety, gun control, gangs.

In providing information about trauma prevention to members of the community, the nurse serves as a healthcare educator, political activist and safety advocate.

Assessment

See 'Interprofessional care' for assessment of the person experiencing trauma.

Nursing diagnoses and interventions

The person experiencing trauma has many complex and interrelated actual or potential alterations in health. The nursing care in this section focuses on person and family problems with respirations, infection, immobility, spirituality and stress. Nursing interventions for decreased cardiac output and altered perfusion are discussed in the section of the chapter on nursing care of the person in shock.

Ineffective maintenance of airway

The person with multiple injuries is at great risk of developing airway obstruction and apnoea. Facial injuries, loose teeth, blood and vomitus increase the risk of aspiration and obstruction. Neurological injuries and cerebral oedema alter the person's respiratory drive and ability to keep the airway clear.

- Assess if airway is patent, maintainable or non-maintainable. Assess for manifestations of airway obstruction: stridor, tachypnoea, bradypnoea, cough, cyanosis, dyspnoea, decreased or absent breath sounds, changes in oxygen levels and changes in level of consciousness. *Assessing the airway and initiating interventions are the first steps in managing the person with multiple injuries.*
- Monitor oxygen saturation by applying a pulse oximeter. Adjust oxygen flow to maintain oxygen saturation above 95%. *Changes in oxygen saturation as measured by the pulse oximeter reflect the effectiveness of the person's ventilation. Pulse oximetry in people who have been exposed to carbon monoxide (i.e. house fires) is unreliable since it cannot differentiate carboxyhaemoglobin from oxyhaemoglobin.*
- Monitor level of consciousness. *An early sign of an ineffective airway is change in the person's behaviour. If the person becomes restless, anxious, combative or unresponsive, airway patency and ventilation effectiveness need to be immediately evaluated and appropriate interventions initiated.*

NURSING CARE PLAN A person with multiple injuries

Jane Souza is a 25-year-old married woman with two children who provides daycare for preschool children in her home. As she is driving on the highway at 100 km per hour, a car crosses the median strip and strikes her vehicle head on. Jane, who is not wearing a seat belt, is thrown forward against the steering wheel. The front of her car is pushed up against her by the car that struck her, entrapping her lower extremities.

After extensive efforts to extricate her from the car, Jane is transported to the local trauma centre. She is still conscious, is receiving high-flow oxygen by mask and has one intravenous line in place. Her vital signs are a palpable systolic blood pressure of 80, a pulse rate of 120 and a respiratory rate of 36. On arrival, she states that she is having difficulty breathing.

ASSESSMENT

- *Airway*: Maintainable with high-flow oxygen in place.
- *Breathing*: Respiratory rate of 36, decreased breath sounds on the right side, equal chest wall movement.
- *Circulation*: No palpable radial pulses; palpable brachial pulses. Cardiac monitor shows sinus tachycardia. No active external bleeding noted. Skin colour pale, cool to the touch and diaphoretic. One intravenous access in place and crystalloid fluids running.
- *Disability*: Moved her fingers when asked; complains of difficulty breathing; denies that she is hurt. Pupils 4 mm, equal and reacting to light. Extremity movement is limited due to broken limbs.

(continued)

NURSING CARE PLAN A person with multiple injuries (continued)

- *Exposure*: Has a broken right arm and an open fracture of the left ankle. Multiple bruising and abrasions on right side of chest.

Because of Jane's respiratory distress, she is intubated and ventilated with 100% oxygen. Another intravenous line is inserted and O-negative blood administered. It is determined that she has sustained a pneumothorax in the right side and an intercostal catheter is inserted.

DIAGNOSES

- *Ineffective breathing pattern* related to multiple bruises and abrasions on the right side of the chest and respiratory difficulty.
- *Deficient fluid volume* related to acute internal blood loss (presumed because no active bleeding can be found).
- *Risk of injury* related to trauma resuscitation.

PLANNING

- Continuously monitor airway and oxygenation.
- Continuously monitor circulatory status.
- Prepare for ongoing care.

Expected outcomes

- Maintain adequate oxygenation.
- Maintain adequate circulating blood volume.

IMPLEMENTATION

- Ensure patency of airway maintained—secure and monitor endotracheal tube.
- Assess and maintain ventilation—monitor ventilatory support, visualise chest expansion, assess air entry through lung auscultation, monitor oxygen saturations.
- Monitor the effects of fluid and blood administration, including any changes in blood pressure, heart rate and rhythm, skin colour and turgor.
- Insert urinary catheter and monitor urine output.
- Prepare for transfer to the operating room for emergency surgery.
- Explain all procedures.
- Keep family informed about her condition.

EVALUATION

- Jane is transferred to the operating room, where it is determined that she has a ruptured spleen and a serious pelvic fracture. Jane's treatment continues in the operating room.

CRITICAL THINKING IN THE NURSING PROCESS

1. Is the nursing diagnosis *Deficient fluid volume* appropriate for Jane Souza? Why or why not?
2. The assessment of a person who has experienced trauma is, in order: A = airway, B = breathing and C = circulation. What is the rationale for this sequence?
3. Following surgery, Jane is moved to the surgical intensive care unit. She is very anxious and restless. What assessments would you perform to identify the cause of her restlessness?
4. Infection is a common complication for a person experiencing trauma. Describe five risks for infection that are present from the time of injury to the time of hospital discharge.

REFLECTION ON THE NURSING PROCESS

1. What communication and education strategies would you use with Jane following surgery?

Risk of infection

Traumatic injuries are considered dirty wounds. Projectiles enter the body through dirty surfaces and clothing, carrying dirt and debris into the wound. Open fractures provide a portal for the entry of bacteria and dirt. Even with surgical intervention, the wounds often remain contaminated.

- Practise effective hand hygiene. *Handwashing remains the single most important factor in preventing the spread of infection.*
- Use standard precautions and aseptic technique when caring for wounds. *Standard precautions are essential to protect the person and the nurse from infection.* In addition:
- Monitor wounds for odour, redness, heat, swelling and copious or purulent drainage.
- Monitor hidden wounds, such as those under casts, by asking the person whether pain has increased and by observing for increased drainage and heat over the area of the wound.
- Ensure that cross-contamination between wounds does not occur. Collect drainage in ostomy bags if it is copious. The skin is the first line of defence against infection; wounds provide a portal of entry for organisms. Risk factors for wound infection include contamination, inadequate wound care and the condition of the wound at the time of closure. *Aseptic techniques used in applying and changing dressings reduce the entry of organisms.*
- Measure and record vital signs, including temperature every 2 to 4 hours. *Vital signs, particularly an elevated body temperature, may indicate the presence of an infection.*
- Provide adequate fluids and nutrition. *Adequate fluids, kilojoules and protein are essential to wound healing.*
- Assess for manifestations of gas gangrene: fever, pain and swelling in traumatised tissues; drainage with a foul odour. *Gas gangrene is usually caused by the organism* Clostridium perfringens. *This bacterium is found in the soil and can be introduced into the body during a traumatic injury. The organism grows in the tissues, causing necrosis; hydrogen and carbon dioxide are released with resultant swelling of tissues. If the infection continues, tissues are progressively destroyed and sepsis and death may result.*
- Assess status of tetanus immunisation and administer tetanus toxoid or human toxin–antitoxin as prescribed. *Tetanus is caused by an exotoxin produced by* Clostridium tetani, *usually introduced through an open wound. The organism is commonly found in the soil.*
- Use strict aseptic technique when inserting catheters, suctioning, administering parenteral medications or performing any other invasive procedure. *Using aseptic technique during invasive procedures reduces the risk of entry of organisms.*

Impaired physical mobility

The person with trauma injuries is often unable to change position independently and is at risk of complications of the integumentary, cardiovascular, gastrointestinal, respiratory, musculoskeletal and renal systems. At greatest risk are those who have had multiple injuries, spinal cord injuries, peripheral nerve injuries and traumatic amputations. Collaborate with the physiotherapist and occupational therapist (if available) to determine the most effective types and schedule of exercises and assistive devices.

The aim of therapy is to ensure the person will maintain joint range of motion and avoid development of contractures and pulmonary complications such as atelectasis.

- If active bleeding or oedema is not present, provide active or passive exercises to affected and unaffected extremities at least once every 8 hours. *Exercise improves muscle tone, maintains joint mobility, improves circulation and prevents contractures.*
- Assist the person to turn, cough and deep breathe, and use an incentive spirometer at least every 2 hours. *Changing positions, coughing, deep breathing and incentive spirometry reduce the risk of integumentary and respiratory complications.*
- If the person is unable to be moved and positioned, consider a specialty bed such as the kinetic continuous rotation bed (see Figure 10.7). *The kinetic continuous rotation bed allows continuous turning of the person; the motion decreases pulmonary complications, venous stasis, postural hypotension, urinary stasis, muscle wasting and bone demineralisation.*
- Monitor the lower extremities each day for manifestations of deep venous thrombosis: heat, swelling and pain. If anti-embolic stockings or intermittent compression stockings are used, remove them for 1 hour during each shift and assess the skin. *Venous stasis results when surrounding muscles are unable to contract and help move the blood through the veins. Thrombus (clot) formation in deep veins is a major risk of pulmonary embolism.*

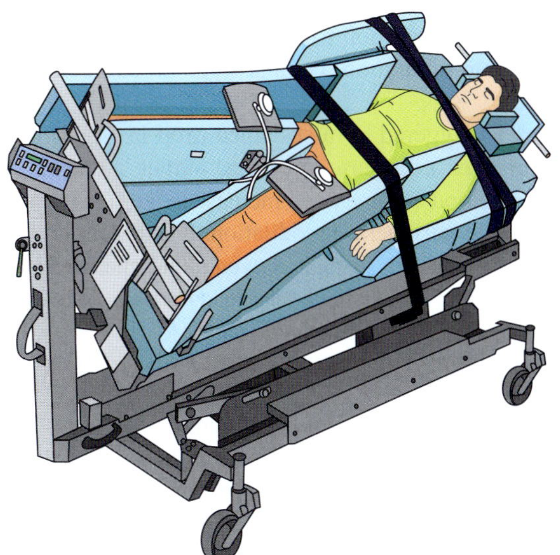

FIGURE 10.7 ***A kinetic continuous rotation bed provides a means of turning the person with multiple injuries to decrease the hazards of immobility***

Spiritual distress

Trauma generally strikes without warning and carries potentially devastating consequences, including severe alterations in the lives of the victim and family, and death. The traumatic death of a loved one may be the most difficult event a family ever experiences. The decision to cease life support systems or to donate organs challenges the family's belief systems and psychological stability. Nursing care of the family (or person) experiencing spiritual distress includes the following:

- Give the family information about the option to donate the person's organs. The decision to donate organs needs to be based on information about the person's condition, prognosis and the criteria by which brain death is determined. *It is important to convey to family members that organ donation is only an option and that they should not feel they are obligated to consent or are doing something wrong if they do not consent.*
- Encourage the family to ask questions and express their feelings about the traumatic event and/or organ donation. *Allowing families to express their feelings may help prevent long-term consequences such as guilt.*
- Refer the family for follow-up care. Long-term follow-up is important for the family facing the sudden death of a loved one. *Grieving is not an overnight process and providing the family with resources that may be used in the future may help prevent future crises and dysfunction.* (For more information see the chapter 'Nursing care of people experiencing loss, grief and death'.)

Post-traumatic stress disorder

Post-traumatic stress disorder is an intense, sustained emotional response to a disastrous event. It is characterised by emotions that range from anger to fear and by flashbacks or psychic numbing. In the initial stage, the person may be calm or may express feelings of anger, disbelief, terror and shock. In the long-term phase, which begins anywhere from a few days to several months after the event, the person often experiences flashbacks and nightmares of the traumatic event. The person may call on ineffective coping mechanisms, such as alcohol or drugs, and withdraw from relationships.

- Assess emotional responses while providing physical care. Observe for excessive crying, sleep problems, suspiciousness and fear during the initial phase of treatment. If the person is unconscious, encourage family members and friends to express their feelings. *These assessments provide valuable information about the person's ability to cope with the trauma.*
- Be available if the person wishes to talk about the trauma and encourage expression of feelings. *The person may initially deny negative feelings; this denial is a coping mechanism in the initial phase of recovery.*
- Teach relaxation techniques such as deep breathing, progressive muscle relaxation or imagery (see the chapter

'Nursing care of people in pain'). *These techniques are often useful in coping when thoughts of the trauma recur.*
- Refer the person and family members for counselling, psychotherapy or support groups as appropriate. *Continued therapy may be necessary in assisting the person and family to resolve the acute and long-term effects of trauma.*

Community-based care

Address the following topics to prepare the person and family for home care:

- the type of home environment to which the person will be returning, including any changes that will be required to let them function in that environment
- medications, dressings, wound care, equipment and supplies
- special diet, if needed
- rehabilitation plan and its effect on the person's family
- follow-up appointments with the general practitioner or at the trauma clinic
- emotional changes that the person may undergo as a result of the trauma
- helpful resources:
  - home healthcare
  - community support groups
  - National Stroke Foundation.

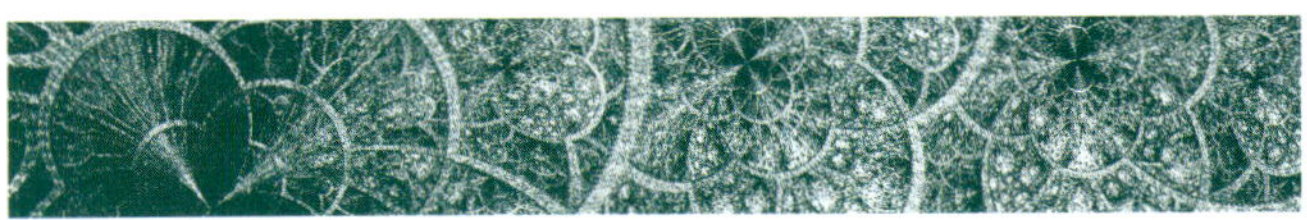

THE PERSON EXPERIENCING SHOCK

Shock is a clinical syndrome characterised by a systemic imbalance between oxygen supply and demand. This imbalance results in a state of inadequate blood flow to body organs and tissues, causing life-threatening cellular dysfunction.

Overview of cellular homeostasis and haemodynamics

To maintain cellular metabolism, cells of all body organs and tissues require a regular and consistent supply of oxygen and the removal of metabolic wastes. This homeostatic regulation is maintained primarily by the cardiovascular system and depends on four physiological components:

1. a cardiac output sufficient to meet bodily requirements
2. an uncompromised vascular system in which the vessels have a diameter sufficient to allow unimpeded blood flow and have good tone (the ability to constrict or dilate to maintain normal pressure)
3. a volume of blood sufficient to fill the circulatory system and a blood pressure adequate to maintain blood flow
4. tissues that are able to extract and use the oxygen delivered through the capillaries.

In a healthy person, these components function as a system to maintain tissue perfusion. During shock, however, one or more of these components are disrupted. An understanding of basic haemodynamics is necessary to understand the pathophysiology of shock:

- **Stroke volume (SV)** is the amount of blood pumped into the aorta with each contraction of the left ventricle.
- **Cardiac output (CO)** is the amount of blood pumped per minute into the aorta by the left ventricle. CO is determined by multiplying the stroke volume (SV) by the heart rate (HR): $CO = SV \times HR$.

> **CONSIDERATION FOR PRACTICE**
> Cardiac output (CO) = stroke volume (SV) × heart rate (HR).

- **Mean arterial pressure (MAP)** is the product of cardiac output and systemic vascular resistance (SVR): $MAP = CO \times SVR$. When CO, SVR or total blood volume rises, MAP and tissue perfusion increase. Conversely, when CO, SVR or total blood volume falls, MAP and tissue perfusion decrease. A MAP of 70 to 110 is normal. A MAP of 60 mmHg is required to maintain adequate perfusion to the brain, heart and kidneys.
- The sympathetic nervous system maintains the smooth muscle surrounding the arteries and arterioles in a state of partial contraction called *sympathetic tone*. Increased sympathetic stimulation increases vasoconstriction and SVR; decreased sympathetic stimulation allows vasodilation which decreases SVR.

Pathophysiology

When one or more cardiovascular components do not function properly, the body's haemodynamic properties are altered. Consequently, tissue perfusion may be inadequate to sustain normal cellular metabolism. The result is the clinical syndrome known as shock. The manifestations of shock result from the body's attempts to maintain vital organs (heart and brain) and to preserve life following a drop in cellular perfusion. However, if the injury or condition triggering shock is severe enough or of long enough duration, cellular hypoxia and cellular death will occur.

Shock is triggered by a sustained drop in MAP. This drop can occur after a decrease in cardiac output, a decrease in the circulating blood volume or an increase in the size of the vascular bed due to peripheral vasodilation. If intervention is timely and effective, the physiological events that characterise shock may be stopped; if not, shock may lead to death. See Table 10.5 for classification of haemorrhagic shock.

Stage I: early, reversible and compensatory shock

The initial stage of shock begins when baroreceptors in the aortic arch and the carotid sinus detect a sustained drop in MAP of less than 10 mmHg from normal levels. The circulating blood volume may decrease (usually to less than 500 mL) but not enough to cause serious effects.

The body reacts to the decrease in arterial pressure. The cerebral integration centre initiates the body's response systems

TABLE 10.5 Classification of haemorrhagic shock and presentation of the person

	COMPENSATED/CLASS I	MILD/CLASS II	MODERATE/CLASS III	SEVERE/CLASS IV
Blood loss	Up to 750 mL	750–1,500 mL	1,500–2,000 mL	> 2,000 mL
Percentage of blood volume loss	Up to 15%	15–30%	30–40%	> 40%
Heart rate (bpm)	< 100	> 100	> 120	> 140
Blood pressure	Normal or increased	Normal	Decreased	Markedly decreased
Pulse pressure	Normal or increased	Decreased	Decreased	Decreased
Capillary refill	Normal	Mild increase	Usually delayed	Delayed
Respiratory rate	Normal	Mild increase	Moderate tachypnoea	Marked tachypnoea
Urine output	> 0.5 mL/kg/hr	> 0.3 mL/kg/hr	< 0.3 mL/kg/hr	Anuria
Mental status	Normal–slightly anxious	Mildly anxious–agitated	Anxious–confused	Lethargic–obtunded

causing the sympathetic nervous system to increase the heart rate and the force of cardiac contraction, thus increasing cardiac output. Sympathetic stimulation also causes peripheral vasoconstriction, resulting in increased SVR and a rise in arterial pressure. The net result is that the perfusion of cells, tissues and organs is maintained.

Symptoms are almost imperceptible during the early stage of shock. The pulse rate may be slightly elevated. If the injury is minor or of short duration, arterial pressure is usually maintained and no further symptoms occur.

Compensatory shock begins after the MAP falls 10 to 15 mmHg below normal levels. The circulating blood volume is reduced by 25% to 35% (1,000 mL or more), but compensatory mechanisms are able to maintain blood pressure and tissue perfusion to vital organs thereby preventing cell damage.

- Stimulation of the sympathetic nervous system results in the release of adrenaline from the adrenal medulla and the release of noradrenaline from the adrenal medulla and the sympathetic fibres. Both hormones rapidly stimulate the alpha- and beta-adrenergic fibres. Stimulated alpha-adrenergic fibres cause vasoconstriction in the blood vessels supplying the skin and most of the abdominal viscera. Perfusion of these areas decreases. Stimulated beta-adrenergic fibres cause vasodilation in vessels supplying the heart and skeletal muscles (beta-1 response) and increase the heart rate and force of cardiac contraction ($beta_2$ response). Further, blood vessels in the respiratory system dilate and the respiratory rate increases ($beta_2$ response). Thus, stimulation of the sympathetic nervous system results in increased cardiac output and oxygenation of these tissues.
- The renin–angiotensin response occurs as the blood flow to the kidneys decreases. Renin released from the kidneys converts a plasma protein to angiotensin II, which causes vasoconstriction and stimulates the adrenal cortex to release aldosterone. Aldosterone causes the kidneys to reabsorb water and sodium and to lose potassium. The absorption of water maintains circulating blood volume, while increased vasoconstriction increases SVR, maintaining central vascular volume and raising blood pressure.
- The hypothalamus releases adrenocorticotropic hormone, causing the adrenal glands to secrete aldosterone. Aldosterone promotes the reabsorption of water and sodium by the kidneys, preserving blood volume and pressure.
- The posterior pituitary gland releases antidiuretic hormone, which increases renal reabsorption of water to increase intravascular volume. The combined effects of hormones released by the hypothalamus and posterior pituitary glands work to conserve central vascular volume.
- As MAP falls in the compensatory stage of shock, decreased capillary hydrostatic pressure causes a fluid shift from the interstitial space into the capillaries. The net gain of fluid raises the blood volume.

Working together, these compensatory mechanisms can maintain MAP for only a short period of time. During this period, the perfusion and oxygenation of the heart and brain are adequate. If effective treatment is provided, the process is arrested and no permanent damage occurs. However, unless the underlying cause of shock is reversed, these compensatory mechanisms soon become harmful and shock perpetuates shock.

Stage II: intermediate or progressive shock

The progressive stage of shock occurs after a sustained decrease in MAP of 20 mmHg or more below normal levels and a fluid loss of 35% to 50% (1,800 to 2,500 mL of fluid). Although the compensatory mechanisms in the previous state remain activated, they are no longer able to maintain MAP at a level sufficient to ensure perfusion of vital organs.

The vasoconstriction response that first helped sustain MAP eventually limits blood flow to the point that cells become oxygen deficient. To remain alive, the affected cells switch from aerobic to anaerobic metabolism. The lactic acid formed as a by-product of anaerobic metabolism contributes to an acidotic state at the cellular level. As a result, adenosine triphosphate, the source of cellular energy, is produced inefficiently. Lacking energy, the sodium–potassium pump fails. Potassium moves out of the cell while sodium and water move inward. As this process continues the cell swells, cell membrane integrity is lost and cell organelles are damaged. Lysosomes within the cell spill out their digestive enzymes which disintegrate any remaining organelles. Some enzymes spread to adjacent cells where they erode and rupture cell membranes.

The acid by-products of anaerobic metabolism dilate the precapillary arterioles and constrict the postcapillary venules. This causes increased hydrostatic pressure within the capillary and fluid shifts back into the interstitial space. The capillaries also become increasingly permeable, allowing serum proteins to shift from the vascular space into the interstitium. The build-up of plasma proteins increases the osmotic pressure in the interstitium, further accelerating the fluid shift out of the capillaries.

Throughout this period, the heart rate and vasoconstriction increase; however, perfusion of the skin, skeletal muscles, kidneys and gastrointestinal organs is greatly diminished. Cells in the heart and brain become hypoxic, while other body cells and tissues become ischaemic and anoxic. A generalised state of acidosis and hyperkalaemia ensues (see the chapter 'Nursing care of people with altered fluid, electrolyte and acid–base balance'). Unless this stage of shock is treated rapidly, the person's chances of survival are poor.

Stage III: refractory or irreversible shock

If shock progresses to the irreversible stage, tissue anoxia becomes so generalised and cellular death so widespread that no treatment can reverse the damage. Even if MAP is temporarily restored, too much cellular damage has occurred to maintain life. Death of cells is followed by death of tissues, which results in death of organs. Death of vital organs contributes to subsequent death of the body.

Effects of shock on body systems

Whatever its causes, shock produces predictable effects on the body's organ systems. (See 'Multisystem effects of shock'.)

CARDIOVASCULAR SYSTEM The perfusion and oxygenation of the heart are adequate in the early stages of shock. As shock progresses, myocardial cells become hypoxic and myocardial muscle function diminishes. Initially, the blood pressure may be normal or even slightly elevated (as a result of compensatory mechanisms) and the heart rate only slightly increased. Sympathetic stimulation increases the heart rate (a sinus tachycardia of 120 beats per minute is common) in an effort to increase cardiac output. As a result of vasoconstriction and decreased blood volume, the palpated pulse is rapid, weak and thready; as shock progresses, peripheral pulses are usually non-palpable.

Tachycardia reduces the time available for left ventricular filling and coronary artery perfusion, further reducing cardiac output. With progressive shock, altered acid–base balance, hypoxia and hyperkalaemia damage the heart's electrical systems and contractility. Consequently, cardiac arrhythmias may develop. Decreased blood volume with decreased venous return also decreases cardiac output, and blood pressure falls.

The blood pressure changes produced by shock are characterised by a progressive decrease in both systolic and diastolic pressures and a narrowing pulse pressure. Auscultation of blood pressure is often difficult or impossible and is an inaccurate reflection of blood pressure status. For this reason, haemodynamic monitoring is usually instituted to follow the person's cardiovascular status accurately.

RESPIRATORY SYSTEM During shock, oxygen delivery to cells may be impaired by a drop in circulating blood volume or, in the case of blood loss, by an insufficient number of red blood cells that carry oxygen. Although the respiratory rate increases because of compensatory mechanisms that promote oxygenation, the number of alveoli that are perfused decreases and gas exchange is impaired. As a result, oxygen levels in the blood decrease and carbon dioxide levels increase. As perfusion of the lungs diminishes, carbon dioxide is retained and respiratory acidosis occurs.

A complication of decreased perfusion of the lungs is acute respiratory distress syndrome (ARDS), or 'shock lung'. The exact mechanism that produces ARDS is unknown, but some contributing factors have been identified. The pulmonary capillaries become increasingly permeable to proteins and water, resulting in non-cardiogenic pulmonary oedema. Production of surfactant (which controls surface tension within alveoli) is impaired and the alveoli collapse or fill with fluid. This potentially lethal form of respiratory failure may result from any condition that causes hypoperfusion of the lungs, but is more common in shock caused by haemorrhage, severe allergic responses, trauma and infection. (ARDS is discussed further in the chapter 'Nursing care of people with gas exchange disorders'.)

GASTROINTESTINAL AND HEPATIC SYSTEMS The gastrointestinal organs normally receive 25% of the cardiac output through the splenic circulation. Shock constricts the splenic arterioles and redirects arterial blood flow to the heart and brain. Consequently, gastrointestinal organs become ischaemic and may be irreversibly damaged.

Gastric mucosa tends to ulcerate when it becomes ischaemic. Lesions of the gastric and duodenal mucosa (called *stress ulcers*) can develop within hours of severe trauma, sepsis or burns (Norris, 2018). Gastrointestinal ulcers may haemorrhage within 2 to 10 days following the original cause of shock. In addition, the permeability of damaged mucosa increases, allowing enteric bacteria or their toxins to enter the abdominal cavity and then progress to the circulation, resulting in sepsis.

Gastric and intestinal motility is impaired during shock and paralytic ileus may result. If the episode of shock is prolonged, necrosis of the bowel may occur. In many cases, alterations in the structure and function of the gastrointestinal tract impair absorption of nutrients such as protein and glucose.

Shock also alters the metabolic functions of the liver. Initially, *gluconeogenesis* (the process of forming glucose from non-carbohydrate sources) and *glycogenolysis* (the breakdown of glycogen into glucose) increase. This process allows blood glucose levels to increase as the body attempts to respond to the stressor; however, as shock progresses, liver functions are impaired and hypoglycaemia develops. Metabolism of fats and protein is impaired and the liver can no longer effectively remove lactic acid, contributing to the development of metabolic acidosis.

The destruction of the liver's reticuloendothelial Kupffer cells (phagocytes that destroy bacteria) causes a further problem. Bacteria may proliferate within the circulatory system, causing overwhelming bacterial infection and toxicity.

Multisystem effects of shock

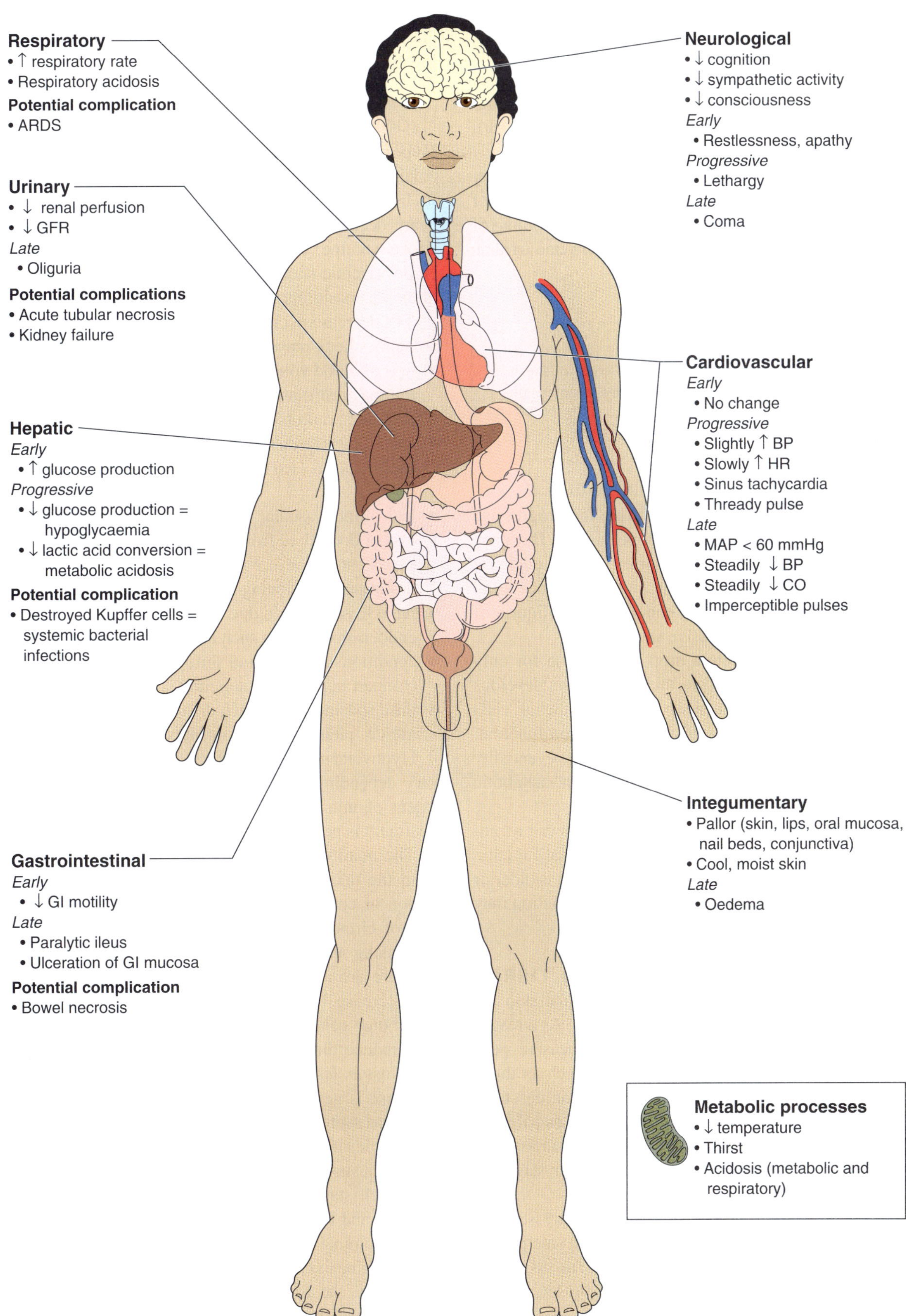

NEUROLOGICAL SYSTEM The primary effects of shock on the neurological system involve changes in mental status and orientation. Cerebral hypoxia produces altered levels of consciousness beginning with apathy and lethargy and progressing to coma. A common early symptom of cerebral hypoxia is restlessness. Continued ischaemia of brain cells eventually causes swelling, resulting in cerebral oedema, neurotransmitter failure and irreversible brain cell damage.

As cerebral ischaemia worsens, the sympathetic activity and vasomotor centres are depressed. This leads to a loss of sympathetic tone, causing systemic vasodilation and pooling of blood in the periphery. As a result, venous return and cardiac output further decrease.

CONSIDERATION FOR PRACTICE

An early sign of shock is a change in the level of consciousness. Late signs of shock include mental status changes, hypotension and marked tachycardia.

RENAL SYSTEM Blood that normally perfuses the kidneys is shunted to the heart and brain during the progressive stage of shock, resulting in renal hypoperfusion. The drop in renal perfusion is reflected in a corresponding decrease in the glomerular filtration rate. Urine output is reduced and the urine that is produced is highly concentrated. Oliguria of < 0.5 mL/kg/hr indicates progressive shock.

Healthy kidneys can tolerate a drop in perfusion for only about 20 minutes; thereafter, acute tubular necrosis develops (Norris, 2018). As tubular necrosis occurs, epithelial cells slough off and block the tubules, disrupting nephron function. The accumulating loss of functional nephrons eventually causes renal failure. Without normal renal function, metabolic waste products are retained in the plasma.

If treatment restores renal perfusion, the kidneys can regenerate the lost epithelial cells in the tubules and renal function usually returns to normal. However, in a person who is older or chronically ill or in sustained shock, loss of renal function may become permanent.

EFFECTS ON SKIN, TEMPERATURE AND THIRST In most types of shock, blood vessels supplying the skin are vasoconstricted and the sweat glands are activated. As a result, changes in skin colour occur. The skin of Caucasian people becomes pale. In people with darker skin (such as those of Indigenous Australian, African or Mediterranean descent), shock-related skin colour changes may be assessed as paleness of the lips, oral mucous membranes, nail beds and conjunctiva. The skin is usually cool and moist and, in the later stages of shock, often oedematous.

The body temperature decreases as shock progresses, the result of a decrease in overall body metabolism. Some people in shock become thirsty, probably a response to decreased blood volume and increased serum osmolality (McCance & Huether, 2018).

Types of shock

Shock is identified according to its underlying cause. All types of shock progress through the same stages and exert similar effects on body systems. Any differences are noted in the following discussion.

Hypovolaemic shock

Hypovolaemic shock is caused by a decrease in intravascular volume of 15% or more (McCance & Huether, 2018). In hypovolaemic shock, the venous blood returning to the heart decreases and ventricular filling drops. As a result, stroke volume, cardiac output and blood pressure decrease. Hypovolaemic shock is the most common type of shock and often occurs simultaneously with other types.

The decrease in circulating blood volume that triggers hypovolaemic shock may result from:

- loss of blood volume from haemorrhage (from surgery, trauma, gastrointestinal bleeding, blood coagulation disorders, ruptured oesophageal varices)
- loss of intravascular fluid from the skin due to injuries such as burns (see the chapter 'Nursing care of people with burns')
- loss of intravascular volume from severe dehydration
- loss of body fluid from the gastrointestinal system due to persistent and severe vomiting or diarrhoea, or continuous nasogastric suctioning
- renal losses of fluid due to the use of diuretics or to endocrine disorders such as diabetes insipidus
- conditions causing fluid shifts from the intravascular compartment to the interstitial space
- third spacing due to such disorders as liver diseases with ascites, pleural effusion or intestinal obstruction.

Hypovolaemic shock affects all body systems. Its effects vary depending on the person's age, general state of health, extent of injury or severity of illness, length of time before treatment is provided and the rate of volume loss.

The manifestations of hypovolaemic shock result directly from the decrease in circulating blood volume and the initiation of compensatory mechanisms (see Figure 10.8). The loss of circulating blood volume reduces cardiac output by decreasing venous return to the heart. As a result, blood pressure drops. The carotid and cardiac baroreceptors sense the decrease in blood pressure and communicate it to the vasomotor centres in the brainstem. The vasomotor centres then induce the sympathetic compensatory responses. If the fluid loss is less than 500 mL, activation of the sympathetic response is generally adequate to restore cardiac output and blood pressure to near normal, although the heart rate may remain elevated.

With a sustained loss of blood volume (1,000 mL or more), the shock stage progresses. Heart rate and vasoconstriction increase and blood flow to the skin, skeletal muscles, kidneys and abdominal organs decreases. Several renal mechanisms and a decline in capillary pressure help conserve blood volume. Eventually, the amount of blood flowing to cells is too low to oxygenate them and sustain production of cellular energy.

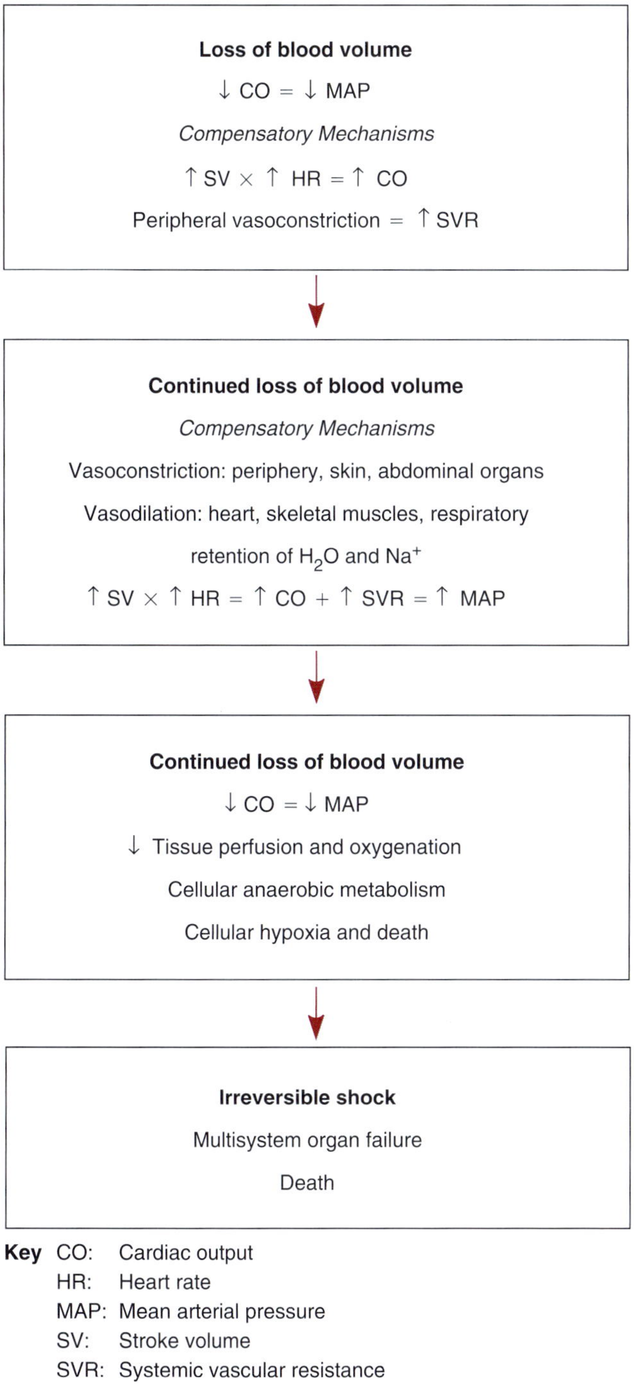

Loss of blood volume

↓ CO = ↓ MAP

Compensatory Mechanisms

↑ SV × ↑ HR = ↑ CO

Peripheral vasoconstriction = ↑ SVR

↓

Continued loss of blood volume

Compensatory Mechanisms

Vasoconstriction: periphery, skin, abdominal organs

Vasodilation: heart, skeletal muscles, respiratory

retention of H_2O and Na^+

↑ SV × ↑ HR = ↑ CO + ↑ SVR = ↑ MAP

↓

Continued loss of blood volume

↓ CO = ↓ MAP

↓ Tissue perfusion and oxygenation

Cellular anaerobic metabolism

Cellular hypoxia and death

↓

Irreversible shock

Multisystem organ failure

Death

Key CO: Cardiac output
HR: Heart rate
MAP: Mean arterial pressure
SV: Stroke volume
SVR: Systemic vascular resistance

FIGURE 10.8 *The stages of hypovolaemic shock*

Anaerobic metabolism begins, producing an acidotic environment for cells. As a result, cells lose their physical integrity. If untreated, shock causes multiple organ failure and death results. Manifestations of various stages of hypovolaemic shock are listed in the 'Manifestations' box.

Cardiogenic shock

Cardiogenic shock occurs when the heart's pumping ability is compromised to the point that it cannot maintain cardiac output and adequate tissue perfusion. Cardiac disorders are discussed in the chapters 'Nursing care of people with coronary heart disease' and 'Nursing care of people with cardiac disorders'; this section focuses only on the effects of shock caused by these disorders.

The loss of the pumping action of the heart may be caused by the following conditions:

- myocardial infarction
- cardiac tamponade
- restrictive pericarditis
- cardiac arrest
- arrhythmias, such as fibrillation or ventricular tachycardia
- pathological changes in the valves
- cardiomyopathies from hypertension, alcohol, bacterial or viral infections, or ischaemia
- complications of cardiac surgery
- electrolyte imbalances (especially changes in normal potassium and calcium levels)
- drugs affecting cardiac muscle contractility
- head injuries causing damage to the cardioregulatory centre.

Myocardial infarction is the most common cause of cardiogenic shock. People admitted to the hospital for treatment of myocardial infarction or cardiac surgery are at risk of

MANIFESTATIONS Hypovolaemic shock

INITIAL STAGE

- *Blood pressure*: normal to slightly decreased
- *Pulse*: slightly increased from baseline
- *Respirations*: normal (baseline)
- *Skin*: cool, pale (in periphery), moist
- *Mental status*: alert and oriented
- *Urine output*: slight decrease
- *Other*: thirst, decreased capillary refill time

COMPENSATORY AND PROGRESSIVE STAGES

- *Blood pressure*: hypotension
- *Pulse*: rapid, thready
- *Respirations*: increased
- *Skin*: cool, pale (includes trunk); poor turgor with fluid loss, oedematous with fluid shift
- *Mental status*: restless, anxious, confused or agitated
- *Urine output*: oliguria (less than 0.5 mL/kg/hr)
- *Other*: marked thirst, acidosis, hyperkalaemia, decreased capillary refill time, decreased or absent peripheral pulses

IRREVERSIBLE STAGE

- *Blood pressure*: severe hypotension (often systolic pressure is below 80 mmHg)
- *Pulse*: very rapid, weak
- *Respirations*: rapid, shallow; crackles and wheezes
- *Skin*: cool, pale, mottled with cyanosis
- *Mental status*: disoriented, lethargic, comatose
- *Urine output*: anuria
- *Other*: loss of reflexes, decreased or absent peripheral pulses

MANIFESTATIONS **Cardiogenic shock**

- *Blood pressure*: hypotension
- *Pulse*: rapid, thready; distension of veins of hands and neck
- *Respirations*: increased, laboured; crackles and wheezes; pulmonary oedema
- *Skin*: pale, cyanotic, cold, moist
- *Mental status*: restless, anxious, lethargic progressing to comatose
- *Urine output*: oliguria to anuria
- *Other*: dependent oedema; elevated central venous pressure (CVP); elevated pulmonary capillary wedge pressure; arrhythmias

cardiogenic shock. The severity and progression of shock are related to the amount of myocardial damage.

Whatever the cardiogenic cause, the decrease in cardiac output causes a decrease in MAP. Heart rate may increase in response to compensatory mechanisms. However, tachycardia increases myocardial oxygen consumption and decreases coronary perfusion. The myocardium becomes progressively depleted of oxygen, causing further myocardial ischaemia and necrosis. The typical sequence of shock is essentially unchanged in cardiogenic shock.

Cyanosis, however, is more common in cardiogenic shock because stagnating blood increases extraction of oxygen from the haemoglobin at the capillary beds. As a result, the skin, lips and nail beds may appear cyanotic. As cardiac failure and cardiogenic shock progress, left ventricular end-diastolic pressure increases. The increase is transmitted to the pulmonary capillary bed and pulmonary oedema may occur. Retention of blood in the right side of the heart increases right atrial pressure which leads to jugular venous distension as a result of backflow through the vena cava. Manifestations of cardiogenic shock are listed in the 'Manifestations' box.

Obstructive shock

Obstructive shock is caused by an obstruction in the heart or great vessels that either impedes venous return or prevents effective cardiac pumping action. The causes of obstructive shock are impaired diastolic filling (e.g. pericardial tamponade or pneumothorax), increased right ventricular afterload (e.g. pulmonary emboli) and increased left ventricular afterload (e.g. aortic stenosis, abdominal distension). The manifestations are the result of decreased cardiac output and blood pressure, with reduced tissue perfusion and cellular metabolism.

Distributive shock

Distributive shock (also called **vasogenic shock**) includes several types of shock that result from widespread vasodilation and decreased peripheral resistance. Because the blood volume does not change, relative hypovolaemia results. Examples of distributive shock include septic, neurogenic and anaphylactic shock. Treatment is based on the underlying pathogenesis.

Septic shock

Septic shock, the leading cause of death for people in critical care units, is one part of a progressive syndrome called *systemic inflammatory response syndrome* (SIRS). This condition is most often the result of Gram-negative bacterial infections (i.e. *Pseudomonas*, *E. coli*, *Klebsiella*) but may also follow Gram-positive infections from *Staphylococcus* and *Streptococcus* bacteria. Gram-negative sepsis has greatly increased in the past 10 years with a 60% mortality rate despite treatment. The pathophysiology of septic shock is complex and not completely understood.

People at risk of developing infections leading to septic shock include those who are hospitalised, have debilitating chronic illnesses or have poor nutritional status. The risk is heightened after invasive procedures or surgery. Others at risk of septic shock include older adults and those who are immunocompromised. Portals of entry for infection that may lead to septic shock are as follows:

- *Urinary system*: catheterisations, suprapubic tubes, cystoscopy.
- *Respiratory system*: suctioning, aspiration, tracheostomy, endotracheal tubes, respiratory therapy, mechanical ventilators.
- *Gastrointestinal system*: peptic ulcers, ruptured appendix, peritonitis.
- *Integumentary system*: surgical wounds, intravenous catheters, intra-arterial catheters, invasive monitoring, decubitus ulcers, burns, trauma.
- *Female reproductive system*: elective surgical abortion, ascending infections from transmission of bacteria during the intrapartal and postpartal periods, tampon use, sexually transmitted infections.

Septic shock begins with *septicaemia* (the presence of pathogens and their toxins in the blood). As pathogens are destroyed, their ruptured cell membranes allow endotoxins to leak into the plasma. The endotoxins disrupt the vascular system, coagulation mechanism and immune system, and trigger an immune and inflammatory response. (See the chapter 'Nursing care of people with infections'.) For this reason, the initial

NURSING CARE OF THE OLDER ADULT **Experiencing hypovolaemia**

With ageing comes a relative decrease in sympathetic activity in relation to the cardiovascular system. Cardiac compliance also decreases with age. Atherosclerosis affects many vital organs' sensitivity to even the slightest reduction in blood flow. Many older adults experience secondary volume depletion due to chronic diuretic use or malnutrition. Also, people prescribed beta-blockers may not present with tachycardia as an early indicator of shock. This important sign can be masked due to beta-adrenergic blockade. This group of people will require early invasive monitoring in order to avoid excessive or inadequate volume restoration. This should be considered early in the treatment phase.

effects of septic shock differ from those of hypovolaemic and cardiogenic shock: cardiac output is high and SVR is low.

Endotoxins directly damage the endothelial lining of small blood vessels first; the small blood vessels of the kidneys and lungs are most susceptible. Cellular damage stimulates the release of vasoactive proteins and activates coagulation factor XII. The vasoactive proteins stimulate peripheral vasodilation and increase capillary permeability; the activation of coagulation factors results in the production of multiple intravascular blood clots.

As a result of the increased capillary permeability and vasodilation, fluid shifts from the intravascular space to the interstitial space. Hypovolaemia results as fluid volume is lost from the circulating blood. Hypovolaemia and intravascular coagulation alter oxygenation and cellular metabolism, leading to anaerobic metabolism, lactic acidosis and cellular death.

Septic shock has an early phase and a late phase (see 'Manifestations' box). In early septic shock (sometimes called the *warm phase*), vasodilation results in weakness and warm, flushed skin, and the septicaemia often causes high fever and chills. In late septic shock (sometimes called the *cold phase*), hypovolaemia and activity of the compensatory mechanisms result in typical shock manifestations including cold, moist skin, oliguria and changes in mental status. Death may result from respiratory failure, cardiac failure or renal failure.

Toxic shock syndrome is an especially virulent form of septic shock occurring most frequently in menstruating women who use tampons. It is thought that bacterial toxins diffuse from the site of infection in the vagina into the circulation. The toxins then trigger a widespread inflammatory response and septic shock. The manifestations of toxic shock syndrome include extreme hypotension, hyperpyrexia, headache, myalgia, confusion, skin rash, vomiting and diarrhoea (McCance & Huether, 2018).

Disseminated intravascular coagulation (DIC), a generalised response to injury, is a potential risk in septic shock. This condition is characterised by simultaneous bleeding and clotting throughout the vasculature. Sepsis injures blood cells, causing platelet aggregation and decreased blood flow. As a result, blood clots form throughout the microcirculation. The clotting slows circulation further while stimulating excess fibrinolysis. As the body's stores of clotting factors are depleted, generalised bleeding begins. DIC is further discussed in the chapter 'Nursing care of people with haematological disorders'.

MANIFESTATIONS Septic shock

EARLY (WARM) SEPTIC SHOCK

- *Blood pressure*: normal to hypotension
- *Pulse*: increased, thready
- *Respirations*: rapid and deep
- *Skin*: warm, flushed
- *Mental status*: alert, oriented, anxious
- *Urine output*: normal
- *Other*: increased body temperature; chills; weakness; nausea, vomiting, diarrhoea; decreased CVP

LATE (COLD) SEPTIC SHOCK

- *Blood pressure*: hypotension
- *Pulse*: tachycardia, arrhythmias
- *Respirations*: rapid, shallow, dyspnoeic
- *Skin*: cool, pale, oedematous
- *Mental status*: lethargic to comatose
- *Urine output*: oliguria to anuria
- *Other*: normal to decreased body temperature; decreased CVP

Neurogenic shock

Neurogenic shock is the result of an imbalance between parasympathetic and sympathetic stimulation of vascular smooth muscle. If parasympathetic overstimulation or sympathetic understimulation persists, sustained vasodilation occurs and blood pools in the venous and capillary beds.

Neurogenic shock causes dramatic reduction in SVR as the size of the vascular compartment increases. As SVR decreases, pressure in the blood vessels becomes too low to drive nutrients across capillary membranes and cellular metabolism is impaired.

The following conditions can cause neurogenic shock by increasing parasympathetic stimulation or inhibiting sympathetic stimulation of the smooth muscle of blood vessels:

- head injury
- trauma to the spinal cord (spinal shock, a form of neurogenic shock, is described in the chapter 'Nursing care of people with cerebrovascular and spinal cord disorders')
- insulin reactions (which cause hypoglycaemia, decreasing glucose to the medulla)
- central nervous system depressant drugs (such as sedatives, barbiturates or narcotics)
- anaesthesia (spinal and general)
- severe pain
- prolonged exposure to heat.

Bradycardia occurs early, but tachycardia begins as compensatory mechanisms are initiated. Central venous pressure drops as veins dilate, venous return to the heart decreases, stroke volume decreases and MAP falls. In early stages, the extremities are warm and pink (from the pooling of blood), but as shock progresses the skin becomes pale and cool. Manifestations of neurogenic shock are listed in the 'Manifestations' box.

Anaphylactic shock

Anaphylactic shock is the result of a widespread hypersensitivity reaction (called *anaphylaxis*). The pathophysiology in this type of shock includes vasodilation, pooling of blood in

MANIFESTATIONS Neurogenic shock

- *Blood pressure*: hypotension
- *Pulse*: slow and bounding
- *Respirations*: vary
- *Skin*: warm, dry
- *Mental status*: anxious, restless, lethargic progressing to comatose
- *Urine output*: oliguria to anuria
- *Other*: lowered body temperature

the periphery and hypovolaemia with altered cellular metabolism. These physiological alterations occur when a sensitised person has contact with an *allergen* (a foreign substance to which an individual is hypersensitive). Many different allergens can cause anaphylactic shock, including medications, blood administration, latex, foods, snake venom and insect stings.

Anaphylactic shock does not occur with the first exposure to an allergen. With the first exposure to a foreign substance (the *antigen*), the body produces specific immunoglobulin E (IgE) antibodies against this antigen. The person is thus sensitised to that specific antigen. With subsequent exposure, the antigen reacts with the already formed IgE antibodies, disrupting cellular integrity. In addition, large amounts of histamine and other vasoactive amines are released and distributed through the circulatory system. These substances cause increased capillary permeability and massive vasodilation resulting in profound hypotension and eventual vascular collapse.

Histamine also causes constriction of smooth muscles in the bladder, uterus, intestines and bronchioles. Respiratory distress, bronchospasm, laryngospasm and severe abdominal cramping result. Serotonin (a neurotransmitter with vasoconstrictive properties) is released, further affecting respiratory status by increasing capillary permeability in the lungs. As a result, plasma leaks into the alveoli, gas exchange is impaired and pulmonary oedema may occur.

Anaphylactic shock begins and progresses rapidly. Manifestations may begin within 20 minutes of contact with an antigen. Unless appropriate intervention is provided, death can occur within a matter of minutes. Because anaphylaxis is rapid and potentially lethal, people with known allergies should carry some form of warning (such as a MedicAlert® bracelet) informing others of their susceptibility. Some patients carry an Epipen® (adrenaline) to use if required. Healthcare providers should be extremely careful to assess and document allergies or previous drug reactions. Manifestations of anaphylactic shock are listed in the 'Manifestations' box.

Similar, but not related, are anaphylactoid reactions that are not humorally mediated and do not require prior exposure to a trigger. These can have similar symptoms and are treated in a similar manner.

MANIFESTATIONS Anaphylactic shock

- *Blood pressure*: hypotension
- *Pulse*: increased, arrhythmias
- *Respirations*: dyspnoea, stridor, wheezes, laryngospasm, bronchospasm, pulmonary oedema
- *Skin*: warm, oedematous (lips, eyelids, tongue, hands, feet, genitals)
- *Mental status*: restless, anxious, lethargic to comatose
- *Urine output*: oliguria to anuria
- *Other*: paraesthesias; pruritus; abdominal cramps, vomiting, diarrhoea

INTERPROFESSIONAL CARE

Medical care for the person in shock focuses on treating the underlying cause, increasing arterial oxygenation and improving tissue perfusion. Depending on the cause and type of shock, interventions include emergency care measures, oxygen therapy, fluid replacement and medications. Emergency care is often the first course of collaborative action taken to arrest shock, as discussed earlier in this chapter.

Diagnosis

The following diagnostic tests can help identify the type of shock and assess the person's physical status. Measurements include:

- *Blood haemoglobin* and *haematocrit* to detect the cell concentration that usually occurs in hypovolaemic shock, which reflects the underlying aetiology. In hypovolaemic shock resulting from haemorrhage, the haemoglobin and haematocrit concentrations are lower than normal. In hypovolaemic shock resulting from intravascular fluid loss, by contrast, the haemoglobin and haematocrit concentrations are higher than normal.
- *Arterial blood gases (ABGs)* to determine oxygen and carbon dioxide levels and pH. The effects of shock and of the body's compensatory mechanisms cause a decrease in pH (indicating acidosis), a decrease in the partial pressure of oxygen (PaO_2) and in total oxygen saturation, and an increase in the partial pressure of carbon dioxide ($PaCO_2$).
- *Serum electrolytes* to monitor the severity and progression of shock. As shock progresses, glucose and sodium levels decrease, and potassium levels increase.
- *Blood urea nitrogen (BUN), serum creatinine levels, urine specific gravity* and *osmolality* to check renal function. As perfusion of the kidneys is decreased and renal function is reduced, the BUN and creatinine levels increase as does urine specific gravity and osmolality.
- *Blood cultures* to identify the causative organism in septic shock.
- *White blood cell (WBC) count* and *differential* in the person with septic or anaphylactic shock. The total WBC count is increased in septic shock. Elevated neutrophils indicate acute infection, increased monocytes indicate a bacterial infection and increased eosinophils indicate an allergic response.
- *Serum cardiac enzymes*, which are elevated in cardiogenic shock: lactate dehydrogenase (LDH), creatine kinase (CK), creatinine kinase MB (CKMB) and troponin levels.

Other diagnostic tests may be ordered to determine the extent of injury or damage, or to locate the site of internal haemorrhage. These tests might include x-ray studies, computed tomography (CT) scans, magnetic resonance imaging (MRI), endoscopic examinations and echocardiograms. Newer diagnostic methods for hypoperfusion include gastric tonometry and sublingual $PaCO_2$. Gastric tonometry measures the partial pressure of carbon dioxide in the gastric lumen. The measurement of sublingual carbon dioxide correlates well with decreased MAP.

Medications

When fluid replacement alone is not sufficient to reverse shock, vasoactive drugs (drugs causing vasoconstriction or vasodilation) and inotropic drugs (drugs improving cardiac contractility) may be administered. When used to treat shock, these drugs increase venous return through vasoconstriction of peripheral vessels; they also improve the pumping ability of the heart by facilitating myocardial contractility and by dilating coronary arteries to increase perfusion of the myocardium.

Drugs used to treat shock are discussed in the 'Medication administration' box. Other drugs that may be administered to the person in shock include:

- diuretics to increase urine output after fluid replacement has been initiated
- sodium bicarbonate to treat acidosis

MEDICATION ADMINISTRATION The person in shock

ADRENERGICS (SYMPATHOMIMETICS)

Vasoconstrictors

Adrenaline
Noradrenaline
Metaraminol (Aramine)

Inotropes

Dopamine
Dobutamine
Isoprenaline

Adrenergic drugs (also called sympathomimetics) mimic the fight-or-flight response of the sympathetic nervous system, selectively stimulating alpha-adrenergic and beta-adrenergic receptors. Many of these drugs have both vasopressor (vasoconstricting) effects and positive inotropic effects. Stimulation of alpha-adrenergic receptors results in vasoconstriction and increased systemic blood pressure. Stimulation of beta-adrenergic receptors increases the force and rate of myocardial contraction.

The physiological effect of these drugs includes improved perfusion and oxygenation of the heart, with increased stroke volume and heart rate and increased cardiac output. Increased cardiac output in turn increases tissue perfusion and oxygenation. The main disadvantage is that increases in stroke volume and heart rate also increase the oxygen requirements of the myocardium. These drugs may be used in the early stages of shock, especially in types of shock characterised by vasodilation.

Nursing responsibilities

- Carefully monitor responses in the older adult, who may be especially sensitive to sympathomimetics and require lower doses.
- Document lung sounds, vital signs and haemodynamic parameters before starting the medication and then according to institutional policy (usually every 5 to 15 minutes).
- When administering these drugs by the subcutaneous route, carefully aspirate the injection site to avoid injecting the drug directly into a blood vessel.
- Use the intravenous route only with continuous infusion pumps. Carefully adjust the dose to accommodate the person's cardiovascular status (as ordered by the doctor or by written protocol).
- Record and monitor urine output. Report output of less than 0.5 mL/kg/hr.
- Be aware that the sympathomimetics are incompatible with sodium bicarbonate or alkaline solutions.
- When administering drugs that cause vasoconstriction, such as noradrenaline and metaraminol, monitor the intravenous insertion site for infiltration. If infiltration does occur, stop the infusion and notify the physician immediately as infiltration may cause ischaemia and necrosis of tissue.

Health education for the person and family

- Because these drugs mimic a physiological reaction to stress, they may cause feelings of anxiety.
- Close monitoring to adjust the dose will be carried out by qualified nurses using written protocols.
- Report heart palpitations or chest pain immediately.

VASODILATORS

Nitroglycerin (Glycerol trinitrate)
Nitroprusside (Nipride)

Drugs that cause vasodilation act directly on smooth muscle affecting both arterioles and veins. Peripheral resistance, cardiac output and pulmonary wedge pressure are all reduced as a result of the vasodilation. These effects decrease the oxygen need of the heart and decrease pulmonary congestion. Vasodilators are used primarily in the treatment of cardiogenic shock and may be combined with a sympathomimetic (e.g. dopamine).

Nursing responsibilities

- Protect these drugs from light by wrapping the intravenous bag in the package that is provided.
- Mix with 5% dextrose only.
- Infuse via an infusion pump and use within 4 hours of reconstitution.
- Do not add other medications to the solution.
- Assess mental status, blood pressure and pulse prior to initiating medication. Thereafter, assess blood pressure and pulse according to institutional policy (usually every 5 minutes initially, then every 15 minutes until stable and then hourly).
- Monitor for confusion, dizziness, tachycardia, arrhythmias, hypotension and adventitious breath sounds. Report these immediately if they occur and slow infusion to a keep-open rate.
- With nitroprusside infusions, monitor for signs of thiocyanate poisoning (nausea, disorientation, muscle spasms, decreased or absent reflexes) if infusion lasts longer than 72 hours.
- Keep the person in bed with side rails up.

Health education for the person and family

- It is important for the person to stay in bed and change positions slowly to avoid dizziness.
- The blood pressure and pulse are taken frequently to adjust the dose of medication.
- Headache is a common side effect.

- calcium to replace calcium lost as a result of blood transfusions
- anti-arrhythmic agents to stabilise heart rhythm
- broad-spectrum antibiotics to suppress organisms responsible for septic shock
- adrenaline, antihistamines, corticosteroids and inhaled beta$_2$ agonists to treat anaphylactic shock
- morphine to dilate veins and decrease anxiety.

Oxygen therapy

Establishing and maintaining a patent airway and ensuring adequate oxygenation are critical interventions in reversing shock. All people in shock (even those with adequate respirations) should receive oxygen therapy (usually by mask or nasal cannula) to maintain the PaO_2 at greater than 80 mmHg during the first 4 to 6 hours of care. If the person's unassisted respiration cannot maintain PaO_2 at this level, ventilatory assistance may be necessary. Care of the person requiring ventilatory assistance is discussed in the chapter 'Nursing care of people with gas exchange disorders'.

Fluid resuscitation

The most effective treatment for the person in hypovolaemic shock is the administration of intravenous fluids or blood. Fluids are also appropriate in the management of septic and neurogenic shock. However, depending on pulmonary artery pressure, the person with cardiogenic shock may require either fluid replacement or restriction.

Various fluids may be administered alone or in combination as part of fluid replacement therapy in treating shock. Fluid replacements are administered through two large-bore cannulae via peripheral intravenous access or through a central line. Current fluid resuscitation guidelines include rapid crystalloid infusion followed by blood transfusion. Whole blood or blood products increase the oxygen-carrying capacity of the blood and thus increase oxygenation of cells. Fluid replacements, such as crystalloid and colloid solutions, increase circulating blood volume and tissue perfusion.

CRYSTALLOID SOLUTIONS Crystalloid solutions contain dextrose or electrolytes dissolved in water; those used for management of shock are either isotonic or hypotonic. Isotonic solutions include normal saline (0.9%) and compound sodium lactate (Hartmann's solution). Hypotonic solutions include one-half normal saline (0.45%) and 5% dextrose in water (D_5W).

All crystalloid solutions increase fluid volume in both the intravascular and the interstitial space. Of the total amount infused, only about 25% remains in the intravascular system; the remaining 75% moves into the interstitial space. Consequently, fluid volume is only minimally expanded and the potential for peripheral oedema is increased when crystalloid solutions are used. However, compound sodium lactate (an electrolyte solution) and 0.9% saline are the fluids of choice in treating hypovolaemic shock, especially in the emergency phase of care while blood is being typed and crossmatched. Large amounts of these solutions may be infused rapidly, increasing blood volume and tissue perfusion.

MEDICATION ADMINISTRATION — Colloid solutions

COLLOID SOLUTIONS (PLASMA EXPANDERS)
Albumin 4% (Albumex 4)
Albumin 20% (Albumex 20)
Gelofusine (GelofuG)
Haemaccel
Stable plasma protein solution (SPPS)

These solutions are blood volume expanders and are used to treat hypovolaemic shock due to surgery, haemorrhage, burns or other trauma. Albumin and plasma protein solutions are prepared from healthy blood donors. Gelofusine and Haemaccel are synthetically prepared large molecules. The solutions promote circulatory volume and tissue perfusion by rapidly expanding plasma volume.

Nursing responsibilities

- Before infusion begins, establish baseline of vital signs, lung sounds, heart sounds and (if possible) CVP and pulmonary artery wedge pressure.
- Start administration of ordered intravenous fluids, using a large-gauge (18- or 19-gauge) infusion needle.
- Take and record vital signs as required by institutional policy (usually every 15 to 60 minutes) and assess status.
- Take and record intake and output every 1 to 2 hours.
- Monitor for manifestations of congestive heart failure or pulmonary oedema (dyspnoea, cyanosis, cough, crackles, wheezes). If these manifestations appear, stop the fluids and notify the physician immediately.
- Monitor for bleeding from new sites; an increase in blood pressure may cause bleeding in severed vessels that did not bleed with decreased blood pressure.
- Monitor for manifestations of dehydration (dry lips; scant, dark-coloured urine; loss of skin turgor). Increased intravenous fluids are usually ordered if the person becomes dehydrated.
- Monitor for manifestations of circulatory overload (jugular vein distension, increase in CVP, increase in pulmonary artery wedge pressure). If these manifestations occur, slow rate of infusion and notify physician.
- Monitor prothrombin time, partial thromboplastin time and platelet counts.
- If administering albumin or plasma protein solution, have adrenaline and antihistamines readily available for any manifestations of a hypersensitivity reaction (fever, chills, rash, headache, wheezing, flushing).
- Maintain the person on bed rest with side rails elevated.

Health education for the person and family

- The solutions are given to replace lost serum protein, which helps maintain the volume of blood.
- The vital signs are taken frequently to ensure the safety of the person.

COLLOID SOLUTIONS Colloid solutions contain substances (colloids) that do not diffuse through capillary walls. Hence, colloids tend to remain in the vascular system and increase the osmotic pressure of the serum. This causes fluid to move into the vascular compartment from the interstitial space, resulting in the plasma volume expanding. Colloid solutions used to treat shock include 5% albumin, 25% albumin, Gelofusine, Haemaccel, plasma protein fraction and Dextran.

Colloid products reduce platelet adhesiveness and have been associated with reductions in blood coagulation. Consequently, the person's prothrombin time (PT), International Normalized Ratio (INR), platelet count and activated partial thromboplastin time (APTT) should be monitored when these solutions are administered. Normal values are as follows:

PT	10–15 seconds
INR	1–1.2 seconds
Platelets	$150 - 400 \times 10^9/L$
APTT	< 35 seconds

See the 'Medication administration' box for further information about colloid solutions and associated nursing responsibilities and teaching.

BLOOD AND BLOOD PRODUCTS If hypovolaemic shock is due to haemorrhage, the infusion of blood and blood products may be indicated. Available blood and blood products include fresh whole blood, stored whole blood, packed RBCs, platelet concentrate, fresh-frozen plasma and cryoprecipitate. Often, packed RBCs are given to provide haemoglobin concentration and are supplemented with crystalloids to maintain an adequate circulatory volume. (See discussion of blood administration earlier in the chapter.)

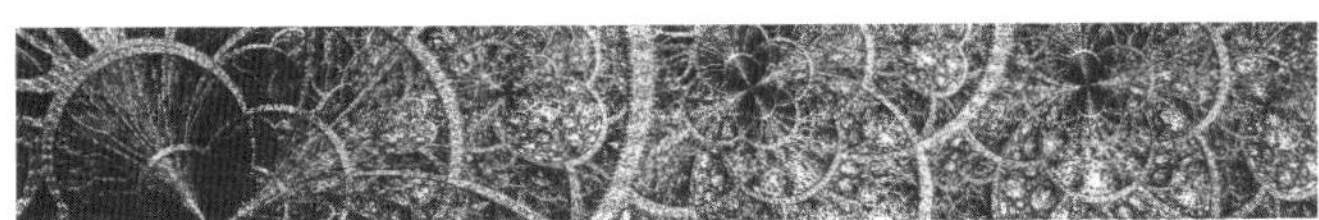

Nursing care

Nursing assessments and interventions to prevent shock are an essential part of the nursing care of every person. The primary nursing interventions to prevent shock are assessment and monitoring.

Health promotion and assessment

Nursing assessments are critical in preventing shock. Identifying people at risk and making focused assessments are essential. Although shock may occur at any age, physiological changes with ageing make the older adult a high-risk population. (See the 'Nursing care of the older adult' box.)

- *Hypovolaemic shock*: people who have undergone surgery, have sustained multiple traumatic injuries or have been seriously burned are most likely to develop hypovolaemic shock. Monitoring fluid status is essential in preventing shock and includes daily assessments of weight, fluid intake by all routes, measurable fluid loss (e.g. urine, vomitus, wound drainage, gastric drainage and chest tube drainage) and fluid loss that must be estimated, such as fluid lost via profuse perspiration and wound drainage. Assessments for the critically ill person are ongoing and include fluid balance, haemodynamic values and vital signs.
- *Cardiogenic shock*: people with left anterior wall myocardial infarctions are at risk of developing cardiogenic shock. Nursing care to prevent the development of cardiogenic shock focuses on maintaining or improving myocardial oxygen supply by providing immediate pain relief, maintaining rest and administering supplemental oxygen.
- *Neurogenic shock*: the risk of neurogenic shock is increased in people who have spinal cord injuries and those who have received spinal anaesthesia. Preventive nursing care includes maintaining immobility of people with spinal cord trauma and elevating the head of the bed 15 to 20 degrees following spinal anaesthesia. Elevations of more than 20 degrees, however, can potentiate headaches following spinal anaesthesia and should be avoided.
- *Anaphylactic shock*: prevent anaphylactic shock by collecting information about allergies and drug reactions during the health history. Note these allergies clearly on all documents and place a special armband on the person. Careful and frequent assessments during blood administration may prevent serious reactions to blood or blood products.
- *Septic shock*: people who are hospitalised, are debilitated, are chronically ill or have undergone invasive procedures or tube insertions are at high risk of septic shock. Nursing care to prevent septic shock includes careful and consistent handwashing, the use of aseptic techniques for procedures (e.g. catheterisations, suctioning, changing dressings, starting and maintaining intravenous fluids or medications) and monitoring for local and systemic manifestations (e.g. WBC and differential counts) of infection.

Nursing diagnoses and interventions

Nursing care for the person in shock focuses on assessing and monitoring overall tissue perfusion and on meeting psychosocial needs of the person and the family. This section discusses nursing diagnoses that are appropriate for the person with hypovolaemic shock. See the 'Nursing care of the older adult' box.

Decreased cardiac output

Decreased cardiac output is the primary problem for the person in shock. Although much of the care related to this diagnosis is collaborative, many independent nursing interventions are critical to the care of the person in shock.

- Assess and monitor cardiovascular function via the following:
  - blood pressure
  - heart rate and rhythm
  - pulse oximetry
  - peripheral pulses
  - haemodynamic monitoring of arterial pressures, pulmonary artery pressures and central venous pressures (CVPs).

NURSING CARE OF THE OLDER ADULT Variations in assessment findings—shock

- Cardiac changes may include a thickened left ventricular wall, decreased elasticity of the myocardium and more rigid valves. These changes result in a decreased stroke volume and cardiac output, thus decreasing responses to shock in general and increasing the risk of cardiogenic shock.
- Decreased arterial wall elasticity and vasomotor tone reduce the ability to respond to a decrease in oxygenation.
- Decreased elasticity and turgor of the skin make assessments of skin turgor more difficult.
- Previous medication and blood administration increase the risk of anaphylactic shock.
- Decreased immune system response increases the risk of septic shock.

A baseline assessment is necessary to establish the stage of shock. If palpable peripheral pulses and audible (to auscultation) blood pressure are lost, inserting central arterial, venous and pulmonary artery catheters is essential to establish progression of shock accurately and to evaluate the person's response to therapy.

- Measure and record intake and output (total output and urinary output) hourly. *A decrease in circulating blood volume with hypotension and the effect of the compensatory mechanisms associated with shock can cause renal failure. Urinary output of < 0.5 mL/kg/hr in an acutely ill adult indicates reduced renal blood flow.*
- Monitor bowel sounds, abdominal distension and abdominal pain. *Decreased splenic blood flow reduces bowel motility and peristalsis; paralytic ileus may result.*
- Monitor for sudden sharp chest pain, dyspnoea, cyanosis, anxiety and restlessness. *Haemoconcentration and increased platelet aggregation may result in pulmonary emboli.*
- Maintain bed rest and provide (to the extent possible) a calm, quiet environment. Place in a supine position with the legs elevated to about 20 degrees, trunk flat, and head and shoulders elevated higher than the chest (see Figure 10.9). *Limiting activity and ensuring rest decreases the workload of the heart. The supine position with legs elevated increases venous return; however, this position should not be used for people in cardiogenic shock. The Trendelenburg position is no longer recommended because it causes the abdominal organs to press against the diaphragm (limiting respirations), decreases filling of the coronary arteries and initiates aortic and carotid sinus reflexes.*

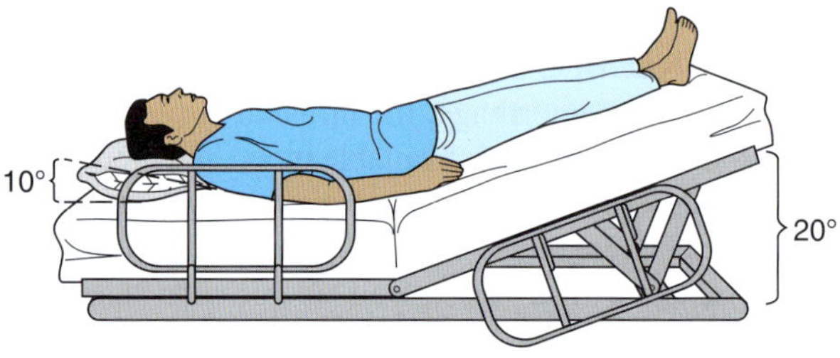

FIGURE 10.9 ***The person in shock should be positioned with the lower extremities elevated approximately 20 degrees (knees straight), trunk horizontal and the head elevated about 10 degrees***

TRANSLATION TO PRACTICE Evidence-based practice for care of ICU people sustaining multiple trauma

Ventilator-associated pneumonia (VAP) is an important person safety issue in critically injured people. The Infectious Diseases Society of America (IDSA) published an evidence-based clinical guideline for the prevention and elimination of VAP in 2016 (IDSA, 2016). The Society recommends the use of a facility-wide VAP infection prevention and control program and overall infection prevention and antimicrobial stewardship. The guideline describes the critical topics of problem identification, surveillance and how it is defined, risk assessment, and the development and use of a surveillance plan and prevention strategies. The guideline also provides examples of documents and reminders that can be used to provide systematic surveillance and management strategies. Research has also been undertaken to include VAP challenges and complications associated with COVID-19 (Giacobbe et al., 2021; Wicky, Niedermann & Timsit, 2021).

IMPLICATIONS FOR NURSING

Recommendations related to prevention of complications in ventilated patients include:

- tracheal tube and cuff design prevent micro-aspiration and bacterial colonisation
- ensuring tracheal cuff pressures are maintained to minimise passage of secretions and mucosal damage
- kinetic therapy—position movements to encourage mucociliary clearance
- strict attention to hand hygiene by staff and visitors
- use of closed-circuit suction systems, heat and moisture exchanges, and limiting ventilator tube changes to when soiled only
- minimisation of reflux and aspiration of gastric contents (Papazian, Klompas & Luyt, 2020)
- challenges and complications associated with COVID-19.

CRITICAL THINKING IN PERSON-CENTRED CARE

1. Considering the information from this guideline, how would you communicate the recommendations to the medical staff for the person with mechanical ventilation?
2. What is the rationale behind the preceding recommendations?

NURSING CARE PLAN A person with septic shock

Huang Mei Lan is a 43-year-old unmarried female who lives alone in a major city. Ms Huang came to Australia 15 years ago from China and now speaks English well. Her family still lives in China. She worked in a neighbourhood sewing shop until 3 years ago when she was diagnosed with breast cancer. Her treatment included mastectomy of the affected breast and follow-up chemotherapy.

Last month, Ms Huang experienced a recurrence of cancer in the lymph glands of the affected side. Surgery to remove the glands was performed and chemotherapy started. Ms Huang has a central line, a urinary catheter and a surgical incision. She is underweight, weak and depressed. Although she has multiple physical problems, she never complains or asks for any kind of medication.

ASSESSMENT

Ms Huang's nurse, Robert O'Brien, enters her room early in the morning to make an initial assessment. He finds Ms Huang huddled in the middle of the bed, shivering violently. Her vital signs are T 40°C, P 110, R 30 and BP 106/66. Her skin is hot, dry and flushed, with poor turgor. She is alert and oriented but is restless and appears anxious. Ms Huang states she is nauseated and suddenly begins vomiting and is incontinent of liquid stool. Laboratory data indicate leucocytosis, respiratory alkalosis and reduced platelet count. Blood cultures, as well as cultures of Ms Huang's sputum, urine and wound drainage, are conducted. She is diagnosed as having septic shock.

Gelofusine is ordered per intravenous line and intravenous broad-spectrum antibiotics are begun until the organism and its portal of entry can be determined. Despite treatment, Ms Huang's condition worsens. Her blood pressure continues to drop, her skin becomes cool and cyanotic, and she begins to have periods of disorientation. She is transferred to the critical care unit. As she is being prepared for the transfer, she begins to cry and asks, 'Am I going to die?'

DIAGNOSES

- *Ineffective breathing pattern* related to rapid respirations and progression of septic shock.
- *Ineffective tissue perfusion* related to progression of septic shock with decreased cardiac output, hypotension and massive vasodilation.
- *Deficient fluid volume* related to vomiting, diarrhoea, high fever and shift of intravascular volume to interstitial spaces.
- *Anxiety* related to feelings that illness is worsening and is potentially life threatening, and to the transfer to the critical care unit.

PLANNING

- Monitor respiratory status, including respiratory rate, rhythm and breath sounds.
- Monitor neurological status, including mental status and level of consciousness.
- Monitor cardiovascular status, including arterial blood pressure; rate, rhythm and quality of pulses; central venous pressure; pulmonary artery pressure and cardiac output.
- Monitor colour and character of skin.
- Monitor body temperature every 2 hours.
- Monitor results of ABGs, blood counts, clotting times and platelet counts.
- Monitor urinary output hourly, reporting any output of < 0.5 mL/kg/hr.

Expected outcomes

- Maintain adequate circulating blood volume.
- Regain and maintain blood gas parameters within normal limits.
- Regain and maintain stable haemodynamic levels.
- Verbalise increased ability to cope with stressors.

IMPLEMENTATION

- Perform hourly neurological assessment, including mental status and level of consciousness.
- Implement continuous cardiac monitoring, including arterial blood pressure; rate, rhythm and quality of pulses; central venous pressure; pulmonary artery pressure and cardiac output.
- Regularly assess colour and character of skin.
- Take samples of blood for ABGs, blood counts, clotting times and platelet counts and report results.
- Assess respiratory status, including respiratory rate, rhythm and breath sounds.
- Assess body temperature every 2 hours.
- Measure urinary output hourly and report output of < 0.5 mL/kg/hr.
- Explain procedures and provide comfort measures (oral care, skin care, turning, positioning).
- Report abnormal findings to medical team.

EVALUATION

Despite intensive nursing and medical care, Ms Huang's condition remains critical. The interventions are continued.

CRITICAL THINKING IN THE NURSING PROCESS

1. Vasoconstrictors may be used in the treatment of septic shock. Explain the rationale for their use.
2. While monitoring Ms Huang's ABGs, the nurse notes that her PaO_2 is < 60 mmHg and her $PaCO_2$ is > 50 mmHg. What do these findings indicate and why have they occurred?
3. Ms Huang has been given large amounts of colloids intravenously. Haemodynamic monitoring indicates a higher than normal CVP and pulmonary artery pressure. What do these findings indicate? What physical assessments would you make to confirm the changes?

REFLECTION ON THE NURSING PROCESS

1. Outline the component of Ms Huang's condition and physical status that posed potential risks for her developing septic shock.
2. What education strategies could have been used to assist Ms Huang to identify and communicate issues prior to her deterioration?

Ineffective tissue perfusion

As shock progresses, diminished tissue perfusion causes ischaemia and hypoxia of major organ systems. As shock worsens, blood flow and oxygenation of the lungs, heart and brain are also impaired. Hypoxia and ischaemia result from decreased tissue perfusion in the kidneys, brain, heart, lungs, gastrointestinal tract and the periphery.

- Monitor skin colour, temperature, turgor and moisture. *Decreased tissue perfusion is evidenced by the skin becoming pale, cool and moist; as haemoglobin concentrations decrease, cyanosis occurs.*
- Monitor cardiopulmonary function by assessing/monitoring the following:
  - blood pressure (by auscultation or by haemodynamic monitoring)
  - rate and depth of respirations
  - lung sounds
  - pulse oximetry
  - peripheral pulses (brachial, radial, dorsalis pedis and posterior tibial); include presence, equality, rate, rhythm and quality. (If unable to palpate pulses, use a device such as a Doppler ultrasound to assess peripheral arterial blood flow.)
  - jugular vein distension
  - central venous pressure measurements.

  Baseline vital signs are necessary to determine trends in subsequent findings. As shock progresses, the blood pressure decreases and the pulse becomes rapid, weak and thready. As perfusion of the lungs decreases, crackles, wheezes and dyspnoea are commonly assessed. Capillary refill is prolonged and peripheral pulses are weak or non-palpable. Neck veins that cannot be seen when the person is in the supine position indicate decreased intravascular volume. CVP is an accurate means of determining fluid status in the person in shock; the findings will be low (5 to 15 cm of water is normal) in hypovolaemic shock because of the decreased blood volume. (See the chapter 'Nursing care of people with altered fluid, electrolyte and acid–base balance' for a discussion of CVP.)
- Monitor body temperature. *An elevated body temperature increases metabolic demands, depleting reserves of bodily energy. It also increases myocardial oxygen demand and may place the person with previous cardiac problems at even greater risk of hypoperfusion.*
- Monitor urinary output per indwelling catheter hourly, using a urine drainage measure bag. *Urine output is a reliable indicator of renal perfusion.*
- Assess mental status and level of consciousness. *The appropriateness of the person's behaviour and responses reflects the adequacy of cerebral circulation. Restlessness and anxiety are common early in shock; in later stages, the person may become lethargic and progress to a comatose state. Altered levels of consciousness are the result of both cerebral hypoxia and the effects of acidosis on brain cells.*

Anxiety

Many people in hypovolaemic shock have experienced some form of major trauma and may have life-threatening, multiple injuries. Following on-the-scene treatment, the person is usually admitted to the healthcare setting through the emergency department. Surgery may be required to treat injuries, followed by care in a critical care unit. Throughout this sequence of crisis events, treatment is invasive and contact with family is minimal. In situations of uncertainty, instability and change people and their families may respond with anxiety, fear and powerlessness. These responses are affected by age, developmental level, cultural and ethnic group, experience with illness and the healthcare system, and support systems.

- Assess the cause(s) of the anxiety and manipulate the environment to provide periods of rest. *Reducing stimuli that cause anxiety is calming and facilitates rest, which is necessary in the person at risk of bleeding.*
- Administer prescribed pain medications on a regular basis. *Pain precipitates and/or aggravates anxiety.*
- Provide interventions to increase comfort and reduce restlessness:
  - Maintain a clean environment.
  - Provide skin and oral care.
  - Monitor the effectiveness of ventilation or oxygen therapy.
  - Eliminate all non-essential activities.
  - Remain with the person during procedures.
  - Speak slowly and calmly, using short sentences.
  - Use touch to provide support.

  Unfamiliar sounds, sights and odours can increase anxiety. Damp skin or a dry mouth increases discomfort. Inadequate gas exchange with a decrease in oxygen or an increase in carbon dioxide in the blood may cause the person to experience a 'feeling of doom'. Activity increases the body's need for oxygen. Listening and touch provide support in an environment in which the person often feels alone and abandoned. Severe anxiety interferes with the ability to understand others and to respond appropriately.
- Provide support for the person and family:
  - Provide time, space and privacy for family members.
  - Allow family members access to the person when feasible.
  - Encourage the expression of feelings and concerns. Provide anticipatory guidance to prepare for recovery or death and to support realistic hope.
  - Acknowledge the beliefs, values and expectations of the person and family.

  Allowing the family access to the person reduces anxiety and gives both the person and the family some feeling of control. If the prognosis is poor, access and involvement allow the family to begin the grieving process. If recovery is expected, contact provides the person and family with a feeling of hope. Supporting the person and family facilitates concrete problem solving, promotes acceptance of the illness and its implications, and helps them begin to establish ways of managing the illness experience.

- Provide information about the current setting to both the person and family; give the family information about available resources (such as pastoral care, social services, temporary housing, meals). *Knowing what to expect and how to control the environment to meet basic needs reduces anxiety.*

Community-based care

Home care for the person who has experienced shock is highly individualised, depending on the cause and the illness or injury that caused shock. Therefore, topics for consideration are not included in this section.

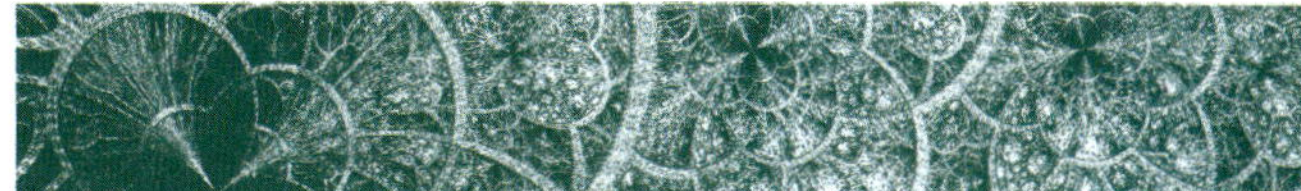

CHAPTER HIGHLIGHTS

- Traumatic injuries affect human tissues and organs resulting from a transfer of energy from the environment. Energy sources can be mechanical, gravitational, thermal, electrical, physical or chemical.
- Trauma types include minor trauma, which causes minimal damage to underlying tissues, or major trauma, which can involve a serious single-system injury or multiple trauma. Trauma is further categorised into blunt and penetrating trauma. Blunt trauma is caused by various forces such as deceleration, acceleration, shearing, compression or crushing. Penetrating trauma occurs when a foreign object enters the body.
- Maintenance of the airway and cervical spine are the highest priority in the trauma victim, with airway assessment superseding all other interventions.
- The primary assessment conducted by the nurse identifies all life-threatening injuries and performance of appropriate interventions. The secondary assessment is when the nurse identifies all injuries in order to prioritise care.
- Shock is a clinical syndrome characterised by a systemic imbalance between oxygen supply and demand. This imbalance results in a state of inadequate blood flow to body organs and tissues, causing life-threatening cellular dysfunction.
- The symptoms of shock arise from the body's attempts to maintain vital organs (heart and brain) and to preserve life in response to a decrease in oxygen delivery to the cells.
- An important early sign of shock is a change in the level of consciousness, with restlessness being a common symptom of cerebral hypoxia.
- Shock is defined in three stages: compensatory (stage 1), an early and reversible stage; progressive (stage 2), occurring after a fluid loss of 35–50% (1,800 to 2,500 mL), where the affected cells switch from aerobic to anaerobic metabolism in order to remain alive; and the final stage is irreversible (stage 3), where tissue anoxia and cellular death become widespread.
- Hypovolaemic shock is the most common type of shock and is caused by a decrease in the circulating blood volume by 15% or greater.
- Cardiogenic shock is caused when the pumping ability of the heart is compromised to the point where adequate cardiac output cannot be maintained.
- Obstructive shock is caused by an obstruction in the heart or great vessels that either impedes venous return or prevents effective cardiac pumping action. Causes can include cardiac tamponade, pneumothorax, pulmonary embolism and aortic stenosis.
- Septic shock is a part of a progressive syndrome called systemic inflammatory response syndrome (SIRS), a condition most often caused by Gram-negative infections.
- Anaphylactic shock is caused by a fulminating hypersensitivity reaction to a foreign substance.

CONCEPT CHECK

1 What is the most common mechanical source of injury in adults of all ages?
1 gunshot wounds
2 fire
3 drowning
4 motor vehicles

2 Severe facial injuries, such as those resulting from going through a windshield, increase the risk of all of the following. Which would you assess first?
1 airway obstruction
2 haemorrhage
3 contusions
4 fractures

3 Which on-the-scene intervention would be a priority?
1 Determine cause of injury.
2 Assess airway patency.
3 Assess peripheral capillary refill.
4 Palpate for internal haemorrhage.

4 You are monitoring blood administration to a trauma victim in shock. Which of the following assessments indicate a dangerous transfusion reaction?
1 red raised areas (wheals) on the skin that itch
2 an increase in body temperature by 3°C
3 decreasing blood pressure and dyspnoea
4 increasing blood pressure and pulse

5 What type of shock causes widespread vasodilation and decreased peripheral resistance?
1 cardiogenic shock
2 septic shock
3 hypovolaemic shock
4 obstructive shock

6 What is the best method to manage uncontrolled bleeding?
1 apply direct pressure
2 clamp a visible vessel
3 apply a tourniquet
4 elevate the injured part

7 Trauma is defined as:
1 injury to human tissues from the transfer of energy
2 result of random chance
3 accidental injury
4 an intentional injury

8 Shock is defined as:
1 a systemic imbalance between oxygen supply and demand
2 sufficient cardiac output
3 haemorrhage
4 abnormal blood pressure

9 Distributive shock is caused by:
1 blood loss
2 widespread vasodilation
3 ineffective cardiac pumping action
4 hypersensitivity reaction

10 What actions should you perform when receiving handover of care immediately postoperative in order to prevent the onset of hypovolaemic shock?
1 Elevate the head of the bed.
2 Provide immediate pain relief.
3 Monitor strict intake and output.
4 Practise careful and consistent hand hygiene.

BIBLIOGRAPHY

American College of Emergency Physicians (2022). *Policy compendium*. Retrieved from https://www.acep.org/

Attorney-General's Department (2022). *Protecting the rights of older adults*. Retrieved from https://humanrights.gov.au

Australian College for Emergency Medicine (2021). *Clinical guidelines*. Retrieved from https://acem.org.au/

Australian Commission on Safety and Quality in Health Care (ACSQHC) (2021). *National Safety and Quality Health Service Standards* (2nd ed.). Sydney: ACSQHC.

Australian Human Rights Commission (2021). *Elder abuse*. Retrieved from https://humanrights.gov.au

Australian Institute of Health and Welfare (AIHW) (2021). *Family, domestic and sexual violence in Australia, 2021*. Retrieved from https://www.aihw.gov.au/

Australian Institute of Health and Welfare (AIHW) (2022). *Injury: Overview*. Retrieved from https://www.aihw.gov.au/

Australian Organ and Tissue Donation and Transplantation Authority Act 2008. Retrieved from https://www.comlaw.gov.au/

Centers for Disease Control and Prevention (2012). Guidelines for field triage of injured patients. *Morbidity and Mortality Weekly Report, 61*(RR–1). Retrieved from https://www.cdc.gov/

Curtis, K., Ramsden, C., Sharban, R. Z., Fry, M. & Considine, J. (2019). *Emergency and trauma care for nurses and paramedics* (3rd ed.). Chatswood, NSW: Elsevier.

de Alencar Domingues, C., Coimbra, R., Poggetti, R. S. et al. (2018). New trauma and injury severity score (TRISS) adjustments for survival prediction. *World Journal of Emergency Surgery, 13*, 12. https://doi.org/10.1186/s13017-018-0171-8

Filipescu, R., Powers, C., Yu, H. et al. (2020). Improving the performance of the revised trauma score using shock index, peripheral oxygen saturation, and temperature: A national trauma database study 2011 to 2015. *Surgery*, *167*(5), 821–828.

Giacobbe, D. R., Battaglini, D., Enrile, E. M. et al. (2021). Incident and prognosis of ventilator-associated pneumonia in critically ill patients with COVID-19: A multicentre study. *Journal of Clinical Medicine*, *10*(4). https://doi.org/10.3390/jcm10040555

Infectious Diseases Society of America (IDSA) (2016). *Management of adults with hospital-acquired and ventilator-associated pneumonia: 2016 clinical practice guidelines by the Infectious Diseases Society of America*. Omaha: Author. Retrieved from https://www.thoracic.org/

Jeong, J. H., Park, Y. J., Kim, D. H. et al. (2017). The new trauma score (NTS): A modification of the revised trauma score for better trauma mortality prediction. *BMC Surgery*, *17*, 77. doi: 10.1186/s12893-017-0272-4

Kaspiew, R., Carson, R., Dow, B., Qu, L., Hand, K., Roopani, D., Gahan, L. & O'Keeffe, D. (2019). *Elder abuse national research*. Retrieved from https://aifs.gov.au/

Kochanek, P. M., Tasker, R., Bell, M. J. et al. (2019). Management of pediatric severe traumatic brain injury: 2019 consensus and guidelines-based algorithm for first and second tier therapies. *Pediatric Critical Care Medicine*, *20*(3), 269–279.

Levett-Jones, T., Dwyer, T., Reid-Searl, K., Heaton, L., Flenady, T., Applegarth, J., Guinea, S. & Andersen, P. (2017). *Patient Safety Competency Framework (PSCF) for Nursing Students*. Sydney. Retrieved from http://psframework.wpengine.com/

McCance, K. L. & Huether, S. E. (2018). *Pathophysiology: The biologic basis for disease in adults and children* (8th ed.). St Louis, MO: Elsevier.

Norris, T. L. (2018). *Porth's pathophysiology: Concepts of altered health states* (10th ed.). Philadelphia: Lippincott Williams & Wilkins.

Papazian, L., Klompas, M. & Luyt, C. E. (2020). Ventilator-associated pneumonia in adults: A narrative review. *Intensive Care Medicine*, *46*, 888–906.

Rabinstein, A. A. (ed.) (2019). Traumatic spinal cord injury. *Neurological emergencies: A practical approach*. New York: Springer.

Wicky, P. H., Niedermann, M. S. & Timsit, J.-F. (2021). Ventilator-associated pneumonia in the era of COVID-19 pandemic: How common and what is the impact? *Critical Care*, *15*. https://doi.org/10.1186/s13054-021-03571-z

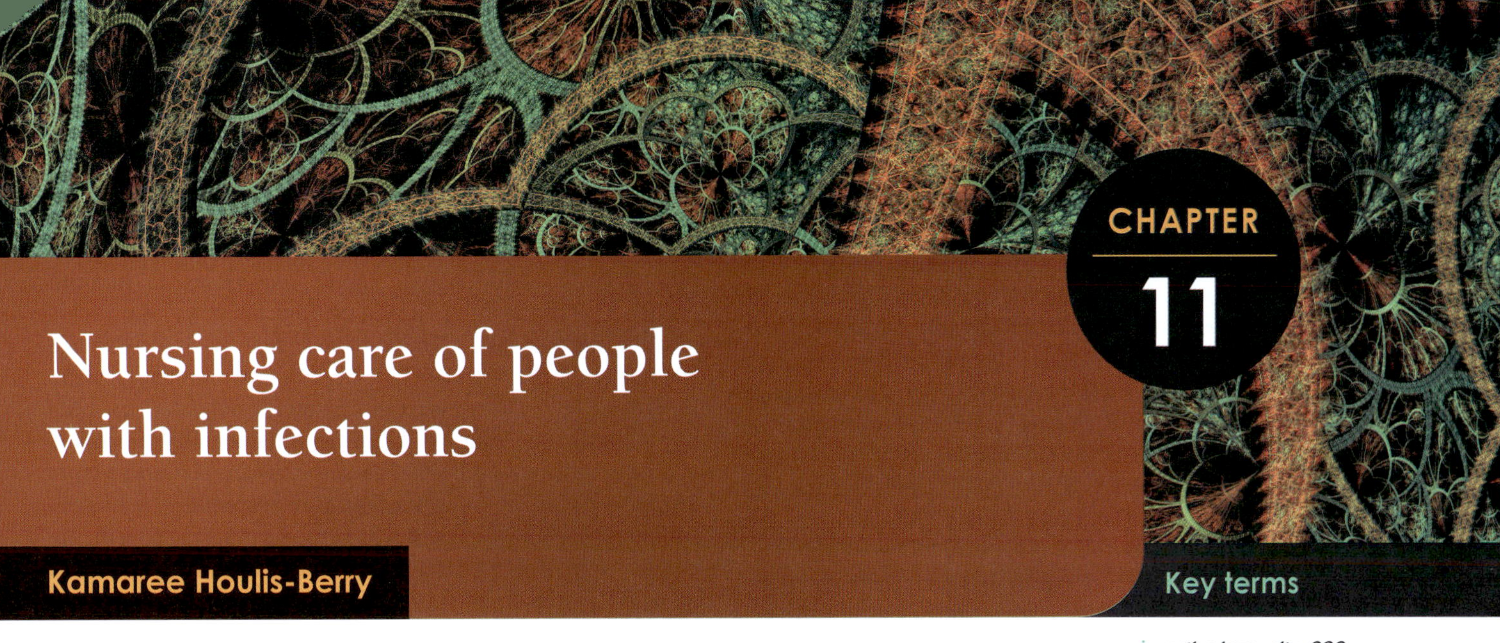

CHAPTER 11

Nursing care of people with infections

Kamaree Houlis-Berry

Learning outcomes

- Discuss the components and functions of the immune system and the immune response.
- Compare antibody-mediated and cell-mediated immune responses.
- Describe the pathophysiology of wound healing, inflammation and infection.
- Identify factors responsible for and the implications of healthcare-associated infections.
- Discuss the nursing implications and health education in the prevention and treatments of inflammation and infection.

Clinical competencies

- Apply standard precautions and evidence-based practices to prevent the spread of infection within the person, to other people in the facility, to members of the interprofessional team and to visitors.
- Provide safe, effective and respectful patient-centred care for patients with inflammation and infection.
- Collaborate with the interprofessional care team to integrate care of people with infection.
- Promote therapeutic levels and completed dosage of anti-inflammatory and anti-infective medication through prompt administration and person and family teaching.
- Assess for hypersensitivities to anti-inflammatories and anti-infectives prior to and during administration.
- Participate in quality improvement processes to reduce the rates and risk of infection.

Key terms

OVERVIEW OF THE IMMUNE SYSTEM

The human body is continually threatened by foreign substances, infectious agents and abnormal cells. The immune system is the body's major defence mechanism against these threats. Recent years have seen the emergence of resistant microorganisms such as methicillin-resistant *Staphylococcus aureus* (MRSA) and altered strains of familiar diseases, such as multiple-drug-resistant tuberculosis. Other diseases have also emerged, including severe acute respiratory syndrome (SARS), *Clostridium difficile*, human immunodeficiency virus (HIV) and coronavirus (COVID-19). Read more about COVID-19 in the COVID Primer.

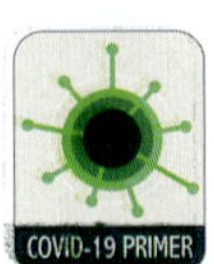

The critical need to prevent healthcare-associated infections and their resulting impact on the patient and healthcare costs is an emerging theme.

A thorough knowledge of the immune system increases understanding of inflammatory responses, resistance to infectious disease and the importance of immunisation. This foundation can help the nurse to promote health by preventing and identifying infections and teaching people and families about recommended treatment regimens.

The immune system is a complex and intricate network of specialised cells, tissues and organs. Cells of the immune system seek out and destroy damaged cells and foreign tissue, yet recognise and preserve host cells. The immune system defends and protects the body from invading pathogens, removes and destroys damaged or dead cells, and identifies and destroys malignant cells, thereby preventing their further development into tumours.

The immune system is activated by minor injuries, such as small lacerations or bruises, or by major injuries, such as burns, surgeries and systemic diseases (e.g. pneumonia). The immune response may be innate or adaptive. **Innate immunity** provides non-specific, generic responses to harmful events. These responses prevent or limit the entry of invaders into the body, thereby limiting the extent of tissue damage and reducing the workload of the adaptive immune system. Inflammation is a non-specific response activated by both minor and major injuries. When the inflammatory process is unable to destroy invading organisms or toxins, a more specific response called the **adaptive immune response** is activated. Adaptive immunity provides a response that is specific to unique organisms. It includes memory that hastens future responses to the organism.

Immune system components

The immune system consists of molecules, cells and organs that produce the immune response (see Table 11.1). These components may be involved in the non-specific inflammatory response, the specific immunological response, or both.

Leucocytes

Leucocytes, or white blood cells (WBCs), are the primary cells involved in both innate and adaptive immune system responses. Like all blood cells, leucocytes derive from stem cells, the haemocytoblasts, in the bone marrow (see Figure 11.1). Leucocytes are not confined to the circulation; they use it to transport themselves to the site of an inflammatory or immune response. As the mobile units of the immune system, leucocytes detect, attack and destroy anything that is recognised

TABLE 11.1 Cells and tissues of the immune system

COMPONENT	LOCATION	FUNCTION
Leucocytes		
Granulocytes		
Neutrophils	Circulation	Phagocytosis and chemotaxis
Eosinophils	Circulation, respiratory tract and gastrointestinal tract	Phagocytosis Protection against parasites Involved in allergic response
Basophils	Circulation	Release of chemotactic substances
Monocytes and macrophages	Circulation (monocytes) and body tissue, such as skin (histocytes), liver (Kupffer cells), alveoli, spleen, tonsils, lymph nodes, bone marrow, brain	Trapping and phagocytising of foreign substances and cellular debris Secretion of interleukin-1 to stimulate lymphocyte growth
Lymphocytes		
T cells (mature in thymus gland)	Circulation, lymph system, tissues	Activation of T and B cells Control of viral infections and destruction of cancer cells Involved in hypersensitivity reactions and graft tissue rejection
B cells (mature in bone marrow)	Circulation, spleen	Production of antibodies (immunoglobulins) to specific antigens
NK (natural killer) cells	Circulation	Cytotoxic; killing of tumour cells, fungi, viral-infected cells and foreign tissue
Lymphoid tissues		
Primary or central lymphoid structures	Bone marrow and thymus gland	Production of immune cells; sites for cell maturation
Secondary or peripheral lymphoid structures	Lymph nodes, spleen, tonsils, intestinal lymphoid tissue, lymphoid tissue in other organs	Sites for activation of immune cells by antigens

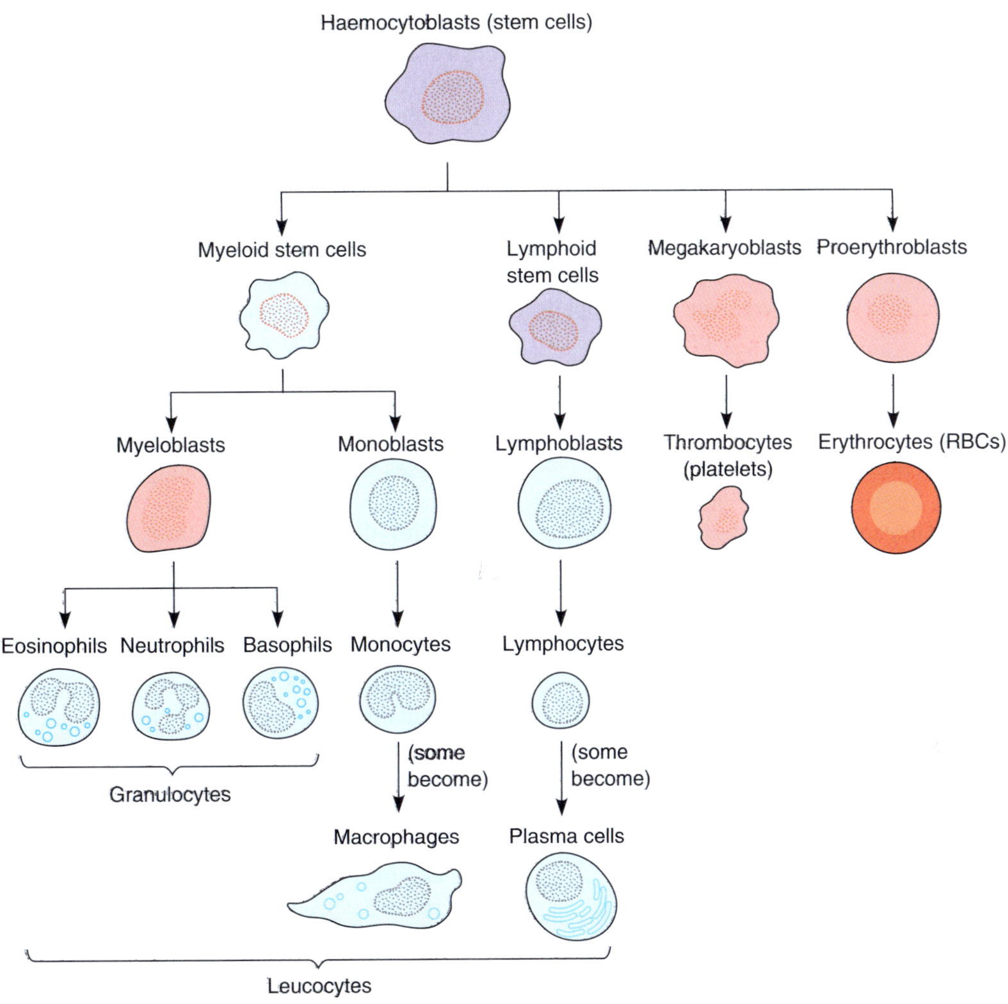

FIGURE 11.1 *The development and differentiation of leucocytes from haemocytoblasts*

as 'foreign'. They are able to move through tissue spaces, locating damaged tissue and infection by responding to chemicals released by other leucocytes and damaged tissue.

The normal number of circulating leucocytes is 4,500 to 10,000 cells per cubic millimetre (mm^3) of blood. Many more leucocytes are marginated. Margination refers to adhesion of leucocytes to vascular epithelial cells along the vessel walls, in other tissue spaces or in the lymph system. Marginated leucocytes migrate into injured areas or areas where pathogens infiltrate as part of the innate immune response. In the presence of an attack such as an infection, additional WBCs are released from the bone marrow, leading to **leucocytosis**, a WBC count of greater than 10,000/mm^3. As WBCs move out of the bone marrow into the blood, the bone marrow increases its production of additional leucocytes. A decrease in the number of circulating leucocytes, known as **leucopenia**, occurs when bone marrow activity is suppressed or leucocyte destruction increases.

Leucocytes are divided into three major groups: granulocytes, monocytes and lymphocytes. The granulocytes and monocytes derive from the myeloid stem cells of the bone marrow and are instrumental in the inflammatory response. Lymphocytes derive from the lymphoid stem cells of the bone marrow and are the primary cells involved in the specific immune response. In laboratory tests, the WBC count indicates the total number of circulating leucocytes. The white cell count (WCC) differential identifies the portion of the total represented by each type of leucocyte.

GRANULOCYTES Granulocytes constitute 60% to 80% of the total number of normal blood leucocytes. Their cytoplasm has a granular appearance and their nuclei are distinctively multi-lobular (see Figure 11.1). Granulocytes have a short life span, measured in hours to days, compared to the lifespan of monocytes, which is measured in months to years. Granulocytes play a key role in protecting the body from harmful microorganisms during acute inflammation and infection. There are three types of granulocytes: neutrophils, eosinophils and basophils.

Neutrophils, also called polymorphonuclear leucocytes (PMNs or polys), are the most plentiful of the granulocytes, constituting 55% to 70% of the total number of circulating leucocytes. Neutrophils are phagocytic cells, responsible for engulfing and destroying foreign agents, particularly bacteria and small particles. Neutrophils are the first phagocytic cells to arrive at the site of invasion, drawn by chemicals released by damaged tissue and invading organisms.

Neutrophils are produced in the bone marrow and released into the circulation when they mature. Segmented neutrophils (or segs) are mature forms and usually account for about 55% of total leucocytes. *Bands* are immature neutrophils and usually comprise 5% of leucocytes. As neutrophils mature, their nucleus changes from round to kidney-bean-shaped (banded) and then the nucleus separates into small, attached segments; thus the designations 'banded' versus 'segmented' neutrophils. It takes about 10 days for a neutrophil to mature and be released into the circulation. Once released, neutrophils have a circulating half-life of 6 to 10 hours. They cannot replicate and must be replaced constantly to maintain adequate numbers in the circulation. They do not return to the bone marrow.

Eosinophils account for 1% to 4% of the total number of circulating leucocytes. They mature in the bone marrow in 3 to 6 days before being released into the circulation. Eosinophils have a circulating half-life of 30 minutes and a tissue half-life of 12 days. They are phagocytic cells but are less efficient at this process than neutrophils. Eosinophils are found in large numbers in the respiratory and gastrointestinal tracts, where they are thought to be responsible for protecting the body from parasitic worms, including tapeworms, flukes, pinworms and hookworms. Eosinophils surround the parasite and release toxic enzymes from their cytoplasmic granules. The parasite, although too large to be phagocytised, is destroyed. Eosinophils are also involved in a hypersensitivity response, inactivating some of the inflammatory chemicals released during the inflammatory response.

Basophils constitute about 0.5% to 1% of the circulating leucocytes. These cells are not phagocytic. Granules within basophils contain proteins and chemicals such as heparin, histamine, bradykinin, serotonin and slow-reacting substances of anaphylaxis (leukotrienes). These substances are released into the bloodstream during an acute hypersensitivity reaction or stress response.

MONOCYTES, MACROPHAGES AND DENDRITIC CELLS Monocytes, macrophages and dendritic cells are the mediators of immunity. They recognise foreign matter (from molecules to cells) and initiate immune responses. *Monocytes* are the largest of the leucocytes and constitute 2% to 3% of circulating leucocytes. After their release from the bone marrow, monocytes circulate in the serum for 1 to 2 days. They then migrate throughout the body, attaching themselves to the tissues, where they remain for months or even years until they are activated. Monocytes mature into **macrophages** after settling into the tissues. Once they have migrated and matured, macrophages are differentiated by the tissues in which they reside. *Histiocytes* are tissue macrophages in loose connective tissue, *Kupffer cells* are found in the liver, *alveolar macrophages* in the lungs and *microglia* in the brain. Tissue macrophages are also found in the spleen, tonsils, lymph nodes and bone marrow. Dendritic cells are star-shaped cells that serve as intermediaries between the innate and adaptive immune systems. Dendritic cells capture antigens, transporting them to lymphoid organs such as regional lymph nodes (Norris, 2018). Monocytes, macrophages and dendritic cells are antigen-presenting cells (APCs) which activate immune responses in both B and T lymphocytes.

Monocytes, macrophages and dendritic cells are actively phagocytic with the capacity to phagocytise large foreign particles and cell debris. Like neutrophils, macrophages are drawn to an inflamed area by chemicals released from damaged tissue in a process known as chemotaxis. Once they are in the tissue, macrophages can multiply to encapsulate and trap foreign matter that cannot be phagocytised. Monocytes and macrophages activate the immune response against chronic infections such as tuberculosis, viral infections and certain intracellular parasitic infections. Dendritic cells have long processes that can capture antigens and migrate to lymphoid tissue. They serve as sentinels for antigens in most organs including the heart, lungs, liver, kidneys and gastrointestinal tract. Dendritic cells activate T cells against cancer, assist B lymphocytes to produce antibodies and down regulate the immune system.

LYMPHOCYTES **Lymphocytes** account for 20% to 40% of circulating leucocytes. Lymphocytes are the principal effector and regulator cells of specific immune responses that protect the body from microorganisms, foreign tissue, and cell mutations or alterations. Through a process known as immune surveillance, lymphocytes monitor the body for cancerous cells and eliminate or destroy them.

Like other leucocytes, lymphocytes derive from the stem cells in the bone marrow (see Figure 11.2). Lymphocytes have 'homing' patterns: they constantly circulate then return to concentrate in lymphoid tissues (the lymph nodes, spleen, thymus, tonsils, Peyer's patches in the submucosa of the distal ileum and the appendix).

The three types of lymphocytes are **T lymphocytes (T cells)**, **B lymphocytes (B cells)** and **natural killer cells (NK cells)**. None of these cells acts independently. Their functions are closely interrelated. T cells mature in the thymus gland, whereas B cells complete their maturation in the bone marrow. T cells and B cells are integral to the adaptive immune response. On contact with an antigen, B lymphocytes are activated and mature into either plasma cells, which secrete antibodies, or memory cells. On contact with APCs, T lymphocytes mature into active helper T cells, cytotoxic T cells or memory T cells. Memory cells stay inactive, sometimes for years, but activate immediately with subsequent exposure to the same antigen. They then proliferate rapidly, producing an intense immune response. Memory cells are responsible for providing acquired immunity.

NK cells are large, granular cells found in the spleen, lymph nodes, bone marrow and blood. They constitute 15% of circulating lymphocytes. NK cells provide immune surveillance and resistance to infection, and they play an important role in the destruction of early malignant cells. Like B cells and T cells, NK cells are cytotoxic; however, unlike T cells, they do not require a specific antigen to become activated and kill cancer cells, virus-infected cells and cells infected with microbes

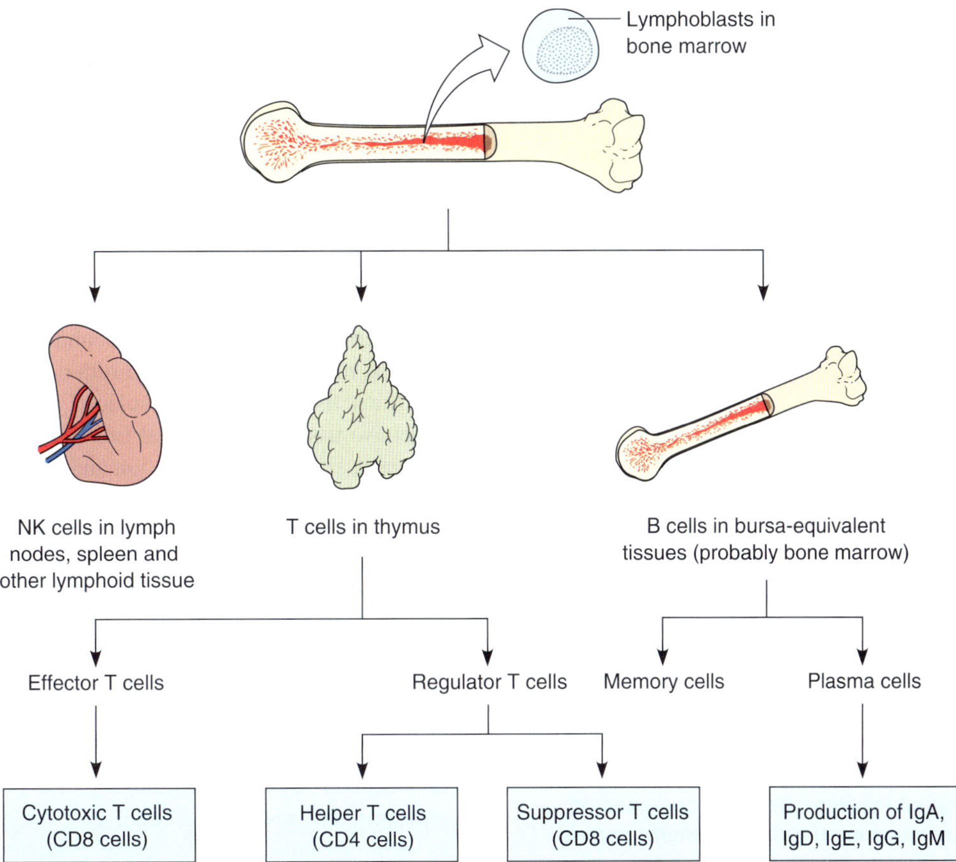

FIGURE 11.2 *The development and differentiation of lymphocytes from the lymphoid stem cell (lymphoblasts)*

(Norris, 2018). Fortunately, NK cells are inhibited when contact is made with normal host cells.

ANTIGENS Substances the immune system recognises as foreign or 'non-self' are called **antigens**. Antigens provoke a specific immune response when introduced into the body. Typically, antigens are large protein molecules found on the cell membrane or cell wall of microorganisms or tissues such as transplanted tissue or organs. Other potentially antigenic substances include pollens, insect venom and the resin of poison ivy (Norris, 2018).

Complete antigens, known as immunogens, have two characteristics: (1) *immunogenicity*, the ability to stimulate a specific immune response, and (2) *specific reactivity*, the stimulation of specific immune system components. In contrast, haptens are small molecules (e.g. chemical toxins or dust) that must link with proteins to evoke an antigenic response. When an antigen is encountered in the body, generation of an effective immune response involves two major groups of cells: lymphocytes and antigen-presenting cells (APCs). Macrophages and dendritic cells function as APCs as they capture, process and present antigens to the lymphocytes. Lymphocyte receptors recognise and respond to specific antigens, generating the immune response. Two separate but overlapping immune responses may occur, depending on the antigen itself and the type of immune cell activated by contact with the antigen. The B cell or humoral branch of the immune system mainly targets extracellular antigens such as bacteria, bacterial toxins and free viruses through the production of **antibodies**, molecules that bind with the antigen and inactivate it. The five classes of antibodies are IgG, IgA, IgM, IgD and IgE. These proteins make up the **antibody-mediated (humoral) immune response**. Intracellular pathogens, such as viral-infected cells, cancer cells and foreign tissue, activate T lymphocytes which are the primary agents of the **cell-mediated (cellular) immune response**. In this immune response, the lymphocytes themselves in the form of helper T cells, cytotoxic T cells and NK cells inactivate the antigen either directly or indirectly.

Lymphoid system

The *lymphoid system* consists of the lymph nodes, spleen, thymus, tonsils, lymphoid tissue scattered in connective tissues and mucosa, and the bone marrow. The thymus and bone marrow, in which T cells and B cells mature, are considered central lymphoid organs. The spleen, lymph nodes, tonsils and other peripheral lymphoid tissue are peripheral lymphoid organs (see Figure 11.3). The lymphoid system recovers proteins such as albumin for the vascular system and protects the bloodstream from invading organisms. Immune cells continuously circulate through lymphoid tissues and organs, identifying and

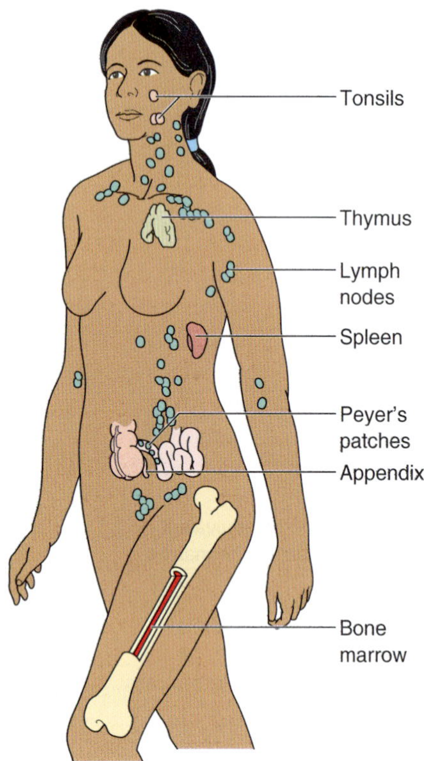

FIGURE 11.3 ***The lymphoid system: the central organs of the thymus and bone marrow, and the peripheral organs, including the spleen, tonsils, lymph nodes and Peyer's patches***

destroying foreign antigens. Lymph nodes, the most numerous elements of the lymphoid system, are small, round or bean-shaped encapsulated bodies that vary in size from 1 mm to 2 cm. Lymph nodes generally occur in groups at the junction of the lymphatic vessels. They can be found in the neck, axillae, abdomen and groin.

Lymph nodes filter foreign products or antigens from the lymph and house and support proliferation of lymphocytes and macrophages. Lymph, a clear, protein-containing fluid transported within lymph vessels, enters the node through afferent lymphatic vessels. Inside the node, the lymph flows through sinuses in the cortex of the lymph node where T and B lymphocytes and macrophages are abundant, then through sinuses of the medulla of the lymph node which contains macrophages and plasma cells. The presence of a foreign antigen stimulates lymphocytes and macrophages to proliferate in the lymph nodes. Macrophages destroy the antigen by phagocytosis. Immune cells and lymph then leave the lymph node through efferent vessels. An abundant blood supply to the node also facilitates lymphocyte movement.

The spleen is the largest lymphoid organ in the body and the only lymphoid organ that can filter blood. The spleen is located in the upper left quadrant of the abdomen. The spleen has two kinds of tissue: white pulp and red pulp. White pulp is lymphoid tissue that serves as a site for lymphocyte proliferation and immune surveillance. B cells predominate in the white pulp. Blood filtration occurs in the red pulp. In blood-filled venous sinuses, phagocytic cells dispose of damaged or aged RBCs and platelets. Other debris and foreign matter, such as bacteria, viruses and toxins, are also removed from the blood. The spleen also stores blood and the breakdown products of RBCs for future use. The spleen is not essential for life. If it is removed because of disease or trauma, the liver and the bone marrow assume its functions.

The *thymus gland* is located in the superior anterior mediastinal cavity beneath the sternum. It reaches its maximum size at puberty, then begins to atrophy slowly. By adulthood, it is difficult to differentiate from surrounding adipose tissue even though it remains active. In the older adult, the vast majority of thymus tissue has been replaced by adipose and fibrous connective tissue. During fetal life and childhood, the thymus serves as a site for the maturation and differentiation of thymic lymphoid cells, the T cells. Thymosin, an immunoregulatory hormone of the thymus, stimulates lymphopoiesis, the formation of lymphocytes or lymphoid tissue.

Bone marrow is soft organic tissue found in the hollow cavity of the long bones, particularly the femur and humerus, as well as the flat bones of the pelvis, ribs and sternum. Bone marrow produces and stores haematopoietic stem cells from which all cellular components of the blood are derived (see Figure 11.1).

Lymphoid tissues are also located at key sites of potential invasion by microorganisms: the submucosa of the genitourinary, respiratory and gastrointestinal tracts and the skin. Plasma cells in these lymphoid tissues defend the body against bacterial invasion at areas exposed to the external environment. In general, these tissues are known as *mucosa-associated lymphoid tissue* (MALT). Diffuse collections of lymphocytes, plasma cells and phagocytes are scattered throughout the respiratory tract, concentrating at bifurcations of the bronchi and bronchioles. Peyer's patches, or gut-associated lymphoid tissue (GALT), comprise the largest collection of immune cells in the body. Ingestion and absorption of solid foodstuffs and liquids continually expose the lining of the gut to resident microflora and infectious pathogens. Unlike peripheral lymph nodes, which respond to pathogens with acute inflammatory responses, GALT processes common intestinal antigens without producing acute inflammation. Collections of immune cells make up the GALT. Intraepithelial lymphocytes fill the spaces between mucosal epithelial cells. Beneath the basement membrane of gut epithelium lie abundant T cells and mature plasma cells, which are sources of IgA. Peyer's patches hold dense collections of lymphocytes in lymphoid nodules. As naive B and T cells migrate through Peyer's patches, they are sensitised to specific antigens. In mesenteric lymph nodes, these sensitised cells proliferate and circulate throughout the vascular tree where they produce secretory IgA. Secretory IgA coats mucosal cells and prevents attachment of intraluminal bacteria in the intestine, upper respiratory tract, bronchi, mammary ducts and salivary glands. Thus the GALT collection of immune cells effectively protects mucosa throughout the body that is exposed to resident and foreign pathogens.

Tonsils and adenoids protect the body from inhaled or ingested foreign agents. Skin-associated lymphoid tissue contains lymphocytes and dendritic cells such as Langerhans cells in the epidermis, which transport antigens to regional lymph nodes for destruction and development of specific immunity to the antigen.

Innate immune response

Innate or natural immunity is the first line of defence against infection. It is non-specific and includes skin and mucosal barriers, vascular and cellular responses and phagocytosis. Cells involved in innate immunity include phagocytic neutrophils and macrophages, and NK cells which target intracellular pathogens. Soluble molecules such as opsonins, cytokines, acute-phase proteins (such as C-reactive protein) and the complement system also are involved in innate immunity.

Barrier protection is the body's first line of defence against infection. Intact skin prevents invasion by external organisms. When the skin is damaged or lost (e.g. as a result of injury, surgery or burns), infection is much more likely. A barrier of mucus, which traps microorganisms and other foreign substances, protects the membranes lining inner surfaces of the body. These can then be removed by other protective mechanisms, such as ciliary movement or the washing action of tears or urine. In addition, many body fluids contain bactericidal substances that provide barrier protection. These include acid in gastric fluid, zinc in prostatic fluid and lysosyme in tears, nasal secretions, saliva and sweat.

When these defences are breached, the resulting tissue damage or foreign material entering the body induces inflammation, another innate defence mechanism. **Inflammation** is a response to injury that brings fluid, dissolved substances and blood cells into the interstitial tissues where the invasion or damage has occurred. The response is *non-specific* as the same events occur regardless of the cause of the inflammatory process. Through the inflammatory reaction, the invader is neutralised and eliminated, destroyed tissue is removed and the process of healing and repair is initiated.

The inflammatory response has two stages: (1) a vascular response characterised by vasodilation and increased permeability of blood vessels, and (2) a cellular response. Phagocytosis sets the stage for healing (tissue repair).

Vascular response

After tissue cells are damaged, local blood vessels briefly constrict. Vasodilation of the capillary arterioles and venules follows almost immediately as inflammatory mediators such as histamine and kinins are released from damaged tissue (see Box 11.1). Increased blood flow causes vasocongestion at the injury site with resultant redness and heat. The congestion also increases local hydrostatic pressure. This, along with increased vessel permeability that results from chemical mediators, moves fluid out of the capillaries and into the interstitial spaces of the tissue. The escaping fluid, called fluid exudate, contains large amounts of protein. This protein increases osmotic pressure in the interstitial spaces, which draws fluid and causes local oedema. Fluid exudate provides protection to the injured tissue by transporting to the tissue certain nutrients needed for tissue healing, diluting bacterial toxins and transporting cells needed for phagocytosis. Exudate may range from *serous*, primarily plasma with some proteins, to *sanguineous* containing large amounts of blood cells. *Fibrinous* exudate forms a thick, sticky meshwork of fibrinogen, in effect 'walling off' inflamed tissues and preventing the spread of infection. In more severe or acute inflammation, the fluid contains fibrin, RBCs and dead and live bacteria. This type of exudate, called *purulent* exudate, has an odour and colour characteristic of the bacteria present.

BOX 11.1 Inflammatory mediators

Many of the manifestations of inflammation are produced by chemicals released as a result of immunological processes or tissue injury or damage. These inflammatory mediators are broadly classified as follows:

- Vasoactive substances (e.g. histamine, prostaglandins, leukotrienes and platelet-activating factor) produce smooth muscle constriction, vasodilation and increased capillary permeability.
- Chemotactic factors (e.g. complement fragments and chemokines) attract leucocytes to the damaged tissue.
- Plasma enzymes (proteases) activate the complement system, the clotting cascade and the vasoactive kinins system, contributing to the vascular phase of the inflammatory response.
- Miscellaneous cell products (e.g. oxygen metabolites and lysosomal enzymes) damage surrounding tissue.

Many of the outward manifestations of inflammation result from vasoactive substances such as histamine, prostaglandins and leukotrienes. Stored in mast cells, basophils and platelets, *histamine* is released when an injury occurs or with stimulation by the immune system. An important component of the early inflammatory response, histamine causes vasodilation and vascular permeability in the affected area. Histamine is also a key factor in many hypersensitivity reactions. The *leukotrienes*, collectively known as slow-reacting substances of anaphylaxis (SRS-A), play a significant vasoactive role in the later stages of the inflammatory response.

Prostaglandins are chemotactic substances that draw leucocytes to the inflamed tissue. In addition, they play a vasoactive role and are pain and fever inducers. Aspirin and other non-steroidal anti-inflammatory drugs (NSAIDs), as well as the glucocorticoids, inhibit prostaglandin synthesis, thereby reducing fever, pain and inflammation.

Plasma proteases activate the clotting cascade, kinin system and complement system. With activation of the clotting cascade, bacteria and other foreign substances are trapped in the area of tissue damage. Fibrin, which has vasoactive by-products, is also released. Activation of the complement system causes vasodilation, increases vessel permeability and facilitates the phagocytic process. Through the release of bradykinin, the kinin system has similar effects. Bradykinin also stimulates pain receptors.

Major chemical mediators of inflammation are summarised in Table 11.2.

TABLE 11.2 Major chemical mediators of inflammation

FACTOR	SOURCE	EFFECT
Histamine	Mast cells, basophils and platelets	Vasodilation and increased capillary permeability producing tissue redness, warmth and oedema
Kinins (bradykinin and others)	Plasma proteins	Histamine-like effects; chemotaxis and pain inducers
Prostaglandins	Formed from arachidonic acid found in cell membranes	Histamine-like effects; chemotaxis, pain, and fever inducers
Leukotrienes	Formed from arachidonic acid	Smooth muscle constriction (especially bronchoconstriction), increased vascular permeability, chemotaxis

The vascular response localises invading bacteria and keeps them from spreading. Increased capillary permeability enhances the release of clotting factors such as fibrinogen, which converts to fibrin threads, entrapping the bacteria and walling them off from contact with the rest of the body.

Cellular response

The cellular stage of the inflammatory process begins within less than an hour after the injury. This stage is marked by changes in the lining of blood vessels and movement of phagocytic blood cells into the damaged tissue.

As serous fluid escapes the capillaries, the viscosity of blood in the area increases and its flow becomes more sluggish. Leucocytes move to the edges of the blood vessels where they accumulate, their movement slows and they begin to adhere to the capillary endothelium. This process is known as *margination*. Leucocyte adhesion causes separation of endothelial cells, allowing leucocytes to transmigrate through the blood vessel wall into the tissue spaces. Within hours, millions of leucocytes immigrate into the area of inflammation.

Once leucocytes have emigrated, they are drawn to the damaged or inflamed tissues by chemotactic signals. Infectious agents, damaged tissues and activated plasma substances such as complement fractions provide chemotaxic signals that attract an army of neutrophils, monocytes and macrophages to the injury site.

The number of neutrophils around the site increases to about 15,000 to 25,000/mm^3 and they begin their role in phagocytosis within a few hours. Monocytes become transient macrophages to augment the activity of the fixed macrophages and dendritic cells; together they engulf dead cells, damaged tissue, non-functioning neutrophils and invading bacteria.

Phagocytosis

Phagocytosis is a process by which a foreign agent or target cell is recognised, engulfed and destroyed. Neutrophils, monocytes and macrophages, known as *phagocytes*, are the primary cells involved in phagocytosis. Once attracted to the inflammatory site, phagocytes select and engulf foreign material.

The following factors or processes help phagocytes differentiate foreign tissue from normal cells:

- *Smooth surface*. Normal tissue has a smooth surface that is resistant to phagocytosis, whereas the rough surface of a foreign agent or target cell promotes phagocytosis.
- *Surface charge*. Healthy body cells present an electronegative surface charge that repels phagocytes. Cellular debris and foreign agents, by contrast, have an electropositive charge that attracts them.
- *Opsonisation*. This immune system process coats the surface of bacteria or target cells with soluble molecules (opsonins) such as complement, lectins and other proteins (see Box 11.2). Opsonisation enables the phagocyte to bind tightly with the foreign tissue, facilitating phagocytosis.

BOX 11.2 The complement system

The *complement system* consists of approximately 20 complex plasma proteins that are activated by a tissue injury or an antigen–antibody reaction. The complement system is involved in both innate and adaptive immune responses. Its activation results in the production of effector molecules that are involved in the processes of inflammation, phagocytosis, and cell lysis or destruction (Norris, 2018). Specifically, complement activation leads to the following:

- *Mediation of the inflammatory response*. When the complement system is activated, chemical mediators such as histamine are released from mast cells and basophils, leading to smooth muscle contraction, increased vascular permeability and oedema, and the attraction of leucocytes.
- *Opsonisation* (or coating) of microbes and antigen–antibody complexes. Opsonisation facilitates recognition of and binding to the antigen by phagocytes, and activation of phagocytosis.
- *Alteration of the cell membrane or viral capsule*. Complement can alter cell membranes, forming pores that cause cell lysis and death. Bacteria and viruses are destroyed; certain normal cells such as RBCs that are damaged or old may also be destroyed through this process.

The complement system has three 'arms', or pathways, of protein and enzyme reactions. The *classic pathway* is activated by antibody-containing immunoglobulins and other substances such as DNA and C-reactive protein. The *alternative* and *lectin pathways* function in innate immunity; they do not require antibodies but are activated by tissue injury, properties of the microbial antigen and proteins produced in response to injury (e.g. C-reactive protein) (Norris, 2018). Complement activation results in mediation of the inflammatory process, attraction of phagocytes, facilitation of phagocytosis and lysis of microbes.

Acute inflammation

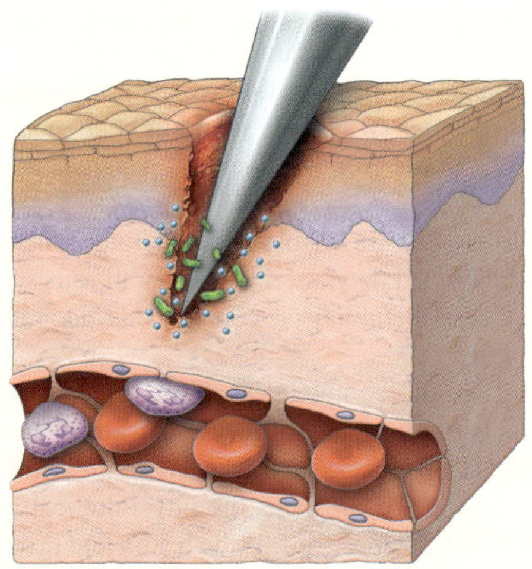

1. Inflammation is a key component of innate immunity, the body's immediate response to tissue damage or invasion of the body by foreign material. The inflammatory response serves to contain, control and eliminate damaged cells and tissue, microorganisms and antigens.

2. Vascular response. Tissue damage causes brief, initial vasoconstriction which is rapidly followed by vasodilation, with resulting redness and warmth. Inflammatory mediators (e.g. histamine, prostaglandins, bradykinins) released in the innate immune response and by damaged tissue dilate local blood vessels and increase the permeability of capillaries in the area. Protein-rich fluid (exudate) accumulates in interstitial spaces, causing swelling and pain. Resulting oedema slows blood flow and, together with activation of clotting in the area, helps localise and prevent microorganisms from spreading.

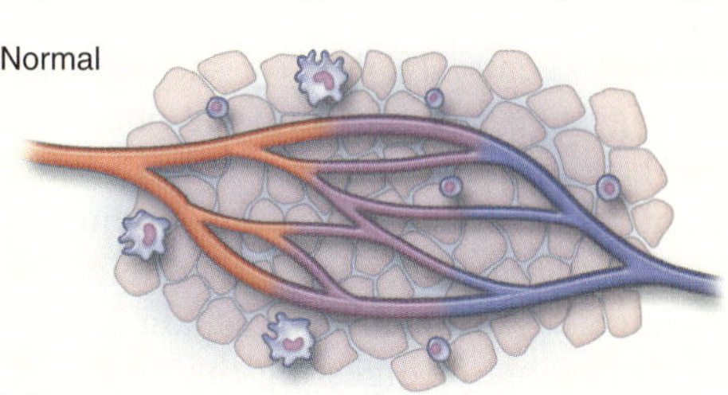

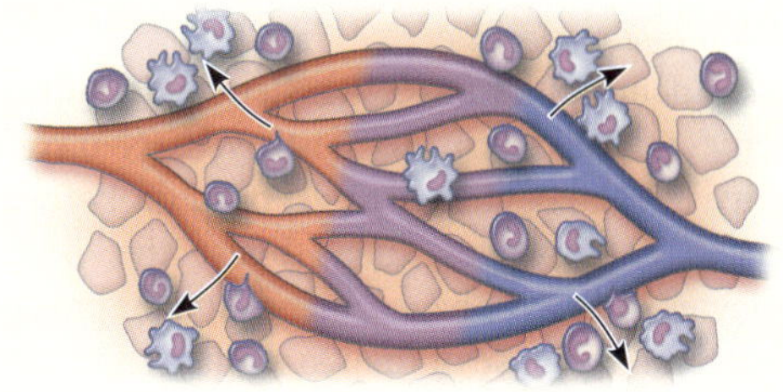

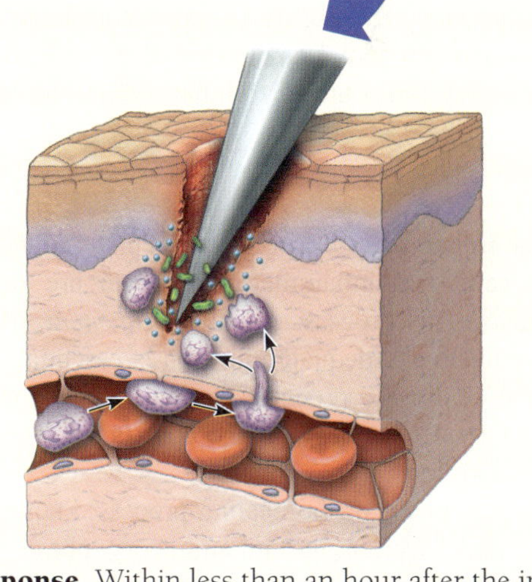

3. Cellular response. Within less than an hour after the injury, the cellular stage of the inflammatory process brings phagocytic blood cells into the damaged tissue. Loss of serous fluid from capillaries increases blood viscosity in the area and slows its flow. Leucocytes marginate, moving to the vessel periphery and adhering to the capillary endothelium. As a result, endothelial cells separate, allowing leucocytes to transmigrate through vessel walls into the tissue spaces. Chemotactic signals draw the leucocytes to the site of the injury or infection.

4. Phagocytosis. Once attracted to the inflammatory site, phagocytes engulf the foreign agent or target cell by projecting pseudopodia ('false feet') in all directions around it. This produces a phagosome containing the antigen, which is ingested into the cytoplasm. Once engulfed, lysosomes fuse with the phagosome, killing any live organism and releasing digestive enzymes, which destroy the antigen.

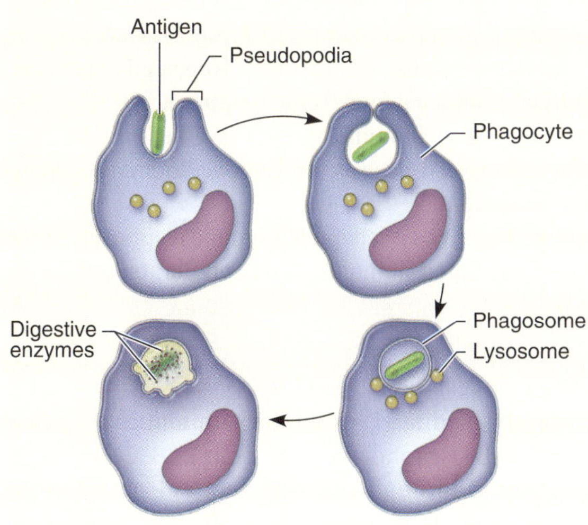

Phagocytes engulf the foreign agent or target cell by projecting pseudopodia in all directions around it. This produces a chamber called a *phagosome* containing the antigen, which is ingested into the cytoplasm. Once the phagosome has been engulfed, lysosomes fuse with the phagosome, releasing antimicrobial molecules and digestive enzymes which destroy the antigen. Phagocytes produce bactericidal agents that kill most pathogens. These agents include toxic oxygen and nitrogen radicals, such as nitric oxide, hydrogen peroxide and hydroxyl ions, as well as digestive enzymes (e.g. lysozyme) that break down bacterial cell walls. They also can produce antimicrobial molecules known as *defensins* (Norris, 2018).

Some antigens, such as the tubercle bacillus, have coats or secrete substances that are resistant to lysosomal and bactericidal agents. To destroy such antigens, lysosomes release digestive enzymes into the phagosome. The lysosomes of neutrophils and macrophages contain an abundance of proteolytic (protein-destroying) enzymes that digest bacteria and other foreign protein components. The macrophage's lysosomes also contain lipases (fat-splitting enzymes) capable of digesting the thick lipid membranes of such bacteria as *Mycobacterium tuberculosis* and *Mycobacterium leprae*.

Once neutrophils have ingested toxic substances to their capacity, they in turn are destroyed. Neutrophils have the capacity to phagocytise 5 to 20 bacteria before they become inactive. Macrophages then digest the dead neutrophils. Monocytes or macrophages are capable of phagocytising up to 100 bacteria. Because of their size, they can ingest larger particles than neutrophils can ingest, such as whole RBCs, necrotic tissue, cell fragments, malarial parasites and dead neutrophils. Dendritic cells are also phagocytic and secrete IL-12, which is an important cytokine in the maturation of helper T cells. Macrophages have the ability to extrude (release) the toxic substances and lysosomal enzymes within their phagosomes. As a result, they can continue to function for months and even years.

Healing

During the inflammatory process, particulate matter, bacteria, damaged cells and inflammatory exudate are removed by phagocytosis. This process, called *debridement*, prepares the wound for healing. Adequate nutrition is essential for inflammation and healing to proceed. Protein, glucose and oxygen are needed by leucocytes for chemotaxis, phagocytosis and intercellular killings.

The second phase of the healing process, known as *reconstruction*, may overlap the inflammatory phase. The ideal result of the healing process is *resolution*, the restoration of the original structure and function of the damaged tissue. Simple resolution occurs when there is no destruction of the normal tissue and the body is able to neutralise and remove the offending agent through the inflammatory process.

Resolution may also occur when the damaged tissue is capable of regeneration. The ability to regenerate or replace lost *parenchyma* (functional tissue) with new functional cells varies by tissue and cell type.

- *Labile cells* continue to regenerate throughout life. These cells are found in tissues where there is a daily turnover of cells—namely, bone marrow and the epithelial cells of the skin, mucous membranes, cervix, gastrointestinal tract and genitourinary tract.
- *Stable cells* normally stop replicating when growth ceases but are capable of regeneration when stimulated by an injury. Osteocytes (which are found in bone) and parenchymal cells of the kidneys, liver and pancreas are stable cells.
- *Permanent* or *fixed cells* are unable to regenerate. When these cells are destroyed they are replaced by fibrous scar tissue. Nerve cells, skeletal muscle cells and cardiac muscle cells are fixed cells.

When regeneration and complete resolution are not possible, healing occurs by replacement of the destroyed tissue with collagen scar tissue. This process is known as *repair*. Although tissue that has undergone repair lacks the physiological function of the destroyed tissue, the scar fills the lesion and provides tensile tissue strength.

Adaptive immune response

The adaptive immune response is a more specific reaction than innate immunity. On the first exposure to an antigen, a change occurs in the host, resulting in a specific and rapid response following subsequent exposures.

The adaptive immune response has the following distinctive properties:

- The immune response typically is directed against materials recognised as foreign (i.e. from outside the body) and is not usually directed against the self (i.e. cells or structures produced by the body). This property is known as *self-recognition*.
- The immune response is *specific*. It is initiated by and directed against particular antigens (such as a specific virus, bacterium or transplanted tissue).
- Unlike a localised inflammatory response, the immune response is systemic. Immunity is not restricted to the initial site of infection or entry of foreign tissue.
- The immune response has memory. Repeated exposures to an antigen produce a more rapid response.

A person whose immune system is able to identify antigens and effectively destroy or remove them is said to be **immunocompetent**.

There are two types of adaptive immune responses: humoral, or antibody-mediated immunity; and cellular, or cell-mediated immunity.

Antibody-mediated immune response

The antibody-mediated (humoral) immune response is produced by B lymphocytes (B cells). B cells are constantly replaced through cell division and proliferation in the bone marrow. It is believed that B cells mature in the bone marrow and then migrate to the spleen to await activation. They normally constitute 10% to 15% of circulating lymphocytes.

B cells are activated by contact with an antigen and by T cells (discussed in the next section). Each B cell has receptor sites for a specific antigen or antigens. When the antigen is encountered, the activated B cell proliferates and differentiates into antibody-producing plasma cells and memory cells (see Figure 11.4). Plasma cells are short-lived, lasting only about 1 day. While alive, however, they can produce thousands of antibody molecules per second. Memory cells retain antibody-producing information, allowing a rapid response if the antigen is again encountered.

An antibody is an **immunoglobulin (Ig)** molecule with the ability to bind to and inactivate a specific antigen. Immunoglobulins fall into five classes: IgG, IgA, IgM, IgD and IgE. Each has a slightly different structure and function. Their roles are summarised in Table 11.3.

Antibodies are Y-shaped molecules with two light and two heavy polypeptide chains (see Figure 11.5). The top portion of the Y, called the *Fab* or *antigen-binding fragment*, is chemically variable and specific to the antigen. The lower portion, the *Fc* or *crystallised fragment*, is constant for its class of immunoglobulin and directs the biological activity of the immunoglobulin (the manner in which it functions). For example, the lower portion of immunoglobulin molecules produced against hepatitis A and hepatitis B are the same (IgG), but the upper portion is different and specific to the virus.

The antibodies produced by B cells (see Figure 11.5) link with the antigen (see Figure 11.6) and inactivate it through one or more of the following processes:

- covering the antigen with antibodies to attract phagocytes, including neutrophils, macrophages and eosinophils
- precipitation—combining with soluble antigens to form an insoluble complex or precipitate that can be captured and destroyed by phagocytes

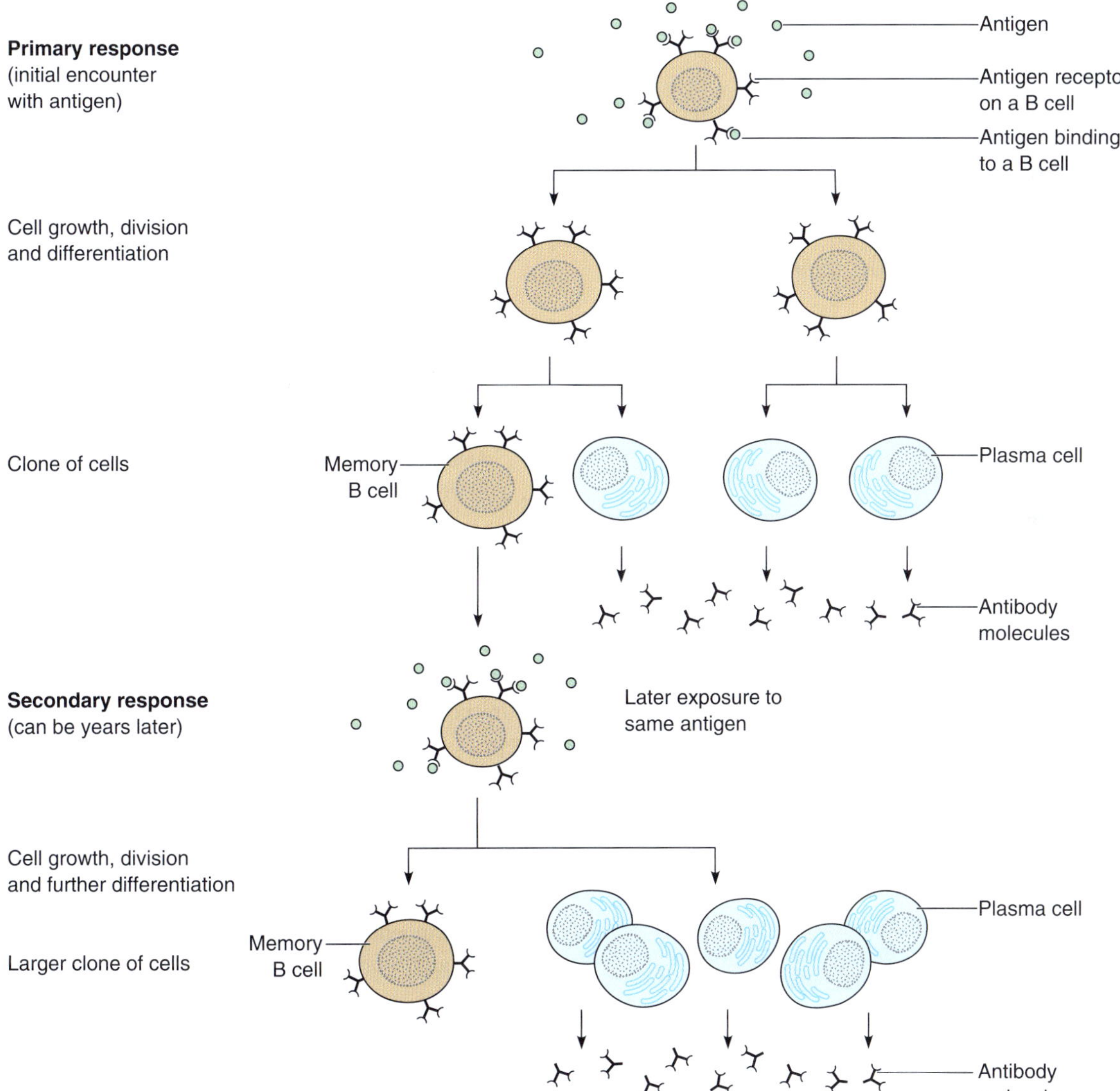

FIGURE 11.4 *Antibody-mediated (humoral) immunity. On initial exposure to the antigen, B cells with appropriate receptor sites are activated to become plasma cells and produce antibodies or memory cells. This is known as the primary response. With subsequent exposures, memory cells respond rapidly with antibody production. This is known as the secondary response*

TABLE 11.3 Immunoglobulin characteristics and functions

CLASS	PERCENTAGE OF TOTAL	CHARACTERISTICS AND FUNCTION
IgG	75%	Most abundant Ig; also known as gamma globulin; found in blood, lymph and intestines Active against bacteria, bacterial toxins and viruses Activates complement and binds to macrophages The only Ig to cross the placenta, providing immune protection to neonates
IgA	10–15%	Found in saliva, tears and bronchial, gastrointestinal, prostatic and vaginal secretions, as well as blood and lymph Provides local protection on exposed mucous membrane surfaces and potent antiviral activity by preventing binding of the virus to epithelial cells Levels decrease during stress
IgM	5–10%	Found in blood and lymph First antibody produced with primary immune response High concentration early in infection decreases within about a week Mediates cytotoxic response and activates complement
IgD	< 1%	Found in blood, lymph and surfaces of B cells Exact function unknown; may be receptor-binding antigens to B-cell surface
IgE	< 0.1%	Found on mast cells and basophils Involved in release of chemical mediators responsible for immediate hypersensitivity (allergic and anaphylactic) response and parasitic infections

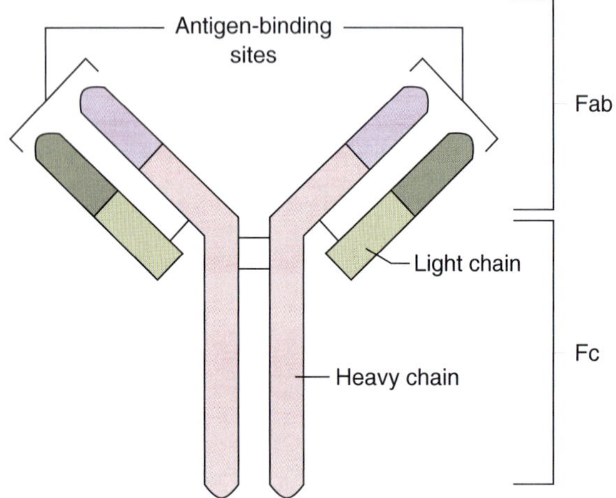

FIGURE 11.5 ***An antibody molecule. The Fab section is unique, providing an antigen-specific binding site. The Fc section is common to each class of immunoglobulin (IgG, IgA, IgM, IgD, IgE)***

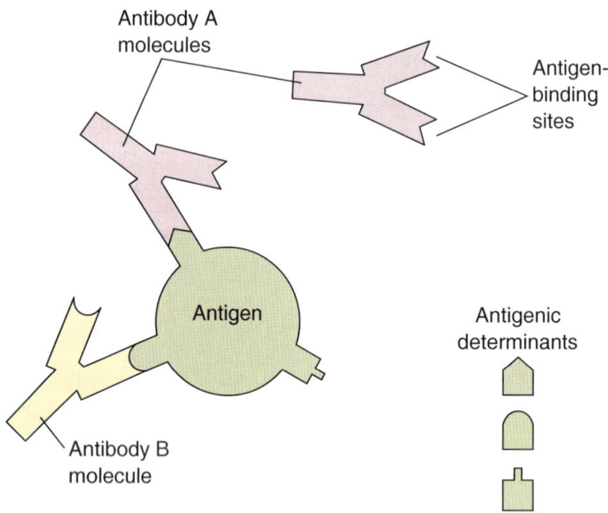

FIGURE 11.6 ***Antigen–antibody binding. The unique Fab site on the antibody binds with specific receptor sites on the antigen. As shown, more than one kind of antibody may be produced for an antigen***

- neutralisation—combining with a virus or toxin to neutralise its effects by preventing it from attaching to cells and tissues; the antigen–antibody complex is then destroyed by the process of phagocytosis
- complement activation and fixation to the antigenic cell surface, leading to cell lysis
- agglutination (clumping) of insoluble antigens (e.g. a cell or virus) to form a large complex
- opsonisation—coating of the antigen with antibodies and complement, making them more susceptible to phagocytosis.

The complete antibody-mediated response occurs in two phases. With initial exposure to an antigen, the primary response develops. B cells are activated to proliferate and begin producing antibodies. There is a latency period of 3 to 6 days before antibodies become detectable in the blood. Levels then continue to rise, peaking at 10 to 14 days after the initial exposure. With many illnesses (e.g. chickenpox), this peak correlates with recovery.

Subsequent exposure to the same antigen elicits a secondary response. Memory cells (see Figure 11.4) formed during the primary response stimulate the production of plasma cells and an almost immediate rise in antibody levels occurs (see Figure 11.7). This rapid secondary response is the basis of acquired immunity and is instrumental in preventing disease. It is also the mechanism through which vaccines provide protection from disease.

Cell-mediated immune response

Many antigens cannot stimulate the antibody-mediated response or are hidden from it because they live inside the body's cells (e.g. viruses and mycobacteria). The cell-mediated immune response, also known as *cellular immunity*, provides protection against these antigens. T lymphocytes (T cells) initiate this type of immune response.

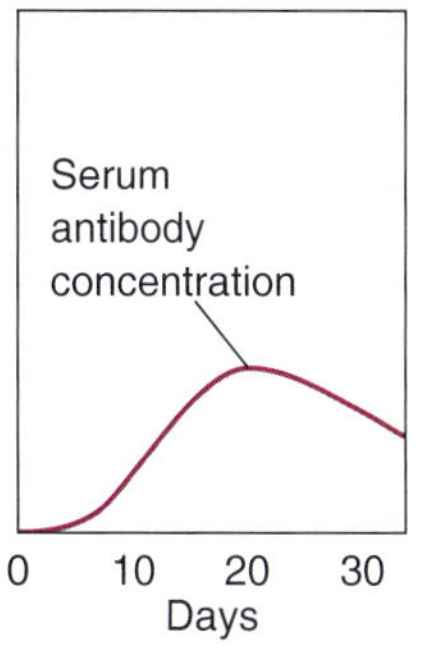

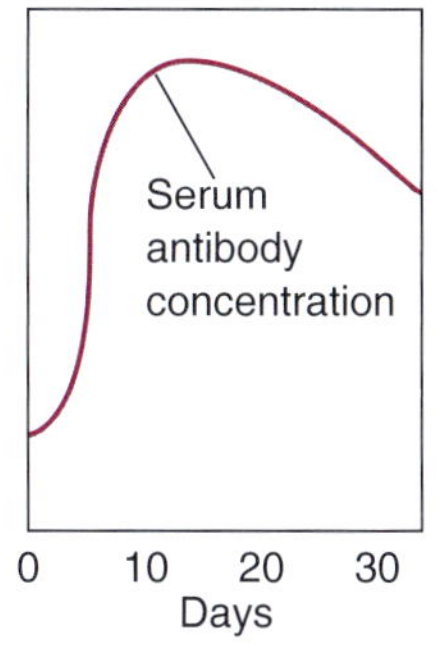

FIGURE 11.7 ***Antibody production in the primary and secondary responses of the antibody-mediated immune response. Note the more rapid and effective production following subsequent exposure***

Approximately 70% to 80% of circulating lymphocytes are T cells. T cells migrate to the thymus during fetal and early life, establishing the lifetime pool of cells. T cells have a lifespan measured in years, maintaining their numbers through proliferation, primarily in the lymph nodes.

T cells are much more complex than B cells. There are two major classes of T cells: CD4 cells and CD8 cells, *differentiated by their cell surface proteins (or markers).*

T cells are antigen-specific; that is, each subset is activated by a particular antigen. The antigens that activate T cells must be presented on another cell surface, such as pieces of virus presented on the surface of an infected cell or the histocompatibility locus antigen on a cell of transplanted tissue. When activated, T cells divide and proliferate, forming antigen-specific *clones* (see Figure 11.8). Activated T cells further differentiate to become *cytotoxic cells, helper cells* or *suppressor cells. Memory cells* are also formed; these remain in reserve for future encounters with the antigen.

The *cytotoxic T cell* (T_C cell), an effector cell with the CD8 markers, seeks out and destroys abnormal cells and cells harbouring anything foreign (e.g. viruses). Cytotoxic T cells bind with cell surface antigens on virus-infected or foreign cells. T_C cells destroy the identified cell by combining with it and then either destroying its cell membrane or releasing cytotoxic substances into the cell. They are vital in the control of viral and bacterial infections.

Helper T cells (T_H cells) develop from T cell populations with the CD4 marker. T_H cells coordinate immune responses to an antigen. They stimulate the proliferation of other T cells, amplify the cytotoxic activity of T_C cells and amplify the innate immune response. T_H cells interact directly with B cells to promote their multiplication and conversion into plasma cells capable of producing antibodies.

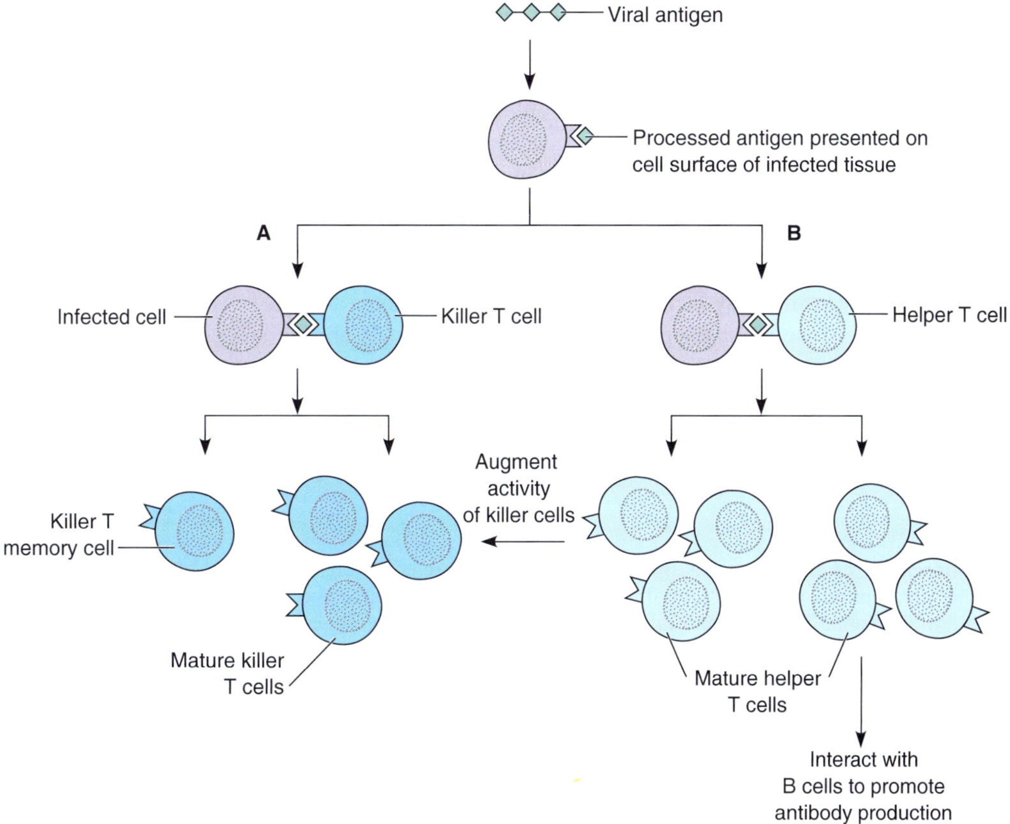

FIGURE 11.8 ***Cellular immune response. A, An infected cell, abnormal cell or phagocyte presents antigen on its surface that binds with a receptor site on a killer T cell or a helper T cell. The killer T cell is activated to proliferate into memory cells or mature cytotoxic cells. B, The helper T cell is activated to augment the cytotoxic response and stimulate the antibody-mediated immune response***

Suppressor T cells (T_S cells), a much smaller subgroup of T cells, are important regulators of immune responses. Suppressor T cells release inhibitory cytokines, which inhibit the activity of other T cells and B cells and limit the extent of the immune response to an antigenic stimulus.

On activation, both effector and regulator T cells synthesise and release soluble proteins known as **cytokines** (see Box 11.3). Cytokines are important in amplifying innate immunity and the specific immune response. They stimulate:

- B cells to become plasma cells and produce antibodies
- attraction and activation of macrophages to become aggressive phagocytes
- proliferation of cytotoxic T cells and memory helper T cells
- cytotoxic T cells to destroy abnormal cells and pathogens.

Although T cells are activated by specific antigens, much of the resulting effect is non-specific—in other words, an enhanced inflammatory response. Like the antibody-mediated response, the cell-mediated response has memory. Subsequent exposures to an antigen result in a more rapid and effective inflammatory response and more effective phagocytosis by macrophages. This memory provides the basis for skin testing. For example, a person previously exposed to tuberculosis develops a more pronounced inflammatory response when minute amounts are injected under the skin.

The person with natural or acquired immunity

Immunity refers to the protection of the body against disease. Immunity to disease may be either natural or acquired, active or passive.

Immunity develops from the activation of the body's immune response. Depending on the antigen, antibody-mediated or cell-mediated responses are activated. The immune response typically involves components of both. In the immunocompetent (having an immune system capable of responding to pathogens and tissue damage) person, these responses inactivate and remove the antigen, allowing recovery to occur or preventing the development of disease. People with suppressed or impaired immune function are more susceptible to disease and require protection from exposure to environmental elements. Isolation techniques are employed to prevent the spread of disease and protect immunosuppressed people.

Pathophysiology

The processes of antibody-mediated and cell-mediated immunity result in the development of **active immunity**. Active immunity occurs when the body produces antibodies or develops immune lymphocytes against specific antigens. Memory cells, which can produce an immediate immune response on re-exposure to the antigen, provide long-term immunity. Active immunity can develop naturally, resulting from contact with the disease-producing antigen and subsequent development of the disease.

For many diseases, however, the potential consequences of a single disease episode for the individual and society make prevention desirable, especially for highly contagious diseases capable of causing epidemics. In these instances, immunisation, or vaccination, is used to provide artificially acquired immunity. The purpose of vaccination is to establish adequate levels of antibody and/or memory cells to provide effective immunity. Vaccination introduces the disease-producing antigen into the body in a manner that will stimulate the immune system to form antibodies and memory cells but will not produce disease. Vaccines may be made of killed organisms or of live organisms that have been attenuated or modified to reduce their disease-producing capability. Typhoid is an example of a killed organism vaccine; the measles-mumps-rubella (MMR) vaccine, by contrast, is made from attenuated organisms. Many newer vaccines use subunits of the antigen; these are portions of the organism that have antigenic properties but are unable to produce disease.

Passive immunity provides temporary protection against disease-producing antigens. Antibodies produced by other people or animals are the source of passive immunity. These acquired antibodies are used up; they either combine with the

BOX 11.3 Cytokines

Cytokines, essential components of an adequate immune response, are hormone-like polypeptides produced primarily by cells of the immune system. Cytokines are produced in small quantities in many different tissues throughout the body. Cytokines act as messengers of the immune system, facilitating communication between the cells to adjust or vary the inflammatory reaction or to initiate immune cell proliferation and differentiation. The major cytokines and their functions are summarised in Table 11.4.

The inflammatory cytokines contribute to illness behaviours. People respond to increases in these chemicals with increased sleep, a need to seek warmth and reduced energy output. These are considered adaptive responses to illness. Interventions to reduce or eliminate the production of certain cytokines are common. Aspirin and NSAIDs to reduce pain and fever are commonly used. Because some cytokines cross the blood–brain barrier, their increase may explain depression and anxiety experienced during illness.

Interferons are a class of cytokine with broad antiviral and anticancer effects. A number of different forms of interferon exist, broadly grouped as alpha, beta and gamma interferons. Interferon is synthesised by cells infected with a virus and secreted into extracellular fluid. It then binds to specific receptors on uninfected neighbouring cells, protecting them from infection. The spread of the virus is thus inhibited and recovery from infection enhanced. It appears that interferons also moderate the activity of NK cells and may be involved in preventing the spread of abnormal malignant cells.

TABLE 11.4 Major cytokines and their functions

CYTOKINE	WHERE PRODUCED	PRIMARY FUNCTIONS
Interleukin-1 (IL-1)	Monocytes, macrophages and dendritic cells	Activates T and B cells Induces fever and tissue catabolism Enhances NK activity Attracts neutrophils, macrophages and lymphocytes Stimulates bone marrow and endothelial cell growth, collagen and collagenases
Interleukin-2 (IL-2)	Helper T cells	Stimulates T and B cell proliferation, aids in discriminating between self and non-self Activates killer T and NK cells
Interleukin-3 (IL-3) Interleukin-4 (IL-4)	T cells	Stimulates growth and differentiation of bone marrow stem cells Stimulates proliferation of T cells Increases IgE secretion by B cells
Interleukin-5 (IL-5)	T cells and activated mast cells	Promotes differentiation of B cells and eosinophils Stimulates production of IgA
Interleukin-6	T cells and macrophages	Is a pro-inflammatory and anti-inflammatory cytokine Induces fever
Interleukin-8	Macrophages	Mediates the innate immune response Induces fever Is angiogenic (stimulates vessel formation)
Gamma interferon	T and NK cells	Stimulates phagocytosis by neutrophils and macrocytes Activates NK cells Augments B cell proliferation, enhancing both cellular and humoral immune responses
Alpha and beta interferons	Virus-infected cells; macrophages	Activate macrophages and endothelial cells; beta interferon induces fever Augment NK cell activity Act at gene level to protect neighbouring cells from invasion by intracellular parasites, such as viruses, rickettsia, malaria
Macrophage inflammatory proteins (MP-1-4CC)	Macrophages, dendritic cells and lymphocytes	Are chemokines (CC), which are small cytokines Promote inflammatory response, chemotaxis and homeostasis (control migration of cells in maintenance and development)
Tumour necrosis factor (TNF)	Activated macrophages, T cells and NK cells	Major chemical mediator of inflammatory response Stimulates T-cell activation, antibody production and accumulation of leucocytes at inflammatory site Directly cytotoxic to some tumour cells Induces fever

antigen or are naturally degraded by the body, and their protection is gradually lost. The transfer of maternal antibodies via the placenta and breast milk to the infant provides naturally acquired passive immunity. Rabies human immune globulin and hepatitis B immune globulin (HBIG) are examples of immunisations used to provide artificially acquired passive immunity. There is no rabies in Australia, but Australian bats carry other viruses in the lyssavirus family, including Australian bat lyssavirus, which is closely related to rabies (Department of Health and Aged Care, 2022).

The types of active and passive immunity are summarised in Table 11.5.

INTERPROFESSIONAL CARE

Interprofessional care is preventive, focusing primarily on assessing the person's immune status and ensuring acquired immunity to prevent disease.

Diagnosis

A number of diagnostic tests can be performed to assess the person's immune status.

- *Serum protein* measures the total protein in the blood, including albumin and globulins. Normal levels for the adult are

TABLE 11.5 Types of acquired immunity

TYPE OF IMMUNITY		HOW DEVELOPED	EXAMPLES
Active immunity	Natural	Acquired by infection with an antigen, resulting in the production of antibodies	Chickenpox
	Artificial	Acquired by immunisation with an antigen, such as attenuated live virus vaccine	MMR, polio, DTP, hepatitis B vaccine
Passive immunity	Natural	Acquired by transfer of maternal antibodies to the fetus or neonate via the placenta or breast milk	Neonate initially protected against MMR if mother immune
	Artificial	Acquired by administration of antibodies or antitoxins in immune globulin	Gamma globulin injection following hepatitis A exposure

62 to 80 g/L; albumin is approximately 60% (32 to 45 g/L) of the total serum protein; and globulins are normally 23 to 34 g/dL. Total protein levels, albumin and globulin are decreased in malnutrition and liver disease. Decreased globulin levels are noted with immunological deficiencies.

- *Protein electrophoresis* analyses protein content, especially for albumin and gamma globulin, and is used to assess immune function. Gamma globulins subjected to further electrophoresis separate into immunoglobulins: IgA, IgD, IgE, IgG and IgM (see Table 11.3). Analysis of specific levels of each provides clues about the immune status of the person. IgG levels are increased during acute infection. Decreased levels of IgG, IgA and IgM are found in malignancies.
- *Antibody testing* is ordered to determine if a person has developed antibodies in response to an infection or immunisation. Antibodies for hepatitis, HIV, rubella, varicella (chickenpox) and certain other diseases can be identified. An elevated titre level for varicella and rubella indicates immunity. Antibody testing may also be used to determine if the person has the disease.
- *Skin testing* can assess cell-mediated immunity. A known antigen such as streptokinase, tuberculin-purified protein derivative or *Candida* protein is injected intradermally. The site is then observed for induration and erythema, which typically peak at 24 to 48 hours. An induration of at least 10 mm in diameter is a positive reaction, indicating previous exposure and sensitisation to the antigen. No reaction to common antigens, or **anergy**, indicates depressed cell-mediated immunity.

Immunisations

Vaccines are suspensions of whole or fractionated bacteria or viruses that have been treated to make them non-pathogenic. Vaccines are given to induce an immune response and subsequent immunity. Although vaccine development has been a major factor in improving public health, no vaccine is completely effective or entirely safe. Table 11.6 outlines the vaccines recommended for the adult person to maintain optimal health and immune status (Centers for Disease Control and Prevention (CDC), 2021).

Adults born before 1966 are generally considered to be immune to measles, mumps and rubella by prior infection. Individuals born after 1966 should have documentation of one or more doses of MMR vaccine unless they have a medical contraindication to the vaccine or laboratory evidence of immunity to the three diseases (CDC, 2021).

Vaccination against diphtheria, tetanus and pertussis (whooping cough), hepatitis B, polio and Hib (haemophilus influenza type b) is part of the National Immunisation Program (NIP) schedule. A combined vaccine is administered in a series of injections at 2 months, 4 months and 6 months. The vaccine stimulates active immunity by inducing the production of antibodies and antitoxins. After an initial series of a three-dose primary schedule as an infant, further separated doses are given at 12 months, 18 months and 4 years of age. *The Australian Immunisation Handbook* (Department of Health, 2022) recommends a further booster dose for diphtheria, tetanus and pertussis in adolescents around 11 to 13 years. It is also recommended that pregnant women in the third trimester of each pregnancy and adults who reach 50 years of age without having a booster dose in the prior 10 years should receive a booster dose.

Hepatitis B (HB) vaccine is given as a series of three immunisations to promote active immunity to hepatitis B. This vaccine is recommended for everyone at high risk of exposure through blood or other body fluids, including healthcare workers, and emergency and essential service workers. Other high-risk populations include intravenous drug users, sexual partners of infected individuals, people on haemodialysis, prison guards, tattooists, body piercers and embalmers. A universal hepatitis B vaccination program was recommended for infants and adolescents in 1996. The adolescent program commenced in 1997 and the universal infant program, with the first dose given at birth, began nationally in 2000.

TABLE 11.6 Recommended immunisations for adults

VACCINE	TYPE	DOSE	INDICATIONS	PRECAUTIONS AND NURSING IMPLICATIONS
Measles-mumps-rubella (MMR)	Live virus	0.5 mL SC	All adults born after 1966, particularly those who are at risk of infection, such as healthcare workers, those working with children, and overseas travellers. MMR vaccination is particularly recommended for males without history of previous infection; rubella vaccination recommended for all seronegative females.	As a live virus vaccine, should not be administered to pregnant women or immunocompromised people. Do not administer to people with a history of anaphylactic reaction to egg protein or neomycin.
Diphtheria, tetanus and pertussis toxoids (Boostrix)	Inactivated toxins	0.5 mL IM	Initial series of 3 injections (minimum intervals of 4 weeks) if never immunised then booster at 10 and 20 years; adults who reach 50 and have not had booster in previous 10 years; following a major or contaminated wound if more than 5 years since last booster.	Do not give in first trimester of pregnancy or to people with a history of anaphylactic reaction to previous dose or any vaccine component; administer deep IM in deltoid of dominant arm.
Hepatitis B (HB)	Inactive viral antigen	1.0 mL IM	Series of 3 doses: initial then at 1 to 2 months, then 2 to 5 months after second dose. Recommended for anyone at risk of exposure and for post-exposure prophylaxis.	Use with caution in pregnant or lactating females, older people and people with active infection.
Influenza	Inactivated virus or viral components	0.5 mL IM	Yearly for all people > 6 months of age; strongly recommended for over age 65, all Aboriginal and Torres Strait Islander people > 15 years of age and those with predisposing conditions to severe influenza, including debilitated people and people with chronic disease.	Do not administer to people who are acutely ill or people with history of anaphylactic reaction to egg protein.
Pneumococcal	Bacterial polysaccharides	0.5 mL IM or SC	One dose for people over age 65, and Aboriginal and Torres Strait Islander people > 50 years of age; and those aged > 10 who are at risk of pneumococcal pneumonia, including people with chronic lung disease or other chronic diseases.	Do not administer to pregnant women.

Influenza vaccine is recommended annually for all adults. The antigenic strains included in the influenza vaccine vary each year according to the predicted predominant strains affecting the population; therefore, yearly re-immunisation is required.

Pneumococcal, rotavirus and meningococcal C vaccine is recommended for all children and is included in the infant immunisation program. Human papillomavirus (HPV) vaccine is recommended for teenagers and is offered through school immunisation programs to 12- or 13-year-olds.

In January 2020, the World Health Organization (WHO) declared a public health emergency—a pandemic—regarding the novel coronavirus (COVID-19) outbreak (WHO, 2022). New vaccines (viral vector and mRNA) were developed to protect against COVID-19. Read more about COVID-19 in the COVID Primer.

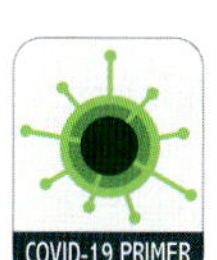

The impact of COVID-19 across a broad spectrum of health-care issues, diagnosis and treatment, including infections, has not been taken into account or fully understood as the full effect will take some years to be understood (Australian Institute of Health and Welfare, 2022).

Indigenous Australians historically have had a very high rate of infectious diseases. In the early period of European colonisation, this was mainly due to a lack of previous exposure, followed by high-density living in newly established settlements. In recent decades, for some diseases such as diphtheria, polio, tetanus, hepatitis B, measles, mumps and rubella, vaccination has been very successful in eliminating or substantially reducing disease in all Australians, significantly contributing to reducing child mortality in Indigenous Australian populations. However, other diseases such as pneumococcal disease, hepatitis A and influenza have a higher rate of illness in Indigenous people compared with non-Indigenous people, and therefore are specifically recommended for administration of vaccine to a broader age group.

In addition to routine immunisations, people travelling outside Australia should receive vaccines against diseases that are endemic in the regions of the world that they intend to visit.

Other immunological substances may be administered as indicated. Immunoglobulins provide passive immunity as protection against a known or potential exposure to an antigen. Normal human immunoglobulin is given to household contacts of people with hepatitis A and people travelling to areas in which it is endemic. HB immunoglobulin contains higher titres of antibody to hepatitis B virus and is used for people exposed by blood or sexual contact. Following confirmed or suspected contact with a pathogen, selected vaccines may be administered to stimulate an immediate immune response.

For most vaccines, a sensitivity test should be performed prior to administration to detect sensitivity to substances such as horse serum or eggs. The substance is injected intradermally; if after 20 minutes there is no evidence of a reaction, the selected vaccine can be administered.

Moderate to severe local reactions may occur following administration of an immunisation. Common reactions include redness, swelling, tenderness and muscle ache. Administering the vaccine in the dominant arm of the person helps minimise local reactions because use and movement of the arm facilitates absorption of the solution. Applying heat to the site is also beneficial. Occasionally local ulcerations occur; when they do, warm wet packs or sterile wet-to-dry dressings may be prescribed.

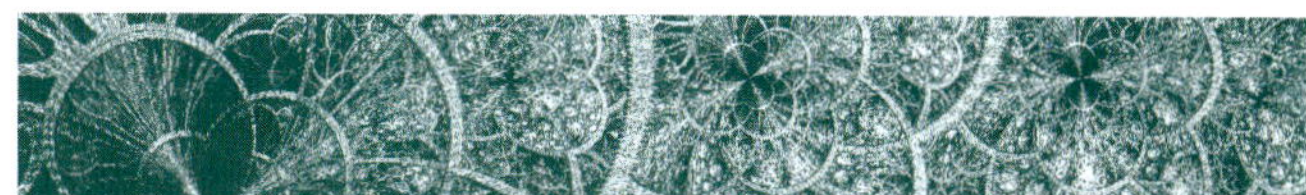

Nursing care

Maintaining a population that is fully immunised against common, potentially epidemic and devastating diseases is a major public health task for nursing. Nurses not only recommend and administer vaccines to individual people and their families, but also plan and implement preventive care for whole communities.

Although this process may appear to be straightforward, multiple issues affect society's ability to immunise the entire population. For some people, for example, religious beliefs may preclude the use of immunisations to prevent disease. Also, people who are not citizens and the medically indigent population have difficulty accessing immunisation services. Lack of immunisation not only puts the individual at increased risk of infectious disease, but also increases the cost of medical services and the possibility of exposing immunocompromised people to disease.

Health promotion

In the public health setting, the nurse looks at the immunisation needs and illness risk of an entire community. Communities include not only cities and localities, but also groups of people, such as university populations and employees in a workplace. Public education needs may be met through presentations to groups of people, feature articles in newspapers and other local publications, advertising, radio presentations, public service announcements, one-to-one discussion and teaching.

Assessment

Collect the following data through the health history and physical examination. Further focused assessments are described with nursing interventions in the next section.

- *Health history*: age, medication use (corticosteroids and antibiotics) and blood transfusion, nutrition, known allergies, pregnancy status, infection, immunisations, autoimmune disorders, chronic diseases such as asthma, diabetes mellitus, cancer.
- *Physical assessment*: skin lesions or rashes, breath sounds, respiratory rate.

Nursing diagnoses and interventions

Nursing care focuses on preventing injury from the immunisation and educating the person. See the accompanying 'Nursing care plan' box.

NURSING CARE PLAN A person with acquired immunity

Terry Adams is a 48-year-old executive who is planning a trip to central Africa. In preparation, he contacts his local healthcare provider to obtain the necessary immunisations. Jane Wong, the Registered Nurse in the clinic, obtains a nursing history of Mr Adams.

ASSESSMENT

Mr Adams' history reveals that he has always been very healthy and active, apart from a mild case of asthma. As an adult he has had little problem with his asthma, 'except for those rare occasions when I am dumb enough to smoke more than one cigarette!'. He is divorced and is not currently in a continuing relationship. He has two grown daughters with whom he has a good relationship. Since contracting hepatitis A several years ago, he drinks alcohol only rarely and never more than one or two drinks at any one time. He confesses to doing little organised exercise but plays golf two or three times a week. He says he is such a hyperactive workaholic that he rarely sits for any length of time. Mr Adams has not seen a doctor since recovering from the hepatitis and is unsure when he last received any immunisations. He does not know if he had all the recommended childhood immunisations but he recalls getting both Salk and Sabin polio vaccines when they became available. His physical examination reveals an alert and healthy individual with no abnormalities noted. His vital signs are as follows: T 37.1°C, P 64, R 14 and BP 142/82.

The doctor orders the following immunisations for Mr Adams:

- measles-mumps-rubella (MMR)
- combined tetanus, diphtheria and pertussis toxoids (Boostrix)
- yellow fever vaccine
- typhoid vaccine
- meningococcal meningitis vaccine.

DIAGNOSES

- *Health-seeking behaviours: immunisation* related to impending international travel.
- *Ineffective health maintenance* related to apparent lapse in immunisation status.
- *Risk of injury* related to adverse response to immunisation.

PLANNING

- Obtain MMR, Boostrix and meningococcal meningitis vaccines for administration.
- Schedule return visit in 1 week for typhoid vaccine.
- Refer Mr Adams to a registered vaccination centre for yellow fever vaccine.
- Ensure instructions are provided for comfort measures to relieve local and systemic adverse effects of vaccines and manifestations that should be reported to the doctor.
- Complete documentation of immunisations on a permanent record at the clinic and for Mr Adams.
- Provide information for ongoing requirements to maintain immunisation status.

Expected outcomes

- Complete necessary immunisations.
- Verbalise a schedule for maintaining up-to-date immunisation status.
- Experience no significant adverse effects from immunisation.

IMPLEMENTATION

- Administer MMR, Boostrix and meningococcal meningitis vaccines prior to discharge from clinic.
- Observe closely for 30 minutes following immunisation for potential adverse responses.
- Schedule return visit in 1 week for typhoid vaccine.
- Provide referral to a registered vaccination centre for yellow fever vaccine and documentation of vaccination.
- Provide instructions for comfort measures to relieve local and systemic adverse effects of vaccines.
- Provide written instructions on signs and symptoms that should be reported to the doctor.
- Document immunisations on a permanent record at the clinic and for Mr Adams.
- Discuss ongoing requirements to maintain immunisation status.

EVALUATION

Terry Adams completes his prescribed immunisations without major adverse effects, although he does complain of fever, malaise and general achiness for several days following the typhoid vaccination. His trip to Africa is successful and he returns to Australia without contracting any infectious diseases.

CRITICAL THINKING IN THE NURSING PROCESS

1. Explain why it is important for adults to continue receiving immunisations throughout their lifespan.
2. If a person says to you, 'I don't believe in immunisations. I hear they are dangerous', how would you respond?
3. When should a person contact the primary caregiver after receiving an immunisation?

REFLECTION ON THE NURSING PROCESS

1. What sources of knowledge or evidence influenced the decision making in this case study?
2. Outline what you have learned from this case study that you could apply in your future practices.

CONSIDERATION FOR PRACTICE

Observe the person for 20 to 30 minutes following vaccine administration to monitor for possible adverse reactions.

Readiness for enhanced immunisation status

For individual people and their families, nurses promote immunocompetence by assessing immune status, recommending appropriate immunisations and administering vaccines as ordered or indicated. Once a person reaches adulthood, routine immunisations often become a neglected part of healthcare.

- Determine knowledge level, understanding, attitudes and religious beliefs about immunisation. *This provides a basis for further education and determines if religious beliefs may contraindicate immunisation.*
- Discuss the value and reasons for recommended immunisations. *Understanding promotes adherence.*
- Reinforce positive health-seeking behaviours. *This will help promote future health maintenance activities.*

- Using recommended immunisation schedules, develop a plan to attain optimal immunisation status. *Adherence with recommended schedules for immunisation is important in preventing disease and disability.*
- Do not administer MMR or influenza vaccine if allergic to eggs, or tetanus antitoxin if sensitive to horse serum. *Vaccines prepared from chicken or duck embryos are contraindicated in people who are allergic to eggs. Tetanus antitoxin is prepared from horse serum. Both will cause a severe allergic reaction.*
- Withhold administration of active immunological products in the presence of an upper respiratory infection or other infection. *Active immunisations can cause a greater inflammatory reaction in the presence of infections.*
- Do not administer oral polio vaccine, MMR or any live virus vaccine to immunosuppressed people or to those who are in close household contact with an immunosuppressed person. *Live virus vaccines can cause disease in the immunosuppressed person. The virus may be transmitted from close household contacts during the initial post-vaccination period.*
- Do not administer vaccines such as MMR, pneumococcal or varicella to women who are pregnant. *Although the risk to the developing fetus is greatest during the first trimester, these vaccines are avoided throughout pregnancy.*
- Do not administer live attenuated virus vaccines and passive immunisations such as gamma globulin simultaneously. *Passive antibodies interfere with the response of the live attenuated virus.*
- Prior to administering the prescribed vaccine, check the expiration date and manufacturer's instructions. *Outdated vaccines cannot provide adequate immunisation protection. Certain injection sites have better absorption than others.*
- Keep adrenaline 1:1,000 readily available for subcutaneous injection when administering immunisations. *Adrenaline causes vasoconstriction and reduces laryngospasm; in acute anaphylaxis, it can be lifesaving.*

Community-based care

Clinically significant medical events including high fever, injection-site hypersensitivity, unspecified rash and injection-site oedema that occur after vaccination should be reported as an adverse event following immunisation (AEFI). Reporting an AEFI is important as it provides a better understanding of the safety issues around vaccines. The ongoing reporting of adverse events following immunisation allows the Therapeutic Goods Administration (TGA) to monitor rates and trends across Australia and assist in identifying issues such as incorrect vaccine administration, manufacture, storage and delivery.

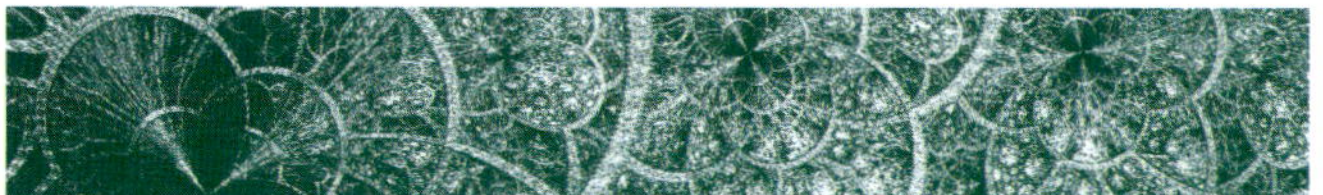

NORMAL IMMUNE RESPONSES

The person with tissue inflammation

Inflammation is a non-specific response to injury that serves to destroy, dilute or contain the injurious agent or damaged tissue. Acute inflammation is a short-term reaction of the body to all types of tissue damage. It is immediate and aimed at protecting the body and preventing further invasion or injury. Acute inflammation usually lasts less than 1 to 2 weeks. Once the injurious agent is removed, the inflammation subsides. Healing with tissue repair or scar formation occurs and the body functions in normal or near-normal capacity.

Chronic inflammation is slower in onset and may not have an acute phase. Its clinical manifestations occur over months or years. While the effects of some chronic inflammatory processes may be evident (such as the joint damage and destruction associated with rheumatoid arthritis), the role chronic inflammation plays in diseases such as asthma, obesity and heart disease has only recently been recognised.

Pathophysiology and manifestations

The tissue damage that evokes an inflammatory response may be caused by specific or non-specific agents. These agents may be *exogenous*, from outside the body, or *endogenous*, from within the body. Causes of inflammation include the following:

- mechanical injuries such as cuts or surgical incisions
- physical damage such as burns
- chemical injury from toxins or poisons
- microorganisms such as bacteria, viruses or fungi
- extremes of heat or cold
- immunological responses, such as hypersensitivity reactions
- ischaemic damage or trauma, such as a stroke or myocardial infarction.

Acute inflammation

Regardless of the cause, location or extent of the injury, the acute inflammatory response follows the previously outlined sequence of vascular response, cellular and phagocytic response, and healing.

Many of the manifestations of inflammation are produced by inflammatory mediators, such as histamine and prostaglandins, released when tissue is damaged (see Box 11.1).

The primary manifestations of inflammation include the following:

- erythema (redness)
- local heat caused by the increased blood flow to the injured area (hyperaemia)
- swelling due to accumulated fluid at the site
- pain from tissue swelling and chemical irritation of nerve endings
- loss of function caused by the swelling and pain.

The degree of functional loss depends on the location and extent of the injury. With increased tissue damage, more fluid exudate is formed, resulting in more swelling, pain and functional impairment. Pain may be immediate or delayed.

Prostaglandins intensify and prolong the pain. Kinins cause irritation to the nerve endings and contribute to the pain sensation.

Dead neutrophils, necrotic tissue and, if the tissue is infected, digested bacteria accumulate as a result of inflammation and phagocytosis, forming *pus*. Pus usually forms and remains until after the infection subsides. Pus may push itself to the surface of the body or become internalised. In the latter case, pus is gradually autolysed (self-digested) by enzymes over a period of days. The end product is then absorbed by the body. On occasion, pus may remain after the infection is resolved. An abscess, or localised collection of pus, may form, necessitating drainage by a surgical procedure.

Systemic responses to inflammation include lymph node swelling (*lymphadenopathy*) due to the proliferation of macrophages within the nodes in response to microorganisms in the lymph. Enlarged lymph nodes are usually noted in the groin, axillae and neck. Fever, often precipitated by inflammatory mediators or bacterial toxins, inhibits the growth of many microorganisms and increases tissue repair functions. Loss of appetite and fatigue may occur in the effort to conserve energy during the inflammatory process. Leucocytosis occurs with increased WBC production to support inflammation and phagocytosis.

Chronic inflammation

Whereas acute inflammation is a self-limiting process lasting less than 2 weeks, chronic inflammation tends to be self-perpetuating, lasting weeks to months or years. Chronic inflammation may develop when the acute inflammatory process has been ineffective in removing the offending agent. Persistent low-grade fever or irritation by chemicals, particulate matter or physical irritants such as talc, asbestos or silica may also result in chronic inflammation.

GRANULOMATOUS INFLAMMATION *Granulomatous inflammation* is characterised by dense infiltration of the site by lymphocytes and macrophages. The macrophages mass to surround the site; they in turn are surrounded by lymphocytes and other immune cells, forming a lesion called a *granuloma*. The granuloma isolates the offending agent from the rest of the body; however, the infectious agent or irritant may not be destroyed and can survive within the granuloma for a long period of time. Chronic inflammation and granuloma formation are common with *Mycobacterium tuberculosis*. The granuloma formed in tuberculosis is called a tubercle. *M. tuberculosis* can survive for many years within the tubercle, emerging when the person's immune system is no longer able to contain it.

NON-SPECIFIC CHRONIC INFLAMMATION *Non-specific chronic inflammation* is implicated in such disorders as pulmonary airway disease (asthma and chronic obstructive lung disease), cardiovascular disease and autoimmune disorders such as inflammatory bowel disease. This type of chronic inflammation is characterised by diffuse accumulation of macrophages and proliferation of fibroblasts in response to ongoing chemotaxis. The fibroblasts and fibrocytes, unique cells formed from monocytes, lead to formation of excessive fibrous connective tissue, disrupting normal tissue functions (Reinhardt & Breuer, 2021). Inflammatory markers such as C-reactive protein, complement fractions and inflammatory cytokines are present in non-specific chronic inflammation and associated disorders (Govindarajan, de Rivero Vaccari & Keane, 2020; Khafagy & Dash, 2021; Snelder et al., 2021).

Complications

Inflammation and wound healing are highly metabolic processes that may be affected by a number of factors. Without adequate nutrition, blood supply and oxygenation, tissues cannot effectively complete the process. Impaired inflammatory and immune processes can interfere with phagocytosis and preparation of the wound for healing. Infection prolongs the inflammatory process and delays healing.

Chronic diseases may also impair healing. High blood glucose levels and small-blood-vessel disease associated with diabetes mellitus impair chemotactic and phagocytic function. Collagen formation and tensile strength of the wound are also impaired. Arterial and venous disorders impair the delivery of oxygen and nutrients to healing tissues, as well as the removal of toxins, bacteria and other waste products from the area. Drug therapy, particularly corticosteroid medications, may suppress the immune and inflammatory responses, delaying healing (Norris, 2018). Other external factors, such as exposure to ionising radiation and wound cleansing agents, can also affect healing. Table 11.7 summarises major factors that affect the inflammatory process and wound healing.

TABLE 11.7 Factors that may impair healing

FACTOR	EFFECT
Malnutrition	
Protein deficit	Prolongs inflammation and impairs healing process
Carbohydrate and kilocalorie deficit	Impairs metabolic processes and promotes catabolism; proteins are used for energy rather than for healing
Fat deficit	Impairs cell membrane synthesis in tissue repair
Vitamin deficiencies	
Vitamin A	Limits epithelialisation and capillary formation
B-complex	Inhibits enzymatic reactions that contribute to wound healing
Vitamin C	Impairs collagen synthesis
Tissue hypoxia	Associated with an increased risk of infection and impaired healing because oxygen is required to support cell function and collagen synthesis
Impaired blood supply	Results in inadequate delivery of oxygen and nutrients to healing tissues and removal of waste products
Impaired inflammatory and immune processes	Results in decreased phagocytosis and wound debridement; increased risk of infection; delayed healing

INTERPROFESSIONAL CARE

Management of the person with inflamed tissue focuses on promoting healing. Care is generally supportive, allowing the person's own physiological processes to remove foreign matter and damaged cells. Wound care may be minimal, involving only simple cleaning, or may require irrigations and debridement. The person is encouraged to rest, to increase fluid intake and to eat a well-balanced, nutritious diet. Antibiotics may be prescribed to help eliminate infectious causes of inflammation.

Diagnosis

The following diagnostic tests may be ordered to identify the source and extent of inflammation.

- *WCC with differential* provides information about the type and extent of inflammatory response. The differential count (the percentage of the total WBC made up by each type of leucocyte) provides further clues about inflammatory processes (see Table 11.8).
- *Erythrocyte sedimentation rate (ESR)* is a non-specific test to detect inflammation. The rate at which RBCs fall to the bottom of a vertical tube is an indicator of inflammation. An increased ESR may indicate acute or chronic inflammation.
- *C-reactive protein (CRP) test* is used to detect CRP. This abnormal glycoprotein is produced by the liver and is excreted into the bloodstream during the acute phase of an inflammatory process. The expected result of this test is negative for CRP. A positive result indicates an acute or chronic inflammatory process.

In addition to these diagnostic tests, cultures of the blood and other body fluids may be ordered to determine if infection is the cause of inflammation.

Medications

Although inflammation is a beneficial process to prepare acutely injured tissue for healing, its manifestations can be distressing. Chronic inflammation can lead to tissue damage and scarring with resulting loss of function. Anti-inflammatory medications may be prescribed to manage these effects. Anti-inflammatory medications fall into three broad groups: salicylates such as aspirin, other NSAIDs and corticosteroids.

Aspirin (acetylsalicylic acid or ASA) is a NSAID with antipyretic, analgesic and antiplatelet effects. Its beneficial effects are largely dose related. Low doses (as little as 75 mg/day) inhibit platelet aggregation and normal blood clotting. A 600 mg dose of aspirin is an effective analgesic and antipyretic dosage. Higher doses (600 to 900 mg, 4 to 5 times per day) are required to produce its anti-inflammatory effects. To relieve pain, aspirin acts primarily on peripheral sensory nerves by inhibiting the synthesis of prostaglandins and kinins, which are chemical stimuli of sensory nerves. As an antipyretic, aspirin acts both centrally and peripherally. It inhibits the formation of pyrogenic substances that raise the hypothalamic thermostat. It also dilates peripheral blood vessels and promotes diaphoresis, increasing the dissipation of heat (Adams, Holland & Urban, 2019).

In therapeutic doses, aspirin mediates the inflammatory process by inhibiting the enzyme cyclooxygenase (COX) and preventing synthesis of prostaglandins. Inflammation is reduced, along with the swelling, redness and impaired function that accompanies it.

The other NSAIDs have activity similar to that of aspirin. They inhibit COX and prostaglandin synthesis, reducing the inflammatory and pain responses. Each NSAID has a slightly different mode of action; sometimes several different agents must be tried before the most effective is identified. Side effects also differ to a certain extent; however, all have a potential cross-sensitivity with aspirin, all irritate the gastrointestinal tract and all are associated with an increased risk of cardiovascular events. NSAIDs are more costly than aspirin, but they have a longer duration of action; therefore, fewer daily doses are required to achieve the desired effect.

For acute hypersensitivity reactions, or for inflammation that cannot be managed using NSAIDs, corticosteroid therapy may be prescribed. The glucocorticoids are hormones produced by the adrenal cortex that have widespread effects on body metabolism and the immune response. Glucocorticoids inhibit inflammation and may be lifesaving in acute fulminating or chronic progressive inflammation. When glucocorticoids are

TABLE 11.8 The white blood cell count and differential

CELL TYPE AND NORMAL VALUE	INCREASED	DECREASED
Total WBCs: 4.5-13.5 $\times$ 10⁹/L	*Leucocytosis*: infection or inflammation, leukaemia, trauma or stress, tissue necrosis	*Leucopenia*: bone marrow depression, overwhelming infection, viral infections, immunosuppression, autoimmune disease, dietary deficiency
Neutrophils (segs, PMNs or polys): 2.0-7.5 $\times 10^9$/L	*Neutrophilia*: acute infection or stress response, myelocytic leukaemia, inflammatory or metabolic disorders	*Neutropenia*: bone marrow depression, overwhelming bacterial infection, viral infection, Addison's disease
Eosinophils (eos): 0.04-0.4 $\times 10^9$/L	Eosinophilia: parasitic infections, hypersensitivity reactions, autoimmune disorders	*Eosinopenia*: Cushing's syndrome, autoimmune disorders, stress, certain drugs
Basophils (basos): $< 0.1 \times 10^9$/L	*Basophilia*: hypersensitivity responses, chronic myelogenous leukaemia, chickenpox or smallpox, splenectomy, hypothyroidism	*Basopenia*: acute stress or hypersensitivity reactions, hyperthyroidism
Monocytes (monos): 0.2-0.8 $\times 10^9$/L	*Monocytosis*: chronic inflammatory disorders, tuberculosis, viral infections, leukaemia, Hodgkin's disease, multiple myeloma	*Monocytopenia*: bone marrow depression, corticosteroid therapy
Lymphocytes (lymphs): 1.5-4.0 $\times 10^9$/L	*Lymphocytosis*: chronic bacterial infection, viral infections, lymphocytic leukaemia	*Lymphocytopenia*: bone marrow depression, immunodeficiency, leukaemia, Cushing's syndrome, Hodgkin's disease, renal failure

prescribed to manage inflammation, the smallest possible effective dose is used. Wherever possible, a local-acting preparation such as a topical agent, metered-dose inhaler or intra-articular injection is prescribed to minimise systemic effects of the drug.

The incidence of potentially harmful side effects increases with higher doses and prolonged therapy. Wound healing is impaired and the metabolism of fats, proteins and carbohydrates is altered. Blood glucose control is impaired. Fat distribution changes, producing a cushingoid appearance with a moon face and increased truncal fat. Fluid retention and hypertension are potential problems, as are osteoporosis, gastrointestinal bleeding and emotional disturbances.

Paracetamol may be administered to reduce the fever and pain associated with inflammation. Paracetamol has no anti-inflammatory effect, and will not reduce the inflammatory process, but can relieve associated symptoms such as fever and pain.

Antibiotics may be used either prophylactically to prevent infection from interfering with the healing process of damaged tissue, or therapeutically to treat the infection. If infection is present, the organism and its response or sensitivity to various antibiotics is used to guide therapy. Antibiotic therapy is presented in greater depth in the section of this chapter on infectious diseases.

Nutrition

Healing depends on cell replication, protein synthesis and the function of specific organs—the liver, heart and lungs, in particular. Malnutrition and protein depletion are risk factors for poor healing and wound complications. Even a few days of severely impaired nutritional intake can noticeably affect healing (Tucker & Dauffenbach, 2019).

The person with an inflammatory process or healing wound requires a well-balanced diet of sufficient kilojoules to meet the metabolic needs of the body (see Table 11.7). Inflammation often produces *catabolism*, a state in which body tissues are broken down. By contrast, healing is a process of *anabolism*, or building up. Without sufficient kilojoules and nutrients, catabolism may predominate, impairing healing.

Adequate protein is necessary for tissue healing and the production of antibodies and WBCs. Lack of adequate protein increases the risk of infection. Complete protein sources, those that provide the essential amino acids, are preferred. Carbohydrates are important to meet energy demands, as well as to support leucocyte function. Care is taken to avoid hyperglycaemia in people with diabetes, as hyperglycaemia interferes with oxygen delivery to the tissues as well as with the chemotactic and phagocytic function of neutrophils, impairing healing. Dietary fats are used in the synthesis of cell membranes.

Vitamins A, B-complex, C and K are also important to the healing process. Vitamin A is necessary for capillary formation and epithelialisation. B-complex vitamins promote wound healing, and vitamin C is necessary for collagen synthesis. Vitamin K provides a vital component for the synthesis of clotting factors in the liver.

Although it has been established that minerals contribute to the inflammatory and healing processes, less is known about required amounts. Minerals serve important roles in maintaining normal cell function and as cofactors in enzyme reactions necessary for cell proliferations. Zinc, a micronutrient, is involved in cell growth and in T-cell development (Tucker & Dauffenbach, 2019).

Oxygen is another important element in healing. It is necessary for collagen synthesis. Phagocytes such as neutrophils and macrophages require oxygen to digest bacteria engulfed in the phagocytic process. Impaired oxygen delivery to the tissues slows healing and increases the risk of infections. Supplemental oxygen administered via nasal cannula or mask improves the oxygen saturation of haemoglobin and its availability to tissues. Hyperbaric oxygen delivery improves leucocyte and fibroblast function as well as the development of new blood vessels, and may be beneficial to promote healing of inflamed ischaemic tissue (Loscalzo et al., 2022).

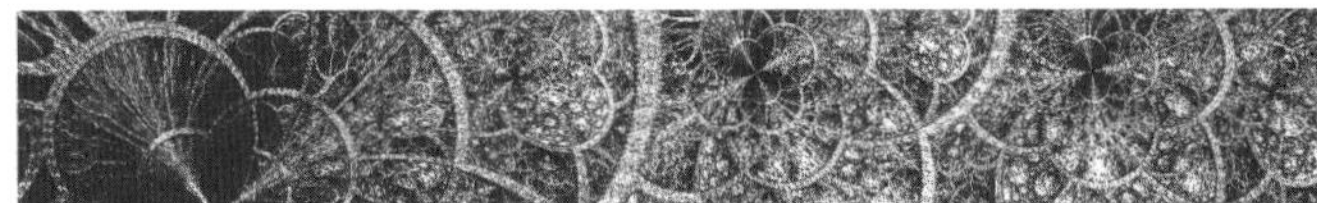

Nursing care

Acute inflammation may be self-limiting, or extensive and require hospitalisation. Nursing care includes teaching people with acute and chronic inflammatory conditions self-management at home.

Health promotion

Health promotion activities to prevent inflammation focus on reducing the risk of accidents and exposure to harmful agents that can result in subsequent injury. It is important to educate the public about potential hazards in both the work and home environments. In addition, safety education guidelines, such as not drinking and driving, wearing a protective helmet when riding a bicycle and using a seat belt in the car, are important areas for discussion. Because most injuries occur at home, it is also important to discuss ways to make the home safer.

Assessment

The following data are collected through the health history and physical examination. Further focused assessments are described with nursing interventions in the next section.

- *Health history*: risk factors, nutrition, medication use (anti-inflammatory and corticosteroids), location, duration and type (redness, heat, pain, swelling and impaired function) of symptoms.
- *Physical assessment*: movement of injured area, circulation, wounds, lymph nodes.

Nursing diagnoses and interventions

The nursing care needs of the person with an inflammatory process are related to the manifestations of inflammation and resulting altered tissue integrity. Nursing care priorities focus on relieving pain, supporting tissue healing and preventing infection.

Acute pain

Along with redness, warmth, swelling and impaired function, pain is one of the primary manifestations of inflammation. Depending on the cause, affected area and degree of inflammation, pain may be acute and immobilising or chronic and demoralising. It is important to remember that pain is a subjective experience and that people's responses to pain vary.

- Assess pain using a scale of 0 to 10, with 0 being no pain and 10 being the worst pain; note the character and location of the pain. *Because pain is subjective, the person provides the most accurate information regarding their pain experience.*
- Use physical and non-verbal cues to further assess the level of pain. *This intervention is especially important if the person is non-verbal or tends to under-report pain.*
- Administer anti-inflammatory medications as prescribed. *These medications help reduce the pain resulting from acute inflammation. Most NSAIDs also have analgesic and anti-pyretic effects, further promoting comfort (Adams et al., 2019).*
- Administer analgesic medications as prescribed. *Moderate to severe pain may require treatment with an analgesic (e.g. opioid). Paracetamol and opioid analgesics act within the CNS to reduce pain. Opioids provide the most effective pain relief overall, activating pain inhibitory neurons and inhibiting pain transmission neurons (Loscalzo et al., 2022).*

> **CONSIDERATION FOR PRACTICE**
> **Because opioids can depress respirations, it is important to monitor oxygen saturation and encourage the person to take deep breaths to maintain adequate oxygen saturation.**

- Provide comfort measures, such as back rubs, position changes or relaxation techniques. *These measures reduce muscle tension, relieve areas of pressure and provide distraction.*
- Encourage activities such as reading, watching television and taking part in social interactions. *Such activities provide distraction from the pain experience.*
- Encourage rest. *Strenuous activity or exercising an inflamed body part may increase discomfort and tissue damage.*
- Provide cold or heat as pain relief measures as ordered. *For an acute injury, cold reduces swelling and relieves pain; after the initial stage, heat increases blood flow to the affected tissue and relieves pain and swelling by promoting absorption of oedema. Do not apply either heat or cold for more than 20 minutes at a time and ensure there is a covering between the skin and the application.*
- Elevate the inflamed area if possible. *Elevation promotes venous return and reduces swelling.*
- Teach about the appropriate use and expected effects of anti-inflammatory medications. *If the person's pain continues after the initial doses of anti-inflammatory medication, they may become discouraged and stop taking the medication before it becomes fully effective.*

> **CONSIDERATION FOR PRACTICE**
> **Use heat or cold application cautiously in older people who have fragile skin and are at risk of tissue injury.**

Impaired tissue integrity

The inflammatory response can either precipitate or result from an impairment in the integrity of skin, support or other tissues.

- Assess general health and nutritional status. *Poor general health or chronic diseases such as diabetes mellitus or renal failure interfere with the healing processes and increase the risk of infection.*
- Assess circulation to the affected area. *Adequate tissue perfusion and oxygenation are necessary for healing (Norris, 2018).*
- Monitor the skin and surrounding tissue for increased signs of inflammation. *Inflammation can spread to adjacent tissues, leading to conditions such as cellulitis.*
- Provide protection and support for inflamed tissue. *This reduces discomfort and decreases the risk of further tissue damage.*
- Clean inflamed tissue gently; if possible, use water, normal saline or non-toxic wound cleansers only. *Soap and harsh cleansers such as povidone-iodine (Betadine) and hydrogen peroxide can cause further drying and tissue damage. Granulation tissue in a healing wound is fragile and easily damaged.*
- Keep the inflamed area dry and expose it to air as much as possible. *This promotes healing and helps prevent infection.*
- Balance rest with activity. *Rest decreases metabolic demands and allows for cell regeneration, while mobility helps to promote oxygenation and perfusion of the tissues.*
- Provide supplemental oxygen as ordered. *Supplemental oxygen improves tissue oxygenation and reduces hypoxia.*
- Provide a well-balanced diet with adequate kilojoules to meet the body's metabolic and healing needs. If the person is allowed nothing by mouth (NBM), suggest parenteral or enteral nutrition. For the person who is unable to consume an adequate diet, consult with a dietitian for between-meal supplements and/or multivitamin supplements. *Careful attention to diet and nutrient intake is important to provide the nutrients necessary for immune function and healing and to prevent catabolism (Tucker & Dauffenbach, 2019).*

Risk of infection

The inflammatory response often indicates that body defence mechanisms have been set in motion to protect against invading microorganisms. The person with a healing wound is at particular risk of infection.

- Assess the wound for specific signs of infection, including purulent drainage, odour and delayed healing. *The normal inflammatory response can indicate infection and, on occasion, mask its presence.*
- Evaluate complete blood counts for adequate WBC response. *Leucocytosis may indicate infection or healthy response to injury and protection from infection. Immune-impaired people may not respond with increased WBCs, and manifestations of inflammation may be diminished in those individuals.*

- Monitor vital signs at least every 4 hours. *In response to the inflammatory process the temperature rises, usually in the range 37.4°C–38.2°C. A temperature of 38.3°C or above usually indicates infection. Fever is usually accompanied by increased heart and respiratory rates.*
- Culture purulent or odorous wound drainage. *Wound culture is used to determine the infectious organism and to direct antibiotic therapy.*
- Apply dry or moist heat to the affected area for no longer than 20 minutes several times a day. Monitor the temperature closely to prevent burns and further damage to the affected area. *Heat increases the circulation of blood to and from the inflamed tissue. Time is limited to prevent burns.*
- Provide and encourage fluid intake of 2,500 mL/day as allowed. *Adequate hydration promotes blood flow and nutrient supply to the tissues and also dilutes and removes waste products from the body.*
- Ensure adequate nutrition. *Adequate nutrition enhances the function and production of T cells and B cells, which are important in the immune response.*
- Use good hand hygiene techniques consistently. *Hand hygiene removes transient microorganisms and is the best mechanism to prevent the spread of infection to a susceptible person.*
- Use aseptic technique when providing wound care. *Using sterile gloves and aseptic technique helps prevent further contamination of the wound and the spread of infection to other people.*

Community-based care

Education for the person and their family enhances understanding of the inflammatory process, its cause and its management. Teaching is also important to prevent further compromise that could result in infection.

Instructions, verbal and written, should include the following:

- Increase fluid intake to 2,500 mL per day.
- Eat a well-balanced diet high in vitamins and minerals and with adequate protein and kilojoules for healing.
- Use good hand hygiene, particularly when caring for wounds or inflamed tissue and after using the bathroom.
- Elevate the inflamed area to reduce swelling and pain.
- Apply heat or cold for no longer than 20 minutes at a time to reduce the risk of tissue damage from burns or frostbite.
- Take all medications as prescribed, notifying the doctor if adverse effects or hypersensitivity responses are noted.
- Rest acutely inflamed tissue; do not engage in strenuous activity until the inflammation has subsided.

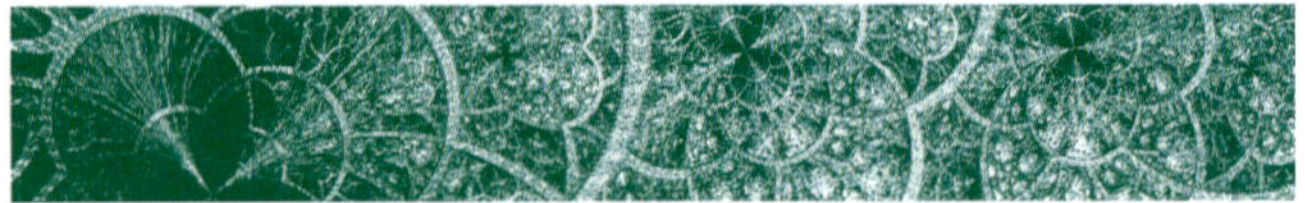

The person with an infection

Microorganisms—including bacteria, viruses, fungi and parasites—often invade the human body and proliferate if undetected and not controlled or eliminated by inflammatory and immune responses. In most cases, contact between humans and microorganisms is incidental and may even be beneficial to both organisms. Resident bacteria of the skin, mucous membranes and gastrointestinal tract are an important part of the body's defence system. However, many microorganisms are virulent; that is, they have the ability to cause disease.

Pathogens are virulent organisms rarely found in the absence of disease. Some microorganisms, known as opportunistic pathogens, rarely cause harm to people with intact immune systems but are capable of producing infectious disease in the immunocompromised host (Norris, 2018).

To a certain extent, modern medicine has contributed to the development of infectious diseases caused by antibiotic-resistant strains of microorganisms. Tuberculosis is on the rise in many countries, partially because organisms have become resistant to standard therapies. People receive immunosuppressive therapy following organ or tissue transplant, or in the treatment of neoplasms, making them more susceptible to infection. Metal and plastic prosthetic devices are implanted, providing potential sites for colonisation by disease-producing organisms. It has also become apparent that many diseases long considered unrelated to microorganisms may actually be infectious; for example, colonisation of the gastric mucosa with *Helicobacter pylori* is the predominant cause of peptic ulcer disease, and oncogenic viruses have the ability to transform normal cells into malignant cells.

Pathophysiology

Infection occurs when an organism is able to colonise and multiply within a host. The host can be any organism capable of supporting the nutritional and physical growth requirements of the microorganism—for example, humans. When the host experiences injury, pathological changes, inflammation or organ dysfunction in response to an infection or from intoxication by cellular poisons produced by a pathogen, the host is said to have an infectious disease.

For a microorganism to cause infection, it must have disease causing potential (virulence), be transmitted from its reservoir and gain entry into a susceptible host. This is known as the chain of infection (see Figure 11.9).

PATHOGENS Pathogens capable of infecting and causing disease in a susceptible host include bacteria, viruses, *Mycoplasma*, *Rickettsia*, *Chlamydia*, fungi and parasites such as protozoa, helminths (worms) and arthropods (see Box 11.4). Each organism causes a different specific reaction in the host.

A number of different mechanisms have evolved in pathogens to facilitate their transmission and increase their ability to invade the host and cause disease. Factors influencing the transmission of an organism include its resistance to drying and to variations in environmental temperature. For example, spore-forming organisms are extremely resistant to drying.

Adhesion factors produced by or incorporated into the cell wall or membrane of the pathogen improve its ability to attach and colonise the host. Pathogens may also produce enzymes to enhance their spread to local tissues, chemicals to block specific immune processes or deplete neutrophils and macrophages, or extracellular capsules to discourage phagocytosis.

Pathogens are often capable of producing toxins that alter or destroy the normal function of host cells and promote colonisation, proliferation and invasion by the pathogen. Toxins often increase the disease-producing capability of the

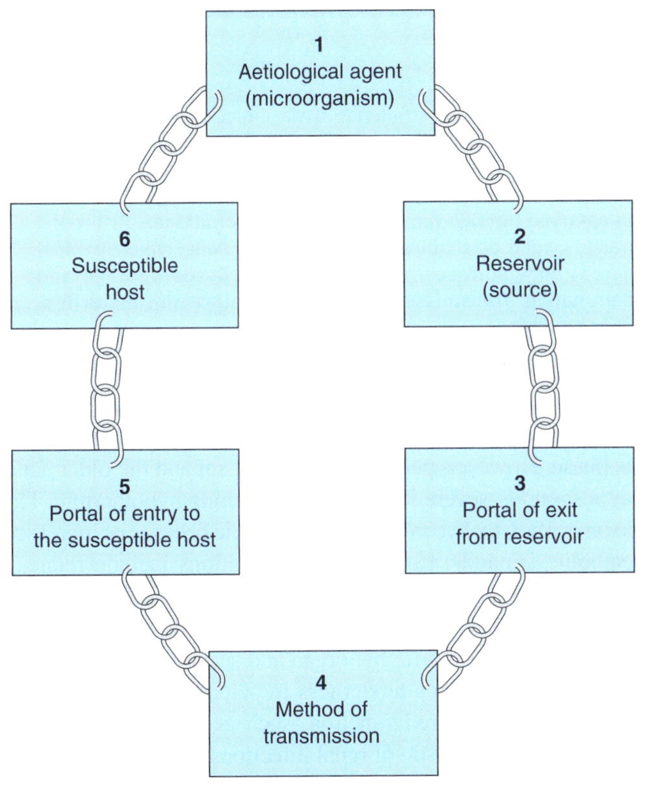

FIGURE 11.9 *The chain of infection*

pathogen and, in some cases, are totally responsible for it; for example, cholera, tetanus and botulism result from bacterial toxins, not from the direct effects of the infection. **Exotoxins** are soluble proteins secreted into surrounding tissue by the microorganism. Exotoxins are highly poisonous, causing cell death or dysfunction. **Endotoxins** are found in the cell wall of Gram-negative bacteria and are released only when the cell is disrupted. Endotoxins have less-specific effects than exotoxins but they act as activators of many human regulatory systems, producing fever, inflammation and, potentially, clotting, bleeding or hypotension when released in large quantities.

RESERVOIR AND TRANSMISSION The reservoir, or source, where the pathogen lives and multiplies, may be either endogenous or exogenous. Organisms that reside on skin or mucosal surfaces of the host are endogenous. Exogenous sources can include other humans, animals, soil, water, intravenous fluid or equipment. Infectious diseases are usually transmitted from human sources—that is, people who have clinical disease or are carriers with subclinical infection. Carriers harbour the pathogen without showing evidence of clinical disease. Pathogens exit human hosts via respiratory secretions, body fluids from the gastrointestinal and genitourinary tracts, skin or mucous membrane lesions, the placenta and blood.

Organisms may be transmitted from the source to the susceptible host by direct or indirect contact, droplet or airborne transmission, or a vector. Direct contact includes person-to-person spread

BOX 11.4 Pathogenic organisms

Bacteria

Bacteria are single-celled organisms capable of autonomous reproduction. Relatively small and simple organisms, they contain a single chromosome. A flexible cell membrane and rigid cell wall surrounds their cytoplasm, giving them a distinctive shape; some also have an extracellular capsule for additional protection. Bacteria have different characteristics and growth requirements: the colonies formed by replicating bacteria differ from one another. *Aerobes* require oxygen for survival, whereas *anaerobes* cannot survive in the presence of oxygen; *Gram-positive* bacteria stain purple when subjected to crystal violet stain, whereas *Gram-negative* bacteria do not stain with crystal violet but turn red when subjected to safranin stain.

Prions

Prions are not independent organisms but small molecules that can modify host proteins. They primarily affect the neurological system, causing neurological degeneration in diseases such as mad cow disease (bovine spongiform encephalopathy) in animals and Creutzfeldt–Jakob disease in humans. These are slowly progressive, non-inflammatory conditions leading to dementia, lack of coordination and death. Prions' entry into the neurological cells makes them resistant to the host immune system and antibacterial and antiviral medications. They enter the host by injections, transplantation of contaminated tissue or medical devices, and possibly food. They are very resistant to disinfection, requiring special procedures for sterilising instruments, especially those used in CNS surgeries (Loscalzo et al., 2022; Rothrock, 2022).

Viruses

Viruses are obligate intracellular parasites that are incapable of reproducing outside of a living cell. Viruses consist of a protein coat around a core of either DNA or RNA. Some viruses are shed continuously from infected cell surfaces; others, after inserting their genetic material into that of the infected cell, remain latent until they are stimulated to replicate. Viruses may or may not cause lysis and death of the host cell during replication. Oncogenic viruses are able to transform normal cells into malignant cells.

Mycoplasma

Although similar to bacteria, *mycoplasma* are smaller and have no cell wall, making them resistant to antibiotics that inhibit cell wall synthesis (e.g. penicillins).

Rickettsia and *Chlamydia*

As obligate intracellular parasites with a rigid cell wall, *Rickettsia* and *Chlamydia* have some features of both bacteria and viruses. Rather than depending on the host cell for reproduction, they use vitamins, nutrients or products of metabolism (e.g. ATP) from the host. *Chlamydiae* are transmitted by direct contact, whereas many *Rickettsiae* infect the cells of arthropods (e.g. fleas, ticks and lice) and are transmitted from these vectors to humans.

Fungi

Fungi are prevalent throughout the world but few are capable of causing disease in humans. Most fungal infections are self-limited,

(continued)

BOX 11.4 Pathogenic organisms (continued)

affecting the skin and subcutaneous tissue. Some fungi, such as *Pneumocystis carinii*, can cause life-threatening opportunistic infections in the immunocompromised host.

Parasites

The term *parasite* is typically applied to members of the animal kingdom that infect and cause disease in other animals. Protozoa, helminths and arthropods are considered parasites. Protozoa are single-celled organisms (e.g. *Giardia lamblia* and *Trichomonas vaginalis*) transmitted via direct or indirect contact or an arthropod vector. Helminths are worm-like parasites: roundworms, tapeworms and flukes are examples. They gain entry into humans primarily through ingestion of fertilised eggs or penetration of larvae through the skin or mucous membranes. Arthropod parasites, such as scabies (mites), lice and fleas, typically infest external body surfaces, causing localised tissue damage and inflammation. Transmission is by direct contact with the arthropod or its eggs.

or contact with infected body fluids, as well as transmission from contaminated food or water. Indirect contact occurs when the infectious agent is contracted by use of inanimate objects such as dirty eating utensils. Sneezing, talking and coughing allow transmission by droplet contact when the host is within 1 metre of the source. Smaller respiratory particles that stay suspended in air and are carried via air currents allow airborne transmission. Vectors are insects and animals such as flies, mosquitoes or rodents that act as intermediate hosts between the source and host. Microorganisms usually first colonise the portal of entry: non-intact skin, wounds, mucous membranes and the respiratory, gastrointestinal or genitourinary tracts.

HOST FACTORS The susceptible host is the final link in the chain of infection. Exposure to pathogens does not automatically cause infection or infectious disease. The outcome of contact with a pathogenic microorganism is determined by the balance of microbial virulence and host resistance. Factors that can enable the host to resist infection include the following:

- physical barriers such as the skin and mucous membranes
- the hostile environment created by acid stomach secretions, urine and vaginal secretions
- antimicrobial factors in saliva, tears and prostatic fluid
- respiratory defences, including humidification, filtration, the mucociliary escalator, cough reflex and alveolar macrophages
- innate and adaptive immune responses to pathogenic invasion.

Stages of the infectious process

When infectious disease develops in the host, it typically follows a predictable course with stages based on the progression and intensity of manifestations.

The initial stage is the *incubation period*, during which the pathogen begins active replication but does not yet cause manifestations. Depending on the organism and host factors, the incubation period may last from hours, as with *Salmonella* infection, to years, as with HIV infection.

The *prodromal stage* follows, during which symptoms first begin to appear. At this stage, manifestations are often non-specific and include general malaise, fever, myalgias, headache and fatigue.

Maximal impact of the infectious process is felt during the *acute phase* as the pathogen proliferates and disseminates rapidly. Toxic by-products of microorganism metabolism and cell lysis, along with the immune response, produce tissue damage and inflammation during this stage (Norris, 2018). Manifestations are more pronounced and specific to the infecting organism and site during the acute stage. Fever and chills may be significant during this phase. However, people with alcoholism and the older adult may respond to severe infection by becoming hypothermic. The person is often tachycardic and tachypnoeic because of increased metabolic demands. Localised manifestations include redness, heat, swelling, pain and impaired function. When the infectious disease affects an internal organ, manifestations are related to inflammatory changes in that organ and surrounding tissue. The person may experience tenderness to palpation over the site or show signs of impaired function, such as the haematuria and proteinuria characteristic of renal infections.

If the infectious process is prolonged, manifestations of the continuing immune response may become apparent. Catabolic and anorexic effects of the infection can lead to loss of body fat and muscle wasting. Immune complexes may be deposited at sites other than the primary infection, resulting in an inflammatory process. Glomerulonephritis (e.g. following strep throat) and vasculitis are possible results. Another possible consequence of prolonged infection and immune response is the triggering of an autoimmune disease process such as rheumatic cardiomyopathy or coeliac disease.

As the infection is contained and the pathogen eliminated, the *convalescent stage* of the disease occurs. During this stage, affected tissues are repaired and manifestations resolve. Resolution of the infection is total elimination of the pathogen from the body without residual manifestations. If a balance between organism and host factors occurs, with neither predominating, chronic disease may develop or the organism may be driven into a protected site such as an abscess. A carrier state develops when host defences eliminate the infectious disease but the organism continues to multiply on mucosal sites.

Complications

Multiple and varied complications are associated with infectious diseases. They are typically specific to the infecting organism and the body system affected.

Acute invasion of the blood by certain microorganisms or their toxins can result in septicaemia and septic shock. Whereas *bacteraemia*, the presence of bacteria in the blood, may not have serious effects, **septicaemia** refers to systemic disease associated with their presence or toxins. Septic shock indicates a state of hypotension and impaired organ perfusion resulting from sepsis, a life-threatening condition that occurs when the body's response to an infection damages its own tissues and organs. Unless treated aggressively, septic shock leads to diffuse cell and tissue injury

FAST FACTS

- Urinary tract infection is the most common type of healthcare-associated infection (HAI), usually associated with indwelling urinary catheters or urological procedures.
- Other common HAIs are bloodstream infections, pneumonia, surgical wound infections and *Clostridium difficile* colitis (National Health and Medical Research Council (NHMRC), 2019; Papadakis, McPhee & Rabow, 2022).
- Pathogens associated with HAI are often different from those causing community-acquired infections and frequently are multidrug resistant, necessitating treatment with multiple, broad-spectrum and potentially toxic antibiotics (Papadakis et al., 2022).

and potentially to organ failure. The ACSQHC Sepsis Clinical Standard, released in June 2022, forms part of the National Sepsis Program that aims to improve early recognition, treatment, outcomes and post-discharge support for people at risk of, or diagnosed with, sepsis in Australia (Australian Commission on Safety and Quality in Health Care (ACSQHC), 2022a).

Healthcare-associated infections

Healthcare-associated infections (HAIs) are acquired in any healthcare setting, such as a hospital or nursing home. Also called *nosocomial* infections, HAIs account for an estimated 200,000 infections, 2 million bed days lost and, for the surgical post-discharge infection subgroup, $21 million in excess healthcare costs annually in Australia. HAIs add hospital days, reduce admissions by occupying available beds and add to the cost of healthcare (ACSQHC, 2009; Mitchell et al., 2017; Russo et al., 2019).

Many HAIs result from the use of invasive devices such as intravascular catheters, urinary catheters and endotracheal tubes for ventilator support. People developing HAIs often are critically ill and among those least able to mount an effective immune defence against infection. HAIs also occur when antibiotic therapy has altered natural defences and impaired resistance to harmful microorganisms. Endogenous organisms outside their normal habitats (such as in *Escherichia coli* in the urinary tract) become a threat to the person. Other pharmacological and therapeutic procedures such as chemotherapy, the use of corticosteroids or radiation therapy also contribute to HAIs. Surgical site infections rank second in frequency of HAIs and add up to 7 to 10 extra days to postoperative hospitalisation (ACSQHC, 2009; Loscalzo et al., 2022). Superficial or deep wounds may be contaminated by endogenous or exogenous sources. Infections in body cavities or those associated with prosthetics are difficult to diagnose and may necessitate removal of the prosthetic device. Box 11.5 lists interventions that should be used to prevent HAIs.

Hospital-acquired pneumonia accounts for 15% of HAIs. It is usually associated with ICU stays and mechanical ventilation. Organisms causing the infection are often resistant to many drugs, not responding to antibiotics usually effective in treating infections acquired outside the hospital. More deaths are associated with hospital-acquired pneumonia than any other site of infections (Loscalzo et al., 2022).

BOX 11.5 Interventions to reduce healthcare-associated infections

- Central venous catheter infections have decreased by using chlorhexidine antiseptic for disinfection and maximal barrier precautions during insertion.
- Ventilator-associated pneumonia is decreased by weaning patients off ventilators as soon as possible, limiting sedation of the patient, positioning patients with the head of the bed elevated to prevent gastric reflux and for maximal ventilation, and using proper hand hygiene and sterile technique for all ventilator-associated care.
- Surgical site infections are reduced by administering a prophylactic antibiotic 1 hour before the incision and discontinuing it within 24 hours after surgery, limiting hair removal (no shaving), controlling perioperative glucose levels (especially in cardiac surgeries) and ensuring normothermia for the patient during the perioperative period (especially in colorectal surgeries).
- Insert urinary catheters only when clearly indicated, using aseptic technique during insertion; minimise manipulation or opening of drainage systems (Loscalzo et al., 2022).

CONSIDERATION FOR PRACTICE

Existing guidelines and literature reviews agree that hand hygiene using alcohol-based hand rubs is more effective against the majority of common infectious agents on hands than hand hygiene with plain or antiseptic soap and water (NHMRC, 2019).

A soap-and-water wash is recommended for visibly soiled hands. Wearing gloves does not eliminate the need to perform hand hygiene.

Prevention is the most important control measure for HAIs. Cross-infection—the spread of pathogens from one person to another on the inadequately cleaned hands of healthcare workers—is one of the primary sources of HAIs (Loscalzo et al., 2022). *Effective hand hygiene is the single most important measure in infection control* (WHO, 2009, 2022) (see Figure 11.10). Although infections may also be transmitted by the airborne route, from contaminated equipment or from the environment, these are less significant causes. Invasive procedures and equipment should be used only when absolutely necessary; for example, it is not appropriate to insert an indwelling catheter when the only indication is incontinence. Peripheral intravenous equipment and sites must be kept clean and changed regularly: intravenous bags and bottles every 24 hours, tubing every 24 to 72 hours and sites every 2 to 3 days according to agency policy.

Antibiotic-resistant microorganisms

Antibiotic-resistant microorganisms are increasing at an alarming rate, primarily due to prolonged or inappropriate use of antibiotic therapy. Although antibiotic therapy is expected to eradicate all targeted microorganisms, sometimes a few bacteria survive, leading to bacteria that reproduce with antibiotic resistance already encoded into their genetic

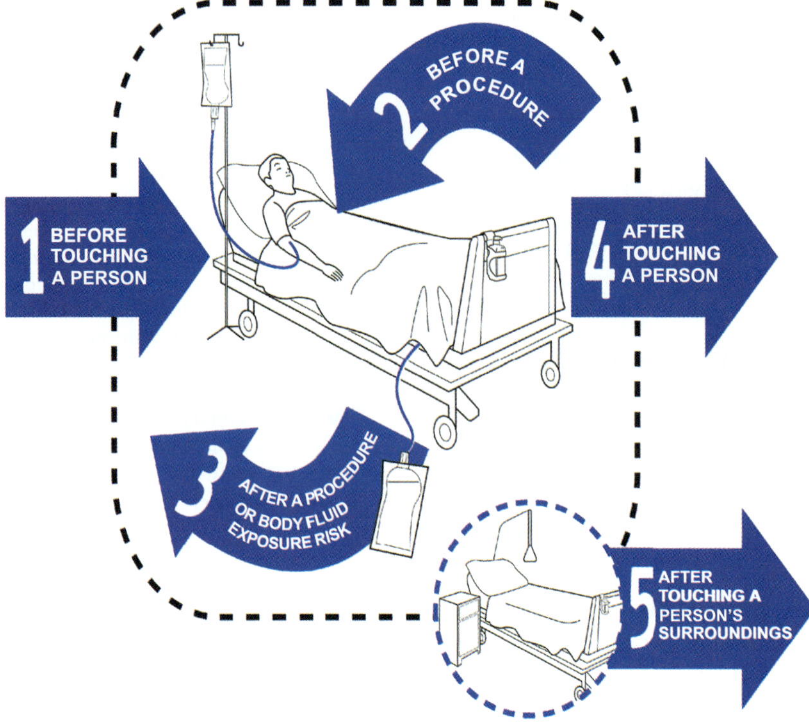

FIGURE 11.10 *5 Moments for Hand Hygiene*

Source: Reprinted from *Hand Hygiene When and How* leaflet, p. 2. © 2009. https://www.who.int/gpsc/5may/background/5moments/en/index.html. © World Health Organization 2009. All rights reserved.

NURSING CARE OF THE OLDER ADULT Infections

Because immune function declines with ageing, older adults are more susceptible to infections. Physiological changes that often occur with ageing place the older adult at greater risk than younger people of acquiring an infection.

- *Cardiovascular changes*: decreased tissue perfusion delays the inflammatory response and healing.
- *Respiratory system changes*: decreased mucociliary clearance, decreased elastic recoil and diminished cough and laryngeal reflexes decrease the clearance of respiratory secretions and increase the risk of pneumonia. The older adult with pneumonia may not present with cough or sputum production due to decreased immune function. The leading causes of pneumonia in older adults include *Streptococcus pneumoniae*, *Haemophilus influenzae* and *Staphylococcus aureus*. Influenza A, a viral infection, is a significant risk factor for secondary bacterial pneumonia in older adults (Eliopoulos, 2021; Vafeas & Slatyer, 2021). Both pneumonia and influenza cause high mortality rates in the older person.
- *Genitourinary changes*: loss of muscle tone, reduced bladder contractility, altered bladder reflexes and prostatic hypertrophy in men increase the risk for incomplete bladder emptying, urinary incontinence and urinary tract infection (UTI). UTI is the most common infection and the leading cause of bacteraemia and sepsis in older adults, particularly those aged 85 and older.
- *Gastrointestinal system changes*: impaired swallow reflex, decreased gastric acidity and delayed gastric emptying increase the risk of aspiration with subsequent pneumonia.
- *Skin and subcutaneous tissue changes*: thinning of skin, decreased cushioning, decreased sensation and decreased vasculature increase the risk of injury, ulceration and infection.
- *Immune changes*: decreased phagocytosis, reduced inflammatory response, diminished antibody-mediated and cellular immune responses, and slowed or impaired healing processes increase the risk for infection. Immunoglobulin levels remain relatively stable, but primary and secondary antibody responses decline with ageing. The thymus gland atrophies and some T-cell populations decrease or decline in function. T-cell activation and the ability to proliferate following activation also decline with advancing age

NURSING CARE OF THE OLDER ADULT **Infections (continued)**

(Norris, 2018). Resistance to antigens such as *Mycobacterium tuberculosis*, influenza and varicella-zoster viruses, malignant cells and tissue grafts is reduced.

Other factors, such as a lower activity level, poor nutrition and an increased risk for dehydration, a higher prevalence of chronic diseases such as diabetes, use of multiple medications and altered mentation contribute to the older adult's risk for infection.

HAIs are more common in older adults. The nurse must steadfastly adhere to principles of infection control. Nursing interventions to reduce the risk of HAIs include: (1) avoiding prolonged bed rest, (2) encouraging patients to take deep breaths, (3) providing adequate fluids, (4) providing regular toileting schedules with good hygiene, and (5) avoiding use of invasive devices such as indwelling catheters unless medically necessary.

The older adult may not exhibit the classic manifestations of inflammation and infection. The manifestations of inflammation—redness, heat and swelling—tend to be diminished or absent in older adults. The classic manifestations of infection—fever and chills—may be absent altogether because of age-related changes in the immune system, loss of central temperature control mechanisms, decreased muscle mass and loss of shivering ability. The older adult may have only subtle manifestations of infection or sepsis, including changes in mental status, disorientation, restlessness and tachypnoea.

Prompt identification and treatment of infection improves outcomes in the older adult. In addition to monitoring for changes in the patient's mental status or behaviour, the nurse should assess fluid intake and urinary output, activity levels, complaints of fatigue and respiratory status. Older adults are at increased risk for dehydration due to diminished thirst sensation and impaired water conservation by the kidneys. Carefully evaluate intake and output to determine if input is adequate.

make-up (ACSQHC, 2022b; Burchum & Rosenthal, 2018). Other bacteria produce enzymes that inactivate drugs, change drug-binding sites or alter their cell membrane to prevent drug absorption.

Standard precautions, most importantly hand hygiene and the use of carefully selected antibiotics, are critical actions for stopping the spread of these diseases. Equipment such as stethoscopes, blood pressure cuffs and thermometers should be restricted to use by each person identified with one of these diseases. Personal protective equipment, used and disposed of appropriately, is an important safeguard.

INTERPROFESSIONAL CARE

The goals of care for the person with an infection are to identify the organ system affected by the infection and the causative agent, and to achieve a cure by the least toxic, least expensive and most effective means. Fortunately, most infectious diseases are self-limiting and will resolve with little or no medical care. However, medical treatment can be lifesaving in an overwhelming infection or immunocompromised host.

The site of the infection is often obvious from the person's history and presenting manifestations. Identifying the affected organ system allows the range of possible infecting organisms to be narrowed to those known to affect that system.

Once the infecting agent has been identified, either positively or by probability, therapy can be specifically tailored to the person's needs. Viral infections often resolve without treatment other than supportive care, such as providing rest and fluids. Skin infections may respond to a topical agent, avoiding the potential adverse effects of one administered systemically.

PATIENT SAFETY COMPETENCY FRAMEWORK

1 Person-centred care

The Patient Safety Competency Framework indicates that nursing students must demonstrate person-centred care by providing holistic care that takes into account reducing the risk of patients acquiring healthcare-associated infections and effectively managing infections if they occur (Levett-Jones et al., 2017).

Diagnosis

To assess the person's response to infection, identify the infecting organism and monitor the progress of therapy, the following diagnostic tests may be ordered:

- *WBC count* provides clues about the infecting organism and the body's immune response to it.
- *WCC differential* is also ordered (see Table 11.8). Neutrophilia, increased numbers of circulating neutrophils (or PMNs), is a common response with infection as the bone marrow responds to an increased need for phagocytes. Along with neutrophilia, a shift to the left is common in acute infection. This means that there are more immature neutrophils in circulation than normal, indicating an appropriate bone marrow response (see Figure 11.11).
- *Procalcitonin (CTpr) and C-reactive protein (CRP)* are diagnostic markers of infection that can be measured in the blood. Blood levels of CTpr and CRP increase dramatically with serious bacterial infection and sepsis, making these markers useful early indicators of systemic infections.

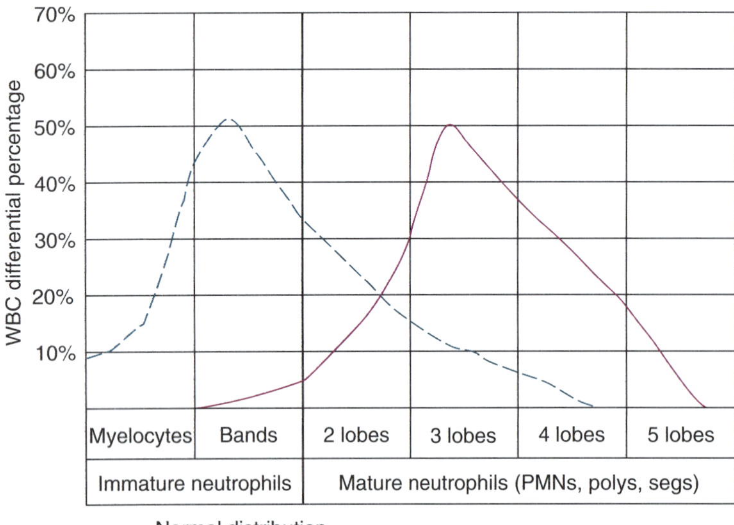

Type of WBC	Normal differential	Shift to left
Myelocytes	0%	Present
Band neutrophils (bands)	3–5%	Increased
Segmented neutrophils (segs, polys, PMNs)	50–65%	May be stable, increased or decreased

FIGURE 11.11 ***Neutrophils by stage of maturity and normal distribution in the blood***

- *Cultures of the wound, blood or other infected body fluids* are used to identify probable microorganisms by their characteristics, such as shape, growth patterns and Gram-staining qualities. After the organism is cultured, it is subjected to various antibiotics known to be effective against its particular strain to determine which antibiotic is likely to be most effective. Generally, 24 to 48 hours are required to grow the organism, potentially delaying the institution of therapy. Because antibiotics can alter the ability to culture an organism, specimens should be obtained before instituting therapy.
- *Serological testing* provides an indirect means of identifying infecting agents by detecting antibodies to the suspected organism. When the antibody titre against a specific organism rises during the acute phase of an infectious disease and begins to fall during convalescence, the diagnosis is supported. Although it is not as accurate as culture, serology is particularly useful for organisms that cannot easily be cultured, such as hepatitis B or HIV.
- *Direct antigen detection methods* use monoclonal antibodies (purified antibody forms) to detect antigens in specimens from the diseased host. The tests offer rapid and accurate identification of the offending microorganism.
- *Antibiotic peak and trough levels* monitor therapeutic blood levels of the prescribed medication(s). The therapeutic range—that is, the minimum and maximum blood levels at which the drug is effective—is known for a given drug. By measuring blood levels at the predicted peak (1 to 2 hours after oral administration, 1 hour after

Links to National Patient Safety Standards

NSQHS: Preventing and Controlling Infections Standard

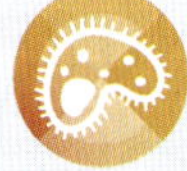

The intention of this standard is to 'reduce the risk of patients acquiring preventable healthcare-associated infections, effectively manage infections if they occur, and limit the development of antimicrobial resistance through prudent use of antimicrobials as part of antimicrobial stewardship' (ACSQHC, 2021, p. 22).

Implementing this standard is achieved by implementing systems to prevent and manage healthcare-associated infections and communicate these to the workforce to achieve appropriate outcomes. This includes governance and systems for infection prevention, control and surveillance; infection prevention and control strategies; infections or colonisations; antimicrobial stewardship (safe and appropriate antimicrobial prescribing); and cleaning, disinfection and sterilisation.

Infection prevention and control is necessary to reduce the development of resistant pathogens and to minimise the risk of transmission by isolating the infectious organism or the patient, and by using standard and transmission-based precautions.

Efficient and appropriate systems are imperative to ensure the safety of not only the person receiving appropriate care, but also any other individual involved in their care.

Effective communication should exist across all individuals involved in a person's care (including the person themself and their significant others).

Source: ACSQHC (2021). *National Safety and Quality Health Service Standards* (2nd ed.). Sydney: ACSQHC.

intramuscular administration and 30 minutes after intravenous administration) and trough (lowest level, usually a few minutes before the next scheduled dose), healthcare personnel can determine that the person is maintaining a level within the therapeutic range at all times, ensuring maximal effect from the drug. It is also possible to determine whether the drug is reaching a toxic or harmful level during therapy, increasing the likelihood of adverse effects.

- *Radiological examination of the chest, abdomen or urinary system* may be ordered to detect organ abnormalities indicating an inflammatory response or tissue damage.
- *Lumbar puncture* is performed to obtain cerebrospinal fluid (CSF) for examination and culture if a central nervous system (CNS) infection, such as meningitis or encephalitis, is suspected.
- *Ultrasonic examination* is a non-invasive diagnostic test such as an echocardiogram or renal ultrasonography to identify an infectious site or evaluate the effects of an infection on organ function.

Medications

After the infecting organism and affected body system have been identified, specific therapy to cure the infectious disease can be instituted.

Antimicrobial preparations are broadly classified as bacteriostatic or bactericidal. **Bacteriostatic agents** inhibit the growth of the microorganism, leaving its destruction to the host's immune system. These agents are generally not indicated for the immunocompromised host. Tetracyclines, erythromycin and chloramphenicol are bacteriostatic preparations. **Bactericidal agents**, including penicillins, cephalosporins and aminoglycoside antibiotics, are capable of killing the organism without immune system intervention.

The activity of antimicrobial agents on bacteria, fungi and viruses falls under five basic mechanisms:

1. impairing cell wall synthesis, leading to lysis and cell destruction
2. inhibiting protein synthesis, causing impaired microbial function
3. altering cell membrane permeability, causing intracellular contents to leak
4. inhibiting the synthesis of nucleic acids
5. inhibiting cell metabolism and growth.

Many microorganisms have the ability to develop resistance to an anti-infective agent; that is, the pathogen continues to live and grow in the presence of the anti-infective. Resistance develops as a result of a chance mutation by the pathogen, allowing a subpopulation of cells to survive. The chance of an organism becoming resistant to an agent is partially related to the dose delivered. Resistance is less likely to occur when a lethal dose is administered; therefore, it is vital that people understand the need to take all doses of the prescribed drug as ordered.

ANTIBIOTICS Medications used to treat bacterial infections are generally known as antibiotics. Most antibiotics are biological substances; that is, substances produced by other microorganisms. Antibiotics fall into classes of drugs with related chemical structure and activity. Some are effective against only Gram-positive bacteria and others are effective against only Gram-negative organisms. Broad-spectrum antibiotics have activity against a wide variety of bacteria including both Gram-positive and Gram-negative forms.

No antibiotic is totally safe. Hypersensitivity responses occur, so always check for allergies before administering the first dose. Some drugs are toxic to organ systems, exhibiting hepatotoxicity, nephrotoxicity, ototoxicity or bone marrow suppression. The antibiotics presented in the 'Medication administration' box are organised according to their antibacterial action.

ANTIVIRALS Most antibiotics have little effect on viruses because the virus has no cell wall and no cytoplasm, produces no enzymes and sequesters itself in a host cell to reproduce. Antiviral agents must be very selective in differentiating normal cellular activity from viral activity. In addition, the immune function of the host is a vital component in fighting viral infections; antiviral therapy may be relatively ineffective in the severely immunocompromised host. Timely diagnosis of viral infections can be an additional problem because viruses are less easily identified using laboratory techniques. Antiviral agents in common use are summarised in the 'Medication administration' box.

MEDICATION ADMINISTRATION Antibiotic therapy

I. Cell wall synthesis inhibitors

PENICILLINS

Penicillin G
Penicillin V
Amoxicillin (Amoxil)
Amoxicillin and clavulanic acid (Augmentin)
Ampicillin (Austrapen)
Dicloxacillin (Diclocil, Distaph)
Flucloxacillin (Staphylex, Floxapen)
Piperacillin and tazobactam (Tazocin)
Ticarcillin and clavulanic acid (Timentin)

Penicillins are bactericidal and interfere with cell wall synthesis and the enzymes involved in cell division and synthesis. They are more effective on Gram-positive than Gram-negative organisms. Penicillins are considered to be safe, effective and of low toxicity. Resistance is now more common among *Streptococci* and *Staphylococci*. Penicillins and related antibiotics such as cephalosporins contain a molecular structure known as a beta-lactam ring. Some bacteria produce enzymes (beta-lactamases or penicillinases) that cleave this ring, making the antibiotics ineffective. To combat this resistance, beta-lactamase or penicillinase inhibitors such as sulbactam

(continued)

MEDICATION ADMINISTRATION Antibiotic therapy (continued)

and clavulanate are combined with some antibiotics to create an antibiotic effective against drug-resistant bacterial strains.

Nursing responsibilities

- Monitor for hypersensitivity responses such as local erythema and itching at the site of injection, skin rashes, urticaria (hives), itching, fever, chills and anaphylaxis.
- Observe people receiving parenteral penicillin for at least 30 minutes.
- Discontinue the drug immediately if any hypersensitivity response occurs. Be prepared to administer antihistamines or corticosteroids for a mild reaction. Anaphylaxis is treated with adrenaline subcutaneously or intravenously and with airway support.
- Do not administer penicillin to anyone with a history of a severe allergic reaction to any form of the drug; a cross-reactivity may occur in people allergic to cephalosporin or carbapenem antibiotics.
- Assess for superinfection (vaginitis, stomatitis or diarrhoea) due to elimination of resident bacteria.

Health education for the person and family

- Notify the doctor if you see white patches on the oral mucosa or if vaginitis develops. An antifungal drug may be prescribed and the antibiotic continued.
- Consuming yoghurt may prevent superinfection. Do not take these products within 1 hour of taking the drug.

CEPHALOSPORINS

1st generation
Cephalexin (Keflex, Ibilex)
Cephazolin (Kefzol)

2nd generation
Cefoxitin (Mefoxin)
Cefaclor (Aclor, Ceclor)

3rd generation
Cefotaxime (Claforan)
Ceftazidime (Fortrum)
Ceftriaxone (Rocephin)

4th generation
Cefepime (Maxipime)

Cephalosporins are structurally similar to the penicillins and also inhibit cell wall synthesis. They are divided into four groups or generations. First-generation cephalosporins act primarily against Gram-positive organisms. Second and third-generation drugs are more effective against Gram-negative organisms than against Gram-positive ones. Fourth-generation cephalosporins act effectively against both Gram-positive and Gram-negative organisms.

Nursing responsibilities

- Monitor for previous hypersensitivity response to cephalosporins or penicillins.
- Assess intravenous site for phlebitis; intramuscular site may cause local pain.
- Monitor laboratory results for adverse response, such as leucopenia and thrombocytopenia, nephrotoxicity (elevated BUN and serum creatinine) or hepatotoxicity (elevated bilirubin, LDH, ALT, AST and alkaline phosphatase).
- Assess for signs of superinfection.

Health education for the person and family

- Take the medication on an empty stomach, 1 hour before or 2 hours after meals.
- Avoid alcohol as alcohol intolerance can develop with these antibiotics. These same drugs intensify bleeding tendencies.
- Space doses of the medication relatively evenly throughout the day and evening hours.
- Increased consumption of yoghurt may prevent intestinal superinfection.

CARBAPENEMS

This class of antibiotics includes only three drugs and all must be given parenterally. Imipenem has the broadest antimicrobial spectrum of any drug (Burchum & Rosenthal, 2018). This makes it especially useful against mixed-organism infections. Imipenem, meropenem and ertapenem cross the meninges and achieve therapeutic doses in CSF; they are effective against methicillin-resistant *Staphylococcus aureus* (MRSA). These antibiotics cause bacterial cell wall lysis and subsequent death of the bacteria. Side effects include nausea and vomiting, diarrhoea, hypersensitivity reactions, occasional superinfections with bacteria or fungi, and, rarely, seizures.

Nursing responsibilities

Ertapenem should not be mixed with dextrose or other drugs containing dextrose. IV infusions should be slow and given over at least 30 minutes.

- Check for history of hypersensitivity to cephalosporins and penicillins and monitor for signs of reactions.
- Assess for signs of superinfection.
- Monitor laboratory indicators of renal function.

Health education for the person and family

- Instruct the person to report any signs or symptoms of allergy such as skin rash, itching or hives.

VANCOMYCIN

This antibiotic inhibits cell wall synthesis and is used for serious infections. It is only effective against Gram-positive bacteria, especially *S. aureus* and *Staphylococcus epidermidis*, including the strains resistant to methicillin. *C. difficile* is also susceptible to this antibiotic, but infection with *C. difficile* is often treated first with metronidazole to delay emergence of resistance to vancomycin.

Nursing responsibilities

- Infuse slowly over 60 minutes or more to avoid 'red man' syndrome. The syndrome is characterised by erythematous rash, flushing, tachycardia and hypotension. People may become dizzy and agitated. The occurrence is usually associated with a first dose of vancomycin and is seen within 4 to 6 minutes of the start of a dose or after completion.
- Ototoxicity is a more serious adverse effect of vancomycin because hearing loss may be irreversible. Notify the doctor immediately if a sensation of fullness in the ears is reported, as this indicates ototoxicity.

II. Bacterial protein synthesis inhibitors

TETRACYCLINES

Tetracycline HCl Minocycline HCl (Minomycin,
Doxycycline (Vibramycin) Akamin)

Tetracyclines are active against many Gram-positive and Gram-negative bacteria, such as *Mycoplasma*, *Rickettsia* and *Chlamydia*. They are bacteriostatic, interfering with microbial

MEDICATION ADMINISTRATION **Antibiotic therapy (continued)**

protein synthesis. Tetracycline binds readily with metal and solid elements in the bowel, limiting its absorption when administered with food; the other preparations are highly soluble in lipids and can be administered with food.

Nursing responsibilities

- Schedule doses 1 hour before or 2 hours after meals. Do not give with milk, milk products or antacids.
- Monitor for signs of superinfection.
- If the person is taking an anticoagulant, monitor prothrombin time and for signs of bleeding.

Health education for the person and family

- Avoid excessive sun exposure to reduce the risk of photosensitivity reactions.
- Tetracyclines can stain the enamel of developing teeth when taken during pregnancy; although deciduous (baby) teeth are affected, permanent teeth are not.

MACROLIDES

Erythromycin (Eryc) **Clarithromycin (Klacid)**
Azithromycin (Zithromax) **Roxithromycin (Rulide)**

Macrolides are bacteriostatic and act effectively against Gram-positive and Gram-negative organisms. Erythromycin is used to treat streptococcal pharyngitis in people who are allergic to penicillin. Azithromycin produces less nausea than erythromycin, increasing patient adherence.

Nursing responsibilities

- Administer erythromycin on an empty stomach or immediately before meals.
- Give the drug with a full glass of water. Do not administer with acidic fruit juice.
- Intravenous doses are very irritating to veins; give slowly (20 to 60 minutes per gram).

Health education for the person and family

- Gastric distress is a common side effect with erythromycin.

AMINOGLYCOSIDES

Amikacin (Amikin) **Gentamicin**
Neomycin (Neosulf) **Tobramycin**

Aminoglycosides are bactericidal, interfering with protein synthesis in the pathogen. They are especially effective against Gram-negative organisms. To provide a broader spectrum of activity, they are often combined with other antibiotics, especially penicillins. Aminoglycosides can be administered in multiple or single daily doses. They are ototoxic and nephrotoxic; the risk is highest for older adults, people with pre-existing renal disease and people receiving other ototoxic or nephrotoxic drugs.

Nursing responsibilities

- Assess renal function before and during aminoglycoside therapy. Monitor intake and output, daily weight, BUN and serum creatinine.
- Assess for adverse effects on hearing such as loss of perception of high tones, tinnitus and vertigo.
- Notify the doctor if the person is receiving other nephrotoxic or ototoxic drugs such as frusemide (Lasix) and ethacrynic acid (Edecrin).
- Administer intravenous preparations separately from other drugs; flush tubing before and after administration.

Health education for the person and family

- Monitor for a sudden weight gain, which may indicate adverse effects on the kidney, and report it to the doctor.

OXAZOLIDINONES

Linezolid is the first antibiotic in the class of oxazolidinones. This antibiotic inhibits protein synthesis and is effective against organisms that are resistant to both vancomycin and methicillin. Because of its usefulness against those organisms, it should be reserved for infections caused by vancomycin-resistant enterococci (VRE) and MRSA (Burchum & Rosenthal, 2018).

Nursing responsibilities

- Monitor for side effects including nausea, diarrhoea, hypertension and headache.
- Monitor platelets if person is at risk for bleeding; this drug may cause thrombocytopaenia.

Health education for the person and family

- It can be taken with or without food.
- Avoid taking adrenaline, pseudoephedrine, methylphenidate or cocaine with this drug as hypertension may develop.

III. Bacterial nucleic acid inhibitors

FLUOROQUINOLONES

Ciprofloxacin (Ciproxin) **Norfloxacin (Noroxin)**
Moxifloxacin (Avelox)

Fluoroquinolones are bactericidal and especially active against Gram-negative and some Gram-positive organisms. They are used to manage infections of the respiratory, gastrointestinal and genitourinary tracts. Rarely, drugs in this class can cause tendon rupture, with the highest risk in people aged 60 and older and in those taking glucocorticoid medications (Adams et al., 2019).

Nursing responsibilities

- Increase fluid intake to 2,000 to 3,000 mL/day, unless contraindicated, to prevent crystalluria.
- Monitor laboratory results for hepatotoxicity (elevated ALT, AST).

Health education for the person and family

- If tendon inflammation or pain develops, stop taking the drug and immediately report to your healthcare provider.
- Drink 6 to 8 glasses of water per day.
- Avoid exposure to sunlight while taking these drugs.

SULFONAMIDES AND TRIMETHOPRIM

Sulfadiazine
Trimethoprim (Alprim)
Timethoprim and Sulfamethoxazole (Bactrim, Septrin)

Sulfonamides are bacteriostatic. Trimethoprim is an antibiotic effective against most Gram-positive and many Gram-negative organisms. It is often combined with sulfamethoxazole to manage urinary tract infections, *P. carinii* pneumonia and otitis media. Skin rashes and pruritus are the most common hypersensitivity reactions. Severe reactions include exfoliative dermatitis and Stevens–Johnson syndrome.

(continued)

MEDICATION ADMINISTRATION Antibiotic therapy (continued)

Nursing responsibilities

- Assess for history of hypersensitivity to sulfonamides and related medications, such as thiazide diuretics and hypoglycaemic preparations.
- Monitor intake and output. Unless contraindicated, maintain a fluid intake of at least 1,500 mL/day.
- Assess for evidence of bleeding, easy bruising or systemic infection, and monitor blood count for possible bone marrow depression.

Health education for the person and family

- Take medication on an empty stomach with a full glass of water. Maintain a fluid intake of at least 2 L per day.
- Protect the skin from excessive sun exposure with clothing and sunscreens to reduce the risk of photosensitivity.

NITROIMIDAZOLES

Metronidazole (Flagyl)
Tinidazole (Fasigyn)

Nitroimidazoles are metabolised to active metabolites that are thought to interfere with DNA synthesis. Metronidazole is effective against anaerobic Gram-negative and Gram-positive bacteria and protozoan infections caused by amoebiasis, giardiasis and trichomoniasis. It is commonly used to prevent and treat infections following intestinal surgery and is the drug of first choice with *C. difficile*.

Nursing responsibilities

- Monitor for CNS effects of dizziness, headache, ataxia, confusion, depression and peripheral neuropathy.
- Administer with food to minimise gastric distress and metallic taste. Infuse intravenous metronidazole over 60 minutes.
- Discontinue the medication and notify the doctor if neurological reactions occur.
- Increase fluid intake to 2,500 mL/day to minimise the risk of nephrotoxicity.

Health education for the person and family

- This medication may turn urine reddish brown; caution the person that this is expected and not harmful.
- Stop taking the drug and notify the doctor if hypersensitivity reaction or adverse effects occur, such as changes in mentation or coordination, painful or frequent urination, painful or difficult intercourse, impotence.
- Do not drink alcohol while taking this medication; an Antabuse-type reaction (flushing, sweating, headache, vomiting and abdominal cramps) may occur.
- Maintain a fluid intake of 2.5 to 3 L per day.
- When the drug is prescribed for *Trichomonas* infections, treatment of both partners is necessary. Use condoms to prevent cross-contamination during intercourse.

MEDICATION ADMINISTRATION Antiviral agents

NEURAMINIDASE INHIBITORS

Oseltamivir (Tamiflu) and zanamivir (Relenza) are used to prevent and treat influenza. They are both active against both influenza A and B. They are generally well tolerated.

ADAMANTANES

Amantadine is used to treat influenza A. When administered within 48 hours of symptom onset, common manifestations are reduced. Generally well tolerated, CNS side effects such as dizziness, anxiety, insomnia and difficulty concentrating may occur.

ACICLOVIR (ZOVIRAX) GANCICLOVIR (CYMEVENE)

Guanine analogues are used primarily in the treatment of herpesviruses. Aciclovir is prescribed mainly in the treatment of genital herpes simplex and varicella. Although it does not kill the virus, it is effective in reducing the severity, duration and frequency of recurrence of symptoms. Ganciclovir is indicated primarily in the treatment of cytomegalovirus infection. Although aciclovir is generally well tolerated with little toxicity, ganciclovir may profoundly suppress bone marrow function.

PROTEASE INHIBITORS

Protease inhibitors prevent viral maturation and replication of HIV. These drugs are used alone or in combination with some taken orally or administered parenterally. Many people are unable to tolerate recommended doses due to adverse effects, including nausea, anorexia, malaise, severe anaemia and granulocytopenia.

INTERFERONS

Interferons (IFNs) are naturally produced cytokines that have antiviral activity. Pegylated interferon is used to treat chronic hepatitis B and hepatitis C, often in combination therapy. Common adverse effects include fatigue, flu-like symptoms, muscle and joint pain, and possible depression and insomnia (Adams et al., 2019; Schwinghammer et al., 2021).

ANTIFUNGALS Antifungal agents are available in both topical and systemic forms. They act by interfering with the cytoplasmic membrane of the fungus. Topical agents include preparations for cutaneous use to treat candidiasis, tineas and ringworm. Vaginal preparations to treat vulvovaginal candidiasis are also available, as are several non-prescription topical and vaginal antifungal agents.

Amphotericin B is a systemic antifungal agent for parenteral administration. It is used to treat severe, life-threatening fungal infections including histoplasmosis, blastomycosis and candidiasis. Another systemic antifungal in current use is flucytosine (Ancobon), which can be administered orally. It is used to treat severe candidiasis infections such as *Candida* septicaemia, endocarditis, pulmonary or urinary tract infections, and *Cryptococcus* meningitis.

Fluconazole (Diflucan) has the broadest use as an antifungal agent. It can be administered either orally or parenterally and is used to treat candidiasis infections as well as *Cryptococcus* meningitis. It is generally better tolerated than other systemic antifungal medications.

Links to National Patient Safety Standards

NSQHS: Medication Safety Standard

The intention of this standard is to 'ensure clinicians are competent to safely prescribe, dispend and administer appropriate medicines and to monitor medicine use' and that 'consumers are informed about medicines and understand their individual medicine needs' (ACSQHC, 2021, p. 30).

Implementing this standard is achieved by organisation-wide systems to support and promote safety for medication management, obtaining the best possible patient medication history, undertaking medication review and providing information about medicines' need and risks, and giving a medicine list to the receiving clinician when handing over care.

Source: ACSQHC (2021). *National Safety and Quality Health Service Standards* (2nd ed.). Sydney: ACSQHC. © Australian Commission on Safety and Quality in Health Care.

PATIENT SAFETY COMPETENCY FRAMEWORK

9 Medication safety

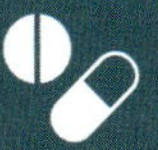

The Patient Safety Competency Framework indicates that nursing students must show medication safety by demonstrating the ability to administer and monitor the therapeutic use of medications and respond appropriately to medication errors and adverse drug effects (Levett-Jones et al., 2017).

ANTIPARASITICS Drugs used to treat parasitic infections are as varied as the organisms that cause them. Generally, agents classified as antiparasitic are both expensive and likely to be toxic. Quinine was one of the first antiparasitic drugs developed in the treatment of malaria. Quinine is highly toxic, but newer forms such as chloroquine, hydroxychloroquine (Plaquenil) and paludrine (Proguanil hydrochloride) are widely used as antimalarial drugs. Metronidazole (e.g. Flagyl) is used to treat infections of protozoan parasites (see the 'Medication administration' box for antibiotic therapy).

Isolation precautions

Controlling the spread of infectious diseases in the hospital or long-term care setting is particularly important in preventing healthcare-associated infections. Hand hygiene remains the single most important factor in preventing the transmission of infections. Most infectious diseases are transmitted by either direct or indirect contact and their spread is prevented through the use of standard precautions. However, diseases such as chickenpox (caricella) are highly contagious and are spread by the airborne route, requiring special precautions to protect other hospitalised patients.

In determining the need for transmission-based precautions, healthcare personnel consider the usual reservoir or source of the microorganism, the mode of transmission and the susceptibility of hospital staff and other people.

Standard precautions

The *Australian Guidelines for the Prevention and Control of Infection in Healthcare* (NHMRC, 2019) describe *standard precautions* as work practices that are applied to everyone, regardless of their perceived or confirmed infectious status. The aim of standard precautions is to prevent or reduce the likelihood of transmission of infectious agents from one person or place to another and to maintain objects and areas as free as possible from infectious agents.

Standard precautions include the following work practices:

- personal hygiene practices, particularly hand hygiene
- use of personal protective equipment (PPE) including gloves, plastic aprons and gowns, masks, face shields and eye protection
- appropriate handling and disposal of sharps
- environmental controls including cleaning and spills management
- appropriate processing of reusable equipment and instruments
- practising respiratory hygiene and cough etiquette
- aseptic non-touch technique
- appropriate handling of waste and linen.

Barrier protection (i.e. use of PPE) is used to prevent exposing skin and mucous membrane surfaces to blood and body fluids. Barrier protection involves using gloves for touching and handling body fluids, and adding other protection such as gowns, masks and goggles if splashing or spraying is likely. Use of aseptic technique, sterile single-use disposable needles and syringes, single-use vials for preparing and administering parenteral medication is emphasised. Needles and other sharp objects are not recapped or bent but are disposed of in puncture-proof containers to prevent inadvertent percutaneous (needle-stick) exposure.

Transmission-based precautions

In addition to the use of hand hygiene and standard precautions, additional work practices are recommended in situations where standard precautions are not sufficient to prevent transmission. Not all infectious diseases spread readily; however, diseases such as chickenpox (varicella) and pulmonary tuberculosis are highly contagious and are spread by the airborne route, requiring special precautions to protect other hospitalised people.

The NHMRC (2019) identifies three types of transmission-based precautions: contact, droplet and airborne precautions. Transmission-based precautions may be combined for diseases that have multiple routes of transmission. Indications for the use of transmission-based isolation precautions and the specific work practices to be taken are outlined in Table 11.9.

TABLE 11.9 Transmission-based precautions

CATEGORY	INFECTIOUS DISEASES	PURPOSE	PRECAUTIONS
Contact precautions	Acute diarrhoea, multidrug-resistant organisms (MROs), intestinal tract pathogens, *C. difficile*, highly contagious skin infections	Reduce risk of transmission by direct or indirect contact. Direct contact transmission involves physical transfer of organisms from skin and blood. Indirect contact involves contact with a contaminated object.	Hand hygiene. Private room with handwashing and toilet facilities. Gown and glove on entry to care areas and remove before leaving to provide barrier protection. Single-use or dedicated devices (or decontamination prior to use on another person).
Droplet precautions	Influenza, pertussis respiratory syncytial virus (RSV), norovirus, meningococcus	Reduce risk of droplet transmission of infectious agents. Droplet transmission involves contact of mucosal surfaces with respiratory droplets generated during coughing, sneezing, talking or procedures such as suctioning.	Hand hygiene. Private room with handwashing and toilet facilities. Surgical mask, goggles or face shields to be worn by everyone entering room.
Airborne precautions	Pulmonary tuberculosis, chickenpox (with contact precautions), measles, SARS	Reduce risk of airborne transmission of infectious agents. Airborne transmission occurs by dissemination of either airborne droplet nuclei or particles containing the infectious agent.	Hand hygiene. Private room with negative pressure or special ventilation not allowing air to circulate to general facility ventilation, with handwashing and toilet facilities. P2 respirators for everyone entering room.

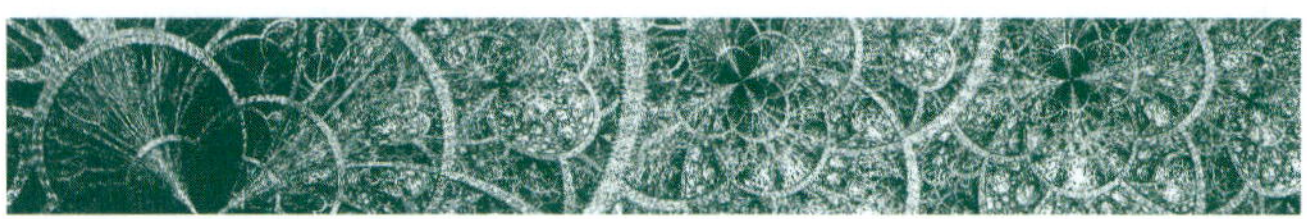

Nursing care

Nursing management related to infectious disease focuses on health promotion, prevention and prompt identification and treatment.

Health promotion

Preventing infection requires education of healthcare personnel and the general public. Education includes understanding the importance of immunisations, guidelines for using antibiotics to prevent the development of drug-resistant microorganisms and how to prevent the spread of infection.

Check immunisation records for all family members and encourage them to keep immunisations up to date. Increase public awareness regarding appropriate antibiotic use. Guidelines for preventing the spread of infection to others include the following:

- Avoid crowds and contact with susceptible people, especially those who are immunosuppressed (e.g. people who have HIV infection, who are undergoing therapy for cancer or who have had an organ transplant).
- Use disposable tissues to contain respiratory secretions when coughing or sneezing.
- Use appropriate food-handling precautions for diseases spread via the faecal–oral route, such as hepatitis A.
- Avoid contact with or sharing of body fluids. For example, do not share needles or razors; use a condom during sexual activity or abstain; have each person clean their own blood spills or wounds, if possible.

Assessment

The following data are collected through the health history and physical examination. Further focused assessments are described with nursing interventions in the next section.

- *Health history*: age, medication use (antipyretics and anti-infectives), nutrition, exposure to infectious people, immunisations, invasive procedures and therapies, chronic diseases such as diabetes mellitus, cancer.
- *Physical assessment*: vital signs, body system(s) where infection is suspected, lymph node enlargement and tenderness.

Nursing diagnoses interventions

People with an infection may be managed in the hospital or at home. During the acute phase, nursing care includes administering prescribed antibiotics, implementing and maintaining aseptic technique and infection control measures, and encouraging a balance of rest and activity, good nutritional intake and other general health measures to support immunological function and healing.

Risk of infection

The spread of infection is a risk in any facility that houses many people. It is a particular risk in hospitals, where many people have at least some degree of immunosuppression and many drug-resistant strains of pathogens are prevalent. It is vital that nurses use good hand hygiene techniques at all times, employ standard precautions in all situations and use transmission-based precautions as indicated to prevent infectious spread to other people, themselves and their families.

- Admit people with known or suspected infections to a private room. *This is important to minimise the risk of infection transmission to others.*
- Practise effective hand hygiene techniques following the '5 moments' (Hand Hygiene Australia, 2022). Utilise alcohol-based hand rubs or, when hands are visibly soiled, wash hands with soap or antibacterial scrub solution and water using a minimum 15-second hand rub. *The appropriate technique for cleansing of hands is as equally important as the selection of correct product.*
- Use standard precautions and personal protective equipment to reduce the risk of transmission. *Gloves, gowns and masks are to be worn whenever there is a risk of skin or mucous membrane contamination by direct contact with infectious material, airborne spread of organisms or droplet nuclei.*
- Explain the reasons for and importance of transmission-based precautions during hospitalisation. *Application of transmission-based precautions may make the person feel neglected, dirty or shunned. Explanation of reasons and procedures can enhance the person's and family's understanding and acceptance.*

- Place a mask on the person and/or cover all infectious lesions or wounds completely when transporting the person to other parts of the facility for diagnostic or treatment procedures. *These measures help minimise air contamination and the risk to visitors and personnel.*
- Collect a culture and sensitivity (C&S) specimen as ordered or indicated by purulent drainage, pyuria or other manifestations of infection. *C&S is performed to determine the presence and type of infectious organisms, as well as the antibiotics most likely to be effective in eradicating them.*
- Administer prescribed anti-infective agents. *Anti-infectives are used to destroy the invading microorganism.*
- Inform all healthcare workers and visitors in contact with the person requiring transmission-based precautions. *Utilise appropriate signage at the entrance to the person's room with appropriate personal protective equipment at hand so that appropriate precautions can be taken.*
- Use appropriate measures for disposing of contaminated tissues, dressings or other material, and for removing soiled linen and equipment from the person's room. *Check hospital policy or published guidelines for appropriate disposal and cleaning procedures.*

CONSIDERATION FOR PRACTICE

Collect the specimen for culture and sensitivity (C&S) before the first dose of antibiotics is administered to ensure adequate organisms for culture.

- Teach the importance of complying with prescribed treatment for the entire course of the regimen. *Because anti-infective agents kill only a portion of the pathogen population with each dose, completion of the entire course of therapy is necessary to reduce the risk of relapse and of creating drug-resistant organisms.*

Anxiety

The person with an infectious disease may experience anxiety related to their manifestations, treatment measures, the prognosis and expected outcome of the disease. The diagnosis of an infection can be traumatic, causing feelings of uneasiness, isolation, guilt (e.g. in regard to sexually transmitted infections), apprehension or depression.

- Assess level of anxiety. *The level of anxiety influences the person's response to and interpretation of the situation and the degree of threat it poses.*
- Discuss the infection, treatments, prognosis and outcomes. *Discussions help to allay fears and misconceptions.*
- Support and enhance the person's coping strategies. *A person uses intrapersonal and interpersonal mechanisms to reduce or relieve anxiety.*
- Include significant others in the plan of care. *Inclusion of family members or significant others promotes understanding and compliance, supporting reassurance and confidence.*
- Explain transmission-based precautions and answer any concerns. *Separation may be necessary to prevent the spread of infection and could cause great anxiety for the person and family members.*
- Provide referrals as needed for continuing care—for example, to home health agencies or for dressing changes or periodic assessment. *Referrals are often necessary to provide ongoing interventions and to maintain continuity of care.*

Hyperthermia

Hyperthermia is an expected consequence of the infectious disease process. Fever may produce mild, short-term effects or, when prolonged, may cause serious life-threatening effects.

- Monitor temperature, especially during episodes of chills; note heart rate and rhythm. *Chills indicate a rising temperature. Hyperthermia can cause arrhythmias.*
- Administer prescribed antipyretic as indicated for elevated temperature. Although antipyretics lower the temperature and enhance comfort for the person, this benefit must be weighed against the possible beneficial effect of an elevated temperature in the immune response. *Fever increases the motility and activity of WBCs, stimulates the production of interferon and activates T cells. In addition, temperatures above the normal range inhibit the growth of many microorganisms (Norris, 2018).*
- Promote body cooling through lowering the room temperature. *Rapid cooling stimulates the hypothalamus to increase the body's temperature; this increases both shivering and metabolic rate.*
- Monitor fluid loss; encourage increased fluid and electrolyte intake either orally or intravenously. *Hyperthermia causes fluid loss from evaporation and may result in dehydration and electrolyte imbalance.*
- If diaphoretic, bathe and provide dry clothing and bedding. *These measures increase comfort and decrease further water evaporation.*
- Promote rest periods. *Rest increases energy reserve that is depleted by an increased metabolic, heart and respiratory rate.*

CONSIDERATION FOR PRACTICE

Use ice packs, cool/tepid baths or fans with caution to prevent unnecessary shivering.

Acute pain

Pain often accompanies infections as part of the inflammatory process or secondary to delayed healing. Increasing pain in a wound may signal infection, especially if accompanied by erythema or purulence. *Keep the wound clean and dry and administer prescribed antibiotics to promote healing and decrease pain.*

Community-based care

Health education for the person and family is directed towards helping the person recover from the infection or disease, preventing its spread to others and preventing life-threatening complications. Instructions should include the following points:

- Promote the use of effective hand hygiene techniques, particularly after touching infected wounds or lesions, coughing, sneezing, blowing the nose or using the bathroom. Wash hands thoroughly before performing any procedures such as dressing changes. Wash hands with soap and water before and after preparing food or eating, using the toilet or handling nappies. Do not share eating utensils.

- Take all prescribed antibiotics as ordered, even after symptoms have subsided. Take the prescription at intervals around the clock as directed.
- Never allow anyone else to use your medications and never use anyone else's prescription even if they appear to be the same.
- Notify your healthcare provider in the following cases:
  - Symptoms do not improve within 24 to 48 hours after antibiotic therapy is instituted, or they worsen.
  - Signs of antibiotic allergy (itching, rash, difficulty breathing or swallowing, swelling of the face or tongue) occur. Discontinue medication and contact prescriber.
  - Adverse responses, such as gastrointestinal distress, that interfere with completion of the prescription.
  - Manifestations of infection that recur after completing prescribed antibiotic.
- Report redness, swelling or drainage around wounds, or persistent high fever.
- Increase fluid intake to at least 2,500 mL per day.
- Report any signs of opportunistic infections: loose, watery and foul-smelling diarrhoea; vaginal discharge or itching; fuzzy growth or white plaques in mouth or on tongue; blood in urine; chills, fever or unusual cough.
- In addition, suggest the following resources:
  - state public health department
  - Department of Health and Aged Care.

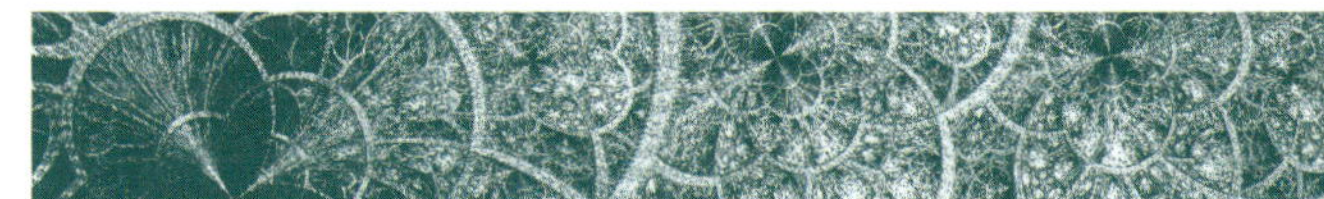

CHAPTER HIGHLIGHTS

- Innate immunity, a non-specific response to tissue injury, and the adaptive immune response, which directly targets invading microorganisms and invading cells, are critical components of the body's defences. Supporting these defences is a key nursing responsibility in promoting patient health.
- Both natural barriers and the immune system prevent the invasion and replication of pathogens.
- The adaptability and specificity of immune responses is possible because immune cells are genetically encoded to capture pathogens, move them to lymph nodes and develop specific immune reactions to destroy them.
- The inflammatory response serves to isolate invading antigens. When it occurs in response to acute injury, inflammation produces discomfort but serves a protective role. In contrast, chronic inflammation can damage affected tissue and may serve no protective function.
- Inflammation is a protective mechanism designed to prevent pathogens from entering the bloodstream and populating functional tissues such as heart, liver and kidney. Pain acts as a signal that tissue has been damaged and stimulates protective responses, such as cleansing wounds and limiting function, while healing progresses. Healing occurs as the inflammatory process isolates the injury and repairs damaged tissue.
- A fully immunised population is an important infection control strategy and a major factor in maintaining the health of individuals and the population as a whole.
- Nurses are instrumental in protecting vulnerable patients from infection, identifying early manifestations of infection, participating with the interprofessional team in treating infection and educating patients and their families about effective treatment of infection.
- Localised infections may damage tissue and create pain, but systemic infections are life threatening. Unfortunately, hospitals are hazardous environments populated with collections of pathogens. Healthcare-associated infections are often introduced into the body by medical procedures.
- Hygiene, protection from harm and nutrition support the immune defences. Antimicrobial medications limit the spread of pathogens but can lose their effectiveness when microbes mutate and develop resistance.

CONCEPT CHECK

1 When a person receives gamma globulin following exposure to hepatitis A, the nurse expects the person to develop:

1 natural active immunity
2 natural passive immunity
3 acquired active immunity
4 acquired passive immunity

2 The nurse is caring for the person with an infection. Which nursing action is a priority when providing the prescribed treatment?

1 Administer prescribed anti-infective.
2 Obtain specimen for culture and sensitivity.
3 Assess for history of hypersensitivities and allergies.
4 Monitor for reaction to prescribed anti-infective.

3 The nurse is providing medications to a patient with an inflammation. Which medication provided by the nurse will inhibit prostaglandin synthesis?

1 aspirin
2 penicillin
3 morphine sulfate
4 warfarin

4 While reviewing a patient's recent complete blood count, the nurse notes a large percentage of banded neutrophils. What does this finding indicate to the nurse?

1 renal failure
2 acute infection
3 hyperthyroidism
4 autoimmune disorder

5 A person is admitted with methicillin-resistant *Staphylococcus aureus* in a draining sacral wound. Which type of precaution should the nurse implement for this person?

1 droplet precautions
2 contact precautions
3 airborne precautions
4 protective precautions

6 A patient with a systemic inflammation is resting in bed, periodically sleeping, and wants additional blankets. Which part of the immune system is responsible for this patient's illness behaviour?
1 interferons
2 phagocytes
3 complement system
4 inflammatory cytokines

7 A patient is diagnosed with neutrophilia. What does this finding indicate to the nurse?
1 a decrease in total white blood cells
2 a decrease in circulating neutrophils
3 an increase in circulating neutrophils
4 an expected average number of white blood cells

8 The nurse is preparing discharge instructions for a person with an inflammation who is at risk for infection. What should the nurse include in the teaching?
1 Limit daily intake of calories.
2 Apply heat for 20 minutes at a time.
3 Resume normal activities of daily living.
4 Take prescribed antibiotics until fever drops.

9 The nurse is caring for an older patient recovering from an acute illness. Which intervention should the nurse implement to reduce the person's risk of developing a healthcare-associated infection?
1 Teach the patient to restrict fluids throughout the day.
2 Coach the patient to breathe deeply and cough frequently.
3 Recommend placement of an indwelling urinary catheter.
4 Wash hands with soap and water before entering the person's room.

10 The nurse is instructing unregistered health workers to use standard precautions when providing morning care to assigned patients. What should the nurse teach them specifically to do?
1 Perform hand hygiene, wear masks and recap needles.
2 Apply a mask and gown and spray working surfaces with disinfectant.
3 Apply gloves, gowns and goggles if coming in contact with body fluids.
4 Wash hands with alcohol-based hand rub for visibly dirty or blood-contaminated hands.

BIBLIOGRAPHY

Adams, M., Holland, N. & Urban, C. (2019). *Pharmacology for nurses: A pathophysiologic approach* (6th ed.). Upper Saddle River, NJ: Pearson.

Australian Commission on Safety and Quality in Health Care (ACSQHC) (2009). *Reducing harm to patients from healthcare-associated infection: The role of surveillance*. Retrieved from https://www.safetyandquality.gov.au

Australian Commission on Safety and Quality in Health Care (ACSQHC) (2021). *National Safety and Quality Health Service Standards* (2nd ed.). Sydney: ACSQHC.

Australian Commission on Safety and Quality in Health Care (ACSQHC) (2022a). *Sepsis*. Retrieved from https://www.safetyandquality.gov.au

Australian Commission on Safety and Quality in Health Care (ACSQHC) (2022b). *Antimicrobial stewardship in healthcare*. Retrieved from https://www.safetyandquality.gov.au

Australian Institute of Health and Welfare (AIHW) (2022). *COVID-19*. Retrieved from https://www.aihw.gov.au/

Burchum, J. & Rosenthal, L. (2018). *Lehne's pharmacology for nursing care* (11th ed.). St Louis, MO: Saunders/Elsevier.

Centers for Disease Control and Prevention (CDC) (2021). *Vaccines and immunizations*. Retrieved from https://www.cdc.gov/

Department of Health (2022). *The Australian immunisation handbook*. Retrieved from https://immunisationhandbook.health.gov.au/

Department of Health and Aged Care (2022). *Rabies*. Retrieved from https://www.health.gov.au/

Eliopoulos, E. (2021). *Gerontological nursing* (10th ed.). Philadelphia: Wolters Kluwer/Lippincott Williams & Wilkins.

Govindarajan, V., de Rivero Vaccari, J. & Keane, R. W. (2020). Role of inflammasomes in multiple sclerosis and their potential as therapeutic targets. *Journal of Neuroinflammation, 17*. https://doi.org/10.1186/s12974-020-01944-9

Hand Hygiene Australia (2022). *5 moments for hand hygiene*. Retrieved from http://www.hha.org.au/

Khafagy, R. & Dash, S. (2021). Obesity and cardiovascular disease: The emerging role of inflammation. *Frontiers in Cardiovascular Medicine, 8*. https://doi.org/10.3389/fcvm.2021.768119

Levett-Jones, T., Dwyer, T., Reid-Searl, K., Heaton, L., Flenady, T., Applegarth, J., Guinea, S. & Andersen, P. (2017). *Patient Safety Competency Framework (PSCF) for Nursing Students*. Sydney. Retrieved from http://psframework.wpengine.com/

Loscalzo, J., Fauci, A. S., Kasper, D. L., Hauser, S. L. & Longo, D. (2022). *Harrison's principles of internal medicine* (21st ed.). New York: McGraw Hill Medical.

Mitchell, B., Shaban, R., MacBeth., D., Wood, C. J. & Russo, P. (2017). *The burden of healthcare-associated infection in Australian hospitals: A systematic review of the literature*. https://doi.org/10.1016/j.idh.2017.07.001

National Health and Medical Research Council (NHMRC) (2019). *Australian guidelines for the prevention and control of infection in healthcare*. Commonwealth of Australia. Retrieved from https://www.nhmrc.gov.au/

Norris, T. L. (2018). *Porth's pathophysiology: Concepts of altered health states* (10th ed.). Philadelphia: Lippincott Williams & Wilkins.

Papadakis, M., McPhee, S. J. & Rabow, M. W. (2022). *Current medical diagnosis and treatment* (61st ed.). New York: McGraw-Hill Education.

Reinhardt, J. W. & Breuer, C. K. (2021). Fibrocytes: A critical review and practical guide. *Frontiers of Immunology, 12*. https://doi.org/10.3389/fimmu.2021.784401

Rothrock, J. C. (2022). *Alexander's care of the patient in surgery* (17th ed.). St Louis, MO: Elsevier.

Russo, P., Stewardson, A. Cheng, A. C. & Mitchell, B. (2019). *The burden of healthcare associated infections in Australia: A modified national point prevalence survey*. Retrieved from https://research.monash.edu/

Schwinghammer, T., DiPiro, J. T., Ellingwood Ringhold, V. & DiPiro, C. V. (2021). *Pharmacotherapy handbook* (11th ed.). New York: McGraw Hill.

Snelder, S. M., Pouw, N., Aga, Y. et al. (2021). Bio, marker profiles in obesity patients and their relation to cardiac dysfunction. *Future Medicine, 15*(14). https://doi.org/10.2217/bmm-2021-0101

Tucker, S. & Dauffenbach, V. (2019). *Nutrition and diet therapy for nurses* (2nd ed.). Upper Saddle River, NJ: Pearson.

Vafeas, C. & Slatyer, S. (2021). *Gerontological nursing: A holistic approach to the care of older people*. Chatswood, NSW: Elsevier.

World Health Organization (WHO) (2009). *WHO guidelines on hand hygiene in health care*. Retrieved from https://www.who.int/

World Health Organization (WHO) (2022). *Coronavirus disease (COVID-19) pandemic*. Retrieved from https://www.who.int/

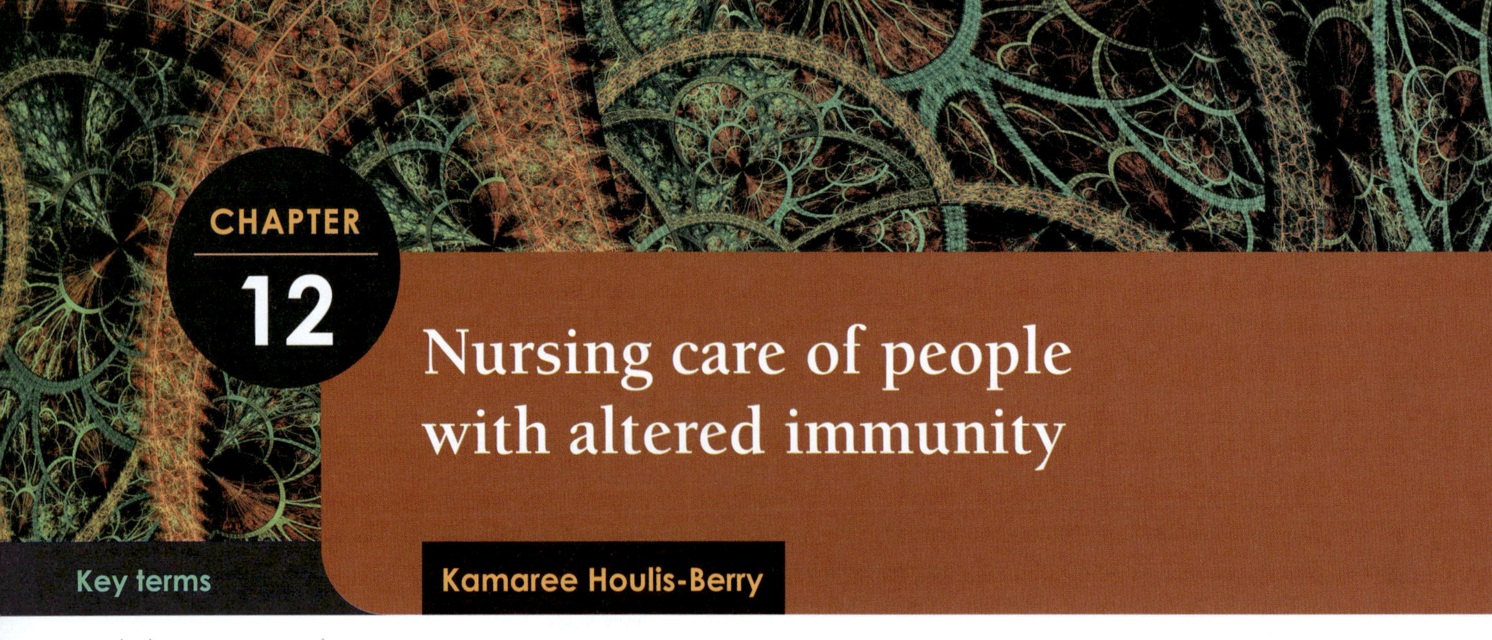

CHAPTER 12

Nursing care of people with altered immunity

Kamaree Houlis-Berry

Key terms

acquired immunodeficiency syndrome (AIDS) 334
allergy 315
allografts 327
anaphylaxis 315
autograft 327
autoimmune disorder 324
histocompatibility 327
human immunodeficiency virus (HIV) 334
hypersensitivity 315
immunosuppression 326
isograft 327
Kaposi's sarcoma (KS) 339
seroconversion 335
xenograft 327

Learning outcomes

- Review the normal anatomy and physiology of the immune system.
- Describe the four types of hypersensitivity reactions.
- Discuss the pathophysiology of autoimmune disorders and tissue transplant rejection.
- Discuss the characteristics of immunodeficiencies.
- Identify laboratory and diagnostic tests used to diagnose and monitor immune response.
- Describe pharmacological and other collaborative therapies used in treating people with altered immunity.
- Correlate the pathophysiological alterations with the manifestations of HIV/AIDS infection.

Clinical competencies

- Assess functional health status of people with altered immunity and monitor, document and report abnormal manifestations.
- Use evidence-based practice to plan and implement nursing care for people with AIDS.
- Assess for hypersensitivities and anticipate treatment if signs and symptoms develop.
- Provide education about hypersensitivities, avoidance of sensitising agents and prophylactic treatment.
- Determine priority nursing diagnoses, based on assessment data, to select and implement individualised nursing interventions and education for people with altered immunity.
- Protect people who are immunosuppressed.
- Recognise manifestations of developing anaphylaxis.
- Recognise manifestations of infection and minimise healthcare-associated exposure.
- Utilise standard precautions to protect self and other people from HIV exposure.
- Recognise the burden and benefit of antiretroviral therapy (ART) for the person with HIV infection.
- Integrate interprofessional care into care of the person with altered immunity.
- Revise plan of care as needed to provide effective interventions to promote, maintain or restore functional health status to people with altered immunity.

OVERVIEW OF THE IMMUNE SYSTEM

Recent years have seen the emergence of new diseases affecting the immune system. These diseases include human immunodeficiency virus (HIV) infection and altered strains of familiar diseases such as multidrug-resistant tuberculosis. At the same time, our understanding of the components of the immune system and specific immune responses is increasing. Therefore, it is vital that today's nurses understand the foundations of the immune system and the immune response.

The immune system functions to protect the body from invasion by foreign antigens, to identify and destroy potentially harmful cells and to remove cellular debris. These functions are accomplished by the lymphoid organs and specifically designed lymphocytes through the processes of antibody-mediated immune response and cell-mediated immune response.

The effectiveness of the immune system depends on its ability to differentiate normal host tissue from abnormal or foreign tissue. Body cells, tissues and fluids have unique antigenic properties recognised by the immune system as 'self'. External agents, such as microorganisms, cells and tissues from other humans or animals and some inorganic substances, have antigenic properties recognised by the immune system as 'non-self'.

Each body cell displays specific cell surface characteristics, or markers, that are unique to each person. These are known as human leucocyte antigens (HLAs). A person's HLA characteristics are coded within a large cluster of genes known as the major histocompatibility complex (MHC), located on chromosome 6. Recall that chromosomes are paired; each person inherits one member of the pair from each parent. A chromosome pair contains multiple genes, each carrying instructions for production of one polypeptide chain. The number of genes in the MHC results in a multitude of HLA combinations. As a result, the possibility of two people having the same HLA type is extremely remote. Identical twins may be the exception and some siblings have very similar HLA patterns. In tissue grafting and organ transplants, matching the HLA type as closely as possible tends to decrease rejection.

Immunocompetent people have an immune system that identifies antigens and effectively destroys or removes them. When the immune system functions improperly, the result may be an overreaction or deficiency, resulting in health problems. Overreaction of the immune system leads to hypersensitivity disorders, such as allergies. When the immune system loses the ability to recognise self, autoimmune disorders may ensue (see Table 12.1). Immunodeficiency diseases or malignancies can develop when the immune system is incompetent or unable to respond effectively, as is the case with acquired immunodeficiency disorder. These alterations in immunity are discussed later in this chapter.

As discussed previously in the chapter 'Nursing care of people with infections', the antibody-mediated immune response is accomplished by B lymphocytes (B cells) that are further divided into memory cells and plasma cells. They are activated by contact with an antigen and by T cells. B cells produce antibodies, also known as immunoglobulins (see Table 11.3), and serve to inactivate an invading antigen. One immunoglobulin in particular, IgM, forms natural antibodies, such as those for ABO blood group antigens, and is an important component of the immune system complexes seen in autoimmune disorders. Memory cells 'remember' an antigen and, when exposed to it a second time, immediately initiate the immune response. This action provides the foundation of acquired immunity.

In contrast, cell-mediated immunity acts at the cellular level by attacking antigens directly and by activating B cells. T lymphocytes comprise the cell-mediated immune response and are subdivided into effector cells and regulator cells. The cytotoxic cell or killer T cell is the primary effector cell. Regulator T cells are divided into two subsets known as helper T cells and suppressor T cells.

Proteins on the surface of the T cell help define its function and also provide a marker that can be used to identify the cell class. These proteins are known as the cluster of differentiation antigen or CD antigen. The two primary CD proteins are CD4 and CD8. Both cytotoxic and suppressor T cells carry the CD8 antigen. Helper T cells have the CD4 antigen and are often called CD4 cells. CD4 cells are the most numerous of the T lymphocytes, making up 70% of the circulating population.

Helper T cells initiate the immune response, whereas suppressor T cells limit it. Helper T cells accomplish their role by promoting growth of additional T cells, by stimulating proliferation of B cells and by activating killer T cells. It is believed that suppressor T cells are important in preventing autoimmune disorders. Proper immune system function depends on the correct balance between helper and suppressor T cells.

In addition to destroying viruses and bacteria, cytotoxic T lymphocytes also attack malignant cells. They also are responsible for the rejection of transplanted organs and grafted tissues.

CHANGES IN IMMUNE FUNCTION IN THE OLDER ADULT

Immune function declines with ageing, although many of the mechanisms leading to this decline are not clear. External factors, such as nutritional status and the effects of chemical exposure, ultraviolet radiation and environmental pollution, affect the older adult's immune status. Internal factors affect it as well, including genetics, the function of the neurological and endocrine systems, chronic and prior illnesses, and individual anatomical and physiological variations. These influences make it difficult to determine the effect of ageing on the immune system. In some older individuals, the immune system is as effective as that of a younger person.

Whereas the antibody response to foreign antigens is diminished, autoantibodies (antibodies that react to the person's own tissues) are more common in older people. The presence of autoantibodies suggests impaired regulation of the immune system, but it is not associated with an increased incidence of autoimmune disorders (Eliopoulos, 2021; Halter et al., 2022; Haynes, 2020; Vafeas & Slatyer, 2021). The hypersensitivity response is also reduced or delayed.

TABLE 12.1 Selected autoimmune disorders

More organ specific	Hashimoto's thyroiditis	A chronic progressive inflammatory disease of the thyroid with lymphocyte infiltration and gradual destruction of the gland. See the chapter 'Nursing care of people with endocrine disorders'.
	Primary myxoedema	Thyroid deficiency resulting from destruction of the thyroid gland due to an autoimmune process, often Hashimoto's thyroiditis. See the chapter 'Nursing care of people with endocrine disorders'.
	Thyrotoxicosis	Hyperthyroidism resulting from thyroid-stimulating immunoglobulins that stimulate activity of the gland. See the chapter 'Nursing care of people with endocrine disorders'.
	Pernicious anaemia	Anaemia resulting from absence of intrinsic factor associated with loss of parietal cells; most people have antibodies to parietal cells. See the chapter 'Nursing care of people with haematological disorders'.
	Addison's disease	Atrophy and hypofunction of the adrenal cortex, probably autoimmune in origin. See the chapter 'Nursing care of people with endocrine disorders'.
	Myasthenia gravis	A disease characterised by episodic muscle weakness caused by antibodies to the acetylcholine receptor of the neuromuscular junction. See the chapter 'Nursing care of people with neurological disorders'.
	Insulin-dependent diabetes mellitus	Impaired insulin secretion, often the result of islet cell destruction by antibodies directed at the cell surface or cytoplasm. See the chapter 'Nursing care of people with diabetes mellitus'.
	Goodpasture's syndrome	A type II hypersensitivity disorder with pulmonary haemorrhage and progressive glomerulonephritis characterised by circulating antiglomerular basement membrane antibodies. See the chapter 'Nursing care of people with kidney disorders'.
	Multiple sclerosis	A probable autoimmune process resulting in disseminated patches of demyelination in the brain and spinal cord and varied neurological manifestations. See the chapter 'Nursing care of people with neurological disorders'.
	Idiopathic thrombocytopenic purpura	A chronic disorder characterised by petechiae, purpura, mucosal bleeding and antibodies against platelets. See the chapter 'Nursing care of people with haematological disorders'.
	Primary biliary cirrhosis	Inflammation and fibrosis of the bile ducts, probably of autoimmune origin. See the chapter 'Nursing care of people with gallbladder, liver and pancreatic disorders'.
	Active chronic hepatitis	A serious liver disease often resulting in hepatic failure and/or cirrhosis; may be autoimmune with infiltration by T cells and plasma cells. See the chapter 'Nursing care of people with gallbladder, liver and pancreatic disorders'.
Less organ specific	Ulcerative colitis	A chronic inflammatory disease of colon mucosa, possibly of autoimmune origin. See the chapter 'Nursing care of people with bowel disorders'.
	Sjögren's syndrome	A systemic inflammatory disorder characterised by dryness of the mouth, eye and other mucous membranes with lymphocyte infiltration of affected tissues. See the chapter 'Nursing care of people with musculoskeletal disorders'.
	Rheumatoid arthritis	A chronic syndrome with inflammation of peripheral joints and generalised manifestations, characterised by infiltration of synovium by lymphocytes and plasma cells. See the chapter 'Nursing care of people with musculoskeletal disorders'.
	Scleroderma	Diffuse fibrosis, degenerative changes and vascular abnormalities of skin, joint structures and internal organs; probably of autoimmune origin. See the chapter 'Nursing care of people with musculoskeletal disorders'.
Non-organ specific	Systemic lupus erythematosus	An inflammatory connective tissue disorder characterised by the presence of antinuclear antibodies. See the chapter 'Nursing care of people with musculoskeletal disorders'.

ASSESSMENT OF ALTERED IMMUNE SYSTEM FUNCTION

Unlike body systems that are composed of a few closely related organs, the immune system is diverse and scattered. Optimal immune function depends on intact skin and mucous membrane barriers, adequate blood cell production and differentiation, a functional system of lymphatics and the spleen, and the ability to differentiate foreign tissue and pathogens from normal body tissue and flora. Because of this diversity of organs and function, assessment of the immune system is often integrated throughout the history and physical examination.

Health history

Prior to interviewing the person, review the biographical data, including age, sex, race and ethnic background. This information can provide valuable clues about possible immunological disorders. For example, many autoimmune disorders are more prevalent in women than in men. Family history is also important because there is a genetic component in the aetiology of many disorders affecting the immune system.

Many interview questions related to the immune system and disorders that affect it are of a sensitive nature. Be sure to provide for privacy prior to the interview. If family members are present, request that they leave as well. Establish a trusting relationship with the person prior to asking the most sensitive questions (e.g. those related to the use of illicit drugs or sexual activity). Epidemiological data show that social and racial groups have peculiar risks for HIV infection; cultural sensitivity is necessary for effective communication.

Physical assessment

The techniques of inspection and palpation are especially important in assessing a person's immune system.

- Assess the general appearance. Note whether the person's stated and apparent age coincide. Evident fatigue or weakness may indicate acute or chronic illness or immunodeficiency. Assess height, weight and body type for apparent weight loss or wasting. Observe ease of movement and note any evident stiffness or difficulty moving. Check vital signs. An elevated temperature may indicate an infection or inflammatory response.

- Inspect the mucous membranes of the nose and mouth for colour and condition. Pale, boggy (oedematous) nasal mucosa is often associated with chronic allergies. Note petechiae, white patches or lacy white plaques in the oral mucosa; they may indicate haemolysis, immunodeficiency or inflammatory injury secondary to inhalation of illicit drugs (Zhang et al., 2017).
- Assess skin colour, temperature and moisture. Pale or jaundiced skin may indicate a haemolytic reaction. Pallor may also indicate bone marrow suppression with accompanying immunodeficiency. Inspect the skin for evidence of rashes or lesions, such as petechiae, numerous bruises, purple or blue patches, or lesions indicative of Kaposi's sarcoma, and wounds that are infected, inflamed or unhealed. Note the location and distribution of any rashes or lesions.
- Inspect and palpate the cervical lymph nodes for evidence of lymphadenopathy (swelling) or tenderness. Palpate the nodes of the axillae and groin as well.
- Assess the musculoskeletal system by inspecting and palpating the joints for redness, swelling, tenderness or deformity. Such changes may indicate an autoimmune disorder such as rheumatoid arthritis or systemic lupus erythematosus. Check joint range of motion as well, including that of the spine. Rule out alternative clinical presentations including gout.

Altered immune responses

Considering the complexity of the immune system, it is not surprising that abnormal or harmful responses occur. Altered immune system responses include those characterised by hyperresponsiveness of the immune system and those characterised by an impaired immune response. Allergies, autoimmune disorders, and reactions to organ or tissue transplants are all examples of hyperresponsive immune function. AIDS and other immunodeficiency disorders result from impairment of the immune system.

THE PERSON WITH A HYPERSENSITIVITY REACTION

Hypersensitivity is an altered immune response to an antigen that results in harm to the person. When the antigen is environmental or exogenous, it is called an **allergy** and the antigen is referred to as an *allergen*. The tissue response to a hypersensitivity reaction may be simply irritating or bothersome, causing a runny nose or itchy eyes, or it may be life threatening, leading to blood cell haemolysis or laryngospasm.

Hypersensitivity reactions are primarily classified by the type of immune response that occurs on contact with the allergen. They may also be classified as immediate or delayed hypersensitivity responses. Anaphylaxis and transfusion reactions are examples of immediate hypersensitivity reactions; contact dermatitis is a typical delayed response. Allergies are sometimes referred to by the affected organ system (e.g. allergic rhinitis) or the allergen involved, as in hay fever. Classification by immunological response is the preferred means of studying allergies. Although more than one type of reaction may occur simultaneously, it is practical and insightful to study and treat allergy by classified types (King et al., 2011). The prevalence of allergy in Australia is one of the highest in the developed world, with more than 5 million Australians living with allergic disease (National Allergy Strategy, 2015, 2022).

Pathophysiology

In a hypersensitivity reaction, an antigen–antibody or antigen–lymphocyte interaction causes a response that is damaging to body tissues. Antigen–antibody responses characterise types I, II and III, also known as immediate hypersensitivity responses. Type IV hypersensitivity is an antigen–lymphocyte reaction, resulting in a delayed hypersensitivity response.

Type I: IgE-mediated hypersensitivity

Common hypersensitivity reactions, such as allergic asthma, allergic rhinitis (hay fever), allergic conjunctivitis, hives and anaphylactic shock, are typical of type I or IgE-mediated hypersensitivity. This type of hypersensitivity response is triggered when an allergen interacts with IgE bound to mast cells and basophils. The antigen–antibody complex prompts release of histamine and other chemical mediators, complement, acetylcholine, kinins and chemotactic factors (see Figure 12.1).

When a potent allergen such as bee or wasp venom or a drug is injected, resulting in widespread antibody–antigen reaction and response to these chemical mediators, a systemic response such as anaphylaxis, urticaria or angio-oedema results.

Anaphylaxis is an acute systemic type I response that occurs in highly sensitive people following injection of a specific antigen. Substances known to trigger anaphylaxis are summarised in Box 12.1. Anaphylaxis rarely follows oral ingestion, although this is possible. The reaction begins within minutes of exposure to the allergen and may be almost instantaneous. The release of histamine and other mediators causes vasodilation and increased capillary permeability, smooth muscle contraction and bronchial constriction. These chemical mediators cause the person to experience the typical manifestations of anaphylaxis. Initially, a sense of foreboding or uneasiness, light-headedness and itching palms and scalp may be noted. Hives may develop, along with angio-oedema (localised tissue swelling) of the eyelids, lips, tongue, hands, feet and genitals. Swelling can also affect the uvula and larynx, impairing breathing. This is further

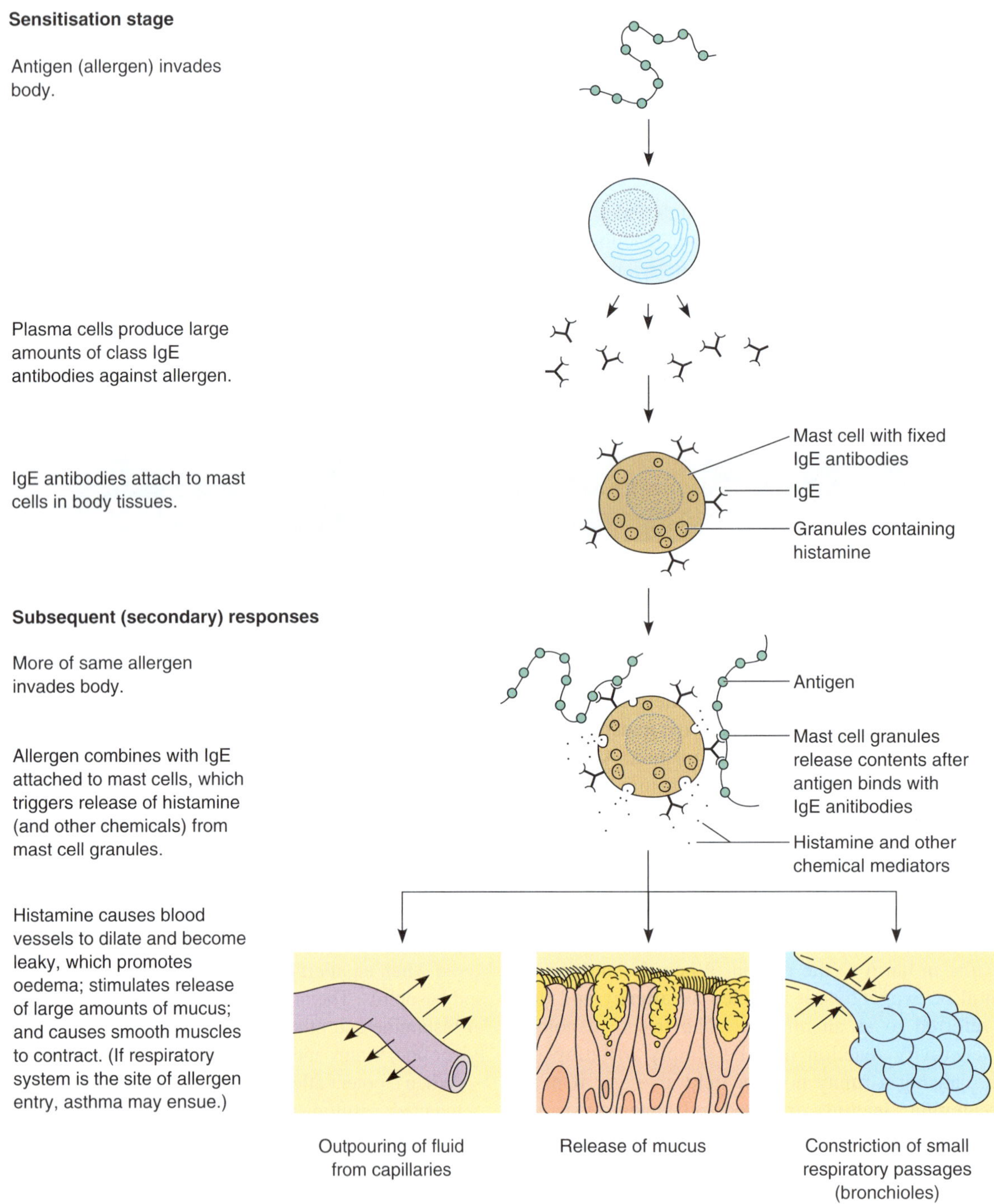

FIGURE 12.1 *Type I or IgE-mediated hypersensitivity response*

complicated by bronchial constriction. The person exhibits air hunger, stridor and wheezing, and a barking cough. These respiratory effects can be lethal if the reaction is severe and intervention is not immediately available. Vasodilation and fluid loss from the vascular system can lead to impaired tissue perfusion and hypotension, a condition known as *anaphylactic shock*.

Fortunately, localised responses are more common manifestations of type I hypersensitivity. These are typically atopic responses; that is, they have a strong genetic predisposition. Atopic reactions are the result of localised, rather than systemic, IgE-mediated responses to an allergen. They are prompted by contact of the allergen with cell-bound IgE in the bronchial tree, nasal mucosa and conjunctival tissues. Chemical mediators are released locally, producing symptoms such as asthma, allergic rhinitis (hay fever), conjunctivitis or atopic dermatitis. Allergens commonly associated with atopic reactions of this type include pollens, fungal spores, house dust mites, animal dander and feathers (Norris, 2018). Food allergens can also cause localised responses such as diarrhoea or vomiting. If the gastrointestinal mucosa is altered by a local allergic response, then the allergen may be absorbed, leading

BOX 12.1 Substances known to trigger anaphylaxis in sensitised people

Hormones
- Insulin
- Vasopressin
- Parathormone

Enzymes
- Trypsin
- Chymotrypsin
- Penicillinase

Pollens
- Ragweed
- Grass
- Trees

Foods
- Eggs
- Seafood
- Nuts
- Grains
- Beans
- Chocolate
- Dairy products
- Royal jelly

Vitamins
- Thiamine
- Folic acid

Insect venom
- Australian native ants (Jack Jumper ant)
- Wasps
- Honey bee
- Hornet
- Tick
- Other arthropods

Occupational agents
- Rubber products
- Industrial chemicals (ethylenes)

Antibiotics
- Penicillins
- Cephalosporins
- Amphotericin B
- Nitrofurantoin

Local anaesthetics
- Procaine
- Lidocaine

Medical diagnostic agents
- Sodium dehydrocholate
- Sulfobromophthalein

Antiserum
- Antilymphocyte gamma globulin

to a systemic reaction. Urticaria (hives) is the most common systemic response to food allergies.

Type II: cytotoxic hypersensitivity

Cytotoxic hypersensitivity reactions are characterised by formation of IgG or IgM antibodies against normal or foreign cells or tissues (Loscalzo et al., 2022; Norris, 2018). A haemolytic transfusion reaction to blood of an incompatible type is characteristic of a type II or cytotoxic hypersensitivity reaction. IgG or IgM type antibodies are formed to a cell-bound antigen such as the ABO or Rh antigen. When these antibodies bind with the antigen, the complement cascade is activated, resulting in destruction of the target cell (see Figure 12.2). Haemolytic disease of the newborn is caused by this type of reaction.

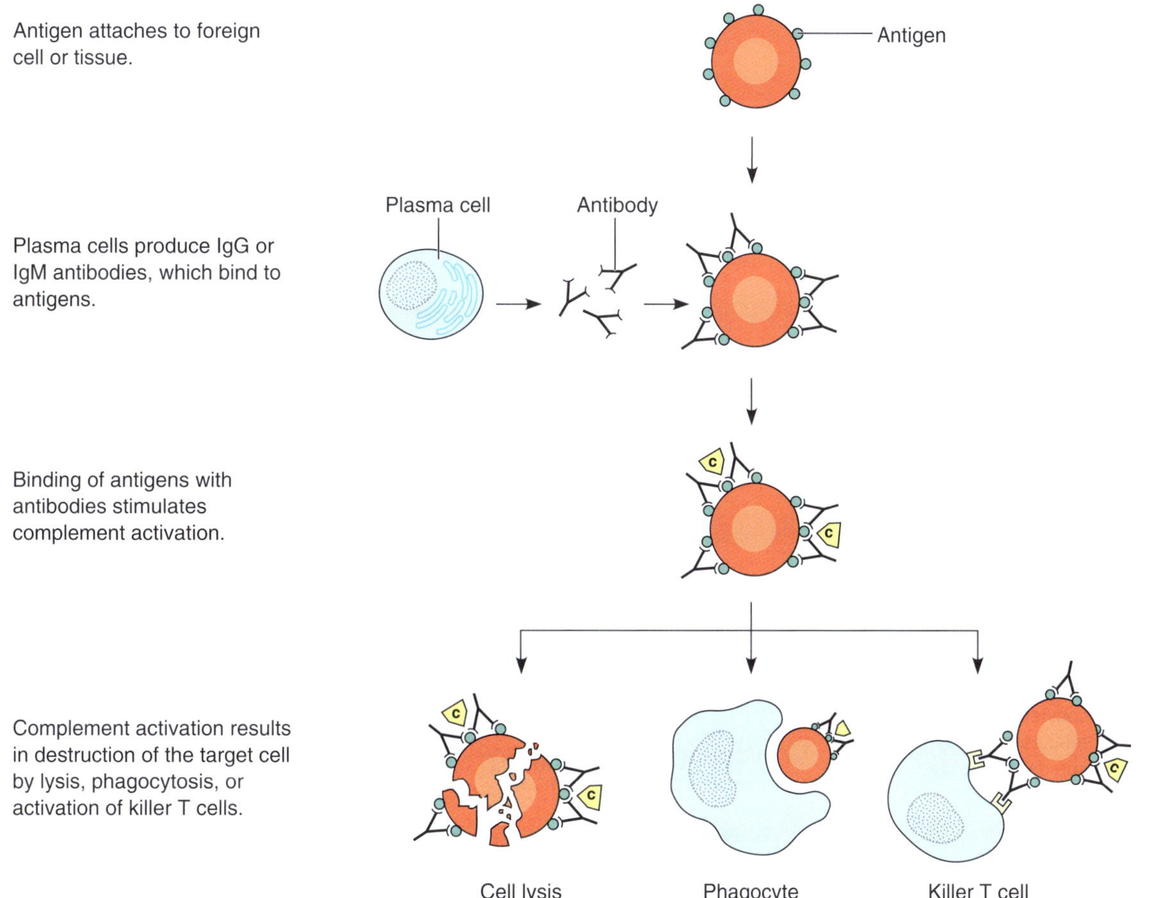

FIGURE 12.2 *Type II or cytotoxic hypersensitivity response*

Type II reactions may be stimulated by an exogenous antigen, such as foreign tissue or cells, or a drug reaction in which the drug forms an antigenic complex on the surface of a blood cell, stimulating the production of antibodies. The affected cell is then destroyed in the resulting antigen–antibody reaction; for example, haemolytic anaemia is sometimes associated with the administration of drugs such as penicillins, cephalosporins and streptomycin. Withdrawal of the drug stops the reaction and cell destruction (Punt et al., 2018).

Endogenous antigens can also stimulate a type II reaction, resulting in an autoimmune disorder such as Goodpasture's syndrome, in which antigens are formed to specific tissues in the lungs and kidneys. Hashimoto's thyroiditis and autoimmune haemolytic anaemia are additional examples of autoimmune type II reactions.

Type III: immune-complex-mediated hypersensitivity

Type III hypersensitivity reactions result from the formation of IgG or IgM antibody–antigen immune complexes in the circulation. When these complexes are deposited in vessel walls and extravascular tissues, complement is activated and chemical mediators of inflammation such as histamine are released. Chemotactic factors attract neutrophils to the site of inflammation. When neutrophils attempt to phagocytise the immune complexes, lysosomal enzymes are released, increasing tissue damage (see Figure 12.3).

Either systemic or local responses may be seen with type III reactions. For example, serum sickness is a systemic response, so named because it was first identified after administration of foreign serum (e.g. horse antitetanus toxin). Although foreign

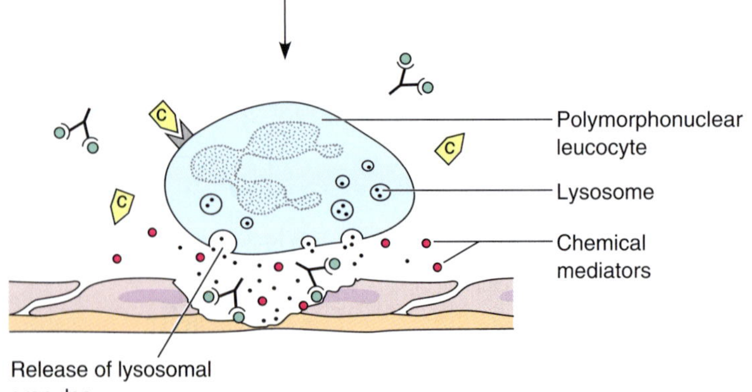

FIGURE 12.3 ***Type III or immune-complex-mediated hypersensitivity response***

serums are no longer administered, serum sickness still occurs in response to some drugs, such as penicillin and sulfonamides. Immune complexes are deposited in walls of small blood vessels, the kidneys and joints. Manifestations of serum sickness include fever, urticaria or rash, arthralgias, myalgias and lymphadenopathy.

Localised responses may occur at a number of different sites. As immune complexes accumulate in the glomerular basement membrane of the kidneys—for example, following a streptococcal infection or with systemic lupus erythematosus—glomerulonephritis develops. When an antigen such as dust from mouldy hay is inhaled, an acute alveolar inflammatory response can occur. This condition can develop in agricultural workers.

Type IV: delayed hypersensitivity

Type IV reactions differ from other hypersensitivity responses in two ways. First, these reactions are cell mediated rather than antibody mediated, involving T cells of the immune system. Second, type IV reactions are delayed rather than immediate, developing 24 to 48 hours after exposure to the antigen. Type IV hypersensitivity responses result from an exaggerated interaction between an antigen and normal cell-mediated mechanisms. This exaggerated interaction results in the release of soluble inflammatory and immune mediators (from the lysozymes within the macrophages) and recruitment of killer T cells, causing local tissue destruction (see Figure 12.4).

Contact dermatitis is a classic example of a type IV reaction. Intense redness, itching and thickening affect the skin in the area exposed to the antigen. Fragile vesicles are often present as well. Many antigens can provoke this response; the gympie-gympie (*Dendrocnide moroides*) (Varnham O'Regan, 2012) is a prime perpetrator. In the healthcare setting, an allergic response to latex can also produce contact dermatitis.

Other examples of cell-mediated responses include a positive tuberculin test and graft rejection episodes.

Latex allergy

Although protective against infection, the repetitive use of latex gloves creates a persistent exposure to latex for

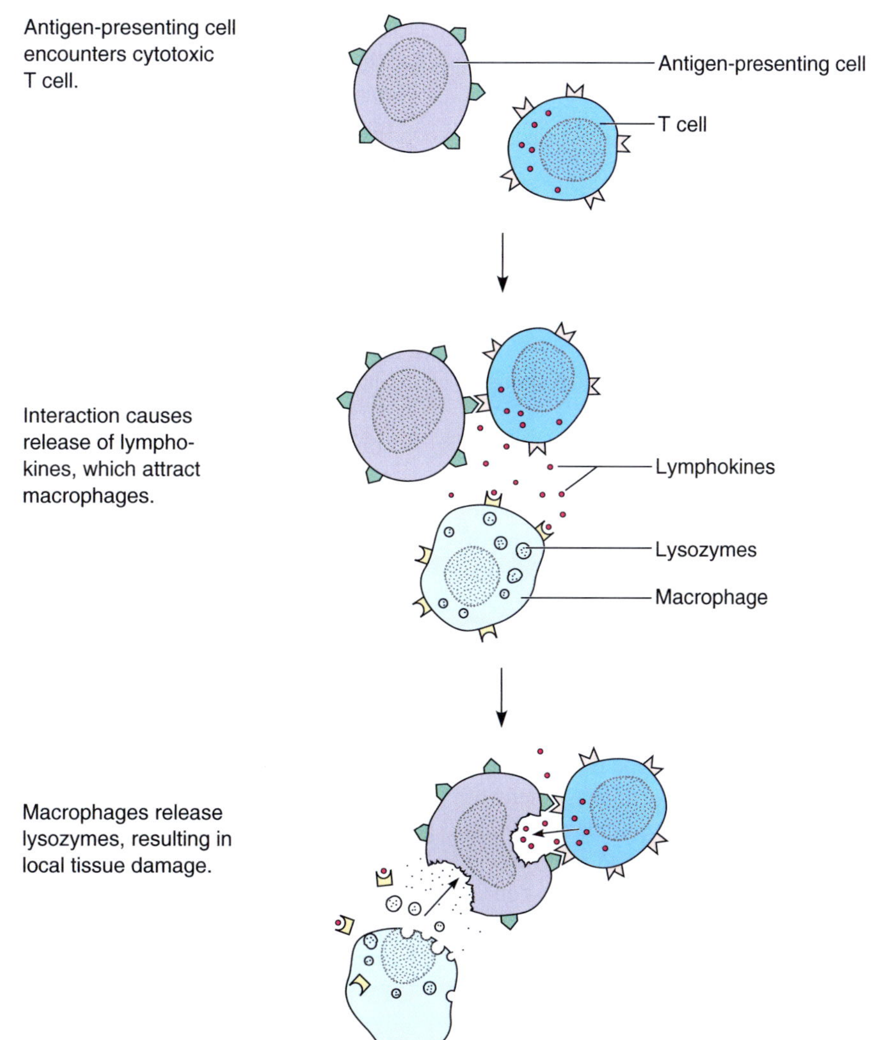

FIGURE 12.4 ***Type IV or delayed hypersensitivity response***

healthcare workers. Latex allergy is a well-recognised occupational issue in healthcare and allergy occurs in up to 30% of workers in this sector (Australasian Society of Clinical Immunology and Allergy (ASCIA), 2019; Parliament of Australia, 2019). Handwashing after using latex products limits exposure. When gloves are powdered with cornflour to facilitate donning and removal, the cornflour particles aerosolise when the gloves are removed. The cornflour includes latex particles. This creates a respiratory exposure as well as dermal exposure to latex. In addition, chemicals used in the manufacture of latex products may be irritating. Products such as balloons, condoms and rubber bands are commonly made of latex.

Sensitivity to latex develops without the user being aware until a rash appears on the hands. Type IV hypersensitivity (contact dermatitis) can progress to type I systemic allergic reactions without previous symptoms signalling an escalation. It is important to protect the person and the healthcare worker who is allergic to latex. Prevention is aided by employers who select products that are free of latex (vinyl, nitrile, neoprene or polyurethane). Non-latex and synthetic gloves must be used. The ASCIA (2017) provides strategies and guidelines for the management of latex-allergy individuals specific to various Australian healthcare settings.

INTERPROFESSIONAL CARE

The focus of care for people with allergic responses is on the following:

- Minimise exposure to the allergen.
- Prevent a hypersensitivity response.
- Provide prompt, effective interventions for allergic responses when they occur.

Identifying allergens for the individual to reduce the likelihood of exposure is a key aspect of management. A complete history of the person's allergies is obtained, including medications, foods, animals, plants and other materials. The type of hypersensitivity response is documented, as is its onset, manifestations and usual treatment.

When a documented or suspected hypersensitivity reaction occurs, the allergen (e.g. intravenous medication or transfusion) is withdrawn immediately. With a type I hypersensitivity response, managing the person's airway takes highest priority, followed by maintenance of cardiac output. Type II hypersensitivity responses may necessitate aggressive management of bleeding or renal failure. A type III (immune complex) reaction is treated by removing the offending antigen and interrupting the inflammatory response. With a hypersensitivity response, supportive care is important to relieve discomfort. This often involves the administration of selected antihistamine or anti-inflammatory medications. Other therapies, such as plasmapheresis, may be prescribed in selected instances, a procedure that involves the continual withdrawal and reinfusion of blood from the patient, during which time the blood is processed to remove the allergic components of the plasma portion.

Diagnosis

To identify possible allergens or hypersensitivity reactions, the following laboratory tests may be ordered:

- *White blood cell (WBC) count with differential* can detect high levels of circulating eosinophils. Normally, eosinophils constitute a very small percentage (1–4%) of the total WBCs. Eosinophilia, however, is often present in people with type I hypersensitivities.
- *Radioallergosorbent test (RAST)* measures the amount of IgE directed towards specific allergens. Test results are compared with control values and used to identify hypersensitivities. RAST poses no risk of an anaphylactic reaction. It is particularly useful in detecting allergies to some occupational chemicals and toxic allergens (Punt et al., 2018).
- *Blood type and crossmatch* are ordered prior to any anticipated transfusions. The person's ABO blood group and Rh status are determined. Two major antigens, designated A and B, may be present on RBCs. People with the A antigen are designated as blood type A; those with blood type B have the B antigen. When neither antigen is found on the RBCs, the person is identified as type O. A third major RBC antigen is the Rh antigen. People with this antigen are called Rh positive; those without are Rh negative. Because a blood transfusion is actually a transplant of living tissue, antigen matching is vital to prevent significant hypersensitivity reactions. Once blood type is determined, a sample of the person's blood is mixed with a sample of matching donor blood and observed for antigen–antibody reactions in the crossmatch portion of this test. Although this procedure greatly reduces the risk of a haemolytic transfusion reaction (type II hypersensitivity), it does not totally eliminate it.
- *Indirect Coombs' test* detects the presence of circulating antibodies (other than ABO antibodies) against RBCs. The person's serum is mixed with the donor's RBCs. If the person's serum contains antibodies to an RBC antigen, agglutination (clumping together) will occur. This is called a positive response. The normal value is negative or no agglutination. This test is also part of the crossmatch of a blood 'type and crossmatch'.
- *Direct Coombs' test* detects antibodies on the person's RBCs that damage and destroy the cells. This is used following a suspected transfusion reaction to detect antibodies coating the transfused RBCs. It can also identify haemolytic anaemia when the cause is unknown. In the direct Coombs' test, the person's RBCs are mixed with Coombs' serum, which contains antibodies to IgG and several complement components. Agglutination will occur if the person's RBCs are coated with antibodies, resulting in a positive test. As with the indirect Coombs' test, the normal test result is negative.
- *Immune complex assays* may be performed to detect the presence of circulating immune complexes in suspected type III hypersensitivity responses. The assays are particularly useful in diagnosing suspected autoimmune disorders. Non-specific assays of IgG-, IgM- and IgA-containing immune complexes, which do not detect specific antibodies,

as well as specific antibody assays, may be done. The normal result is a test negative for circulating immune complexes. A negative test does not, however, rule out an immune complex hypersensitivity response. In some cases, a negative result may indicate that the disease process has reached a later stage, in which complexes are no longer circulating but have initiated extensive tissue damage, such as glomerulonephritis (Loscalzo et al., 2022).

- *Complement assay* is also useful in detecting immune complex disorders. In these disorders, complement is, in effect, used up by the development of antigen–antibody complexes. Decreased levels are seen on examination. Both total complement level and amounts of individual components of the complement cascade can be determined.

SKIN TEST FOR ALLERGIES Skin tests are also used to determine causes of hypersensitivity reactions. These tests are used to identify specific allergens to which a person may be sensitive. Allergens for testing are selected according to the person's history. Test solutions made from extracts of inhaled, ingested or injected materials, such as pollens, mites, venoms or some drugs, are used for the prick test and intradermal testing. Epicutaneous testing (prick testing) is generally done first to avoid a systemic reaction; it is followed by intradermal testing of allergens with a negative response to prick testing (Papadakis, McPhee & Rabow, 2022).

If the large-dose intradermal tests were done initially, individuals highly allergic to a substance would be at increased risk of an anaphylactic reaction. Substances that cause a reaction to the prick test should not be tested intradermally.

- *Skin prick (epicutaneous or puncture) test*: a drop of diluted allergenic extract is placed on the skin and the skin is then pricked or punctured through the drop. With a positive test, a localised pruritic wheal and erythema occur. The response is maximal at 15 to 20 minutes.
- *Intradermal*: a small amount (just enough to create a wheal) of allergen extract at a 1:500 or 1:1,000 dilution is injected on the forearm or intrascapular area. If several allergens are being tested, injections are spaced 0.7 to 1.25 cm apart. As control measures, plain diluent (negative control) and histamine (positive control) are also injected. If there is no response to a particular allergen at 15 to 20 minutes, the test is negative. The appearance of a wheal (inflamed, usually circular) and erythema, with a wheal diameter at least 5 mm greater than that produced by the control, indicates a positive response (see Figure 12.5). Intradermal is not recommended for routine use for aeroallergens and food allergens, as it carries a greater risk of anaphylaxis (ASCIA, 2019).
- *Patch*: a 2.5 cm patch impregnated with the allergen (e.g. perfume, cosmetics, detergents or clothing fibres) is applied to the skin for 48 hours. Absence of a response indicates a negative test result. Positive responses are graded from mild (erythema in the exposed area) to severe (erythema, papules, vesicles or ulceration).
- *Food allergy testing* is performed when a food allergy is suspected but the source or implicated food item has not been clearly identified. Food allergy symptoms are typically demonstrated within hours of eating. Initially, the person is asked to keep a diary of foods consumed and allergic responses for a week. An elimination diet is then prescribed. The diet excludes most common food allergens and all suspected foods for 1 week. Any foods that may contain allergens in combination, such as breads, are also eliminated. If symptoms do not improve, a different variation of the elimination diet is prescribed. If symptoms are relieved, foods are reintroduced to the diet one at a time until symptoms recur, indicating allergy to that food.

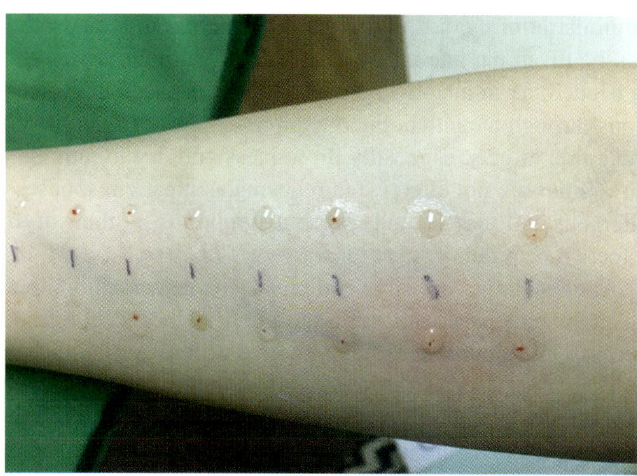

FIGURE 12.5 ***Positive allergy skin test***

Source: © Hunna/Shutterstock.

Medications

When it is impossible to avoid the offending allergen and allergic manifestations are severe or disrupt the person's activities of daily living (ADLs), pharmacological intervention is prescribed. *Immunotherapy*, also called hyposensitisation or desensitisation, consists of injecting an extract of the allergen(s) in gradually increasing doses. Immunotherapy is used primarily for allergic rhinitis or asthma related to inhaled allergens. It has also been shown to be effective in preventing anaphylactic responses to insect venom. With weekly or biweekly subcutaneous injections of the allergen, the person develops IgG antibodies to the allergen that appear to block effectively the allergic IgE-mediated response. Once a therapy plateau is reached, injections are continued indefinitely either monthly or bimonthly.

Antihistamines are the major class of drugs used in treating the symptoms of hypersensitivity responses, type I in particular. They are also useful to some extent in relieving manifestations (such as urticaria) of some type II and type III reactions.

Antihistamines block H_1-histamine receptors, acting as a competitive antagonist to histamine, but they do not affect the production or release of histamine. The prototype antihistamine is diphenhydramine (Benadryl). It and other antihistamines alleviate the systemic effects of histamine such as urticaria and angio-oedema. They are also useful in relieving allergic rhinitis, although they are not effective in all people. Antihistamines are available in both prescription and non-prescription preparations. The preferred route of administration is oral, although diphenhydramine and others can be given parenterally, particularly when immediate action is needed, as in anaphylaxis. They also dry respiratory secretions through an anticholinergic effect. Their use is limited by their side effects, especially drowsiness and dry mouth. Antihistamines are not effective in relieving asthmatic responses to allergens and may actually worsen symptoms by their drying effect on respiratory secretions.

Antihistamines are often combined with a sympathomimetic agent such as pseudoephedrine to improve their decongestant activity and counteract their sedative effect. Antihistamines and decongestants are discussed further in the chapter 'Nursing care of people with upper respiratory disorders'.

The immediate treatment for anaphylaxis is parenteral adrenaline, an adrenergic agonist (sympathomimetic) drug that has both vasoconstricting and bronchodilating effects. These qualities, combined with its rapid action, make adrenaline ideal for treating an anaphylactic reaction. For mild reactions with wheezing, pruritus, urticaria and angio-oedema, preferably an intramuscular injection of 0.3 to 0.5 mg (adults) of 1:1,000 adrenaline is generally sufficient and can be repeated every 5 minutes if required as per the organisational protocol. Intravenous adrenaline using a 1:100,000 concentration may be used in the person with a more severe anaphylactic reaction. Refer to the organisational protocols, guidelines and doctor's orders.

People who have experienced an anaphylactic reaction to insect venom or other potentially unavoidable allergens should wear a Medic-Alert® pendant or bracelet identifying allergy triggers. They should also carry an adrenaline autoinjector kit for immediate treatment of future exposures. The adrenaline autoinjector kit contains a prefilled syringe of adrenaline (epinephrine), allowing prompt self-treatment or, in an emergency, administration by a person who has not been medically trained.

Cromolyn sodium is a drug used to treat allergic rhinitis and asthma. Cromolyn sodium acts by stabilising the mast cell membrane, thus preventing chemical mediator release (Burchum & Rosenthal, 2018). It is most effective when applied directly to involved tissue by inhaler or nasal spray. It has few side effects and a wide margin of safety, making it a good choice for people in whom it is effective (Papadakis et al., 2022).

Glucocorticoids (corticosteroids) are used in both systemic and topical forms for many types of hypersensitivity responses. Their anti-inflammatory effects, rather than their immunosuppressive effects, are of most benefit. A short course of corticosteroid therapy is often used for severe asthma, allergic contact dermatitis and some immune-complex disorders: alternate day dosing is preferred in long-term use (Papadakis et al., 2022). Corticosteroids in topical forms or delivered by inhaler may be used for longer periods of time with few side effects; however, systemic absorption can occur.

Other therapies

Other treatments used for hypersensitivity responses are generally dictated by the severity of the response and the organ system affected. Airway management takes highest priority for the person with an acute anaphylactic reaction. Insertion of an endotracheal tube or emergency tracheostomy may be required to maintain airway patency with severe laryngospasm. Because anaphylaxis places the person at risk of vasomotor collapse and significant hypotension, it is necessary to insert an intravenous line and initiate fluid resuscitation with an isotonic solution such as compound sodium lactate (Hartmann's solution).

Plasmapheresis, removal of harmful components in the plasma, may be used to treat immune complex responses such as glomerulonephritis and Goodpasture's syndrome. Plasma and the glomerular-damaging antibody–antigen complexes are removed by passing the person's blood through a blood cell separator. The RBCs are then returned to the person along with an equal amount of albumin or human plasma. This procedure is usually done in a series rather than as a one-time treatment. It is not without risk and informed consent is required. Potential complications of plasmapheresis include those associated with intravenous catheters, shifts in fluid balance and alteration of blood clotting.

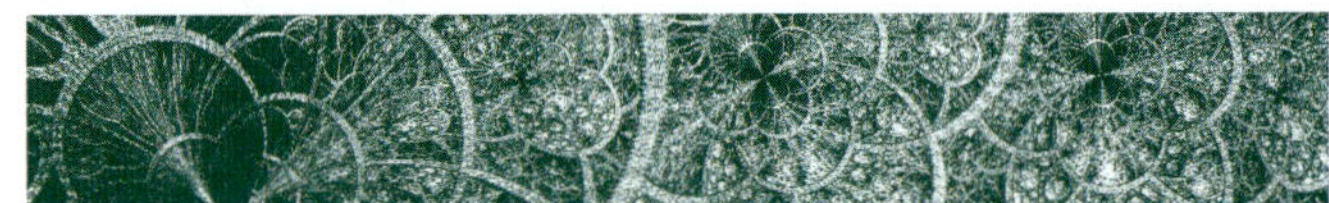

Nursing care

Nursing care related to hypersensitivity reactions is primarily directed towards prevention, early identification and providing prompt, effective treatment.

Health promotion

Health promotion activities include helping people to identify possible allergens that prompt a hypersensitivity response and discussing possible strategies to avoid these allergens. Anyone with severe food allergies may need assistance from a dietitian to discuss necessary dietary changes and ways to continue meeting nutrient needs. It is important that people with hypersensitivities inform healthcare personnel of all allergens. People who experience anaphylactic reactions should wear a MedicAlert® bracelet or pendant at all times to identify the substance(s) that provokes this response. Patients who have experienced an anaphylactic reaction to insect venom or other potentially unavoidable allergens may also be required to carry an adrenaline autoinjector (commonly known as an Epipen®) on their person at all times. The need to carry the adrenaline autoinjector is on a prescription basis and is only offered in conjunction with a full anaphylaxis management plan (ASCIA, 2019).

Assessment

Collect the following data through the health history and physical examination. Further focused assessments are described with nursing interventions in the next section.

- *Health history*: risk factors, hypersensitivities (medications, household dust, bee stings, etc.), reaction (rash, hives, difficulty breathing), type of treatment for hypersensitivity reactions; allergy skin testing; asthma, hay fever or dermatitis.
- *Physical assessment*: mucous membranes of nose and mouth, skin for lesions or rashes, eyes (tearing and redness), respiratory rate and adventitious breath sounds.

Nursing diagnoses and interventions

Priority nursing diagnoses will vary according to the type of hypersensitivity reaction experienced by the person. Because nurses are most likely to become involved with a person experiencing a type I or type II response, this section focuses on diagnoses for these people. Airway, breathing and circulation (the ABCs) are of greatest importance for people with an anaphylactic reaction. When a haemolytic reaction to an incompatible blood transfusion occurs, the person is at risk of injury.

> **CONSIDERATION FOR PRACTICE**
> **Anaphylaxis is a life-threading emergency. Maintain ABC (airway, breathing, circulation) and, if alone, call for help.**

Ineffective airway clearance

In anaphylactic reactions, the airway may be obstructed due to facial angio-oedema, bronchospasm or laryngeal oedema. Establishing and maintaining a patent airway is of highest priority.

- Administer oxygen via nasal prongs at a rate of 2 to 4 L/min or facemask at a rate of > 6 L/min. Apply oxygen and obtain a doctor's order for oxygen administration as per the organisational protocol. *Oxygen administration increases the alveolar oxygen and its availability to cells of the body.*
- Assess respiratory rate and pattern, level of consciousness and anxiety, nasal flaring, use of accessory muscles of respiration, chest wall movement, audible stridor; palpate for respiratory excursion; auscultate lung sounds and any adventitious sounds, such as wheezes. *Extreme anxiety or agitation, nasal flaring, stridor and diminished lung sounds indicate air hunger and possible airway obstruction, necessitating immediate intervention.*
- Position in Fowler's to high Fowler's *to promote optimal lung expansion and ease of breathing.*
- Insert a nasopharyngeal or oropharyngeal airway if required and arrange for immediate intubation as indicated. *Ensuring an adequate airway is vital to preserve life.*
- Administer intramuscular adrenaline 1:1,000, 0.3 to 0.5 mL, as prescribed. This may be repeated if necessary as per the prescribed protocol. Administer parenteral antihistamine (deep intramuscular or intravenous) as prescribed. *Adrenaline is a potent vasoconstrictor and bronchodilator, counteracting the effects of histamine. An antihistamine (e.g. promethazine hydrochloride) blocks histamine receptors and their effect. These medications can be effective in rapidly reversing manifestations of anaphylaxis.*
- Provide calm reassurance. Hypoxaemia and air hunger are terrifying for the person. *Anxiety can impair the person's ability to cooperate with treatment and can increase the respiratory rate, making breathing less effective.*

Decreased cardiac output

Peripheral vasodilation and increased capillary permeability from the release of histamine can significantly impair cardiac output. When it falls to the degree that tissue perfusion becomes impaired and hypoxia results, a state of anaphylactic shock exists.

- Monitor vital signs frequently, noting fall in blood pressure, decreasing pulse pressure, tachycardia and tachypnoea. *These vital sign changes may be early indicators of shock.*
- Assess skin colour, temperature, capillary refill, oedema and other indicators of peripheral perfusion. *As cardiac output falls, peripheral vessels constrict and tissue perfusion is impaired.*
- Monitor level of consciousness. *A change in level of consciousness (lethargy, apprehension or agitation) is often the first indicator of decreased cardiac output.*
- Insert one or more large-bore (18-gauge or larger) intravenous catheters. *It is important to insert intravenous catheters as soon as possible to provide sites for rapid fluid replacement.*
- Administer intravenous solutions of normal saline 0.9% or compound sodium lactate, as prescribed. These isotonic solutions help maintain intravascular volume. *Warmed solutions are used to prevent hypothermia from the rapid administration of large amounts of fluid at room temperature (about 21.1°C).*
- Insert an indwelling catheter and monitor urinary output frequently. As the cardiac output drops, the glomerular filtration rate (GFR) falls. *With an output of less than 30 mL/h, the person is at risk of acute renal failure from ischaemia.*
- Once breathing is established safely and maintained, place the person flat with the legs elevated. *This position enhances perfusion of the central organs, such as the brain, heart and kidneys.*

> **CONSIDERATION FOR PRACTICE**
> **Aggressive fluid therapy may lead to hypervolaemia and acute cardiogenic pulmonary oedema; assess for shortness of breath and crackles in the lungs.**

Risk of injury

As noted, the potential for hypersensitivity responses is high in people subjected to medical treatments. Because a blood transfusion is a transplant of living tissue, the risk of adverse immunological response and injury is particularly significant.

- Obtain and record a thorough history of previous blood transfusions and any reactions experienced, *no matter how mild.* Alert the doctor if previous transfusion reactions have occurred. *The person who has received prior blood transfusions is at increased risk of a hypersensitivity reaction, because antibody production may have been stimulated by prior exposure to antigens.*

> **CONSIDERATION FOR PRACTICE**
> **Begin a blood transfusion within 30 minutes of its delivery from the blood bank to reduce bacterial contamination.**

- Check for a signed informed consent as per organisational protocol to administer blood or blood products. *It is important to obtain informed consent for this invasive and risky procedure.*
- Using two registered healthcare professionals, double-check the person's identity, blood type, Rh factor, crossmatch and expiration date for all blood and blood components received from the blood bank with the person's data. *Check bag for signs of leakage, clots and discolouration. This is an important safety measure to reduce the risk of a haemolytic transfusion reaction due to incompatible blood types.*
- Take and record vital signs within 15 minutes prior to initiating the blood infusion. *This provides a baseline for evaluating any changes related to the blood transfusion.*
- Infuse blood into a site separate from any other intravenous infusion. Use at least a 20-gauge cannula for the infusion to promote flow. This reduces the risk of damage to the blood cells due to incompatibility with other intravenous solutions or physical trauma. *When blood is administered with dextrose solutions (e.g. dextrose 5%, dextrose 5% and normal saline 0.9%), blood cell haemolysis and aggregation occur; administration with Hartmann's can cause agglutination of cells. Administer with normal saline to prime intravenous tubing.*
- Remain with the person for the first 15 minutes of the transfusion (from when the blood enters the vein) and observe for reactions. *Reactions generally occur within the first 15 minutes.*
- During transfusion, monitor observations as per organisational protocol and monitor for complaints of back or chest pain, an increase in the temperature of more than 1°C, chills, tachycardia, tachypnoea, wheezing, hypotension, hives, rashes or cyanosis. *These signs may indicate an adverse reaction to the blood transfusion.*
- Stop the blood transfusion immediately if a reaction occurs, no matter how mild. Remove the blood bag and the tubing with blood in it. Flush new intravenous tubing with normal saline, keeping the intravenous line open. Notify the doctor and the transfusion service provider.
- If a reaction is suspected, send the blood and administration set to the transfusion service provider with a freshly drawn blood sample and urine specimen from the person. *These will be used to identify the cause of the reaction as well as its effect on the person.*
- If no adverse reaction occurs, administer the transfusion over 2 hours to a maximum of 4 hours as ordered. *This time frame is important to limit the risk of bacterial growth.*

Community-based care

The vast majority of hypersensitivity responses are appropriately treated by the person or family members with little or no medical intervention. Teaching, therefore, is a vital component of care. If the person is at risk of anaphylaxis, involving the family in teaching is essential because the response may occur with such rapidity that the person will be unable to provide self-care.

Include the following points in teaching the person and family about managing hypersensitivities:

- Importance of following the anaphylaxis action plan prepared by a general practitioner.
- When and how to use an anaphylaxis autoinjector pen containing adrenaline and antihistamines in injectable, inhaler and oral forms.
- When to seek medical attention.
- Use of and adverse reactions to prescription and non-prescription antihistamines and decongestants.
- Advantages of autologous blood transfusion if future surgery is scheduled.
- Preventing an immune complex reaction such as glomerulonephritis.
- Skin care to prevent contact dermatitis, including:
  - Expose affected areas to air and sun as much as possible.
  - Avoid direct contact with people who have an infection.
  - Wear cool, light, non-restrictive clothing made of natural fibres, such as cotton, to avoid irritating affected areas.
  - Avoid exposure to extremes of heat or cold.
  - Use bath oils or plain water instead of soaps and detergents.
  - Take baths in cool to lukewarm water rather than showers.
  - To decrease pruritus, maintain a cool environment and avoid exercising.
  - Trim fingernails to reduce the risk of skin damage.
- Helpful resources:
  - Australasian Society of Clinical Immunology and Allergy
  - Allergy and Anaphylaxis Australia
  - Asthma Foundation—Asthma Australia.

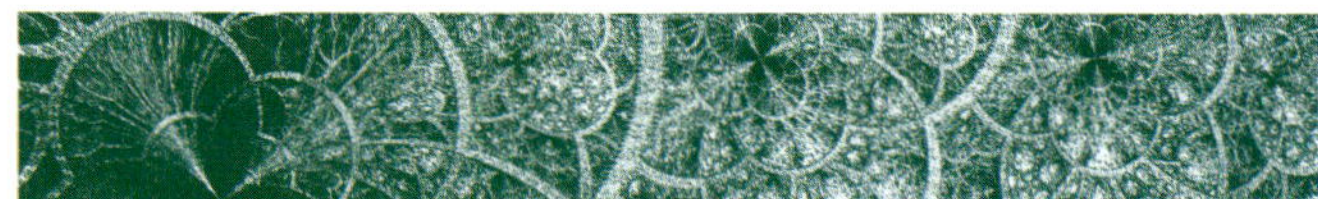

THE PERSON WITH AN AUTOIMMUNE DISORDER

Maintaining optimal health and preventing disease depends not only on the immune system's ability to recognise and destroy foreign tissues and other antigens, but also on the immune system's ability to recognise self. When this self-recognition is impaired and immune defences are directed against normal host tissue, the result is an **autoimmune disorder**.

Autoimmune disorders can affect any tissue in the body. Some are tissue or organ specific, affecting particular tissue or a particular organ. Hashimoto's thyroiditis is an example of an organ-specific autoimmune disorder. Circulating antibodies are formed to certain thyroid components, resulting ultimately in destruction of the gland. In other disorders, autoantibodies are formed that are not tissue specific, but tend to accumulate and cause an inflammatory response in certain tissue; for example, the renal glomerulus or the hepatic small bile ductules.

Additional factors are believed to contribute to the development of autoimmune disorders including age, gender and environmental elements—for example, infectious agents (Loscalzo et al., 2022). Autoimmune disorders may also be systemic, with neither antibodies nor the resulting inflammatory lesions confined to any one organ. Rheumatological disorders, such as rheumatoid arthritis and systemic lupus erythematosus (SLE), are characteristic of systemic autoimmune disorders (Punt et al., 2018). A list of selected autoimmune disorders is included in Table 12.1.

Pathophysiology

The mechanism that causes the immune system to recognise host tissue as a foreign antigen is not clear. The following factors are under study as possible contributors to the development of autoimmune disorders:

- the release of previously 'hidden' antigens into the circulation, such as DNA or other components of the cell nucleus, which elicit an immune response
- chemical, physical or biological changes in host tissue that cause self-antigens to stimulate the production of autoantibodies
- the introduction of an antigen, such as a bacteria or virus, whose antigenic properties closely resemble those of host tissue, resulting in the production of antibodies that target not only the foreign antigen but also normal tissue. Heart damage in rheumatic fever and encephalitis following rabies vaccination are examples of the development of antibodies against normal tissue (Norris, 2018)
- a defect in normal cellular immune function that allows B cells to produce autoantibodies unchecked
- initiation of the autoimmune response by very-slow-growing mycobacteria.

Although the exact mechanism producing autoimmunity is unclear, several characteristics of autoimmune diseases are known. It is apparent that genetics plays a role because a higher incidence is seen in family members of people with autoimmune disorders. Autoimmune disorders are far more prevalent in females than in males. The disorders tend to overlap, so that the person with one autoimmune disorder may develop another or some manifestations of another. The onset of an autoimmune disorder is frequently associated with an abnormal stressor, either physical or psychological. Autoimmune disorders are frequently progressive relapsing–remissing disorders characterised by periods of exacerbation and remission.

Specific autoimmune disorders are discussed in the sections of this text related to the affected organ systems or functional disruption.

INTERPROFESSIONAL CARE

For the most part, the diagnosis of an autoimmune disorder is based on the person's clinical manifestations. Serum assays are useful to identify autoantibodies. Other diagnostic tests are generally specific to the suspected disorder and to identifying the degree of tissue damage and destruction. Although the manifestations of these disorders can often be managed, a cure typically is not possible unless the affected target tissue is removed (e.g. colectomy for the person with ulcerative colitis).

Diagnosis

Serological assays are used to identify and measure antibodies directed towards host tissue antigens or normal cellular components. Many detectable autoantibodies are not specific to a single autoimmune disorder and are used to establish the autoimmune process rather than the specific disorder. Although healthy people often have low levels of autoantibodies, levels are much higher in people affected by an autoimmune disorder. The following serological assays may be ordered:

- *Antinuclear antibody (ANA)* detects antibodies produced to DNA and other nuclear material. These antibodies can cause tissue damage characteristic of autoimmune disorders, such as SLE. The person's serum is combined with nuclear material and tagged antihuman antibody to detect ANA–antihuman antibody complexes. Titres are not necessarily comparable between laboratories; refer to the laboratory reference levels. This test is not specific for SLE because high levels of ANA may be present in rheumatoid arthritis (RA) and cirrhosis of the liver; nevertheless, 95% of people with SLE have a positive ANA titre.
- *Lupus erythematosus (LE) cell test* is also used to detect SLE and monitor its treatment. Neutrophils that contain large masses of phagocytised DNA from the nuclei of PMNs are called LE cells. Like the ANA, the LE cell prep is non-specific for SLE. A positive result may also be seen in RA or with medications such as isoniazid, penicillin, phenytoin, procainamide, streptomycin, tetracycline, oral contraceptives or sulfonamide drugs.
- *Rheumatoid factor (RF)* is an immunoglobulin present in the serum of approximately 80% of people with rheumatoid arthritis. Low titre levels may be present in the elderly. An RF titre 1:80 or higher indicates RA. A titre between 1:20 and 1:80 could indicate SLE, scleroderma or liver cirrhosis (Pagana, Pagana & Pagana, 2020). Reference factors are variable; refer to the laboratory reference range.
- *Complement assay* may also be useful in identifying autoimmune disorders. In these disorders, complement may be consumed in the development of antigen–antibody complexes. Decreased levels are seen on examination. Both total complement level and amounts of individual components of the complement cascade can be determined.
- *CCP (also known as anti-CCP antibody test)* is a blood test for RA. It measures cyclic citrullinated peptide antibody in the blood. This is a specific test to identify RA from other forms of arthritis.

Medications

Various approaches are used in the treatment of autoimmune disorders. Anti-inflammatory medications such as aspirin, nonsteroidal anti-inflammatory drugs (NSAIDs) and corticosteroids may be prescribed to reduce the inflammatory response and minimise tissue damage. (Refer to the chapter 'Nursing care of people in pain' for additional detail on these drugs.) When these agents are not effective or well tolerated by the person, slow-acting anti-inflammatory medications may be prescribed. Slow-acting or antirheumatic drugs include such medications as gold salts, hydroxychloroquine and penicillamine. Their use is further detailed in the chapter 'Nursing care of people with musculoskeletal disorders'. Cytotoxic drugs may be used in combination with plasmapheresis in treating many autoimmune disorders. Cytotoxic drugs are discussed in further detail in the next section of this chapter. Disease-modifying antirheumatic drugs (DMARDs) reduce signs and symptoms, reduce or prevent joint damage, and preserve the structure and function of the joints in people with RA. These drugs may reduce health costs for people with RA and allow them to remain active and productive. The most common DMARDs in current use are methotrexate, sulfasalazine, hydroxychloroquine, leflunomide and cyclosporin.

Another class of antirheumatic drugs, referred to as *biologicals* or *biological response modifiers*, consists of laboratory-produced proteins that decrease the inflammatory process. These antibodies bind tumour necrosis factor alpha (TNF-α) and interleukin-1, both inflammatory elements. These medications include infliximab or adalimumab, etanercept and anakinra.

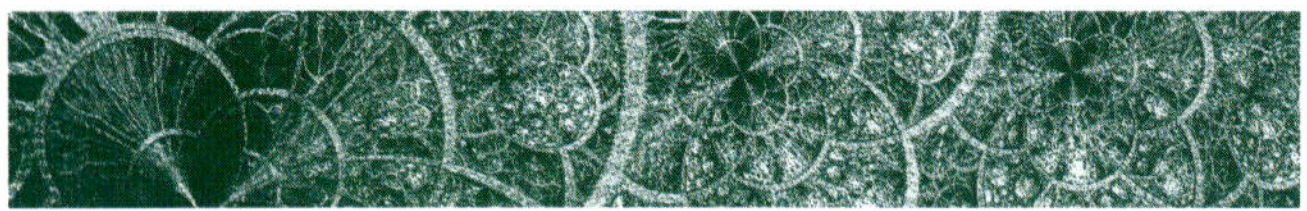

Nursing care

Nursing interventions for the person with an autoimmune disorder are individualised and tailored to needs dictated by manifestations of the disorder. Nurses will often be involved with the person in an outpatient setting such as an office or home, evaluating the person's response to therapy and self-care management.

Consider the following nursing diagnoses in planning care for the person with an autoimmune disorder:

- *Risk of activity intolerance* related to inflammatory effects of autoimmune disorder.
- *Risk of ineffective coping* related to chronic disease process.
- *Risk of interrupted family processes* related to lack of understanding about autoimmune disorder and its effects.
- *Risk of ineffective protection* related to disordered immune function.
- *Risk of ineffective therapeutic regimen management* related to lack of understanding.

Community-based care

Because many autoimmune disorders are chronic, educating the person and family about the disorder and its management is a key nursing care component. The person may be taking drugs with multiple side effects or long-term effects, necessitating effective education. People with autoimmune disorders often do not appear to be ill, making it difficult for friends and families to understand their care needs. The chronicity of these disorders also puts the person at high risk of unproven remedies and quackery. Provide psychological support, listening and teaching. In addition, suggest resources such as local support groups.

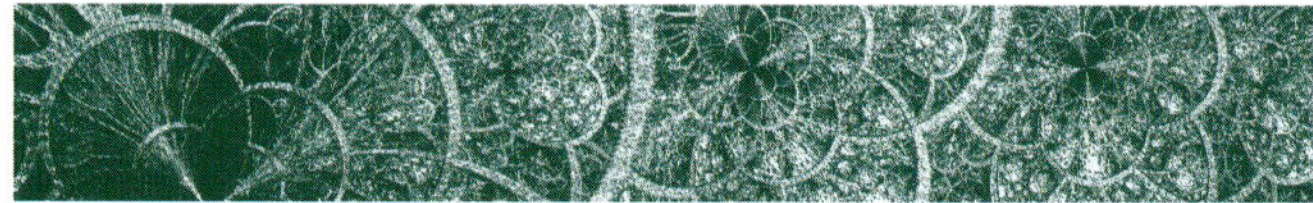

THE PERSON WITH A TISSUE TRANSPLANT

Since the first kidney transplant was performed from one identical twin to the other in 1954, organ and tissue transplantation have become increasingly popular and viable treatment options. The transplantation of avascular tissues, such as skin, cornea, bone and heart valves, is considered routine, with little need for tissue matching and **immunosuppression**. Transplants of organs (e.g. the kidney, heart, heart and lung, liver and bone marrow) are increasingly common and are no longer considered experimental or extraordinary procedures. In 2021, 421 deceased organ donors and 203 live organ donors gave 11,174 Australians a new chance at life, the highest number since the commencement of Australian record keeping (Australian Government Organ and Tissue Authority, 2021). Common organ transplants are outlined in Table 12.2.

TABLE 12.2 Organ transplants

ORGAN	GRAFT TYPE	INDICATIONS FOR TRANSPLANT	SUCCESS RATE
Kidney	Allograft; may be isograft	End-stage renal disease	81.1% at 5 years
Heart	Allograft	End-stage cardiac disease refractory to medical management	74.4% at 5 years
Lung	Allograft	Pulmonary hypertension, cystic fibrosis, pulmonary fibrosis, chronic obstructive pulmonary disease	52.6% at 5 years
Liver	Allograft	Severe liver dysfunction due to chronic active hepatitis, primary biliary cirrhosis, sclerosing cholangitis	73.6% 5-year survival
Bone marrow	Autograft or allograft	Leukaemia, aplastic anaemia, congenital immunological defects	30–70% cure
Skin	Autograft, allograft or xenograft	Severe burns, plastic surgery	> 95% at 5 years
Cornea	Allograft	Corneal ulceration and opacification	> 95% at 5 years
Pancreas	Allograft	Pancreatic insufficiency, diabetes	88.1%
Islet cells	Allograft (multiple donor)	Type 1 diabetes mellitus	100% > 2 years

Source: US Department of Health and Human Services (2020). OPTN/Scientific registry of transplant recipients, *2020 Annual Report: Transplant Data Report*. Retrieved from https://optn.transplant.hrsa.gov/data/view-data-reports/annual-report/.

Transplant success is closely tied to obtaining an organ with tissue antigens as close to those of the recipient as possible. As noted earlier in this chapter, every body cell has cell surface antigens known as human leucocyte antigens that are unique to the individual. Although identical twins may have the same HLA type, the chance is reduced to 1 in 4 for siblings and less than 1 in several thousand for unrelated individuals (Papadakis et al., 2022). Matching the HLA type of the donor and recipient as closely as possible decreases the potential for rejection of the transplanted organ or tissue but does not eliminate it.

Pathophysiology

An **autograft**, a transplant of the person's own tissue, is the most successful type of tissue transplant. Skin grafts are the most common example of autografts. Increasingly, autologous bone marrow transplants and blood transfusions are being used to reduce immunological responses. When the donor and recipient are identical twins, the term **isograft** is used. Because of the high likelihood of an HLA match, the success of these grafts is good and rejection episodes are mild.

Few people, however, have an identical twin to provide tissue for donation and when the need is for an organ such as the heart, liver or lungs, a living donor transplantation is not possible. Most often organ and tissue transplants are **allografts**, which are grafts between members of the same species but who have different genotypes and HLA. Allografts may come from living donors; examples are bone marrow, blood and a kidney. Most often, however, organs for transplantation are obtained from a cadaver. Donors are typically people who meet the criteria for brain death, are less than 65 years old, and are free of systemic disease, malignancy or infection, including HIV, hepatitis B or hepatitis C. The organ is removed immediately before or after cardiac arrest and preserved until it is transplanted into the waiting recipient. Finally, **xenograft** is a transplant from an animal species to a human. These transplants are the least successful but may be used in selected instances, such as the use of pigskin as a temporary covering for a massive burn.

Tissue typing is used to determine **histocompatibility**, the ability of cells and tissues to survive transplantation without immunological interference by the recipient. Tissue typing is performed in an attempt to match the donor and recipient as closely as possible for HLA type and blood type (ABO, Rh) and to identify preformed antibodies to the donor's HLA.

Both antibody-mediated and cell-mediated immune responses are involved in the complex process of transplant rejection. Host macrophages process donor antigen, presenting it to T and B lymphocytes. Activated lymphocytes (B and T cells) produce both antibody- and cell-mediated effects. Killer T cells bind with cells of the transplanted organ, resulting in cell lysis. Helper T cells stimulate the multiplication and differentiation of B cells, and antibodies are produced to graft endothelium. Complement activation or antibody-dependent cell-mediated cytotoxicity leads to transplant cell destruction. Rejection typically begins after the first 24 hours of the transplant, although it may present immediately. Rejection episodes are characterised as hyperacute, acute or chronic, as summarised in Table 12.3.

Hyperacute tissue rejection occurs immediately to 2 to 3 days after the transplant of new tissue. Hyperacute rejection is due to preformed antibodies and sensitised T cells to antigens in the donor organ. Hyperacute rejection is most likely to occur in people who have had a previous organ or tissue transplant, such as a blood transfusion. Hyperacute rejection may be evident even before the transplant procedure is completed. The grafted organ initially appears pink and healthy, but soon becomes soft and cyanotic, as blood flow is impaired. Organ function deteriorates rapidly and symptoms of organ failure develop.

Acute tissue rejection is the most common and treatable type of rejection episode. It occurs between 4 days and 3 months after the transplant. Acute rejection is mediated primarily by the cellular immune response, resulting in transplant cell destruction. The person experiencing acute rejection demonstrates manifestations of the inflammatory process, with fever, redness, swelling and tenderness over the graft site. Signs of impaired function of the transplanted organ may be noted (e.g. elevated blood urea nitrogen (BUN) and creatinine, liver enzyme and bilirubin elevations, or elevated cardiac enzymes and signs of cardiac failure).

Chronic tissue rejection occurs from 4 months to years after transplant of new tissue. Chronic rejection is most likely the result of antibody-mediated immune responses. Antibodies and complement are deposited in transplant vessel walls, causing narrowing and decreased function of the organ due to ischaemia. The gradual deterioration of transplanted organ function is seen with chronic tissue rejection.

Graft-versus-host disease (GVHD) is a frequent and potentially fatal complication of bone marrow transplant. When there

TABLE 12.3 Transplant rejection episodes

TYPE	CAUSE	PRESENTATION	TREATMENT
Hyperacute	Pre-existing antibodies to donor ABO or HLA antigens	Occurs within minutes to hours or days of the transplant Rapid deterioration of organ function	The transplant usually cannot be saved; prevent with crossmatch and use antimetabolites or anti-inflammatory drugs before surgery
Acute	Primarily a cell-mediated immune response to HLA antigens; antibody-mediated response may also contribute	Occurs within days to months after the transplant Signs of inflammation and impaired organ function	Increase immunosuppression using steroids, cyclosporin, monoclonal antibodies or antilymphocyte globulins
Chronic	Probably antibody-mediated response; may also involve inflammatory damage to vessel endothelium	Occurs 4 months to years after the transplant Gradual deterioration of organ function	None; loss of graft will occur, requiring retransplant

is no close match between donor and recipient HLA, immunocompetent cells in the grafted tissue recognise host tissue as foreign and mount a cell-mediated immune response. If the host is immunocompromised, as is often the case when a bone marrow transplant is performed, host cells are unable to destroy the graft and instead become the targets of destruction. Of people with very closely matched bone marrow, 30% to 60% nevertheless develop GVHD. Acute GVHD occurs within the first 100 days following a transplant and primarily affects the skin, liver and gastrointestinal tract. The person develops a maculopapular pruritic rash beginning on the palms of the hands and soles of the feet. The rash may spread to involve the entire body and lead to desquamation. Gastrointestinal manifestations include abdominal pain, nausea and bloody diarrhoea. GVHD that lasts longer than 100 days is said to be chronic. If it is limited to the skin and liver, the prognosis is good. If multiple organs are involved, the prognosis is poor (Norris, 2018).

INTERPROFESSIONAL CARE

Pre-transplant and post-transplant care are directed towards reducing the risk that transplanted tissue will be rejected or result in GVHD. Diagnostic studies are directed first at identifying a suitable donor, then at monitoring the immune response to the transplant. Immunosuppressive therapy with medications is a vital part of post-transplant care. Indeed, the development of effective immunosuppressive drugs is responsible for the success of organ transplants using allografts.

Diagnosis

The following diagnostic tests may be ordered prior to organ or tissue transplantation:

- *Blood type and Rh factor* of both the donor and recipient are determined. Although there is some question about the benefit of histocompatibility testing prior to transplant of a cadaver organ, there is no question about the need for ABO blood group compatibility.
- *Crossmatching* of the person's serum against the donor's lymphocytes is performed to identify any preformed antibodies against antigens on donor tissues. If present, these antibodies would likely result in an immediate or hyperacute graft rejection with probable loss of the transplant.
- *DNA sequencing* is made on blood cells to determine histocompatibility. Sequencing can be completed quickly. Quick response is important to minimise cold ischaemia in cadaverous organs. Diagnostic testing for recipients can be done less urgently.
- *HLA histocompatibility testing* identifies donors with an HLA type close to that of the recipient. It is used primarily to identify living donors for bone marrow and kidney transplant. Because of GVHD, histocompatibility tests to identify an identical or very close HLA match are particularly important in bone marrow transplant. HLA tests are performed using lymphocytes from a blood sample. The sample should not be obtained within 72 hours of a blood transfusion because this will interfere with results.
- *Mixed lymphocyte culture (MLC) assay tests* also are used to determine histocompatibility between the donor and the recipient. This test identifies whether mononuclear cells of the recipient will react against the potential donor's leucocyte antigens. The disadvantage of this test is that results cannot be obtained until 7 to 10 days later (Chernecky & Berger, 2012). If the intended recipient is severely immunocompromised, the results may be falsely negative. People treated with chemotherapy within 2 weeks of specimen collection are potentially immunocompromised.
- *Ultrasonography* or magnetic resonance imaging (MRI) of the transplanted organ may be performed to evaluate its size, perfusion and function.
- *Tissue biopsies* of the transplanted organ are performed routinely to assess for evidence of tissue rejection.

Medications

Prior to transplantation, several antibiotic and antiviral drugs may be prescribed, including the following:

- trimethoprim-sulfamethoxazole, which decreases the incidence of gram-negative bacterial infections
- aciclovir, which prevents the development of the herpes simplex virus and pneumonia in bone marrow transplant recipients
- ganciclovir, which prevents the development of cytomegalovirus (CMV) pneumonia in bone marrow transplant recipients.

The mainstays of drug therapy for people following a tissue or organ transplant are immunosuppressive agents. Varying regimens of these drugs are used, depending on the transplanted tissue and the medical centre; however, a combination of corticosteroids and cyclosporin is common for maintenance therapy (see Figure 12.6). Antilymphocyte therapy and the use of monoclonal antibodies are increasingly common in the immediate post-transplant period and for treating steroid-resistant rejection episodes.

Corticosteroids, primarily prednisone and methylprednisolone, were among the first medications used to prevent transplant rejection and they remain important agents today. Although the exact anti-inflammatory and immunosuppressive activity of corticosteroids is unknown, they are known to suppress production of interleukin-1 and -2, decrease monocyte migration and suppress proliferative and cytotoxic T-cell activity. Although they are very effective, large doses of corticosteroids used post-transplant are associated with significant adverse effects. Wound healing is impaired and the metabolism of fats, proteins and carbohydrates is altered. Blood glucose increases with steroid use, impairing glucose control. Fat distribution changes, producing a cushingoid appearance with moon face, increased truncal fat and 'buffalo hump'. Fluid retention and hypertension are potential problems, as are osteoporosis, gastrointestinal bleeding and emotional disturbances.

Azathioprine has been in use as an immunosuppressant for more than 25 years and continues to be a component of many regimens. Azathioprine inhibits both cell-mediated and antibody-mediated immunity, although its activity is more

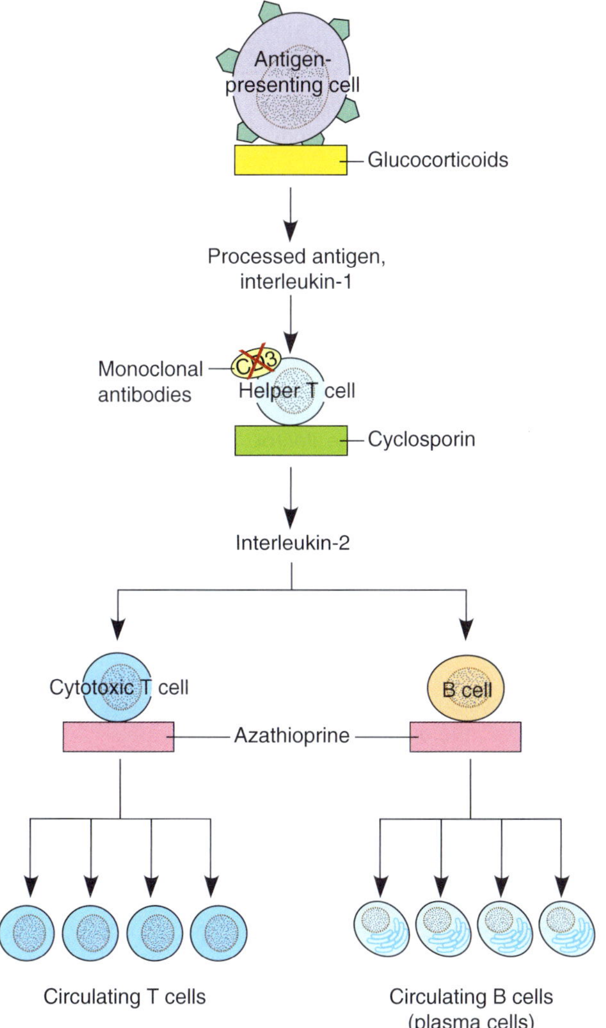

FIGURE 12.6 ***Sites of action of immunosuppressive agents***

specific for T cells than B cells. Because it is rapidly metabolised by the liver, azathioprine can be given to people with impaired renal function but may not be effective in people with impaired hepatic function. Bone marrow suppression is the most common adverse effect of this drug, necessitating frequent evaluation of the full blood count (FBC). Hepatotoxicity, pancreatitis and increased risk of neoplasm are also associated with azathioprine administration. Nursing responsibilities related to azathioprine are listed in the 'Medication administration' box. People who cannot tolerate azathioprine may receive a newer immunosuppressant, mycophenolate mofetil. Primarily, it is prescribed following renal and cardiac transplants.

Cyclosporin inhibits T-cell function and the normal cell-mediated immune response. The incidence of cyclosporin toxicity and side effects is related to blood levels, so blood levels are monitored closely. Cyclosporin is both nephrotoxic and hepatotoxic, especially at high doses. Observable toxic effects include hypertension and CNS symptoms such as flushing or tingling of the extremities, confusion, visual disturbances and seizures or coma.

Muromonab-CD3, also known as OKT3, is the first monoclonal antibody produced for therapeutic use in humans. As a monoclonal antibody, OKT3 is specific to T cells, blocking their generation and function. It binds with a surface antigen on T cells, inactivating and removing them from circulation. It also blocks killer T cells attached to the graft. Because of significant side effects, the use of OKT3 is limited primarily to treatment of steroid-resistant rejection. Two newer monoclonal antibodies, basiliximab (Simulect) and daclizumab (Zenapax), are a combination of mouse and human antibodies and cause fewer side effects.

Polyclonal antilymphocyte antibodies are also used as adjunctive immunosuppressant therapy. These are administered as antilymphocyte globulin (ALG) or antithymocyte globulin (ATG). These globulins contain antibodies against both T and B cells, as well as other mononuclear leucocytes. When administered, they deplete circulating lymphocytes, platelets and granulocytes.

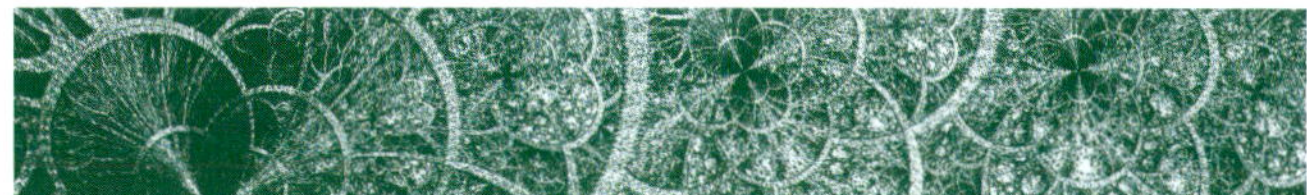

Nursing care

The person who has an organ or tissue transplant has both immediate and long-term nursing care needs. Both the person and the family must be considered in providing nursing care.

Health promotion

Health promotion activities focus partly on preventing the need for a tissue transplant. It is important to increase public awareness regarding unhealthy lifestyle behaviours, such as excessive alcohol consumption and illegal drug use, and their relationship to organ failure. People with chronic diseases such as diabetes mellitus and hypertension must understand that inadequate management of these disorders could lead to end-stage renal disease. Other risk factors may simply relate to a person's heredity; it is important to understand how heredity could affect future health and might influence the person's lifestyle choices.

Assessment

Assessment data collected following a tissue transplant focus on identifying potential rejection episodes. Further focused assessments are described with nursing interventions in the next section.

Nursing diagnoses and interventions

Because of the continuing risk of transplant rejection and the need for immunosuppression, *Ineffective protection* and *Risk of impaired tissue integrity* are priority nursing care foci. The person's underlying disease process, the transplant and the continuing need for immunosuppressive drug therapy also have emotional and psychological consequences. Many nursing diagnoses, such as *Powerlessness* or *Ineffective coping*, may be appropriate. The diagnosis *Anxiety* related to potential transplant rejection is considered in this section.

MEDICATION ADMINISTRATION Immunosuppressive agents

T-CELL SUPPRESSORS

Cyclosporin
Tacrolimus
Sirolimus

These drugs inhibit T-cell development and activation. They are given concurrently with a glucocorticoid and in combination with other immunosuppressants and inhibit immune system activity and organ rejection.

Nursing responsibilities

- Monitor BUN and creatinine for evidence of nephrotoxicity.
- Teach the signs and symptoms of infection unique to immunosuppressed individuals. A temperature of 38.1°C is significant evidence of infection. A sore throat may be a manifestation. Other signs and symptoms of inflammation and infection may be absent.
- Teach people good hygiene to avoid infection, with special emphasis on handwashing and avoiding infected individuals.
- Monitor blood pressure and availability and use of antihypertensive medications.
- Teach to avoid grapefruit juice, which can raise cyclosporin levels by 50% to 200% and increase the risk of toxicity. Sirolimus should not be taken with grapefruit juice. Sirolimus increases cholesterol and triglycerides. Lipid-lowering drugs may be necessary to prevent hyperlipidaemias.

CYTOTOXIC AGENTS

Azathioprine
Cyclophosphamide
Methotrexate
Mycophenolate

Certain drugs that are identified as cytotoxic or antineoplastic agents are effective as immunosuppressive agents. They act by decreasing the proliferation of cells within the immune system and are widely used to prevent rejection following a tissue or organ transplant. They are usually administered concurrently with corticosteroid therapy, allowing lower doses of both preparations and resulting in fewer side effects.

Nursing responsibilities

- Monitor blood count, with particular attention to the WBC and platelet counts. Notify the doctor of decreases in WBCs or platelet counts.
- Monitor renal and liver function studies, including creatinine, BUN, creatinine clearance and liver enzymes. Report abnormal levels to the doctor.
- Administer the drug as ordered. Administer oral preparations with food to minimise gastrointestinal effects. Antacids may be ordered.
- Have the person increase fluids to maintain good hydration and urinary output, void frequently and avoid taking the drug in the evening, which promotes dwelling of the drug in the bladder overnight.
- Monitor intake and output.
- Monitor for signs of abnormal bleeding, bleeding gums, bruising, petechiae, joint pain, haematuria and black or tarry stools.
- Use meticulous handwashing and other appropriate measures to protect the person from infection. Assess for signs of infection.
- Pulmonary fibrosis is a rare ($< 1\%$) potential adverse effect of cyclophosphamides. Therefore, monitor respiratory function using pulmonary function studies, and monitor for clinical signs of dyspnoea or cough.

Health education for the person and family

- Avoid large crowds and situations where exposure to infection is probable.
- Report signs of infection—such as chills, fever, sore throat, fatigue or malaise—to the doctor.
- Use contraceptive measures to prevent pregnancy while on immunosuppressive therapy; these drugs are teratogenic.
- Avoid the use of aspirin or ibuprofen while taking these drugs. Report any signs of bleeding to the doctor. Many over-the-counter products contain aspirin; check labels for aspirin.
- With cyclophosphamide, amenorrhoea may occur. The menses will resume after the drug is discontinued.
- If taking cyclophosphamide, report any difficulty breathing or cough to the doctor.

MONOCLONAL ANTIBODY

Muromonab-CD3 or OKT3

This monoclonal antibody against T cells is formed by immunising a mouse with an antigen to produce a specific antibody. Lymphocytes producing the antibody, OKT3, are cloned and the antibody is harvested. When injected into humans, OKT3 binds with a surface antigen on T cells, removing them from circulation and inactivating those bound to allograft cells. Due to the high incidence of adverse effects, refer to the organisational protocol regarding the administration of initial and subsequent doses of OKT3 and to observation protocols following the administration of OKT3.

Nursing responsibilities

- Be sure a chest x-ray has been performed within 24 hours preceding initiation of OKT3 therapy and that no congestion is present. The risk of anaphylaxis is greater in the person with fluid overload.
- Premedicate as ordered with hydrocortisone, paracetamol and diphenhydramine to reduce potential adverse effects.
- Position the emergency trolley and/or emergency medications in the person's room or in proximity to it. Refer to the organisational protocol.
- Monitor vital signs following administration of OKT3 as per organisational protocols.
- Refer to the organisational protocols for administration of initial and subsequent doses of OKT3 and administer as per guidelines.
- Observe closely for potential adverse effects, including chills and fever; tachycardia; headache and tremor; hypertension or hypotension; nausea, vomiting and diarrhoea; chest pain, dyspnoea and wheezing.
- OKT3 can also cause anaphylaxis; observe for evidence of urticaria, angio-oedema, laryngeal oedema, wheezing or other signs of anaphylactic reaction.

MEDICATION ADMINISTRATION Immunosuppressive agents (continued)

- Monitor FBC for evidence of leucopenia or pancytopenia.
- Assess for infection. Remember that typical signs of infection, including symptoms such as fever and inflammation, may be masked or reduced by immunosuppressive therapy.

Health education for the person and family
- Teach about the drug and its purpose.
- Discuss potential adverse and side effects and emphasise the need to report symptoms promptly.
- Inform the person that adverse effects are most likely to occur following the first two doses, necessitating close observation at that time. Reassure the person that this is standard protocol for this medication.

ANTILYMPHOCYTE GLOBULINS
Antithymocyte globulin or ATG (ATGAM)
Antilymphocyte globulin or ALG

These globulins containing antilymphocyte antibodies are produced by immunising horses (the main source), rabbits or sheep with human lymphocytes to stimulate production of antibodies (see figure). Serum from the animal is then recovered and the active IgG fraction is isolated, purified and administered parenterally to the person. It binds with peripheral lymphocytes and mononuclear cells, removing them from circulation.

ATG or ALG is used both to induce immunosuppression immediately following a transplant and to treat steroid-resistant rejection episodes. As with monoclonal antibody, multiple side effects are associated with ATG or ALG.

Nursing responsibilities
- Ensure a skin test for sensitivity to horse serum has been carried out prior to initial dose. Report any positive reaction to the doctor and hold administration until desensitisation therapy has been completed.
- Premedicate as ordered with paracetamol and diphenhydramine prior to each dose. Steroids may also be administered before the initial dose. Have adrenaline and hydrocortisone injections available at the bedside in case of anaphylactic reaction.
- Administer by intravenous infusion into a central line over 4 to 6 hours as per organisational protocol.
- Monitor vital signs during infusion as per organisational protocol.
- Assess for adverse effects, including chills and fever, erythema and pruritus. Notify the doctor; these may be treated symptomatically.
- Monitor FBC daily; notify the doctor if WBC or platelet count decrease. The medication may be stopped or reduced.
- Assess renal function studies to monitor for serum sickness. Report complaints of joint pain.

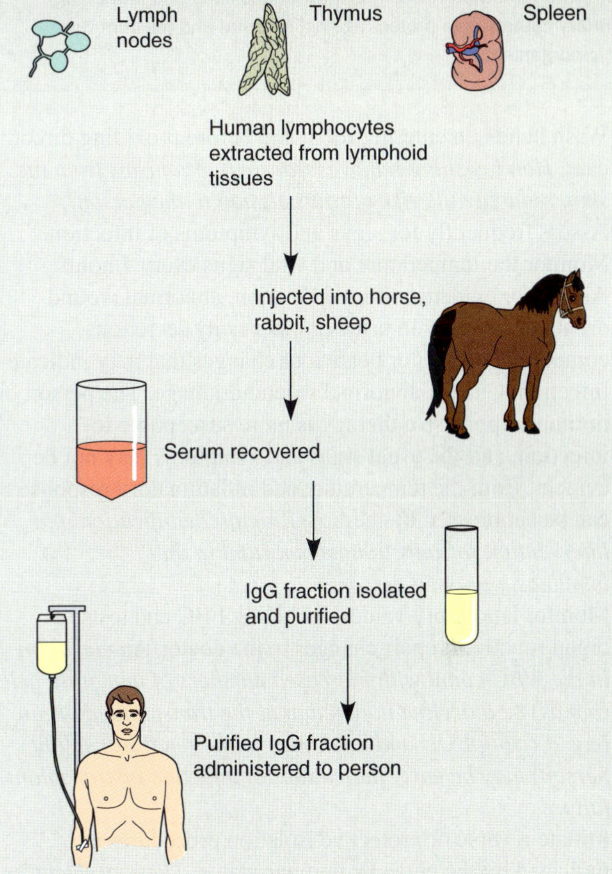

A horse is inoculated with washed human lymphocytes, stimulating the production of immunoglobulin with polyclonal antilymphocyte antibodies. These are then extracted from horse serum, purified, and administered intravenously to the person

- Monitor for signs of infection and report any signs promptly.

Health education for the person and family
- Explain the need for special precautions and close monitoring while this drug is being administered.
- Instruct the person to report any adverse effects, including malaise or joint pain, promptly.
- Ask the person to report any evidence of easy bruising, bleeding gums or black stools.
- Teach family members about the importance of not exposing the person to other people with infectious diseases.

Ineffective protection

Ineffective protection is a problem for the transplant person at all stages. Before the transplant occurs, failure of the affected organ may put the person at risk of infection and other multisystemic problems. Incisions and invasive perioperative procedures impair skin and mucous membrane protection from infectious organisms and other antigens. Immunosuppressive drugs given postoperatively to prevent graft rejection disarm the immune response to a certain extent, increasing the risk of infections and neoplastic growths.

CONSIDERATION FOR PRACTICE

Use strict aseptic technique in changing dressings and caring for invasive catheters such as intravenous lines and indwelling urinary catheters to protect against external and resident host microorganisms.

- Wash hands on entering room and before providing direct care. *Handwashing removes transient organisms from the skin, reducing the risk of transmission to the person.*
- Assess frequently for signs and symptoms of infection. Monitor the temperature and vital signs every 4 hours. Assess for evidence of inflammation, abnormal wound drainage, changes in urine or other body secretions, complaints of pain or behaviour changes that may indicate infection. Culture abnormal wound drainage. The person on immunosuppressive therapy is more susceptible to infection, and the usual signs and symptoms may not be evident. Both the temperature and inflammatory response can be suppressed by therapy. *Prompt identification and intervention for infection is important in the immunosuppressed person.*
- Monitor laboratory values, including FBC and tests of organ function; report changes to the doctor. *An elevation in the WBC count with increased numbers of immature cells (bands) or a decline in function of the transplanted organ (e.g. a rising BUN and creatinine in the renal transplant person) may be early indications of infection or transplant failure.*
- Initiate reverse or protective isolation procedures as indicated by the person's immune status. *These procedures further protect the severely immunocompromised person from infection.*
- Instruct ill family members and visitors to avoid contact with the person. *A 'minor' upper respiratory infection can be a significant illness in the immunocompromised host.*
- Help ensure adequate nutrient intake, offering supplementary feedings as indicated or maintaining parenteral nutrition if necessary. *Adequate nutrition is important for healing and immune system function.*
- Change intravenous bags and tubing as per organisational protocol, generally every 24 hours, and change peripheral intravenous sites every 48 to 72 hours, unless contraindicated. Remove invasive catheters and lines as soon as they are no longer necessary. *Changing lines and sites is important to reduce bacterial contamination. Fewer invasive lines provide fewer sites for bacterial invasion of the body.*
- Emphasise the importance of washing hands thoroughly after using the bathroom and before eating. *This reduces the risk of infection with endogenous organisms.*
- Provide good mouth care. *Good mouth care reduces the population of oral microorganisms and helps maintain an intact mucous membrane lining.*
- Monitor for potential adverse effects of medications:
  - thrombocytopenia and possible bleeding
  - fluid retention with oedema and possible hypertension
  - loss of bone density, osteoporosis and possible pathological fractures
  - renal or hepatic toxicity
  - cardiac effects, particularly in the presence of fluid retention and hypervolaemia.

  Medications used to maintain immunosuppression and preserve the allograft have many potential adverse effects that can alter normal protective and homeostatic mechanisms.

Risk of impaired tissue integrity: allograft

As noted, the risk of transplant rejection is highest in the initial postoperative period, but it is never completely eliminated for the person who has had an allograft. The person who has had a bone marrow transplant has the additional risk of developing GVHD, which can affect the integrity of skin, mucous membranes and other organs.

- Administer immunosuppressive therapy as prescribed. *Suppression of the immune response is necessary to reduce the risk of graft destruction by normal immune responses and to preserve the graft's function.*
- Assess for evidence of graft rejection, including tenderness, erythema and swelling over the site; sudden weight gain, oedema and hypertension; chills and fever; malaise and an increased WBC count and sedimentation rate. Report any changes immediately. *Early identification of rejection allows adjustment of medication regimens and, possibly, preservation of the graft.*
- Monitor results of laboratory studies for function of the transplanted organ. *With a functional graft, results (e.g. renal or liver function studies) will improve; a functional decline may be an early indicator of rejection.*
- Assess for and report signs of GVHD immediately, including maculopapular rash, erythema of the skin and possible desquamation, hair loss, abdominal cramping and diarrhoea, or jaundice with elevated bilirubin and liver enzymes (AST, ALT). *GVHD is a potentially lethal complication in the immunosuppressed person and necessitates immediate intervention.*
- Stress the importance of maintaining immunosuppressive therapy and reporting signs of graft rejection promptly to the doctor. *Continued immunosuppression and prompt treatment of rejection are vital to preserving graft function.*

Anxiety

The person who undergoes organ or tissue transplantation often faces the unwelcome choices of death from organ failure or receiving an organ that their body will likely attempt to reject. In most cases, the person understands that to receive this transplant, someone else must die and be willing to give up an organ. When the transplant (bone marrow or kidney) comes from a living donor, the person may not only worry about themself but also about the condition of the donor. Fear of rejection and guilt may be even greater in this instance.

- Assess level of anxiety by noting such cues as expressions of apprehension, fear or inadequacy; facial expression, tension or shakiness; difficulty focusing; helplessness; poor eye contact and restlessness. *People may have difficulty identifying or verbalising feelings of fear and anxiety. Non-verbal cues are often useful in recognising states of anxiety.*

- Provide opportunities to express feelings. Use opening statements such as, 'Facing an organ transplant must be very stressful.' Listen attentively. *Encouragement and active listening allow the person to express feelings of anxiety or fear.*
- Arrange tasks to allow as much time with the person as possible. When leaving, tell the person when you will return. *Time spent with the person facilitates the development of trust.*
- Provide clear, concise directions. *Highly anxious people have difficulty focusing and retaining information.*
- Encourage involvement in care, but do not request unnecessary decisions. *The person needs to feel a sense of control but may become irritated if asked to make decisions unrelated to the situation.*
- Encourage family members to remain with the person as much as possible. *This can help reduce the person's anxiety.*
- Encourage the use of coping behaviours that have been effective for the person in the past. *Coping mechanisms and behaviours help lower anxiety to a more acceptable level.*
- Reduce or eliminate environmental stressors to the extent possible. *This gives the person a better sense of control.*
- Assist with stress reduction and relaxation techniques, such as guided imagery, meditation and muscle relaxation. *These techniques help the person gain control over physical responses to anxiety.*
- Refer to a counsellor or mental health specialist to work with the person. *Counselling can help the person identify and deal with their feelings.*
- Assess the person's preference and desire for spiritual counselling prior to transplant. *Because there is a risk of death if the transplant fails, the person may want to discuss their concerns with a spiritual counsellor.*

Community-based care

Teaching of the person and family regarding an organ or tissue transplant begins well before the transplant and continues throughout hospitalisation and follow-up treatment.

Initial teaching focuses on the options, risks and potential benefits of the transplant itself. Include the procedure by which the organ is selected and obtained, as well as the procedure by which it is transplanted into the person. If a living related donor is an option, discuss the risks and benefits for both the person and the donor. Outline the post-transplant treatment regimen, including any lifestyle changes that may be necessary.

Following the transplant, provide verbal and written instructions, including the following:

- manifestations of transplant rejection and the importance of notifying the doctor
- immunosuppressive drug regimen and side effects
- wound care
- avoiding exposure to infectious diseases, particularly respiratory infections and wearing a mask when going outside
- meticulous personal hygiene, handwashing technique and frequent mouth care
- wearing a MedicAlert® bracelet or pendant
- follow-up visits to the doctor or clinic
- helpful resources:
  - Transplant Australia
  - Donate Life—Australian Government Organ and Tissue Authority
  - ShareLife—an Outcomes Australia project
  - local and state support groups and organisations related to the specific organ transplant.

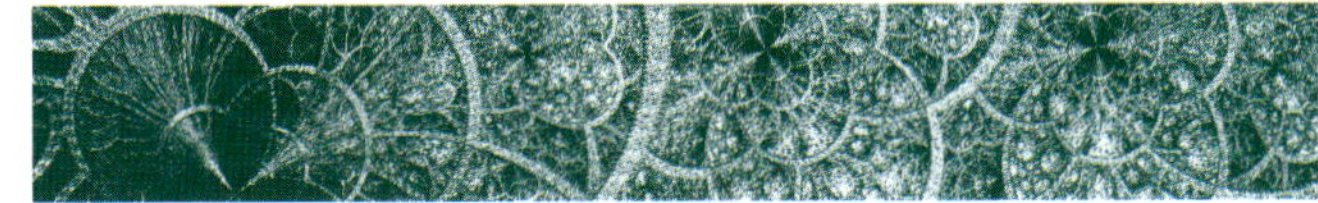

Impaired immune responses

Disorders of impaired immune system responses may be either congenital or acquired. Often the function of either T or B cells is impaired, reducing the body's ability to defend against foreign antigens or abnormal host tissue.

No matter what the cause, people with immunodeficiency disorders demonstrate an unusual susceptibility to infection. When the antibody-mediated response is primarily affected, the person is at particular risk of severe and chronic bacterial infections. These people also do not develop long-lasting immunity to such diseases as chickenpox and are prone to recurrent cases. People with a defect of cell-mediated immunity tend to develop disseminated viral infections such as herpes simplex and CMV. Candidiasis and other fungal infections are also common. Because T cells are involved with activating antibody-mediated immune responses as well, overwhelming bacterial infections may occur. Immunodeficiency in its most severe form occurs when both antibody-mediated and cell-mediated responses are impaired. People with combined immunodeficiency are susceptible to all varieties of infectious organisms, including those not normally considered to be pathogens.

Most immunodeficiency diseases are genetically determined and rare. They affect children more than adults. The noted exception is AIDS, an infectious disease caused by a virus.

THE PERSON WITH HIV INFECTION

In 1981, five cases of *Pneumocystis carinii* pneumonia (PCP) and 26 cases of a rare cancer, Kaposi's sarcoma, were diagnosed in young, previously healthy homosexual males in Los Angeles and New York. The term **acquired immunodeficiency syndrome (AIDS)** was ascribed to this new phenomenon to describe the immune system deficits associated with these opportunistic disorders. Prior to this, both PCP and Kaposi's sarcoma had been seen only in older people or debilitated or severely immunodeficient people. Other groups at risk of AIDS were soon identified: injection drug users, people with haemophilia, recipients of blood transfusions and those engaging in unsafe sexual practices.

Research to identify the cause of this apparently new disease progressed feverishly and, in 1983, a common antibody was identified in people with AIDS. The **human immunodeficiency virus (HIV)** was isolated in 1984. It then became apparent that AIDS was the final, fatal stage of HIV infection.

It began, like so many epidemics, with a few isolated cases and has become a worldwide plague (see the accompanying 'Focus on cultural diversity' box). AIDS invades our lives in ways we never imagined—testing our scientific knowledge, probing our private values and eluding a vaccine or a cure. Progression of HIV-positive disease to AIDS has slowed because of the effectiveness of antiretroviral therapy (ART) (Centers for Disease Control and Prevention (CDC), 2020). This change in progression to AIDS makes monitoring of AIDS less useful as an indicator of infected cases. For that reason, the CDC (2022a) developed new surveillance methods based on infection rates in high-risk populations.

Although the incidence of HIV has levelled and mortality due to AIDS has declined, the epidemic is far from over.

Incidence and prevalence

In comparison with other countries, the overall incident rates of HIV/AIDS in Australia are low. In Australia, there are approximately 29,090 living with HIV and 2,610 people suspected to be living with HIV but not currently diagnosed. HIV prevalence is at 0.14% and, while HIV transmission among sex workers and people who inject drugs has been virtually eliminated, it continues to be high among gay and bisexual men (Australian Federation of AIDS Organisations (AFAO), 2022). Funding is provided to professional and community organisations to assist in research and provision of education programs aimed at increasing knowledge and awareness within the community.

A continued decline in deaths is dependent on access to quality care and treatment and continued development of treatments for those already heavily treated (Papadakis et al., 2022).

In Australia, HIV risk criteria and indicators include sharing syringes, STI diagnosis or other clinical indicators of HIV, occupational or non-occupational exposure to HIV, unprotected intercourse with an HIV-positive person, unprotected intercourse between males and being born in or travelling to countries with a high HIV prevalence. Routine HIV testing is provided to antenatal women. Mandatory testing is carried out for specific visas; upon entry to the Australian Armed Forces; for all organ, tissue or blood donations; and in some legal or insurance requirements (Australasian Society for HIV, Viral Hepatitis and Sexual Health Medicine (ASHM), 2020).

The risk factors for HIV infection are behavioural. In 2020, 58% of HIV notifications involved sexual contact between homosexual partners, 24% involved heterosexual contacts, 10% related to injecting drug use and sexual contact between men, 3% related to injecting drug use and 5% were noted as other/unspecified. Of those HIV notifications in 2020 related to homosexual contact as their risk exposure, 45% were overseas-born men. Co-factors that increase the risk of transmission include the presence of ulcerative or inflammatory sexually transmitted diseases, trauma, menses and lack of male circumcision (Papadakis et al., 2022; UNAIDS, 2021).

For the haemophilia community, who require large amounts of intravenous clotting factors, transfusion-related infections have been a significant cause of morbidity and mortality in the past. Ongoing diagnosis, counselling, treatment and monitoring

FOCUS ON CULTURAL DIVERSITY HIV/AIDS

In 2020, HIV notifications were 2.2 per 100,000 for Aboriginal and Torres Strait Islander people and 2.3 per 100,000 for non-Indigenous Australians. Although a decrease has been noted, it is important that a cautious approach be taken and culturally appropriate education and prevention programs are offered to support the populations that need them (AFAO, 2022; Kirby Institute, 2018; Ward, Gilles & Russel, 2021).

HIV/AIDS worldwide

There are an estimated 37.7 million people living with HIV worldwide, with virtually every country in the world reporting cases of AIDS. Of those infected, 81% know that they are HIV positive, 2 out of 3 are on ART and 59% of those have undetectable levels of the virus (UNAIDS, 2020). New HIV infections have been reduced by 52% since they peaked in 1997. In 2020, key populations and their sexual partners accounted for 65% of HIV infections globally (with 93% of new HIV infections outside sub-Saharan Africa and 39% in sub-Saharan Africa) (UNAIDS, 2021).

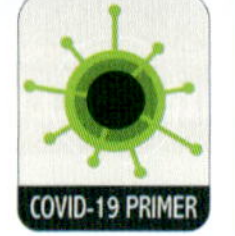

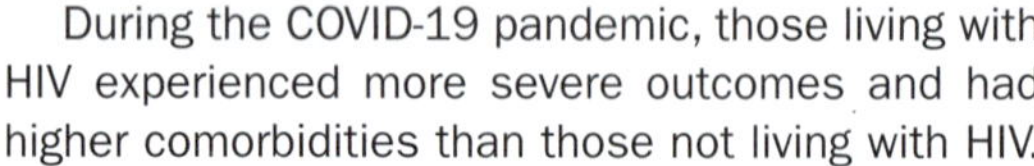

During the COVID-19 pandemic, those living with HIV experienced more severe outcomes and had higher comorbidities than those not living with HIV. Not having access to COVID-19 vaccines doubled their risk of dying compared with the general population (UNAIDS, 2021). The COVID-19 pandemic saw a significant decline and disruption in HIV notifications and testing (AFAO, 2022).

Critical thinking in person-centred care

1 Identify specific ways in which an HIV/AIDS prevention program focusing on injection drug use might be tailored to Aboriginal and Torres Strait Islander people.
2 What additional areas for research might further knowledge and guide strategies for HIV prevention in high-risk groups?

of complications is in place (Australian Haemophilia Centre Directors' Organisation (AHCDO), 2016).

Declining immune system function and other associated comorbidities in older adults significantly increases their risk of contracting HIV/AIDS, along with the belief that they cannot be affected by it. Just as younger people with HIV/AIDS contract the diseases primarily through sexual intercourse, so does the older population. Because older adults are beyond childbearing years, they often fail to use condoms when engaging in sexual activity. Manifestations may be overlooked by healthcare professionals, leading to a delayed diagnosis and increased severity of the disease.

HIV is a retrovirus transmitted by direct contact with infected blood and body fluids. The risk of acquiring HIV varies depending on the type of exposure and behaviour (CDC, 2019a). Significant concentrations of the virus are present in blood, semen, vaginal and cervical secretions and cerebrospinal fluid (CSF) of infected individuals. It is also found in breast milk and saliva. Sexual contact is the primary mode of transmission. HIV is also transmitted through contact with infected blood via needle sharing during injection drug use or by blood transfusion (CDC, 2019a). Approximately 13% to 40% of infants born to HIV-positive mothers are infected perinatally. Breastfeeding is a route of transmission and should be avoided (Papadakis et al., 2022). HIV is not transmitted by casual contact, nor is there any evidence of its transmission by vectors such as mosquitoes.

A small but real occupational risk exists for healthcare workers. Percutaneous exposure to infected blood or body fluids through a needle-stick injury or non-intact skin is the primary route of transmission. Documented evidence indicates that parenteral exposure poses a 0.3% risk of becoming HIV positive. Mucosal exposures, such as splashing in the eyes or mouth, pose a much smaller risk (Papadakis et al., 2022).

Pathophysiology and manifestations

As mentioned, HIV is a retrovirus, meaning it carries its genetic information in RNA. On entry into the body, the virus infects cells that have the CD4 antigen. Once inside the cell, the virus sheds its protein coat and uses an enzyme called *reverse transcriptase* to convert the RNA to DNA (see Figure 12.7). This viral DNA is then integrated into host cell DNA and duplicated during normal processes of cell division. Within the cell, the virus may remain latent or become activated to produce new RNA and to form *virions*. The virus then buds from the cell surface, disrupting its cell membrane and leading to destruction of the host cell.

Although the virus may remain inactive in infected cells for years, antibodies are produced to its proteins, a process known as **seroconversion**. These antibodies are usually detectable 6 weeks to 6 months after the initial infection. Helper T or CD4 cells are the primary cells infected by HIV. It also infects macrophages and certain cells of the CNS. Helper T cells play a vital role in normal immune system function, recognising foreign antigens and infected cells and activating antibody-producing B cells. They also direct cell-mediated immune activity and influence the phagocytic activity of monocytes and macrophages. The loss of these helper T cells leads to the immunodeficiencies seen with HIV infection (Norris, 2018). Figure 12.8 illustrates the typical course of HIV infection.

The clinical manifestations of HIV infection range from no symptoms to severe immunodeficiency with multiple opportunistic infections and cancers (see the 'Manifestations' box). It appears that the majority of people develop an acute mononucleosis-type illness within days to weeks after contracting the virus. Typical manifestations include fever, sore throat, arthralgias and myalgias, headache, rash and lymphadenopathy. Pathological changes are also noted in the CNS of many infected individuals, although the mechanism of neurological dysfunction is unclear. The person may also experience nausea, vomiting and abdominal cramping. The person often attributes this initial manifestation of HIV infection to a common viral illness such as influenza, upper respiratory infection or stomach virus.

Following this acute illness, people enter a long-lasting asymptomatic period. Although the virus is present and can be transmitted to others, the infected host has few or no symptoms. Clearly, the majority of HIV-infected people are in this stage of the disease. The length of the asymptomatic period varies widely, but its mean length is estimated to be 8 to 10 years.

Some people with few other symptoms develop persistent generalised lymphadenopathy. This is defined as enlargement of two or more lymph nodes outside the inguinal chain, with no other illness or condition to account for the lymphadenopathy.

The move from asymptomatic disease or persistent lymphadenopathy to AIDS is often not clearly defined. The person may complain of general malaise, fever, fatigue, night sweats and involuntary weight loss. Persistent skin dryness and rash may be a problem. Diarrhoea is common, as are oral lesions such as hairy leucoplakia, candidiasis, gingival inflammation and ulceration. The development of advanced HIV typically occurs 10 to 11 years after initial infection; this varies according to the viral load, rate of disease progression and the development of resistance to ART (Justiz Vaillant, Guilick & Pinto, 2022). With the development of significant constitutional disease, neurological manifestations or opportunistic infections or cancers, the person has manifestations that are characteristic of AIDS and a very poor prognosis. HIV infection and AIDS may be classified by using the revised CDC's HIV stage-based approach combining the adult and paediatric criteria for a confirmed case of HIV infection. This classification specifies the different criteria for staging across three age groups ($<$ 1 year, 1–5 years and $\geq$ 6 years to adult). Under this system, HIV disease is determined by both laboratory (preferable) and clinical evidence to adapt to recent changes in diagnostic criteria (see Box 12.2) (Battistini Garcia & Guzman, 2021; CDC, 2014, 2022b; Reeves et al., 2021).

When clinical manifestations develop, the outcome varies. With ART, many people are living longer after being diagnosed with AIDS. Today, PCP is most commonly diagnosed in those who are undiagnosed or have a late diagnosis of HIV infection, or who fail to take prophylactic antibiotics when their CD4 count is $<$ 200. ART is credited with decreasing the incidence of opportunistic infections and improving survival (Healthdirect, 2020). The time of survival has increased from

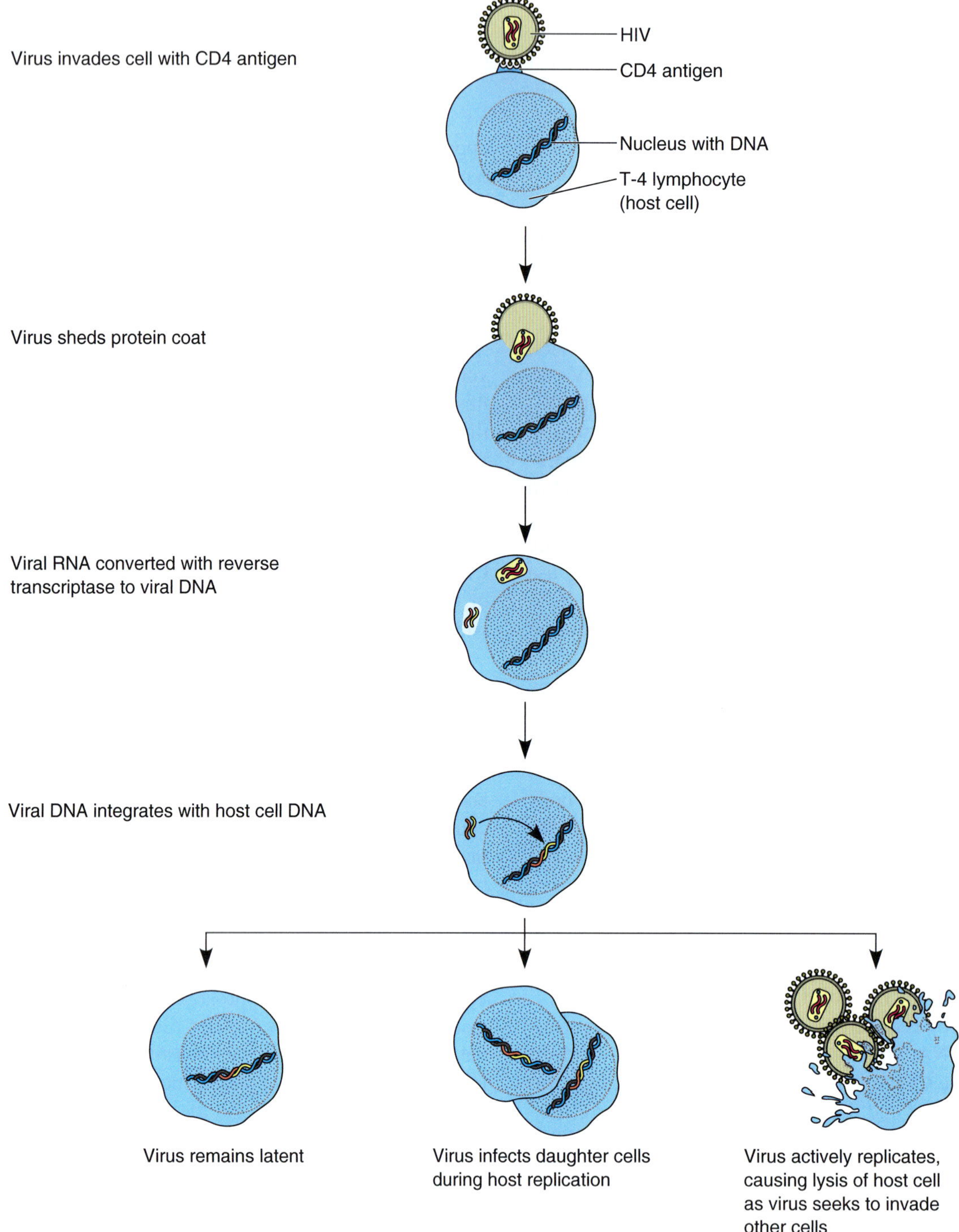

FIGURE 12.7 ***How HIV infects and destroys CD4 cells***

about 13 months at the start of the AIDS epidemic; however, survival after diagnosis of HIV-related lymphomas still averages less than 8 months.

AIDS dementia complex and neurological effects

Neurological manifestations of HIV are common, affecting 40% to 60% of people with AIDS. Included among the manifestations are dementia, delirium and seizures. They result from both the direct effects of the virus on the nervous system and opportunistic infections. AIDS dementia complex is the most common cause of mental status changes for people with HIV infection. This dementia results from a direct effect of the virus on the brain and affects cognitive, motor and behavioural functioning. Fluctuating memory loss, confusion, difficulty concentrating, lethargy and diminished motor speed are typical manifestations of AIDS dementia complex. People become

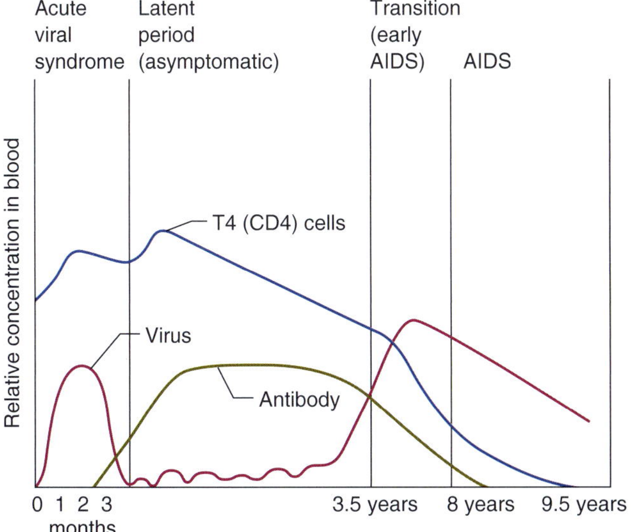

FIGURE 12.8 ***The progression of HIV infection. Acute illness develops shortly after the virus is contracted, corresponding with a rapid rise in viral levels. Antibodies are formed and remain present throughout the course of infection. Late in the disease, viral activation results in a marked increase in virus while CD4 (T4) cells diminish as they are destroyed with viral replication. Antibody levels gradually decrease as immune function is impaired***

apathetic, losing interest in work and social and recreational activities. As the complex progresses, the person develops severe dementia with motor disturbances such as ataxia, tremor, spasticity, incontinence and paraplegia (Loscalzo et al., 2022; Norris, 2018).

Infections and lesions common with AIDS may also affect the CNS. Toxoplasmosis and non-Hodgkin's lymphoma are space-occupying lesions that may cause headache, altered mental status and neurological deficits. Cryptococcal meningitis and CMV infection also are common in people with AIDS. CNS complications have declined with the use of ART therapy (Papadakis et al., 2022).

Peripheral nervous system manifestations are also common in HIV-infected people. Sensory neuropathies with manifestations of numbness, tingling and pain in the lower extremities affect about 30% of people with AIDS. A Guillain–Barré type of inflammatory demyelinating polyneuropathy can also occur, resulting in progressive weakness and paralysis.

Opportunistic infections

Opportunistic infections are the most common manifestations of AIDS, often occurring simultaneously. The risk of opportunistic infections is predictable by the T4 or CD4 cell count. The normal CD4 cell count is 500 to 1,500/mm^3. When the CD4 count falls to less than 500/mm^3, manifestations of immunodeficiency are seen. With a count of less than 250/mm^3, opportunistic infections and cancers are likely.

***PNEUMOCYSTIS CARINII* PNEUMONIA** *Pneumocystis carinii* pneumonia is the most common opportunistic infection affecting people with AIDS. Approximately 75% to 80% of people develop PCP at some point in their disease (Papadakis et al., 2022). It tends to be recurrent and is the cause of death in about 20% of people with AIDS. PCP is caused by a common environmental fungus that is not pathogenic in people with intact immune systems.

Unlike many pneumonias, the manifestations of PCP are non-specific and may progress insidiously. People often present with fever, cough, dyspnoea, tachypnoea and tachycardia. Complaints of mild chest pain and sputum may also be present. Breath sounds may initially be normal. With severe disease, the person may present with cyanosis and significant respiratory distress.

BOX 12.2 Surveillance case definitions for HIV infection

Stage	Laboratory evidence: Age on date of CD4+ T-lymphocyte test						Clinical evidence
	< 1 year		1–5 years		≥ 6 years to adult		
	Cells/mm^3	%	Cells/mm^3	%	Cells/mm^3	%	
0	Early infection, recognised by a negative HIV test within 6 months *and* after 6 months of HIV diagnosis						None required unless opportunistic infections (AIDS-defining conditions) have been diagnosed, then Stage 3 or laboratory confirmation of HIV infection
1	≥ 1,500	≥ 34	≥ 1,000	≥ 30	≥ 500	≥ 26	None required (but no AIDS-defining condition)
2	750-1,499	26-33	500-599	22-29	200-499	14-25	None required (but no AIDS-defining condition)
3	< 750	< 26	< 500	< 22	< 200	< 14	or documentation of an AIDS-defining condition (with laboratory confirmation of HIV infection)
Unknown	Laboratory confirmation of HIV infection *and* no information on CD4+ T-lymphocyte or percentage						and no information on presence of AIDS-defining conditions

Sources: Adapted from CDC (2008). *Revised surveillance case definitions for HIV infection among adults, adolescents, and children aged <8 months and for HIV infection and aids among children aged 18 months to <3 years—United States, 2008.* Retrieved from https://www.cdc.gov/; CDC (2014). *Revised surveillance case definition for HIV infection—United States 2014.* Retrieved from https://www.cdc.gov/; Reeves et al. (2021). British HIV Association guidelines for the management of HIV-2 2021. *HIV Medicine, 22*(S4). https://doi.org/10.1111/hiv.13204.

MANIFESTATIONS HIV infection and AIDS

I. Acute retroviral syndrome (ARS) or primary HIV infection
- Fever
- Sore throat
- Arthralgias and myalgias
- Headache
- Rash
- Nausea, vomiting and abdominal cramping

II. Asymptomatic infection
- None; converts to seropositive status

III. Persistent generalised lymphadenopathy
- Enlargement of two or more extrainguinal sites for more than 3 months

IV. Other acute disease symptoms
- General malaise, fatigue
- Low-grade fever
- Night sweats
- Involuntary weight loss
- Skin dryness or rashes

V. Other diseases and AIDS
  A. *AIDS dementia complex*
  B. *Secondary infectious diseases*
  - *Pneumocystis carinii* pneumonia
  - *Mycobacterium* tuberculosis
  - *Mycobacterium avium* complex
  - Candidiasis
  - Cryptosporidiosis
  - Cryptococcosis
  - Toxoplasmosis
  - Herpes simplex or herpes zoster
  - Cytomegalovirus

  C. *Secondary cancers*
  - Kaposi's sarcoma
  - Non-Hodgkin's lymphoma
  - Cervical dysplasia and cervical cancer

  D. *Other conditions*
  - Pelvic inflammatory disease
  - Human papillomavirus

TUBERCULOSIS In some people, active tuberculosis results from reactivation of a prior infection. In other people, it is a new, primary disease facilitated by impaired immune function. Rapid progression, diffuse pulmonary infiltrates and disseminated disease occur more commonly in people with AIDS. Multidrug-resistant strains of tuberculosis present a significant problem (Papadakis et al., 2022).

People with pulmonary tuberculosis present with a productive cough of purulent sputum, fever, fatigue, weight loss and lymphadenopathy. Disseminated disease affects the bone marrow, bone, joints, liver, spleen, CSF, skin, kidneys, gastrointestinal tract, lymph nodes, brain and other sites.

CANDIDIASIS *Candida albicans* infection is a common opportunistic infection in people with AIDS. It is usually manifested as oral thrush or oesophagitis. In women, vaginal candidiasis is frequent and often recurrent. Oral thrush presents as white, friable plaques on the buccal mucosa or tongue and, in the HIV-infected person, is often the first indication of progression to AIDS. People with oesophagitis have difficulty swallowing and substernal pain or burning that increases with swallowing.

***MYCOBACTERIUM AVIUM* COMPLEX** *Mycobacterium avium* complex (MAC) affects up to 25% of people with AIDS, typically occurring late in the course of the disease when CD4 cell counts are less than 100/mm^3. MAC is more common in women than men. MAC is caused by organisms commonly found in food, water and soil. It is a major cause of 'wasting syndrome' in people with AIDS (see Figure 12.9). Manifestations of MAC include chills and fever, weakness, night sweats, abdominal pain and diarrhoea, and weight loss. Nearly every organ can be infected and most people with MAC develop disseminated disease.

OTHER INFECTIONS Herpesvirus infections are common in people with AIDS and may be severe. CMV can affect the retina, the gastrointestinal tract or lungs. Disseminated herpes simplex or herpes zoster may occur, although severe mucocutaneous manifestations are more common.

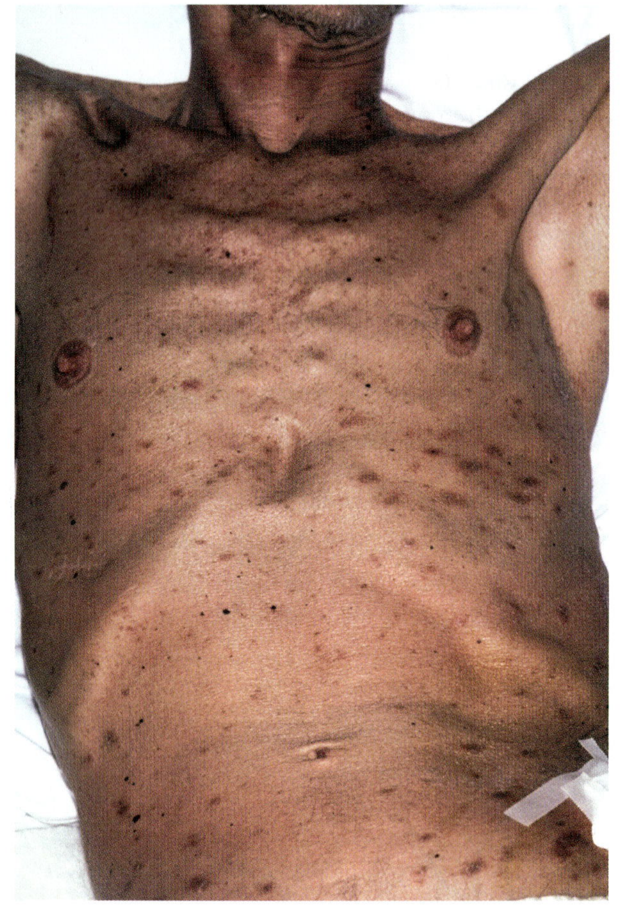

FIGURE 12.9 ***Wasting syndrome in a person with AIDS***

Source: Dept of Medical Photography, St Stephen's Hospital, London/Science Photo Library/Alamy Stock Photo.

Parasitic infections with *Toxoplasma gondii* and *Cryptococcus neoformans* commonly affect the CNS. Toxoplasmosis occurs as encephalitis or an intracerebral mass lesion. Changes in mental status, focal neurological signs and seizures may result. *Cryptococcus* infection may present as either meningitis or disseminated disease primarily affecting the lungs. *Cryptosporidium*, a protozoon affecting the gastrointestinal tract, is an important cause of prolonged diarrhoea in people with AIDS. Bacterial *Salmonella* infections are also a relatively common cause of diarrhoea.

Women with AIDS have a high incidence of pelvic inflammatory disease (PID). Although the pathogens appear to be the same as those in PID affecting non-HIV-infected women, the disease is more severe. Inpatient treatment with intravenous antibiotics is often necessary.

Secondary cancers

As cell-mediated immune function declines, the risk of malignancy increases. The CDC classification of AIDS currently includes four cancers: Kaposi's sarcoma, non-Hodgkin's lymphoma, primary lymphoma of the brain and invasive cervical carcinoma.

KAPOSI'S SARCOMA **Kaposi's sarcoma (KS)** is often the presenting symptom of AIDS. It remains the most common cancer associated with the disease. Kaposi's sarcoma is caused by a virus called the Kaposi-sarcoma-associated herpesvirus, also known as human herpesvirus 8. Men who have sex with men not only have a risk of HIV infection but are also more likely to be infected with the virus responsible for KS. Women who have sex with these men also have a risk of HIV and KS. The virus associated with KS appears to be mainly transmitted through sexual contact and oral contact (via saliva), although cases have also been reported in injection drug users. People whose immune system is suppressed because they have received an organ transplant have a 1 in 200 risk of developing KS (World Health Organization, 2021). It is estimated that in 2020, over 15,000 people died from KS globally (Cancer.Net, 2022).

A tumour of the endothelial cells lining small blood vessels, KS presents as vascular macules, papules or violet lesions affecting the skin and viscera (see Figure 12.10). The face is a common site for skin lesions, especially the tip of the nose and pinnae of the ears. Common sites for visceral disease include the gastrointestinal tract, lungs and lymphatic system.

The lesions of KS are usually painless initially but may become painful as the disease progresses. Internally, the tumours may obstruct organ function or cause bleeding. When the lungs are involved, gas exchange may be severely impaired, resulting in pulmonary haemorrhage. KS is an indicator of late-stage HIV disease, with an average survival time of 18 months after diagnosis. The disease may progress slowly or rapidly. Rapidly progressing KS is treated with chemotherapy; milder forms may improve with the initiation of ART therapy (Papadakis et al., 2022).

LYMPHOMAS Lymphomas are malignancies of the lymphoid tissue, including lymphocytes, lymph nodes and the lymphoid organs such as the spleen and bone marrow. In

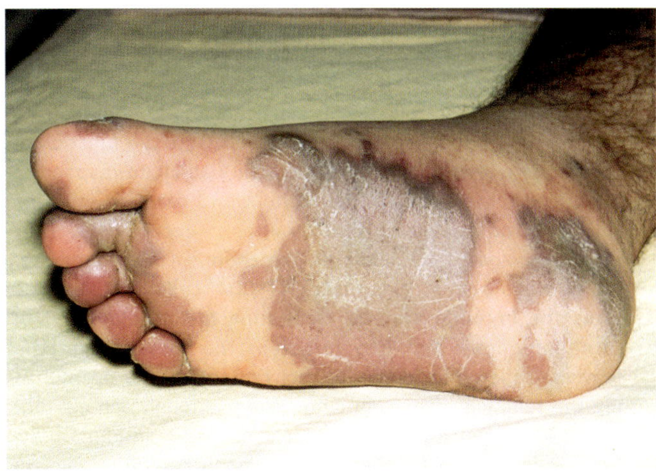

FIGURE 12.10 ***Kaposi's sarcoma lesions***

Source: St Mary's Hospital Medical School/Science Photo Library/Alamy Stock Photo.

AIDS, two lymphomas are common: non-Hodgkin's lymphoma (including Burkitt's lymphoma) and primary lymphoma of the brain. Hodgkin's disease also occurs five times more frequently in people with HIV infection than in those without. The CNS is the usual site for these lymphomas, although they may be found in the bone marrow, gastrointestinal tract, liver, skin and mucous membranes. They are aggressive tumours, growing and spreading rapidly. Headache and changes in mental status are common early symptoms of lymphomas affecting the CNS.

CERVICAL CANCER Of women with HIV infection, 40% have cervical dysplasia. Cervical cancer develops frequently and tends to be aggressive. Women with concurrent HIV infection and cervical cancer usually die of the cervical cancer, not AIDS. Because of this, it is recommended that women with HIV infection have cervical screening tests every 6 months and aggressive treatment of cervical dysplasia with colposcopic examination and cone biopsy, as per the National Cervical Screening Program introduced by the Australian Government in 2017.

INTERPROFESSIONAL CARE

Although multiple research studies to identify a cure for HIV infection and AIDS are under way, no cure is currently available. This fact, plus the apparent universally fatal nature of the disease, makes prevention a vital strategy in HIV care. New treatments are under investigation (see Box 12.3).

The goals of care for the person with HIV disease are as follows:

- early identification of the infection
- promoting health-maintenance activities to prolong the asymptomatic period as long as possible
- prevention of opportunistic infections
- treatment of disease complications, such as cancers

BOX 12.3 Investigational immune-based treatment for HIV

HIV infection progressively alters the function of and destroys $CD4^+$ lymphocytes. $CD4^+$ cells are essential to the function of the immune system, including the body's ability to respond to infections. These cells initiate, direct and regulate immune responses and may also directly attack infected cells. They also are a source of cytokines, the chemical messengers of the immune system. Destruction of $CD4^+$ cells by HIV devastates the immune system, facilitating the development of fatal infections and neoplasms in the infected person. Immune-based treatments indirectly affect the HIV by improving the function of the immune system through actions that inhibit cytokines, replenish cytokines or restore immune function. These treatments, used alone or in combination with antiretroviral drugs, are being investigated for use in the treatment of HIV.

Inhibiting cytokines

Tumour necrosis factor alpha (TNF-α) is a cytokine secreted by activated monocytes and macrophages in response to infection, infestation or tumour growth. It causes a proliferation of B cells and T cells. However, high levels of this cytokine may actually facilitate the development of disease by blocking the normal inflammatory response. It is believed that blocking the effect of TNF-α can suppress HIV production, although caution must be used.

Replenishing cytokines

Some cytokines (interleukin-2, interleukin-12 and interferon alpha) may be helpful in treating HIV by stimulating the production of killer cells as well as increasing the function of lymphocytes. The interferons are part of the body's first line of defence against viruses. All of these agents have toxic side effects, requiring careful nursing assessment and care.

Restoring immune system function

HIV infection not only destroys $CD4^+$ cells, but also eventually destroys the lymphoid organs, such as bone marrow and the thymus gland. Lymphocytes, including the $CD4^+$ cells, are derived from stem cells in bone marrow and mature in the thymus. Two investigational treatments to restore the immune system are bone marrow transplant and thymus transplant. Bone marrow transplants have been used to correct other types of immune disorders (such as leukaemia or lymphoma) but have yet to be effective in people with HIV. A few thymus transplants have been done in HIV-infected people but they have provided only temporary benefits.

- access to a broad spectrum of services including condoms, oral pre-exposure prophylaxis (PrEP), post-exposure prophylaxis (PEP), Treatment as Prevention (TasP), testing facilities
- providing emotional and psychosocial support.

Diagnosis

Diagnostic testing is used to screen and identify the infection, as well as to monitor the person's disease and immune status. The following diagnostic tests may be ordered. The likelihood that a positive screening test truly indicates the presence of HIV infection decreases as HIV prevalence in the tested population becomes lower. Therefore, false-positive HIV test results are more likely in settings where the tested population prevalence is lower than in settings where the tested population prevalence is higher. When a preliminary, positive rapid test is explained to people, phrases like 'a good chance of being infected' or 'very likely infected' can be used to indicate the likelihood of HIV infection and can be qualified based on the HIV prevalence in the setting and the person's individual risk.

Further testing is always required to confirm a reactive screening test result.

- *HIV rapid antibody tests* are available in many countries including Australia.
- *Enzyme-linked immunosorbent assay (ELISA)*, also called the HIV antigen/antibody test, is the most widely used screening test for HIV infection. The ELISA test was developed in 1985 to screen blood donors. ELISA tests for HIV antibodies; it does not detect the virus. Therefore, a person may have a negative ELISA test early in the course of infection, before detectable antibodies have developed. The test has a 99.5% or higher sensitivity when performed at least 13 weeks after infection. This means that more than 99.5% of tests performed on blood containing HIV antibodies will show a positive result. False positives can occur; therefore, an initial positive result is always tested repeatedly and confirmed using a different method of antibody detection, usually the Western blot.
- Immediate notification is critical because many people tested for HIV do not return to learn the results; many cannot be located to give the test results and educate about safe behaviours, whether they are positive or negative for HIV. Although confirmation of results is dependent on testing with a second source, ELISA or Western blot test, learning results immediately gives the person more information to make wise choices about their behaviours and self-care.
- *Western blot antibody testing* is more reliable but more time-consuming and more expensive than ELISA. When combined with ELISA, however, a specificity of greater than 99.9% is achieved. Specificity is a measure of the probability that a negative test result indicates that no antibodies are present. In this test, the person's serum is mixed with HIV proteins to detect reaction. If antibodies to HIV are present, a detectable antigen–antibody response will occur.
- *HIV viral load tests* measure the amount of actively replicating HIV. Levels correlate with disease progression and response to antiretroviral medications. Public health guidelines state treatment should be considered for asymptomatic people with HIV with viral loads greater than 5,000 to

100,000 copies/mL. HIV viral load testing is used in conjunction with CD4 cell count to inform treatment decisions.

- *FBC* is performed to detect anaemia, leucopenia and thrombocytopenia, which are often present in HIV infection. Lymphopenia (or low levels of lymphocytes) is especially common in this disease.
- *CD4 cell count* is the most widely used test to monitor the progress of the disease and guide therapy. The CD4 cell count correlates very closely with the immunodeficiency disorders seen in AIDS. AIDS is now defined not only by the presence of opportunistic infections and other diseases indicative of immunodeficiency, but also by HIV-seropositive status; the CD4 count goes down as the disease progresses. The standard reference range for CD4 count is dependent on many factors. The doctor monitors the pattern for changes over several months to determine strategies for optimal treatment.

In addition to these widely used tests, several other diagnostic tests may be performed:

- *Blood culture for HIV* provides the most specific diagnosis but is an expensive and cumbersome test that is not widely available.
- *Immune-complex-dissociated p24 assay* is a test for p24 (HIV) antigen in the blood. This antigen indicates active reproduction of HIV and tends to be positive prior to seroconversion and with advanced disease. It is most useful in monitoring disease progression and the antiviral activity of experimental medications (Pagana et al., 2020; Papadakis et al., 2022).

Other diagnostic tests are used primarily to detect secondary cancers and opportunistic infections in the person with HIV. Tests ordered are both general and specific to the person's manifestations and may include the following:

- *tuberculin skin testing* to detect possible tuberculosis infection
- *MRI* of the brain to identify lymphomas
- *specific cultures and serology examinations for opportunistic infections* such as PCP, toxoplasmosis and others
- *cervical screening tests* every 6 months for early detection of cervical cancer in women with cervical dysplasia (Papadakis et al., 2022).

Medications

Pharmacological management of the person with HIV disease has four primary foci:

1. to suppress the infection itself, decreasing symptoms and prolonging life
2. to provide prophylaxis of opportunistic infections
3. to stimulate haematopoietic response
4. to treat opportunistic infections and malignancies.

Effectiveness of treatment is monitored by viral load and CD4 cell counts; positive results are indicated by a reduction in viral load along with preserving the CD4 count above 350/mm^3. Treatment is recommended when the CD4 count falls below 200/mm^3. People with symptoms of severe disease are treated regardless of their CD4 level or viral load, so monitoring these individuals may reveal higher levels of CD4 or lower viral load. Initiating therapy in asymptomatic individuals with higher CD4 levels has not shown a protective effect and is thought to perhaps increase viral resistance. Today the drugs have been combined and dosing schedules simplified, which helps people adhere to medication administration schedules. There have been significant advances in ART drug regimens which not only prevent drug resistance by the viral organisms but also transform HIV from a life-limiting condition to a manageable chronic disease (Dharan et al., 2019; Raubinger, Lee & Pinto, 2022).

Types of antiretroviral treatment include nucleoside reverse transcriptase inhibitors (NRTIs), non-nucleoside reverse transcriptase inhibitors (NNRTIs), protease inhibitors (PIs), integrase inhibitors (IIs), CCR5 antagonist, fusion inhibitors and entry inhibitors. ART involves a combination of these antiretroviral drugs based on individual needs, including reducing the incidence of drug resistance and drug interactions.

Combination therapies increase the likelihood of decreasing viral load and symptoms but also burden people with complicated and expensive medication schedules. People beginning the ART protocol must understand the benefits, risks, costs and effects on daily life. ART does not eradicate HIV infection but can reduce the risk of HIV transmission (HIVinfo, 2021). ART medications are expensive, particularly the newer triple combinations such as Trizivir. These medications are scheduled for specific times throughout the day; therefore, leading a normal life becomes a challenge. In addition, as with most chronic diseases, all ART medications cause major adverse reactions leading to less than perfect adherence; however, in this case, the outcome could be fatal.

Each person must be able to adhere to the treatment regimen. It may be preferable to delay initiating therapy until the person is able to agree to adherence so that irregular dosing does not lead to viral resistance. Some providers gauge a person's ability to follow the ART regimen by their success with prophylaxis for an opportunistic infection.

Several methods to promote and ensure adherence are being used and studied, including the development of the HIV Care Continuum (HIVgov, 2022), a public health model outlining the steps taken by people from diagnosis to maintaining viral suppression. Intentional and non-intentional barriers to treatment regimen adherence continue to be a factor due to a person's personal and/or cultural beliefs, cognitive abilities, psychosocial issues, comorbidities and other factors. The role of nurses, allied health and other HIV care support providers is critical in identifying these barriers and providing strategies, education and behavioural goals to support the person to improve adherence (CDC, 2019b; Wagner et al., 2016).

NUCLEOSIDE REVERSE TRANSCRIPTASE INHIBITORS

The NRTIs (also called nucleoside analogues) inhibit the action of viral reverse transcriptase, a retroviral enzyme that catalyses the substrates for conversion and copying of viral RNA to DNA sequences. This enzyme is necessary for viral integration into cellular DNA and replication. The nucleoside analogues act as a chemical decoy for building blocks of the formation of the

DNA copy, preventing the RNA from being copied into DNA. Each drug substitutes for a particular nucleoside base at different points on the chain. See the 'Medication administration' guidelines for this group of drugs. Zidovudine (Retrovir, AZT) was the first antiretroviral agent approved for use with HIV infection. It remains in widespread use and has been shown to decrease symptoms and prolong the lives of people with AIDS. Zidovudine is often given to people with a CD4 cell count of less than 500/mm^3 because of evidence that it slows the progression to severe disease (Papadakis et al., 2022). Zidovudine may also be used prophylactically following a documented parenteral exposure to HIV. It is used in combination with ddI, ddC or 3TC.

- Didanosine (ddI, Videx) also inhibits reverse transcriptase and viral replication. It is used in combination therapy with zidovudine.
- Stavudine (d4T, Zerit) is a retroviral inhibitor that has been shown to increase CD4 cell counts and decrease serum p24 antigen levels. Current use is for people who are intolerant of zidovudine.
- Lamivudine (3-TC, Combivir) is used for low CD4 cell counts or symptomatic disease as a first-line treatment in combination with zidovudine.
- Abacavir (Ziagen) is a potent inhibitor of reverse transcriptase; however, it may cause serious hypersensitivity reactions.
- Zidovudine plus lamivudine (Combivir) is a combination drug in use to decrease HIV zidovudine-resistant strains.

PROTEASE INHIBITORS Protease is a viral enzyme necessary for the formation of specific viral protein needs for viral assembly and maturation. Protease inhibitors bond chemically with protease to block the function of the enzyme and result in the production of immature, non-infectious viral particles. When combined with other antiviral drugs, these chemicals increase the chance of eliminating the virus by interfering with different stages of its life cycle. However, viral resistance occurs rather quickly. PIs inhibit and induce metabolism of other drugs, so their use with other medications and the dose of those medications must be carefully planned. Some drugs will circulate longer because their metabolism is inhibited; others will be speedily metabolised and eliminated.

Protease inhibitors and nucleoside analogues are associated with serious metabolic derangements. These include elevated cholesterol and triglycerides, insulin resistance and diabetes mellitus, and changes in body fat composition, which are particularly distressing to the person. These body fat changes are primarily abdominal obesity and skeletal wasting. This set of symptoms is referred to as lipodystrophy (Papadakis et al., 2022). Elevated cholesterol should be treated with pravastatin or atorvastatin. Lovastatin and simvastatin react to PIs, so they need to be avoided. Dietary sources of cholesterol should be reduced.

- Saquinavir is used in combination with nucleoside analogues to treat progression of the disease.
- Ritonavir is used in combination with nucleoside analogues to treat progression of the disease.
- Indinavir is used in combination with nucleoside analogues to treat progression of the disease.
- Nelfinavir is used in cases of failure of or intolerance to other protease inhibitors.
- Amprenavir is the newest protease inhibitor.
- Lopinavir/ritonavir is the first combination of protease inhibitors active against some HIV strains resistant to other protease inhibitors.

MEDICATION ADMINISTRATION Antiretroviral nucleoside analogues

ZIDOVUDINE (AZT, AZIDOTHYMIDINE)

Zidovudine is the first antiretroviral agent developed to treat HIV infection. It interferes with reverse transcriptase, thus inhibiting replication of the virus. The usual dose is 250 mg twice daily. It is administered orally. Dose-limiting side effects are anaemia and neutropenia.

Nursing responsibilities

- Assess for possible contraindications to therapy, including allergic response or a CD4 count of greater than 350/mm^3.
- Administer by mouth, instructing the person to swallow capsules whole.
- Assess for adverse effects. Nausea and headache are common. They may be self-limiting, decreasing with time, or significant and continuing, necessitating a change of therapy. Nausea and neutropenia are treated with erythropoietin and G-CSF.
- Assess FBC with differential and creatinine phosphokinase. Notify the doctor of significant changes.

Health education for the person and family

- Antiretroviral medications will not cure HIV infection but slow its progress and reduce significant symptoms.
- Take the drug according to the directions for administration at least 0.5 hour before or 1 hour after meals, if tolerated.
- With this and all antiretroviral drugs, it is important to emphasise that the person is still infective and can pass the infection to others. Use safer sex practices and other measures to prevent transmission to partners. Do not donate blood or breastfeed.
- Notify the doctor if signs of an infection or adverse response to the medication develop: sore throat, swollen lymph glands, fever; unusual fatigue or weakness; easy bruising, bleeding gums or an injury that will not heal; persistent or intractable nausea; muscle pain or wasting.
- Continue all scheduled follow-up visits and laboratory studies to monitor for drug toxicity.
- Check with the doctor before taking any prescription or over-the-counter drug.

MEDICATION ADMINISTRATION **Antiretroviral nucleoside analogues (continued)**

DIDANOSINE (DDI, VIDEX)

As with zidovudine, didanosine does not kill HIV but inhibits its replication within the cells. Its activity is similar to that of zidovudine. Didanosine has been shown to increase CD4 cell counts and lower p24 antigen levels (Papadakis et al., 2022). Didanosine is used alone for people who are intolerant or resistant to zidovudine. It is also being used with zidovudine in combination therapy regimens. Didanosine does not cause the anaemia associated with zidovudine, but it may cause neutropenia. Didanosine is also associated with an increased risk of pancreatitis, peripheral neuropathy, development of diabetes mellitus and dry mouth.

Nursing responsibilities

- Assess for possible contraindications to didanosine therapy, including previous episodes of pancreatitis and impaired renal or liver function.
- Administer as directed and refer to the product information for administration instructions.
- Administer with caution to people taking vincristine, rifampin, pentamidine, ethambutol, allopurinol, stavudine or metronidazole; the action of both drugs may be affected by concurrent administration.
- Intravenous pentamidine and trimethoprim-sulfamethoxazole taken concurrently may increase the risk of acute and fatal pancreatitis.
- Didanosine interferes with the absorption of ketoconazole and dapsone. Doses of these drugs should be scheduled at least 2 hours apart from didanosine doses.
- Evaluate for therapeutic response and possible adverse effects. Notify the doctor if manifestations of peripheral neuropathy, diarrhoea, depression, agitation or other adverse effects develop.
- Stop the drug and notify the doctor immediately if the person develops manifestations of pancreatitis or hepatic failure, including nausea and vomiting, severe abdominal pain, elevated bilirubin or elevated serum enzymes (e.g. amylase, AST, ALT).

Health education for the person and family

- Take the drug as directed. The prescribed dose must always be taken to get the required amount of antacid to prevent the drug from being destroyed by stomach acid.
- Take on an empty stomach, at least 1 hour before or 2 hours after meals.
- Do not drink alcohol while taking didanosine; alcohol may increase the risk of pancreatitis.
- Stop the drug and call the doctor immediately if nausea, vomiting, abdominal pain or diarrhoea develops. These may indicate pancreatitis.
- Call the doctor if extremity pain, weakness, numbness or tingling occurs. These side effects usually disappear when didanosine is discontinued.
- Other side effects to report to the doctor include unusual bleeding or bruising, fatigue, weakness, fever or persistent sore throat.

ABACAVIR

Abacavir is a nucleoside analogue with activity against some HIV strains resistant to other nucleoside drugs. It is prepared in combination with zidovudine and lamivudine (Trizivir) and is taken as prescribed. This combination drug is composed exclusively of nucleoside analogues, lacking NNRTIs or PIs. As such, it is less effective at decreasing viral load and allowing immune system enhancement, but the ease of administration makes it a useful drug for people who cannot adhere to more complex regimens. The main toxicity is a hypersensitivity response in approximately 5% of people, manifested as flu-like symptoms and hypotension. Avoid repeated use in those individuals.

Nursing responsibilities

- Assess for possible hypersensitivity reactions, anaemia and neutropenia.
- Evaluate for desired effect of increased CD4 counts and lower blood levels of p24 antigen.
- Notify the doctor if the person develops evidence of pancreatitis, impaired hepatic function or painful peripheral neuropathy.

Health education for the person and family

- Take without regard to food or water.
- Check with the doctor before taking any other prescription or over-the-counter medication.
- Report all signs and symptoms of hypersensitivity to the drug.
- Report to the doctor signs of infection, flu-like symptoms or changes in condition.

NON-NUCLEOSIDE REVERSE TRANSCRIPTASE INHIBITORS Nevirapine, delavirdine and efavirenz are NNRTIs that may be used in combination with nucleoside analogues and protease inhibitors. However, one limitation to NNRTIs is the high incidence of cross-resistance to NRTIs. Some studies have shown that nevirapine and efavirenz may significantly reduce serum levels of the protease inhibitors. Only one NNRTI should be used at the same time (HIVgov, 2021).

ENTRY INHIBITORS: ENFUVIRTIDE (FUZEON) This class of drugs became available in 2003. These fusion and CCR5 (a key cell-surface receptor for HIV) inhibitors prevent HIV from entering target cells by binding to the protein envelope that surrounds the virus. When bound to the drug, the virus cannot morph in order to fit and adhere to cell membranes (ASHM, 2019a; HIVinfo, 2022). Adding this new class of drug to the regimen of heavily pre-treated individuals improves CD4 counts and lowers viral loads (Papadakis et al., 2022). However, tests can sometimes return false positives or higher counts.

OTHER MEDICATIONS Other agents may also be administered in combination with ART. Interferons, which are naturally occurring lymphokines, have been used alone and in combination. Interferon alpha may be used to treat KS and in combination with zidovudine to slow disease progression. Interferon gamma is also used. As more drugs become available, the burden to choose the best regimen increases for the healthcare provider. The most important limiting factor when choosing a regimen is a person's adherence. Second to that is selecting an effective combination of drugs without overlapping toxicities or toxicities so debilitating that adherence will be further impaired.

As global ART is changing, with new medications fast becoming the first choice in HIV/AIDS treatment, some people undergoing ART are developing body composition changes and metabolic abnormalities associated with the therapy, especially the PIs. Increased fat deposition in the midsection, breasts and neck, with atrophy in the face, buttocks and extremities, describes the body composition changes; metabolic abnormalities include increased low-density lipoprotein cholesterol and triglycerides and insulin resistance. The combination of changes is consistent with metabolic syndrome, which increases the risk of cardiovascular disease and diabetes. These conditions are commonly treated with medications along with changes to diet and exercise (Bai et al., 2022).

A number of pharmacological agents are used to prevent and treat opportunistic infections and malignancies in the person with HIV. These agents are outlined in Table 12.4.

Many people at some point require a central venous access device, such as a Groshong catheter, to facilitate blood sampling, intravenous medication administration, transfusions and parenteral nutrition. See the chapter 'Nursing care of people with cancer' for nursing care of the person with a central venous catheter.

It is recommended that all HIV-infected people receive pneumococcal, influenza, hepatitis B, *Haemophilus influenzae* b and COVID-19 vaccines. People with a positive PPD and negative chest x-ray are given prophylactic isoniazid. When the person's CD4 cell count falls to less than 200/mm^3, prophylactic treatment for PCP is begun, usually with trimethoprim-sulfamethoxazole. People with a CD4 count of less than 100/mm^3 are started on prophylactic treatment for MAC.

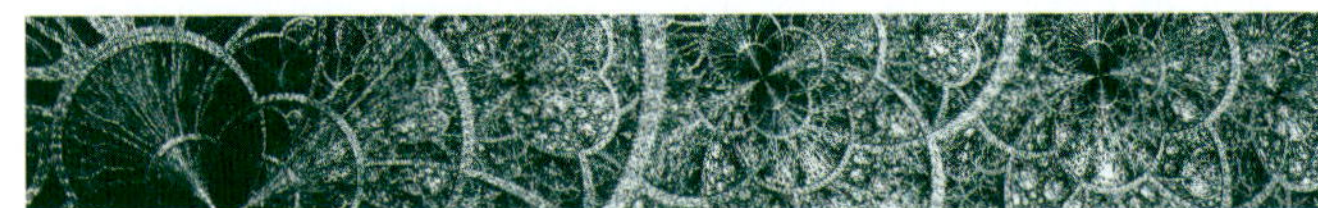

Nursing care

The person with HIV and AIDS has many care needs, including both physical and psychosocial support (see the 'Translation to practice' box). Because there is as yet no cure or effective treatment for HIV disease, many of these needs fall within the realm of nursing to promote knowledge and understanding, self-care, comfort and quality of life. As with many diseases that have an ultimately fatal outcome, the course of HIV infection may well

TABLE 12.4 Pharmacological treatment of common opportunistic infections and malignancies in HIV disease

CONDITION	TREATMENT	POTENTIAL ADVERSE EFFECTS
Infections		
Pneumocystis carinii pneumonia	Trimethoprim/sulfamethoxazole Pentamidine	Rash, neutropenia, anaemia, thrombocytopenia, Stevens-Johnson syndrome Hypotension, altered blood glucose levels, hypocalcaemia, anaemia and leucopenia, liver and renal toxicity, pancreatitis
Tuberculosis	Combination drug therapy using isoniazid, rifampicin, ethambutol, pyrazinamide or streptomycin	Multiple; see the chapter 'Nursing care of people with ventilation disorders'
Candidiasis	Clotrimazole troches	Few toxic responses noted
Oral thrush	Nystatin suspension	
Oesophagitis or recurrent vaginitis	Ketoconazole Fluconazole Amphotericin B	Hepatitis, adrenal insufficiency Hepatitis Bone marrow toxicity, acute renal or hepatic failure; nausea, vomiting; chills, fever, headache
Mycobacterium avium complex	Combination therapy using • Clarithromycin, plus • Clofazimine • Ethambutol • Rifampin • Ciprofloxacin • Amikacin	 • Hepatitis, nausea, diarrhoea • Diarrhoea, nausea, vomiting; skin discolouration, pruritus, rash • Thrombocytopenia, hepatitis, optic euritis • Bone marrow depression, renal failure, hepatitis • Nausea, rash • Bone marrow depression, renal failure, ototoxicity, hepatitis
Cytomegalovirus	Ganciclovir	Bone marrow depression, fever
	Foscarnet	Renal failure, electrolyte imbalances, seizures
Herpes simplex or herpes zoster	Aciclovir	Nausea, vomiting, diarrhoea; CNS effects; renal failure
Toxoplasmosis	Pyrimethamine, plus sulfadiazine or clindamycin and folinic acid	Bone marrow depression, rash; respiratory failure; nausea, vomiting, abdominal pain; haematuria
Malignancies		
Kaposi's sarcoma	Intralesional vinblastine	Inflammation and pain at injection site
Lymphoma	Combination chemotherapy	Nausea, vomiting; bone marrow toxicity; alopecia

TRANSLATION TO PRACTICE Evidence-based practice and nurses' willingness to care for people with AIDS

As reported by the CDC in the United States (2020), the number of deaths from AIDS has declined. This is believed to be the result of both the slowing of the epidemic and of improved treatment, which has lengthened the lifespan of people with AIDS. However, as treatment continues to improve survival, a key challenge will be the increasing number of people living with HIV and AIDS and the additional resources needed for services, treatment and care.

Several studies have found that some professional nurses and students are resistant to caring for people with AIDS, from prevention and testing through to long-term management and palliative care. The ethical issues may be extremely complex and difficult to resolve as they are related to personal and professional values and beliefs (ASHM, 2019b).

While the introduction of the 90-9-90 targets (UNAIDS, 2020) has showcased many ways nurses can lead in this area, few studies have been conducted that address both nursing willingness and reluctance to treat people with HIV infection. Nursing education certainly increases knowledge and awareness of the science of HIV infection, but it may not modify individual attitudes or behaviours of both faculty and students (Leyva-Moral et al., 2019).

A study by Valois et al. (2001) researched the impact of persuasive messages on nursing students' beliefs and attitudes about caring for HIV-positive people. According to the underlying theory of the research, individuals who receive evidence-based persuasive messages may develop favourable beliefs that will alter their willingness to perform a given behaviour. Three main types of beliefs were considered in this study: behavioural belief (related to the expected consequences of adopting a behaviour); normative belief (related to perceived social pressures by significant others resulting from adopting a behaviour); and control belief (related to resources or barriers that seem to facilitate or hamper adoption of the behaviour).

In three sessions, the student nurses in the experimental group were given positive persuasive messages about caring for HIV-infected people. The persuasive messages were compelling and specific to caring for people with HIV; case studies provided opportunities for the students to discuss the elements of the case within the framework of the persuasive messages. Students in the control group studied the science of caring for people with HIV but did not receive the persuasive messages. When beliefs and attitudes about caring for HIV-positive people were compared, the researchers found significantly greater willingness to provide care in the experimental group. Nursing students proved to be well prepared and motivated to receive this information.

IMPLICATIONS FOR NURSING

To increase nurses' willingness to care for people with AIDS, students need to be better socialised into their roles and responsibilities. Incorporating education about HIV/AIDS into the undergraduate curriculum; analysing and defining effective nursing care in cases based on evidence-based framework; and utilising the standards of professional nursing all support the development of positive attitudes. Discussions within the classroom and clinical settings provide a safe means of bringing fears into the open and sharing experiences. Student groups can serve as support groups, improving communications, decreasing isolation and anxiety, and improving self-esteem and morale. Within the work setting, perceived support from colleagues and administrators as well as increased contact with people with AIDS are important factors in making caring a rewarding and positive experience.

CRITICAL THINKING IN PERSON-CENTRED CARE

1. These studies were of student nurses and Registered Nurses. What differences do you think might have been found between the two groups today?
2. Carefully consider each of the following people with AIDS and write a brief paragraph about how you would feel if you were assigned to care for them:
   a. a heterosexual female, aged 25
   b. a homosexual male, aged 35
   c. a newborn baby girl
   d. a 40-year-old single mother of three teenagers
   e. a 30-year-old homeless drug user
   f. a 17-year-old male with haemophilia, infected by blood transfusions.

be affected by the person's social support systems, control, perceived self-efficacy in management and coping mechanisms.

As the epidemic continues, nurses are providing care for increasing numbers of people with HIV infection at various stages of disease. These people are not only in special care settings but also in general units, maternal–child units, hospice and home settings. As people with HIV disease live longer, nurses will increasingly encounter people in whom HIV disease is a secondary diagnosis, with another primary diagnosis—for example, seizures, heart disease, diabetes mellitus or an operative procedure.

Prevention

To date, no safe immunisation to protect against HIV infection has been developed. Education, counselling and behaviour modification are the primary tools for AIDS prevention. The benefit of education and behaviour modification is evident in the homosexual male population. The incidence of new HIV infections in this population has declined dramatically in high-prevalence cities. Nurses play a vital role in providing education about this epidemic and infection prevention for individuals and communities.

All sexually active individuals need to know how HIV is spread. Following are the only *totally* safe sex practices:

- no sex
- long-term mutually monogamous sexual relations between two uninfected people
- mutual masturbation without direct contact.

People who do engage in sexual activity need to know and practise safer sex (see Box 12.4). Reducing the number of sexual partners—for example, by entering into and remaining in a long-term mutually monogamous relationship with an

BOX 12.4 Guidelines for safer sex

- Practise mutual monogamy; if you are not in a mutually monogamous relationship, limit the number of sexual partners.
- Do not engage in unprotected sex, especially if the HIV status of your partner is unknown. (Remember that a person may be infected and infective for up to 6 months before converting to seropositive status.)
- When entering into a new monogamous relationship, both partners should undergo HIV testing initially. If both are negative, practise abstinence or safer sex for 6 months, followed by re-testing. If results still indicate that both partners are negative, sexual activity can probably be considered safe.
- Use dental dams or latex condoms for oral, vaginal or anal intercourse; avoid natural or animal-skin condoms, which allow passage of HIV.
- For vaginal or anal sex, lubricate the condom with the spermicidal agent nonoxynol-9 for additional protection.
- Do not use an oil-based lubricant such as petroleum jelly, which can result in condom damage; water-based lubricants are acceptable.
- Women should carry and use a female condom.
- Remember that use of other means of birth control, such as oral contraceptives, provide no protection against HIV; barrier protection with a condom is necessary.
- Engage in safer sexual practices that are less damaging to sensitive tissues (e.g. mutual masturbation, avoiding anal or oral sex).
- Do not use drugs or alcohol.
- Do not share needles, razors, toothbrushes, sexual toys or other items that may be contaminated with blood or body fluids.
- Use PrEP medication for people at risk of getting HIV (PrEP does not prevent other STIs).
- If HIV positive:
  a. Do not engage in unprotected sexual activity.
  b. Inform all current and former sexual partners of HIV status.
  c. Inform all healthcare personnel—primary care providers, doctors and dentists, in particular—of HIV status.
  d. Continue to take medications as prescribed.
  e. Do not donate blood, plasma, blood products, sperm organs or tissue.
  f. If female, do not become pregnant.
  g. If already pregnant, speak to a doctor about ART to prevent infection being passed onto the baby during pregnancy, childbirth and/or breastfeeding.

uninfected partner—reduces the risk. People should not engage in unprotected sex, especially if the HIV status of the partner is unknown. Latex condoms have been shown to reduce the risk of transmitting HIV. Their effectiveness is improved when nonoxynol-9, a spermicide, is used for lubrication; however, it may cause genital ulcers, which can facilitate HIV transmission. To be effective, condoms must be used with every sexual encounter involving vaginal, oral or anal intercourse. They also need to be applied and removed properly. A female condom is also available for use.

Healthcare workers exposed to HIV infection or adults who experience a high-risk exposure to HIV may choose post-exposure prophylaxis. Risk of exposure for healthcare workers may be through needle sticks or cuts with a sharp object, contact with mucous membranes or non-intact skin, semen, vaginal secretions, fluids contaminated with visible blood and possibly CSF, synovial fluid and pleural, peritoneal, pericardial or amniotic fluids. CDC guidelines recommend treatment with ART, which includes two NRTIs for lower-risk exposures and the addition of a third drug for higher-risk exposure (CDC, 2019b). A PEP 4-week course of treatment is recommended and should be started within 72 hours, preferably within 2 to 3 hours of exposure (Healthdirect, 2021). The most difficult group of high-risk people to reach and educate has been injection drug users. People in this group should never share needles, syringes or other drug paraphernalia. Australian cities have established needle-exchange programs, providing a sterile needle and syringe in exchange for a used one. It is important also to teach people in this population about safer sex practices, because most heterosexual HIV transmission occurs between injection drug users and their partners.

Australia's blood screening ensures one of the safest blood supplies in the world. Screening of voluntary blood donors and donated blood supplies commenced in 1985 and has reduced the risk of transmission of HIV/AIDS by transfusion, with no transmission via transfusion since 1985. Because current blood-screening methods use antibody testing, receiving donated blood continues to carry a small risk. People in the *window period* between contraction of the virus and the development of detectable antibodies are able to transmit the virus to others, even though they do not yet test positive for HIV. This window period usually lasts from 6 weeks to 6 months; rarely, it lasts up to 1 year. When possible, encourage people to use autologous transfusion, donating their own blood prior to an anticipated surgery. Seeking donations from family members is not encouraged for several reasons. Family members may have engaged in high-risk behaviours but lie about their risk because of embarrassment or fear of discovery. Furthermore, the family member may have a different blood type or have other contraindications to donating.

Encourage HIV-positive people to abstain from donating blood organs or sperm. They should understand tactics to avoid exchange of body fluids by not sharing needles or other drug paraphernalia, not sharing razors and not obtaining a tattoo. Stress the importance of informing all medical personnel providing direct care (especially anyone performing a dental, surgical or obstetric procedure) about the diagnosis.

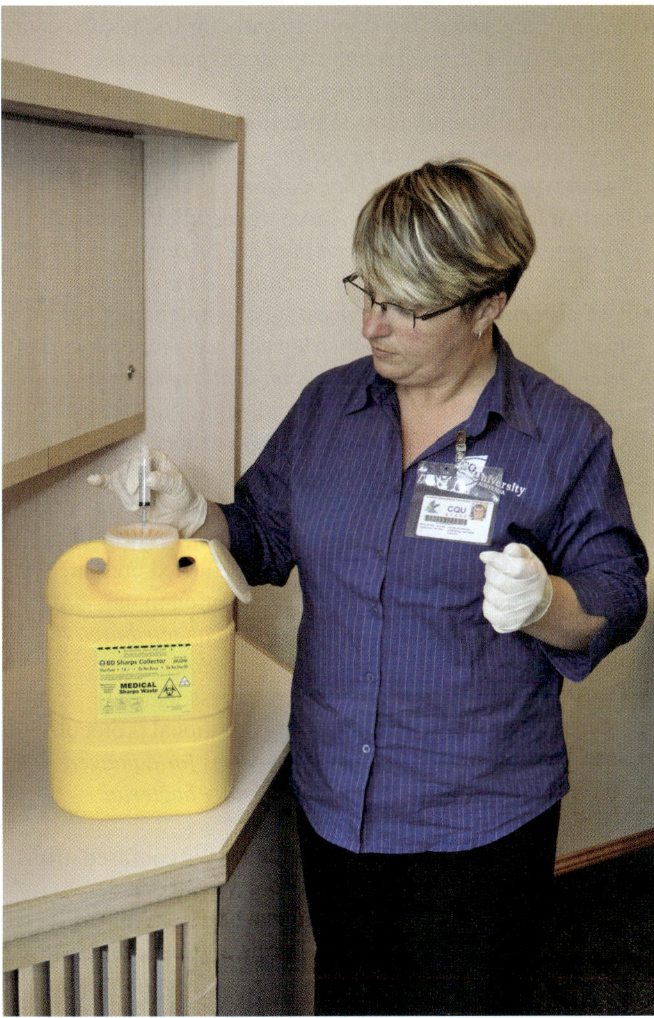

FIGURE 12.11 ***This nurse is disposing of a needle and syringe in a special container, a necessary practice to avoid the transmission of HIV through needle sticks with contaminated needles***

Source: Courtesy of Tracy Levett-Jones.

Healthcare workers can prevent most exposures to HIV by using standard precautions (see Figure 12.11). Testing to determine HIV status remains voluntary and relies on the use of antibody-screening methods. It is therefore impossible to identify every person who is HIV positive. With standard precautions, all people are treated alike, eliminating the need to know the person's HIV status. All high-risk body fluids are treated as if they are infectious and barrier precautions are used to prevent skin, mucous membrane or percutaneous exposure to them. Counselling and testing are provided to healthcare workers with a documented needle-stick exposure. Some clinicians and facilities recommend prophylactic AZT therapy after needle-stick or splash exposure; however, it must be initiated immediately and its effectiveness has yet to be established.

Assessment

Collect the following data through health history and physical examination. Further focused assessments are described with nursing interventions.

- *Health history*: risk factors (transfusion, unprotected sex, needle exposure), infections (sexually transmitted infections, hepatitis, tuberculosis), medications, recreational drug use, foreign travel, pets.
- *Physical assessment*: height, weight, nutrition, skin and mucous membranes, vision, lymph nodes, breath sounds, abdominal tenderness, motor strength, coordination, cranial nerves, gait, deep tendon reflexes, genitourinary examination, mental status. Remember that symptoms must be interpreted and reported by the person. Like pain, the presence and severity of dyspnoea are determined and reported by the person. We must believe what the person tells us. Assessment is the basis for differential diagnosis; fitting appropriate treatment to the correct aetiology is critical. For example, delirium is an acute confusional state and, unlike dementia, is reversible. There are effective nursing interventions for these conditions (Justiz Vaillant et al., 2022).

Nursing diagnoses and interventions

Nursing care needs for the person with HIV infection change over the course of the disease. Preventive healthcare measures, health maintenance activities, education and support of coping mechanisms are important in the early stages of the disease. Counselling the person with a new diagnosis of HIV infection is vital. HIV infection and AIDS continue to carry a social stigma that may interfere with the person's usual support systems and coping mechanisms. As the disease progresses and the person experiences more physical symptoms, direct care needs become more important while the need for psychosocial support continues. Acute exacerbation of opportunistic infections may necessitate hospitalisation, but typically the person is managed at home. See the 'Nursing care plan'.

Ineffective coping

On receiving the test results indicating HIV seropositive status, the person with HIV infection is faced with multiple issues rarely affecting other people. First and foremost, HIV is a disease for which there is no known cure and which is, at this time, thought to be almost universally fatal. Social support systems, family relationships, the ability to obtain and retain useful work, and health insurance may be disrupted by the disease. The person may experience guilt about their lifestyle and how the disease was contracted. As the disease progresses, social isolation, fatigue, body image changes, medication side effects and multiple other issues affect the person's ability to cope.

- Assess social support network and usual methods of coping. *This will help both the nurse and the person identify people and mechanisms that can help the person cope more effectively with the disease.*
- If possible, assign a primary nurse, whether the setting is community-based, hospice or acute care. *This helps promote the development of a therapeutic and trusting relationship and provides for continuity of care.*

- Plan for consistent, uninterrupted time with the person. *Time and a consistent presence encourage the person to express feelings and work through issues related to HIV infection.*
- Interact at every opportunity outside of providing specific nursing care treatments. *This purposeful interaction communicates caring and acceptance without fear of HIV disease.*
- Support the person's social network. Non-traditional families may offer more support than the traditional family. *This in turn may necessitate a liberal interpretation of the term 'family' if unit policy is 'immediate family' only.*
- Promote interaction between the person, significant others and family. *Hospitalisation and manifestations of HIV disease may bring about isolation from others and decrease the person's ability to cope.*
- Encourage involvement in making care decisions. *This gives the person a greater sense of self-worth and control over the situation, increasing coping abilities.*
- Set and maintain limits on manipulative and other destructive behaviours. *The person who is unable to limit inappropriate behaviours needs the external control established by setting limits.*
- Assist to accept responsibility for actions without blaming others. *Effective coping cannot occur without accepting responsibility for one's actions.*
- Support positive coping behaviours, decisions, actions and achievements. *As self-esteem is enhanced, coping improves (Banerjee et al., 2022).*

Impaired skin integrity

Dryness, malnutrition, immobility from fatigue and skin lesions on pressure sites contribute to impaired integrity of the skin for the person with HIV disease. Maintaining skin integrity is important because of the progressive and debilitating nature of the disease. It is also a consideration both as the first line of defence against infection in an immunosuppressed person and as a site for secondary manifestations such as KS and herpes.

- Monitor and assess the skin frequently for lesions and areas of breakdown. *Early identification of impaired skin integrity allows prompt intervention.*
- Monitor lesions for signs of infection or impaired healing. *Infection or poor tissue perfusion not only impairs healing but may lead to further skin breakdown.*
- Turn at least every 2 hours, more frequently if necessary. *Turning decreases unrelieved pressure on bony prominences and improves circulation to the tissues.*
- Use pressure-relieving devices, such as alternating air mattresses and overlays, or sheep skin pads for elbows and heels. *These devices provide prophylactic relief of pressure.*
- Keep skin clean and dry using mild, non-drying soaps or oils for cleansing. Night sweats and diarrhoea, if present, can cause breakdown and damage to the skin. *Frequent cleansing with non-drying products discourages bacterial growth, thus reducing the risk of infection.*
- Gently massage around, but not over, affected pressure sites or bony prominences to increase circulation to the surrounding tissue. *Massaging over the affected area or bony prominences can cause skin breakdown.*
- If blisters are noted, leave intact and dress with a hydrocolloid dressing or as per organisational protocol. *Blisters provide natural sterile coverings for damaged tissue, improving healing and preventing bacterial invasion.*
- Caution against scratching. If the person is confused, trim fingernails and use mitts or soft restraints to prevent scratching. Check for circulation of hands and fingers frequently if mitts or restraints are used. *Scratching and skin damage allow bacteria to be introduced into lesions, increasing the risk of infection. Tight or restrictive restraints or mitts may compromise circulation.*

CONSIDERATION FOR PRACTICE

Applying protective creams to reddened areas in the rectal area protects skin from the caustic effects of diarrhoea.

NURSING CARE PLAN A person with HIV infection

Sara Lu is a 26-year-old primary school teacher who lives with her parents and two younger sisters. Ms Lu is very close to her parents and sisters; they share everything with each other. During a routine medical check-up, Ms Lu tells her doctor that lately she has felt fatigued. She also states that she has had a persistent sore throat, intermittent bouts of diarrhoea and mild shortness of breath for about a month. She takes no routine medications other than a daily multivitamin and an occasional paracetamol tablet for a headache. She is active in a drama club in her community and she jogs 5 km three to four times a week. She is engaged to be married; her wedding date is 6 months away. Her fiancé is the only person with whom she has had sexual relations. Her sexual activity has been unprotected. Ms Lu has a history of open-heart surgery 7 years ago to correct a congenital valve defect. She has been physically healthy since that time, until about a month or two ago. The doctor orders a mononucleosis test, ELISA, Western blot analysis, CD4 T-cell count, a p24 antigen test and an erythrocyte sedimentation rate (ESR). Ms Lu has been asked to return in 1 week for follow-up.

ASSESSMENT

On Ms Lu's follow-up visit, Carole Kee, RN, obtains her nursing history. Ms Lu continues to have flu-like symptoms but has improved somewhat. She states that she has not been as active as usual and is worried about her health. Her appetite has decreased because of soreness in her mouth, and she has noted some whitish patches on her tongue and cheeks.

NURSING CARE PLAN A person with HIV infection (continued)

A chest x-ray film reveals no abnormality. The results of her laboratory tests are as follows:

- ELISA: positive for antibodies against HIV
- Western blot analysis: positive for antibodies against HIV
- p24 antigen test: positive for circulating HIV antigens
- ESR: increased to 55 mm/h (normal for women is 15 to 20 mm/h; normal for men is 10 to 15 mm/h)
- CD4 T-cell count: 499/mm^3 (normal range is 500–1,550/mm^3).

Ms Lu's physical examination reveals that she has enlarged lymph nodes in her neck and white patches on her oral mucosa. Her skin is warm to the touch. Her vital signs are as follows: T 37.7°C, P 84, R 20 and BP 120/78.

Ms Lu is told of the results of her laboratory tests and the medical diagnosis of HIV infection. Ms Lu is obviously distressed and wants to know how this happened, its meaning, whether she has infected her loved ones and whether she will get better.

DIAGNOSES

- *Imbalanced nutrition* related to soreness of mouth and throat as evidenced by nutritional intake being less than body requirements.
- *Risk of deficient fluid volume* related to decreased fluid intake and diarrhoea as evidenced by fluid intake being less than body requirements.
- *Risk of infection* related to altered immune protection as evidenced by elevated ESR.
- *Risk of anxiety* and fear related to diagnosis as evidenced by distress.
- *Knowledge deficit* related to the HIV disease process as evidenced by questions asked.

PLANNING

- Plan time to educate Ms Lu on the importance of nutritionally balanced diet and maintaining adequate fluid intake.
- Identify strategies for coping with anorexia and nausea.
- Referral for dietary consultation.
- Plan time for discussion of concerns and coping strategies.

Expected outcomes

- Maintain adequate nutrition for optimal body and cellular function.
- Consume at least 2,500 mL of fluid per day.
- Remain free of infections and their complications.
- Verbalise anxiety and use appropriate coping mechanisms.
- Verbalise and demonstrate knowledge of HIV disease.
- Verbalise measures to prevent HIV transmission to others, including safer sex practices.

IMPLEMENTATION

- Monitor for signs of dehydration, such as poor skin turgor, oliguria and orthostatic hypotension.
- Monitor daily weight and intake and output.
- Monitor dietary habits and serum albumin levels.
- Assess bowel sounds and monitor elimination pattern.
- Administer anti-emetic and antimotility medications as ordered.
- Increase fluid to 2,500 mL daily.
- Use strict aseptic technique for all invasive procedures.
- Teach Ms Lu to avoid exposure to infection and people with known illnesses.
- Monitor response to prescribed medications.
- Encourage regular physical exercise.
- Provide opportunities for Ms Lu to verbalise her feelings.
- Avoid false reassurances.
- Provide appropriate and adequate information about HIV/AIDS.
- Teach safer sex practices and other measures to prevent HIV transmission.
- Teach anxiety-controlling techniques, such as deep breathing and meditation.

EVALUATION

Ms Lu is eager to learn about her illness and wants her family to come with her for further explanation. She states that she is sure her fiancé will be available as well. Ms Lu is taking home antifungal medication, diet plans and a schedule for increased exercise. She will return in 1 week for counselling and in 1 month for a follow-up medical.

CRITICAL THINKING IN THE NURSING PROCESS

1. How does age affect the body's response to fighting HIV? What other factors affect the risk of HIV infection and its progression?
2. Are the laboratory results for Ms Lu a true indication that she is HIV positive? What additional tests might be ordered?
3. What is the most likely source of Ms Lu's infection? What measures are used to reduce this risk and how did she contract HIV? What is another possible source of Ms Lu's HIV infection?
4. Ms Lu says that her fiancé would like to have a child. How will you counsel her regarding pregnancy and childbearing?

REFLECTION ON THE NURSING PROCESS

1. Outline what you have learned from this case study that you will apply to your future practice.
2. What communication and education strategies could you use when caring for a person newly diagnosed with HIV?

- Avoid the use of heat or occlusive dressings. *Heat can further dry and damage the skin; occlusive dressings may impair circulation and lead to ulceration.*
- Prevent skin shearing by using a slide sheet and adequate personnel when repositioning. *Shearing causes tissue trauma that can lead to decubitus ulcers.*
- Encourage ambulation if possible; if the person is confined to bed, encourage active or passive range-of-motion exercises. *Activity increases circulation, decreases pressure and skin breakdown, and helps maintain muscle tone.*
- Monitor nutritional intake and albumin levels. *Maintenance of optimal nutrition decreases the risk of tissue breakdown and improves resistance to infection.*

Imbalanced nutrition: less than body requirements

Many factors associated with HIV disease, including manifestations of the disease itself, put the person at risk of altered nutrition and weight loss. Nausea and anorexia may be manifestations of the disease or the result of ART. Chronic diarrhoea is a common manifestation of constitutional HIV disease. Wasting syndrome is also common. It is manifested by involuntary weight loss of greater than 10% to 15% of baseline weight, severe diarrhoea, fever, and chronic fatigue and weakness. The exact cause of wasting syndrome is unclear, but the diarrhoea and fatigue contribute, as does the increased metabolic rate associated with fever. Oral and oesophageal candidiasis and KS of the gastrointestinal tract may cause painful swallowing, making eating difficult and thereby contributing to anorexia. Poor nutritional status in the person with HIV can ultimately result in altered comfort, a change in body image, muscle wasting, increased risk of infection, and higher mortality and morbidity.

- Assess nutritional status, including weight; body mass; kilojoule intake, and laboratory studies such as total protein and albumin levels, haemoglobin and haematocrit. *These factors provide a baseline to determine the effectiveness of interventions.*
- Identify possible causes of altered nutrition. *Identification of causes provides direction for planned interventions.*
- Administer prescribed medications for candidiasis and other manifestations as ordered. Eliminating this opportunistic infection improves comfort and facilitates food intake. *Topical viscous anaesthetic can help to reduce pain and improve oral intake.*
- Administer antidiarrhoea medications after stools and anti-emetics prior to meals. Provide antipyretics as needed to control fever. Reducing diarrhoea will improve nutrient absorption; preprandial medication with an anti-emetic reduces nausea and improves food intake. *Reduction of fever lowers the body's metabolic demands.*
- Provide a diet high in protein and kilojoules. *A high-protein, high-kilojoule diet provides the necessary nutrients to meet metabolic and tissue healing needs.*
- Offer soft foods and serve small portions. *Soft foods are easily digested. Small portions are more appealing to the anorectic or nauseated person.*

CONSIDERATION FOR PRACTICE

High-fibre foods can increase intestinal motility and the incidence of diarrhoea.

- Involve in meal planning and encourage significant others to bring favourite foods from home. *The person is more likely to consume adequate amounts of preferred foods. Allowing food choices enhances the person's sense of control.*
- Assist with eating as needed. *Fatigue and weakness can prevent the person from eating an adequate amount of food.*
- Provide supplementary vitamins and supplements, such as Ensure. *This improves nutritional status and kilojoule intake.*
- Provide or assist with frequent oral hygiene. *Oral hygiene improves comfort and appetite and reduces the risk of mucosal lesions.*
- Administer appetite stimulants, such as megestrol or dexamethasone, as ordered. *Both drugs may increase appetite and promote weight gain.*

Ineffective sexuality patterns

The diagnosis of HIV infection can significantly alter the person's expressions of sexuality. Guilt over the diagnosis may interfere with libido. The person may be angry with a significant other or partner if that person was the probable source of infection. The person may fear spreading the disease to others via sexual relations. As the disease progresses, its manifestations can affect body image and self-esteem, impairing sexuality. Other symptoms, such as nausea, fatigue and weakness, may also interfere with libido and sexual satisfaction.

- Examine your feelings about sexuality, your role in dealing with a person's sexuality, the person's lifestyle and sexual preferences. *To deal effectively with the person's concerns, it is vital that the nurse is comfortable with their own feelings of sexuality and is able to accept the person's lifestyle. Referring the person to another nurse or counsellor may be necessary.*
- Establish a trusting, therapeutic relationship through the use of time, active listening, caring and self-disclosure. Maintain a non-threatening, non-judgmental attitude towards the person. *Sexuality is a private issue that will be uncomfortable or impossible for the nurse and person to discuss without a mutually trusting relationship.*
- Provide factual information about HIV infection and its effects. *This helps the person separate fears and myths from reality.*
- Discuss safer sex practices, including hugging, cuddling, non-sexual contact, the use of latex condoms and spermicidal lubricant, and mutual masturbation. *Alternative forms of sexual activity and expressing affection can allow the person and significant other to remain close throughout the course of the disease.*
- Encourage discussion of fears and concerns with significant other. *Open communication helps them to deal with issues related to sexuality.*
- For the person without a significant other, stress the need to continue to meet people and develop social relationships while practising safer sex. *The risk of isolation is high in the person with HIV infection, and relationships with others help the person to cope with the disease.*
- Refer the person and significant other to local support groups for people and partners of people with HIV. *Support groups provide a social and support network of people facing the same issues.*

Community-based care

Teaching needs for both the person and significant others are extensive. The primary need is information about the disease, its spread and its expected course. The person and family need current factual information to plan realistically and to combat myths, misperceptions and prejudices. At the same time, it is important to include information about current research and progress in treating the disease to maintain a sense of hopefulness.

The following topics should be discussed with the person and family to prepare for home care:

- guidelines for safer sex practices
- nutrition, rest and exercise, stress reduction, lifestyle changes and maintaining a positive outlook
- infection prevention and transmission, including handwashing and wearing gloves when handling people's secretions or excretions
- importance of regular medical follow-up and monitoring of immune status
- signs and symptoms of opportunistic infections and malignancies, as well as other symptoms that should be reported
- medications and adverse effects
- use and care of central venous access devices, total parenteral nutrition, intravenous pumps and continuous medication delivery systems, and intravenous or aerosolised medications
- cessation of smoking, alcohol and recreational or illicit drug use
- community health services
- hospice and respite care services
- community resources, such as support groups, social agencies and counsellors
- helpful resources:
  - National Association of People with AIDS
  - ACON (https://www.acon.org.au)
  - Australian Federation of AIDS Organisations (AFAO)
  - Multicultural HIV/AIDS and Hepatitis C Service (MHAHS).

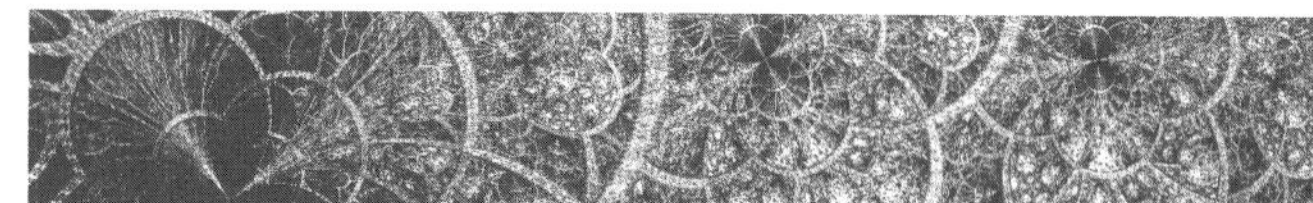

CHAPTER HIGHLIGHTS

- The immune system is a complex combination of cellular and humoral components that protect against disease. Immunity develops when the body recognises foreign proteins as 'non-self' and develops non-specific inflammatory responses and specific cellular responses to each foreign antigen.
- People suffer when the immune system is excessively or inadequately responsive or when recognition of self fails and reactions escalate against self. The latter occurs in autoimmune diseases.
- With ageing, there is a general decline in the sensitivity and regulation of the immune system, often resulting in autoimmune disease.
- Hypersensitivities are excessive responses to antigens that result in harm to the person. These range from benign to severely life-threatening. Damage to host tissue is caused by chemicals of the immune response, destruction of cells or creation of large antigen–antibody complexes that accumulate in the kidney glomerular capillaries.
- Allergic reactions are treated pharmacologically to prevent or moderate allergic responses. Another method of dampening allergic responses is by desensitisation, a weekly process of introducing increasing amounts of known allergens subdermally.
- People must be taught that the safest practice is to avoid contact with all known allergens.
- Latex allergy is a problem for healthcare professionals. Repeated exposure to latex-containing equipment and gloves results in delayed hypersensitivity.
- Any type of allergic reaction has the potential to escalate to anaphylaxis. Respiratory arrest and cardiac failure are risks with full-blown allergic reactions. Nurses must recognise early signs and symptoms and immediately signal for emergency care.
- Intentional immunosuppression is an essential step in preventing transplant rejection. The person receiving a transplanted organ will be treated with immune-suppressing drugs to prevent initial rejection, to maintain the transplant and to halt any rejection process that may develop. People will take the immune-suppressing, antirejection drugs for their lifetime. The drugs prevent cytokine production that up-regulates an immune reaction and targets the transplanted organ. Most immunosuppressing drugs are nephrotoxic; immunosuppression places people at greater risk of infection and cancers.
- HIV/AIDS continues to spread and many people are unaware they have the virus. AIDs is a profoundly immunosuppressed condition that results from viral destruction of cellular components of host immunity.
- A major change in the AIDS epidemic is the disease profile, which has benefited from ART. ART is a combination of drugs that limits viral replication and host susceptibility to opportunistic infections and cancer. People are living much longer with the disease without progression to AIDS. 'Pill burden' refers to the number of pills the person must take daily to maintain immune function; side effects of the combination of drugs which make up ART are appearing as people live longer. In addition to increased susceptibility to infections and cancers, people suffer from a dementia peculiar to AIDS.

CONCEPT CHECK

1 Which one of the following conditions is caused by a type I IgE-mediated hypersensitivity reaction?

1 autoimmune haemolitic anaemia
2 systemic lupus erythematosus
3 graft rejection
4 anaphylaxis

2 A person received a liver transplant 1 day ago. If the person were to develop an acute transplant rejection episode, when should the nurse expect to see the manifestations?

1 approximately 4 days to 3 months later
2 approximately 2 days later
3 within the first 24 hours
4 within the first 8 hours

3 The nurse notes a cough, shortness of breath and tachypnoea in a person with AIDS. Which opportunistic infection is probably causing these manifestations?

1 *Toxoplasma gondii*
2 Cytomegalovirus
3 *Pneumocystis carinii*
4 *Cryptococcus neoformans*

4 Which of the following explanations should the nurse give to a person who has tested positive for HIV?
1 'You have been diagnosed with AIDS.'
2 'At this point, AIDS is not active in your blood.'
3 'This means that you will not develop AIDS in the future.'
4 'Antibodies to the AIDS virus are present in the blood.'

5 People taking zidovudine should be monitored for which of the following adverse reactions?
1 cardiotoxicity
2 leucopenia
3 nephrotoxicity
4 polycythaemia

6 The order of administering antigens in allergy testing is based on prevention of anaphylaxis. Which method should be used first?
1 inhalation
2 prick test
3 intradermal injection
4 subcutaneous injection

7 If a hypersensitivity response is suspected when blood products are infusing, the nurse should:
1 discard the product immediately
2 replace all tubing and attach a new line with normal saline
3 backflush the line and run normal saline attached at the Y tubing
4 remove the intravenous catheter and establish access distal to the site

8 Protease inhibitors and nucleoside analogues share correlations to metabolic abnormalities, including:
1 lactose intolerance
2 diabetes mellitus
3 Hashimoto's thyroiditis
4 systemic lupus erythematosus

9 The priority when initiating or changing HIV drug therapy regimens is:
1 cost of therapy
2 access to dental care
3 toxicities associated with each drug
4 the person's willingness to adhere to the drug regimen

10 People receiving kidney transplants will receive immunosuppressant therapy. The agent used to induce immunosuppression immediately following a transplant is often:
1 azathioprine
2 corticosteroids
3 muromonab-CD3
4 antithymocyte globulin

BIBLIOGRAPHY

Australasian Society for HIV, Viral Hepatitis and Sexual Health Medicine (ASHM) (2019a). *Antiretroviral drugs and other therapies in HIV patients*. Retrieved from https://hivmanagement.ashm.org.au/

Australasian Society for HIV, Viral Hepatitis and Sexual Health Medicine (ASHM) (2019b). *HIV management for nurses and midwives: Nursing ethics in the care of people with HIV*. Retrieved from https://hivmanagement.ashm.org.au/

Australasian Society for HIV, Viral Hepatitis and Sexual Health Medicine (ASHM) (2020). *National HIV testing policy*. Retrieved from https://testingportal.ashm.org.au/

Australasian Society of Clinical Immunology and Allergy (ASCIA) (2017). *Guidelines for the management of latex-allergic individuals*. Retrieved from https://www.allergy.org.au/

Australasian Society of Clinical Immunology and Allergy (ASCIA) (2019). *Latex allergy: Information for patients, consumers and carers*. Retrieved from https://www.allergy.org.au/s

Australian Federation of AIDS Organisations (AFAO) (2022). *HIV in Australia 2022*. Retrieved from https://www.afao.org.au

Australian Government Organ and Tissue Authority (2021). Retrieved from https://www.donatelife.gov.au

Australian Haemophilia Centre Directors' Organisation (AHCDO) (2016). *Guidelines for the management of haemophilia in Australia*. Retrieved from https://www.blood.gov.au/

Bai, R., Lv, S., Wu, H. & Dai, L. (2022). Effects of different integrase strand transfer inhibitors on body weight with HIV/AIDS: A network meta-analysis. *BMC Infectious Diseases, 22*(18). https://doi.org/10.1186/s12879-022-07091-1

Banerjee, N., Goodman, Z. T., McIntosh, R. & Ironson, G. (2022). Cognition, coping and psychological distress in HIV. *AIDS and Behaviour, 26*. https://doi.org/10.1007/s10461-021-03462-y

Battistini Garcia, S. A. & Guzman, N. (2021). *Acquired immune deficiency syndrome CD4⁺ count*. Retrieved from https://www.ncbi.nlm.nih.gov/

Burchum, J. & Rosenthal, L. (2018). *Lehne's pharmacology for nursing care* (11th ed.). St Louis, MO: Saunders/Elsevier.

Cancer.Net. (2022). *Sarcoma—Kaposi: Statistics*. Retrieved from https://www.cancer.net/

Centers for Disease Control and Prevention (CDC) (2008). *Revised surveillance case definitions for HIV infection among adults, adolescents, and children aged <8 months and for HIV infection and aids among children aged 18 months to <3 years—United States, 2008*. Retrieved from https://www.cdc.gov/

Centers for Disease Control and Prevention (CDC) (2014). *Revised surveillance case definition for HIV infection—United States 2014*. Retrieved from https://www.cdc.gov/

Centers for Disease Control and Prevention (CDC) (2019a). *HIV risk behaviours*. Retrieved from https://www.cdc.gov/

Centers for Disease Control and Prevention (CDC) (2019b). *ART adherence*. Retrieved from https://www.cdc.gov/

Centers for Disease Control and Prevention (CDC) (2020). *New HIV diagnoses and people with diagnosed HIV in the US and dependent areas by area of residence*. Retrieved from https://www.cdc.gov/

Centers for Disease Control and Prevention (CDC) (2022a). *HIV surveillance*. Retrieved from https://www.cdc.gov/

Centers for Disease Control and Prevention (CDC) (2022b). *Terms, definitions and calculation used in CDC HIV surveillance publications*. Retrieved from https://www.cdc.gov/

Chernecky, C. C. & Berger, B. M. (2012). *Laboratory tests and diagnostic procedures* (6th ed.). Philadelphia: W. B. Saunders/Elsevier.

Dharan, N. J., Radovich, T., Che, S. et al. (2019). HIV treatment regimens and adherence to national guidelines in Australia: An analysis of dispensing data from the Australian pharmaceutical benefits scheme. *BMC Public Health, 19*(13). https://doi.org/10.1186/s12889-018-6325-5

Eliopoulos, E. (2021). *Gerontological nursing* (10th ed.). Philadelphia: Wolters Kluwer/Lippincott Williams & Wilkins.

Halter, J. B., Ouslander, J. G., High, K. P. et al. (2022). *Hazzard's geriatric medicine and gerontology* (8th ed). New York: McGraw-Hill Medical.

Haynes, L. (2020). Aging of the immune system: Research challenges to enhance the health span of older adults. *Frontiers in Ageing, 1*. https://doi.org/10.3389/fragi.2020.602108

Healthdirect (2020). *HIV and AIDS medication (antiretrovirals)*. Retrieved from https://www.healthdirect.gov.au/

Healthdirect (2021). *HIV infection and AIDS*. Retrieved from https://www.healthdirect.gov.au/

HIVgov (2021). *Drug database: Nevirapine*. Retrieved from https://clinicalinfo.hiv.gov/

HIVgov (2022). *HIV Care Continuum*. Retrieved from https://www.hiv.gov/

HIVinfo (2021). *HIV treatment: The basics*. Retrieved from https://hivinfo.nih.gov/

HIVinfo (2022). *HIV overview: FDA-approved HIV medicines*. Retrieved from https://hivinfo.nih.gov/

Justiz Vaillant, A. A., Guilick, P. G. & Pinto, K. M. (2022). *HIV disease current practice (nursing)*. Retrieved from https://www.ncbi.nlm.nih.gov/

King, H. C., Mabry, R. L., Mabry, C. S. et al. (2011). *Allergy in ENT practice: The basic guide* (2nd ed.). New York: Thieme Medical Publisher.

Kirby Institute (2018). *Bloodborne viral and sexually transmissible infections in Aboriginal and Torres Strait Islander people: Annual surveillance report*. Retrieved from https://www.kirby.unsw.edu.au

Leyva-Moral, J. M., Dominguez-Cancino, K. A., Guevara-Vasquez, G.M. et al. (2019). Faculty attitudes about caring for people living with HIV/AIDS: A comparative study. *Journal of Nursing Education, 58*(12), 712–717. doi: 10.3928/01484834-20191120-06

Loscalzo, J., Fauci, A. S., Kasper, D. L., Hauser, S. L. & Longo, D. (2022). *Harrison's principles of internal medicine* (21st ed.). New York: McGraw Hill Medical.

National Allergy Strategy (2015). *National Allergy Strategy*. Retrieved from https://nationalallergystrategy.org.au/

National Allergy Strategy (2022). *Australia leading the world: Federal funding secured for allergy prevention and management*. Retrieved from https://nationalallergystrategy.org.au/

Norris, T. L. (2018). *Porth's pathophysiology: Concepts of altered health states* (10th ed.). Philadelphia: Lippincott Williams & Wilkins.

Pagana, K. D., Pagana, T. J. & Pagana, T.N. (2020). *Mosby's diagnostic and laboratory test reference* (15th ed.). St Louis, MO: Elsevier Health Sciences.

Papadakis, M., McPhee, S. J. & Rabow, M. W. (2022). *Current medical diagnosis and treatment* (61st ed.). New York: McGraw-Hill Education.

Parliament of Australia (2019). *Overview of allergies and anaphylaxis in Australia*. Retrieved from https://www.aph.gov.au/

Punt, J., Stranford, S., Jones, P. & Owen, J. A. (2018). *Kuby immunology* (8th ed.). New York: Macmillan Learning.

Raubinger, S., Lee, F. J. & Pinto, A. N. (2022). HIV: The changing paradigm. *Internal Medicine Journal*, *52*(4). https://doi.org/10.1111/imj.15739

Reeves, I., Cromarty, B., Deayton, J. et al. (2021). British HIV Association guidelines for the management of HIV-2 2021. *HIV Medicine*, *22*(S4). https://doi.org/10.1111/hiv.13204

UNAIDS (2020). *90-90-90: Treatment for all*. Retrieved from http://www.unaids.org/

UNAIDS (2021). *Global HIV and AIDS statistics—2021 fact sheet*. Retrieved from http://www.unaids.org/

US Department of Health and Human Services (2020). OPTN/Scientific registry of transplant recipients, *2020 Annual Report: Transplant Data Report*. Retrieved from https://optn.transplant.hrsa.gov/

Vafeas, C. & Slatyer, S. (2021). *Gerontological nursing: A holistic approach to the care of older people*. Chatswood, NSW: Elsevier.

Valois, P., Turgeon, H., Godin, G. et al. (2001). Influence of a persuasive strategy on nursing students' beliefs and attitudes toward provision of care to people living with HIV/AIDS. *Journal of Nursing Education*, *40*(8), 354–358.

Varnham O'Regan, S. (2012). *Australia's most poisonous plants*. Australian Geographic. Retrieved from https://www.australiangeographic.com.au/

Wagner, G. J., Linnermayr, S., Gosh-Dastiar, B. et al. (2016). Supporting treatment adherence readiness through training (START) for patients with HIV on antiretroviral therapy: Study protocol for a randomized controlled trial. *Trials*, *17*, 162. doi 10.1186/s13063-016-1287-3

Ward, J., Gilles, M. & Russel, D. (2021). *HIV infection in Aboriginal and Torres Strait Islander people*. Retrieved from https://hivmanagement.ashm.org.au/

World Health Organization (WHO) (2021). *HIV/AIDS*. Retrieved from https://www.who.int/

Zhang, D., Patel, K. B., Cass, L. M., Foster, A. E., Guntupalli, L. & Brunworth, J. D. (2017). Heroin-induced nasal necrosis and septal perforation. *Acta Oto-Laryngolgica Case Reports*, *2*(1), 145–149.

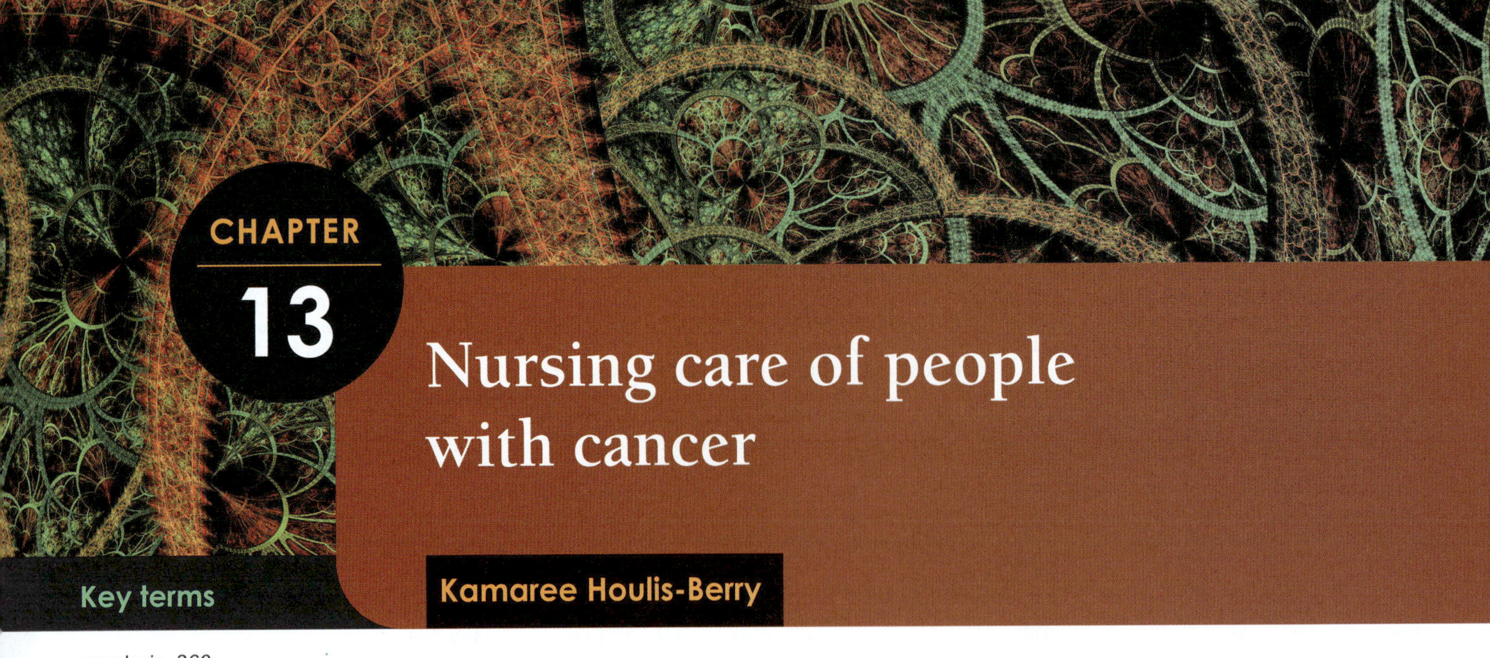

CHAPTER 13

Nursing care of people with cancer

Kamaree Houlis-Berry

Key terms

anaplasia 360
biotherapy 382
cachexia 366
cancer 355
carcinogen 360
carcinogenesis 360
cell cycle 359
chemotherapy 375
differentiation 360
dysplasia 360
hospice care 398
hyperplasia 360
metaplasia 360
metastasis 364
neoplasm 362
oncogene 360
oncology 355
radiation therapy 381
tumour marker 369
xerostomia 395

Learning outcomes

- Define cancer and theories of carcinogenesis and differentiate benign from malignant neoplasms.
- Explain known carcinogens and identify risk factors for cancer.
- Compare the mechanisms and characteristics of normal cells with those of malignant cells.
- Describe physical and psychological effects of cancer.
- Describe and compare laboratory and diagnostic tests for cancer.
- Discuss and compare the role of surgery, chemotherapy and classification of chemotherapeutic agents, radiation therapy and biotherapy in the treatment of cancer.
- Identify causes and discuss the nursing interventions for common oncological emergencies.
- Develop an appropriate care plan for people with cancer and their families regarding cancer diagnosis, treatment and coping strategies.

Clinical competencies

- Assess functional health status of people with cancer and monitor, document and report abnormal manifestations.
- Incorporate evidence-based practice and research into the plan of nursing care for people with cancer.
- Prioritise nursing diagnosis based on assessment data and implement appropriate nursing interventions for people with cancer during cancer diagnosis, treatment and rehabilitation.
- Safely administer chemotherapeutic medications and other medications for pain, nausea and vomiting, mucositis or anaemia.
- Use the nursing process as a framework for planning and providing individualised care and integrating interprofessional care for people with cancer to meet their healthcare needs.
- Include cultural variation and diverse values in designing and implementing individualised plans of care for people with cancer.
- Design and provide individualised education to the person and family to restore, promote and maintain the person's functional status.
- Revise the plan of care as needed to provide effective interventions for people with cancer and their families.

CANCER AND THEORIES OF CARCINOGENESIS

Cancer is a group of complex diseases with various manifestations, depending on which body system is affected and the type of tumour cells involved. Cancer can affect people of any age, gender, ethnicity or geographical region. Although the incidence and mortality rates of cancer have continued to decline since 1990, it remains one of the most feared diseases. In Australia in 2021, the number of deaths from cancer was estimated at 49,221 people (27,600 males and 21,621 females) (Cancer Australia, 2021). The fear engendered by even the suggestion of a cancer diagnosis often evokes feelings of hopelessness and helplessness (Bradt et al., 2021).

This chapter focuses on the general pathogenesis, pathophysiology and aetiology of cancer; identifies current diagnostic and treatment modalities; and discusses nursing care appropriate for people with cancer. Discussions of cancers that affect specific body systems (e.g. leukaemia, lung cancer) can be found in corresponding body system chapters in the text.

Cancer results when normal cells mutate into abnormal, deviant cells that proliferate and spread within the body. Cancer can affect any body tissue. Nursing care of the person with cancer is holistic and comprehensive, focusing on cancer not as one disease but as a constellation of many diseases. The nurse recognises that cancer is a disruptive and life-threatening process that affects the person who has the diagnosis, their family and their significant others. Nursing interventions are based on the understanding that cancer is a chronic disease that has acute episodes, and that the person is usually treated with a combination of therapeutic modalities within the home or community setting. Equally important, the nurse recognises that caring for the person with cancer involves prevention, early detection, treatment, supportive care, education, rehabilitation, long-term follow-up and end-of-life care (International Society of Nurses in Cancer Care (ISNCC), 2022; Oncology Nursing Society, 2022).

Oncology is the study of cancer. The term is derived from the Greek word *oncoma* ('bulk'). Oncologists specialise in caring for people with cancer. They may be medical doctors, surgeons, radiologists, immunologists or researchers. The oncology nurse is an important and significant member of the multidisciplinary team who has received specialised training in cancer care and treatment. Oncology nurses have specialised skills and knowledge to assist the person and family with the psychosocial issues associated with cancer and terminal illness. Collaboration among healthcare professionals (e.g. surgeons, oncologists, nurses, social workers) ensures a multidisciplinary approach in implementing the most effective care and treatment for the person with cancer.

INCIDENCE AND MORTALITY

In Australia in 2021, 150,800 new cases of cancer were diagnosed (on average 413 new diagnoses daily), with an estimated 49,200 cancer-related deaths (Australian Institute of Health and Welfare (AIHW), 2021). Cancer is the second leading cause of death in Australia, with a mortality rate of 1 in 5 before 85 years of age, with a higher incidence rate in males. Mortality rates for different cancers vary. Lung cancer remains the leading cause of all cancer deaths in both men and women in Australia, followed by colorectal cancer, prostate cancer in males and breast cancer in females, and pancreatic cancer. In regards to COVID-19, 'the full effect of the pandemic on cancer diagnosis and outcomes, while expected to become clearer over time, will likely not be fully understood and enumerated for some years' (AIHW, 2021, p. 4).

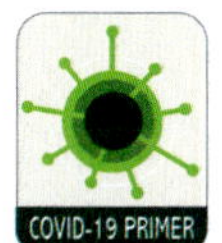

During 1989–2021, it was identified that cancer mortality rates decrease as socioeconomic status increases; and for cervical cancer, lung cancer and cancer with an unknown primary site, the cancer mortality rates increase with the remoteness of the area in which the person resides (AIHW, 2021).

Due to advances in cancer prevention, early detection and treatment, at the end of 2012, 410,530 people were alive who had been diagnosed with cancer in the previous 5 years. The combined survival rate has increased from 48% in 1984–1988 to 68% in 2009–2013 (AIHW, 2021).

Indigenous Australians have a lower 5-year survival rate following a cancer diagnosis and a higher mortality rate than non-Indigenous Australians (Cancer Australia, 2020; Morris et al., 2017). During 2015–2019, 3,612 Indigenous Australians died due to cancer, accounting for 23.4% of all deaths. Cancer has a greater impact on Indigenous Australians (at 1.4 times the rate of non-Indigenous Australians), who are more likely to live in a remote area of Australia with limited access to health infrastructures and are less likely to have an early diagnosis and receive adequate treatment, such as preventive, curative and palliative services. It has been identified that Indigenous Australians have a lower incidence of skin melanoma, lymphoma, bladder and kidney cancer; however, they have a higher incidence of cancers that have poorer prognosis but are largely preventable, such as lung, liver, cervix, lip and oropharynx cancers. The patterns of cancer are related to the higher prevalence of health risk behaviours such as smoking in conjunction with the barriers created by inadequate health systems (AIHW, 2022).

For information about diversity and cancer risk and incidence, see the 'Focus on cultural diversity' box.

FOCUS ON CULTURAL DIVERSITY Cancer in Indigenous Australians

- The incidence of cancer is lower, but mortality rates are significantly higher, for Indigenous people.
- Indigenous Australians have a higher incidence of cancers of the lung and cervix, and cancer with an unknown primary site.
- Lower incidence rates have been identified for bowel cancer, lymphoid cancer, melanoma of the skin and breast cancer in Indigenous females and prostate cancer in Indigenous males.
- Indigenous Australians have a lower 5-year post-cancer survival rate than non-Indigenous Australians.
- Mortality rate is higher in Indigenous Australians for breast cancer, lung cancer and cancer with an unknown primary site, but lower for melanoma of the skin.

Source: AIHW (2021). *Cancer in Australia 2021.* Cat. no. CAN 144. Canberra: AIHW.

FAST FACTS

Cancer in Australia

- Breast cancer is the most commonly diagnosed cancer in women, with an incidence of 19,866 cases in 2021.
- Prostate cancer is the most commonly occurring cancer in men, with an incidence of 18,110 cases during 2021.
- In 2021, the second most common cancer in males was melanoma of the skin (9,869 cases) and the third most common cancer was colorectal cancer (8,247 cases).
- The second leading cancer for females was colorectal cancer (7,293 cases) followed by melanoma of the skin (7,009 cases).
- It is estimated that the number of cancers will continue to increase.
- In 2019–2020, although the five most common cancers were non-melanoma skin cancer, prostate cancer, cancer of secondary site, colorectal cancer and breast cancer, the five most common causes of death were lung cancer (8,693), colorectal cancer (5,295), pancreatic cancer (3,391), prostate cancer (3,323) and breast cancer (3,198).
- The impact of COVID-19 on cancer diagnosis and treatment has not been taken into account or fully understood and the full effect will likely take years to be enumerated.

Sources: Cancer Australia (2021). *All cancers in Australia*. Australian Government. Retrieved from https://canceraustralia.gov.au/; AIHW (2021). *Cancer in Australia 2021*. Cancer series no. 133. Cat. no. CAN 144. Canberra: AIHW.

PATIENT SAFETY COMPETENCY FRAMEWORK

5 Clinical reasoning

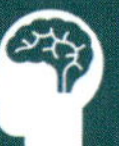

The Patient Safety Competency Framework indicates that nursing students must demonstrate clinical reasoning through the ability to accurately assess, interpret and respond to individual patient data in a systematic and timely way (Levett-Jones et al., 2017).

Risk factors

Risk factors make an individual or a population vulnerable to a specific disease or other unhealthy outcome. Risk factors can be divided into those that are controllable and those that are not controllable. Knowledge and assessment of risk factors are especially important in counselling people and families about measures to prevent cancer.

Genetics and heredity

It is estimated that 5% to 10% of cancers may have a hereditary component. Even though the majority of people will not have an inherited form of cancer, it is important to determine which people have a genetic predisposition. The familial pattern of some breast and colon cancers has been well documented. Lung, ovarian and prostate cancers have also shown some familial relationships. Recurring patterns of cancer within a family are a risk factor for a hereditary component, but do not necessarily indicate that a specific gene or mutation is the cause. An increased rate of cancer between relatives can be due to genetics as well as shared environmental exposures, lifestyle and other non-genetic risk factors. The Human Genome Project, which concluded in 2003, identified new cancer-linked genes (Garvan Institute of Medical Research, 2021; Nogrady, 2020), leading to the formation the International Cancer Genome Consortium and The Cancer Genome Atlas in 2006 (National Cancer Institute, 2021a). Familial cancers generally occur during old age, whereas hereditary cancers usually happen at a younger age (Jorde, Carey & Barnshad, 2019). For most cancers, research has yet to distinguish true genetic transfer from environmental causes. Although further research is needed to identify cancers that are due to the inheritance of defective genes, familial predisposition to malignancies should be counted among risk factors so that people at risk can reduce behaviours that promote cancer. For example, a person with a family history of lung cancer should be counselled to avoid smoking, to avoid areas where smoking is allowed and to avoid working in an occupation that may expose them to inhaled carcinogens.

Age

Cancer is a disease associated with ageing; the risk of being diagnosed with cancer before the age of 75 years is 1:3, and before 85 years is 1:2 (AIHW, 2021). A number of factors are associated with this increased risk in older adults. One possible factor is that at least five cycles of genetic mutations seem necessary to cause permanent damage to the afflicted cells. In addition, long-term exposure to high doses of promotional agents is usually necessary to allow the cancer to take hold. Also, the immune response alters with ageing, its actions becoming more generalised and less specific (Ebeling et al., 2021; Eliopoulos, 2021). Another problem is that free radicals (molecules resulting from the body's metabolic and oxidative processes) tend to accumulate in the cells over time, causing damage and mutation.

However, nature versus heritability is not fully understood; therefore, ageing impacted on by environment and heritability cannot be fully blamed when gene mutation can cause cancer (Ebeling et al., 2021).

Hormonal changes that occur with ageing can be associated with cancer. Postmenopausal women receiving exogenous oestrogen may have an increased risk of breast and uterine cancers. Older men are at risk of prostate cancer, possibly due to breakdown of testosterone into carcinogenic forms. See the 'Nursing care of the older adult' box for a discussion about older adults and cancer.

Severe and/or cumulative losses also are implicated in promoting cancer (Fabi et al., 2020). These losses, which are common to older adults, include the death of a spouse or friends, loss of position and status in society and a decline in physical abilities. These repeated stressors are related to changes in the immune system that may lead to the development of cancer.

NURSING CARE OF THE OLDER ADULT Older adults with cancer

Nurses need to be aware of how cancer and cancer treatments affect older adults. Cancer is the fourth leading cause of death in people over 75. The incidence of cancer increases with advancing age, probably as a result of the accumulated exposure to carcinogens and to age-related declines in the action of the immune system. The most commonly seen cancers in women are breast, colorectal and lung cancers, and melanoma of the skin. In men, prostate, lung and colorectal cancers, and melanoma of the skin, occur most frequently.

The importance of screening and early detection of cancer does not diminish with age. Unfortunately, older adults may be less likely to undergo cancer screening or seek treatment for cancer due to fear, depression, cognitive impairments, poor access to healthcare or financial constraints. Some older adults (and healthcare providers) mistake cancer symptoms for normal age-related changes. Believing that little can be done, they do not seek healthcare for their symptoms. Fear of the cancer diagnosis also keeps older adults from seeking appropriate healthcare. When they do seek treatment, chronic conditions frequently seen in older adults may make the diagnosis of cancer more difficult by masking or confounding the usual symptoms associated with cancer.

Older adults are at greater risk of side effects associated with cancer treatment because of age-related physiological changes and chronic conditions associated with ageing. This is particularly true for the side effects of chemotherapeutic agents. The incidence of toxic effects on the heart and central nervous system is increased. The side effects of chemotherapy can contribute to fatigue and cause problems related to immobility and functional decline. Alterations in the function of the immune system are also more frequent in older adults, increasing their risk of developing infection.

The problems associated with chemotherapy do not rule out its use, but the nurse must be aware of potential problems and monitor the person closely for the development of side effects. The nurse needs to consider the effect of ageing on responses to the disease and its treatment.

HEALTH EDUCATION FOR THE PERSON AND FAMILY

- Discuss signs and symptoms of cancer.
- Stress the importance of seeking healthcare if any of the warning signs develop.
- Stress the importance of having an annual physical examination.
- For women, teach how to perform a monthly breast self-exam (BSE) and emphasise the importance of continuing BSE and regular mammography, available free from age 40 onwards.
- Teach men the early signs of prostate cancer and encourage them to have an annual digital rectal exam.

Gender

Gender is a risk factor for certain types of cancer. Breast cancer is the most frequently diagnosed cancer in women and prostate cancer in men. The incidence of laryngeal cancer is three times higher in men than in women (AIHW, 2021). Cancer of the peritoneum and the thyroid occurs more commonly among females (AIHW, 2021). See the chapters 'Nursing care of men with reproductive system and breast disorders' and 'Nursing care of women with reproductive system and breast disorders' for more information on gender-specific cancers.

Poverty

The poor are at a higher risk of cancer than the population in general. Inadequate access to healthcare, especially preventive screening and counselling, may be a major factor. Other factors that may be involved, such as diet and stress, usually come under the category of controllable risks; however, these risks are frequently uncontrollable in this population.

Stress

Continuous unmanaged stress that keeps hormones such as adrenaline (epinephrine) and cortisol at high levels can result in systematic 'fatigue' and impaired immunological surveillance. When the body attempts to adapt to physiological and psychological stressors, it goes through a series of stages called the general adaptation syndrome (Fabi et al., 2020). First, the 'alarm reaction' occurs, in which adrenal hormones increase allowing the body to cope with the stressor. Eventually the body reaches the 'stage of resistance', in which the stress hormones are significantly reduced, indicating that adaptation has occurred. If the physiological adaptation is supported by appropriate coping strategies, the stressor is considered managed and the body systems return to pre-alarm functioning. However, if adaptation continues and the stress hormones remain elevated, the 'stage of exhaustion' sets in. This stage will maintain life but at great expense to body systems, resulting in general wear and tear and depression of the immune system (Antoni et al., 2012).

Diet

Some foods are considered genotoxic, such as the nitrosamines and nitrous indoles found in preserved meats and pickled, salted foods. Other foods, such as high-fat, low-fibre foods—the mainstay of many Australian diets—promote colon, breast and sex-hormone-dependent tumours. When fish and meat are excessively fried or grilled, potent carcinogenic compounds can form that may cause tumours in the mammary glands, colon, liver, pancreas and bladder. Also, repeatedly using fat to fry foods at high temperatures produces high levels of polycyclic hydrocarbons, which increase cancer risk considerably. Although many people profess to have changed their dietary habits, one only has to observe the large number of people who still lunch on hamburgers and chips (and teach their children to do the same) to realise that much more educational and motivational work is needed in this area. Other food-related substances believed to increase cancer risk include sodium saccharine, red food dyes and both regular and decaffeinated coffee.

TABLE 13.1 Chemical carcinogens and relationship to occupation

CHEMICAL AGENT	ACTION	OCCUPATION AFFECTED
Polycyclic hydrocarbons (smoke, soot, tobacco, smoked foods)	Genotoxic	Miners, coal/gas workers, migrant workers
Benzopyrene		
Arsenic	Genotoxic	Pesticide manufacturers, mining
Vinyl chloride polymers	Promotional	Plastics workers Artists
Methylaminobenzine	Genotoxic	Fabric workers Rubber and glue workers
Asbestos	Promotional	Construction workers, workers in old, run-down buildings with asbestos insulation, insulation makers
Wood and leather dust	Promotional	Woodworkers, carpenters, leather toolers
Chemotherapy drugs	Genotoxic	Drug manufacturers, pharmacists, nurses

Occupation

Occupational risk might be considered to be either controllable or uncontrollable. For many people, both education and ability limit their choice of occupation, particularly during times of high unemployment. Moreover, changing one's occupation because it poses risk factors may not be a viable option. Federal standards are designed to protect workers from hazardous substances, but many believe that these standards are not strict enough and that inspections are not frequent enough to prevent violations.

Specific risks vary according to the occupation. For example, outdoor workers such as farmers and construction workers are exposed to solar radiation; healthcare workers such as x-ray technicians and biomedical researchers are exposed to ionising radiation and carcinogenic substances; and exposure to asbestos is a problem for people who work in old buildings with asbestos insulation in the walls. Table 13.1 correlates known carcinogens and occupations.

Infection

As a number of viruses have been linked to some cancers, avoiding those specific infections will decrease risk. Although some infections may be unavoidable (e.g. Epstein–Barr) others, such as genital herpes and papillomavirus-induced genital warts, can often be avoided by following safer sex practices (e.g. using condoms) or obtaining the human papillomavirus (HPV) vaccine. The HPV vaccine is currently given to 12–13-year-old females and males as part of the Australian National Immunisation program (Cancer Council, 2021).

Tobacco use

Lung cancer is considered highly preventable because of its relationship to smoking. The genotoxic carcinogenic substances in tobacco are considered weak; therefore, stopping smoking can reverse the damage it causes. However, many other substances in tobacco are highly promotional, so that the larger the dose and longer the use, the higher the risk of developing cancer. Research has shown a significantly lower lung cancer death risk of former smokers compared to current smokers. Smokers who quit before middle age avoid more than 90% of the risk of lung cancer that can be attributed to tobacco.

Tobacco is also related to other forms of cancer. Smokers face an increased risk of oropharyngeal, oesophageal, laryngeal, gastric, pancreatic and bladder cancers. Pipe and cigar smokers are especially susceptible to oropharyngeal and laryngeal cancers. Oral and oesophageal cancers are more common among those who chew tobacco or use snuff. Smokers who have a genetic decrease in alpha$_1$-antitrypsin (an enzyme that protects lung tissue) that results in emphysema face an even higher cancer risk than smokers without this defect.

Additional research has documented the deleterious effects of second-hand tobacco smoke. Tobacco-specific nitrosamines were recovered in the urine of children living with smokers. It is now accepted that non-smokers exposed to tobacco smoke over long periods of time, whether in the workplace or the home, have an increased risk of lung or bladder cancer. Current research on e-cigarettes and their potential links to cancer is limited.

Alcohol use

Alcohol promotes cancer by enhancing the contact between carcinogens, such as those in tobacco, and the stem cells that line the oral cavity, larynx and oesophagus (Norris, 2018). People who smoke and drink a considerable amount of alcohol daily have an increased risk of oral, oesophageal and laryngeal cancers.

Recreational drug use

Recreational drug use often promotes an unhealthy lifestyle that increases general cancer risk; for example, drug users often do not maintain adequate nutrition. Furthermore, recreational drugs are implicated as promoters because of their suppressive effect on the immune system. Although it has not been directly implicated in cancer development, marijuana has been demonstrated to cause chromosomal damage that may over time also result in cancer-causing DNA damage and genetic mutations. Marijuana smoke is also much more injurious to lung tissue than tobacco smoke.

Obesity

Excessive body fat has been linked to an increased risk of hormone-dependent cancers. Because sex hormones are synthesised from fat, obese people often have excessive amounts of the hormones that feed hormone-dependent malignancies of the breast, bowel, ovary, endometrium and prostate.

Sun exposure

As the protective ozone layer thins, more of the sun's damaging ultraviolet radiation reaches the earth. As a consequence, the rate of skin cancers has increased. Australia has one of the highest rates of skin cancer in the world, with the majority of skin cancers being caused by exposure to UV radiation in sunlight. Around 95% to 99% of skin cancers in Australia can be attributed to sun exposure (Cancer Council, 2007). Sun-related skin cancers are considered to be a problem for all people, regardless of skin colour, but people with very fair skin, blue or green eyes, and light-coloured hair are most vulnerable. Older people with decreased pigment are also more at risk, even those with darker skin. By the age of 70 years, 2 out of every 3 Australians will be diagnosed with skin cancer due to solarium use, which is now banned in Australia (Cancer Council, 2007).

Figure 13.1 summarises the interaction of factors that promote cancer.

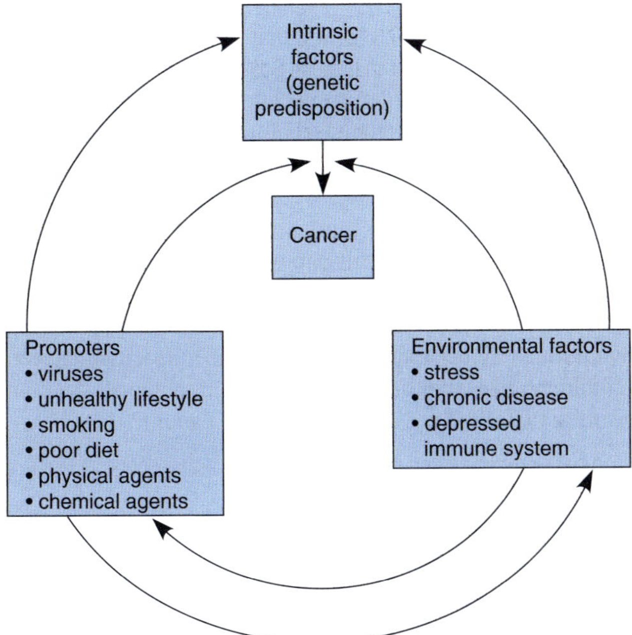

FIGURE 13.1 *Interaction of factors that promote cancer. Most people have immune systems that are competent enough to resist the establishment of cancer from an initiated cell. Cancer takes hold when a number of promotional factors occur together and over enough time to weaken immune resistance. Like factors are grouped together for ease of presentation but may occur in any combination*

PATHOPHYSIOLOGY

Cancer is a complex disease with hundreds of agents that can contribute to its pathogenesis. Advances in research have greatly increased the understanding of how cancer develops. It is now known that the development of cancer is a process in which normal cells are changed and acquire malignant properties. Before moving on to discuss the various theories of the causes of cancer, it is useful to review how normal cells divide and adapt to changing conditions.

Normal cell growth

Mature normal cells are uniform in size and have nuclei that are characteristic of the tissue to which the cells belong. Within the nucleus of normal cells, chromosomes containing deoxyribonucleic acid (DNA) molecules carry the genetic information that controls the synthesis of polypeptides (proteins). Genes are subunits of chromosomes and consist of portions of DNA that specify the production of particular sets of proteins. Thus, genes control the development of specific traits. The genetic code in the DNA of every gene is translated into protein structures that determine the type, maturity and function of a cell. Any change or disruption in a gene can result in an inaccurate 'blueprint' that can produce an aberrant cell, which may then become cancerous. Box 13.1 lists some of the functions of DNA.

The cell cycle

Two coordinated events are responsible for cellular reproduction. Reproduction occurs as the result of replication of cellular DNA and mitosis, when the cell divides into two daughter cells with identical DNA.

The **cell cycle** consists of four phases. In the gap 1 or G_1 phase, the cell enlarges and synthesises proteins to prepare for DNA replication. During this phase, the cell prepares to replicate and enter into the synthesis phase. During the synthesis (S) phase, DNA is replicated and the chromosomes in the cell are duplicated. During the next phase, gap 2 (G_2), the cell prepares itself for mitosis. Finally, with all preparation complete, the cell begins mitosis (M). This phase culminates in the division of the parent cell into two exact copies called daughter cells, each having identical genetic material. The cells then immediately enter G_1 where they begin the cell cycle again or divert into a resting phase called G_0. The cell cycle is controlled by cyclins, which combine with and activate enzymes called cyclin-dependent kinases. Some cyclins cause a 'braking' action and prevent the cycle from proceeding (Lan, Chen & Wei, 2021). Checkpoints in the cell cycle ensure that it proceeds in the correct order.

BOX 13.1 Functions of DNA

- Orders production of enzymes
- Instructs cells to produce specific chemicals
- Instructs cells to develop specific structures
- Determines individual traits and characteristics
- Controls other DNA by telling a cell to 'switch on' and use some portion of the genetic information stored in it

A malfunction of any of these regulators of cell growth and division can result in the rapid proliferation of immature cells. In some cases, these cells are considered cancerous (malignant). Knowledge of cell cycle events is used in the development of chemotherapeutic drugs, which are designed to disrupt the cancer cells during different stages of their cell cycle. These drugs and their use are discussed later in the chapter.

Differentiation

Differentiation is a normal process occurring over many cell cycles that allows cells to specialise in certain tasks. For example, some epithelial cells lining the lungs develop into tall columnar cells with cilia. These columnar cells sweep potentially dangerous debris out of the lungs. When adverse conditions occur in body tissues during differentiation, protective adaptations can produce alterations in cells. Some of these alterations are helpful, but in other cases the cells mutate beyond usefulness and become liabilities (Norris, 2018). Following are potentially unproductive cellular alterations that occur during cell differentiation:

- **Hyperplasia** is an increase in the number or density of normal cells. Hyperplasia occurs in response to stress, increased metabolic demands or elevated levels of hormones. Examples include the hyperplasia of myocardial cells in response to a prolonged increase in the body's demand for oxygen and hyperplasia of uterine cells in response to rising levels of oestrogen during pregnancy. Hyperplastic cells are under normal DNA control.
- **Metaplasia** is a change in the normal pattern of differentiation such that dividing cells differentiate into cell types not normally found in that location in the body. The metaplastic cell is normal for its particular type, but it is not in its normal location. Some metaplastic cells are less functional than the cells they replace. Metaplasia is a protective response to adverse conditions. Metaplastic cells are under normal DNA control and are reversible when the stressor or other disruptive condition ceases.
- **Dysplasia** represents a loss of DNA control over differentiation occurring in response to adverse conditions. Dysplastic cells show abnormal variation in size, shape and appearance, as well as a disturbance in their usual arrangement. Examples of dysplasia include changes in the cervix in response to continued irritation, such as from the human papillomavirus or leucoplakia on oral mucous membranes in response to chronic irritation from smoking.
- **Anaplasia** is the regression of a cell to an immature or undifferentiated cell type. Anaplastic cell division is no longer under DNA control. Anaplasia usually occurs when a damaging or transforming event takes place inside the dividing, still undifferentiated cell, leading to loss of useful function. Anaplasia may occur in response to overwhelmingly destructive conditions inside the cell or in surrounding tissue (Norris, 2018).

Although hyperplasia, metaplasia and dysplasia often reverse after the irritating factor is eliminated, they can lead to malignancy under certain conditions. This is especially true of dysplasia, which represents a loss of DNA control. Anaplasia is not reversible, but the degree of anaplasia determines the potential risk of cancer.

Theories of carcinogenesis

Factors that cause cancer are both external (chemicals, radiation and viruses) and internal (hormones, immune conditions and inherited mutations). Causal factors may act together or in sequence to initiate or promote **carcinogenesis**. Ten or more years often pass between exposures or mutations and detectable cancer.

Central to these theories are two important concepts about the aetiology of cancer. First, damaged DNA, whether inherited or from external sources, sets up the necessary initial step for cancer to occur. Second, impairment of the human immune system, from whatever cause, lessens its ability to destroy abnormal cells.

Cellular mutation

The theory of cellular mutation suggests that carcinogens cause mutations in cellular DNA. It is believed that the carcinogenic process has three stages: initiation, promotion and progression. The initiation stage involves permanent damage in the cellular DNA as a result of exposure to a carcinogen (e.g. radiation, chemicals) that was not repaired or had a defective repair. Promotion may last for years and includes conditions, such as smoking or alcohol use, that act repeatedly on the already affected cells. In the progression stage, further inherited changes acquired during the cell replication develop into a cancer.

Oncogenes

Oncogenes are abnormal genes that promote cell proliferation and are capable of triggering cancerous characteristics. Oncogenes can be classified according to their overall function. Several oncogenes and their relationship to human cancers have been identified. For example, BRCA-1 and BRCA-2 are associated with breast cancer.

A decrease in the body's immune surveillance may allow the expression of oncogenes; this can occur during times of stress or in response to certain carcinogens. For example, people with AIDS, who have a decreased number of helper T lymphocytes, have a much higher than normal incidence of certain cancers, including non-Hodgkin's lymphoma and Kaposi's sarcoma (Portilla-Tamarit et al., 2021; Schwetz & Fauci, 2019).

Tumour suppressor genes

Tumour suppressor genes normally suppress oncogenes. They can become inactive by deletion or mutation. Inherited cancers have been associated with tumour suppressor genes. An example is *p53*, a suppressor gene that has been associated with sarcoma and cancer of the breast and brain.

Known carcinogens

A number of agents are known to cause cancer, or at least are strongly linked to certain kinds of cancers. These known carcinogens include viruses, drugs, hormones and chemical and physical agents.

Carcinogens can be categorised into two groups: genotoxic carcinogens directly alter DNA and cause mutations, and promoter substances cause other adverse biological effects, such as cytotoxicity, hormonal imbalances, altered immunity or chronic tissue damage. Promoter substances do not cause cancer in the absence of previous cell damage (initiation) and often require high-level and long-term contact with the altered cells (see Table 13.1). Although everyone comes into contact with a vast number of substances that are considered carcinogenic, not everyone develops cancer. Other factors, such as genetic predisposition, impairment of the immune response and repeated exposure to the carcinogen, are necessary for a cancer to develop.

Viruses

Several viruses have been associated with the development of cancer. They damage cells and induce hyperplastic cell growth. Viral infection may play a role in cell mutation that can progress to malignant cells. Most people are able to suppress this progression (Rubin, 2001). Box 13.2 identifies these viruses and the cancers with which they are associated.

In addition, viruses play a significant role in weakening immunological defences against neoplasms. For example, human immunodeficiency virus (HIV), which infects helper T lymphocytes and monocytes, impairs the person's protection against certain cancers such as lymphoma and Kaposi's sarcoma (Portilla-Tamarit et al., 2021; Schwetz & Fauci, 2019).

Other viruses have also been associated with human malignancies. Hepatitis B virus integrates its DNA with liver cell DNA and is believed to cause primary hepatocellular carcinoma. Papillomaviruses cause plantar, common and flat warts, which are benign and usually regress spontaneously; however, they also cause genital warts and laryngeal papillomas, which are associated with malignant melanoma and cervical, penile and laryngeal cancers. Retroviruses have been found to cause cancer in animals. Adult T-cell leukaemia is the only human cancer known to be associated with a retrovirus (Rubin, 2001).

Vaccines to prevent virus-induced cancers are being investigated. Currently readily available vaccines include the human papilloma vaccine (HPV) and the hepatitis B vaccine.

BOX 13.2 Cancers associated with different viruses

Herpes simplex virus types I and II (HSV-1 and HSV-2)
- Carcinoma of the lip
- Cervical carcinoma
- Kaposi's sarcoma

Human cytomegalovirus (HCMV)
- Kaposi's sarcoma
- Prostate cancer

Epstein–Barr virus (EBV)
- Burkitt's lymphoma

Human herpesvirus-6 (HHV-6)
- Lymphoma

Hepatitis B virus (HBV)
- Primary hepatocellular cancer

Papillomavirus
- Malignant melanoma
- Cervical, penile and laryngeal cancers

Human T-lymphotropic viruses (HTLV)
- Adult T-cell leukaemia and lymphoma
- T-cell variant of hairy-cell leukaemia
- Kaposi's sarcoma

Drugs and hormones

Certain drugs can be either genotoxic or promotional. For example, chemotherapeutic drugs used to disrupt the cell cycle of malignant cells can be genotoxic for normal cells. They can also be promotional: by drastically reducing the number of leucocytes, they impair immune function. Examples of these chemotherapeutic drugs include busulfan, chlorambucil and cyclophosphamide. Some recreational drugs also are implicated as carcinogens. These include the genotoxic betel nut chewed by many Pacific Islanders and the immunosuppressant promoters heroin and cocaine.

Hormones are also potential genotoxic carcinogens or promoters. Gonadotropic hormones often mediate cancers of the reproductive organs. Oestrogen, both natural and synthetic, and diethylstilbestrol (DES) have been linked to cervical, endometrial and breast cancers. Oestrogen-containing contraceptive pills have been implicated in breast cancer but have also been shown to decrease the risk of ovarian cancer. Investigators have not reached a final conclusion about the cancer risk posed by contraceptives. Newer research suggests that alterations in the molecular structure of testosterone in older men may promote the development of prostate cancer. Also, glucocorticosteroids (cortisone) and anabolic steroids may act as promoters by altering the immune response or endocrine balance.

Chemical agents

Many chemicals have been demonstrated to be both genotoxic and promotional. As many of these substances are encountered in the workplace, they constitute occupational hazards. Examples of industrial and environmental carcinogens include polycyclic hydrocarbons, found in soot; benzopyrene, found in cigarette smoke; and arsenic, found in pesticides. These chemicals have some genotoxic action, with some altering DNA replication. Other industrial and environmental chemicals are considered promotional agents. These include wood and leather dust, polymer esters (used in plastics and paints), carbon tetrachloride, asbestos and phenol.

Natural substances in the body may also be carcinogenic or promotional. For example, end products of metabolism that are produced in excess amounts or are ineffectively eliminated, such as bile acids from a high-fat diet, may promote cancer.

Some foods contain carcinogens added during preparation or preservation. Examples include the sugar substitute sodium saccharine, and nitrosamines and nitrous indoles, which are found in pickled, salted foods. In some cases, food contaminants produce carcinogenic chemicals. The *Aspergillus* fungi produce aflatoxin, a highly potent carcinogen. These organisms grow on improperly stored vegetable products, such as grains and peanuts.

Polycyclic aromatic hydrocarbons, nitrosamines, phenols and other chemicals in tobacco act as either carcinogens or promoters of cancer (see Table 13.1).

Physical agents

It has been well documented that excessive exposure to radiation causes increased rates of cancer by damaging the DNA in cells, by activating other oncogenetic factors or by suppressing antitumour activity (protein inhibitors). Both solar radiation from ultraviolet rays and ionising radiation from industrial or medical sources are carcinogenic. This fact has implications for workers exposed to these agents and for the population in general. Radon, a naturally formed radioactive gas that can be found in the basements of some buildings, is also a known carcinogen. People who have lived in areas where nuclear weapons have been tested or whose groundwater has been polluted by nuclear wastes are at risk of developing cancers. The effects of high-dose radiation exposure and subsequent cancer development have been demonstrated in the survivors of the atomic bombs at Nagasaki and Hiroshima and in workers exposed to radiation during the clean-up of nuclear disaster sites, such as Chernobyl. The full effects of the 2011 Fukushima nuclear plant disaster have yet to be documented.

Types of neoplasms

A **neoplasm** is a mass of new tissue (a collection of cells) that grows independently of its surrounding structures and has no physiological purpose. The term *neoplasm* is often used interchangeably with *tumour*, from the Latin word meaning 'swelling'. Neoplasms are said to be autonomous because they grow at a rate uncoordinated with the needs of the body, they share some of the properties of the parent cells but with altered size and shape and they do not benefit the host and in some cases are actively harmful.

Neoplasms are not completely autonomous, as they require a blood supply with nutrients and oxygen to sustain their growth. Neoplasms are typically classified as benign or malignant on the basis of their potential to damage the body and on their growth characteristics.

Benign neoplasms

Benign neoplasms are localised growths. They form a solid mass, have well-defined borders and are frequently encapsulated. Benign neoplasms tend to respond to the body's homeostatic controls. Thus, they often stop growing when they reach the boundaries of another tissue (a process called *contact inhibition*). They grow slowly and often remain stable in size. Since they are usually encapsulated, benign neoplasms are often easily removed and tend not to recur.

Although typically harmless, benign neoplasms nevertheless can be destructive if they crowd surrounding tissue and obstruct the function of organs. For example, a benign meningioma (from the meninges of the brain and spinal cord) can cause severely increased intracranial pressure (ICP), which progressively impairs the person's cerebral function. Unless the meningioma can be successfully removed, the steadily rising ICP will eventually lead to coma and death.

Malignant neoplasms

In contrast to benign neoplasms, malignant neoplasms grow aggressively and do not respond to the body's homeostatic controls. Malignant neoplasms are not cohesive and present with an irregular shape. Instead of slowly crowding other tissues, malignant neoplasms cut through surrounding tissues, causing bleeding, inflammation and necrosis (tissue death) as they grow. This invasive quality of malignant neoplasms is reflected in the word origin of *cancer*, from the Greek *karkinos*, meaning 'crab'. Healthcare professionals are referring to a malignant neoplasm when they use the term *cancer*.

TABLE 13.2 Comparison of benign and malignant neoplasms

BENIGN	MALIGNANT
Local	Invasive
Cohesive	Non-cohesive
Well-defined borders	Does not stop at tissue border
Pushes other tissues out of the way	Invades and destroys surrounding tissues
Slow growth	Rapid growth
Encapsulated	Metastasises to distant sites
Easily removed	Not always easy to remove
Does not recur	Can recur

Malignant cells from the primary tumour may travel through the blood or lymph to invade other tissues and organs of the body and form a secondary tumour called a *metastasis*. This term also refers to the process by which such spreading of malignant neoplasms—perhaps their most destructive trait—occurs. Malignant neoplasms can recur after surgical removal of the primary and secondary tumours and after other treatments. Table 13.2 compares benign and malignant neoplasms.

Malignant neoplasms vary in their degree of differentiation from parent tissue. Highly differentiated cancer cells try to mimic the specialised function of the parent tissue, but undifferentiated cancers, consisting of immature cells, have almost no resemblance to the parent tissue and therefore no useful function. To make matters worse, undifferentiated cancers rob the body of its energy and nutrition as they grow. Undifferentiated anaplastic cells have little structural or functional relationship to the parent cells and are the basis of many malignant neoplasms. The degree of differentiation of anaplastic cells is a consideration in the classification and staging of neoplasms, discussed later in this chapter.

Characteristics of malignant cells

Malignant neoplasms may be identified by the following predictable cellular characteristics:

- *Loss of regulation of the rate of mitosis.* This results in rapid cell division and growth of the neoplasm.
- *Loss of specialisation and differentiation.* Malignant cells do not perform typical cellular functions. Many produce hormones and enzymes similar to those of the parent tissue but usually in excessive amounts, possibly revealing their presence.
- *Loss of contact inhibition.* Malignant cells do not respect other cellular boundaries. They easily invade and destroy other tissues.
- *Progressive acquisition of a cancerous phenotype.* Cellular mutation seems to be a sequential process involving successive generations of cells, with each generation becoming more deviant than the previous one. Additionally,

malignant cells seem to be 'immortal' in that they do not stop growing and die, as do normal cells, which have a genetically determined lifespan.

- *Irreversibility.* The transformation into a malignant cell is irreversible. Rarely does a malignant neoplasm revert to a benign state.
- *Altered cell structure.* Cytological examination of malignant cells reveals distinct differences in the cell nucleus and cytoplasm, as well as an overall cell shape that differs from that of normal cells of the particular tissue type.
- *Simplified metabolic activities.* The work of malignant cells is simpler than that of normal cells. They show an increased synthesis of substances needed for cell division and they have no need to create proteins for the specialised functions of the tissues they invade.
- *Transplantability.* Malignant cells often break away from the primary tissue site and travel to other locations in the body, where they establish new growths.
- *Ability to promote their own survival.* Malignant cells may create ectopic sites to produce the hormones they need for their growth. By their very presence and their ability to initiate vascular permeability, malignant cells promote the development of non-neoplastic stroma, a connective tissue framework consisting of collagen and other components, which then supports the neoplasm. They may also create their own blood supply. Through a process called angiogenesis, tumour cells secrete a polypeptide angiogenic growth factor that stimulates blood vessels from surrounding normal tissue to grow into the tumour. Finally, malignant cells divert nutrition from the host to meet their own needs, by diffusion when the tumour is less than 1 mm and thereafter by means of the newly formed blood vessels. If unchecked, malignant cells eventually destroy their host.

BOX 13.3 Characteristics of malignant cells

- **Loss of regulation of mitotic rate**
- **Loss of cell specialisation**
- **Loss of contact inhibition**
- **Progressive acquisition of a cancerous phenotype and immortality**
- **Irreversibility of cancerous phenotype to greater aggressiveness**
- **Altered cell structure: differences in cell nucleus and cytoplasm**
- **Simplified metabolic activity**
- **Transplantability (metastasis)**
- **Ability to promote own survival**

The characteristics of malignant cells are summarised in Box 13.3.

Tumour invasion and metastasis

The ability of cancer cells to invade adjacent tissues and travel to distant organs is considered their most ominous characteristic. This quality makes treatment a considerable challenge.

Invasion

Aggressive tumours possess several qualities that facilitate invasion (see Figure 13.2):

- *Ability to cause pressure atrophy.* The pressure of a growing tumour can cause atrophy and necrosis of adjacent tissues. The malignancy then moves into the vacated space.

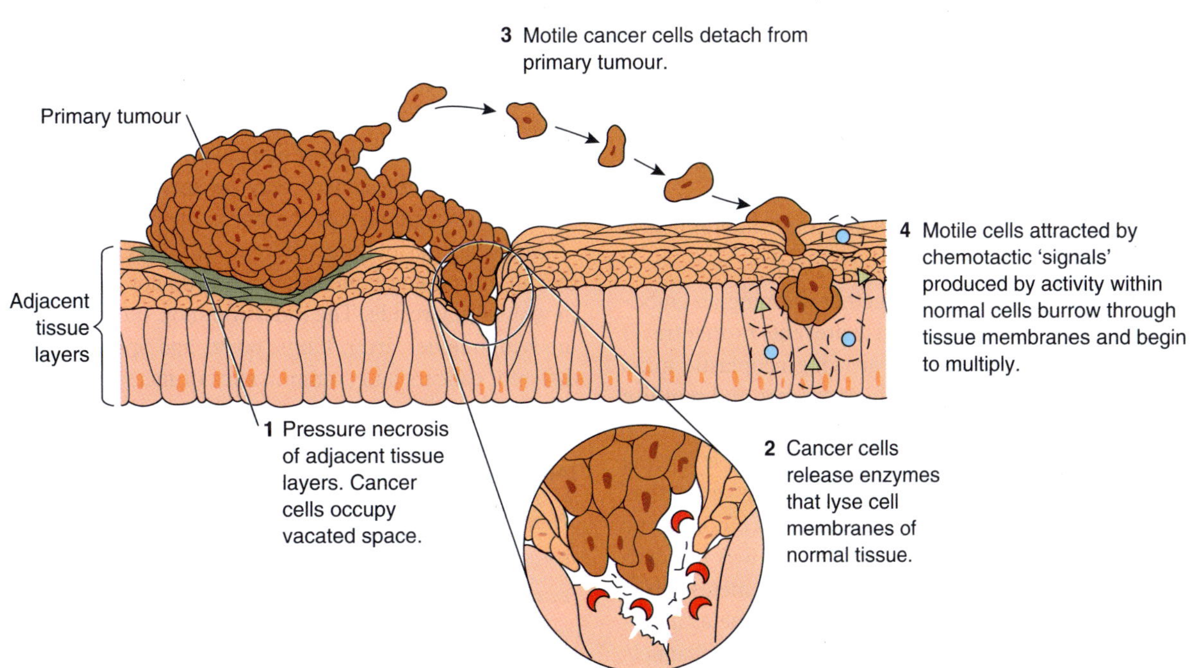

FIGURE 13.2 *How cancer cells invade normal tissue*

- *Ability to disrupt the basement membrane of normal cells.* Many cancer cells can bind to elements of the basement membrane and secrete enzymes that degrade that physical barrier, thus facilitating their movement into normal tissues, lymph and blood circulation.
- *Motility.* Because malignant cells are less tightly bound to each other than normal cells (reduced adhesiveness), they easily separate from the neoplasm and move into surrounding body fluids and tissues.
- *Response to chemical signals from adjacent tissues.* Chemotaxis (the movement of cells in response to a chemical stimulus) calls the tumour cells into the normal tissues, possibly as a result of the degrading of the basement membranes of the normal cells. This breakdown of normal cellular membranes releases the chemical stimulus physiologically designed to draw normal phagocytic cells to clean up the debris. (See the chapter 'Nursing care of people with infections', on the inflammatory response, for more information on chemotaxis.) Malignant cells are also known to respond chemotactically to the end product of cellular metabolism. Some cancer cells even produce a substance called autocrine motility factor, which calls other malignant cells to a normal tissue. The first invading cells produce this substance, which then actively draws other malignant cells from the primary tumour into the invaded normal tissue.

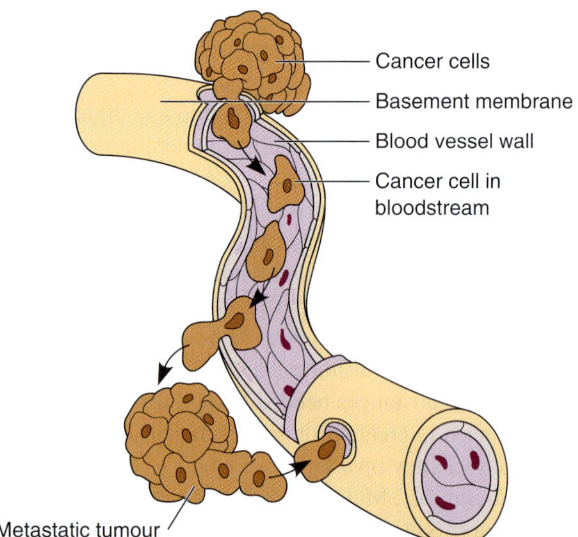

FIGURE 13.3 ***Metastasis through the bloodstream. Cancer cells secrete enzymes and a motility factor that disrupt the basement membrane in the blood vessel. In this way, the cancer cells gain access to the circulation. Once in the blood, only about 1 cell in 1,000 escapes immune detection, but that can be enough. Undetected cells move out of the blood, again secreting enzymes and cutting through the vessel wall into new tissue. The tissue selected for establishing a new tumour may be downstream from the original tumour or a chemical attraction may cause the malignant cells to target a specific site. Once in the new site, the malignant cells multiply and establish a metastatic tumour***

Metastasis

The factors that favour invasion also contribute to the process of metastasis. **Metastasis** can occur by means of one or more mechanisms including embolism in the blood or lymph or spread by way of body cavities.

A blood or lymph-borne metastasis allows a new tumour to be established in a distant organ. Figure 13.3 shows metastasis through the bloodstream. A tumour's ability to metastasise in this manner requires the following steps:

1. Intravasation of malignant cells through blood or lymphatic vessel walls and into the circulation.
2. Survival of the malignant cells in the blood. (To survive, the cells must escape the notice of the body's immune surveillance; only about 1 in 1,000 cells does so.)
3. Extravasation from the circulation and implantation in a new tissue.

The tumour cells tend to clump together, forming an embolus, and continue growing until their size prevents further travel in the vessel or lymph channel. The growing neoplastic mass then uses its invasive abilities (secreting enzymes and motility factor) to move into the nearest organ.

About 60% of metastatic lesions tend to occur in a schema reflecting the pattern of blood or lymph circulation. However, it has been demonstrated that some malignant cells defy a blood-borne pattern and actually target specific organs to which they prefer to metastasise. For example, lung cancer frequently metastasises to the adrenal glands, and breast cancer frequently metastasises to bone. Malignant cells that gain access to the lymph channels may travel to a preferred organ and then move into it the same way they emigrate through blood vessels. Alternatively, the malignant cells may become trapped in the lymph node and continue to grow. Eventually, the malignant cells replace the node's tissues. At this point, emboli from the cancerous node disseminate to other nodes, creating a cascade reaction. The malignant cascade causes widespread transfer of the tumour to uncharacteristic sites.

A malignant tumour may break through the walls of the organ in which it is primarily housed, shedding cells into the nearby body cavity. The cells are then free to establish new tumours in a distant area of that cavity. For example, malignant cells from a colon cancer may be seeded into the peritoneal cavity, establishing a new tumour in the mesenteric epithelium.

Metastatic lesions are differentiated from primary neoplasms by cell morphology: metastatic cells do not resemble the tissue in which they reside. The most common sites of metastasis are the lymph nodes, liver, lungs, bones and brain. Table 13.3 lists different cancers and common sites of metastasis.

TABLE 13.3 Various cancers and sites of metastases

PRIMARY TUMOUR	COMMON METASTATIC SITES
Bronchogenic (lung)	Spinal cord, brain, liver, bone
Breast	Regional lymph nodes, vertebrae, brain, liver, lung, bone
Colon	Liver, lung, brain, ovary, bone
Prostate	Bladder, bone (especially vertebrae), liver
Malignant melanoma	Lung, liver, spleen, regional lymph nodes, brain

BOX 13.4 Factors that may weaken or alter the immune response

- Accumulated stress
- Depression
- Increased age
- Pregnancy
- Chronic disease
- Chemotherapy treatment for the primary cancer

For metastasis to occur, the cancerous cells must avoid detection by the immune system. Thus, impairment of the immune system is a major factor in the establishment of metastatic lesions. Cells may escape detection in several different ways:

- Aggressive cancer cells may compile a large mass (greater than 1 cm) so rapidly that the immune system is unable to overcome the tumour before it takes hold in a new tissue.
- For tumour cells to be recognised as foreign by the immune system, they must display on their surface a special antigen called tumour-associated antigen (TAA). TAA marks tumour cells for destruction by the lymphocytes. Some oncogenic viruses depress the expression of TAA on infected cells. Also, some tumours in advanced stages of growth no longer display TAA. Thus, such tumour cells escape detection as they travel through the blood or lymph.
- If the person's immune response is weakened or altered, then a metastatic tumour may take hold with little opposition. Factors that may weaken or alter the immune response are listed in Box 13.4.

An estimated 50% to 60% of all cancers have already metastasised by the time the primary tumour is identified. This may account for the current 50% death rate and certainly supports the need to educate people to facilitate early diagnosis. The time it takes for metastasis to occur is extremely variable and often difficult to predict. Some cancers, such as basal cell carcinomas, do not metastasise. The aggressiveness and location of the tumour and the state of the person's immune system determine how rapidly and whether metastasis will take place.

PHYSIOLOGICAL AND PSYCHOLOGICAL EFFECTS OF CANCER

Much of the nursing care for people with cancer is related to the generalised effects of cancer on the body and the side effects of the treatments used to remove or destroy the cancer. Although pathophysiological effects of the cancer vary with the type and location of the cancer, the following effects usually are observed.

Disruption of function

Physiological functioning can be upset by obstruction or pressure. For example, a large tumour in the bowel can stop intestinal motility, resulting in a bowel obstruction. Prostate tumours can obstruct the bladder neck or urethra, resulting in urine retention. Intracranial pressure can be dangerously increased by a glioma. Obstruction or pressure can cause anoxia and necrosis of surrounding tissues, which in turn cause a loss of function of the involved organ or tissue. For example, a kidney tumour may progress to renal failure. Pressure against the superior vena cava from an adjacent lung tumour or tumour-infiltrated lymph nodes can interrupt the blood flow to the heart.

In the liver, either a primary hepatocellular cancer or metastatic lesion can have several significant effects:

- In liver parenchymal tissue, it impairs the multiple life-sustaining functions of the liver, such as carbohydrate metabolism, synthesis of plasma proteins, detoxification and immunological functions. These functional impairments result in severe nutritional, hormonal, haematological and immunological problems. (See the chapter 'A person-centred approach to assessing the gastrointestinal system' for a more complete discussion of liver functions and effects of disruption.)
- Because more than 1 L of blood per minute passes through the liver via the portal vein, obstruction to this flow by a tumour can cause portal hypertension. This results in backup of fluid and increased pressure in the splanchnic circulation. The end result is ascites (third-spaced fluid in the peritoneal cavity) and varices (friable, over-distended blood vessels) of the oesophageal, gastric, mesenteric and haemorrhoidal vessels.

Haematological alterations

Haematological alterations can impair the normal function of blood cells. For example, in leukaemia, a malignant proliferative disease of the haematopoietic (blood-cell-producing) system, the immature leucocytes cannot perform the normal protective phagocytic functions and immunity is compromised. The excessive numbers of immature leucocytes in the bone marrow diminish erythrocyte and thrombocyte (platelet) production, resulting in secondary anaemia and clotting disorders.

Other examples of haematological alteration include the following:

- Gastrointestinal tumours disrupt the absorption of vitamin B_{12} and iron.
- Growing tumours need purines and folate and have a unique ability to accumulate and store these substances. Thus, the tumour deprives the bone marrow of these substances, which are needed for erythropoiesis (red blood cell production).
- Renal cell carcinoma produces its own erythropoietin hormone, which causes an excessively large number of red blood cells to be produced and dumped into the bloodstream. The resulting polycythaemia causes viscous blood, which impairs circulation, plugs small capillaries and promotes thrombus formation.

Infection

If the tumour invades and connects two incompatible organs, such as the bowel and bladder, and thus creates a fistula, infection becomes a serious problem. As they destroy viable tissue and thus their source of nutrition, tumours may become necrotic and septicaemia may result. Some tumours are less efficient in creating capillaries and, as a consequence, the centre of the tumour may become necrotic and infected. When a tumour grows near the surface of the body, it may erode through to the surface, thus breaking down the natural defences of intact skin and mucous membranes and providing a site for the entry of microorganisms. Any malignant involvement of the organs or tissues of immunity—such as the liver, bone marrow, Peyer's patches in the small intestine, spleen or lymph nodes—can seriously impair the immune response, allowing infections to develop in vulnerable tissues.

Haemorrhage

Tumour erosion through blood vessels can cause extensive bleeding, giving rise to severe anaemia. Haemorrhage can be serious enough to cause life-threatening hypovolaemic shock.

Anorexia–cachexia syndrome

A characteristic feature of cancer is the wasted appearance of its victims, called **cachexia**. In many cases, unexplained rapid weight loss is the first symptom that brings the person to a healthcare provider. This can be due to a variety of problems associated with cancer, such as pain, infection, depression or the side effects of chemotherapy and radiation. However, usually the emaciation, malnutrition and loss of energy are attributed to the anorexia–cachexia syndrome.

This syndrome is specific to cancer because of the effect of cancer cells on the host's metabolism. The neoplastic cells divert nutrition to their own use while causing changes that reduce the person's appetite. Early in the disease, glucose metabolism is altered, causing an increase in serum glucose levels. Through the process of negative feedback, anorexia (loss of appetite) results. In addition, the tumour secretes substances that decrease appetite by altering taste and smell and producing early satiety. Pain, infection and depression also contribute to anorexia. Some types of cancers cause specific food aversions, such as to red meat, coffee or chocolate.

Avaricious cancer cells support their growth through widespread catabolism of the body's tissue and muscle proteins. This catabolism, coupled with inadequate nutrient intake, results in the typical cachexia. Normally, a starvation state reduces the body's basal metabolic rate. However, in many people with cancer, the metabolic rate is increased, probably because of the hyperactive metabolic and reproductive activities of the malignant cells. One theory suggests that cytokinins the body produces in response to the tumour are responsible for both early satiety and cachexia. One specific cytokine—called tumour necrosis factor alpha, or cachectin—is believed to enhance the increased metabolic consumption of nutrients. Cancers of the gastrointestinal system further promote anorexia–cachexia by decreasing absorption and use of nutrients; the side effects of some treatment modalities enhance this effect. Figure 13.4 shows the characteristic appearance of a cachectic person.

Paraneoplastic syndromes

Paraneoplastic syndromes are indirect effects of cancer. They may be early warning signs of cancer or indicate complications or return of a malignancy. The most frequently occurring paraneoplastic syndromes are endocrine, occurring when

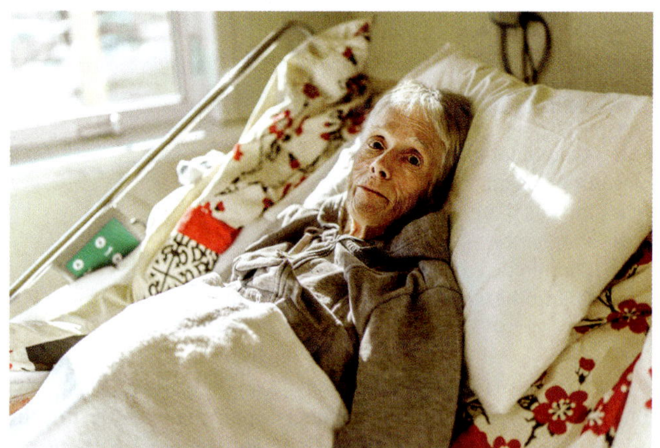

FIGURE 13.4 ***A cachectic person. Cancer robs its host of nutrients and increases body catabolism of fat and muscle to meet its metabolic needs***

Source: Louis-Paul st-onge Louis/Alamy Stock Photo.

cancers set up ectopic sites of hormone production (Norris, 2018). Table 13.4 lists laboratory indicators of ectopic functioning.

These ectopic sites produce excessive amounts of the hormone, which harm the host. Consider the following examples:

- Breast, ovarian and renal cancers may set up ectopic parathyroid hormone sites, causing severe hypercalcaemia.
- Oat cell and other lung cancers may produce ectopic secretions of insulin (causing hypoglycaemia), parathyroid hormone (PTH), antidiuretic hormone (ADH, which causes excessive fluid retention, hypertension and peripheral oedema) and adrenocorticotropic hormone (ACTH). See the chapter 'Nursing care of people with endocrine disorders' for a description of the multiple problems caused by excessive secretions of cortisone.

Other paraneoplastic syndromes include haematological abnormalities such as anaemia, thrombocytopenia and coagulation abnormalities; nephrotic syndrome; cutaneous syndromes and neurological syndromes, such as distant tumours that produce increased ICP.

TABLE 13.4 Laboratory indicators of ectopic functioning

HORMONE	SPECIFIC LABORATORY TEST
Antidiuretic hormone (ADH)	Serum and urine osmolality
Adrenocorticotropic hormone (ACTH)	Plasma ACTH ACTH suppression test ACTH stimulation test Urine catecholamines
Calcitonin	Serum calcitonin
Insulin	Serum glucose Glucose tolerance test
Parathyroid hormone (PTH)	Serum PTH Serum calcium
Thyroxine	Serum thyroid-stimulating hormone (TSH), T_3, T_4

Pain

Pain is ranked as one of the most serious concerns of people with cancer, their families and oncology healthcare professionals. Despite extensive progress in the scientific understanding of pain, more than 60% of people with cancer experience moderate to severe pain at some time during their illness. Because pain management for people with cancer has a reputation for being ineffective, the anticipation of pain may engender fear in even the most stoic people. Most people fear pain and suffering even more than possible death, although pain management strategies have improved tremendously. The findings from a 10-year study of more than 2,000 people in a palliative care program are encouraging. Following the World Health Organization (WHO) guidelines for cancer pain relief, 88% of people reported good to satisfactory pain relief (WHO, 2018). Research on pain, with its devastating statistics, has led to great improvement in pain management strategies (Anekar & Cascella, 2022; Yoong & Poon, 2018).

Types of cancer pain

Cancer pain can be divided into two main categories, acute and chronic, with subgroupings. These classifications serve to indicate appropriate therapeutic approaches. Acute pain has a well-defined pattern of onset, exhibits common signs and symptoms, and is often identified with hyperactivity of the autonomic system. Chronic pain, which lasts more than 6 months, frequently lacks the objective manifestations of acute pain, primarily because the autonomic nervous system adapts to this chronic stress. Unfortunately, chronic pain often results in personality changes, alterations in functional abilities and lifestyle disruptions that can seriously affect compliance with treatment and the quality of life.

Most people with cancer who cite acute pain as the primary symptom that led to the diagnosis tend to associate pain with the introduction to their disease. If these people experience pain during the illness or after therapy, they often perceive the pain as introducing another cancer or as a recurrence of the original cancer. Other people report experiencing pain as a component of cancer therapy. These people are often able to endure the pain in anticipation of a successful outcome of treatment (Sitarz & Spencer, 2022; Smith et al., 2019).

Chronic pain may be related to treatment or may indicate progression of the disease. Identifying the pain as treatment-related rather than tumour-related is extremely important because it has a definite effect on the person's psychological outlook. For the person whose pain is due to the advancement of the disease, psychological factors play an even more important role. Hopelessness and fear of impending death intensify physiological pain and contribute to overall suffering, which goes well beyond just physical pain.

Three other categories used to classify people with cancer pain are worth mentioning: people with pre-existing pain, those with a history of drug abuse and people dying with cancer-related pain. The first two groups may have altered perceptions of pain and may not have the anticipated response to pain medication. For the dying person, pain is strongly associated with both the person and their family's confrontation of issues of hopelessness and death. Confronting these issues can intensify the perception of pain (see the chapter 'Nursing care of people experiencing loss, grief and death').

Causes of cancer pain

Direct tumour involvement is the primary cause of the pain experienced by people with cancer. This includes metastatic bone disease, nerve compression and involvement of visceral organs. The pain from tumour involvement is believed to be mechanical, resulting from stretching of tissues and compression. Chemicals from ischaemia or tumour metabolites and toxins that activate and sensitise nociceptors and mechanoreceptors are also responsible for tumour pain. See the chapter 'Nursing care of people in pain' for a more complete discussion of the mechanics of pain.

Side effects or toxic effects of cancer therapies (e.g. surgery, radiation and chemotherapy) may also cause cancer pain. These are usually the result of traumatised tissue; one example of this is the oropharyngeal ulcerations that occur with some types of chemotherapy. However, these therapies may also be used to manage pain, such as radiation to decrease pain associated with bone metastasis.

Physical stress

When the immune system discovers a neoplasm, it tries to destroy it using the resources of the body. The body mounts an all-out assault on the foreign invader, calling on many resources including chemical mediators, hormones and enzymes, blood cells, antibodies, proteins and inflammatory and immune responses.

These protective responses also mobilise fluid, electrolytes and nutritional systems. This massive effort requires tremendous energy. See the chapters 'Nursing care of people with altered fluid, electrolyte and acid–base balance' and 'Nursing care of people with nutritional disorders' for specific information on these systems. If the neoplasm is small enough (i.e. microscopic), the immune system can destroy it and a tumour will never manifest. A neoplasm of 1 cm is large enough to overwhelm most immune systems; however, the body will continue to try to fight it until it reaches the stage of exhaustion and is no longer capable (Selye, 1984). Thus, many people with cancer present with fatigue, weight loss, anaemia, dehydration and altered blood chemistries (e.g. decreases in electrolytes) (Fabi et al., 2020; Smith et al., 2019).

Psychological stress

People confronted with the diagnosis of cancer exhibit a variety of psychological and emotional responses. Some people see cancer as a death sentence and experience overwhelming grief, often giving up. Others may feel guilt, considering the cancer a punishment for past behaviours, such as smoking or unhealthy eating habits, or for delaying diagnosis or treatment. The person may experience anger, especially if they believe that they had been practising a healthy lifestyle; beneath that anger may reside feelings of powerlessness. Fear is common: fear of the outcome of the illness, fear of the effects of treatment, fear of pain, fear of death. Some people feel isolated because of the stigma of cancer and old beliefs of contagion. Body image

BOX 13.5 Physiological and psychosocial effects of cancer

- Disruption of function (due to obstruction or pressure)
- Haematological alterations
  a. Decreased leucocytes, erythrocytes and thrombocytes
  b. Altered erythropoiesis
- Infections
  a. Fistula between non-compatible organs
  b. Necrosis of tumour centre
  c. Malignant involvement of organs of immunity
- Haemorrhage (caused by erosion of neoplasm through blood vessels or surface of skin)
- Anorexia–cachexia syndrome
  a. Hyperglycaemia
  b. Catabolism of tissue and muscle proteins
  c. Altered taste and smell
- Creation of ectopic sites of hormones
  a. PTH
  b. Insulin
  c. ADH
  d. ACTH
- Paraneoplastic syndromes
  a. Deep venous thrombosis
  b. Peripheral nerve problems
  c. Increased intracranial pressure
  d. Anorexia–cachexia syndrome
  e. Nephrotic syndrome
- Pain
  a. Acute and chronic
  b. Caused by direct tumour involvement or side effects of therapy
- Physical stress
  a. Increased general adaptation syndrome activity
  b. Increased immunological activity
  c. Increased inflammatory response activity
  d. Nutritional, fluid and electrolyte alterations
- Psychological stress
  a. Grief
  b. Hopelessness
  c. Guilt
  d. Anger
  e. Fear
  f. Isolation
  g. Body image concerns
  h. Sexual dysfunction

Note: Manifestations depend on the type and location of the cancer.

concerns and sexual dysfunction may be present but often unexpressed, especially if the cancer is of the breast or sexual organs or causes visible body changes. Box 13.5 summarises the physiological and psychosocial effects of cancer.

INTERPROFESSIONAL CARE

Interprofessional care for the person with cancer begins with a variety of specialised laboratory and diagnostic tests.

Diagnosis

Several procedures are used to diagnose cancer. X-ray imaging, computed tomography (CT), ultrasonography and magnetic resonance imaging (MRI) can locate abnormal tissues or tumours. However, only microscopic histological examination of the tissue reveals the type of cell and its structural difference from the parent tissue. Tissue samples are acquired through biopsy, shedded cells (e.g. cervical screening test) or collections of secretions (e.g. sputum). Lymph nodes are also biopsied to determine whether metastasis has begun. Simple screening procedures can be used to pick up substances secreted by the tumour, such as the prostatic-specific antigen (PSA) blood test which is being used to identify early prostatic cancers. Increases in enzymes or hormones released by normal tissues when they are damaged can also contribute to the diagnosis. Increased alkaline phosphatase noted in bone metastases and osteosarcoma is one example of an enzyme increase associated with cancer. Tumour markers are used for early diagnosis, for tracking responses to therapy and for devising immunological treatments.

Some investigators studying chemical mediators of the immune system have noted that there seems to be communication between the chemical mediators and the emotional centres of the brain. A person who states 'I feel I have cancer' should be listened to and the complaint investigated thoroughly.

CLASSIFICATION To help standardise diagnosis and treatment protocols, an elaborate identification system has been developed. This consists of naming the tumour (classification) and describing its aggressiveness (grading) and spread within or beyond the tissue of origin (staging).

Tumours are classified and named by the tissue or cell of origin. Tumour nomenclature often incorporates the Latin stem identifying the tissue from which the tumour arises. For example, a carcinoma arises from epithelial tissue; adjectives are added to further specify the location. A glandular malignancy arising from epithelial tissue is classified as an adenocarcinoma. A tumour arising from supportive tissues is called a sarcoma; the specific type of tissue is added as a prefix. For example, a cancer of fibrous connective tissue is called fibrosarcoma and a smooth muscle cancer is a leiomyosarcoma. A tumour from seminal or germ tissue is called a seminoma. Table 13.5 compares the nomenclature of benign and malignant neoplasms.

Other names for tumours incorporate the name of the discoverer of that particular cancer, such as Burkitt's lymphoma or Hodgkin's disease. Haematopoietic malignancies (also known as 'liquid tumours') are usually named by the type of immature blood cell that predominates. An example is

TABLE 13.5 Nomenclature for benign and malignant neoplasms

	TISSUE OF ORIGIN	BENIGN	MALIGNANT
Ectoderm/endoderm	Epithelium	Papilloma	Carcinoma
	Gland	Adenoma	Adenocarcinoma
	Liver cells	Hepatocellular adenoma	Hepatocellular carcinoma
	Neuroglia	Glioma	Glioma
	Melanocytes	Melanoma	Malignant melanoma
	Basal cells		Basal cell carcinoma
	Germ cells	Tetroma	Seminoma
Mesoderm	*Connective tissue*		
	Adipose tissue	Lipoma	Liposarcoma
	Fibrous tissue	Fibroma	Fibrosarcoma
	Bone tissue	Osteoma	Osteosarcoma
	Cartilage	Chondroma	Chondrosarcoma
	Muscle		
	Smooth muscle	Leiomyoma	Leiomyosarcoma
	Striated muscle	Rhabdomyoma	Rhabdomyosarcoma
	Neural tissue		
	Nerve cells	Ganglioneuroma	Neuroblastoma
	Endothelial tissues		
	Blood vessels	Haemangioma	Angiosarcoma
			Kaposi's sarcoma
	Meninges	Meningioma	Malignant meningioma
Haematopoietic tissues	Granulocytes	Granulocytosis	Leukaemia
	Plasma cells		Multiple myeloma
	Lymphocytes		Lymphoma

myelocytic leukaemia, named for the immature form of the granulocyte that is predominant in this malignancy.

GRADING AND STAGING Grading evaluates the amount of differentiation (level of functional maturity) of the cell and estimates the rate of growth based on the mitotic rate. Cells that are the most differentiated—that is, most like the parent tissue and therefore the least malignant—are classified as grade 1 and are associated with a better prognosis. Grade 4 is reserved for the least differentiated and most aggressively malignant cells. Because of the differences inherent in tumour appearance and biological behaviour, grading criteria may vary with different locations and types of tumours.

Staging is used to classify solid tumours and refers to the relative size of the tumour and extent of the disease. The TNM classification system is an internationally recognised staging system: T stands for the relative tumour size, depth of invasion and surface spread; N indicates the presence and extent of lymph node involvement; and M denotes the presence or absence of distant metastases. Table 13.6 shows the basic outline of the TNM system; however, other systems are also used to differentiate types and locations of tumours (e.g. melanomas, cervical cancer, Hodgkin's disease).

CYTOLOGICAL EXAMINATION For malignant tissues to be identified by name, grade and stage, they must first be subjected to histological and cytological examination by light or electron microscope. Specimens are collected by three basic methods:

1. *Exfoliation from an epithelial surface.* Examples include scraping cells from the cervix (cervical screening test) or bronchial washings.
2. *Aspiration of fluid from body cavities or blood.* Examples include white blood cells for evaluation of haematopoietic cancers, pleural fluid and cerebrospinal fluid.
3. *Needle aspiration of solid tumours.* This could include the breast, lung or prostate.

Cytological examination is also carried out on specimens from biopsied tissues or tumours and on collected body secretions, such as sputum or urine.

After collection, specimens are spread on a glass slide, fixed and stained if necessary. The morphological features of the cells are examined, with special attention to the nucleus and cytoplasm. Other special pathological procedures can be carried out on the specimen, but they must be ordered ahead of time if special preparations of the specimen are necessary. Several special diagnostic cytological procedures, such as cytogenetics, are proving useful in diagnosing and monitoring a person's response to treatment.

TUMOUR MARKERS A **tumour marker** is a protein molecule detectable in serum or other body fluids. This marker is used as a biochemical indicator of the presence of a malignancy. Small amounts of tumour marker proteins are found in normal body tissues or benign tumours and are not specific for malignancy. However, high levels are suspicious and mandate follow-up diagnostic studies. Tumour marker tests are most useful for monitoring the person's response to therapy and

TABLE 13.6 TNM staging classification system

	STAGE	MANIFESTATIONS
Tumour	T_0	No evidence of primary tumour
	T_{IS}	Tumour in situ
	T_1, T_2, T_3, T_4	Ascending degrees of tumour size and involvement
Nodes	N_0	No abnormal regional nodes
	N_{1a}, N_{2a}	Regional nodes–no metastasis
	N_{1b}, N_{2b}, N_{3b}	Regional lymph nodes–metastasis suspected
	N_x	Regional nodes cannot be assessed clinically
Metastasis	M_0	No evidence of distant metastasis
	M_1, M_2, M_3	Ascending degrees of metastatic involvement of the host including distant nodes

for detecting residual disease. However, one marker, PSA, is a detector of prostate cancer. As a result, many healthcare practitioners recommend screening for it in men aged over 40, much as cervical screening tests and mammograms are recommended for women.

Tumour markers fall into two general categories: those derived from the tumour itself and those associated with host (immune) response to the tumour. Examples of tumour markers include the following:

- *Antigens.* These are present in fetal tissue but are normally suppressed after birth. Thus, their presence in large amounts may reflect an anaplastic process in tumour cells. Alpha-fetoprotein (AFP) and carcinoembryonic antigen (CEA) are oncofetal antigens.
- *Hormones.* Hormones are, of course, present in considerable amounts in human blood and tissues, but very high levels not related to other conditions may signify the presence of a hormone-secreting malignancy. Some common hormones seen as tumour markers include human chorionic gonadotropin (HCG), antidiuretic hormone (ADH), parathyroid hormone (PTH), calcitonin and catecholamines.
- *Proteins.* These narrow down the type of tissue that may be malignant, although they can also be increased in hyperplastic disorders. Examples of tissue-specific proteins include serum immunoglobin and beta-2 microglobulin.
- *Enzymes.* Rapid, excessive growth of a tissue may cause some of the enzymes and isoenzymes normally present in that particular tissue to spill into the bloodstream. Elevated levels can point to either hyperplasia of the tissue or cancer. Prostatic acid phosphatase (PAP) and neuron-specific enolase (NSE) are examples. Table 13.7 compares selected tumour-derived markers with their presence in neoplasms and other conditions.

ONCOLOGICAL IMAGING Because physical assessment usually cannot detect cancer until the tumour has reached a size that poses a major risk of metastasis, radiological examination is extremely important in early diagnosis. This diagnostic process may involve routine x-ray imaging (usually for screening only), CT, MRI, ultrasonography, nuclear imaging, angiography and positron emission tomography.

X-ray imaging Considered the least expensive and least invasive diagnostic procedure, film screen imaging (standard x-ray imaging) is the method of choice for screening such body areas as the breast (mammography), lung and bone to identify changes in tissue density that may indicate malignancies. X-ray studies are limited in that they do not easily

TABLE 13.7 Tumour-derived markers associated with specific neoplasms

	TUMOUR MARKER	ASSOCIATED NEOPLASM
Oncofetal antigens	Carcinoembryonic antigen (CEA)	Adenocarcinomas of colon, lung, breast, ovary, stomach, pancreas
	Alpha-fetoprotein (AFP)	Hepatocellular carcinoma, gonadal germ-cell tumours (seminoma)
Hormones	Human chorionic gonadotropin (HCG)	Gonadal germ-cell tumours
	Calcitonin	Medullary cancer of thyroid
	Catecholamines/metabolites	Pheochromocytoma
Isoenzymes	Prostatic acid phosphatase (PAP)	Adenocarcinoma of prostate
	Neuron-specific enolase (NSE)	Small-cell lung carcinoma, neuroblastoma
Specific proteins	Prostate-specific antigen (PSA)	Adenocarcinoma of prostate
	Immunoglobin	Multiple myeloma
	CA 125	Epithelial ovarian cancer
	CA 19-9	Adenocarcinoma of pancreas, colon
	CA 15-3	Breast cancer

Source: Adapted from American Cancer Society (1995). *American Cancer Society textbook of clinical oncology*, pp. 75–95. Atlanta: American Cancer Society.

distinguish between calcifications, benign cystic growths and true malignancies. However, as a screening tool, x-ray imaging can usually reassure the person if findings are negative or encourage follow-up studies if findings are suspicious. X-ray imaging is still the method of choice for lung cancer. Unfortunately, it does not usually reveal tumours until they have reached about 1 cm in size, which is late in their development.

Computed tomography CT has vastly advanced the effectiveness of traditional x-ray methods. CT allows the visualisation of cross-sections of the anatomy and can reveal subtle differences in tissue densities; they provide much greater accuracy in tumour diagnosis. This procedure is useful in the screening for some cancers such as renal cell and most gastrointestinal tumours. CT scans are especially useful to evaluate possible lymph node involvement.

Magnetic resonance imaging MRI involves computerised mathematical technology. The person is placed within a strong magnetic field, pulsed radio waves are directed at the person and transmitted signals, based on tissue characteristics, are analysed by a computer. Related diagnostic imaging procedures—positron emission tomography (PET) and single photon emission computed tomography (SPECT)—create visible images by measuring electrical impulses from different body structures. MRI is the diagnostic tool of choice for both screening and follow-up of cranial and head and neck tumours.

Some people become claustrophobic during the MRI procedure because they must be placed inside the diagnostic imaging machine. The machines make loud thumping sounds that can be frightening if the person is not informed beforehand that this is normal.

Ultrasonography Ultrasonography measures sound waves as they bounce off various body structures, giving an image of normal anatomy as well as revealing abnormalities that indicate tumours. Ultrasonography has been adapted for diagnosing some specific tumours. For example, transrectal ultrasonography has provided excellent imaging of early prostate cancers and is used to guide needle biopsy. Ultrasound imaging is also more useful for detecting masses in the denser breast tissue of young women.

Nuclear imaging Nuclear imaging involves the use of a special scintillation scanner in conjunction with the ingestion or injection of specific radioactive isotopes. This is an invasive but usually safe diagnostic method for identifying tumours in various body tissues. This procedure is often used to check for possible bone or other organ metastases. This evaluation helps the healthcare provider determine appropriate treatment.

The procedure is usually minimally distressing for people. Drinking the isotope solution is not pleasant but is tolerable; some anxious people may have difficulty lying still during the scan. Anti-anxiety medication may help. Some people may experience nausea from drinking the isotope and require antiemetic drugs to complete the procedure. Preparation for the person may include allowing nothing by mouth or clear fluids only after midnight.

Angiography An expensive and invasive procedure, angiography is used infrequently for tumour diagnosis. Angiography is performed when the precise location of the tumour cannot be identified or there is a need to visualise the tumour's extent prior to surgery. The procedure involves injecting a radiopaque dye into a major blood vessel proximal to the organ or tissue to be examined. The movement of the dye through the vasculature of the organ or tissue is then traced by means of fluoroscopy or serial x-ray films. In some cases, small catheters are threaded through the vein under fluoroscopy to ensure the specific placement of the dye. Blockage to the flow of the dye indicates the tumour's location. Dye may also be used to identify blood vessels supplying a tumour, allowing the surgeon to know where to safely ligate vessels. Angiography requires preparation similar to that for minor surgery. This includes ensuring that the person takes in only fluids on the day of the examination, performing skin preparation at the insertion site and administering sedative medications prior to the procedure. People should be informed that injection of the dye used to enhance imaging may cause a hot, flushing sensation or nausea and vomiting. Although angiography is usually done on an outpatient basis, the person will be kept in a short-stay unit for several hours and monitored for such complications as bleeding at the catheter insertion site.

DIRECT VISUALISATION Direct visualisation procedures are invasive but do not require the use of radiography. Examples include the following:

- sigmoidoscopy (viewing the sigmoid colon with a fibre-optic flexible sigmoidoscope)
- cystoscopy (viewing the urethra and bladder)
- endoscopy (viewing the upper gastrointestinal tract)
- bronchoscopy (inspecting the tracheobronchial tree).

These methods allow the visual identification of the organs within the limits of the scope and usually permit biopsy of suspicious lesions or masses. Flexible fibre-optic scopes may be more useful because they allow deeper penetration than do traditional scopes. These procedures all require the person to complete some preparation, cause moderate to considerable discomfort and may require sedation or even anaesthesia, as in the case of bronchoscopy. Some procedures, such as sigmoidoscopy and cystoscopy, may be performed in the doctor's surgery and therefore cost less, making them more accessible screening procedures.

Preparation of the person includes a thorough bowel cleansing prior to sigmoidoscopy and cystoscopy; the person may ingest only liquids the morning of the procedure. Because anaesthesia may be required, people undergoing bronchoscopy and endoscopy may be instructed to have nothing by mouth from midnight until the procedure. These procedures are discussed in greater detail in later chapters of this textbook. When the tumour is exposed, a sample of tissue (biopsy) is sent to the pathology laboratory for a 'frozen-section' histological examination. This can be done rapidly while the person remains on the operating table under anaesthesia. If the initial report is negative, the benign mass is usually removed to prevent further symptoms. If the report is positive for cancer, the tumour and, often, adjacent lymph nodes are resected, along with any other suspicious tissue. The tumour, nodes and any other specimens are sent to the pathology laboratory for more in-depth analysis. The person then receives the usual postoperative care.

LABORATORY TESTS Most laboratory tests of blood, urine and other body fluids are used to rule out nutritional disorders and other non-cancerous conditions that may be causing the person's symptoms. For example, a full blood count (FBC) helps screen for such problems as anaemia, infection and impaired immunity. Blood chemistries can point out nutritional disturbances and electrolyte imbalances. In conjunction with other diagnostic studies, some laboratory tests can be quite useful either in screening for other pathological conditions or for validating the cancer diagnosis (LeFever Kee, 2018). These tests include evaluating levels of enzymes such as alanine aminotransferase (alT), aspartate aminotransferase (AST) and lactic dehydrogenase (LDH) for liver metastases. Special protein tumour markers such as PSA for prostate cancer and CEA for colon cancer are also used. Table 13.8 identifies some useful laboratory tests, their normal values and their possible indications. This is an evolving area, with new methods and tests being developed (Burki, 2018).

TABLE 13.8 Laboratory tests used for cancer diagnosis*

TEST	REFERENCE VALUE	ABNORMALITY INDICATED
Acid phosphatase (ACP)		No longer used for prostatic cancer diagnosis
Adrenocorticotropic hormone (ACTH)	8-80 pg/mL	Decreased in adrenal cancer Elevated in pituitary cancer or with tumour that secretes ACTH (bronchiogenic cancer)
Alanine aminotransferase (alT)	Female: <35 u/L Male: <40 u/L	Moderate elevation in liver cancer
Albumin	35-40 g/L	Decreased in malnutrition, metastatic liver cancer
Alkaline phosphatase (alP)	Adult: 35-135 u/L	Elevated in cancer of liver, bone, breast and prostate, in leukaemia and in multiple myeloma
Alpha-fetoprotein (AFP)	Male and non-pregnant female: <11 ng/mL	Elevated in germ-cell tumours (e.g. seminoma), testicular cancer
Aspartate aminotransferase (AST)	<42 u/L	Elevated in liver cancer
Bilirubin	<20 mg/dL	Elevated in liver and gallbladder cancer
Bleeding time	Ivy method: 2-9 minutes	Prolonged in leukaemia and metastatic liver cancer
Blood urea nitrogen (BUN)	3.0-8.0 mmol/L	Decreased in malnutrition; increased in renal cancer
Calcitonin	Male: <40 pg/mL Female: <20 pg/mL	Elevated to 7,500 pg/mL in thyroid medullary cancer, breast cancer and lung cancer
Calcium (Ca)	2.15-2.65 mmol/L	Elevated in bone cancer and ectopic parathyroid hormone production (paraplastic syndrome)
Carcinoembryonic antigen (CEA)	2.5 ng/mL in non-smokers 5 ng/mL in smokers: >12 ng/mL neoplasms	Elevated with GI cancers, lung, breast, bladder, kidney, cervical cancers and leukaemias. Used to evaluate effectiveness of cancer treatment
Chloride (Cl)	95-108 mmol/L	Decreased in vomiting, diarrhoea, syndrome of inappropriate antidiuretic hormone (SIADH)
C-reactive protein	<10 mg/L	Elevated in metastatic cancer and Burkitt's lymphoma
Creatinine	Male: 50-110 µmol/L Female: 40-80 µmol/L	Decreased in malnutrition; elevated in most cancers
Dexamethasone suppression test	>50% reduction in plasma cortisol	Non-suppression in adrenal cancer and ACTH-producing tumours, severe stress
Oestradiol	Female: 20-300 pg/mL Menopausal female: <20 pg/mL Male: 15-50 pg/Ml	Elevated in oestrogen-producing tumours and testicular tumours
Fibrinogen	2.0-4.0 g/L	Decreased in leukaemia and as a side effect of chemotherapy
Gamma glutamyltransferase (GammaGT)	Male: <60 u/L Female: <40 u/L	Elevated in cancer of liver, pancreas, prostate, breast, kidney, lung and brain
Fasting blood sugar	3.5-5.5 mmol/L	Decreased in malnutrition, cancer of stomach, liver and lung

TABLE 13.8 Laboratory tests used for cancer diagnosis* (continued)

TEST	REFERENCE VALUE	ABNORMALITY INDICATED
Haptoglobin	0.3–2.0 g/L	Elevated in Hodgkin's disease and cancer of lung, large intestine, stomach, breast and liver
Haemoglobin (Hgb)	Male: 132–170 g/L Female: 115–155 g/L	Decreased in anaemia, many cancers, Hodgkin's disease, leukaemia and malnutrition, and as a side effect of chemotherapy
Human chorionic gonadotropin (HCG)	Non-pregnant female: $<$0.01 international unit/L	Elevated in choriocarcinoma
Insulin	5–25 microunit/mL	Elevated in insulinoma (islet cell tumour) and insulin-secreting cancers (e.g. lung cancer)
Lactic dehydrogenase (LDH)	200–400 u/L	Elevated in liver, brain, kidney, muscle cancers, acute leukaemia, anaemia
Occult blood	Negative	Positive in gastric and colon cancers
Serum osmolality	280–300 mOsm/kg H_2O	Decreased in SIADH
Urine osmolality	50–1,200 mOsm/kg H_2O	Increased in SIADH
Parathyroid hormone (PTH)	1.5–6.5 pg/mL	Increased in PTH-secreting tumours
Platelet (thrombocyte) count	150–400 ($\times 10^9$/L)	Decreased in bone, gastric and brain cancer, in leukaemia and as a side effect of chemotherapy
Potassium (K)	3.4–5.5 mmol/L	Decreased in vomiting and diarrhoea, and in malnutrition
Prostatic-specific antigen (PSA)	Age-dependent 2.5–6.5 mg/L	Elevated from 10 to 120+ in prostate cancer
Total protein	60–80 g/L	Decreased in malnutrition, gastrointestinal cancer, Hodgkin's disease; elevated in vomiting, diarrhoea, multiple myeloma
Red cell count (RBCs)	Male: 4.5–5.5 million/mm^3 Female: 3.8–4.8 million/mm^3	Decreased in anaemia, leukaemia, infection, multiple myeloma
Sodium (Na)	134–146 mmol/L	Decreased in SIADH, vomiting; elevated in dehydration
Uric acid	Male: $<$0.44 mmol/L Female: $<$0.38 mmol/L	Increased in leukaemia, metastatic cancer, multiple myeloma, Burkitt's lymphoma and after vigorous chemotherapy
White blood cells (WBC)		
Total leucocytes	4,500–10,000/mm^3	Elevated in acute infection, leukaemias, tissue necrosis; decreased as a side effect of chemotherapy
Neutrophils	50–70%	Elevated in bacterial infection and Hodgkin's disease; decreased in leukaemia and malnutrition, and as a side effect of chemotherapy
Eosinophils	1–3%	Elevated in cancer of bone, ovary, testes and brain
Basophils	0.4–1.0%	Elevated in leukaemia and healing stage of infection
Monocytes	4–6%	Elevated in infection, monocytic leukaemia and cancer; decreased in lymphocytic leukaemia and as a side effect of chemotherapy
Lymphocytes	25–35%	Elevated in lymphocytic leukaemia, Hodgkin's disease, multiple myeloma, viral infections and chronic infections; decreased in malnutrition, cancer and other leukaemias, and as a side effect of chemotherapy

*All values refer to serum values unless otherwise indicated. Values are approximate; check the reference standards specified by your own organisation's laboratory.

PSYCHOLOGICAL SUPPORT DURING DIAGNOSIS Preparing for and awaiting the results of diagnostic tests can create extreme anxiety. Many people compare the experience to that of a prisoner awaiting trial and sentencing: after they know what the 'sentence' is, they can then prepare for the future. In addition to coping with the possibility of having a life-threatening disease or at least a life-altering one, people often also face the prospect of uncomfortable, even painful, diagnostic procedures. They have important decisions to make that depend on the outcome of those tests. Many unspoken questions may exist, including the following:

- Do I have cancer?
- If so, what kind and how serious?
- Has it spread?
- Will I survive?
- What kind of treatment is needed?
- How will this affect my lifestyle?
- How will this affect my family members and friends?

Denial or intellectualisation serves some people well, but others display signs of anxiety and stress as they attempt to cope. The nurse can provide valuable support during this very difficult stage by helping people become actively involved in managing their life and disease. Talk with the person as soon as they enter the healthcare system, asking what they know already about what is going to happen and soliciting questions from them. Taking this approach and encouraging people to share what knowledge and experience they have allows them to maintain control. From there, the nurse can provide the information needed.

It is essential that people thoroughly understand the preparation required for their tests, especially if they will be preparing at home. They also need to be informed of any unusual effects that may occur as a result of the procedure, such as nausea from radioactive dye. If possible, a phone call the evening before to verify the person's understanding of the procedure and to answer questions can be helpful and supportive.

As the person begins to feel more comfortable with the nurse, they may express concerns, fears and other emotions. The nurse should actively listen and be supportive, but avoid giving advice and false reassurance, providing appropriate information when needed. For people who are not ready to discuss their concerns, or for those who appear angry, being non-judgmental and providing non-verbal support may facilitate more open communication. An atmosphere of calmness, warmth, caring and respect can ease the tension and often unspoken terror of this initial period.

Support of and communication with the person's significant others is extremely important. Often they try to be strong for the person but have many fears and emotional concerns that they do not feel comfortable expressing. The nurse needs to be available to the family while the person is undergoing diagnostic procedures. Allowing them to talk without the need to edit for the person's benefit can help them manage their own difficulties in coping with their loved one's potential cancer diagnosis.

Cancer treatment

The goals of cancer treatment are aimed at cure, control or palliation of symptoms. These goals may overlap. Cancer may be treated through surgery, chemotherapy, radiation therapy, biotherapy, photodynamic therapy, bone marrow and stem cell transplants, and complementary therapies. Once cancer is diagnosed, the initial focus is on surgical and medical treatment. The goals of treatment are:

- eliminating the tumour or malignant cells
- preventing metastasis
- reducing cellular growth and the tumour burden
- promoting functional abilities and providing pain relief to those whose disease has not responded to treatment.

SURGERY Surgery was once considered the only treatment for cancer before the mechanisms of cancer were understood. Today, surgery remains an important approach in cancer care. Surgical resection is used for diagnosis and staging of more than 90% of all cancers and for primary treatment of more than 60% of cancers. The goals of surgery have also expanded to include prophylaxis, diagnosis, treatment, reconstruction and palliation.

Prophylactic surgery aims to remove tissues or organs that are likely to develop cancer. Advances in identification of genetic markers make prophylactic surgery an option for individuals with a strong family history and genetic predisposition for the development of cancer. For example, a woman with a strong history of breast cancer, positive findings of BRCA-1 or BRCA-2 and abnormal finding on mammography may consider prophylactic mastectomy as one of the selective options. Other examples of prophylactic operations include colectomy and oophorectomy. With limited research on the long-term physiological and psychological effects on individuals undergoing prophylactic surgery for cancer, it is vital for nurses and other healthcare professionals to discuss the potential risks and postoperative outcomes of the prophylactic surgery thoroughly with the person and their family prior to the surgery. Nurses should respect the person's decision whether or not to pursue the prophylactic surgery. For those people who choose prophylactic surgery as a preventive measure for cancer, comprehensive preoperative teaching and counselling should be provided and long-term postoperative follow-up should be ensured to monitor the person's physiological and psychological adjustment to the surgery.

Diagnostic surgery aims to ensure histological diagnosis and staging of cancer through biopsy, endoscopy, laparoscopy and open surgical exploration. Table 13.9 provides information about common surgical diagnostic procedures.

As a primary treatment for cancer, the goal of surgery is to remove the entire tumour and involved surrounding tissue and

TABLE 13.9 Surgical diagnostic procedures

PROCEDURE	EXPLANATION
Fine-needle biopsy	Use of a very thin needle to aspirate a small amount of tissue from the tumours
Needle core biopsy	Use of a slightly larger needle than that used for a fine-needle biopsy to extract a small amount of tissue from tumours that cannot be aspirated by fine-needle aspiration
Incisional biopsy	Removal of part of a larger tumour by cutting through the skin
Excisional biopsy	Removal of an entire tumour through operation
Endoscopy	Use of a small viewing lens or video camera through natural body openings to view tumours such as cancer of the oesophagus, stomach or colon
Laparoscopy	Use of a small viewing lens or video camera through a small incision in the abdominal wall

lymph nodes as much as possible and feasible. This sometimes necessitates mutilation of the body and the creation of new structures to assume the function of the lost structures. For example, removal of the distal sigmoid colon and rectum requires a new means of bowel elimination, so the remaining healthy segment of the bowel is brought out through a created opening (stoma) in the abdominal wall, resulting in a permanent colostomy (see the chapter 'Nursing care of people with bowel disorders'). In like manner, when the bladder is removed, the ureters are transplanted into a created pouch just under the abdominal wall. This serves as a continent ileostomy, a substitute reservoir for urine (see the chapter 'Nursing care of people with urinary tract disorders'). Surgery can also destroy sensitive nerve plexuses, resulting in alteration or loss of normal functioning; for example, prostate surgery may result in incontinence and impotence. Surgical removal of involved regional lymph nodes can also lead to long-term lymphoedema (swelling in the affected area) that greatly impacts on cancer survivors' quality of life; for instance, lymphoedema following surgery for breast cancer and melanoma (Norman et al., 2009).

Not all surgery results in such radical changes in functioning. The following surgeries can eliminate cancer successfully with less distressing results:

- removing a non-essential portion of the organ or tissue containing the tumour, such as in situ small-bowel tumours
- removing an organ whose function can be replaced chemically, such as the thyroid
- resecting one of a pair of organs when the unaffected organ can take over the function of the missing one, such as a lung.

Although the removal of any major body part has physiological and psychological consequences, the alternative—terminal disease—is usually less desirable.

If the tumour is in a non-resectable location or deeply invasive with metastases, surgery may be a palliative measure to allow the involved organs to function as long as possible, to relieve pain and provide comfort, or to bypass an obstruction. Surgery may also be done to reduce the bulk of the tumour in advanced disease, both at primary and metastatic sites. Decreasing the tumour size enhances the ability to control the remaining disease through other modalities. Surgery is often used in conjunction with other treatments to effect a cure. In cases when extensive removal of tissue is contraindicated (e.g. in surgical removal of a brain tumour), radiation may be used prior to surgery in an attempt to shrink the tumour before it is removed.

Surgical intervention may also be used for reconstruction and rehabilitation to achieve more desirable functional and cosmetic effects after curative or radical surgery. One example is the construction of transabdominal myocutaneous (TRAM) flaps in conjunction with or following modified radical mastectomy (see the chapter 'Nursing care of women with reproductive system and breast disorders'). For surgical interventions for cancers affecting specific body systems, refer to later chapters.

Surgical oncologists are working with researchers to identify premalignant disease earlier in high-risk populations and to conduct studies on ways to reverse oncogenic cell activity. Surgeons also work with molecular biologists using sophisticated techniques to develop monoclonal antibodies. Laser technology is being explored for use in different types of cancer surgery because it minimises blood loss, reduces deformity, increases the accuracy of tissue resection and enhances healing. Lasers are currently being used to treat radical prostatectomy in order to preserve urinary continence and sexual functioning. Another collaborative strategy under development is intraoperative radiation therapy, in which radiosensitive, non-diseased organs that may be damaged by radiation therapy are moved away from the radiation field and shielded. Radiation is then administered while the person is on the operating table. This technique allows more penetrating radiation to be directed to the malignant tumour with less trauma to normal, vulnerable tissues or organs.

Nursing responsibilities focus on preparing the person physically and psychologically for the specific surgery, as well as teaching routine postoperative care in which the person is expected to participate. For example, the nurse teaches the person about respiratory care and deep breathing to improve postoperative ventilation, about early ambulation to prevent circulatory problems and about how the person will receive fluids and nutrition (intravenously or orally, depending on the type of surgery). In addition, the nurse explains the specific surgical procedure and any anticipated alterations to the person's body, especially those that require major lifestyle adjustments, such as a colostomy. Before surgery, the nurse should give the person the opportunity to ask questions and to discuss concerns and fears. In some cases, the person may want to discuss alternative treatment options. In the latter case, the nurse should contact the oncologist and the surgeon and set up a conference for the person before surgery.

CHEMOTHERAPY **Chemotherapy** involves the use of cytotoxic medications to cure some cancers, such as leukaemias, lymphomas and some solid tumours; to decrease tumour size, adjunctive to surgery or radiation therapy; or to prevent or treat suspected metastases. Chemotherapy may also be used in conjunction with biotherapy. All chemotherapy has side effects or toxic effects. The type and severity depend on the drugs used.

Chemotherapy disrupts the cell cycle in various phases by interrupting cell metabolism and replication. It also works by interfering with the ability of the malignant cell to synthesise vital enzymes and chemicals. Phase-specific drugs work during only some phases of the cell cycle; non-phase-specific drugs work through the entire cell cycle. Figure 13.5 lists some of the drugs useful in each phase of the cell cycle.

Most chemical treatment involves combinations of drugs in specific protocols given over varying periods of time. One protocol for adult acute lymphocytic leukaemia (alL) uses the acronym DVPA: daunorubicin given on days 1 to 3; vincristine given on days 1, 8, 15 and 22; prednisone given on days 1 to 28 and asparaginase given on days 17 to 28. The treatment regimen is given in cycles with rest periods allowed, especially if toxic effects such as liver dysfunction or severe neutropenia occur. The treatment is continued until the disease goes into remission. If the disease progresses, the particular protocol is abandoned and a new one may be tried.

The cell-kill hypothesis explains why several courses of chemotherapy are necessary. A 1 cm tumour contains about

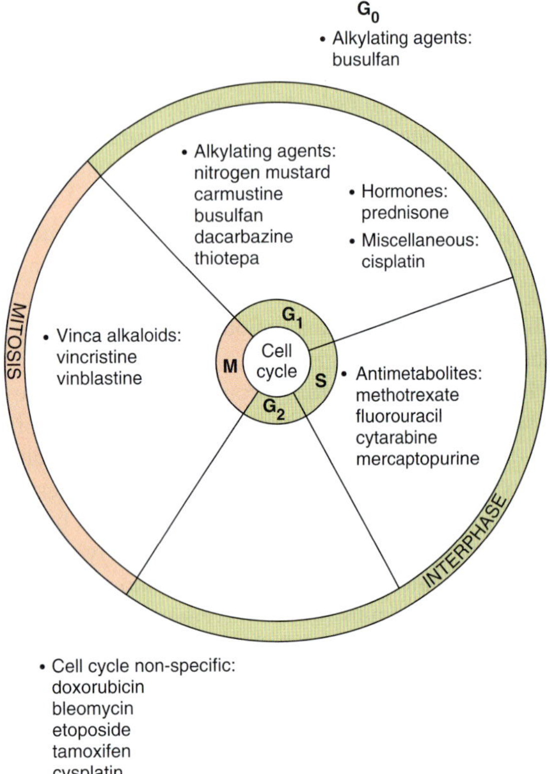

FIGURE 13.5 ***Chemotherapeutic drugs useful in each phase of the cell cycle. Based on their chemical make-up and biological activity, different drugs used for cancer treatment act in specific phases and subphases of the cell cycle. Some drugs, called non-phase-specific drugs, are generalised and act throughout the cycle. Chemotherapy often involves combinations of drugs designed to attack the cancer cells at many different times in the cycle and thus to enhance effectiveness***

10^9 (10 billion) total cells, most of which are viable. During each cell cycle, the chemotherapy kills a fixed percentage of cells, always leaving some behind. With each reduction, the tumour burden of cells decreases until the number of viable, clonogenic cells (i.e. those that are able to clone daughter cells) becomes small enough to allow the body's immune system to finish the job. Oncologists usually give the maximum amount of chemotherapy tolerated by the person. High-dose chemotherapy remains controversial.

Classes of chemotherapy drugs Chemotherapeutic agents can be classified either by the effects of the agent on the cell or by the pharmacological properties of the agent. According to the effects of the agent on the cell, chemotherapeutic agents can be divided into cell-cycle-specific and cell-cycle-non-specific agents. Cell-cycle-specific agents are effective at a specific phase (e.g. S and M phases) in the cell cycle to prevent cell replication by damaging cellular DNA and blocking production of protein necessary for DNA and RNA synthesis. Cell-cycle-non-specific agents are effective throughout all the phases of the cell cycle, including the resting phase. Both cell-cycle-specific and cell-cycle-non-specific agents are effective in rapidly dividing cells to prohibit the growth of fast-growing tumours.

The most common way of classifying chemotherapeutic agents is based on pharmacological properties of the agent. The classifications include alkylating agents, antimetabolites, antitumour antibiotics, mitotic inhibitors, hormones and hormone antagonists, and miscellaneous agents.

Alkylating agents Alkylating agents are not phase specific and basically act on preformed nucleic acids by creating defects in tumour DNA. They cause crosslinking of DNA strands, which can permanently interfere with replication and transcription.

Alkylating agents work with both proliferating and non-proliferating cells (those in the G_0 phase). Their toxicity relates to their ability to kill slowly cycling stem cells and manifests in delayed, prolonged or permanent bone marrow failure. Toxicity can also cause a mutagenic effect on bone marrow stem cells, culminating in a treatment-resistant form of acute myelogenous leukaemia. Because of the alkylating agents' effect on stem cells, they also cause irreversible infertility. Other common adverse effects include nephrotoxicity and haemorrhagic cystitis.

The several subclasses of alkylating agents include nitrogen mustard (mechlorethamine), nitrosoureas (carmustine), alkyl sulfonates (busulfan), triazines (dacarbazine), ethyleneimines (thiotepa) and cisplatin. Cisplatin is an alkylating agent containing platinum and chlorine atoms. It is most active in the G_1 subphase, but it is also not phase specific. Cisplatin binds to DNA and acts much like alkylating agents by forming intrastrand DNA crosslinks (gluing strands of DNA together so that they cannot separate). Its major toxic effect is reversible renal tubular necrosis. Cisplatin may be used alone or in combination with other chemotherapeutic drugs for testicular and ovarian cancers.

Antimetabolites The different types of antimetabolites include folic acid analogues (methotrexate), pyrimidine analogues (5-fluorouracil), cytosine arabinoside (ARA-C) and purine analogues (6-mercaptopurine). Antimetabolites are phase specific, working best in the S phase and having little effect in G_0. They interfere with nucleic acid synthesis by either displacing normal metabolites at the regulatory site of a key enzyme or by substituting for a metabolite that is incorporated into DNA or RNA molecules. Toxic effects usually do not occur until very high levels of the drug are administered. Toxicity is also more likely when the drugs accumulate in third-spaced fluid, such as pleural fluid (a characteristic that also makes them useful in treating malignant pleural effusions). Because the drug diffuses out slowly from the third-spaced fluid, exposure of the tissue to the drug is prolonged. Most toxic effects relate to rapidly proliferating cells, such as cells in the gastrointestinal tract, hair and skin, and white blood cells (WBCs). Signs and symptoms include nausea and vomiting, stomatitis, diarrhoea, alopecia and leukopenia. Some of the drugs can also cause liver and pulmonary toxicity.

Antitumour antibiotics Antitumour antibiotics are derived from natural sources that are generally too toxic to be used as antibacterial agents. They are not phase specific and act in several ways: they disrupt DNA replication and RNA transcription; create free radicals, which generate breaks in DNA and other forms of damage; and interfere with DNA repair. These drugs bind to cells and kill them, probably by damaging the cell membrane. Their main toxic effect is damage to the cardiac muscle. This limits the amount and duration of treatment. Examples of these antibiotics include actinomycin D, doxorubicin, bleomycin, mitomycin-C and mithramycin.

Mitotic inhibitors Mitotic inhibitors are drugs that act to prevent cell division during the M phase. Mitotic inhibitors include the plant alkaloids and taxoids. Plant alkaloids consist of medications extracted from plant sources: vinca alkaloids (e.g. vincristine and vinblastine) and etoposide (also called VP-16). The vinca alkaloids are phase specific, acting during mitosis. They bind to a specific protein in tumour cells that promotes chromosome migration during mitosis and serves as a conduit for neurotransmitter transport along axons. The toxicity of these drugs is characterised by depression of deep tendon reflexes, paraesthesias (pain and altered sensation), motor weakness, cranial nerve disruptions and paralytic ileus. Etoposide acts in all phases of the cell cycle, causing breaks in DNA and metaphase arrest. Although etoposide may cause bone marrow suppression and nausea and vomiting, the most common toxic effect is hypotension resulting from too rapid intravenous administration.

The taxoids act during the G_2 phase to inhibit cell division. Paclitaxel is used for the treatment of Kaposi's sarcoma and metastatic breast and ovarian cancer. Taxotere is used for breast cancer. Toxicities associated with these drugs include alopecia, bone marrow depression and severe hypersensitivity reactions (e.g. hypotension, dyspnoea and urticaria).

Hormones and hormone antagonists The main hormones used in cancer therapy are the corticosteroids (e.g. prednisone), which are phase specific (G_1). These act by binding to specific intracellular receptors, repressing transcription of mRNA and thereby altering cellular function and growth. Corticosteroids have multiple side effects such as impaired healing, hyperglycaemia, hypertension, osteoporosis and hirsutism.

Hormone antagonists work with hormone-binding tumours, usually those of the breast, prostate and endometrium. They block the hormone's receptor site on the tumour and prevent it from receiving normal hormonal growth stimulation. These drugs do not cure, but do cause regression of the tumour in about 40% of breast and endometrial tumours, and 80% of prostate tumours. Tamoxifen competes with oestradiol receptors in breast tumours. Raloxifene blocks oestrogen in the breast. Diethylstilbestrol competes with hormone receptors in endometrial and prostate tumours. Antiandrogen (Flutamide) and luteinising-hormone-releasing hormones block testosterone synthesis in prostate cancers. The main side effects of these drugs are alterations of the secondary sexual characteristics.

Miscellaneous agents Several miscellaneous agents act at different phases in the cell cycle. L-Asparaginase and hydroxyurea are examples of miscellaneous agents.

Effects of chemotherapeutic drugs As described, the side effects and toxic effects of chemotherapy vary with the drug used and the length of treatment. Because most of these drugs act on fast-growing cells, the side effects are manifestations of damage to normal rapidly dividing somatic cells. The side effects of hormones express the action of the hormone used or suppression of the normal hormone, such as the masculinising effects of male hormones administered for ovarian cancers.

Tissues usually affected by cytotoxic drugs include the following:

- Mucous membranes of the mouth, tongue, oesophagus, stomach, intestine and rectum. This may result in anorexia, loss of taste, aversion to food, erythema and painful ulcerations in any portion of the gastrointestinal tract, nausea, vomiting and diarrhoea.
- Hair cells, resulting in alopecia.
- Bone marrow depression affecting most blood cells (e.g. granulocytes, lymphocytes, thrombocytes and erythrocytes). This results in an impaired ability to respond to infection, a diminished ability to clot blood and severe anaemia.
- Organs, such as heart, lungs, bladder, kidneys. This kind of damage is related to specific agents, such as cardiac toxicity with doxorubicin or pneumonitis with bleomycin.
- Reproductive organs, resulting in impaired reproductive ability or altered fetal development.

Table 13.10 gives the classifications of chemotherapeutic drugs, common examples, target malignancies, adverse effects and side effects, and nursing implications. Consult current pharmacology textbooks for additional drugs and for new combination therapies as they are developed.

Preparation and administration Australia has legislative Acts and regulations that govern the handling, labelling, transport, waste disposal, documentation and the designation, training and employee health monitoring of staff engaged in duties with the potential for exposure to radiation (including, but not limited to, *Occupational Health and Safety Act (OH&S) 2000*, OH&S Regulations 2001, *Poisons & Therapeutic Goods Act 1966, Cytotoxic Drugs & Related Waste: Risk Management Guide 2008* and Australian Radiation Protection and Nuclear Safety Agency—Radiation Protection Series Codes and Guides). Organisations are required to have procedures in place to minimise risk to staff (environmental and personal protective equipment) when preparing, administering and disposing of chemotherapeutic drugs, and individuals are required to demonstrate duty of care and to follow legislative and organisational guidelines. Refer to your organisation's policy/procedures. It is the nurse's responsibility to ensure they are working within their NMBA standards. The nurse is required to teach people to dispose of their own body fluids safely. Oral medications pose a lesser risk of exposure, but a risk nonetheless, primarily through excretion in the urine.

Chemotherapeutic drugs, such as cyclophosphamide and chlorambucil, can be administered orally. Other drugs, such as hormones or hormone-blocking agents, may also be given intramuscularly. However, many drugs require intravenous infusion or direct injection into intraperitoneal or intrapleural body

TABLE 13.10 Classifications of chemotherapeutic drugs

DRUG CLASSIFICATION	COMMON DRUGS	TARGET MALIGNANCIES	ADVERSE EFFECTS OR SIDE EFFECTS	NURSING IMPLICATIONS
Alkylating agents	Mechlorethamine	Hodgkin's disease Lymphosarcoma Lung cancer Chronic leukaemia	Nausea and vomiting Leucopenia Thrombocytopenia Hyperuricaemia	Maintain good hydration. Alkalinise urine. Administer anti-emetics prior to chemotherapy. Monitor WBC, uric acid. Assess for infection.
	Busulfan	Chronic myelogenous leukaemia	Leucopenia Thrombocytopenia Renal failure Pulmonary fibrosis	Monitor WBCs, BUN. Maintain adequate fluid intake. Assess for infection. Assess lungs for fibrotic (coarse, loud) rales.
	Cyclophosphamide	Lymphomas Multiple myeloma Leukaemias Adenocarcinoma of lung and breast	Haemorrhagic cystitis Renal failure Alopecia Stomatitis Liver dysfunction Infertility	Encourage daily fluid intake of 2 to 3 L during treatment. Monitor WBCs, BUN, liver enzymes. Teach ways to manage hair loss.
Antimetabolites	Methotrexate	Acute lymphoblastic leukaemia Osteosarcoma Gestational trophoblastic carcinoma	Oral and gastrointestinal ulcerations Anorexia and nausea Leucopenia Thrombocytopenia Pancytopenia	Monitor CBC, WBC differential, BUN, uric acid, creatinine. Assess oral mucous membranes; treat ulcers prn. Assess for infection, bleeding.
	5-fluorouracil (5-FU)	Colon carcinoma Rectal carcinoma Breast carcinoma Gastric carcinoma Pancreatic cancer	Stomatitis Alopecia Nausea and vomiting Gastritis Enteritis Diarrhoea Anaemia Leucopenia Thrombocytopenia Red sore peeling hands and feet	Monitor CBC with differential, BUN, uric acid. Administer anti-emetics prn. Assess for bleeding; check stool occult blood. Evaluate hydration and nutrition status. Teach oral care for stomatitis. Assess for infection. Teach care for hair loss.
Antitumour antibiotics	Doxorubicin	Acute lymphoblastic leukaemia (ALL) Acute myeloblastic leukaemia Neuroblastoma Wilms' tumour Breast, ovarian, thyroid, lung cancer	Stomatitis Alopecia Nausea and vomiting Gastritis Enteritis Diarrhoea Anaemia Leucopenia Thrombocytopenia Cardiac toxicity	Monitor ECG; assess for arrhythmias, gallops and congestive heart failure (CHF). Monitor CBC with differential, BUN, uric acid. Administer anti-emetics prn. Assess for bleeding; check stool for occult blood. Evaluate hydration and nutrition status. Teach oral care for stomatitis. Assess for infection. Teach care for hair loss.
	Bleomycin	Squamous cell carcinoma Lymphosarcoma Reticulum cell sarcoma Testicular carcinoma Hodgkin's disease	Mucocutaneous ulcerations Alopecia Nausea and vomiting Chills and fever Pneumonitis and pulmonary fibrosis	Check for fever 3 to 6 hours after administration. Have chest x-ray films taken every 2 to 3 weeks. Assess respiratory status and check for coarse rales. Evaluate hydration and nutrition status. Teach oral care for stomatitis. Assess for infection. Teach care for hair loss.

TABLE 13.10 Classifications of chemotherapeutic drugs (continued)

DRUG CLASSIFICATION	COMMON DRUGS	TARGET MALIGNANCIES	ADVERSE EFFECTS OR SIDE EFFECTS	NURSING IMPLICATIONS
Plant alkaloids	Vincristine	Combination therapy for acute leukaemia, Hodgkin's and non-Hodgkin's lymphomas, rhabdomyosarcoma, neuroblastoma, Wilms' tumour	Areflexia Peripheral neuritis Constipation Paralytic ileus Mild bone marrow Depression	Assess neuromuscular function. Monitor FBC with differential. Evaluate gastrointestinal function. Manage constipation.
	Vinblastine	Combination therapy for Hodgkin's disease, lymphocytic and histocytic lymphoma Kaposi's sarcoma, advanced testicular carcinoma, unresponsive breast cancer	Areflexia Alopecia Nausea and vomiting Bone marrow depression Tingling and numbness of fingers and toes	Assess neuromuscular function. Monitor FBC with differential. Administer anti-emetics prn. Teach ways to manage hair loss.
	Etoposide, also called VP-16	Non-responsive testicular tumours Small-cell lung cancer	Alopecia Hypotension with rapid infusion Facial flushing Sweating Difficulty breathing/ wheezing	Hydrate adequately before administration. Administer for 60 minutes. Monitor vital signs every 15 minutes during administration and every 2 to 4 hours thereafter. Teach ways to manage hair loss.
	Prednisolone	Combination therapy for many tumours Leukaemia Lymphoma	Fluid retention Hypertension Steroid diabetes Emotional lability Silent bleeding ulcers Increased risk of infection Euphoria or insomnia	Monitor vital signs. Administer diuretics prn. Check blood glucose regularly. Evaluate mental status. Administer oral medications with food. Administer hydrogen ion antagonist drugs (antacids) as ordered. Monitor WBC with differential. Check for signs of systemic infection.
	Diethylstilbestrol (DES)	Advanced breast and prostrate cancers	Fluid retention Feminisation Uterine bleeding	Monitor vital signs. Administer diuretics prn as ordered. Explain reason for feminisation to men, bleeding to women. Monitor for excessive bleeding.
	Tamoxifen	Breast cancer	Hot flashes Nausea and vomiting	Explain reason for hot flashes. Teach ways to manage hot flashes. Administer anti-emetics as ordered.
Miscellaneous drugs	Cisplatin (CDDP) (Platinol)	Combination and single therapy for metastatic testicular and ovarian cancers, advanced bladder cancer, head and neck tumours, non-small-cell lung carcinoma, osteogenic sarcoma, neuroblastoma	Bone marrow depression: leucopenia and thrombocytopenia Renal tubular damage Deafness	Monitor WBC with differential and platelets, BUN, creatinine, uric acid. Watch for bleeding. Monitor for signs of infection. Evaluate hearing; check for tinnitus. Ensure that person is well hydrated before drug is administered. Encourage 2 to 3 L of fluid intake daily.

cavities. Intravenous preparations can be given through large peripheral veins, but the risk of extravasation or irritation to the vein may preclude this method for long-term therapy. Many people now receive central venous access devices (CVADs), especially if their treatment requires several cycles over weeks or months. CVADs are also useful for adjunctive parenteral nutrition in the person who needs continuous intravenous infusions to manage pain or frequent blood drawing to monitor blood counts. Different types of CVADs are available:

- Catheters inserted non-surgically by threading them through a large peripheral vein into the vena cava. Called *peripherally inserted central catheters (PICCs)*, they have multiple lumens that facilitate blood drawing. Placement is usually monitored by fluoroscopy.
- Catheters tunnelled under the skin on the chest into a major vein, such as the subclavian vein. Hickman or Groshong catheters may be used.
- Surgically implanted ports, placed under the skin with a connected catheter inserted into a major vein. These are accessed by means of a special needle with a 90-degree angle inserted through the skin directly into the rubber dome of the port, which has a hard plastic back to prevent tissue damage.

Figure 13.6 shows examples of different catheters and vascular access ports.

Risk of infection, catheter obstruction and extravasation are the main problems associated with CVADs. Nurses therefore must teach people and family members to observe for redness, swelling, pain or exudate at the insertion site, which may indicate infection; to observe for swelling of the neck or skin near the CVAD for extravasation and infiltration; and to flush catheters and provide site care (cleaning and dressing changes) on a regular basis. During each encounter with the person, the nurse always inspects the site; observes for infection, infiltration and catheter occlusion, and provides site care when necessary.

Management of people receiving chemotherapy In addition to providing the previously mentioned nursing interventions, nurses help identify and manage toxic effects or side effects of the drugs and provide psychosocial support. Careful assessment and monitoring of the person's signs and symptoms, including appropriate laboratory tests, alert the nurse to the onset of toxicity. Nausea and vomiting, diarrhoea, inflammation and ulceration of oral mucous membranes, hair loss, skin changes, anorexia and fatigue require specific medical and nursing actions. These actions are discussed later in this chapter under the appropriate nursing diagnoses. Indicators of organ toxicities, such as nephrotoxicity, neurotoxicity or cardiac toxicity, must be reported immediately to the doctor. Another aspect of managing people undergoing chemotherapy is to teach them how to care for access sites and to dispose of used equipment and excretions safely. Nurses also teach people to increase fluid intake to flush out the drugs; to get extra rest, which can both assist therapy and help the person avoid other illnesses; to identify major complications of their particular drug protocol; to know when to call the doctor or emergency medical services; and, if their WBC count is low, to limit their exposure to other people, especially children or those with infections.

During chemotherapy, a number of psychological issues that can cause moderate to severe emotional distress may arise. The need to plan activities around chemotherapy treatments and their side effects can impair the person's ability to work, manage a household or care for family members, function sexually or participate in social and recreational activities. Weight loss and alopecia may prompt feelings of powerlessness and depression. The nurse can assist by carefully evaluating symptoms, providing specific interventions as indicated and allowing people opportunities to express their fears, concerns and feelings. People should be encouraged to participate in their

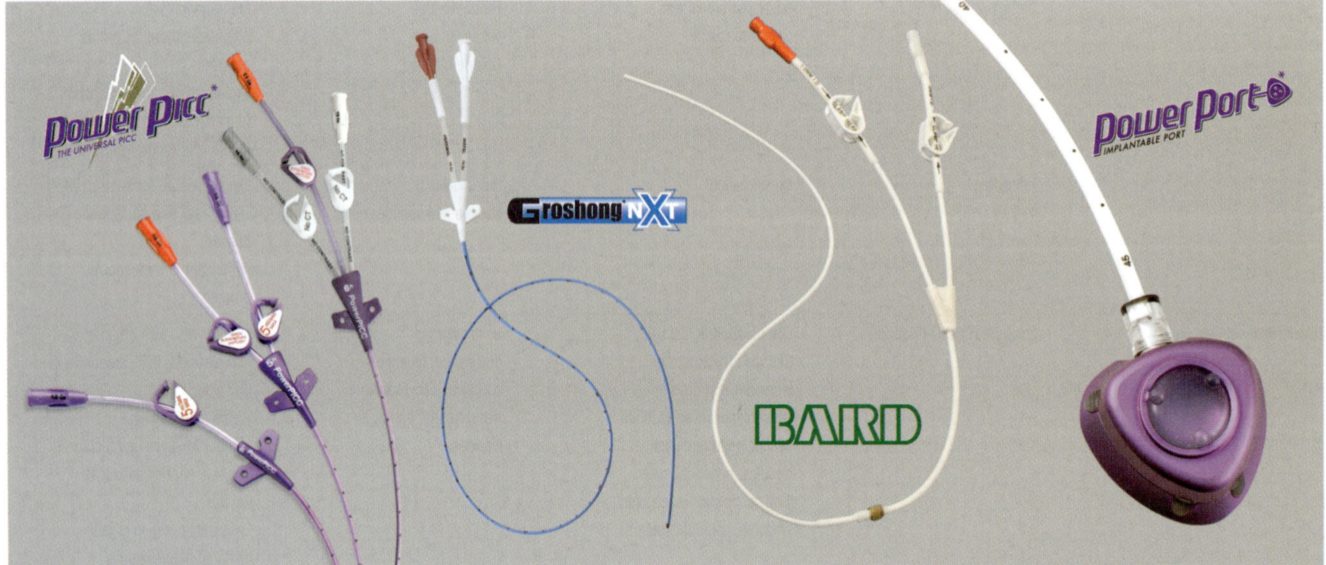

FIGURE 13.6 ***Vascular access devices: peripherally inserted central catheters (single, dual and triple lumen PowerPICC and dual lumen Groshong), tunnelled central venous catheter (dual lumen Hickman) and implantable port (PowerPort)***

Source: Courtesy and © Becton, Dickinson and Company. Reprinted with permission.

care and maintain control over their life as much as possible. Specific interventions are discussed later in the chapter under the appropriate nursing diagnoses. Table 13.10 includes nursing implications for specific adverse effects of common chemotherapy drugs.

RADIATION THERAPY Still the treatment of choice for some tumours or by some oncologists, radiation may be used to kill the tumour, reduce its size, decrease pain or relieve obstruction. Lymph nodes and adjacent tissues are irradiated when beginning metastasis is suspected. **Radiation therapy** consists of delivering ionising radiations of gamma and x-rays in one of two ways:

1. *External radiation*, also known as teletherapy, involves delivery of radiation from a source at some distance from the person. A relatively uniform dosage is delivered to the tumour.
2. *Brachytherapy*. In brachytherapy, the radioactive material is placed directly into or adjacent to the tumour, a technique that delivers a high dose to the tumour and a lower dose to the normal tissues. This allows delivery of high doses of radiation to the tumour while sparing adjacent tissue. Brachytherapy is also referred to as internal, interstitial or intracavitary radiation.

For many common neoplasms, a combination of these two therapies is used.

Lethal injury to DNA is believed to be the primary mechanism by which radiation kills cells, especially cells in faster-growing tumours and tissues. As a result, when given over time, radiation can destroy not only rapidly multiplying cancer cells but also rapidly dividing normal cells, such as those of the skin and mucous membranes. A malignant tumour is considered cured when there are no surviving tumour stem cells. The goal of radiation therapy is to achieve maximum tumour control with a minimum of damage to normal tissue.

Implanted or ingested radiation can be dangerous for those living with, taking care of or treating the person. Caregivers must use protection by shielding themselves from the source of radiation, limiting the time of exposure to the person, increasing the distance from the person and using specific safety procedures for handling secretions. Box 13.6 identifies safety principles to be followed by those caring for people undergoing internal radiation.

PATIENT SAFETY COMPETENCY FRAMEWORK

9 Medication safety

The Patient Safety Competency Framework indicates that nursing students must demonstrate medication safety (Levett-Jones et al., 2017).

BOX 13.6 General safety principles for radiation

Guidelines from the 2008 Australian Radiation Protection and Nuclear Safety Agency (ARPANSA) include:

- a radiation management plan that must be reviewed every 5 years to support updates and changes
- storage, handling and disposal of radioactive materials
- protection of employees, patients and members of the public who care for, support or comfort patients
- protection of health professionals, other than those trained in nuclear medicine, who may have close contact with patients
- accidental, abnormal or unplanned exposures to radiation
- relevant regulatory requirements that need to be satisfied.

Post procedure, a risk assessment should be completed and the following care introduced:

- A single room should be used to minimise exposure to staff and other people.
- Nursing staff carrying out procedures with the possibility of contamination should wear suitable gloves and gowns at all times.
- Essential care should be clustered together to limit patient interaction.
- Readily identified signage needs to be posted on the patient's room to keep clinicians and visitors safe during the initial exposure period.
- It is preferable to assign staff who are unlikely to be pregnant.
- Staff should be subject to monitoring by personal monitors or an approved device. Records should be kept and available upon request.
- Nursing staff should never touch a radioactive source with the fingers. Special forceps or other remote-control equipment should be used to handle radioactive sources.
- Specific precautions should be used to reduce the risk of spill of body fluids that are radioactive.
- Handle bed linen and clothing with care and according to the organisation's protocol.
- Dispose of crockery and cutlery in radioactive waste (due to possible contamination).
- Patient transfer(s) must include a clear handover of the treatment plan, and current precautions must be advised to the receiving unit.
- In life-threatening situations, the patient's medical management will always take precedence over radiation safety considerations, with only essential staff involved. Patient ventilation should be via mask-bag system only.
- Consult the organisation's radiation therapy department for any questions or problems in caring for people with radioactive implants.

Source: ARPANSA (2008). *Safety guide: Radiation protection in nuclear medicine*. Radiation protection series no. 14.2. Canberra: ARPANSA.

BOX 13.7 Degree of radiosensitivity for selected cancers

Very radiosensitive
- Neuroblastoma
- Lymphomas
- Chronic leukaemia

Moderately radiosensitive
- Bronchogenic carcinoma
- Oesophageal carcinoma
- Squamous cell carcinoma
- Prostate carcinoma
- Cervical carcinoma
- Testicular carcinoma

Non-radiosensitive
- Many adenocarcinomas
- Fibrosarcoma
- Osteogenic carcinoma

Tumours have differing sensitivities to radiation. Tumours that have the greatest number of rapidly proliferating cancer cells usually exhibit the best early response to radiation. The decision to use radiation rather than other modalities is based on balancing the probability of controlling the tumour against the probability of causing complications, such as tissue damage. The decision is usually made by risk–benefit analysis. Planning for radiation therapy includes assessing the disease site, tumour size and histological findings. Treatment schedules vary based on these factors. Box 13.7 lists the degree of radiosensitivity for selected cancers.

The person receiving external radiation may experience skin changes such as blanching, erythema, desquamation, sloughing or haemorrhage. Ulcerations of mucous membranes may cause severe pain; in addition, oral secretions can decrease, making the person more vulnerable to infection and dental caries. Gastrointestinal effects include nausea and vomiting, diarrhoea or bleeding. Lungs may develop interstitial exudate, a condition called radiation pneumonia. Occasionally, external radiation therapy may cause fistulas or necrosis of adjacent tissues. Implanted radioactive materials can lead to similar problems; moreover, the excretory products of these people are usually considered dangerous and need special disposal. See the accompanying 'Nursing care' box for nursing implications for people receiving radiation therapy.

BIOTHERAPY **Biotherapy** modifies the biological processes that result in malignant cells, primarily through enhancing the person's own immune responses. The development of this therapy was based on the immune surveillance hypothesis. Although it has been established that a competent immune system is the body's most important defence against any disease, the role that various immune cells play in combatting different types of malignancies continues to be investigated. Currently, biotherapy is used for both haematological malignancies, such as lymphoma and hairy-cell leukaemia, and solid tumours, such as renal cancer and melanoma (Fox et al., 2013; Poust, Woolery & Green, 2013).

Tumour immunology has the following applications: detection screening in high-risk groups, differential diagnosis and classification of tumour cells, monitoring the course of the disease, with early detection of recurrence and active therapies to halt or limit the disease. The theory underlying tumour immunology is that most tumour cells have a structural appearance recognisable by the immune cells. Tumour-associated antigens (TAAs) exist on tumour cells but not on normal cells. TAAs elicit an immune response that, in a person with a competent immune system, destroys or inhibits tumour growth. Thus, TAAs can be isolated from serum and used for both diagnosis and various treatment modalities. The PSA is one such TAA currently in successful diagnostic use.

Tumour cells are often in a stage of arrested development (i.e. in the differentiation stage) for the cell type they represent; thus, they express antigens characteristic of that particular stage of development. The immaturity of the cells provides the doctor with information about the relative aggressiveness of the cancer.

Another aspect of immunotherapy is the development of monoclonal antibodies that enhance the immune system's ability to fight the cancer. Monoclonal antibodies are developed by inoculating an animal with the tumour antigen and recovering the specific antibodies produced. The antibodies are then given to the person with that cancer to assist in the destruction of the tumour. Monoclonal antibodies are also re-created or cloned in the genetic laboratory by recombining DNA to produce the specific antibody. Techniques involving recombinant DNA have been used to combine these antibodies with toxins and drugs that are then delivered selectively to the tumour sites.

A number of cytokines (normal growth-regulating molecules) with antitumour activity have been synthesised. Alpha interferon (IFN-α), bacillus Calmette-Guérin (BCG, which has been used for many years as an inoculation against tuberculosis) and interleukin-2 (IL-2) have shown some therapeutic benefit in eliciting increased immune responses. Combination strategies have also helped stimulate the function of macrophages.

A promising discovery has been the natural killer (NK) cells. These cells are like large granular lymphocytes but they have a cell surface phenotype different from that of T lymphocytes or macrophages. They have demonstrated a spontaneous cytotoxic effect on some types of cancer cells. They also provide a strong resistance to metastasis and secrete cytokines. When augmented by biological response modifiers such as IL-2, they show increased tumour destructive activity (Battiato & Wheeler, 2018).

The use of haematopoietic growth factors (HGFs) has been one of the most successful in biotherapy. HGFs, such as granulocyte colony-stimulating factor and erythropoietin, offset the suppression of granulocytes and erythrocytes that results from chemotherapy (Battiato & Wheeler, 2018).

Since the early 1990s, the combination of cytokines, particularly IFN-α and IL-2, with chemotherapy has been used in people with metastatic melanoma with promising results. Such a combination is referred to as either biochemotherapy or chemoimmunotherapy (Anderson et al., 1998; Cohen & Falkson, 1998; Legha et al., 1998). The rationale for biochemotherapy is based on the independent antitumour activity of both IFN-α and IL-2 against melanoma and their lack of cross-resistance with cytotoxic chemotherapy. Although the precise mechanism of the antitumour effect of biochemotherapy regimens is less well understood, two hypotheses have been proposed: (1) chemotherapy enhances the antitumour effect of biological agents, and (2) the biological agents enhance the antitumour cytotoxic effect of chemotherapy (Anderson et al., 1998; Legha et al., 1998).

As promising as these biotherapies or biochemotherapies are, they are accompanied by serious side effects and toxicities (Legha et al., 1998; Smith et al., 2019). IL-2 can cause acute alterations in renal, cardiac, liver, gastrointestinal and mental functioning. IFN-α causes mental slowing, confusion and lethargy, and when used in combination with 5-fluorouracil or IL-2, severe flu-like symptoms—chills and fever of 39.4°C to 41.1°C, nausea, vomiting, diarrhoea, anorexia, severe fatigue and stomatitis—may result. The toxic effects are probably exaggerations of the normal systemic effects that these substances cause when fighting infection. For example, IL-2 is known to raise body temperature substantially in an attempt to create a hostile environment for foreign invaders.

The accompanying 'Nursing care' box discusses nursing implications for people receiving immunotherapy. For nursing care of specific problems, refer to the appropriate nursing diagnoses later in this chapter.

NURSING CARE OF THE PERSON receiving radiation therapy

NURSING RESPONSIBILITIES FOR EITHER EXTERNAL OR INTERNAL RADIATION THERAPY

- Assess and manage any complications, usually in collaboration with the radiation oncologist.
- Assist in documenting the results of the therapy; for example, people receiving radiation for metastases to the spine will show improved neurological functioning as tumour size diminishes.
- Provide emotional support, relief of physical and psychological discomfort, and opportunities to talk about fears and concerns. For some people, radiation therapy is a last chance for cure or even just for relief of physical discomfort.

EXTERNAL RADIATION

Prior to the start of treatments, the treatment area will be specifically located by the radiation oncologist and marked with coloured semi-permanent ink or tattoos. Treatment is usually given 5 days per week for 15 to 30 minutes per day over 2 to 7 weeks.

Nursing responsibilities

- Monitor for adverse effects: skin changes, such as blanching, erythema, desquamation, sloughing or haemorrhage; ulcerations of mucous membranes; nausea and vomiting, diarrhoea or gastrointestinal bleeding.
- Assess lungs for rales, which may indicate interstitial exudate. Observe for any dyspnoea or changes in respiratory pattern.
- Identify and record any medications that the person will be taking during the radiation treatment.
- Monitor white blood cell counts and platelet counts for significant decreases.

Health education for the person and family

- Wash the skin that is marked as the radiation site with plain water only, no soap; do not apply deodorant, lotions, medications, perfume or talcum powder to the site during the treatment period. Take care not to wash off the treatment marks.
- Do not rub, scratch or scrub treated skin areas. If necessary, use only an electric razor to shave the treated area.
- Apply neither heat nor cold (e.g. heating pad or ice pack) to the treatment site.
- Inspect the skin for damage or serious changes and report these to the radiologist or doctor.
- Wear loose, soft clothing over the treated area.
- Protect skin from sun exposure during treatment and for at least 1 year after radiation therapy is discontinued. Cover skin with protective clothing during treatment; once radiation is discontinued, use sun-blocking agents with a sun protection factor (SPF) of at least 15.
- External radiation poses no risk to other people for radiation exposure, even with intimate physical contact.
- Be sure to get plenty of rest and eat a balanced diet.

INTERNAL RADIATION

The radiation source, called an implant, is placed into the affected tissue or body cavity and is sealed in tubes, containers, wires, seeds, capsules or needles. An implant may be temporary or permanent. Internal radiation may also be ingested or injected as a solution into the bloodstream or a body cavity or be introduced into the tumour through a catheter. The radioactive substance may transmit rays outside the body or be excreted in body fluids.

Nursing responsibilities

- Place the person in a private room.
- Limit visits to 10 to 30 minutes and have visitors sit at least 2 metres from the person.
- Monitor for side effects such as burning sensations, excessive perspiration, chills and fever, nausea and vomiting, or diarrhoea.
- Assess for fistulas or necrosis of adjacent tissues.

Health education for the person and family

- While a temporary implant is in place, stay in bed and rest quietly to avoid dislodging the implant.
- For outpatient treatments, avoid close contact with others until treatment has been discontinued.
- If the radiologist indicates the need for such measures, dispose of excretory materials in special containers or in a toilet not used by others.
- Carry out daily activities as able; get extra rest if feeling fatigued.
- Eat a balanced diet; frequent, small meals often are better tolerated.
- Contact the nurse or doctor about any concerns or questions after discharge.

PHOTODYNAMIC THERAPY Photodynamic therapy is a method of treating certain kinds of superficial tumours. It is known by several different names: phototherapy, photoradiation and photochemotherapy. People suffering from tumours growing on the surface of the bladder, peritoneal cavity, chest wall, pleura, bronchus or head and neck are candidates for this treatment. The person is given an intravenous dose of a photosensitising compound, Photofrin, which is selectively retained in higher concentrations in malignant tissue. This drug is activated by a laser treatment that is started 3 days after the drug injection and administered for 3 days. The drug interacts with oxygen molecules in the tissue to produce a cytotoxic oxygen molecule called singlet oxygen.

At the time of the first intravenous injection, people are observed for adverse hypersensitivity reactions, such as nausea, chills and hives. Systemic or long-term toxicities are rare. The main side effects are local skin reactions and temporary photosensitivity, transiently elevated liver enzymes and inflammatory responses of the tissues being treated, such as peritoneal or pleural tissues. This treatment has been used successfully with early-stage lung cancer with response rates as high as 90% (Madsen, 2016; National Cancer Institute, 2021b).

The major nursing responsibilities associated with photodynamic therapy are to address the person and family's anxiety about undergoing a relatively new treatment procedure and to educate them in managing side effects. The drug remains in the subcutaneous tissues for 4 to 6 weeks after injection. Any direct or indirect exposure to the sun activates the drug, resulting in a chemical sunburn. People are taught to protect themselves from sunlight (even on cloudy days) by covering themselves from head to toe in opaque clothing, including a wide-brimmed hat, gloves, shoes and stockings, and sunglasses with 100% ultraviolet block. Long-term care of treated skin includes moisturising lotions and protection from trauma or irritation.

BONE MARROW AND PERIPHERAL BLOOD STEM CELL TRANSPLANTATIONS Bone marrow transplantation (BMT) is an accepted treatment to stimulate a non-functioning marrow or to replace marrow. BMT is given as an intravenous infusion of bone marrow cells from donor to person. Most commonly used in leukaemias, this therapy is being expanded to include treatment of other cancers including melanoma and testicular cancer. the chapter 'Nursing care of people with haematological disorders' provides an in-depth discussion of this procedure. Peripheral blood stem cell transplantation (PBSCT) is the process of removing circulating stem cells from the peripheral blood through apheresis and returning these cells to the person after dose-intensive chemotherapy. PBSCT has fewer side effects, shorter hospitalisation and decreased cost compared to BMT.

COMPLEMENTARY THERAPIES Although advances in cancer treatment have increased 5-year survival rates, the uncertainty of cure of cancer and cancer reoccurrence often compel some people to look for complementary therapies. It is estimated that approximately 30% to 50% of people with cancer may have had the experience of using some kind of complementary therapy. Complementary therapies are those that people choose as a complement to medical treatment. Common complementary therapies for cancer can be categorised into botanical agents, nutritional supplements, dietary regimens, mind–body modalities, energy healing, spiritual approaches and miscellaneous therapies. Box 13.8 provides detailed information about complementary therapies.

To provide sensitive nursing care, nurses should be knowledgeable about common complementary therapies. Nurses should use ethical principles of autonomy, beneficence, nonmaleficence and justice to guide their professional practice and care for people who choose to use complementary therapies. It

NURSING CARE OF THE PERSON receiving immunotherapy

Immunotherapy can consist of various substances used alone, such as IL-2, or combination biotherapy, such as IFN-α with 5-fluorouracil. The nurse's role is to enhance the person's quality of life.

NURSING RESPONSIBILITIES

- Monitor for side effects: IFN-α may cause mental slowing, confusion and lethargy; combination therapy of 5-fluorouracil or IL-2 and IFN-α may cause severe flu-like symptoms, with chills and fever of 39.4°C to 41.1°C, nausea, vomiting, diarrhoea, anorexia, severe fatigue and stomatitis; erythropoietin may cause acute hypertension.
- Monitor enzymes and other appropriate biochemical indicators for acute alterations in renal, cardiac, liver or gastrointestinal functioning, which can be side effects of IL-2.
- Evaluate response to therapy by conducting a thorough evaluation of the person's symptoms.
- Assess the person's coping behaviours and teach new strategies as needed.
- Manage fatigue and depression.
- Encourage self-care and participation in decision making.
- Provide close supervision for people with altered mental functioning, either by caretakers or through frequent nursing visits to the person's home.
- If the person is unable to manage alone, teach medication administration and care of equipment to caregivers.

HEALTH EDUCATION FOR THE PERSON AND FAMILY

- Minimise symptoms by managing fever and flu-like symptoms: increase fluid intake, take analgesic and antipyretic medications, and maintain bed rest until symptoms abate.
- Seek help for serious problems not managed by usual means, such as dehydration from diarrhoea.
- Use correct techniques for providing subcutaneous injections.
- Identify how to work and care for ambulatory pumps when medication is administered through an intercatheter or vascular access device.

BOX 13.8 Common complementary therapies for cancer

Type	Description
Botanical agents	Herbs are believed to be the most 'natural' and 'safe' plants ingested with the hope for a cure of cancer. Commonly used botanical agents include echinacea, essiac, ginseng, green tea, pau d'arco and hoxsey. The safety of many of these botanical agents has not been proven, especially as a complement to medical treatment.
Nutritional supplements	Chemical compounds include vitamins, minerals, enzymes, amino acids and essential fatty acids or proteins (such as shark cartilage). They are believed to have the ability to promote health and to help cure cancer. The safety of certain compounds such as vitamins has been established; however, in megadoses, many of the compounds can be toxic and have potential interactions with some therapeutic agents used for cancer, such as chemotherapy.
Dietary regimens	The ingestion of only natural substances is believed to have the effect of purifying the body and slowing down the growth of cancer. Popular regimens include the grape diet, the carrot juice diet and garlic, onions and liver intake. However, the effectiveness of these dietary regimens remains to be established.
Mind–body modalities	The harmony of mind and body is believed to facilitate physiological and psychological healing. Such modalities include relaxation, meditation or imagery. Recent research has shown that these modalities have helped individuals with cancer adjust to the experience of cancer.
Energy healing	The human body is believed to be an energy field and cancer might be the result of a disturbed energy field. Energy therapies, such as therapeutic touch and healing touch, can affect the energy field of the human body and promote physiological healing. Therapeutic touch uses the hands on or near the body with the intent to promote healing. Healing touch uses energy healing techniques to heal by restoring the harmony and balance of the body. Clinical practice and research on energy healing have shown positive findings of energy healing in a variety of people.
Spiritual approaches	Faith in God or a higher power of the universe is believed to help cancer healing. Spiritual approaches include faith healing, prayer to God, prayer groups and chain prayer. Research has shown that faith in God or a higher power also helped individuals with cancer to adjust to the experience of cancer.
Miscellaneous therapies	Aromatherapy has been used for people with cancer to relieve nausea, vomiting or retching, and to decrease anxiety. However, aromatherapy might not be appropriate for people who are highly sensitive to strong fragrance. Music, art and humour therapies have also been used to help people with cancer to reduce anxiety, to express feelings of loss and to promote optimism.

is also important for nurses to provide truthful, non-judgmental responses to the questions or inquiries about complementary therapies from people with cancer. Nurses should encourage people to report the use of any complementary therapies to their oncologist to prevent potential interactions of the complementary therapies with their medical treatment.

Pain management

Pain management is an important component of oncology care and is considered a crucial part of the collaborative treatment plan. It is estimated that more than 50% of people with early-stage cancer and up to 95% of people with advanced cancer experience pain that requires analgesia (Anekar & Cacella, 2022; Piotrowska, Leppert & Majkowicz, 2019; Yoong & Poon, 2018). There are three main categories of pain syndromes in people with cancer, and the category influences the type of treatment:

1. *Pain associated with direct tumour involvement.* The most common causes are metastases to bone, nerve compression or infiltration, and involvement of hollow visceral organs.
2. *Pain associated with treatment.* This may include postsurgical incisional or wound pain; peripheral neuropathy, ulceration of mucous membranes and pain from herpes zoster outbreaks secondary to chemotherapy; and pain in nerve plexuses, muscles and peripheral nerves from radiation therapy.
3. *Pain from a cause not related to either the cancer or therapy,* such as diabetic neuropathy.

The goal of pain therapy is to provide relief that allows people to function as they wish and, in the case of terminally ill people, to die relatively free of pain. Drug therapy with opioid and non-opioid analgesics as well as adjuvant medications (those that enhance the effect of the analgesic) is the basis of most doctor-guided pain management. Other therapies include injection of anaesthetic drugs into spinal cord or specific nerve plexuses, surgical severing of nerves, radiation to reduce tumour size and pressure, and behavioural approaches. Pharmacological pain management follows these steps:

- Conduct careful initial and ongoing assessment of the pain.
- Evaluate the person's functional goals.
- Establish a plan with combinations of non-narcotic drugs (such as aspirin or ibuprofen) with adjuvants (such as corticosteroids or antidepressants).
- Evaluate the degree of pain relief.
- Progress to stronger drugs as needed, from mild narcotics, such as oxycodone or propoxyphene, to strong narcotics, such as morphine or hydromorphone, and monitor side effects.

- Continue to try combinations and escalate dosages until maximal pain relief balanced with the person's need to function is achieved.

Medication is usually administered by the oral route as long as this route continues to be effective. Medication is given on a regular time schedule (e.g. every 4 hours), with additional medication prescribed to cover breakthrough pain. When the oral route alone becomes inadequate, the primary narcotic can be administered intramuscularly, subcutaneously or rectally on an intermittent schedule or continuously by transdermal patches, or intravenously by a continuous drip, usually controlled by an infusion pump. Some pumps are portable, deliver medication continuously and allow people to control their breakthrough pain with a limited number of boluses. When narcotic doses are increased gradually, there is no limit to the amount the person can receive, as long as adverse reactions can be managed. People have received up to 4,800 mg daily (200 mg per hour) of morphine sulfate with up to six 200–400 mg breakthrough doses daily without major ill effects and with good pain control. The body develops tolerance to the sedative after a short period and most people are able to tolerate the level of medication needed to control the pain. Other side effects, such as constipation, nausea and vomiting, and itching, can be managed through the usual means and are discussed under the appropriate nursing diagnoses. If the person has persistent untoward side effects that do not respond to treatment, or if the person does not get adequate relief from the narcotic, different narcotics and combinations are tried. Morphine sulfate and transdermal fentanyl are the most commonly used drugs for relief of cancer pain (Brant, 2022; Piotrowska et al., 2019).

People receiving high-dose narcotics should not have the medication abruptly stopped, because withdrawal symptoms will occur. If the drug needs to be stopped, it must be tapered gradually. For more information on pain management, and on alternative therapies in particular, see the chapter 'Nursing care of people in pain'.

BOX 13.9 Cancer Council: signs and symptoms to look for

- **Lumps, sores or ulcers that do not heal.**
- **Coughs that persist or show blood, or a hoarseness that hangs around.**
- **Unexplained weight loss.**
- **Moles that have changed shape, size or colour or an inflamed skin sore that has not healed.**
- **Blood in a bowel motion.**
- **Persistent changes in toilet habits.**

Men

- **Unusual changes in your testicles—changes in shape, consistency or lumpiness.**
- **Urinary problems or changes.**

Women

- **Unusual changes in your breasts—lumps, thickening, unusual discharge, nipples that suddenly turn inwards, change in shape, colour or unusual pain.**
- **Blood loss between or following periods.**
- **Persistent abdominal pain or bloating.**

These symptoms are often related to more common, less serious health problems. However, if you notice any unusual changes, or these symptoms persist, visit your doctor.

Source: Cancer Council (2022a). *Common cancer symptoms*. Retrieved from https://www.cancer.org.au.

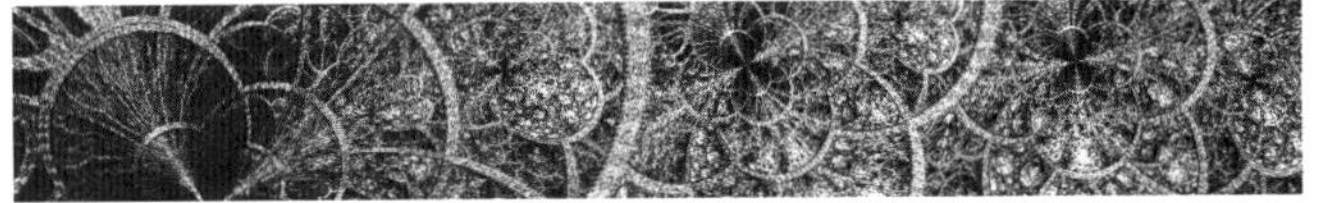

Nursing care

Nurses face a major challenge in educating people about preventive measures and lifestyle changes to reduce the risk of cancer. At the same time, people with cancer must be reassured that they are not responsible for having acquired cancer.

Once a cancer diagnosis is established, nurses help people recover and support them during the rehabilitation phase. In cases of terminal cancer, nurses provide comfort and facilitate positive growth for the person and significant others.

Health promotion

Early detection and treatment are considered the most important factors influencing the prognosis of those who have cancer. However, many people do not seek early diagnosis and treatment because of denial, fear and anxiety, stigma or the absence of specific early signs such as pain or weight loss (which usually are late signs). For this reason, screening procedures such as mammograms, PSA, occult blood stool tests and sigmoidoscopy may be lifesaving.

The Cancer Council advises the Australian Government on policy and practices to help in the prevention, detection and treatment of cancer. The Cancer Council undertakes and funds cancer research as well as advocates for the rights of people with cancer to receive the best treatment, care and support. Recommendations on reducing preventable risk factors and early screening strategies are outlined in the *National Cancer Prevention Policy 2007–2009* by the Cancer Council (2007). The Cancer Council highlights that one-third of cancer deaths in Australia can be attributed to known avoidable risk factors (Cancer Council, 2007). The Cancer Council provides cancer-smart lifestyle fact sheets that provide information on common signs and symptoms that may indicate cancer. The signs and symptoms to look for (see Box 13.9) are helpful in promoting awareness but do not substitute for medical advice.

If a person is at special risk due to heredity, environment, occupation or lifestyle, special tests or more frequent examinations may be necessary. A routine cancer check-up should include counselling to improve health behaviours and physical examination with related tests of the breast, uterus, cervix, colon, rectum, testes, prostate, skin, thyroid and lymph nodes. Box 13.10 lists the recommendations for screening. Nurses have a special role in public education and should encourage all with whom they come into contact to schedule cancer check-ups. Nurses must be familiar with the cancer guidelines so that they can advise people, their families and significant others.

BOX 13.10 National Cancer Prevention Policy: cancer screening recommendations

Cervical screening

- Routine cervical screening tests from the age of 25.

Breast cancer

- If you are over 40, you can have a free BreastScreen Australia mammogram (breast x-ray) every 2 years.
- Regular mammograms can reduce your risk of breast cancer death by 25%, particularly women in the 50–69 age group, for whom the benefit is highest.

Bowel cancer

- The Cancer Council recommends all Australians aged over 50 have a faecal occult blood test (FOBT) every 2 years to screen for bowel cancer.

Source: Cancer Council (2022b). *Early detection of breast cancer*. Retrieved from https://www.cancer.org.au/ cancer-information/causes-and-prevention/early-detection-and-screening/early-detection-of-breast-cancer. For more information visit https://www.cancer.org.au.

Assessment

Focused interview

During this initial phase of the nursing process, collect the following significant data about the person:

- history of the person's disease, including the signs and symptoms that led the person to seek healthcare
- other concurrent diseases, such as diabetes
- current physical or psychological problems resulting from the cancer, such as pain or depression
- understanding of the treatment plan
- expectations of the treatment plan
- functional limitations due to illness or treatment (see Box 13.11)
- effect of the disease on current lifestyle
- reliable support systems or caretakers for the person
- coping strategies and how well they are working.

INTERVIEW QUESTIONS The following are appropriate questions to ask the person during the initial interview and at subsequent assessments:

- *'What brought you in to see the doctor?'* Asking this question allows people to tell their story in their own way, which may elicit more information than asking specific questions. The answer should elicit not only data about the signs and symptoms but also fears or concerns. If the cancer was discovered during a routine physical examination or check-up, the person may have some difficulty accepting the disease, especially if there were no symptoms. For people who offer insufficient information in response to this open-ended question, more specific questions may be necessary, such as 'Did you have pain or any specific physical problems that caused you to seek healthcare?'
- *'Do you have any other medical conditions or problems that are troubling you at this time?'* It may be necessary to ask about specific diseases to help the person focus. For example, 'Do you have high blood pressure?' or 'Are you having any problems with your lungs?' Information gained from these questions can help you anticipate problems and formulate potential nursing diagnoses related to other diseases that may interact with the cancer.
- *'What kinds of physical problems are you having at this time? Do you have pain? Are you nauseated? Have you lost a great deal of weight? Are you so tired you have difficulty carrying on your daily activities? Are you feeling depressed or discouraged because of your illness?'* For each positive response, ask follow-up questions to narrow down or define the exact nature of the problem. Again, these data help identify what nursing diagnoses should be included in the care plan.
- *'What options has your doctor suggested for treating your cancer?'* The answer will indicate the person's knowledge about their treatment and, possibly, their communication with the doctor. Often, under the stress of a cancer diagnosis, people do not hear or understand what the doctor is saying and are afraid to ask questions. Lack of knowledge indicates a need to collaborate with the doctor to explain the information to the person so that the person can absorb and understand it. If the person has a good understanding of the treatment plan, discussing how they feel about it can be useful in exposing fears, concerns and emotional responses.
- *'What do you expect to happen as a result of this treatment?'* The answer may reveal unrealistic

BOX 13.11 Example of an instrument for assessing functional status for cancer patients (Australia-modified Karnofsky Performance Scale (AKPS))

Score	Description
100	Normal; no complaints; no evidence of disease.
90	Able to carry on normal activity; minor signs or symptoms of disease.
80	Normal activity with effort; some signs or symptoms of disease.
70	Cares for self; unable to carry on normal activity or to do active work.
60	Able to care for most needs but requires occasional assistance.
50	Considerable assistance and frequent medical care.
40	In bed more than 50% of the time.
30	Almost completely bedfast.
20	Totally bedfast and requiring extensive nursing care by professionals and/or family.
10	Comatose or barely rousable.
0	Dead.

Source: Abernethy et al. (2005). The Australia-modified Karnofsky Performance Status (AKPS) Scale: A revised scale for contemporary palliative care clinical practice [electronic version]. *BioMed Central Palliative Care*, 4(7), 1–12, Table 1. http://creativecommons.org/licenses/by/2.0/.

expectations or lack of understanding of consequences of the treatment.

- *'What effect is the disease and/or treatment having on your ability to carry on with your usual daily activities?'* Additional questions may also be needed to pinpoint the types of limitations. The response to this question should provide information on the person's functional status, such as those shown in Box 13.11. This information can also be used to identify the need to collaborate with professionals from other disciplines. For example, if the person is the sole financial support of the family and is unable to work, a social worker may be able to help with resources; if the person is extremely weak, referral to a physiotherapist may help with energy conservation strategies and strengthening exercises.
- *'Who is available to help you at home and run errands for you? Who can provide transportation for you to get to your appointments or treatments? Who can you rely on to be a good listener when you're sad or just to be a comfortable companion? Is there someone you would like to make healthcare decisions for you if there is a time when you are unable to make them for yourself?'* It often seems that the person with cancer is the one who takes care of everyone else; asking for help may be difficult for this person. This information can identify how much support and help the person has access to. The last question introduces the concept of advance directives and enduring power of attorney regarding healthcare (see the chapter 'Nursing care of people experiencing loss, grief and death').
- *'How do you manage your stress or your feelings of discomfort? What helps you feel better? Do you think these measures work well for you?'* The responses to these questions provide information about the person's coping strategies and may identify maladaptive strategies such as alcohol or drug use. Lack of appropriate coping methods can interfere with the person's response to treatment and decrease overall quality of life.

Other assessment questions may be useful at different stages of the person's illness. For example, if the person is not expected to survive the cancer, it is important to ask whether the person has made decisions about last wishes (e.g. for a funeral and burial), whether these have been discussed with significant others and whether the person has made out a will.

BOX 13.12 Factors to consider in assessing hydration status

- Intake and output
- Rapid weight changes
- Skin turgor and moisture
- Venous filling
- Vital sign changes
- Tongue furrows and moisture
- Eyeball softness
- Lung sounds
- Laboratory values

Physical assessment

As soon as the person is admitted to the healthcare service or organisation, conduct a complete physical assessment to establish a baseline against which to evaluate later changes. It is especially important to document the nutritional status of the person using anthropomorphic measurements (i.e. frame size, height, weight, body fat and muscle mass) and to evaluate laboratory results and note any specific signs and symptoms. Table 13.11 compares the manifestations of good nutrition with those of malnutrition.

It is also important to assess the person's hydration status, especially if the person is not taking oral food and fluids well or is having bouts of vomiting. Box 13.12 lists specific assessments for hydration status. Other recommended assessments are discussed under the specific nursing diagnoses that follow. They can also be found in other chapters that address specific body systems affected by the cancer.

Nursing diagnoses and interventions

Nursing goals focus on supporting the whole person and managing specific problems such as pain, poor nutrition, dehydration, fatigue, adverse emotional responses, altered individual and family coping, and the side effects of medical treatment. Nursing

TABLE 13.11 Signs of nutritional status

SYSTEM	GOOD NUTRITION	POOR NUTRITION
General	Alert, energetic, good endurance, psychologically stable Weight within range for height, age, body size	Withdrawn, apathetic, easily fatigued, irritable Over- or underweight
Integumentary	Skin glowing, good turgor, smooth, free of lesions Hair shiny, lustrous, minimal loss	Skin dull, pasty, scaly-dry, bruises, multiple lesions Hair brittle, dull, falls out easily
Head, eyes, ears, nose and throat	Eyes bright, clear, no fatigue circles Oral mucous membranes pink-red and moist Gums pink, firm Tongue pink, moderately smooth, no swelling	Eyes dull, conjunctiva pale, discolouration under eyes Oral mucous membranes pale Gums red, spongy and bleed easily Tongue bright to dark red, swollen
Abdomen	Abdomen flat, firm	Abdomen flaccid or distended (ascites)
Musculoskeletal	Firm, well-developed muscles Good posture No skeletal changes	Flaccid muscles, wasted appearance Stooped posture Skeletal malformations
Neurological	Good attention span, good concentration, astute thought processes Good reflexes	Inattentive, easily distracted, impaired thought processes Paraesthesias, reflexes diminished or hyperactive

also focuses on improving the quality of life by promoting rehabilitation for survivors of cancer and helping those who succumb to the disease maintain their dignity in the dying process. Because cancer affects the whole family, nursing care includes everyone involved with the person from the onset of diagnosis through the entire disease and treatment process and the ultimate outcome. Many diagnoses are pertinent to people with cancer; this section addresses only the most common diagnoses. See the accompanying 'Nursing care plan'. (Diagnoses specific to individual diseases can be found in their respective chapters.)

NURSING CARE PLAN A person with cancer

James Casey, aged 72, is of northern European heritage. He has been receiving medical care for chronic obstructive pulmonary disease, chronic bronchitis, post myocardial infarction and type I diabetes mellitus for over 15 years. He reports that he lost his wife to lung cancer 5 years ago and still 'misses her terribly'. He describes his bad habits as smoking two packets of cigarettes a day for 52 years (104 packs/year), one to two six-packs of beer a week, one 'bourbon and water' a night and 'a lot of sugar-free junk food, like chips'. He assures the nurse that he quit smoking 2 years ago, when he could no longer walk a block without considerable shortness of breath, and just quit drinking alcohol a few weeks ago at his doctor's insistence. About a year ago, he had a basal cell carcinoma removed from his right ear. Six months ago, cancerous tumours were discovered in his bladder and he underwent two 6-week chemotherapy courses of bladder instillations of BCG. His latest report indicates that the tumours have grown back and no further chemotherapy would be useful. The urologist had considered surgery but believed that Mr Casey's other medical problems would compromise his chances of survival. Mr Casey decides to let the disease run its course and to be managed at home through hospice care. Because he lives alone in a modest home, he asks his daughter, Mary, and her family to move in with him to provide care and support during his final months. His daughter accepts, saying she is glad to be able to spend this time with her father; she has been informed of the physical and emotional stress this will entail.

ASSESSMENT

Glynis Jackson, RN, the hospice nurse assigned as case manager for James Casey, completes a health history and physical examination during her first two visits in his home, 1 day apart. She gathers this information over 2 days to conserve his strength and allow more time for Mr Casey and his daughter to talk about their concerns.

During the physical assessment, Glynis notes that Mr Casey is pale with pink mucous membranes, thin with a wasted appearance and has a strained, worried facial expression. He complains of severe back pain no longer adequately relieved by oxycodone and Panadeine Forte alternating every 2 to 4 hours. His blood pressure is 90/50, right arm in the reclining position with no significant orthostatic change; his apical pulse is 102, regular and strong; respiratory rate 24 and unlaboured; breath sounds are clear but diminished in the bases; oral temperature is 36°C.

A tunnelled Groshong catheter as a CVAD is present in the right anterior chest. There is no drainage, redness or swelling at the site. The catheter was placed last week when Mr Casey was being evaluated at the anaesthetist's office for pain management, but no medication is running via the CVAD. Mary reports that his urinary output is adequate. Approximately 200 mL of yellow, cloudy, non-malodorous urine is present in the urinal at the bedside from his last voiding.

Mr Casey states that he spends most of his time either in bed or sitting up in a chair in his room. He reports that he has no energy anymore and is unable to walk to the bathroom unassisted, dress himself or take care of his own personal hygiene. Glynis rates Mr Casey's functional level at ECOG level 4: capable of only limited self-care, confined to bed or chair 50% or more of waking hours (Karnofsky 10 to 20). Mr Casey tells the nurse that his daughter 'is working day and night to help me and is looking awfully tired'.

Mary reports that Mr Casey is eating very poorly: he usually eats a small bowl of oatmeal with milk for breakfast and vegetable soup and crackers for lunch, but he tells her that he is too tired for dinner and wants only fruit juice. Mr Casey tells the nurse that he has no appetite and eats just to please Mary. He does drink at least three to four glasses of water a day plus juice. His blood sugar levels remain within normal range.

His current weight is 54.6 kg at 170 cm tall, down from 81.8 kg 2 months ago.

Available laboratory values from his visit with the doctor show the following:

Total protein: 41 g/L (normal range: 62 to 8.0 g/L)
Albumin: 22 g/L (normal range: 35 to 50 g/L)
Haemoglobin: 102 g/L (normal range: 132 to 170 g/L)
Haematocrit: 30.5% (normal range: 40.0–54.0%)
BUN: 30 mml/L (normal range: 5 to 25 mm/L, slightly higher in older people)
Creatinine: 116 μmol/L (normal range: 50 to 110 μmol/L).

DIAGNOSES

- *Imbalanced nutrition related to dietary intake being less than body requirements* as evidenced by loss of appetite and weight loss.
- *Risk of caregiver role strain* related to severity of her father's illness and lack of help from other family members as manifested by physical exhaustion and emotional stress.
- *Chronic pain* related to progression of the disease process as evidenced by increased frequency of analgesia with limited effect.
- *Impaired physical mobility* related to pain, fatigue and beginning of neuromuscular impairment as evidenced by lack of energy and inability to ambulate without assistance.
- *Risk of impaired skin integrity* related to decreased physical mobility and malnourished state as manifested by skin breakdown.

PLANNING

- Plan to have a home health aide come to the home, give Mr Casey a shower or bed bath daily and assist his daughter with some of the household chores.

(continued)

NURSING CARE PLAN A person with cancer (continued)

- Plan for a volunteer to spend up to 4 hours a day, twice a week with Mr Casey so that Mary can attend to outside activities and chores.
- Order a hospital bed with electronic controls to be delivered to the house.
- Order a special foam pad for bed and chair, and a bedside commode from the medical supply house.
- Request a physiotherapy consultation to evaluate current level of functioning and determine how to maintain current level.

Expected outcomes

- Increase oral intake and show improvement in serum protein values.
- Minimal pain for the rest of his life.
- Able to continue his current activity level.
- Maintain skin integrity.
- Daughter will be able to maintain supportive caretaking activities as long as Mr Casey needs them.

IMPLEMENTATION

- Talk with the doctor about prescribing a medication to help stimulate the appetite.
- Ask about favourite foods and ask Mary to offer a small portion of one of these foods each day.
- Encourage drinking up to four cans of liquid nutritional supplement with fibre a day, sipping them throughout the day.
- Discuss a pain control program with the specialist, using the CVAD and a CADD-PCA infusion pump with a continuous morphine infusion.
- Call a community nurse to set up the equipment and supplies (including the medication) for the morphine infusion.
- Teach Mary how to use the pump and about the side effects of the morphine infusion, including those that require a call to the nurse for assistance. Teach which untoward effects should be reported.
- Instruct Mary to allow ample rest periods for her father between activities.
- Instruct Mary and the community carer to inspect skin daily, give good skin care with emollient lotion after bathing and report any beginning lesions immediately to the nurse.
- Talk with Mary about having her adult son and daughter relieve her of the housework and stay with Mr Casey so that she can get out of the house occasionally. Offer to talk with them if she is uncomfortable doing so.

EVALUATION

James Casey did increase his oral intake a little, sometimes eating the special treats his daughter prepared and drinking one or two cans of liquid nutritional supplement a day. However, his weight did not increase; it stayed at about 54.6 kg until his death 2 weeks later. His daughter was very grateful for the extra help from the community carers and the volunteer, although she could not bring herself to ask her son and daughter for help and did not want the nurse to do so. She did become more rested and reported that 'Dad and I had some wonderful 3 am talks when he couldn't sleep'.

Mr Casey was started on 20 mg of morphine per hour with boluses of 10 mg 4 times a day, for breakthrough pain. This medication relieved his pain quite well; after 2 days he was alert enough most of the time to carry on a normal conversation and still walk to the bathroom with help up until 2 days before he died.

The hospital bed simplified Mr Casey's care and made it much easier for him to rest comfortably and change position. His skin remained intact and in good condition.

Mary reported that Mr Casey died peacefully in his sleep, about 2 weeks after care was started. She said that spending the last weeks of his life with him was a healing experience for both of them.

CRITICAL THINKING IN THE NURSING PROCESS

1. What other tests could be done to evaluate James Casey's nutritional status?
2. Mr Casey had severe back pain. What were the possible pathophysiological reasons for his pain?
3. One of the specified interventions was to consult the doctor regarding medication to increase Mr Casey's appetite. What medications might fulfil that function? What side effects might they have that would contraindicate these medications for him?
4. If Mr Casey had developed signs and symptoms of sepsis, what manifestations would you expect to see? As the nurse making the home visits, what would be your nursing actions and in what order of priority?

REFLECTION ON THE NURSING PROCESS

1. What support strategies could you recommend to assist Mr Casey and his family with anticipatory grieving?
2. Outline what you have learned from this case study that you can implement in your future practice.

Anxiety

Early in the disease process—for example, during diagnosis and treatment—threats to or changes in health status, physical comfort, role functioning or even socioeconomic status can cause anxiety. Later, anxiety may result from the anticipation of pain, disfigurement or the threat of death. In particular, people whose coping skills have been poor in the past (e.g. in managing anger) may find themselves at a loss to manage this current crisis. The person may manifest overt signs of anxiety: trembling, restlessness, irritability, hyperactivity, stimulation of the sympathetic nervous system (increased blood pressure, pulse, respiration, excessive perspiration, pallor), withdrawal, worried facial expressions and poor eye contact. The person may report insomnia and feelings of tension and apprehension, or express concerns regarding perceived changes brought about by the disease and fear of future events.

- Carefully assess the person's level of anxiety (moderate anxiety, severe anxiety or panic) and the reality of the threats represented in the person's current situation. The level of anxiety and the reality of the perceived threat influence the type of intervention that is appropriate for the person. *A person in panic may need medical intervention with appropriate medications, whereas those with moderate or severe anxiety are often managed by the nurse through counselling and teaching new coping skills.*

- Establish a therapeutic relationship by conveying warmth and empathy and using non-judgmental and effective listening. *A person who feels safe in the relationship with the nurse more readily expresses their thoughts and feeling. The person will be able to develop trust in the nurse and perhaps be willing to try new behaviours as suggested. The amount of time this relationship may take to develop depends on the person's current emotional and mental state and the stage of the disease process.*
- Encourage the person to acknowledge and express feelings, no matter how inappropriate they may seem to the person. *Just by expressing their feelings, people often can significantly diminish anxiety. Expressing feelings also allows the person to direct energy towards healing and thus has a positive therapeutic effect. Moreover, by acknowledging feelings, especially those the person considers unacceptable, the person can lay the groundwork for new coping behaviours.*
- Review the coping strategies the person has used in the past and build on past successful behaviours, introducing new strategies as appropriate. Explain why inappropriate strategies, such as repressing anger or turning to alcohol, are not helpful. *The person will be more willing to make changes that build on what has already worked in the past. The person will also be more willing to reject inappropriate strategies if they are given a persuasive reason why they have not had the desired effect in managing previous crises.*
- Identify resources in the community, such as crisis hotlines and support groups that can help the person manage anxiety-producing situations. *The person may not have support systems available or the person's significant others may be having their own difficulties in dealing with the cancer diagnosis. The Cancer Council provides programs, support groups and counselling in all states and territories throughout Australia.*
- Provide specific information for the person about the disease, its treatment and what may be expected, especially for those people with obvious misinformation. *Knowing what is to come gives the person a sense of control and enables them to make decisions. Also, knowing that every effort will be made to keep the person as free of pain as possible can do a great deal to relieve anxiety.*
- Provide a safe, calm and quiet environment for the person in panic. Remain with the person and administer anti-anxiety medications as ordered. *Staying with the person and displaying calmness and confidence can protect the person from injury and prevent further panic. If the panic does not subside with the nurse's presence and support, referral to the doctor for medication management may be necessary.*
- Use crisis intervention theory to promote growth in the person and their significant others, regardless of the outcome of the disease. *During a major crisis, people can, with assistance, transform the experience from one that causes defeat and despair to one that enhances personal and spiritual growth. If you are not skilled in this area, a referral to an appropriate mental health professional may be helpful to the person and their family.*

Disturbed body image

Cancer and cancer treatments frequently result in major physiological and psychological body image changes. See the 'Manifestations' box for manifestations of cancer. Loss of a body part (e.g. amputation, prostatectomy or mastectomy), skin changes and hair loss from chemotherapy or radiation therapy, disfigurement of a body part (e.g. lymphoedema in the affected upper and lower extremities) or the creation of unnatural openings on the body for elimination (e.g. colostomy or ileostomy) may have a major effect on the person's self-image. The gaunt, wasted appearance of the cachectic person, or draining, malodorous lesions that result when cancer breaks through the skin, are other significant aetiologies of body image disturbance. This may also give rise to fear of rejection, which plays a major role in sexual dysfunction. In addition to all of the other afflictions that cancer brings about, the person may undergo major changes in appearance and function. The person may exhibit a visible physical alteration of some portion of the body, verbalise negative feelings about the body and/or fear of rejection by others, refuse to look at the affected site and depersonalise the body change or lost part (e.g. by calling the colostomy 'that thing').

- Discuss the meaning of the loss or change with the person. *Doing so helps the nurse discover the best approach for this particular person and involves the person more actively in interventions. A small, seemingly trivial loss may have a big impact, especially when viewed in light of the other changes that are occurring in the person's life. Likewise, a major loss may not be as important as the nurse might imagine. To ensure more appropriate and individualised care, evaluate each situation in terms of the reactions of the specific person.*
- Observe and evaluate interaction with significant others. *People who are important to the person may unintentionally reinforce negative feelings about body image; on the other hand, the person may perceive rejection where none exists.*
- Allow denial, but do not participate in the denial; for example, if a person does not want to look at the wound, the nurse may say, 'I am going to change the dressing to your breast incision now'. *During the initial stage of shock at the loss of a body part, denial is a protective mechanism and should not be challenged, nor should it be promoted. A matter-of-fact approach and an empathetic attitude will go far to facilitate the eventual acceptance of the change.*

MANIFESTATIONS Cancer

- Hair loss
- Depression
- Fever
- Bleeding gums
- Oropharyngeal ulcerations
- Stomatitis
- Anorexia
- Nausea and vomiting
- Diarrhoea
- Emaciation
- General weakness
- Flaccid muscles
- Stooped posture
- Pallor
- Excessive bruising
- Radiation burns
- Visible tumour (abdomen)
- Odour of decay
- Hypotension

- Assist the person and significant others to cope with the changes in appearance:
  a. Provide a supportive environment.
  b. Encourage the person and significant others to express feelings about the situation.
  c. Give matter-of-fact responses to questions and concerns.
  d. Identify new coping strategies to resolve feelings.
  e. Enlist family and friends in reaffirming the person's worth.

  A supportive, safe environment in which feelings are respected and new coping strategies can be tried promotes acceptance, as does reaffirming that the person's worth is not diminished by any physical changes.
- Teach the person or significant others to participate in the care of the afflicted body area. Provide support and validation of their efforts. *Active involvement in providing care, such as changing a dressing or emptying a colostomy bag, empowers the person and/or significant others. This intimate involvement also desensitises feelings about disfigurement and promotes acceptance. Involving significant others reduces the risk of them rejecting the person and can promote closeness. Positive reinforcement from the nurse encourages them to continue these behaviours.*
- Teach strategies for minimising physical changes, such as providing skin care during radiation therapy and dressing to enhance appearance and minimise change in the body part. *Early intervention can limit the negative side effects of treatment and actually promote recovery. Involving the person provides an additional way for the person to be in control of a difficult situation.*
- Teach ways to reduce the alopecia that results from chemotherapy and to enhance appearance until the hair grows back:
  a. Discuss the pattern and timing of hair loss. *This allows the person to cope with changes and incorporate them into daily activities.*
  b. Encourage wearing cheerful, brightly coloured head coverings; assist in colour coordinating them with usual clothing. *Attractive head coverings protect the bald head while allowing the person to feel stylish and well dressed.*
  c. Refer to a good wig shop before hair loss is experienced. *Hair colour and texture can be matched to minimise obvious changes in appearance.*
  d. Refer to support programs such as cancer support workshops that are provided by the Cancer Council in each state and territory. *A support group can diminish feelings of isolation and provide practical tips for managing problems. For a list of community resources available to people with cancer or for confidential information and support, contact the Cancer Council Helpline on 13 11 20. (The cost is that of a local phone call from anywhere in Australia.)*
  e. Reassure that hair will grow back after chemotherapy is discontinued, but also inform that the colour and texture of the new hair may be different. Hair loss has been identified as the most distressing symptom by many people (Cancer Council, 2019; Sitarz & Spencer, 2022). *Interventions to reduce that loss can have a significant impact on body image concerns. Moreover, knowing what to expect may decrease anxiety and distress.*

Anticipatory grieving

Anticipatory grieving is a response to loss that has not yet occurred. Overall, only 50% of people with cancer fully recover, and certain types of cancer have a much higher death rate; thus, the person with cancer is often confronted with facing death and making preparations for it. This can be a healthy response that allows the person and family to work through the dying process and achieve growth in the final stage of life. Perceived changes in body image and lifestyle can also prompt anticipatory grieving. The person or significant others may show sorrow, anger, depression or withdrawal, expressing distress at the potential loss or verbalising concern about unfinished life business. (See the chapter 'Nursing care of people experiencing loss, grief and death' for more on nursing care of the person who is grieving or dying.)

- Use the therapeutic communication skills of active listening, silence and non-verbal support to provide an open environment for the person and significant others to discuss their feelings realistically and to express anger or other negative feelings appropriately. *This helps the person and family to get in touch with feelings and confront the possibility of the loss or death.*
- Answer questions about illness and prognosis honestly, but always encourage hope. *This allows for realistic appraisal of the situation and planning and helps to combat feelings of hopelessness and depression.*
- Encourage the dying person to make funeral and burial plans ahead of time and to be sure the will is in order. Make sure the necessary phone numbers can be easily located. *This gives a sense of control and relieves family members of these*

concerns at a time when the person is most in need of their support and when they themselves are extremely stressed.

- Encourage the person to continue taking part in activities they enjoy, including maintaining employment as long as possible. *This gives a sense of continuity of life even in the face of severe losses.*

Risk of infection

Malnutrition, impaired skin and mucous membrane integrity, tumour necrosis and suppression of the white blood cells (WBC) from chemotherapy or radiation may contribute to the risk of infection. Anorexia, as well as the disease itself, deprives the body of nutrients needed for healing, while impaired integrity of skin and mucous membranes (a result of chemotherapy and/or radiation therapy) compromise the first lines of defence against microbial invasion. Cells in the centre of large or not very vascular tumours may die from malnutrition, eventually eroding through tissues to increase the risk of sepsis. Bone marrow depression resulting from the effects of certain types of cancers and from chemotherapy undermine the body's ability to respond to infection. The person may exhibit the classic signs of infection: lassitude, fever, anorexia, pain in the affected area and physical evidence of infection, such as a purulent, draining lesion or wound. If the bone marrow is compromised, the usual signs and symptoms of infection may be absent or reduced.

- Monitor vital signs. *Fever and sympathetic nervous system responses, such as increased pulse and respiration, are usual early signs of infection. However, severely immunosuppressed people may be unable to mount a fever; therefore, the absence of fever cannot rule out infection.*
- Monitor WBC counts frequently, especially if the person is receiving chemotherapy known to cause bone marrow suppression. *This allows the nurse to notify the doctor at the first sign of diminishing WBC counts so that corrective action can be taken.*
- Teach the person to avoid crowds, small children and people with infections when WBC count is at nadir (lowest point during chemotherapy) and to practise scrupulous personal hygiene. *During periods of leucopenia, the person may lose immunity to his or her own natural flora. Careful attention to hygiene reduces the risk of infection. Crowds, which promote contact with a greater variety of infectious agents, and friends with minor infections can be very dangerous for the immunosuppressed. Small children should be avoided because they often have microbes to which most people are usually immune but which the person with cancer may not be able to resist.*
- Protect skin and mucous membranes from injury. Teach appropriate skin care measures, such as good hygiene, use of a moisturising lotion to prevent dryness and cracking, frequent changes of position for the bed-bound and immediate attention to skin breaks or lesions. *Ensuring intact skin strengthens the first line of defence against infection.*
- Encourage the person to consume a diet high in protein, minerals and vitamins, especially vitamin C. *Improving nutrition decreases the risk of infection. Vitamin C has been shown to help prevent certain types of infection, such as colds.*

Risk of injury

In addition to infection, cancer can pose a risk of injury from, for example, obstruction by a large tumour or one located in a limited body space (e.g. in the brain, bowel or bronchial airways). If the cancer is one that creates ectopic sites of hormones, elevated levels of hormones that are not under the control of the pituitary gland can injure the person in a variety of ways. Signs of obstruction depend on the organ involved: bowel obstruction presents with pain, distension and cessation of bowel activities; obstruction in the brain gives signs of increased intracranial pressure or personality/behavioural change; bronchial obstruction manifests as respiratory distress, cyanosis and altered arterial blood gases. Ectopic production of parathyroid hormone manifests as high serum calcium levels as well as signs of hypercalcaemia; ectopic production of antidiuretic hormone causes fluid retention and manifests as hypertension and peripheral and pulmonary oedema.

- Assess frequently for signs and symptoms indicating problems with organ obstruction. *Early detection of major problems allows the nurse to seek medical help before the problem evolves into a physiological crisis.*
- Teach to differentiate minor problems from those of a serious nature. Encourage the person to consult with the nurse or doctor if in doubt, or to call 000 if they become very ill. Box 13.13 provides guidelines to help people identify serious problems. *Having guidelines for when to call the doctor*

BOX 13.13 When to call for help

Instruct the person or family member to call the nurse or doctor if any of the following signs or symptoms occurs:

- Oral temperature greater than 38.6°C.
- Severe headache; significant increase in pain at usual site, especially if the pain is not relieved by the medication regimen; or severe pain at a new site.
- Difficulty breathing.
- New bleeding from any site, such as rectal or vaginal bleeding.
- Confusion, irritability or restlessness.
- Withdrawal, greatly decreased activity level or frequent crying.
- Verbalisations of deep sadness or a desire to end life.
- Changes in body functioning, such as the inability to void or severe diarrhoea or constipation.
- Changes in eating patterns, such as refusal to eat, extreme hunger or a significant increase in nausea and vomiting.
- Appearance of oedema in the extremities or significant increase in oedema already present.

Instruct the person or family member to call 000 if the person:

- is having much difficulty breathing or if the face or lips have a bluish tinge
- becomes unconscious or has a convulsion
- exhibits unmanageable behaviour, such as being physically abusive, hurting self or engaging in uncontrollable activity.

provides an anxiety-reducing safety net for the person and family and promotes early detection of complications.

- Monitor laboratory values that may indicate the presence of ectopic functioning and report abnormal findings to doctors immediately. (See Table 13.4 for laboratory indicators of ectopic functions.) *Early detection promotes early medical intervention and prevents serious consequences from the ectopic secretion.* Refer to the chapters 'Nursing care of people with altered fluid, electrolyte and acid–base balance', 'Nursing care of people with endocrine disorders' and 'Nursing care of people with diabetes mellitus' for specific signs and symptoms of electrolyte imbalances and endocrine disorders.

Imbalanced nutrition: less than body requirements

The anorexia–cachexia syndrome (described earlier in this chapter) is a common cause of malnutrition in people with cancer. Metabolism increases in response to increased cancer cell production, while the cancer's parasitic activity reduces the nutrients available to the body. Loss of appetite, food aversion, nausea and vomiting, and painful oral lesions from chemotherapy or radiation may contribute to impaired nutrition. Tumours of the gastrointestinal tract that affect absorption also contribute to the problem. Manifestations include wasted appearance, considerable weight loss over a relatively short period of time, anthropometric measurements below 85% of standard for fat and muscle tissue, decreases in serum proteins and negative responses to antigen testing.

- Assess current eating patterns, including usual likes and dislikes, and identify factors that impair food intake. *This allows for a more individualised plan based on needs and preferences.*
- Evaluate degree of malnutrition:
  a. Check laboratory values for total serum protein, serum albumin and globins, total lymphocyte count, serum transferrin, haemoglobin and haematocrit. *These values represent the laboratory values that are most likely to decrease with malnutrition.*
  b. Calculate nitrogen balance and creatinine height index. Calculate skeletal muscle mass and compare findings to normal ranges. *Urinary creatinine is an index of lean body mass and decreases in malnutrition. Lean muscle mass is catabolised for energy in people with cancer.*
  c. Take anthropometric measurements and compare them to standards: height, weight, elbow breadth, arm circumference, triceps skinfold thickness and arm muscle mass. *This estimates the degree of wasting; findings below 85% of standard are considered malnutrition.*
- Teach the principles of maintaining good nutrition and adapting the diet to medical restrictions and current preferences. *This tailors the food plan to the person's needs and thereby promotes compliance.*
- Manage problems that interfere with eating:
  a. Encourage eating whatever is appealing and consider adding nutritional supplements such as Ensure Plus or Isocal to the diet. *It is better to eat something even if it is not nutritionally balanced.*
  b. Eat small, frequent meals. *These are more easily digested and absorbed and are usually better tolerated by the person with anorexia.*
  c. Encourage trying icy cold foods (such as ice-cream) or those that are more highly seasoned if food has no taste. *Chemotherapy and radiation therapy may harm taste buds and prevent distinguishing the taste of foods. Strong seasonings and coldness make food more enjoyable to the person with diminished taste. However, spicy foods are not recommended for people with stomatitis.*
  d. Encourage cold and bland semi-soft and liquid foods with painful oropharyngeal ulcers; use a non-alcohol anaesthetic mouthwash prior to eating. *These foods are less irritating to sensitive mucous membranes; deadening the pain can make chewing and swallowing easier.*
  e. Manage nausea and vomiting by administering anti-emetic drugs. (Around-the-clock medication may be an effective preventive measure.) Encourage the person to eat small, frequent, low-fat meals with dry foods such as crackers and toast, to avoid liquids with meals and to sit upright for an hour after meals. Remove emesis basins and encourage oral hygiene before eating. *Dry, low-fat foods are more readily tolerated when nauseated. Removing vomiting cues, such as odour and supplies associated with vomiting, can reduce nausea.*
- Teach to supplement meals with nutritional supplements such as Ensure Plus or Isocal and to take multivitamin and mineral tablets with meals. Suggest increasing kilojoules by adding ice-cream or frozen yoghurt to the liquid supplement or commercial protein–carbohydrate powders to milk or fruit juice. *Because the food intake is usually less than that needed to maintain or gain weight, these supplements can add kilojoules in a manner often tolerated.*
- Teach to keep a food diary to document daily intake. If the person can see how little is being consumed, they may eat more. *A food diary also helps the nurse keep a kilojoule count and alert the doctor if more drastic nutritional measures, such as a feeding tube or parenteral nutrition, need to be instituted.*
- Teach to administer parenteral nutrition via a central line or other CVAD. Teach safety measures and care of the CVAD and explain how the pump delivering the solution works. Provide an emergency phone number for help with administration problems. (See the chapter 'Nursing care of people with nutritional disorders' for safety guidelines for administering parenteral nutrition.) *The person with chronic or terminal cancer requiring parenteral nutrition is usually managed at home, so information on how to manage the entire process may be needed.*

Impaired tissue integrity

The most common impairment of tissue integrity occurs in the oral–pharyngeal–oesophageal mucous membranes. It is secondary to the effects of some chemotherapeutic drugs and radiation treatment to the head and neck. The oral–pharyngeal–oesophageal tissues are lined with cells with a high mitotic turnover rate and are therefore vulnerable to many chemotherapeutic drugs. Leukaemias, bone marrow transplants and herpes viral infections are other aetiological factors in the disruption of oral–pharyngeal–oesophageal tissue. Manifestations of this problem may include the following:

- Small ulcers occur on the tongue and mucous membranes in the mouth and throat.
- Herpes simplex type 1 lesions or vesicles evolve into ulcerations.
- Fungal infections, such as thrush (due to *Candida* infections), are manifested by a white, yellow or tan coating with dry, red, fissured tissue underneath.
- Red, swollen, friable gums bleeding with minimal or no trauma.
- **Xerostomia** is excessive dryness of the mucous membranes (due to chemotherapy or radiation).

Manage such problems with the following interventions:

- Carefully assess and evaluate the type of tissue impairment present. Identify possible sources, such as chemotherapy or radiation therapy to head and neck. *This allows the nurse to implement corrective measures appropriate to the type of problem.*
- Implement and teach measures for preventing oropharyngeal infection:
  a. Observe for systemic signs of infection. Be suspicious of any fever that has no apparent cause. *This facilitates early identification of an infection before it spreads.*
  b. Encourage cleaning teeth gently and using a non-alcohol mouthwash several times a day. This can be done after waking in the morning, after any oral intake and before bedtime. Soak dentures nightly in hydrogen peroxide and floss gently with waxed floss after meals and bedtime; this measure may be contraindicated for people with leukaemia or thrombocytopenia. *Disrupted mucous membranes allow the normal oral bacterial flora into the systemic circulation, which can result in sepsis in the immunocompromised person. Reducing the oral flora by frequent hygiene decreases the risk of infection.*
  c. Culture any oral lesions and report the problem to the doctor. *Herpes lesions may not follow a typical pattern in immunosuppressed people. Identifying the cause of the infection, whether viral, fungal or bacterial, allows the doctor to prescribe the appropriate treatment.*
- Implement and teach measures for reducing trauma to delicate tissues:
  a. Counteract dry mouth (xerostomia) with lubricating and moisturising agents, such as Gatorade, sugarless gum and Blistex. *This protects mucous membranes from infection and trauma.*
  b. Avoid putting sharp instruments in the mouth. Use smooth plastic spoons and forks for eating, especially with a bleeding disorder. Dental work should be done by dental oncologists.
  c. Brush teeth with a very soft toothbrush and obtain a new toothbrush monthly. If gums are friable and bleeding, clean teeth with a soft cloth or toothpaste over finger. Chlorhexidine mouthwash (Savacol) may be used. This protects gums from trauma and decreases risk of haemorrhage.
- Administer specific medications as ordered to control infection and/or pain:
  a. Aciclovir is often used to treat viral infections.
  b. Systemic antibiotics are used to treat bacterial infections.
  c. Nystatin or clotrimazole solution for 'swish and swallow' or lozenges that dissolve slowly in the mouth are used for fungal infections.
  d. Use viscous xylocaine or various combination mouthwashes before meals and as needed. These agents reduce pain and inflammation. See Box 13.14 for the ingredients of combination mouthwashes. *Knowing the contents of each mouthwash can prevent hypersensitivity reactions (e.g. lignocaine) and assist when teaching.*

BOX 13.14 Combination mouthwashes for oropharyngeal pain control

Kaiser mouthwash
- Nystatin
- Hydrocortisone
- Tetracycline

Stanford mouthwash
- Nystatin
- Tetracycline
- Lignocaine
- Hydrocortisone

Xyloxylin suspension
- Benylin syrup
- Lignocaine
- Maalox suspension

Stomafate suspension
- Sucralfate
- Sterile water
- Benylin syrup
- Maalox suspension

Nursing interventions for oncological emergencies

In caring for people with cancer, nurses may encounter a number of emergency situations in which their role may be pivotal to the person's survival. Most of these emergencies require astute observations, accurate judgments and rapid action once the problem has been identified. A brief description of the more common oncological emergencies with nursing interventions follows. In all cases, immediate notification of the doctor or emergency team is the first step.

Pericardial effusions and neoplastic cardiac tamponade

Malignant pericardial effusion is an accumulation of excess fluid in the pericardial sac that compresses the heart, restricts heart movement and results in a cardiac tamponade. The signs of cardiac tamponade are caused by compression of the heart, which leads to decreased cardiac output and impaired cardiac function. Signs include hypotension, tachycardia, tachypnoea, dyspnoea, cyanosis, increased central venous pressure, anxiety, restlessness and impaired consciousness.

Interventions include the following:

- Start oxygen and alert respiratory therapy for other respiratory support as needed.
- Insert an intravenous cannula if one is not already in place.

- Monitor vital signs and initiate haemodynamic monitoring.
- Prepare vasopressor drugs as ordered.
- Bring emergency cart to bedside.
- Set up for and assist doctor with a pericardial tap (pericardiocentesis).
- Reassure the person.

Superior vena cava syndrome

The superior vena cava can be compressed by mediastinal tumours or adjacent thoracic tumours. The most common cause is small-cell or squamous cell lung cancers. Occasionally the problem is caused by thrombus around a central venous catheter that then plugs up the vena cava, resulting in obstruction and backup of the blood flowing into the superior vena cava.

Obstruction of the venous system causes increased venous pressure, venous stasis and engorgement of veins that are drained by the superior vena cava. Signs and symptoms may develop slowly; facial, periorbital and arm oedema are early signs. As the problem progresses, respiratory distress, dyspnoea, cyanosis, tachypnoea, altered consciousness and neurological deficits may occur. Figure 13.7 illustrates the superior vena cava syndrome.

Emergency measures include the following:

- Provide respiratory support with oxygen and prepare for tracheostomy.
- Monitor vital signs.
- Administer corticosteroids (e.g. dexamethasone) to reduce oedema.
- If the disorder is due to a clot, administer antifibrinolytic or anticoagulant drugs.
- Provide a safe environment, including seizure precautions.

After the emergency is managed, the person often receives radiation or chemotherapy to reduce the tumour size.

Sepsis and septic shock

Tumour necrosis, immune deficiency, antineoplastic therapy, malnutrition and comorbid conditions can lead to the development of sepsis. Bacteria gain entrance to the blood, grow rapidly and produce septicaemia. Because malignant tumours are more likely to use anaerobic metabolic pathways, the bacteria of tumour sepsis are usually Gram-negative and damage the body through a combination of bacterial endotoxins and an uncontrolled immune reaction. Gram-negative sepsis progresses to systemic shock and eventually results in multisystem failure. Signs and symptoms appear in two phases. The first phase is characterised by vasodilation with vascular dehydration, high fever, peripheral oedema, hypotension, tachycardia, tachypnoea, hot flushed skin with creeping mottling beginning in the lower extremities and anxiety or restlessness. Without treatment, the shock progresses to the second phase, which shows the more classic signs of shock: hypotension, rapid thready pulse, respiratory distress, cyanosis, subnormal temperature, cold clammy skin, decreased urinary output and altered mental state. Identifying the problem while the person is still in the hyperdynamic state is crucial to the person's survival. See the chapter 'Nursing care of people experiencing trauma and shock' for further discussion of septic shock.

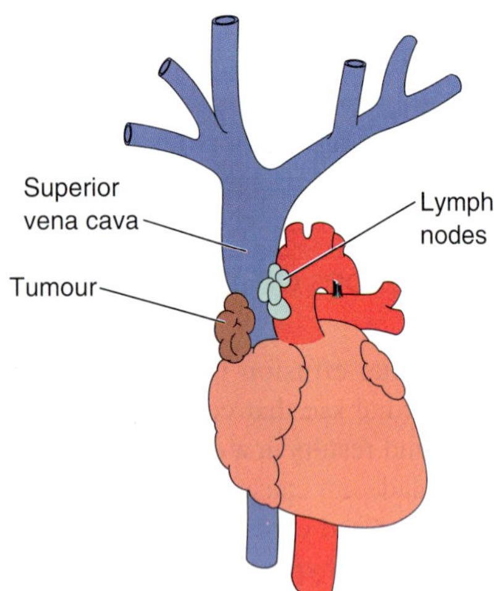

FIGURE 13.7 ***The superior vena cava syndrome. The enlargement of a tumour adjacent to the superior vena cava (usually in the lung or mediastinum) compresses that major blood vessel, which leads into the right atrium of the heart. As a result, blood backs up into the venous system behind the obstruction, diminishing blood flow into the heart***

Spinal cord compression

Spinal cord compression is most commonly associated with pressure from expanding tumours of the breast, lung or prostate, and with lymphoma or metastatic disease. Spinal cord compression constitutes an emergency because of the potential for irreversible paraplegia. Back pain is the initial symptom in 95% of the cases of spinal cord compression. This may progress to leg pain, numbness, paraesthesias and coldness. Later, bowel and bladder dysfunction occur; finally, neurological dysfunction progresses from weakness to paralysis. Treatment often consists of radiation or surgical decompression, but early detection is essential. See the chapter 'Nursing care of people with cerebrovascular and spinal cord disorders' for further discussion of spinal cord compression.

Obstructive uropathy

People with intra-abdominal, retroperitoneal or pelvic malignancies, such as prostate, cervical or bladder cancers, may experience obstruction of the bladder neck or the ureters. Bladder neck obstruction usually manifests as urinary retention, flank pain, haematuria or persistent urinary tract infections, but ureteral obstruction is often not evident until the person is in renal failure. See the chapters 'Nursing care of people with urinary tract disorders' and 'Nursing care of people with kidney for further discussion of obstructive uropathy.

Hypercalcaemia

Hypercalcaemia in people with cancer results from the excessive ectopic production of parathyroid hormone and is most commonly associated with cancers of the breast, lung, oesophagus, thyroid, head and neck, and with multiple myeloma. Bone metastases may also cause hypercalcaemia. When the rate of calcium mobilisation from the bone exceeds the renal threshold for excretion, serum calcium levels can become dangerously elevated. People with hypercalcaemia often present with non-specific symptoms of fatigue, anorexia, nausea, polyuria and constipation. Neurological symptoms include muscle weakness, lethargy, apathy and diminished reflexes.

Without treatment, hypercalcaemia progresses to alterations in mental status, psychotic behaviour, cardiac arrhythmias, seizures, coma and death (see the chapter 'Nursing care of people with altered fluid, electrolyte and acid–base balance').

Hyperuricaemia

Hyperuricaemia usually is a complication of rapid necrosis of tumour cells after vigorous chemotherapy for lymphomas and leukaemias. Hyperuricaemia may be related to increased uric acid production or to the tumour lysis syndrome associated with Burkitt's lymphoma. Uric acid crystals are deposited in the urinary tract, causing renal failure and uraemia. People with hyperuricaemia manifest with nausea, vomiting, lethargy and oliguria.

Syndrome of inappropriate antidiuretic hormone secretion

Occurring in only about 2% of people with cancer, syndrome of inappropriate antidiuretic hormone secretion (SIADH) is related to an ectopic secretion of antidiuretic hormone that is usually associated with small-cell lung carcinoma, but also occasionally with prostate and adrenal cancers. The kidney secretes an excessive amount of sodium and conserves a disproportionate amount of free water, causing profound hyponatraemia. Signs and symptoms include anorexia, nausea, muscle aches and subtle neurological symptoms that can progress to lethargy, confusion, seizures and coma from cerebral oedema.

Tumour lysis syndrome

Tumour lysis syndrome (TLS) is a life-threatening emergency for people with cancer. TLS is characterised by a combination of two or more metabolic abnormalities, including hyperuricaemia, hyperphosphataemia, hyperkalaemia and/or hypocalcaemia (Gupta & Moore, 2018; Webster & Kaplow, 2021). The syndrome develops because of massive and rapid destruction or death of cancer cells caused by cytotoxic treatment such as chemotherapy, radiation, biological therapy, hormonal therapy, steroids or surgery, or any combination of these. It can also occur spontaneously with sudden death of tumour cell. A high incidence of TLS occurs in people with bulky, highly proliferating and chemosensitive tumours such as high-grade lymphomas (Burkitt's lymphoma) and acute lymphoblastic leukaemia (ALL). Although the incidence of TLS in solid tumours is rare, cases of TLS following chemotherapy have been reported in people with small-cell lung cancer, breast cancer, neuroblastoma, melanoma and ovarian cancer.

The major cause of TLS is chemotherapy to tumours with a high proliferative rate, a relatively large tumour burden and high sensitivity to cytotoxic agents, which leads to massive and rapid cell death. Usually, within a week of initiating chemotherapy, the body no longer can excrete the large amount of metabolic by-products from the cell death, resulting in the release of intracellular contents and metabolic by-products (such as potassium, phosphorus and nucleic acid) into the bloodstream (Gupta & Moore, 2018; Webster & Kaplow, 2021). As a result, a combination of metabolic derangements occurs, including hyperkalaemia, hyperuricaemia and hyperphosphataemia with secondary hypocalcaemia. These metabolic abnormalities put people at risk of cardiac malfunction and renal failure.

Clinical manifestations of TLS include nausea, vomiting, lethargy, oedema, fluid overload, congestive heart failure, cardiac dysrhythmias, seizures, muscle cramps, tetany, syncope and possible sudden death. Diagnosis of TLS mainly depends on laboratory tests and clinical signs and symptoms.

Prevention is crucial in management of TLS. People at risk of TLS include those with bulky chemosensitive cancer such as high-grade lymphomas and acute leukaemia, elevated serum uric acid, potassium, phosphorus and renal deficiency. Preventive and management measures include identifying people at risk, administration of allopurinol to inhibit the conversion of nucleic acid to uric acid, hydration and diuretic therapy to promote urinary excretion of uric acid and phosphate, urine alkalinisation to promote the urinary excretion of uric acid, administration of oral phosphate binder such as aluminium hydroxide to promote the excretion of phosphate through the bowel, administration of sodium polystyrene sulfonate (Kayexalate) to promote the excretion of potassium through the bowel and initiation of haemodialysis to people unresponsive to standard approaches to hyperkalaemia, hyperuricaemia or hyperphosphataemia.

Health education for the person and family

Prevention

The Cancer Council (2022c, 2022d) promotes strategies to reduce cancer risk in addition to the screening measures discussed earlier in this chapter. Based on these strategies, nurses teach people and families to decrease risk factors by:

- quitting smoking
- eating healthy foods (see Box 13.15)
- staying in shape
  - maintain a healthy body weight range and body mass index
  - waist circumference below 94 cm for men and 80 cm for women
- being sun smart
  - slip on protective clothing
  - slop on SPF 30+ or SPF 50 sunscreen (20 minutes before going outside and re-apply every 2 hours)
  - slap on a broad-brimmed, legionnaire or bucket-style hat
  - seek shade
  - slide on some sunglasses
- limiting alcohol
  - limit intake—no more than two standard drinks per day
  - choose low-alcohol drinks
  - avoid binge drinking
  - have at least 2 alcohol-free days per week
  - eat some food when you drink
- moving your body
  - only 30 minutes of moderate intensity exercise each day is good for your health and 60 minutes can reduce your risk of developing cancer
  - increase walking—at lunchtime, park your car further away, take the stairs.

Sources: Cancer Council (2022c). *Maintain a healthy weight*. Retrieved from https://www.cancer.org.au; Cancer Council (2022d). *Food and nutrition*. Retrieved from https://www.cancer.org.au.

In addition, encourage people to report to the public health department any known leaking of chemicals or radioactive materials into the water or air and any noted increase in the incidence of cancer, especially of one specific type, in their communities.

BOX 13.15 Cancer Council: strategies for eating healthy foods

Eat two serves of fruit and five serves of vegetables per day.
Eat cereals—preferably wholegrain.
Limit cured meats.
Red meat three to four times a week only and on other days eat fish, poultry, beans and lentils.
Choose foods low in salt, sugars and saturated fats.

Sources: Cancer Council (2022c). *Maintain a healthy weight*. Retrieved from https://www.cancer.org.au; Cancer Council (2022d). *Food and nutrition*. Retrieved from https://www.cancer.org.au. For more information visit https://www.cancer.org.au.

Rehabilitation and survival

Rehabilitation from cancer not only involves regaining strength, recovering from surgery or chemotherapy and learning to live with an altered body part or appliance, but also entails recovering from associated psychological and emotional turmoil.

Rehabilitation centres provide physiotherapy, occupational therapy, speech pathology, job retraining and an opportunity to recuperate before resuming full responsibilities. In addition, many people go home to convalesce and receive in-home support in the form of nursing supervision, direct care and teaching. Hygiene and home maintenance can be provided by home and community care organisations. Physiotherapists and occupational therapists provide muscle strengthening and mobility training (especially with prostheses) and home safety teaching.

Psychological rehabilitation of cancer survivors addresses quality-of-life issues. Three 'seasons of cancer survival' have been described (Mullan, 1985). The first starts with diagnosis but is dominated by treatment. The second stage is one of extended survival, which occurs when treatment ends and the watchful waiting period begins. This period is characterised by fear of recurrence. Permanent survival is said to begin when the survival period has gone on long enough that the risk of recurrence is small. In this period, the person has to deal with secondary problems related to health and social issues resulting from the cancer experience. Employment may be a problem, private health insurance may be cancelled and life insurance may be difficult to get. Relationships may have suffered from the strain of the illness on significant others and the essential self-focusing required for recovery. However, both the person and significant others may have undergone a personal and spiritual growth that ushers in a new and enriching period of their lives.

New self-help groups are emerging in many communities to support others through their 'seasons of survival'. Many cancer survivors speak to groups about assisting other cancer survivors. People and families need to be informed about the many resources available through community agencies as well as the survivor support groups.

Community-based care

Before the person is discharged, teach both the person and significant others or caregivers to manage the person at home. Discuss problems that may result from the type of cancer and the treatment received and provide information on how to manage these problems and when to call the doctor.

- Teach wound care to the person with an open wound or draining lesion and provide a referral to a community nurse to monitor progress.
- Explain special diets clearly or refer the person to a dietitian before discharge.
- Carefully review the doctor's instructions with the person and family, making sure they understand the medications to be taken, any other treatments and when to see the doctor for follow-up care.
- Provide or order equipment and supplies needed for home care, especially any specialised bed or equipment to aid mobility and ensure safety in the home.
- For the person who will need complex care, such as parenteral nutrition, provide a referral to the community nurse before discharge.

Because the hospital stay is often short, the person and family will benefit from follow-up phone calls at home for several days. People do not learn well under the stress of going home; give the person and family a number to call if they have concerns or questions.

Hospice care

More and more people with terminal disease are electing to die at home. This decision has been made easier by the increased availability of hospice programs. When a person and family or significant others elect **hospice care**, they are usually precluding additional hospitalisations other than those required to manage reversible problems. People in hospice care also refuse resuscitation measures (CPR and other extraordinary measures).

Many hospice services are connected with an inpatient respite care unit, where the person can receive 24-hour care for up to several weeks. This source provides the necessary care to the person if a family member becomes ill or needs to be relieved temporarily of the tremendous burden of caring for a dying loved one. Hospice care involves a multidisciplinary team and is designed to give the person comfort and to assist in a peaceful death with support to caretakers. The team usually consists of a nurse case manager, a doctor, an anaesthetist or pharmacist, an infusion therapist, a social worker, a physiotherapist, a home health aide and volunteers.

Studies of families that have participated in hospice services have found that family members were very positive about the experience (Aparicio et al., 2017; Coyle & Ferrell, 2016; Palliative Care Australia, 2022). The aspects of hospice care they most appreciated were the 24-hour accessibility and availability of the healthcare team and the quality of communication from all team members. Family members emphasised that 'the nurses listened, answered questions honestly and prepared us for changes in the patient's condition'. Team members were rated as very professional, but more relaxed and friendly than hospital staff; they talked with the family and displayed accepting, non-judgmental attitudes. Team members were also seen as well informed, knowledgeable and competent with excellent problem-solving skills. the chapter 'Nursing care of people experiencing loss, grief and death' provides more information on hospice care.

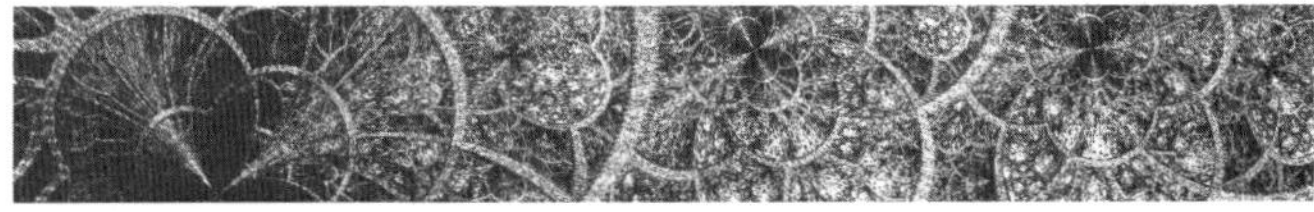

CHAPTER HIGHLIGHTS

- Lung cancer was the leading cause of all cancer deaths in both men and women in Australia in 2018, accounting for 18.9% of all cancer deaths. Cancer can affect people of any age, gender, ethnicity or geographical region.
- The incidence of cancer increases with advancing age. The most commonly seen cancers in women are breast, colorectal and lung cancer, and melanoma of the skin. In men, prostate, lung and colorectal cancer, and melanoma of the skin occur most frequently.
- Oncogenes are genes that promote cell proliferation and are capable of triggering cancerous characteristics. Several oncogenes, such as BRCA-1 and BRCA-2, are associated with breast cancer.
- Tumour suppressor genes, which normally suppress oncogenes, can become inactive by deletion or mutation. Inherited cancers have been associated with tumour suppressor genes, such as *p53*, a suppressor gene that has been associated with sarcoma and cancer of the breast and brain.
- The diagnosis and treatment of cancer is a pivotal life-changing event that prompts individuals to make immediate and ongoing adjustment to this life-threatening illness.
- Effective physical and psychosocial adjustment to cancer diagnosis and treatment has been shown to lead to successful completion of treatment, enhancement of the person's ability to cope with disease, improvement of the person's quality of life and, ultimately, improvement of survival.
- The goals of cancer treatment are cure and control of cancer, as well as management of cancer-related and treatment-related symptoms.
- Chemotherapy uses cytotoxic medications to cure or control cancer by interrupting cell metabolism and replication and by interfering with the ability of the malignant cell to synthesise vital enzymes and chemicals.
- Pain management is an important component of care for people with cancer. It is estimated that 20% to 50% of people with early-stage cancer and up to 95% of people with advanced cancer experience pain.
- Complementary therapies are therapies that people choose as a complement to medical treatment. Common complementary therapies for cancer include botanical agents, nutritional supplements, dietary regimens, mind–body modalities, spiritual approaches and miscellaneous therapies.
- Tumour lysis syndrome (TLS), a combination of two or more metabolic abnormalities, is a life-threatening emergency for people with cancer. People at risk of TLS include those with bulky chemosensitive cancer such as high-grade lymphomas and acute leukaemia, elevated serum uric acid, potassium and phosphorus, and renal deficiency.

CONCEPT CHECK

1 Mr Lawrence has a history of colon cancer. He has been advised that the cells from the colon tumour have travelled to his liver. This process is called:

1 carcinogenesis
2 dysplasia
3 metastasis
4 mutation

2 A person diagnosed with lung cancer reports they are having difficulty sleeping and often feel tense. The most appropriate initial nursing intervention would be to:

1 encourage the person to express his feelings about the cancer diagnosis
2 document the person's report of difficulty sleeping and tenseness in the chart
3 obtain an order for medication for sleep from the doctor
4 offer an anti-anxiety drug such as Ativan (lorazepam)

3 Mr Palacci is receiving external radiation for treatment of lung cancer. Educating Mr Palacci to care for his skin in the marked area includes:

1 apply antibacterial ointment daily
2 avoid contact with others
3 avoid rubbing or scratching treated skin areas
4 cleanse the skin with plain water

4 Ms Hernandez complains of nausea and vomiting following her daily chemotherapy treatment. The most appropriate nursing intervention would be to:

1 keep Ms Hernandez on nil orally until her daily chemotherapy is completed
2 provide anti-emetic medication 30 to 40 minutes prior to each treatment
3 provide clear liquids until the chemotherapy is completed
4 schedule chemotherapy administration for bedtime

5 Mrs Smith experiences bone marrow depression as a result of chemotherapy. Which of the following would the nurse expect to find?

1 alopecia
2 nausea and vomiting
3 platelet count 50
4 temperature 38.9°C

6 Mr Wu, a 46-year-old businessman with a diagnosis of metastatic lung cancer, is going to have chemotherapy tomorrow. To help Mr Wu better understand chemotherapy, you have provided him with education about the role of the chemotherapeutic agents being used to treat his cancer. You determine that your teaching is effective when Mr Wu states:

1 'Chemotherapy uses drugs that promote the normal growth of cells while killing the cancer cells.'
2 'Chemotherapy only uses a single drug to treat cancer because drug resistance is rare.'
3 'Chemotherapy includes drugs that attack not only cancer cells but also normal rapidly dividing cells.'
4 'Chemotherapy is a preferred therapy because it has fewer adverse effects than radiation therapy.'

7 During training for new radiation nurses, you have learned that the delivery of high-energy radiation (e.g. electrons, x-rays, photons) to kill cancer cells by using a machine to focus a beam of radiation on the body is called:

1 external radiation therapy
2 internal-beam radiation therapy
3 brachytherapy
4 biochemotherapy

8 You are taking care of a person who just received the first cycle of chemotherapy for acute leukaemia 2 days ago. As an oncology nurse, you are closely monitoring the person's laboratory tests of uric acid, potassium, phosphorus and calcium as you are aware the person is at risk of:

1 spinal cord compression
2 tumour lysis syndrome
3 septic shock
4 superior vena cava syndrome

9 In which phase of the cell cycle does the DNA replicate to form two sets of chromosomes?
1 G_1
2 G_2
3 S
4 M

10 Oncogenes are genes that:
1 promote cell growth when activated
2 block cell growth
3 stimulate a complex signalling process
4 are strictly regulated

BIBLIOGRAPHY

Abernethy, A. P., Shelby-James, T., Fazekas, B. S., Woods, D. & Currow, D. C. (2005). The Australia-modified Karnofsky Performance Status (AKPS) Scale: A revised scale for contemporary palliative care clinical practice [electronic version]. *BioMed Central Palliative Care*, *4*(7), 1–12.

American Cancer Society (1995). *American Cancer Society textbook of clinical oncology*. Atlanta: American Cancer Society.

Anderson, C. M., Buzaid, A. C., Sussman, J. J. et al. (1998). Nitric oxide and neopterin levels and clinical response in stage III melanoma patients receiving concurrent biochemotherapy. *Melanoma Research*, *8*(2), 149–155.

Anekar, A. A. & Cascella, M. (2022). *WHO analgesic ladder*. Retrieved from https://www.ncbi.nlm.nih.gov/

Antoni, M. H., Lutgendorf, S. K., Blomberg, B., Carver, C. S., Lechner, S., Diaz, A. & Cole, S. W. (2012). Cognitive-behavioral stress management reverses anxiety-related leukocyte transcriptional dynamics. *Biological Psychiatry*, *71*(4), 366–372.

Aparicio, M., Centeno, C., Carrasco, J. M. et al. (2017). What are families most grateful for after receiving palliative care? Content analysis of written documents received: A chance to improve the quality of care. *BMC Palliative Care*, *16*(47). doi: 10.1186/s12904-017-0229-5.

Australian Institute of Health and Welfare (AIHW) (2021). *Cancer in Australia 2021*. Cancer series no. 133. Cat. no. CAN 144. Canberra: AIHW. Retrieved from https://www.aihw.gov.au/

Australian Institute of Health and Welfare (AIHW) (2022). *Indigenous and Torres Strait Islander health performance framework: 1.08 Cancer*. Retrieved from https://www.indigenoushpf.gov.au/

Australian Radiation Protection and Nuclear Safety Agency (ARPANSA) (2008). *Safety guide: Radiation protection in nuclear medicine*. Radiation Protection Series No. 14.2. Canberra: ARPANSA.

Battiato, L. A. & Wheeler, V. S. (2018). Biotherapy. In C. H. Yarbro, M. H. Frogge, M. Goodman et al. (eds), *Cancer nursing: Principles and practice* (8th ed., pp. 543–579). Boston: Jones & Bartlett.

Bradt, J., Dileo, C., Myers-Coffman, K. & Biondo, J. (2021). Music interventions for improving psychological and physical outcomes in people with cancer. *Cochran Database of Systematic Reviews*. https://doi.org/10.1002/14651858.CD006911.pub4

Brant, J. M. (2022). The assessment and management of acute and chronic cancer pain syndromes. *Seminars in Oncology Nursing*, *38*. https://doi.org/10.1016/j.soncn.2022.151248

Burki, T. K. (2018). New cancer blood test developed. *The Lancet*, *19*(3), 140.

Cancer Australia (2020). *A guide to implementing the optimal care pathway for Aboriginal and Torres Strait Islander people with cancer*. Retrieved from https://canceraustralia.gov.au/

Cancer Australia (2021). *All cancers in Australia*. Retrieved from https://canceraustralia.gov.au/

Cancer Council (2007). *National cancer prevention policy—2007–2009*. Retrieved from https://www.cancer.org.au

Cancer Council (2019). *Hair loss: Information for people affected by cancer*. Retrieved from https://www.cancer.org.au

Cancer Council (2021). *The HPV vaccine*. Retrieved from http://www.hpvvaccine.org.au/

Cancer Council (2022a). *Common cancer symptoms*. Retrieved from https://www.cancer.org.au

Cancer Council (2022b). *Early detection of breast cancer*. Retrieved from https://www.cancer.org.au

Cancer Council (2022c). *Maintain a healthy weight*. Retrieved from https://www.cancer.org.au

Cancer Council (2022d). *Food and nutrition*. Retrieved from https://www.cancer.org.au

Cohen, G. L. & Falkson, C. I. (1998). Current treatment options for malignant melanoma. *Drugs*, *55*(6), 791–799.

Coyle, N. & Ferrell, B.R. (2016) (eds). *Social aspects of care*. New York: Oxford University Press.

Ebeling, M., Rau, R., Malstrom, H., Ahlbom, A. & Modig, K. (2021). The rate by which mortality increases with age is the same for those who experienced chronic disease as for the general population. *Age and Ageing*, *50*(5), 1633–1640. https://doi.org/10.1093/ageing/afab085

Eliopoulos, E. (2021). *Gerontological nursing* (10th ed.). Philadelphia: Wolters Kluwer/Lippincott Williams & Wilkins.

Fabi, A., Bhargava, R., Fatigoni, S. et al. (2020). Cancer-related fatigue: ESMO clinical practice guidelines for diagnosis and treatment. *Annals of Oncology*, *31*(6), 713–723. Retrieved from https://www.annalsofoncology.org/

Fox, M. C., Lao, C. D., Schwartz, J. L., Frohm, M. L., Bichakjian, C. K. & Johnson, T. M. (2013). Management options for metastatic melanoma in the era of novel therapies: A primer for the practicing dermatologist: Part II: Management of stage IV disease. *Journal of the American Academy of Dermatologists*, *68*(1), 13–e1.

Garvan Institute of Medical Research (2021). *Genomic cancer medicine program*. Retrieved from https://www.garvan.org.au/

Gupta, A. & Moore, J. A. (2018). Tumor lysis syndrome. *Journal of American Medical Association (JAMA) Oncology*, *4*(6), 895. doi: 10.1001/jamaoncol.2018.0613

International Society of Nurses in Cancer Care (ISNCC) (2022). *Position statements*. Retrieved from https://www.isncc.org/

Jorde, L. B., Carey, J. C. & Barnshad, M. J. (2019). *Medical genetics* (6th ed.). Philadelphia: Mosby.

Lan, T., Chen, L. & Wei, X. (2021). Inflammatory cytokines in cancer: Comprehensive understanding and clinical progress in gene therapy. *Cells*, *10*(1). doi: 10.3390/cells10010100. Retrieved from https://www.ncbi.nlm.nih.gov/

LeFever Kee, J. L. (2018). *Laboratory & diagnostic tests with nursing implications* (10th ed.). Upper Saddle River, NJ: Pearson.

Legha, S., Ring, S., Eton, O. et al. (1998). Development of a biochemotherapy regimen with concurrent administration of cisplatin, vinblastine, dacarbazine, interferon alfa and interleukin-2 for patients with metastatic melanoma. *Journal of Clinical Oncology*, *16*(5), 1752–1759.

Levett-Jones, T., Dwyer, T., Reid-Searl, K., Heaton, L., Flenady, T., Applegarth, J., Guinea, S. & Andersen, P. (2017). *Patient Safety Competency Framework (PSCF) for Nursing Students*. Sydney. Retrieved from http://psframework.wpengine.com/

Madsen, S. (2016). Photochemical internalisation for solid malignancies. *The Lancet Oncology*, *17*(9), 1173–1174.

Morris, B. A., Anderson, K., Cunningham, J. & Garvey, G. (2017). Identifying research priorities to improve cancer control for Indigenous Australians. *Public Health Research & Practice*, *27*(4). https://doi.org/10.17061/phrp2741735

Mullan, F. (1985). Seasons of survival: Reflections of a doctor with cancer. *New England Journal of Medicine*, *313*, 270–273.

National Cancer Institute (2021a). *The cancer genome atlas program*. Retrieved from https://www.cancer.gov/

National Cancer Institute (2021b). *Photodynamic therapy to treat cancer*. Retrieved from https://www.cancer.gov/

Nogrady, B. (2020). Cancer diagnosis: How cancer genomics is transforming diagnosis and treatment. *Nature*, *579*, s10–s11. Retrieved from https://media.nature.com/

Norman, S., Localio, A., Potashnik, S., Simoes Torpey, H., Kallan, M., Weber, A. & Solin, L. (2009). Lymphedema in breast cancer survivors: Incidence, degree, time course, treatment, and symptoms. *Journal of Clinical Oncology*, *27*(3), 390–397.

Norris, T. L. (2018). *Porth's pathophysiology: Concepts of altered health states* (10th ed.). Philadelphia: Lippincott Williams & Wilkins.

Oncology Nursing Society (2022). *Oncology Nursing Society position paper: Access to quality cancer care*. Retrieved from https://www.ons.org/

Palliative Care Australia (2022). *How can I support my friend/family member?* Retrieved from https://palliativecare.org.au/

Piotrowska, W., Leppert, W. & Majkowicz, M. (2019). Comparison of analgesia, adverse effects, and quality of life in cancer patients during treatment of procedural pain with intravenous morphine, fentanyl nasal spray, and fentanyl buccal tablets. *Cancer Management and Research*, *11*. Retrieved from https://www.ncbi.nlm.nih.gov/

Portilla-Tamarit, J., Reus, S., Portilla, I. et al. (2021). Impact of advanced HIV disease on quality of life and morality in the era of combined antiretroviral treatment. *Journal of Clinical Medicine*, *10*(4). https://doi.org/10.3390/jcm10040716

Poust, J. C., Woolery, J. E. & Green, M. R. (2013). Management of toxicities associated with high-dose interleukin-2 and biochemotherapy. *Anti-Cancer Drugs*, *24*(1), 1–13.

Rubin, P. (2001). *Clinical oncology: A multidisciplinary approach for doctors and students* (8th ed.). Philadelphia: W. B. Saunders.

Schwetz, T. A. & Fauci, A. S. (2019). The extended impact of human immunodeficiency virus/AIDS research. *The Journal of Infectious Diseases*, *1*(1), 6–9. https://doi.org/10.1093/infdis/jiy441

Selye, H. (1984). *The stress of life* (rev. 2nd ed.). New York: McGraw-Hill.

Sitarz, J. & Spencer, C. (2022). Chemotherapy-induced alopecia: Examining patient perceptions and adherence to home haircare recommendations. *Clinical Journal of Oncology Nursing*, *26*(2), 190–197. doi: 10.1188/22.CJON.190-197

Smith, T. G., Troeschel, A. N., Castro, K. M. et al. (2019). Perceptions of patients with breast and colon cancer of the management of cancer-related pain, fatigue, and emotional distress in community oncology. *Journal of Clinical Oncology*, *37*(19), 1666–1676.

Webster, J. S. & Kaplow, R. (2021). Tumor lysis syndrome: Implications for oncology nursing practice. *Seminars in Oncology Nursing*, *37*(2). https://doi.org/10.1016/j.soncn.2021.151136

Yoong, J. & Poon, P. (2018). Principles of cancer pain management: An overview and focus on pharmacological and interventional strategies. *Australian Journal of General Practice*, *47*(11), 758–762.

World Health Organization (WHO) (2018). *WHO guidelines for the pharmacological and radiotherapeutic management of cancer pain in adults and adolescents*. Retrieved from https://www.who.int/

UNIT 3 BUILDING CLINICAL COMPETENCE

Pathophysiology and patterns of health

Clinical scenario

You have been assigned to work with the following four people for the 0700 shift on a medical–surgical unit. Significant data obtained during report are as follows:

- Allen Barber is a 55-year-old with diabetes mellitus who is 4 days postoperative abdominal surgery with an inflammation of the incision site. Vital signs are T 38.3°C, P 94, R 24, BP 138/82. The abdominal incision appears red with warmth and oedema around the incision. Mr Barber states that his pain level is 8 on a pain scale of 1 to 10. Labs and wound cultures have been ordered.
- Tamra Sanders is a 22-year-old with Down syndrome. She is admitted in sickle cell crisis with T 38.9°C, P 90, R 30 and shallow and BP 110/84. Tamra is complaining of severe chest pain with shortness of breath. She states that her pain scale level is 10 of 10. She has an order to begin morphine PCA.
- Mia Windham is a 26-year-old who was admitted yesterday with a maculopapular rash on the hands and feet that is spreading to the arms and legs. This morning she is complaining of abdominal pain, nausea and bloody diarrhoea. She has a history of having a bone marrow transplant 3 months ago as treatment for leukaemia.
- Harry Anderson is a 40-year-old in the late stages of AIDS. He is confused, incontinent and has severe spasticity. He is on seizure precautions. He needs to be turned every 2 hours to prevent pressure sores. He is currently yelling that he needs help.

Critical-thinking questions

1 In what order would you visit these people after report?

1. ______________________________
2. ______________________________
3. ______________________________
4. ______________________________

2 What would you prioritise as the two most important nursing diagnoses for each of the people presented above? Can you explain, if asked, the rationale for your choices?

	Priority nursing diagnosis #1	Priority nursing diagnosis #2
Allen Barber		
Tamra Sanders		
Mia Windham		
Harry Anderson		

3 In which position does the nurse place the person with hypovolaemic shock?

1. semi-Fowler's position with legs straight
2. Trendelenburg position with legs elevated 10 degrees
3. left lateral position with legs bent towards chest
4. supine position with legs elevated 20 degrees

4 Tamra Sanders' family asks the nurse how sickle cell anaemia is transmitted from one family member to another. Which statement by the nurse is the correct response?

1. 'The mother carries the gene for sickle cell anaemia and passes it to the children.'
2. 'The father carries the gene for sickle cell anaemia and passes it to the children.'
3. 'Both parents carry the gene for sickle cell anaemia and children have a 25% chance of getting the disease process.'
4. 'One parent has the disease and one parent carries the affected gene and they have a 50% chance of passing it to the children.'

5 Mr Anderson, who has AIDS, has experienced weight loss. The dietitian teaches him meal planning in which type of diet?

1. high protein, high fibre
2. high protein, high kilojoule
3. low fibre, low protein
4. high carbohydrate, high vitamins

6 The nurse performs wound cleansing with which procedure?

1. Cleanse the wound with soap and water.
2. Use normal saline to cleanse the wound.
3. Cleanse the wound with povidone-iodine.
4. Hydrogen peroxide (half strength) is used to cleanse the wound.

7 Prior to administering cytotoxic agents, such as cyclophosphamide (Cytoxan), the nurse needs to notify the doctor of which lab results?

1. haemoglobin of 108 g/L, haematocrit of 35%
2. potassium of 3.4 mmol/L, sodium of 130 mmol/L
3. creatinine of 2 mg/dL, blood urea nitrogen of 3.0 mmol/L
4. white blood cell count of $3.9(\times 10^9/L)$, platelets of $74(\times 10^9/L)$

8 Due to diarrhoea, Ms Windham's arterial blood gas results are pH, 7.30, $PaCO_2$, 35 mmHg; PaO_2, 90 mmHg, HCO_3^-, 19 mEq/L. The nurse interprets these results as indicating the person has:

1. metabolic acidosis
2. metabolic alkalosis
3. respiratory acidosis
4. respiratory alkalosis

9 Which laboratory studies would you expect to draw on a person who is 4 days postoperative with an inflammation of the incision site?

1. white blood cell count/differential, erythrocyte sedimentation rate, C-reactive protein
2. troponins, metabolic panel for electrolytes, cultures of wound site
3. blood cultures, haematocrit and haemoglobin, blood glucose level
4. full blood count, alkaline phosphatase, urine creatinine and blood urea nitrogen

10 The person is admitted to the emergency department for a severe anaphylactic reaction to aspirin. Which medication is ordered to be administered?

1. 0.5 mL of 1:1,000 adrenaline subcutaneously
2. 0.3 mL of 1:10,000 adrenaline subcutaneously
3. intravenous infusion of 1:10,000 adrenaline
4. intravenous infusion of 1:100,000 adrenaline

11 When administering a blood transfusion, which manifestations indicate a haemolytic reaction to the blood being administered?

1. abdominal cramps and diarrhoea
2. bradycardia and hypertension
3. dyspnoea and hypotension
4. diaphoresis and tachycardia

12 The nurse educates people and families to decrease risk factors of cancer by following which cancer prevention recommendations? (Select all that apply.)

1. Avoid tobacco and excessive alcohol use.
2. Eat a diet low in fat and high in carbohydrates.
3. Increase intake of vitamins A, D, E and K.
4. Limit exposure in sun from 11 am to 4 pm.
5. Increase fruit and vegetables in the diet.
6. Eat meats grilled over a charcoal fire instead of fried.

Case study

Mr Johnson is a 60-year-old construction worker who has presented at the doctors complaining of dull chest pain, shortness of breath, swelling of his hands and feet, weight loss, fatigue and weakness. On physical assessment, vital signs are temperature 37.7°C, pulse 84, respirations 24, blood pressure 168/92. His height is 180.3 cm and weight is 79.5 kg. Mr Johnson states that this is a loss of 15.9 kg during the past 3 months. Wheezing is heard when breath sounds are auscultated. Coughing is noted with deep breathing. The remainder of the physical assessment is unremarkable. He has a medical history of high blood pressure for which he takes diltiazem and ramipril. He has a history of smoking 1 to 2 packets of cigarettes a day since he was 15 years old. He states he has been exposed to asbestos in his employment. Mr Johnson's nutrition assessment indicates that his diet consists of fried meats (especially chicken), green vegetables cooked in pork fat, eggs and bacon for breakfast, and during breaks he eats biscuits. His fluid intake consists of coffee for breakfast and during breaks, soft drinks at lunch, and 3 to 4 beers at night.

Blood is drawn for a full blood count, electrolytes, blood glucose, calcitonin, CEA, haptoglobulin, GGT and creatinine. A sputum specimen is sent to the laboratory. A chest x-ray and CT scan are done. Based on the results of the chest x-ray, bronchoscopy and needle aspiration biopsies are performed to confirm a diagnosis of lung cancer. The oncologist recommends an initial treatment plan of radiation therapy followed by combination chemotherapy to reduce the tumour size prior to surgical resection of the tumour.

Based on Mr Johnson's medical diagnosis and treatment plan, *Readiness for enhanced therapeutic regimen management* is identified as the priority nursing diagnosis at this time.

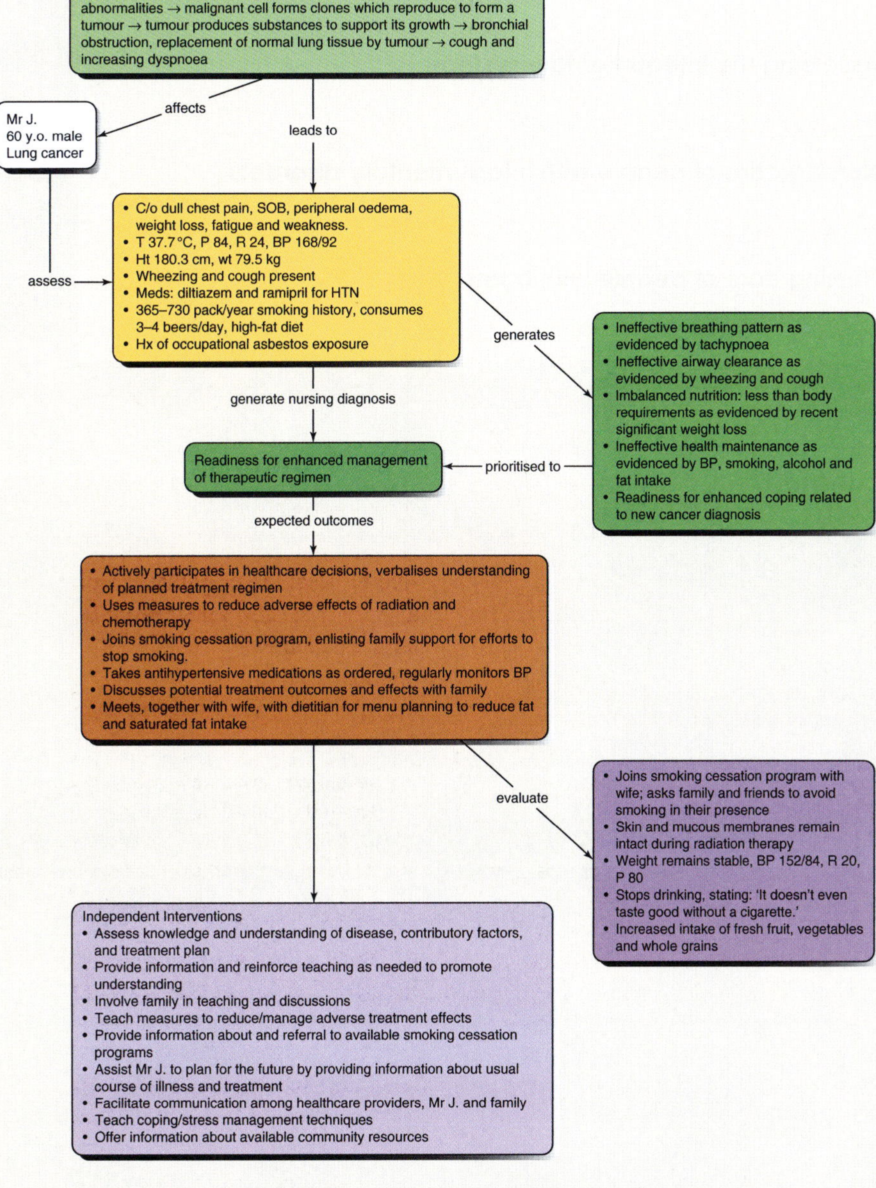

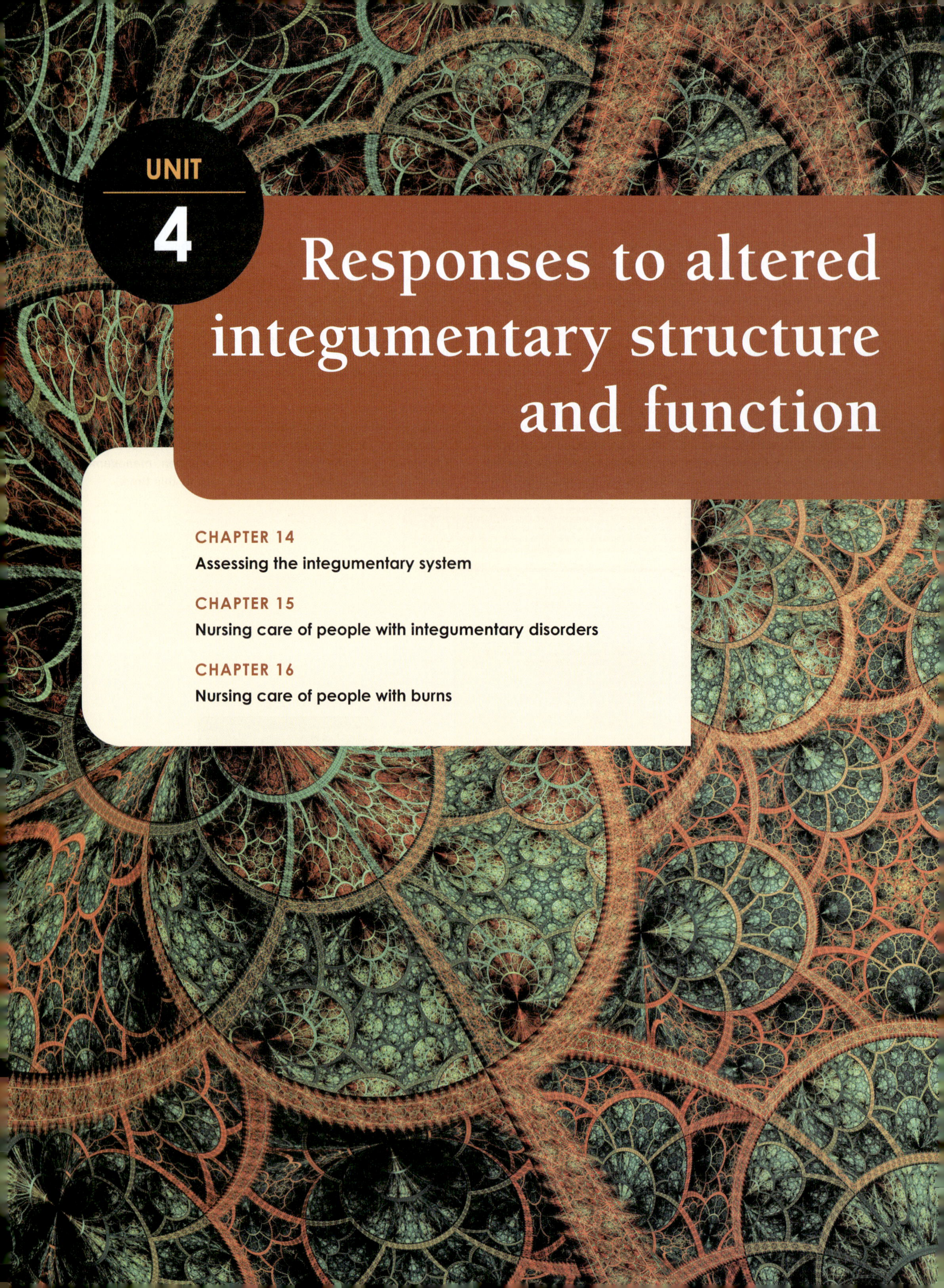

UNIT 4

Responses to altered integumentary structure and function

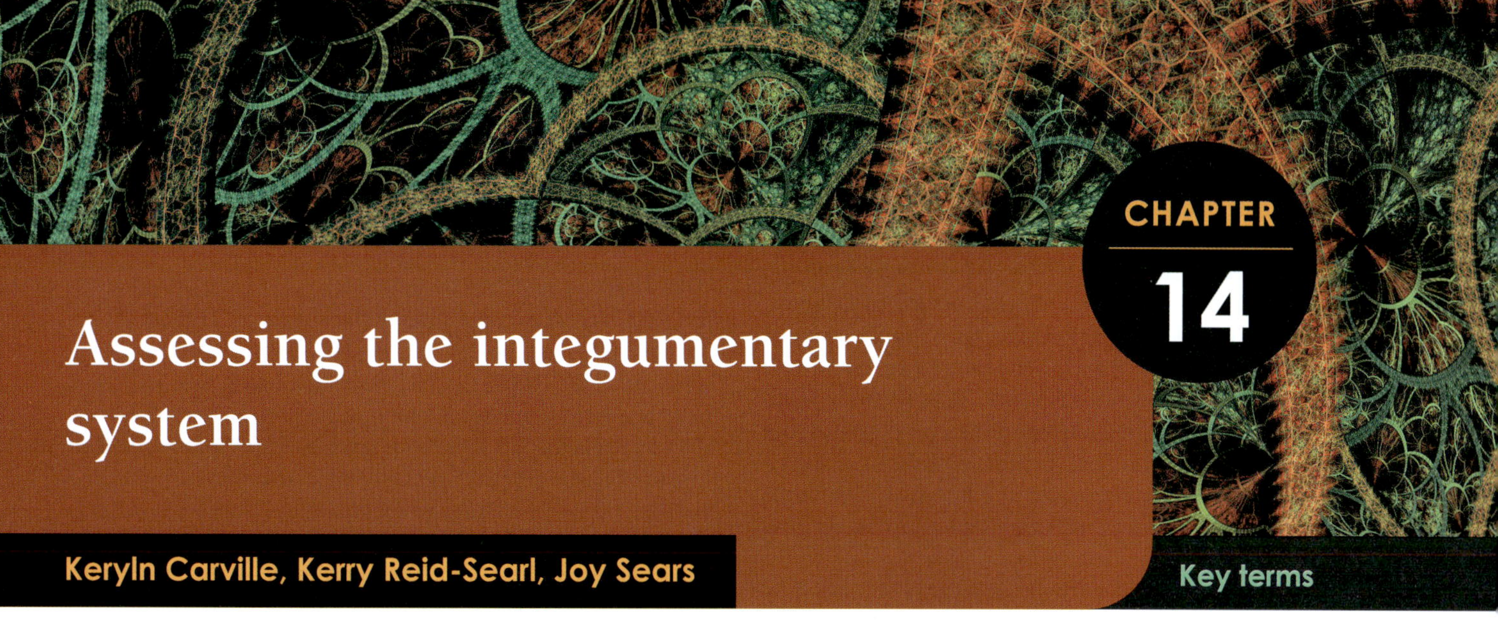

Chapter 14 Assessing the integumentary system

Keryln Carville, Kerry Reid-Searl, Joy Sears

Key terms

Learning outcomes

- Describe the anatomy, physiology and functions of the skin, hair and nails.
- Explain the integumentary assessment process, including conducting a comprehensive and focused nursing assessment.

Clinical competencies

- Conduct and document a health history for people who have or are at risk of alterations in the skin, hair or nails.
- Conduct and document a comprehensive and focused assessment of the integumentary system.
- Monitor the results of diagnostic tests and report abnormal findings.

Equipment needed

- Disposable gloves
- Ruler
- Torch or good light source

The skin and its accessory appendages, which include hair, nails and sebaceous, sudoriferous and ceruminous glands, make up the integumentary system. The skin, the largest organ of the body, provides an external covering for the body, separating and protecting the body's organs and tissues from the external environment. Compared with all other body organs, it is the most exposed to infection and injury. In the average adult, the skin receives one-third of the circulating blood volume. The pH of the skin is slightly acidic, ranging from 4.2 to 6, which ensures an 'acid mantle' for protective purposes and maintenance of normal skin flora. Functions of the skin and its accessory structures are summarised in Table 14.1. The nurse should understand the normal functioning to apply the process of clinical reasoning.

Disorders of the integumentary structures may be caused by a variety of factors including environmental factors, allergies, infection, infestation, disease, malignancy, trauma and genetic influences.

PATIENT SAFETY COMPETENCY FRAMEWORK

5 Clinical reasoning

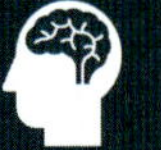

The Patient Safety Competency Framework indicates that nursing students should demonstrate the ability to accurately assess, interpret and respond to individual patient data in a systematic and timely way (Levett-Jones et al., 2017).

ANATOMY, PHYSIOLOGY AND FUNCTIONS OF THE INTEGUMENTARY SYSTEM

The skin

The skin has an average total surface area of 7,600 cm^2. An average male may be covered by 16,000 cm^2 of skin (Nash, Matts & Ertel, 2007). It has been estimated that in 1 cm^2 there is almost 1 metre of blood vessels, 4 metres of nerves, 100 sweat glands, 15 sebaceous glands, 3,000 sensory cells at the end of nerve fibres, 25 pressure apparatuses to record tactile stimuli, 200 nerve endings to record pain, 2 sensory apparatus for cold, 12 sensory apparatus for heat, 300,000 epidermal cells and 10 hairs (Klein, 1988). The appearance of the integumentary system is dependent upon age, ethnicity, general health and wellbeing, and cultural and occupational pursuits. Structurally, the skin consists of the epidermis, the dermis and the hypodermis (see Figure 14.1).

The epidermis

The epidermis, which comprises the surface or outermost part of the skin, consists of stratified squamous epithelium. It is avascular and is approximately 0.04 mm thick (Carville, 2017). The epidermis receives its nutrients from the dermal layer beneath it. The epidermis regenerates itself, and the normal epidermal turnover time of epidermal cells as they migrate from the stratum germinativum to the stratum corneum and are then shed averages 28 days. The epidermis has either four or five layers, depending on its anatomical location; there are five layers over the palms of the hands and the soles of the feet, and four layers over the rest of the body.

TABLE 14.1 Functions of the skin and its appendages

STRUCTURE	FUNCTIONS
Epidermis	Protects tissues from physical, chemical and biological damage.
	Prevents water loss and serves as a water-repellent layer.
	Stores melanin, which protects tissues from harmful effects of ultraviolet radiation in sunlight.
	Converts cholesterol molecules to vitamin D when exposed to sunlight.
	Contains phagocytes, which prevent bacteria from penetrating the skin.
Dermis	Contains blood vessels, which supply nutrients to the stratum germinativum of the epidermis and the skin appendages.
	Regulates body temperature by dilating and constricting capillaries.
	Contains specialised sensory receptors and nerves, which transmit sensation signals to the central nervous system.
Hypodermis	Main support system for the skin.
	Protective layer for underlying organs and structures.
	Participates in temperature regulation.
	Storage depot for fat.
Sebaceous (oil) glands	Secrete sebum, which lubricates skin and hair. Play a role in maintaining the pH of the skin.
Eccrine sweat glands	Present at birth and regulate body heat by excretion of perspiration.
Apocrine sweat glands	Remnant of sexual scent gland, activated at pubescence.
Ceruminous glands	Modified apocrine glands which, together with sebaceous glands, produce cerumen—ear wax.
Hair	Cushions the scalp. Eyelashes and cilia protect the body from foreign particles. Provides insulation in cold weather.
Nails	Protect the fingers and toes, aid in grasping and allow for various other activities, such as scratching the skin, picking up small items and so on.

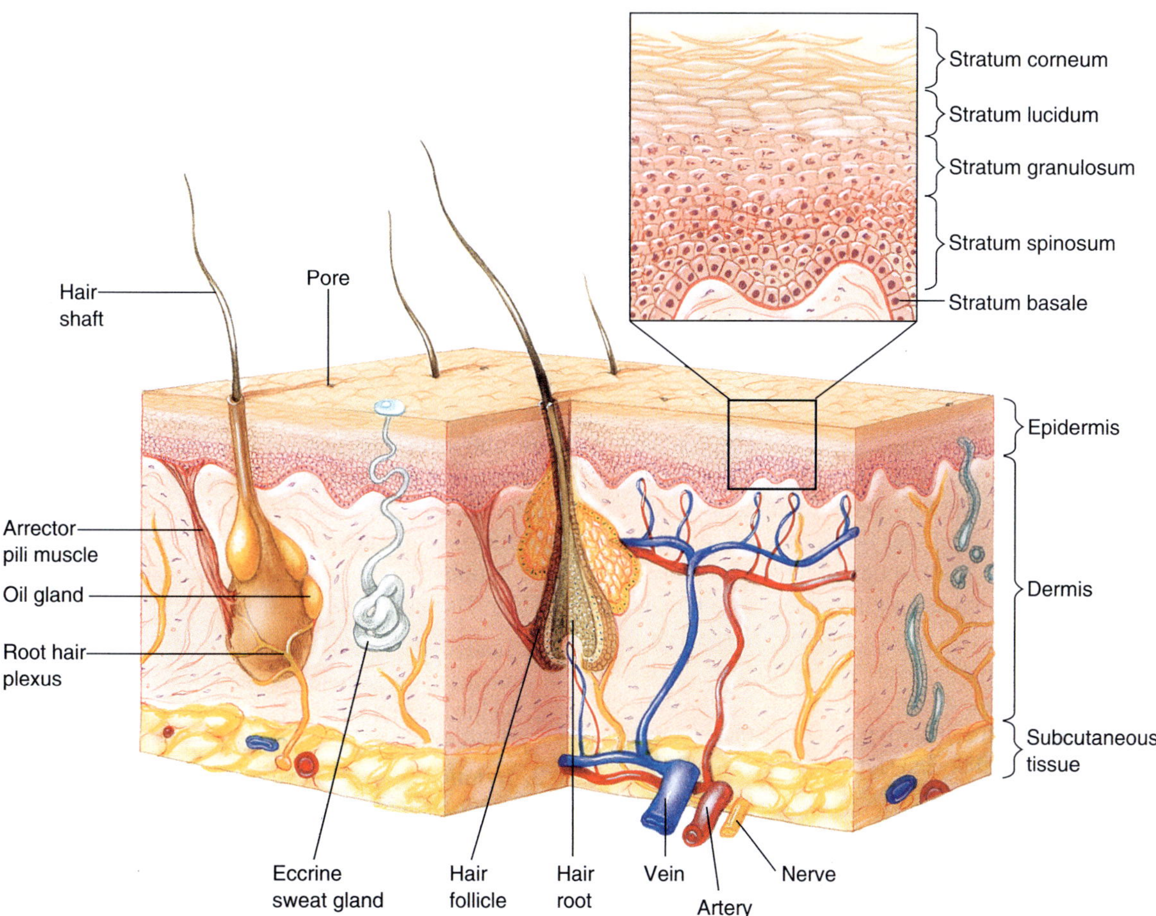

FIGURE 14.1 ***Anatomy of the skin***

The stratum germinativum, also known as the stratum basale, is the deepest layer of the epidermis. It is comprised of a single layer of basal cells that are mitotically active and constantly dividing. It contains melanocytes, cells that produce the pigment **melanin**, and keratinocytes, which produce **keratin**. Melanin forms a shield to protect the keratinocytes and the nerve endings in the dermis from the damaging effects of ultraviolet light. Melanocyte activity probably accounts for the difference in skin colour in humans. Keratin is a fibrous, water-repellent protein that gives the epidermis its tough, protective quality. As keratinocytes mature, they move upwards through the epidermal layers, eventually becoming dead cells at the surface of the skin. Millions of these cells are worn off by abrasion each day; simultaneously millions more are produced in the stratum germinativum.

The next layer of the epidermis is the stratum spinosum or prickle cell layer, which is composed of several stratified layers of polygonal cells that are attached by desmosomes, which appear as spiny processes. Mitosis occurs at this layer, although not as abundantly as in the stratum germinativum.

The stratum granulosum, the next layer, is two to three cells thick. The cells of the stratum granulosum contain a glycolipid that slows water loss across the epidermis. As cells migrate from stratum spinosum to stratum granulosum the nucleus is destroyed by enzymes, the cells flatten and cellular contents are converted into tough, insoluble keratin. Keratinisation, a thickening of the cells' plasma membranes, begins in the stratum granulosum.

The stratum lucidum is a transparent layer with no visible nuclei and is present only in areas of thick skin—for example, on the soles or palms. The outermost layer of the epidermis, the stratum corneum, is also the thickest, making up about 75% of the epidermis' total thickness. It consists of about 20 to 30 layers of dead cells called corneocytes, which are filled with keratin fragments arranged in 'shingles' that flake off as dry skin.

THE BASEMENT MEMBRANE The basement membrane is an acellular, non-vascular and non-innervated membrane that separates the epidermis from the dermis. The basement membrane serves as an adherent and mechanical support layer between the epidermis and the dermis (Martini, Nath & Bartholomew, 2018). It is also thought to play a role in regulating the transfer of proteins, oxygen, and nutrients across the dermal–epidermal junction (Carville, 2017).

The dermis

The dermis is attached to the basement membrane, but is often referred to as the second, deeper layer of skin. Made of a flexible connective tissue, this layer is richly supplied with blood cells, nerve fibres and lymphatic vessels. The hair follicles, sebaceous glands and sweat glands are located in the dermis, although they are derived from the epidermal layer. The dermis consists of a papillary (upper layer) and a reticular layer (deeper layer). The papillary layer contains reti ridges that indent the overlying epidermis. It also contains capillaries and receptors for pain and touch. The deeper, reticular layer contains blood vessels, sweat and sebaceous glands, deep pressure receptors and dense bundles of collagen fibres. The regions between these bundles form lines of cleavage in the skin, which are referred to as Langer's lines. Surgical incisions parallel to these lines of cleavage heal more easily and with less scarring than incisions or traumatic wounds across cleavage lines.

The hypodermis

The hypodermis (also called the subcutaneous layer) contains large blood vessels that supply the skin. Additionally, it serves as a storage depot for fat and thus contains adipose tissue as well as connective tissue. The function of the hypodermis is to insulate, afford protection to underlying structures and regulate temperature. The hypodermis plays a significant role as it acts as a support framework for the skin. This is because the fibres that extend from the dermis anchor the skin to the hypodermis, which then attaches to the underlying fascia (the connective tissue around muscles and bones) (Jenkins & Tortora, 2013).

Skin appendages

Appendages of the skin include the glands (sebaceous, sudoriferous and ceruminous), the hair and the nails. The following sections explain each appendage.

Glands of the skin

The skin contains sebaceous (oil) glands, sudoriferous (sweat) glands and ceruminous (cerumen or earwax) glands. Each of these glands has a different function.

Sebaceous glands enter halfway up the hair follicle; thus, they are found all over the body except on the palms, soles, lips and nipples where there are no hair follicles. These glands secrete an oily substance called **sebum**, which is usually ducted into a hair follicle. Sebum softens and lubricates the skin and hair and decreases water loss from the skin in low humidity. Sebum and sweat influence the pH of the skin, and the 'acid mantle' or slightly acidic pH protects the body against opportunistic infection. The secretion of sebum is stimulated by hormones, especially androgens. If a sebaceous gland becomes blocked, a pimple or whitehead appears on the surface of the skin; as the material oxidises and dries, it forms a comedone or blackhead. Acne vulgaris is an inflammation of the sebaceous glands.

There are two types of sweat glands: eccrine and apocrine. Eccrine sweat glands are present at birth and are more numerous on the forehead, palms and soles. The gland itself is located in the dermis; the duct to the skin rises through the epidermis to open in a pore at the surface. The secretion of the eccrine glands is composed mostly of water, but it also contains sodium, antibodies, small amounts of metabolic wastes, lactic acid and vitamin C. The production of sweat is regulated by the sympathetic nervous system and serves to maintain normal body temperature. Sweating also occurs in response to emotions.

Apocrine sweat glands are activated at pubescence. Most apocrine sweat glands are located in the axillary, anal and genital areas. The secretions from apocrine glands are similar to those of eccrine sweat glands, but they also contain fatty acids and proteins. Apocrine glands are a remnant of sexual scent glands.

Ceruminous glands are modified apocrine sweat glands. Located in the skin of the external ear canal, they secrete yellow-brown waxy cerumen. This substance provides a sticky trap for foreign materials.

The hair

Hair is distributed all over the body, except the lips, nipples, parts of the external genitals, the palms of the hands and the soles of the feet. Hair is composed of keratin. It is produced by a hair bulb and its root is enclosed in a hair follicle (see Figure 14.2). The exposed part, called the shaft, consists mainly of dead cells. Hair follicles extend into the dermis and in some places, such as the scalp, below the dermis. Many factors, including nutrition and hormones, influence hair growth. Humans have three types of hair. They are:

1. lanugo, the fine hair found on the body of premature neonates that is usually shed within weeks of birth
2. vellus, the fine, lightly coloured body hair that grows to 1 cm, found on the arms, legs or female face
3. terminal hair, which is found on the scalp, face of males, pubic region and armpits, and can grow to 50 cm.

Hair in various parts of the body has protective functions: the eyebrows and eyelashes protect the eyes; hair in the nose helps keep foreign materials out of the upper respiratory tract; and hair on the head protects the scalp from heat loss and sunlight. On average, an adult loses 50–100 head hairs a day. Scalp hair can last 2–4 years and eyelashes tend to last 3–5 months.

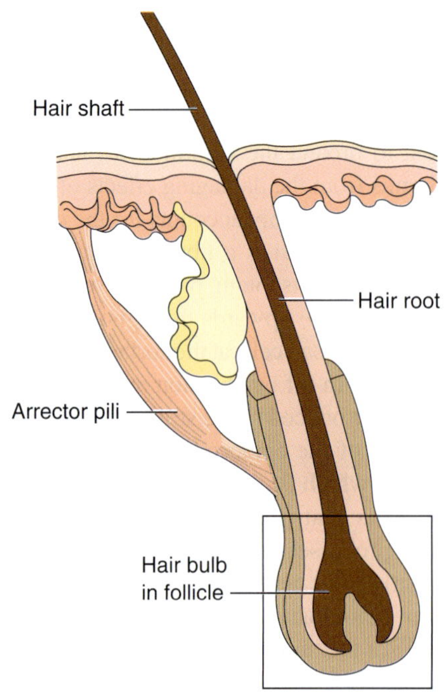

FIGURE 14.2 ***Anatomy of a hair follicle***

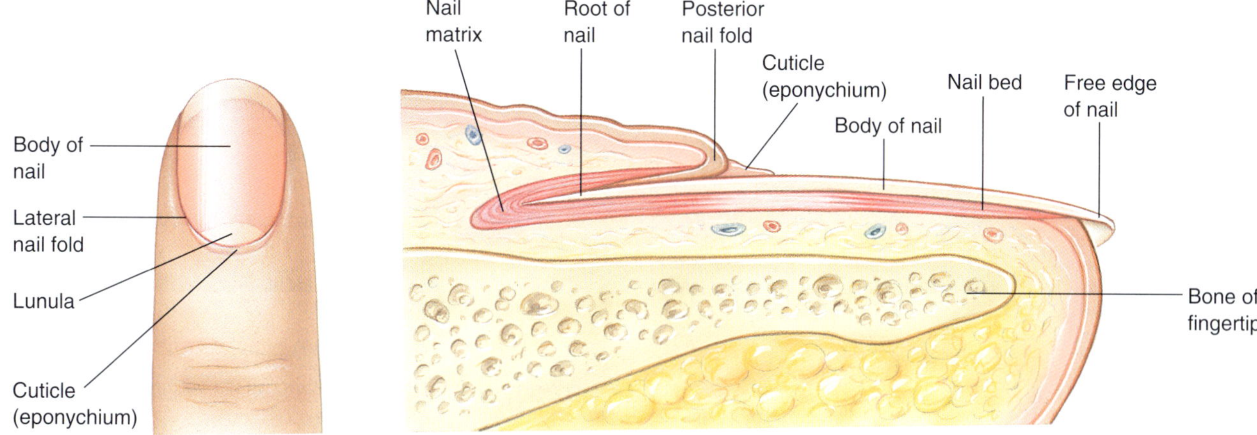

FIGURE 14.3 *Anatomy of a nail (frontal and side views)*

The nails

A nail is composed of keratin. Like hair, nails consist mainly of dead cells. They arise from the stratum germinativum of the epidermis. The body of the nail rests on the nail bed (see Figure 14.3). The nail matrix is the active, growing part of the nail. The proximal visible end of the nail has a white crescent, called a lunula. The sides of the nail are overlapped by skin, called nail folds. The proximal nail fold is thickened and is called the eponychium or cuticle. Nails form a protective coating over the dorsum of each digit on the fingers and toes.

Skin colour

Skin colour varies among individuals and among people of different races, ranging from a pinkish white to various shades of brown and black. Areas of the skin that are normally exposed to the sun and environment, such as the face and hands, may have a slightly different colour from areas that are usually covered with clothing. Special care must be taken when assessing changes in skin colour in people with darker skin, such as people who are Aboriginal or Torres Strait Islander, Pacific Islander, Asian, of Mediterranean descent and Caucasian who are deeply suntanned.

Skin colour is the result of varying levels of pigmentation. Melanocytes produce melanin, a yellow-to-brown pigment, which is predominately responsible for skin tone and protects against damage from ultraviolet rays. All races have the same number of melanocytes, but melanin is produced in greater amounts in people with dark skin colour. Exposure to the sun causes a build-up of melanin and a darkening or tanning of the skin in people with light skin. Carotene, a yellow-to-orange pigment, is found mostly in areas of the body where the stratum corneum is thickest, such as the palms of the hands. Carotene is more abundant in the skins of people of Asian ancestry and, together with melanin, accounts for their golden skin tone. The epidermis in Caucasian skin has very little melanin and is almost transparent. Thus, the colour of the haemoglobin found in red blood cells (RBCs) circulating through the dermis shows through, lending Caucasians a pinkish skin tone. The Fitzpatrick skin type classification (Fitzpatrick, 1988) is a validated tool for assessing skin colour in individuals (see Table 14.2).

Skin colour is influenced by emotions and pathological disorders. **Erythema**, a reddening of the skin, may occur with embarrassment (blushing), fever, hypertension or inflammation. It may also result from a drug reaction, sunburn, acne rosacea or other factors. A bluish discolouration of the skin and mucous membranes, called **cyanosis**, results from poor oxygenation of haemoglobin. **Pallor**, or paleness of skin, may occur with shock, fear or anger, or be a sign of anaemia and hypoxia. **Jaundice**, a yellow-to-orange colour visible in the skin and mucous membranes, is most often the result of a hepatic disorder or physiological jaundice in the newborn. Table 14.3 further defines these terms and compares and contrasts skin colour changes in people with light and dark skin.

TABLE 14.2 Fitzpatrick skin type

SKIN TYPE	CHARACTERISTICS	SCORE
Type I Pale white skin	Extremely sensitive skin, always burns never tans. As seen in people with red hair and freckles.	0-6
Type II White skin	Very sensitive skin, burns easily, tans minimally. As seen in fair-skinned, fair-haired Caucasians, northern Asians.	7-13
Type III Light brown skin	Sensitive skin, sometimes burns, slowly tans to light brown. As seen in darker Caucasians and some Asians.	14-20
Type IV Moderate brown skin	Mildly sensitive, burns minimally, always tans to moderate brown. As seen in Mediterranean and Middle Eastern Caucasians and Southern Asians.	21-27
Type V Dark brown skin	Resistant skin, rarely burns, tans well. As seen in some Hispanics, some Africans.	28-34
Type VI Deeply pigmented dark brown to black skin	Very resistant skin, never burns, deeply pigmented. As seen in darker Africans, Indigenous Australians.	35+

Source: Fitzpatrick (1988). The validity and practicality of sun reactive skin types I through VI. *Archives Dermatology*, *124*(6), 869–871.

TABLE 14.3 Skin colour assessment variations in people with light and dark skin

DISORDER AND CAUSE	CHANGE IN LIGHT SKIN	CHANGE IN DARK SKIN
Pallor: *a decrease or absence in skin colour as the result of a decrease in tissue perfusion; a decrease in shape, size or amount of red blood cells (RBCs); or absence of melanin (local or generalised).*		
Anaemia (decreased or abnormal size and shape of RBCs)	Generalised paleness	Brown skin is dull and has a yellow cast; black skin is dull and has an ashen grey cast
Haemorrhage (decreased amount of circulating RBCs)	Generalised paleness	Brown skin is dull and has a yellow cast; black skin is dull and has an ashen grey cast
Shock (decreased amount of circulating RBCs or decreased perfusion)	Generalised paleness	Brown skin is dull and has a yellow cast; black skin is dull and has an ashen grey cast
Arterial insufficiency (trauma, acute arterial occlusion or arteriosclerosis)	Local paleness	Dull, ashen grey
Vitiligo (patchy loss of melanocytes)	Patches of white spots, most often found over skin of the face, hands or groin	Patches of white spots, most often found over skin of the face, hands or groin
Albinism (total absence of melanin)	White/pink	Light tan, cream or white
Cyanosis: *a bluish discolouration of the skin and mucous membranes resulting from a local or generalised excess of deoxygenated haemoglobin or a structural defect in the haemoglobin molecule.*		
Acute and chronic disorders of the structure and function of the heart and lungs (arterial insufficiency or respiratory distress). Peripheral cyanotic changes may also be due to exposure to cold or hypothermia	Dusky blue (may be generalised or local, depending on cause)	Skin may appear darker, but will be dull; cyanosis is more readily assessed in the nail beds, oral mucous membranes and conjunctivae
Erythema: *redness of the skin or mucous membranes that is the result of dilatation and congestion of superficial capillaries.*		
Hyperaemia (inflammation, increased body temperature, hot environmental temperature, embarrassment, alcohol ingestion)	Red or bright pink	Difficult to assess; skin may have dark red cast
Carbon monoxide poisoning (carbon monoxide displaces oxygen on the haemoglobin molecule, causing hypoxia, carboxyhaemoglobinaemia)	Cherry red in face and upper torso	Cherry red lips, oral mucous membranes and nail beds
Pressure injury	Dusky red	Difficult to assess; may be warm to touch or bluish tint
Reactive hyperaemia (a compensatory erythema in response to tissue pressure that fades when tissues are compensated)		
Non-reactive hyperaemia does not blanch after 30 minutes pressure relief and indicates a stage 1 pressure injury		
Jaundice: *yellowish discolouration of the skin, mucous membranes and sclerae of the eyes, caused by increased amounts of bilirubin or other pigments such as elevated carotene in the blood.*		
Increased serum bilirubin to >2–3 mg/100 mL or other pigments such as elevated carotene in haemolysis, such as following blood transfusion, severe burns or infections	Yellowing of skin follows yellowing of sclerae and mucous membranes; may also be assessed in the fingernails and palms of the hands	Yellowing is best assessed at the junction of the hard palate and the soft palate or on the palms of the hands. Sclerae may be yellow near the limbus (do not confuse with normal yellow eye pigmentation)
Uraemia (retained urochrome pigments in the blood)	Orange-green or grey cast to skin. Yellowing of skin follows yellowing of sclerae and mucous membranes; may also be assessed in the fingernails and palms of the hands	Difficult to assess; may appear as yellowish green colour in the sclera
Physiological jaundice occurs in newborns around the third to fourth day and is due to haemolysing excess red cells	Obvious yellowing of the skin and sclerae	Yellowing is best assessed at the junction of the hard palate and the soft palate or on the palms of the hands. Sclerae may be yellow

ASSESSING THE INTEGUMENTARY SYSTEM

The functions of the integumentary system (skin, glands, hair and nails) are assessed by a health assessment interview to collect subjective data, a physical assessment to collect objective data, and findings from diagnostic tests. Nurses have a responsibility to undertake a comprehensive and focused assessment that is supported by thorough documentation in an electronic or hard copy format.

See the 'Sample documentation' box for sample documentation of an assessment of the integument.

Health assessment interview

A health assessment interview to determine problems with the integumentary system may be conducted as part of a health screening or total health assessment, or it may focus on a chief complaint (such as itching or a rash). Like all assessments, the nurse needs to first establish effective communication, both verbally and non-verbally, with the

Links to National Patient Safety Standards

NSQHS: Comprehensive Care Standard

One of the key criteria for this standard is developing and delivering a comprehensive care plan. The plan is developed in collaboration with the patient and family, and specific risks of harm are identified in order to 'prevent and manage harm' (Australian Commission on Safety and Quality in Health Care (ACSQHC), 2021). Many of the NSQHS Standards apply here because if a patient is assessed as having challenges or concerns with their integumentary system, it may put them at greater risk of harm from pressure or falls, in addition to being at risk from complications relating to infection control and administration of medications. However, meaningful implementation of the Comprehensive Care Standard ensures a patient's individual risks are identified and managed appropriately, reducing the likelihood of harm.

Source: ACSQHC (2021). *National Safety and Quality Health Service Standards* (2nd ed.). Sydney: ACSQHC. © Australian Commission on Safety and Quality in Health Care.

SAMPLE DOCUMENTATION

Assessment of the skin post-allergic reaction

21/01/2023 NURS 0900 hrs — A 27-year-old male, Jimmy Fascer, with no history of skin lesions, hair loss or disorders of the nails. Jimmy reports that he took an antibiotic for a respiratory infection approximately 10 days ago which resulted in the appearance of a fine, raised, red, itchy rash on his trunk and arms. Jimmy further reports that he presented to the doctor, who prescribed an antihistamine and the rash cleared in 3 days. Upon current assessment the person's skin is light brown, warm, dry and supple. Patches of vitiligo are present over the dorsum of his hands. No lesions or oedema are noted. Jimmy has a healed scar on his lower left abdomen (an appendectomy as a young adult). He has clean, dark brown hair which is greying at the temples. His nails are smooth, hard and immobile.________________ K Simpson

(KATE SIMPSON, RN)

PATIENT SAFETY COMPETENCY FRAMEWORK

2 Therapeutic communication

The Patient Safety Competency Framework indicates that nursing students should demonstrate the ability to use verbal and non-verbal communication to convey respect and empathy and be able to develop therapeutic relationships while maintaining professional boundaries (Levett-Jones et al., 2017).

patient in order to proceed with the interview. A therapeutic relationship is the goal, and in order to achieve this the nurse needs to be empathetic to the patient's needs and be respectful. When assessing skin colour it is advisable to use a validated tool such as the Fitzpatrick skin type classification (Fitzpatrick, 1988).

If the person has a skin problem, analyse its onset, characteristics and course, severity, precipitating and relieving factors, and note the timing and circumstances of any associated symptoms. For example, ask the person:

- When did the itching begin and how severe was it?
- When did you first notice a change in this mole?
- Did you change to any different kinds of shampoo or other hair products just before you started to lose your hair?

Ask about any change in health, rashes, itching, colour changes, dryness or oiliness, growth of or changes in warts or moles, and the presence of lesions. Precipitating causes, such as medications, the use of new soaps, skin care agents, cosmetics, pets, travel, stress or dietary changes, must also be explored. In assessing hair problems, ask about any thinning or baldness, excessive hair loss, change in distribution of hair, use of hair care products, diet and dieting. When assessing nail problems, ask about nail splitting or breakage, discolouration, change in shape, infection, diet and exposure to chemicals.

It is necessary to observe patient behaviours and ask the person about their habitual history or their habits or tics, such as biting of finger nails, twisting or pulling of hair, picking at skin lesions.

The person's medical history is important. Questions focus on identifying previous problems, allergies and the presence of lesions. Skin problems may be manifestations of other disorders, such as cardiovascular disease, endocrine disorders, hepatic disease and haematological disorders. The occupational and social history may provide cues to skin problems. It is important to ask the person about travel, exposure to toxic substances at work or socially, their use of alcohol and responses to stress. Family history may provide insight into hereditary-linked disorders such as atopic eczema or dermatitis (these terms are used interchangeably). Assess the presence of risk factors for skin cancer carefully. These include male gender; aged over 50; family history of skin cancer; extended exposure to sunlight; tendency to sunburn; history of sunburn or other skin trauma; light-coloured hair or eyes; residence in high altitudes or near the equator; and exposure to radiation, x-rays, coal, tar or petroleum products.

It is also important to explore the risk factors for malignant melanoma. These include the presence of a large number of moles, the presence of atypical moles, a family history of melanoma, prior melanoma, repeated severe sunburns, ease of freckling and sunburning, or inability to tan.

See the 'Functional health pattern interview' box. Responses should be documented in the person's medical record.

FUNCTIONAL HEALTH PATTERN INTERVIEW Integumentary system

FUNCTIONAL HEALTH PATTERN	INTERVIEW QUESTIONS AND LEADING STATEMENTS
Health perception–Health management	■ Describe your current problem. How long has it lasted? What have you done to treat it?
	■ Describe any past skin problems or injuries you have had. How were these treated?
	■ Did you undergo any surgical procedures and, if so, why and when?
	■ List prescribed or over-the-counter medications, herbs and vitamins you currently take.
	■ Do you have allergies to plants, chemicals or pets?
	■ Describe what you do each day to care for your skin, hair and nails.
Nutritional–Metabolic	■ Describe the type and amount of food and drink you consume in a 24-hour period.
	■ Do you have a history of food allergies? If so, describe what you are allergic to and how you respond.
	■ Have you recently eaten any new foods?
Integumentary condition	■ Is your skin and scalp dry, oily or itchy?
	■ Have you noticed swelling around your eyes or ankles?
	■ Have you noticed any changes in your hair or nails?
	■ Do you perspire a lot?
	■ Do you bruise easily?
	■ How well do your cuts and scratches heal?
Activity–Exercise	■ Describe your physical activities in a typical day.
	■ Do you use a sunscreen when you are outside? If so, what SPF?
	■ Do you visit tanning salons?
Sleep–Rest	■ How many hours do you sleep each night?
	■ Do you have trouble sleeping because of itching or sweating?
Pain and discomfort	■ Do you have any of the following: pain, discomfort, itching, tingling, burning, tenderness or numbness? If so, where?
Self-perception–Self-concept	■ How does this condition make you feel about yourself?
Role–Relationships	■ How does this condition affect your relationships with others?
	■ Is there anything in your work environment that may have caused this condition?
Sexuality–Reproductive	■ Has this condition interfered with your usual sexual activities?
	■ If you use a birth control method, could it have caused this condition?

FUNCTIONAL HEALTH PATTERN INTERVIEW **Integumentary system (continued)**

FUNCTIONAL HEALTH PATTERN	INTERVIEW QUESTIONS AND LEADING STATEMENTS
Coping–Stress tolerance	■ Have you experienced any type of stress that may have worsened this condition?
	■ Has this condition created stress for you?
	■ Describe what you do when you feel stressed.
Value–Belief	■ Tell me how specific relationships or activities help you cope with this condition.
	■ Describe specific cultural beliefs or practices that affect how you care for and feel about this condition.
	■ Are there any specific treatments that you would not use to treat this condition?

Physical assessment

Physical assessment of the skin, hair and nails may either be performed as part of a total assessment, or it may be a focused assessment of the integument for people with known or suspected problems. Physical assessment of the skin, hair and nails is conducted using inspection and palpation techniques. Assess the skin for colour, presence and characteristics of lesions (observable changes from normal skin structure), temperature alterations, texture, moisture, turgor and presence of oedema (see Table 14.4).

Characteristics of lesions are described in Table 14.5.

Common skin lesions found on older adults are outlined in Box 14.1. Examine the hair for hygiene status, infestations, colour, texture, quality and distribution, and the presence of scalp

TABLE 14.4 Age-related skin changes

AGE-RELATED CHANGE	SIGNIFICANCE
Epidermis: reduced thickness and miotic activity	• Skin is more fragile and at greater risk of tears or injury • Delayed wound healing • Hyperkeratoses and skin cancers in sun-exposed areas are more evident
Epidermis: increased permeability, reduced Langerhans cells	• Increased risk of reactions to irritants • Decreased inflammatory response
Epidermis: reduced number of active melanocytes	• Increased susceptibility to sun exposure
Epidermis: hyperplasia of melanocytes, especially in sun-exposed areas	• Small areas of hyperpigmentation (solar lentigines or 'liver spots')
Epidermis: impaired vitamin D production	• Increased risk of osteomalacia, osteoporosis
Epidermis: dermal–epidermal junction flattens	• Increased risk of skin tears, purpura and pressure injures
Dermis: reduced perfusion	• Decreased sensation (pain, touch, temperature and peripheral vibration) • Increased risk of injury
Dermis: reduced vasomotor response	• Greater risk of hyperthermia and hypothermia
Dermis: collagen and elastic fibres degenerate	• Decreased tone and elasticity, with wrinkle formation
Dermis: proliferation of capillaries	• Cherry haemangiomas are common
Subcutaneous skin layer: thins	• Greater risk of hypothermia • Increased risk of pressure injuries
Subcutaneous skin layer: adipose tissue is redistributed	• Cellulite forms • Bags over and under the eyes • Double chin forms • Abdominal fat increases • Breasts sag • Skin returns to normal more slowly when pinched (tenting)
Glands: reduced eccrine and apocrine activity	• Dry skin is common
Glands: reduced sebaceous gland activity	• Reduced or absent perspiration • More susceptible to dry skin • Skin pH is higher

TABLE 14.5 Lesion characteristics

Configuration and shape	Single, grouped cluster, linear, annular (ring-shaped) or round, artiform (bite)
Appearance	Dimensions, raised, indented, flush, colour, mobile, non-mobile
Edges	Raised, rolled, undermined, coloured
Fluid-filled lesion or draining exudate	Colour, type, amount, consistency, odour

BOX 14.1 Common skin lesions of older adults

- Skin tags: soft brown or flesh-coloured benign papules
- Keratoses: horny growth of keratinocytes; may be seborrhoeic (benign) or actinic (premalignant)
- Lentigines ('liver' or 'age' spots): brown or black benign macules with a defined border
- Angiomas (haemangioma): benign vascular tumours with dilated blood vessels, found in the middle to upper dermis
- Telangiectases: single dilated blood vessels, capillaries or terminal arteries
- Venous lakes (phlebectases): small, dark blue, slightly raised benign papules that usually occur on sun-exposed areas
- Photoageing: wrinkling, mottling, pigmented areas, loss of elasticity, benign or malignant lesions

lesions. Determine the shape, colour, contour and condition of the nails. Terminology of skin lesions with examples is outlined in Table 14.6.

The examination should be conducted in a warm, private room. Cultural considerations are important in terms of protecting the person's modesty; however, in order to undertake a comprehensive examination, the areas to be examined should be fully exposed. Ideally, the person should remove all clothing and put on a gown. The person may be standing, sitting or lying down at various times of the examination. The assessor should adhere to infection prevention and control measures by practising hand hygiene and donning disposable gloves when undertaking a skin assessment including palpating open lesions, skin surfaces suspicious of infections or infestations, or discharge from lesions of the skin and mucous membranes. A disposable ruler is used to measure the size of lesions. A torch is used to better visualise lesions.

TABLE 14.6 Terminology of skin lesions with associated disorders

LESION	EXAMPLES OF DISORDERS
Pigmented	Freckle, seborrhoeic keratosis, naevus, melanoma
Scaly	Psoriasis, dermatitis, xerosis, tinea, actinic keratoses
Pustular	Acne vulgaris, folliculitis, candidiasis
Vesicular	Herpes simplex, herpes zoster, scabies
Nodular	Warts, basal cell carcinoma, acne
Weepy, crusted	Acute contact allergic dermatitis, impetigo
Figurate (shaped) erythema	Urticaria, cellulitis
Bullous	Pemphigus, toxic epidermal necrolysis
Pruritic	Xerosis, scabies, pediculosis
Ulcerated	Pressure injury, skin cancer, herpes simplex

Diagnostic tests

The results of diagnostic tests of the structure and function of the integumentary system are used to support the diagnosis of a specific injury or disease, to provide information to identify or modify the appropriate medication or treatments used to treat the disease and to help nurses monitor the person's responses to nursing care interventions. Diagnostic tests to assess the integumentary system are described later and summarised in the 'Integumentary assessments' section. More information is given in the chapters 'Nursing care of people with integumentary disorders' and 'Nursing care of people with burns'.

The use of laboratory tissue analysis, exudate cultures or skin scrapings will not be routine for all wounds but is restricted to situations when clinical assessment indicates infection to be the cause of delayed healing. Conditions that indicate the need for investigation include:

- acute or chronic wounds that demonstrate signs of infection (erythema, swelling, heat, pain and increased exudate or purulence) and that are not responding to standard management
- a clinical diagnosis of infection has been made and drug sensitivities are required to ensure correct coverage for the organisms in the wound
- infected chronic wounds are deteriorating, despite appropriate debridement and antimicrobial treatment
- local surveillance is required to identify drug-resistant organisms (International Wound Infection Institute, 2016; Sussman, 2016; Young, 2012). There are several recognised methods for collecting a tissue or fluid sample for diagnosing infection. A wound swab can be collected using a sterile swab for microscopy culture and this will identify the species and semi-quantitatively the number of organisms (normally reported as scant, low, moderate or heavy growth). This method does not accurately identify organisms in deeper tissues, and surface contamination results in over-reporting of organisms.

Although there are several methods reported for collecting a wound swab, there is no single, universally accepted method. Methods include:

- *Random swab sampling*: risks contamination with surrounding skin and topical isolates.
- *Levine method*: a swab is rotated over a 1 cm^2 area (necrotic tissue is debrided prior to this) with sufficient pressure to express fluid from within the wound tissue (Levine et al., 1976).
- *Zig-zag stroke method*: rotation of the collection swab between the fingers as the swab is manipulated from close to wound margin to margin in a 10-point zig-zag (Z) fashion (Angel et al., 2011; Cuzzell, 1993).

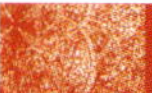

INTEGUMENTARY ASSESSMENTS

Technique/normal findings	Abnormal findings
Inspect skin colour and note any odours coming from the skin. *Skin colour should be even, appropriate to the age and race of the person, without foul odours.*	■ A strong odour of perspiration may indicate poor hygiene and a need for health education. A foul odour may indicate a disorder of the sweat glands. ■ Pallor and/or cyanosis are seen with exposure to cold and with decreased perfusion and oxygenation. In cyanotic dark-skinned people, skin appears dull. Cyanosis may be more visible in the mucous membranes and nail beds of these people. ■ In dark-skinned people, jaundice may be most apparent in the sclerae of the eyes. ■ Redness, swelling and pain are seen with various rashes, inflammations, infections and burns. Superficial burns cause areas of painful erythema and swelling. Red, painful blisters appear in superficial partial-thickness burns, whereas white or blackened areas are common in deep partial-thickness or full-thickness burns. ■ **Vitiligo**, an abnormal loss of melanin in patches, typically occurs over the face, hands or groin. Vitiligo can occur at any age and is thought to be an autoimmune disorder.
Inspect the skin for lesions and alterations, including calluses, scars, tattoos and piercings. Include inspection of skin creases and folds. *Skin should be intact without abnormal lesions.*	Primary, secondary and vascular lesions are described and shown in Tables 14.7 to 14.9. ■ Pearly edged nodules with a central ulcer are seen in basal cell carcinoma. ■ Scaly, red, fast-growing papules are seen in squamous cell carcinoma. ■ Dark, asymmetric, multicoloured patches (sometimes moles) with irregular edges appear in malignant melanoma. ■ Circular lesions are usually present in ringworm and in tinea versicolor. ■ Grouped vesicles may be seen in contact dermatitis. ■ Linear lesions appear in poison ivy contact and herpes zoster. ■ **Urticaria** (hives) appears as patches of pale, itchy wheals in an erythematous area. ■ In psoriasis, scaly red patches appear on the scalp, knees, back and genitals. ■ In herpes zoster, vesicles appear along sensory nerve paths, turn into pustules and then crust over. ■ Bruises (**ecchymoses**) are raised bluish or yellowish vascular lesions. Multiple bruises in various stages of healing suggest trauma or abuse.
Palpate skin temperature. *Skin should be warm.*	■ Skin is warm and red in inflammation and is generally warm with elevated body temperature. ■ Decreased blood flow decreases the skin temperature; this may be generalised, as in shock, or localised, as in arteriosclerosis.
Palpate skin texture. *Skin should be smooth.*	■ Changes in the texture of the skin may indicate irritation or trauma. ■ The skin is soft and smooth in hyperthyroidism and coarse in hypothyroidism.
Palpate skin moisture. *Skin should be dry.*	■ Excessively dry skin often is present in older adults and people with hypothyroidism. ■ Oily skin is common in adolescents and young adults. Oily skin may be a normal finding or it may accompany a skin disorder such as acne vulgaris. ■ Excessive perspiration may be associated with shock, fever, increased activity or anxiety.

(continued)

TABLE 14.7 Primary skin lesions

Lesion	Description	Lesion	Description
Macule, patch 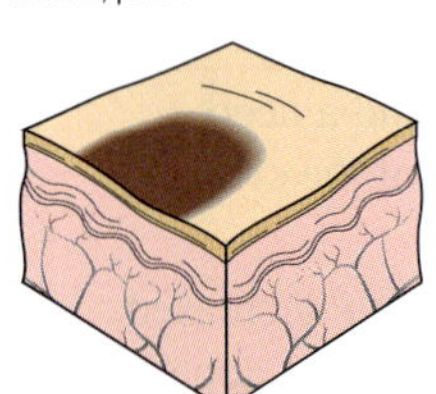	Flat, non-palpable change in skin colour. Macules are smaller than 1 cm, with a circumscribed border, and patches are larger than 1 cm and may have an irregular border. **Examples** Macules: freckles, measles and petechiae. Patches: Mongolian spots, port-wine stains, vitiligo and chloasma.	Vesicle, bulla 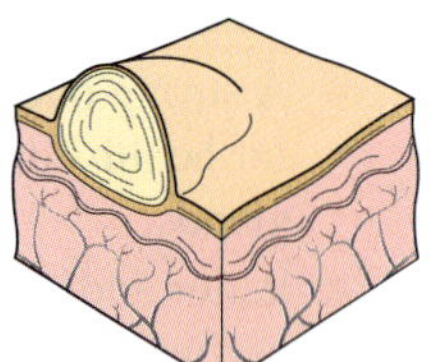	Elevated, fluid-filled, round or oval shaped, palpable mass with thin, translucent walls and circumscribed borders. Vesicles are smaller than 0.5 cm; bullae are larger than 0.5 cm. **Examples** Vesicles: herpes simplex/zoster, early chickenpox and small burn blisters. Bullae: contact dermatitis, friction blisters and large burn blisters.
Papule, plaque 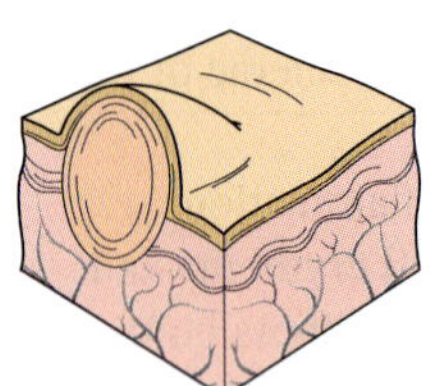	Elevated, solid, palpable mass with circumscribed border. Papules are smaller than 0.5 cm; plaques are groups of papules that form lesions larger than 0.5 cm. **Examples** Papules: elevated moles, warts and lichen planus. Plaques: psoriasis, actinic keratosis and lichen planus.	Wheal 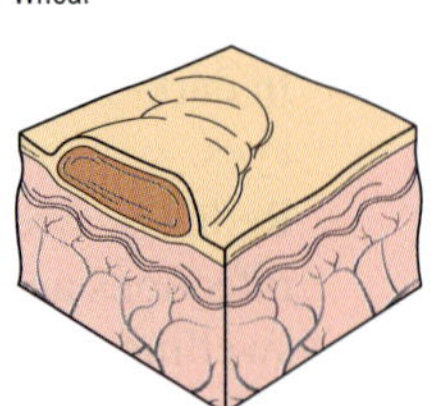	Elevated, often reddish area with irregular border caused by diffuse fluid in tissues rather than free fluid in a cavity, as in vesicles. Size varies. **Examples** Insect bites and hives (extensive wheals).
Nodule, tumour 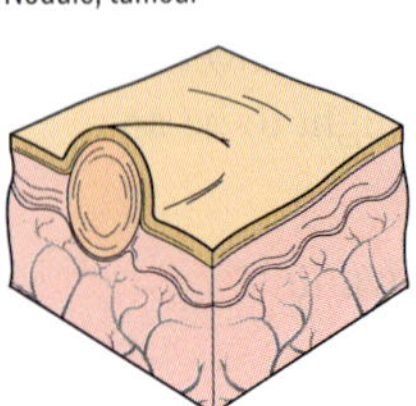	Elevated, solid, hard or soft palpable mass extending deeper into the dermis than a papule. Nodules have circumscribed borders and are 0.5 to 2 cm; tumours may have irregular borders and are larger than 2 cm. **Examples** Nodules: small lipoma, squamous cell carcinoma, fibroma and intradermal nevi. Tumours: large lipoma, carcinoma and haemangioma.	Pustule 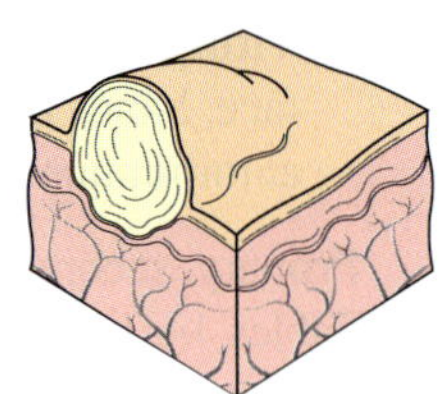	Elevated, pus-filled vesicle or bulla with circumscribed border. Size varies. **Examples** Acne, impetigo and carbuncles (large boils).
		Cyst 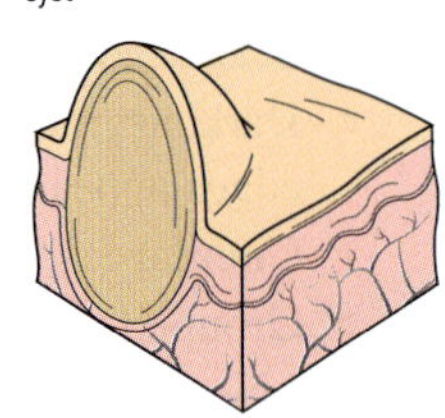	Elevated, encapsulated, fluid-filled or semisolid mass originating in the subcutaneous tissue or dermis, usually 1 cm or larger. **Examples** Varieties include sebaceous cysts and epidermoid cysts.

TABLE 14.8 Secondary skin lesions

Lesion	Description	Lesion	Description
Atrophy 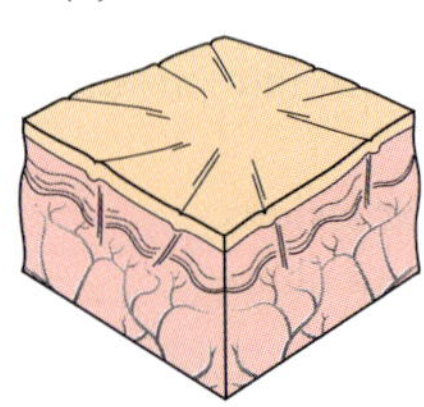	A translucent, dry, paper-like, sometimes wrinkled skin surface resulting from thinning or wasting of the skin due to loss of collagen and elastin. **Examples** Striae, atrophie blanche	Ulcer 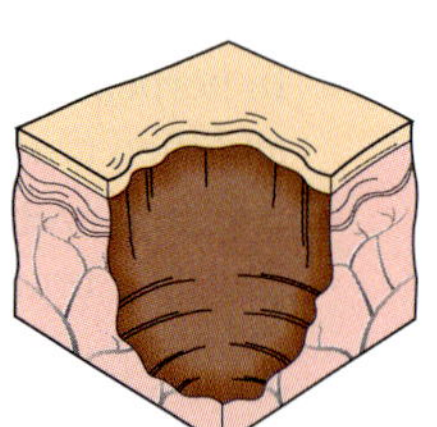	Deep, irregularly shaped area of skin loss extending into the dermis or subcutaneous tissue. May bleed. May leave scar. **Examples** Pressure injuries, venous stasis ulcers, chancres.
Erosion 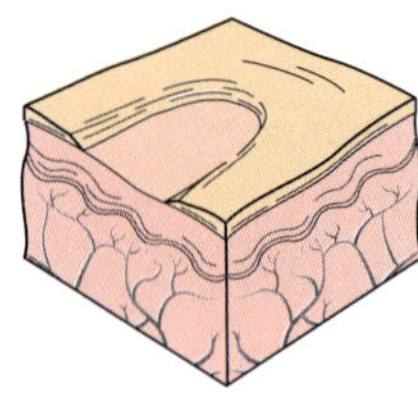	Wearing away of the superficial epidermis causing a moist, shallow depression. Because erosions do not extend into the dermis, they heal without scarring. **Examples** Scratch marks, ruptured vesicles.	Fissure 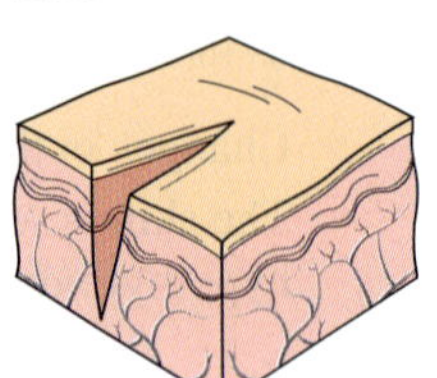	Linear crack with sharp edges, extending into the dermis. **Examples** Cracks at the corners of the mouth or in the hands, athlete's foot.
Lichenification 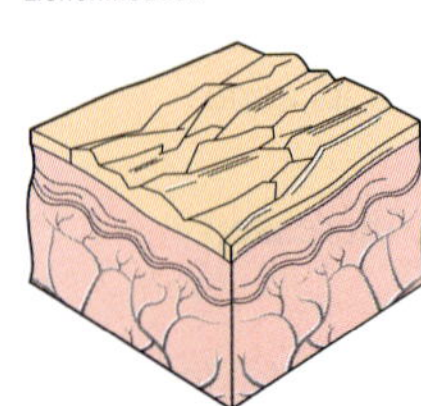	Rough, thickened, hardened area of epidermis resulting from chronic irritation such as scratching or rubbing. **Example** Chronic dermatitis.	Scar 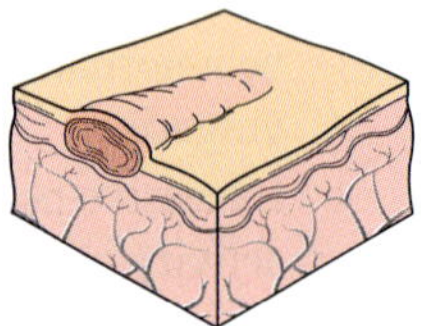	Flat, irregular area of connective tissue left after a lesion or wound has healed. New scars may be red or purple; older scars may be silvery or white. **Examples** Healed surgical wound or injury, healed acne.

TABLE 14.8 Secondary skin lesions (continued)

Scales 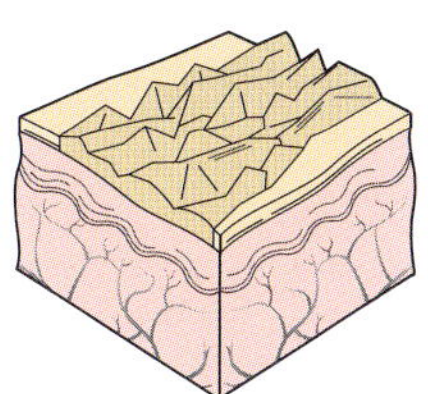	Shedding flakes of greasy, keratinised skin tissue. Colour may be white, grey or silver. Texture may vary from fine to thick. **Examples** Dry skin, dandruff, psoriasis and eczema.	Keloid 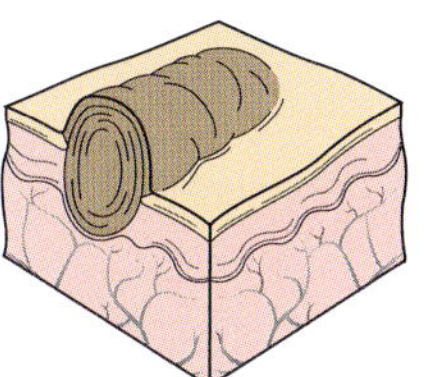	Elevated, irregular, darkened area of excess scar tissue caused by excessive collagen formation during healing. Extends beyond the site of the original injury. Higher incidence in people of African descent. **Examples** Keloid from ear piercing or surgery.
Crust 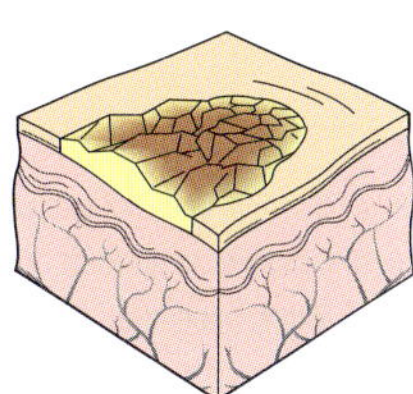	Dry blood, serum or pus left on the skin surface when vesicles or pustules burst. Can be red-brown, orange or yellow. Large crusts that adhere to the skin surface are called scabs. **Examples** Eczema, impetigo, herpes or scabs following abrasion.	Hypertrophic scar 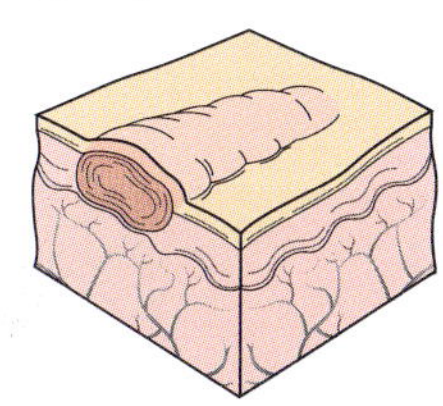	Elevated excessive scar that remains within the original wound site. **Example** Post-burn scar

TABLE 14.9 Vascular skin lesions

Spider angioma	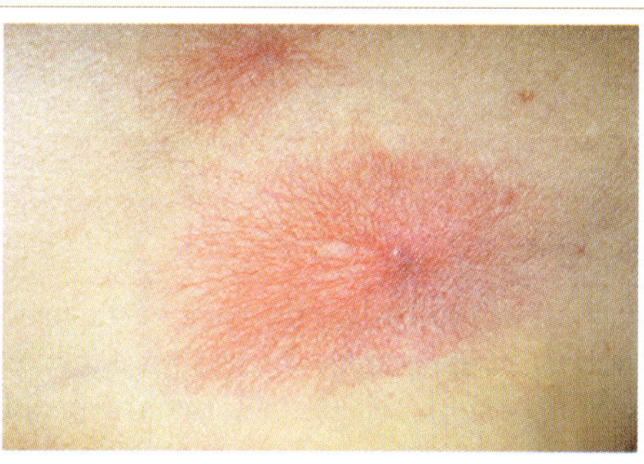 *Source*: Mediscan/Alamy Stock Photo.	A flat, bright red dot with tiny radiating blood vessels ranging in size from a pinpoint to 2 cm. It blanches with pressure. **Cause** A type of telangiectasis (vascular dilatation) caused by elevated oestrogen levels, pregnancy, oestrogen therapy, vitamin B deficiency or liver disease, or may not be pathological. **Localisation/distribution** Most commonly appear on the upper half of the body.
Venous star	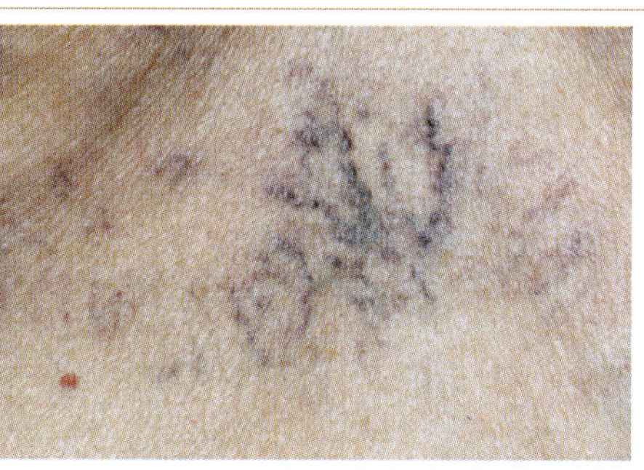 *Source*: Southern Illinois University/Science Source.	A flat blue lesion with radiating, cascading or linear veins extending from the centre. It ranges in size from 3 to 25 cm. **Cause** A type of telangiectasis (vascular dilatation) caused by increased intravenous pressure in superficial veins. **Localisation/distribution** Most commonly appear on the anterior chest and the lower legs near varicose veins.
Petechiae	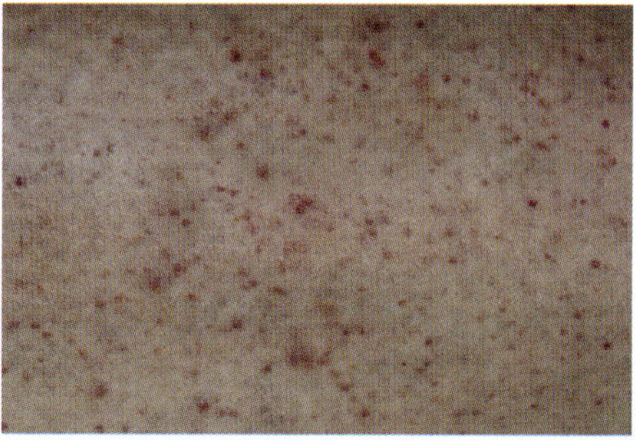 *Source*: © CLS Digital Arts/Shutterstock.	Flat red or purple rounded freckles approximately 1 to 3 mm in diameter. Difficult to detect in dark skin. Do not blanch. **Cause** Minute haemorrhages resulting from fragile capillaries, petechiae are caused by septicaemias, liver disease or vitamin C or K deficiency. They may also be caused by anticoagulant therapy. **Localisation/distribution** Most commonly appear on the dependent surfaces of the body (e.g. back, buttocks). In the person with dark skin, look for them in the oral mucosa and conjunctivae.

(continued)

TABLE 14.9 Vascular skin lesions (continued)

Purpura	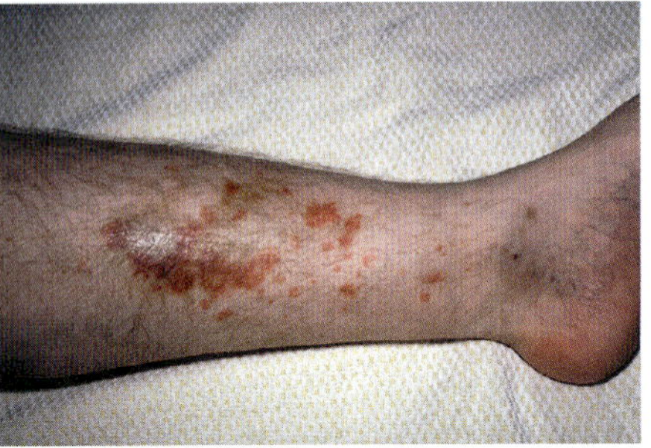 *Source*: Mediscan/Alamy Stock Photo.	Flat, reddish blue, irregularly shaped extensive patches of varying size. **Cause** Bleeding disorders, scurvy and capillary fragility in the older adult (senile purpura). **Localisation/distribution** May appear anywhere on the body, but are most noticeable on the legs, arms and backs of hands.
Ecchymosis	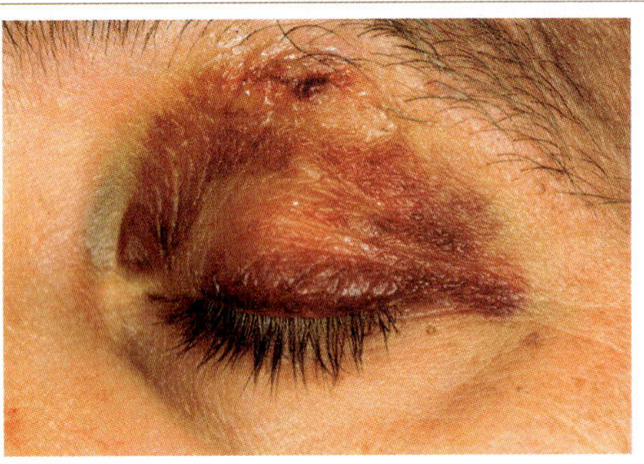 *Source*: Scott Camazine/Science Source.	A bruise. A flat, irregularly shaped lesion of varying size with no pulsation. Does not blanch with pressure. In light skin, it begins as a bluish-purple mark that changes to greenish yellow. In brown skin, it varies from blue to deep purple. In dark skin, it appears as a darkened area. **Cause** Release of blood from superficial vessels into surrounding tissue due to trauma, haemophilia, liver disease or deficiency of vitamin C or K. **Localisation/distribution** Occurs anywhere on the body at the site of trauma or pressure.

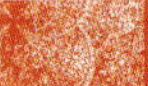

INTEGUMENTARY ASSESSMENTS (continued)

Technique/normal findings	Abnormal findings
Palpate skin turgor. *Skin fold should return rapidly to normal position.*	■ Pinch the person's skin gently over the back of the hand or collarbone. Tenting, in which the skin remains pinched for a few moments before resuming its normal position, is common in older people who are thin (see Figure 14.4). ■ Skin turgor is decreased in dehydration. It is increased in oedema and scleroderma. 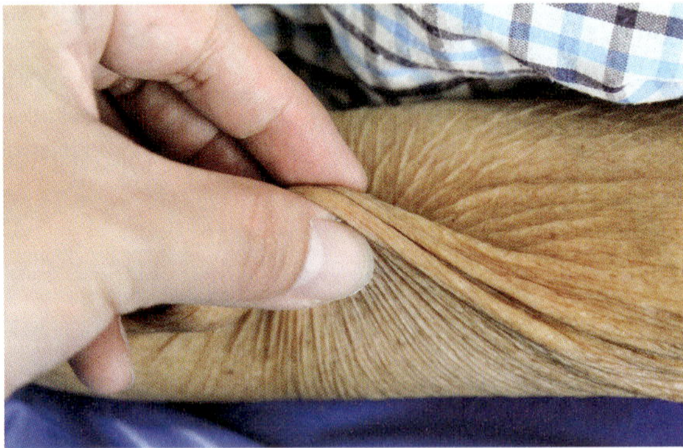 **FIGURE 14.4** ***Tenting in an older person*** *Source*: © Akkalak Aiempradit/Shutterstock.
Assess for oedema. *No oedema should be present.*	■ Assess **oedema** (accumulation of fluid in the body's tissues) by depressing the person's skin (see Figure 14.5). Record findings as follows: 1 + Slight pitting, no obvious distortion 2 + Deeper pit, no obvious distortion 3 + Pitting is obvious; extremities are swollen 4 + Pitting remains with obvious distortion. ■ Oedema is common in cardiovascular disorders, renal failure and cirrhosis of the liver. It also may be a side effect of certain drugs.

INTEGUMENTARY ASSESSMENTS (continued)

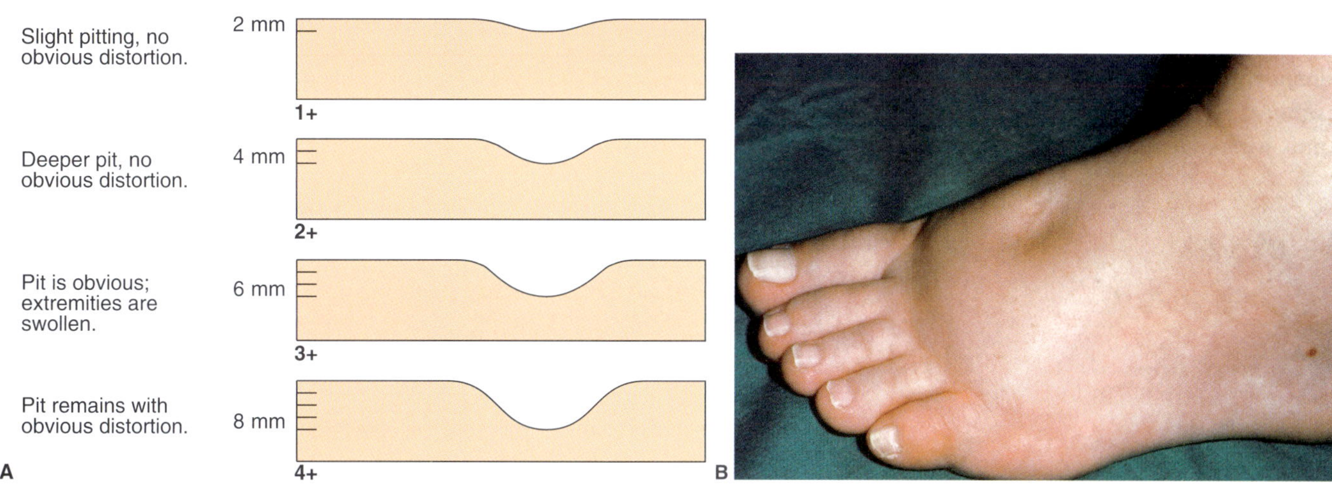

FIGURE 14.5 *A, Degrees of pitting in oedema. B, 4+ pitting*

Source: B, © Dr P. Marazzi/Science Source.

Technique/normal findings	Abnormal findings
Inspect distribution and quality of hair. *Hair should be evenly distributed for person's gender.*	■ A deviation in the normal hair distribution in the male or female genital area may indicate an endocrine disorder. **Hirsutism** (increased growth of coarse hair, usually on the face and trunk) is seen in Cushing's syndrome, acromegaly and ovarian dysfunction. **Alopecia** (hair loss) may be related to changes in hormones, chemical or drug treatment, or radiation. In adult males whose hair loss follows the normal male pattern, the cause is usually genetic.
Palpate hair texture. *Hair should be of even texture.*	■ Some systemic diseases change the texture of the hair. For instance, hypothyroidism causes the hair to coarsen, whereas hyperthyroidism causes the hair to become fine.
Inspect the scalp for lesions. *There should be no lesions on the scalp.*	■ Mild dandruff is normal, but excessive, greasy flakes indicate seborrhoea requiring treatment. ■ Hair loss, pustules and scales appear on the scalp in tinea capitis (scalp ringworm). ■ Red, swollen pustules appear around infected hair follicles and are called folliculitis. ■ Head lice may be seen as oval nits (eggs) adhering to the base of the hair shaft. Head lice are usually accompanied by itching.
Inspect nail curvature. *Nails should not be excessively curved.*	■ Clubbing (see Figure 14.6), in which the angle of the nail base is greater than 160 degrees, is seen in respiratory disorders, cardiovascular disorders, cirrhosis of the liver, colitis and thyroid disease. The nail becomes thick, hard, shiny and curved at the free end.

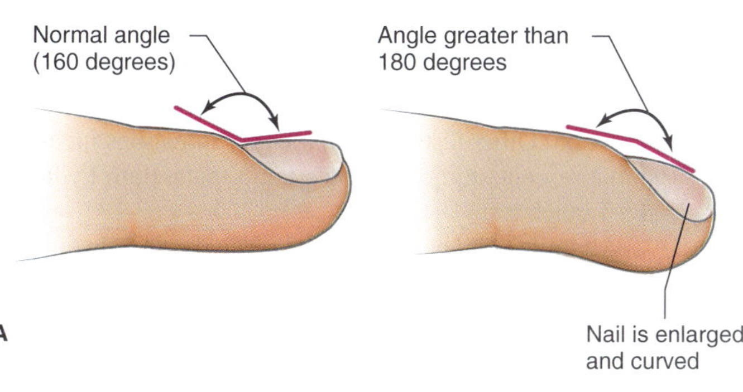

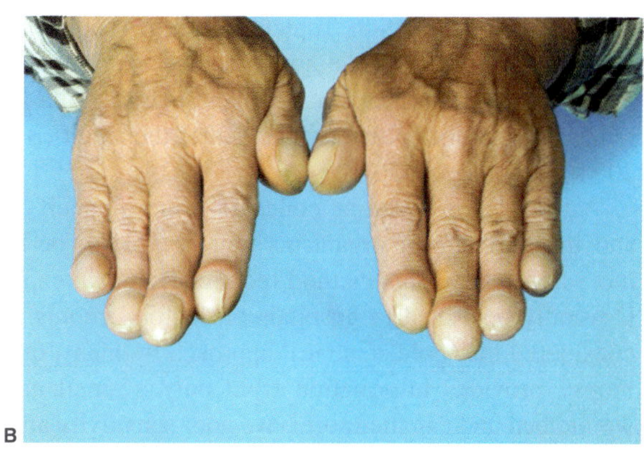

FIGURE 14.6 *A, Assessing clubbing of the nails. B, Hand with nail clubbing.*

Source: B, Science Photo Library/Alamy Stock Photo.

(continued)

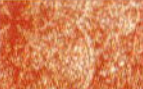

INTEGUMENTARY ASSESSMENTS (continued)

Technique/normal findings	Abnormal findings
Inspect the surface of the nails. *Nail surfaces should be smooth and nail folds firm, without redness.*	■ The nail folds become inflamed and swollen and the nail may loosen in paronychia, an infection of the nail fold. ■ Inflammation and transverse rippling of the nail are associated with chronic paronychia and/or eczema. ■ The nail plate may separate from the nail bed in trauma, psoriasis and *Pseudomonas* and *Candida* infections. This separation is called oncolysis. ■ Nail grooves may be caused by inflammation, by lichen planus or by nail biting. ■ Nail pitting may be seen with psoriasis. ■ A transverse groove (Beau's line) may be seen in trachoma and/or acute diseases. ■ Thin spoon-shaped nails (see Figure 14.7) may be seen in anaemia. 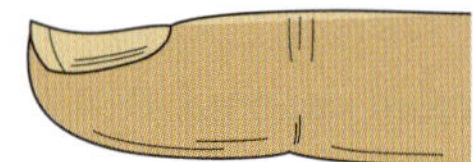 **FIGURE 14.7** ***Spoon-shaped nails***
Inspect nail colour. *Nail colour should be even.*	■ The sudden appearance of a pigmented band may indicate melanoma in Caucasians. ■ Yellowish nails are seen in psoriasis and fungal infections. ■ Dark nails occur with trauma, *Candida* infections and hyperbilirubinemia. ■ Blackish-green nails are apparent in injury and in *Pseudomonas* infection. ■ Red splinter longitudinal haemorrhages may be seen in injury and/or psoriasis.
Inspect nail thickness. *Nails should not be excessively thick.*	■ Trauma to the nails usually causes thickening. Other causes of thick nails include psoriasis, fungal infections and decreased peripheral vascular blood supply. ■ Thinning of the nails is seen in nutritional deficiencies.

The Levine technique is considered to be superior to the Z technique because of possible sampling of a greater concentration of microorganisms from both the surface and slightly below the surface of the wound (Angel et al., 2011; Rondas et al., 2013).

The wound should be cleaned with sterile water or normal saline prior to taking any wound swab in order to minimise the risk of contamination. Topical antiseptics should be avoided prior to taking the wound swab as they may alter the result. Avoid the use of topical anaesthetics such as Emla which can reduce the number of bacteria and alter the result (Batai et al., 2004; Purcell et al., 2017).

A tissue biopsy can be collected using a punch or scalpel, and the numbers of organisms will be able to be quantified more accurately. This method requires technical expertise and is usually restricted to hospitals or doctors' rooms. Although considered the 'gold standard' approach by many, quantitative biopsy provides information from only a small area of the wound bed and can therefore have poor sensitivity and reliability in large wounds (Angel et al., 2011; Gjødsbøl et al., 2012; Rondas et al., 2013; Sibbald et al., 2003).

A needle aspiration of adjacent tissues for tissue fluid can be collected to identify tissue organisms. This method also requires technical expertise and, like biopsy, is usually restricted to hospitals and doctors' rooms. Increased pain can be associated with this technique, and it can underestimate the number of organisms when compared to biopsy (Bowler, Duerden & Armstrong, 2001; Kingsley, 2003). There is however some recent research that suggests fine-needle aspiration could still be considered for first-line pathological investigations as it can be a highly accurate and less expensive technique, especially if rapid onsite evaluation (ROSE) is available (Khan et al., 2017; Nagar et al., 2012).

Skin scrapings may be collected for diagnosing fungal infection. Other tests used to identify infections include immunofluorescent studies, Wood's lamp, potassium hydroxide and the Tzanck test.

Allergies may be determined through analysis of patch tests or scratch tests.

Some studies are conducted to identify bacterial carriers. For example, if people have repeated bacterial skin infections or if a healthcare unit or agency experiences numerous bacterial infections of people, nasal cultures may be performed to determine if the people or the healthcare workers are carriers of the bacteria. Regardless of the type of diagnostic test, the nurse is responsible for explaining the procedure and any special preparation needed; for assessing for medication use that may affect the outcome of the tests; for supporting the person during the examination as necessary; for documenting the procedures as appropriate; and for monitoring the results of the tests.

Genetic considerations

When conducting a health assessment interview and physical assessment, it is important for the nurse to consider genetic and ageing influences on the health of the adult.

Ascertain age and, during the health assessment interview, ask about integumentary disorders or abnormalities among immediate family members. During the physical assessment, assess for any manifestations that indicate a possible genetic disorder. If data are found that indicate genetic risk factors or alterations, ask about genetic testing and refer for appropriate genetic counselling and evaluation. The chapter 'Genetic implications of adult health nursing' provides further information about genetics in medical–surgical nursing.

DIAGNOSTIC TESTS The integumentary system: tissue biopsy

There are several methods to obtain a tissue biopsy.

NAME OF TEST Punch biopsy **PURPOSE AND DESCRIPTION** Used to obtain a tissue sample for histological study. Helpful in diagnosing pathology which lies in the epidermis, dermis and subcutaneous tissue. Best biopsy technique for undiagnosed rashes and suspected neoplasms. Punch biopsy instrument is used to remove a small section of epidermis, dermis and subcutaneous tissue. Depending on the size of the biopsy removed, the incision may need to be sutured.	**RELATED NURSING CARE** Explain procedure to the person and ensure a consent form is signed (if required). Assist with procedure. Apply appropriate dressing and provide information about self-care. If sutures are used, advise the person when to return for suture removal. Document procedure and send labelled specimen to the laboratory.
NAME OF TEST Incisional skin biopsy **PURPOSE AND DESCRIPTION** Used to excise a section of tissue from the wound bed and wound edge. Incision is made using a scalpel extracting a block of tissue, quadrangular at the skin surface. Biopsy rarely needs to be more than 5 mm deep. The incision is closed with sutures.	**RELATED NURSING CARE** As for a punch biopsy.
NAME OF TEST Excisional skin biopsy **PURPOSE AND DESCRIPTION** Incision is made using a scalpel and the *entire* skin lesion or tumour is removed for analysis. Excision is closed with sutures.	**RELATED NURSING CARE** As for a punch biopsy.
NAME OF TEST Shave biopsy **PURPOSE AND DESCRIPTION** Helpful in diagnosing diseases where the pathology is in or near the epidermis. Lumps and bumps as opposed to rashes are best biopsied with the shave technique. Using a scalpel or curette, a slice of the top layer of the raised area is taken. Stitches are not usually required.	**RELATED NURSING CARE** Individual should be advised to clean wound with tap water and apply dressing to keep the wound moist. Change as required generally twice a week initially, then weekly until healed.
NAME OF TEST Skin scrapings **PURPOSE AND DESCRIPTION** Useful where fungal infections and some parasite infestations are suspected. Scalpel is used to collect the sample and the sample is transported dry.	**RELATED NURSING CARE** As for a punch biopsy.
NAME OF TEST Immunofluorescent slides **PURPOSE AND DESCRIPTION** Used to identify IgG antibodies (present in pemphigus vulgaris) and to identify varicella in skin cells (for herpes zoster). Skin or blood samples collected in a sterile specimen container. Procedure should be documented, and specimen clearly labelled and sent to the laboratory where it will be placed on a slide and examined microscopically for analysis.	**RELATED NURSING CARE** As for a punch biopsy.

(continued)

DIAGNOSTIC TESTS The integumentary system: tissue biopsy (continued)

NAME OF TEST Wood's lamp **PURPOSE AND DESCRIPTION** Used in the clinical setting and uses an ultraviolet light that causes certain organisms to fluoresce (such as *Pseudomonas* organisms and fungi). Skin is examined under a special lamp.	**RELATED NURSING CARE** Explain the procedure to the person. Document the procedure.
NAME OF TEST KOH (potassium hydroxide) preparation **PURPOSE AND DESCRIPTION** Used to examine for a fungal infection. Specimen of hair or nails is obtained, placed in a sterile specimen-labelled container and sent with the supporting documentation to the laboratory for analysis. In the laboratory the specimen is placed on a slide, potassium hydroxide solution is added and the specimen is examined microscopically.	**RELATED NURSING CARE** Explain the procedure to the person. Assist with or obtain the specimen, document the procedure and send the labelled specimen to the laboratory for analysis.
NAME OF TEST Tzanck test **PURPOSE AND DESCRIPTION** Used to diagnose herpes infections, but it does not differentiate herpes simplex from herpes zoster. Fluid and cells from the vesicles are obtained, sent to the laboratory where they are put on a slide, stained and examined microscopically.	**RELATED NURSING CARE** Explain the procedure to the person. Use sterile procedure to assist with or obtain the specimen. Document the procedure and send the labelled specimen to the laboratory for analysis.
NAME OF TEST Patch test, scratch tests **PURPOSE AND DESCRIPTION** Used to determine a specific allergen. Small amount of the suspected material is placed on the skin under an occlusive bandage. Patch tests generally detect delayed allergic reactions. In a scratch test, a needle is used to prick a small amount of a suspected allergen into the skin of the forearm. The type of allergen is selected from the patient's history. A positive reaction will usually occur within 20–30 minutes after exposure in the form of itchy, raised red wheals.	**RELATED NURSING CARE** Explain the procedure to the person, including the need to return, usually in 48 hours, to have the patched area or scratched areas evaluated. Document the procedure.

CHAPTER HIGHLIGHTS

- Intact structure and function of the integumentary system is vital to the protection of the body's organs from the external environment.
- Manifestations of dysfunction, injury and disorders affecting the integumentary system may be detected during a general health assessment as well as during focused integumentary assessments.

CONCEPT CHECK

1 Which layer of the skin contains most of the hair follicles, sebaceous glands and sweat glands?
1 epidermis
2 dermis
3 hypodermis
4 stratum lucidium

2 What pigment is responsible for skin tanning?
1 carotene
2 red blood cells
3 melanin
4 sebum

3 Which of the four assessment techniques are used during assessment of the integumentary system? (Select all that apply.)
1 inspection
2 palpation
3 percussion
4 auscultation

4 Superficial skin damage that involves the epidermis only is referred to as:
1 ulceration
2 erosion
3 atrophy
4 lichenification

5 You are assessing a person who is complaining of severe itching. What would be an appropriate interview question?
1 'Tell me how this itch feels.'
2 'Why do you keep scratching it?'
3 'Have you used a new soap?'
4 'Describe your daily fluid intake.'

6 You are assessing the skin of an older person for dehydration. What finding would indicate this condition?
1 decreased turgor
2 increased moisture
3 presence of lesions
4 pallor or cyanosis

7 What part of the body would you commonly palpate to assess oedema due to chronic venous insufficiency?
1 scalp
2 fingers
3 clavicle
4 ankle/foot

8 You are assessing a person with chronic dermatitis and note that they have rough, thickened areas of skin. You document these areas as:
1 ulcers
2 papules
3 atrophy
4 lichenification

9 On assessment you observe clubbing of the fingernails. What disorders could this be related to?
1 cirrhosis of the liver
2 cardiovascular disorders
3 emphysema
4 excessive vitamin C intake

10 While assessing the hair, you note small white eggs on the hair shaft. What type of infestation are you assessing?
1 bacterial
2 viral
3 head lice
4 head lichens

BIBLIOGRAPHY

Angel, D. E., Lloyd, P., Carville, K. & Santamaria, N. (2011). The clinical efficacy of two semi-quantitative wound-swabbing techniques in identifying the causative organism(s) in infected cutaneous wounds. *International Wound Journal*, *8*(2), 176–185. doi: 10.1111/j.1742-481X.2010.00765.x

Australian Commission on Safety and Quality in Health Care (ACSQHC) (2021). *National Safety and Quality Health Service Standards* (2nd ed.). Sydney: ACSQHC.

Batai, I., Juhasz, V., Batai, R. & Kerenyi, M. (2004). The antibacterial effect of EMLA-cream on skin flora compared to an alcohol containing skin disinfectant: A-42. *European Journal of Anaesthesiology (EJA)*, *21*, 11.

Bowler, P. G., Duerden, B. I. & Armstrong, D. G. (2001). Wound microbiology and associated approaches to wound management. *Clinical Microbiology Reviews*, *14*(2), 244–269.

Carville, K. (2017). *Wound care manual* (7th ed.). Osborne Park, WA: Silver Chain Foundation.

Cuzzell, J. Z. (1993). The right way to culture a wound. *American Journal of Nursing*, *93*(5), 48–50.

Fitzpatrick, T. B. (1988). The validity and practicality of sun-reactive skin types I through VI. *Archives of Dermatology*, *124*(6), 869–71. doi: 10.1001/archderm.124.6.869. PMID: 3377516

Gjødsbøl, K., Skindersoe, M. E., Christensen, J. J. et al. (2012). No need for biopsies: Comparison of three sample techniques for wound microbiota determination. *International Wound Journal*, *9*(3), 295–302. doi: 10.1111/j.1742-481X.2011.00883.x

International Wound Infection Institute (2016). *Wound infection in clinical practice.* Wounds International. Retrieved from http://www.woundinfection-institute.com/

Jenkins, G. & Tortora, G. J. (2013). *Anatomy and physiology: From science to life* (3rd ed.). Hoboken, NJ: John Wiley & Sons.

Khan, M., Grimm, I., Ali, B., Nollan, R., Tombazzi, C., Ismail, M. & Baron, T. (2017). A meta-analysis of endoscopic ultrasound–fine-needle aspiration compared to endoscopic ultrasound–fine-needle biopsy: Diagnostic yield and the value of onsite cytopathological assessment. *Endoscopy International Open*, *5*(5), E363–E375.

Kingsley, A. (2003). Audit of wound swab sampling: Why protocols could improve practice. *Professional Nurse*, *18*(6), 338–343.

Klein, L. (1988). Maintenance of healthy skin. *Journal of Enterostomal Therapy*, *15*(6), 227–231.

Levett-Jones, T., Dwyer, T., Reid-Searl, K., Heaton, L., Flenady, T., Applegarth, J., Guinea, S. & Andersen, P. (2017). *Patient Safety Competency Framework (PSCF) for Nursing Students.* Sydney. Retrieved from http://psframework.wpengine.com/

Levine, N. S., Lindberg, R. B., Mason, A. D. et al. (1976). The quantitative swab culture and smear: A quick, simple method for determining the number of viable aerobic bacteria on open wounds. *Journal of Trauma*, *16*(2), 89–94.

Martini, F. H., Nath, J. L. & Bartholomew, E. F. (2018). *Fundamentals of anatomy and physiology* (11th ed.). San Francisco: Pearson Education.

Nagar, S., Iacco, A., Riggs, T., Kestenberg, W. & Keidan, R. (2012). An analysis of fine-needle aspiration versus core needle biopsy in clinically palpable breast lesions: A report on the predictive values and a cost comparison. *The American Journal of Surgery*, *204*(2), 193–198.

Nash, J., Matts, P. & Ertel, K. (2007). Maintenance of healthy skin: Cleansing, moisturization, and ultraviolet protection. *Journal of Cosmetic Dermatology*, *6*(1), 7–11.

Purcell, A., Buckley, T., Fethney, J., King, J., Moyle, W. & Marshall, A. (2017). The effectiveness of EMLA as a primary dressing on painful chronic leg ulcers: Effects on wound healing and health-related quality of life. *The International Journal of Lower Extremity Wounds*, *16*(3), 163–172.

Rondas, A. A., Schols, J. M., Halfens, R. J. & Stobberingh, E. E. (2013). Swab versus biopsy for the diagnosis of chronic infected wounds. *Advances in Skin and Woundcare*, *26*(5), 211–219.

Sibbald, G. R., Orsted, H., Schultz, G. S. et al. (2003). Preparing the wound bed 2003: Focus on infection and inflammation. *Ostomy Wound Management*, *49*(11), 24–51.

Sussman, G. (2016). Antimicrobial resistance relating to wound management and infection. *Wound Practice & Research: Journal of the Australian Wound Management Association*, *24*(4), 224–227.

Young, L. (2012). Identifying infection in chronic wounds. *Wound Practice & Research*, *20*(1), 38–44.

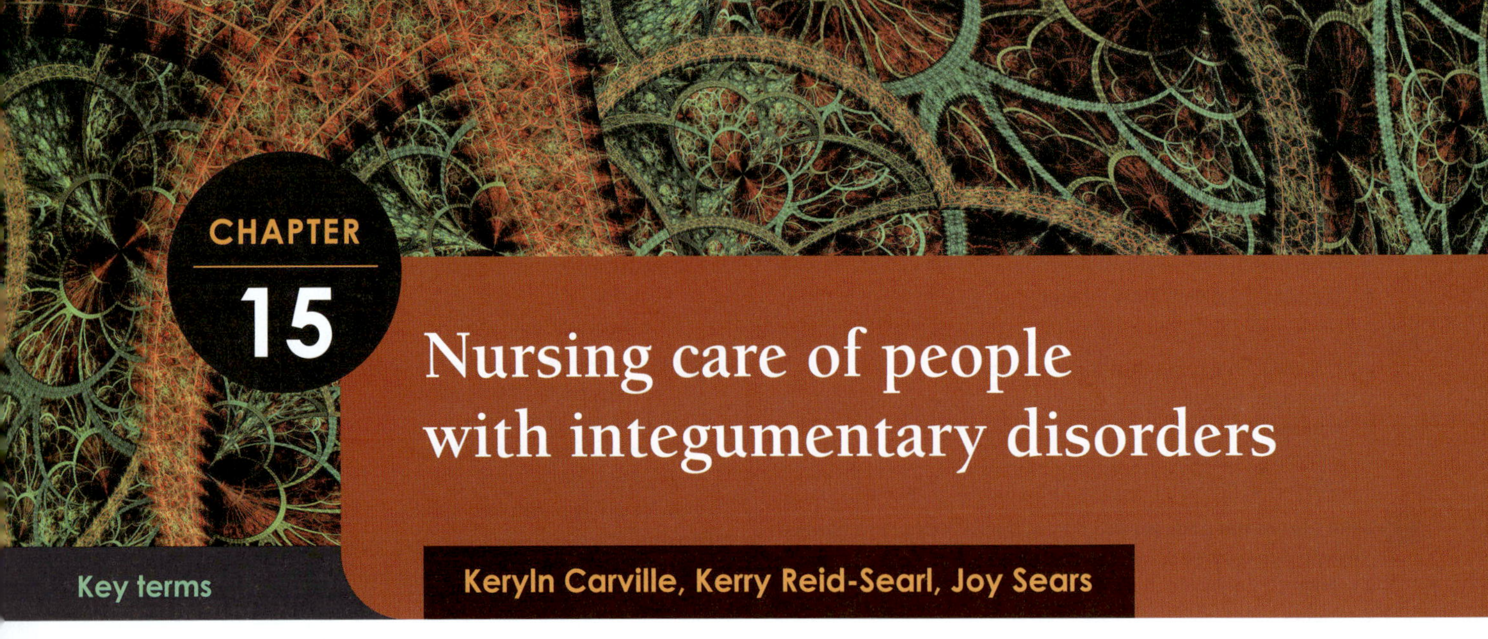

CHAPTER 15

Nursing care of people with integumentary disorders

Keryln Carville, Kerry Reid-Searl, Joy Sears

Key terms

acne 443
actinic keratosis 445
angioma 428
basal cell carcinoma 446
biofilm 461
candidiasis 434
carbuncle 432
cellulitis 432
comedone 443
cyst 427
dermatitis 440
dermatophytoses 434
erysipelas 433
folliculitis 432
furuncle 432
herpes simplex 437
herpes zoster 437
impetigo 433
keloid 427
keratosis 428
malignant melanoma 449
naevi 427
pediculosis 439
pressure injury 455
pruritus 425
psoriasis 428
scabies 439
skin tear 463
squamous cell carcinoma 447
wart 436
xerosis 425

Learning outcomes

- Describe the manifestations and nursing care, including the effects of treatment and medications, of common skin problems and lesions.
- Compare and contrast the aetiology, pathophysiology, interprofessional care and nursing care of people with infections and infestations of the skin.
- Compare and contrast the aetiology, pathophysiology, interprofessional care and nursing care of people with inflammation disorders of the skin.
- Differentiate between the various malignant skin conditions, including the nursing implications and treatment options for people with these conditions.
- Explain the risk factors for, pathophysiology of and nursing interventions to prevent and care for skin trauma.

Clinical competencies

- Assess functional health status of people with integumentary disorders and monitor, document and report abnormal manifestations.
- Use evidence-based research to plan and implement nursing care for people with pressure injuries and skin tears.
- Determine priority nursing diagnoses, based on assessed data, to select and implement individualised nursing interventions for people with integumentary disorders.
- Administer topical, oral and injectable medications used to treat integumentary disorders knowledgeably and safely.
- Integrate interprofessional care into care of people with integumentary disorders.
- Provide teaching appropriate for prevention and self-care of disorders of the integumentary system.
- Revise plan of care as needed to provide effective interventions to promote, maintain or restore functional health status to people with disorders of the integument.

The integumentary system is comprised of the skin and its accessory structures: hair, nails and glands (sebaceous, sudoriferous and ceruminous). The skin is the largest body organ and provides protection by serving as a barrier between the internal and external environments. As described in the chapter 'Assessing the integumentary system', the functions of the skin are many, as the skin contains receptors for touch and sensation, helps regulate body temperature and maintains fluid and electrolyte balance. The skin also provides cues to determining health and wellbeing, ethnic background and plays a major role in determining self-concept and cosmesis.

There are many disorders of the integument. Many of them are treated in an outpatient or community setting or by self-care. This chapter discusses disorders of the skin, hair and nails; the chapter 'Nursing care of people with burns' discusses the person with burns. Primary and secondary skin lesions are described and illustrated in Tables 14.6 and 14.7. The terms from these tables are used throughout this and the chapter 'Nursing care of people with burns'.

Common skin problems and lesions

The disorders discussed in this section are those experienced by many people. Although they considered minor health problems in terms of healthcare, they may cause major problems, such as impaired learning ability and earning potential for the person experiencing a high level of discomfort and loss of quality of life (Metz et al., 2013).

THE PERSON WITH PRURITUS

Pruritus is a subjective itching sensation that produces an urge to scratch. Pruritus may occur in a small, circumscribed area or it may involve a widespread area; it may or may not be associated with a rash. Pruritus is believed to result from either stimulation of itch receptors in the skin or as a response to the stimulation of skin receptors for pain and touch. The central nervous system (CNS) interprets these stimuli as an itch through central summation (Grossman & Porth, 2014).

Intrinsic and extrinsic factors can predispose a person to pruritus. Ingestion of foods or medications, contact with insects, animals, plants, fabrics or metals, allergic responses and even emotional distress are among the most common causes. Pruritus also may occur as a secondary manifestation of systemic disorders, such as certain types of cancer, diabetes mellitus, hepatic disease and renal failure. Although the exact physiology is unknown, it is known that heat and prostaglandins trigger pruritus and that histamine and morphine exacerbate the itch response.

The pathophysiological response of pruritus to stimulation or irritation follows a similar pathway, regardless of cause. The irritating agent stimulates receptors in the junction between the epidermis and dermis and may also trigger the release of histamine and other chemical mediators that either further stimulate or mediate the itch response. The response of the person experiencing the itch is to scratch or rub the affected area. This may irritate the skin and cause further inflammation, which in turn sets off a cycle of increasingly intense itching and scratching, called the *itch–scratch–(itch) cycle* (Wolz & Burge, 2014).

Secondary effects of pruritus include skin excoriation, erythema, wheals, changes in pigmentation and infections. Persistent pruritus may interrupt sleep patterns because the itching sensation is often more intense at night. Long-term pruritus may be debilitating and increases the risk of infection as excoriation occurs. In children, chronic pruritus has been shown to increase the risk of depression, anxiety and suicidal thoughts (Metz et al., 2013). Although not the most prevalent symptom in palliative care patients, pruritus remains the most puzzling. It can cause discomfort and has a major impact on the person's quality of life.

Treatment for this cohort remains challenging and requires an individualistic approach (Xander et al., 2013). Management of pruritus focuses on identifying and eliminating the cause and the topical application or the use of systemic medications to relieve the itch. Control of pruritus is crucial in breaking the itch/scratch cycle and preventing damage to the skin (excoriation and lichenification). A cool environment may cause vasoconstriction and decrease itching. Antihistamines may relieve pruritus in some people. Tranquillisers may be prescribed to provide sedation, which may in turn relieve the emotional stress associated with pruritus. Systemic antibiotics are used to treat any infection resulting from the scratching and excoriation. Topical medications that contain corticosteroids are often used to relieve the pruritus and inflammation. Other topical preparations that contain menthol, camphor or phenol can be used to numb the itch receptors. Those with generalised itch may benefit from phototherapy (de Menezes, 2016). This is particularly useful for individuals with chronic renal failure on dialysis and eosinophilic infiltrations (de Menezes, 2016). Therapeutic baths or soaks with antipruritic agents such as cornflour, oatmeal, baking soda or coal tar concentrates may prove effective. Therapeutic baths are discussed in the 'Medication administration' box. Table 15.1 lists examples of topical agents used to treat skin disorders. Creams containing a topical anaesthetic or antibiotic may also be prescribed.

THE PERSON WITH DRY SKIN (XEROSIS)

Dry skin, also called **xerosis**, is most often a problem in the older adult, as sebaceous and sweat gland activity reduces with ageing and this reduces the skin's lubrication and moisture retention. However, dry skin may occur at any age from overexposure to low humidity, sunlight, wind, excessive bathing and a decreased intake of liquids.

TABLE 15.1 Topical agents used to treat skin disorders

TYPE	USE	EXAMPLES
Creams and lotions	Moisturise the skin Cool the skin	Sorbolene Alpha Keri™ Ego QV™ skin lotion Calamine lotion (contains phenol which cools the skin, but limit use to a few days)
Ointments	Lubricate the skin Retard water loss	Urea Vaseline
Topical anaesthetics	Relieve itching	Xylocaine
Topical antibiotics (use prudently and only as prescribed)	Treat infection	Mupirocin (eye and nose mucous membrane) Silver sulfadiazine
Corticosteroids (use prudently and only as prescribed)	Suppress inflammation Relieve itching	Dexamethasone Hydrocortisone Betamethsone

MEDICATION ADMINISTRATION Therapeutic baths

AGENTS USED IN THERAPEUTIC BATHS

Saline or tap water

Antibacterial agents: potassium permanganate, Pinetarsol™ bath oil, hexachlorophene

Food substances: colloidal oatmeal, cornflour, sodium bicarbonate

Coal tar derivatives: Polytar™ and Alpha Keri™ tar bath preparations

Emollients: Alpha Keri™ and Ego QV™ bath oils

Coal tar preparations are not recommended for use under occlusive products, except under the direction and supervision of a doctor; and coal tar preparations can cause skin irritation, rashes and skin photosensitivity (MIMS Online, 2022).

Therapeutic baths have a variety of uses in treating skin disorders. Depending on the agent used, therapeutic baths soothe the skin, lower the skin bacteria count, clean and hydrate the skin, loosen scales and relieve itching.

Nursing responsibilities

- Ensure that the bath water is at a comfortable tepid temperature that is neither too hot nor too cool, usually 45°C to 46°C.
- Fill the bath one-third to one-half full.
- Mix the agent well with the water.
- Assist the person into and out of the bath to prevent falls.
- Dry the person by blotting with the towel and avoid rubbing the skin.

Health education for the person and family

- Use a non-slip bath mat in the bath because the medications may cause the bath to become slippery.
- Keep the bathroom warm but adequately ventilated.
- If using a prescribed medication, follow directions carefully for the amount of medication to use in the bath.
- Fill the bath one-third to one-half full of water that is at a comfortable temperature.
- Stay in the bath for 20 to 30 minutes and immerse the areas to be treated.
- Do not get the medicated bathwater in your eyes.
- Dry by blotting (not rubbing) with the towel.
- If the medications cause staining, use old towels or linen.
- If the itching is not relieved or the skin becomes excessively dry, call your healthcare provider.

Two types of severe dry skin are xeroderma and ichthyosis. Xeroderma is a chronic skin condition characterised by dry, rough skin. Ichthyosis is an inherited dermatological condition in which the skin is dry, fissured and hyperkeratotic; the surface of the skin has the appearance of fish scales.

The primary manifestation of dry skin is pruritus. Other manifestations include visible flaking of surface skin and an observable pattern of fine lines over the area. If the skin has been excessively dry and pruritic for a long period, the person may have secondary skin lesions and lichenification (roughened thick epidermis with accentuated skin markings).

Nursing care focuses on teaching the person and family how to reduce the dry skin and relieve the pruritus, as outlined in Box 15.1.

THE PERSON WITH BENIGN SKIN LESIONS

The skin is subject to many different types and kinds of benign skin lesions, including cysts, hypertrophic scars, keloids, naevi, angiomas, skin tags and keratoses. Although these benign lesions are often considered more of a nuisance than an illness, they do require monitoring for malignant changes or an increase in size that interferes with the skin's appearance or function.

Most benign skin lesions do not require treatment, although excision or laser surgery may sometimes be desired or necessary for cosmetic or functional purposes. Cysts may enlarge, skin tags may become irritated and bleed, naevi may change in appearance or any of the lesions may cause discomfort with appearance.

BOX 15.1 Teaching to reduce dry skin and relieve pruritus

- Wash clothing in a mild detergent and rinse twice; do not use fabric softeners.
- Avoid using perfumes and lotions containing alcohol.
- Apply skin moisturisers after a bath to help retain moisture.
- Soaps and hot water are drying. Clean the skin with tepid water and either a pH-neutral cleanser or mild soap. If soap is used, rinse it off thoroughly.
- It is not necessary to take a bath every day.
- If bath oils are used, add them to the bathwater at the end of the bath (the moist skin is more likely to retain the oil). Be careful not to slip in the bath.
- Pat the skin lightly and immediately apply a moisturising lotion or cream after bathing.
- Use a humidifier to humidify the air if the environment is very dry.
- Apply creams and lotions when the skin is slightly damp after bathing.
- Increase fluid intake.
- Keep nails trimmed short, wear loose clothing and keep the environment cool.
- A brief application of pressure or cold may relieve pruritus.
- Cotton gloves may be worn at night if scratching during sleep causes skin excoriation.
- Distraction or relaxation techniques may prove helpful.

Cysts

Cysts of the skin are benign closed sacs in or under the skin surface that are lined with epithelium and contain fluid or a semisolid material. Epidermal inclusion cysts and pilar cysts are the most common types.

Epidermal inclusion cysts may occur anywhere on the body, but are most often found on the head and trunk. Although they are painless, they may grow so large that they become irritated by contact with clothing (e.g. if located on the back of the neck) or cause obstruction (e.g. if located on the nose). The cysts contain a semisolid material composed mainly of keratin. Pilar cysts are painless and are found on the scalp and originate from sebaceous glands. Both types of cysts rarely require treatment unless they become large and bothersome.

Hypertrophic scar

Hypertrophic scars are characterised by an excess of collagen in the healed wound that results in excessive elevated scar. They are contained within the perimeter of the original wound (Bullock & Hales, 2019). Hypertrophic scars can form following intentional or accidental trauma such as burns. Hypertrophic scarring is aberrant or abnormal wound healing (Carville, 2017). The mechanism and reasons for hypertrophic scarring are not fully understood, but such scarring commonly occurs following burn trauma. The use of custom-made pressure garments for the prevention and treatment of hypertrophic scarring is considered standard care. Although it is not definitively understood how pressure garments impact on scar formation, studies demonstrate that they do improve scar appearance and cause a scar to be softer and thinner (Monstrey et al., 2014). Pressure garments are often used in conjunction with silicone sheets or gels, which appear to aid in keeping the scar hydrated and softer as they reduce moisture vapour transmission (Stavrou et al., 2010).

Keloids

Keloids are elevated, irregularly shaped, progressively enlarging scars that extend outside the perimeters of an original wound. Like hypertrophic scars, keloid formation is aberrant wound healing. They arise from excessive amounts of collagen in the stratum corneum during scar formation in connective tissue repair. These lesions are more common in young adults and appear within 1 year of the initial trauma.

This abnormal response most often occurs in people of African and Asian descent who sustain burns of the skin, but even seemingly minor trauma such as infection or an injection site can result in keloid formation (Bullock & Hales, 2019). There is a familial tendency to develop keloids. Other risk factors for keloid formation include excessive tension on a wound and poor alignment of skin edges following accidental or intentional skin trauma. Certain skin surfaces are also more likely to develop keloids: the chin, ears, shoulders, back and lower legs.

The excessive scar formation is associated with increased metabolic activity of fibroblasts and increased type III collagen. The principal cells of the keloids are myofibroblasts, which have characteristics of both fibroblasts and smooth muscle cells. The swollen appearance of the keloids is the result of an excess of extracellular material.

The keloids first appear as red, firm, rubbery plaques that persist for several months after the initial trauma (see Figure 15.1). Uncontrolled overgrowth over time causes the keloids to extend beyond the original scar. Eventually, the keloid becomes smooth and hyperpigmented. Intralesional steroid injections and excision may be tried to control keloid formation; however, they can recur following these treatments.

Naevi

Naevi, more commonly called *moles*, are flat or raised macules or papules with rounded, well-defined borders (see Figure 15.2). Naevi arise from melanocytes during early childhood, with the cells initially accumulating at the junction of the dermis and epidermis. Over time, the cluster of cells moves into the dermis and the lesion becomes visible. Almost all adults have naevi.

Naevi range from flesh coloured to black and occasionally contain hair. They can occur on any skin surface of the body and may arise as single lesions or in groups. Some pigmented naevi

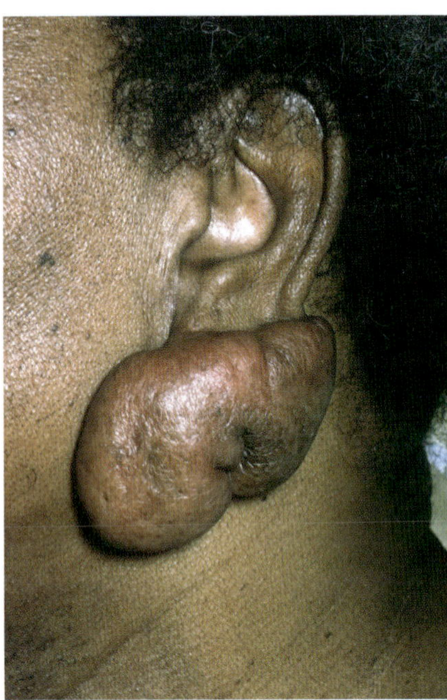

FIGURE 15.1 ***Keloids form as a result of deposits of excessive amounts of collagen during scar formation***

Source: Mediscan/Alamy Stock Photo.

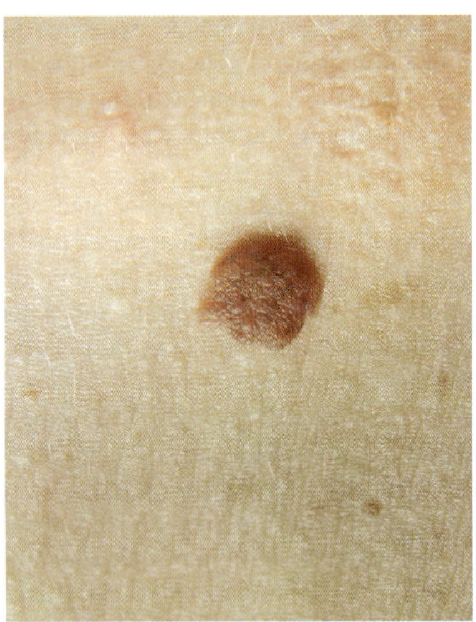

FIGURE 15.2 ***Naevi (moles) arise from melanocytes and are common in all adults***

Source: Nathalie Speliers Ufermann/Shutterstock.

can transform into malignant lesions. Australian malignant melanoma rates are on the rise. The whole-body naevi count, when increased, is an independent risk factor for melanoma (Mar, Wolfe & Kelly, 2011). It is important to monitor naevi for changes in size, thickness, colour, bleeding or itching. If any of these changes occur, the person should seek immediate professional assessment.

Angiomas

Angiomas, also called *haemangiomas*, are benign vascular tumours. They appear in the adult in different forms:

- Naevus flammeus (port-wine stain) is a congenital vascular lesion that involves the capillaries. The lesions tend to occur on the upper body or face as macular patches that range from light red to dark purple. These lesions are present at birth and grow proportionately with the child into adulthood.
- Cherry angiomas are small, rounded papules that may occur at any age, but they most commonly arise in the forties and gradually increase in number. The lesions range in colour from bright red to purple. These lesions are often found on the trunk. They are also called senile angiomas or de Morgan spots, named after Campbell de Morgan, a 19th century British surgeon who first described them (Watkins, 2012).
- Spider angiomas are dilated superficial arteries. They are common in pregnant women and in people with hepatic disease. Spider angiomas occur most often on the face, neck and upper chest. The lesions are usually small, bright red papules with radiating lines, and they blanch with pressure.
- Telangiectases are single dilated capillaries or terminal arteries that appear often on the cheeks and nose. These lesions are most common in older adults and result from photoaged skin. The lesions look like broken veins.

Skin tags

Skin tags are soft papules on a pedicle. They can be as small as a pinhead or as large as a pea and are most often found on the front or side of the neck and in the axillae, as well as in areas where clothing (such as underwear) rubs the skin. These lesions have normal skin colour and texture.

Keratoses

A **keratosis** is any skin condition in which there is a benign overgrowth and thickening of the cornified epithelium. These lesions most often appear in adults after age 50. *Seborrhoeic keratoses* appear as superficial flat, smooth or warty-surfaced growths, 5 to 20 mm in diameter, most often on the face and trunk. The lesions may be tan, waxy yellow, dark brown or flesh coloured and they often appear greasy. They are most often seen in the older adult and do not appear to be related to damage from sun exposure.

THE PERSON WITH PSORIASIS

Psoriasis is a chronic immune skin disorder characterised by raised, reddened, round circumscribed plaques covered by silvery white scales (see Figure 15.3). The size of these lesions varies. The lesions may appear anywhere on the body, but they are most commonly found on the scalp, extensor surfaces of the arms and legs, elbows, knees, sacrum and around the nails. As with any chronic illness, the skin manifestations may occur and disappear throughout life, with no discernible pattern to the recurrence (Oakley, 2014).

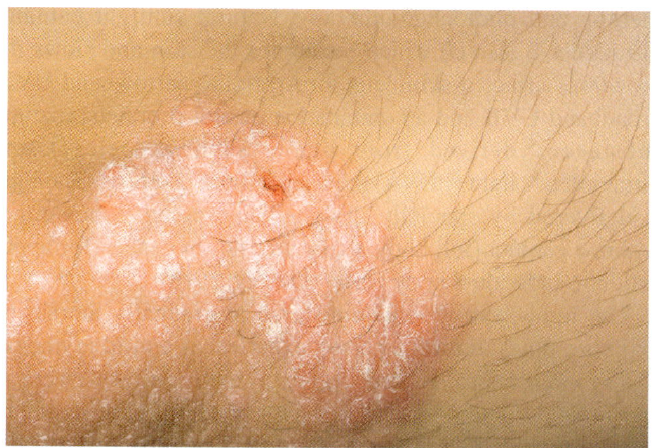

FIGURE 15.3 *The characteristic lesions of psoriasis are raised, red, round plaques covered with thick, silvery white scales*

Source: © olavs/Shutterstock.com.

The incidence of psoriasis is lower in warm, sunny climates. Onset usually occurs in the person's twenties, but it may occur at any age. Psoriasis occurs more often in Caucasians; men and women are affected equally. Sunlight, stress, seasonal changes, hormone fluctuations, steroid withdrawal and certain drugs (such as alcohol, corticosteroids, lithium and chloroquine) appear to exacerbate the disorder. Evidence suggests that psoriasis is linked to genetic susceptibility (Witte & Sabat, 2014). About one-third of people have a family history of psoriasis. Trauma to the skin from such events as surgery, sunburn or excoriation is also a common precipitating factor; lesions that result from trauma are called Koebner phenomenon (Bullock & Hales, 2019; Luo, 2014).

Pathophysiology

Normally, the keratinocyte (an epidermal cell making up 95% of the epidermis) migrates from the basal cell to the stratum corneum (the outer skin layer) in about 14 days and is sloughed off 14 days later. Psoriatic skin cells, by contrast, have a shorter cycle of growth, completing the journey to the stratum corneum in only 4 to 7 days, a condition called *hyperkeratosis*. These immature cells produce an abnormal keratin that forms thick, flaky scales at the surface of the skin. The more rapid cell metabolism stimulates increased vascularity, which contributes to the erythema of the lesions. As part of the abnormal process, certain immune cells become overactive and release proteins called cytokines. One of the cytokines is tumour necrosis factor (TNF); in psoriasis, TNF causes inflammation, further contributing to plaque formation.

Psoriasis vulgaris is the most common form of psoriasis. The lesions can be found anywhere on the skin but most commonly involve the skin over the elbows, knees and scalp. Initially, the lesions are papules that form into well-defined erythematous plaques with thick, silvery white scales. The plaques in people with darker skin may appear purple.

Permanent remission of psoriasis is rare. The prognosis depends on the type, extent and severity of the initial attack. Age at onset is also a factor; early-onset disease is usually more severe.

Manifestations

The characteristic lesions in psoriasis are well-demarcated regions of erythematous plaques that shed thick, silvery white flakes. Pruritus is common over the psoriatic lesions. If the lesions are located in an intertriginous zone, such as between the toes, under the breasts or in the perianal region, the psoriatic scales may soften, allowing painful fissures to form. When psoriasis affects the nails, pitting and a yellow or brown discolouration result. The nail may separate from the nail bed, thicken and crumble. The involved nails, which are more often fingernails than toenails, are at high risk of infection. The person may also exhibit manifestations of psoriatic arthritis, seen most often in the distal interphalangeal joints, especially if the fingernails are involved.

INTERPROFESSIONAL CARE

Treatment is based on the type of psoriasis, the extent and location of the lesions, the age of the person and the degree of disfigurement or disability.

Diagnosis

Skin biopsy may be done if the person presents with atypical manifestations or to differentiate psoriasis from other inflammatory or infectious skin disorders. In addition, an ultrasound may reveal typical psoriatic changes in the stratum corneum and inflammation of the dermis.

Medications

A variety of medications and treatments may be prescribed, including topical medications and photochemotherapy. Although there is no cure, treatment decreases the severity and pain of the lesions.

Topical medications are administered to decrease inflammation, prolong the maturity time of keratinocytes and increase remission time. Corticosteroids, tar preparations, anthralin and the retinoids are typically used. Box 15.2 outlines general guidelines for teaching the person to apply topical medications.

Topical corticosteroids decrease inflammation, suppress mitotic activity of psoriatic cells and delay the movement of keratinocytes to the surface of the skin. The most effective topical corticosteroids are potent preparations that are well absorbed through the skin and are used under an occlusive dressing. Corticosteroids may also be taken systemically or injected directly into the lesions. However, corticosteroids rarely cause a lasting remission and may cause the psoriasis to become unstable (Papadakis, McPhee & Rabow, 2018). They are therefore used for repeated short periods of treatment and combined with other measures, such as tar preparations, occlusions or a topical retinoid.

Tar preparations (such as Psor-Asist™) suppress mitotic activity and are also anti-inflammatory. Tar preparations are made from distillation of coal and wood, and they can stain clothing and have a pungent odour. The exact mechanism of action of tar preparations is unknown, but they are effective in

BOX 15.2 General guidelines for applying topical medications

Each time a medication is applied, the skin surface must be clean and dry. Remove any medication from the previous application. Remove creams by washing the skin with tap water and a pH-neutral skin cleanser or mild soap.

- ***To apply gels, creams and pastes*: squeeze about 1 to 2.5 cm of the gel or cream into the gloved palm of the hand. Rub the hands together until they are covered. Apply gels and creams to the affected areas with long gentle strokes until the skin is thinly covered. Differences from these general guidelines follow:**
  a. **Corticosteroids are usually applied two to three times a day in small amounts and rubbed directly on to the lesions. Apply the medication after a bath; it can be covered with an occlusive dressing if prescribed.**
  b. **Apply medications containing tar in the direction of hair growth. Do not apply these medications to the face, to the genitals or in skin folds. If the tar is water-based or oil-based, it will stain clothing.**
  c. **Wear gloves when applying as dithranol stains.**
- ***To apply lotions*: shake the bottle of lotion well. Pour a small amount into the palm of the gloved hand and pat the medication on to the skin. If the lotion is thin, apply it with a gauze pad.**
- ***To apply sprays*: hold the container about 15 cm from the skin and apply the medication in a short spray.**
- ***To apply medicated shampoo*: apply the shampoo, massage into the hair and over the scalp carefully and allow it to remain for the prescribed time. Rinse.**
- ***To apply pastes*: use enough paste on an applicator (such as a wooden tongue depressor) to cover the lesion thinly.**

removing scales and increasing remission time; however, they can make a person more sun sensitive.

Topical dithranol, which is extracted from tree bark, inhibits the mitotic activity of epidermal cells and is effective in some cases of chronic, localised psoriasis that do not respond to other topical agents. The medication is applied to the plaque patches at bedtime and left in place for 8 to 12 hours. The person should be tested for sensitivity to the drug before use and it should not be applied to inflamed or open areas of skin.

Calcipotrial (Daivovex™, a vitamin D analogue) has been effective and safe in both the short-term and long-term treatment of psoriasis. It inhibits cell proliferation in the epidermis and facilitates cell differentiation. Although a derivative of topical vitamin D, calcipotrial does not seem to affect bone or calcium metabolism; however, periodic monitoring is prudent if used in children or large doses (Pharmaceutical Society of Australia, 2018).

Ultraviolet light therapy

Psoriasis that is widespread (i.e. involves more than 30% of the body surface) is difficult to treat with topical medications. Treatments for generalised psoriasis include ultraviolet light therapy and photochemotherapy. Natural sunlight contains ultraviolet-B (UVB) which penetrates the skin and slows the growth of affected skin cells. In Australia, narrowband UVB, broadband UVB and a combination of oral psoralens (natural substances derived from plants such as celery) and ultraviolet-A light (PUVA) are used to treat psoriasis. The light is delivered by specially designed fluorescent tubes either within a cabinet (full body application) or in panels (for application to individual body parts) (Oakley, 2018).

The light therapy is administered in gradually increasing exposure times, until the person experiences a mild erythema, like a mild sunburn. Treatments are given three times a week as an outpatient and are measured in seconds of exposure. The eyes are shielded during the treatment. The erythema response occurs in about 8 hours. Careful assessment is necessary to prevent more severe burning, which could exacerbate the psoriasis. In the person with extensive psoriasis, UVB treatments may be combined with tar preparations, which increase the photosensitivity of the skin.

PHOTOCHEMOTHERAPY In photochemotherapy, a light-activated form of the drug methoxsalen is used. This drug is an antimetabolite that inhibits DNA synthesis and thereby prevents cell mitosis, decreasing hyperkeratosis. Exposure to ultraviolet-A (UVA) rays activates methoxsalen; it is administered orally and the person is exposed to UVA 2 hours later. The eyes are covered by dark glasses during the treatment. Treatments are administered two to three times a week; usually, 10 to 20 total treatments are given over 1 to 2 months. Treatment causes tanning and direct sunlight must be avoided for 8 to 12 hours thereafter. If the person exhibits erythema, the treatments are stopped until the redness and swelling resolve.

Photochemotherapy has had a high success rate in achieving remission of psoriasis, but it can accelerate ageing of exposed skin, induce cataract development, alter immune function and increase the risk of melanoma.

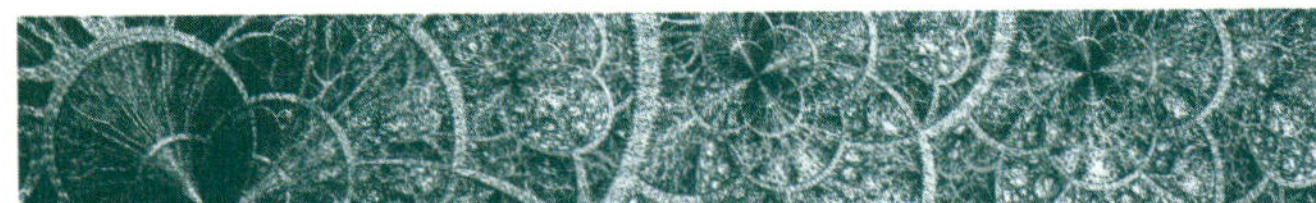

Nursing care

The person with psoriasis requires nursing care to meet physical and psychological responses to the illness. The nurse provides teaching for self-care and emotional support through non-judgmental acceptance.

Nursing diagnoses and planning

The nursing care discussed in this section focuses on the diagnoses of:

- *Impaired skin integrity* related to psoriasis as evidenced by open lesions on lower legs and lower arms.
- *Disturbed body image* related to psoriasis as evidenced by reluctance to wear clothing that may expose lesions.

Impaired skin integrity related to psoriasis

Psoriatic lesions range from several scales to large, open areas. Typical psoriatic skin lesions increase the risk of infection, which can further compromise healing. In addition, certain treatments (e.g. the use of UVA or retinoids) may cause erythema or peeling of the skin, further altering skin integrity.

- Teach methods to reduce injury to the skin when taking therapeutic baths or treatments:
  - Use warm, not hot, water.
  - Gently rub lesions with a soft washcloth, using a circular motion.
  - Dry the skin with a soft towel, using a blotting or patting motion.
  - Keep the skin always lubricated.
- Explain application of topical medications:
  - Apply the medication as prescribed in a thin layer, using gloved hands, wooden tongue depressors or a gauze pad.
  - Avoid getting medications in the eyes, on mucous membranes or in skin folds.
  - Apply a covering such as an occlusive dressing over the medicated areas if prescribed. Topical corticosteroids are often covered with occlusive dressings or wraps to increase absorption and thus facilitate treatment. However, constant occlusion may increase the effects of the medications to undesired levels and also increases the risk of infections.
- Teach manifestations of infection and how to contact the healthcare provider if these occur: elevated temperature, increased swelling, redness, pain, increase in drainage and any change in the colour of the drainage.
- Teach manifestations of the complications of treatment: excoriation, increased erythema, increased peeling and blister formation. The topical medications or treatments may damage cells through chemical burns or excessive exposure to ultraviolet light.

Disturbed body image related to psoriasis

The chronic skin lesions of psoriasis often cause people to isolate themselves from social contacts, withdraw from normal roles and responsibilities, and feel helpless or powerless.

- Establish a trusting relationship by expressing acceptance of the person, both verbally and non-verbally. For example, touch the person during social communications, demonstrating that the lesions are not contagious or offensive.
- Encourage the person to verbalise feelings about self-perception in view of the chronic nature of psoriasis and to ask questions about the disease and treatment.
- Promote social interaction through family involvement in care and by referral to support groups of people with psoriasis or other chronic skin conditions.

Community-based care

Person and family teaching focuses on treatments and skin care needs. The following topics should be addressed:

- The chronic nature of the disease, factors that may precipitate an exacerbation and methods to reduce stress.
- Interventions for pruritus and dry skin and specific care for psoriasis:
  - Expose the skin to sunlight but avoid sunburn.
  - Avoid trauma to the skin (e.g. do not scrub off scales and use only an electric razor).
  - Avoid exposure to contagious illnesses such as influenza and colds.
  - Discuss current medications with the healthcare provider. Certain drugs (such as indomethacin (Indocin™), lithium and beta-adrenergic blocking agents) are known to precipitate exacerbations of psoriasis.
  - Suggest contact with resources such as Psoriasis Australia www.psoriasisaustralia.org.au.

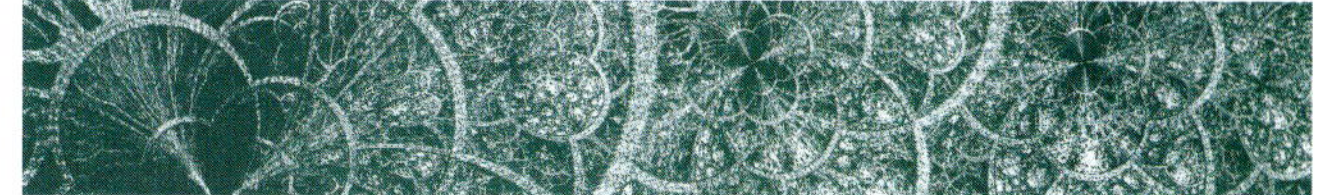

Infections and infestations of the skin

The skin's resistance to infections and infestations is provided by protective mechanisms, including skin flora, sebum and the immune response. Although the skin is normally resistant to infections and infestations, these disorders may occur as a result of a break in the skin surface, a virulent agent, and/or decreased resistance due to a compromised immune system. This section discusses skin disorders resulting from bacterial infections, fungal infections, parasitic infestations and viral infections.

THE PERSON WITH A BACTERIAL INFECTION OF THE SKIN

A number of bacteria normally inhabit the skin and do not cause an infection. However, when a break in the skin allows invasion by pathogenic bacteria, an infection may occur. The most common bacterial infections are caused by Gram-positive organisms commonly found on the skin, such as *Staphylococcus aureus*.

Bacterial infections of the skin may be primary or secondary. Primary infections are caused by a single pathogen and arise from normal skin; secondary infections develop in injured or diseased skin.

Most bacterial infections are treated by a primary care provider within the home environment. If the infection becomes more serious, however, inpatient care may be required. In addition, nosocomial infections of wounds or open lesions in hospitalised people are often the result of bacterial infections, especially by methicillin-resistant *Staphylococcus aureus* (MRSA).

Pathophysiology

Bacterial infections of the intact skin arise from the hair follicle, where bacteria can accumulate and grow and cause localised infection. The bacteria also can invade deeper tissues and cause systemic infection, a potentially life-threatening disorder. Various types of bacterial infections involve the skin, including folliculitis, furuncles, carbuncles, cellulitis, erysipelas and impetigo.

Folliculitis

Folliculitis is a bacterial infection of the hair follicle, most commonly caused by *Staphylococcus aureus*. The infection begins at the follicle opening and extends down into the follicle. The bacteria release enzymes and chemical agents that cause an inflammation. The lesions appear as pustules surrounded by an area of erythema on the surface of the skin (see Figure 15.4). The lesions are accompanied by discomfort ranging from slight burning to intense itching. A major complication is abscess formation. Folliculitis is found most often on the scalp and extremities. It is also often seen on the face of bearded men (called sycosis barbae), on the legs of women who shave and on the eyelids (called a stye). Folliculitis can also present on peristomal skin that has been irritated by stomal effluent and the aggressive removal of ostomy appliances.

Although folliculitis may appear without any apparent cause, contributing factors include poor hygiene, poor nutrition, prolonged skin moisture, tight heavy fabrics on the upper legs, shaving and trauma to the skin.

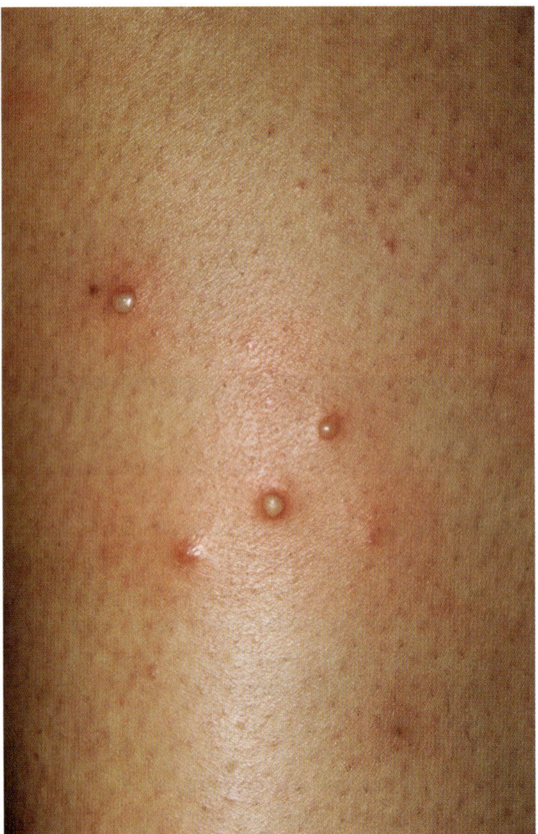

FIGURE 15.4 ***The lesions of folliculitis are pustules surrounded by areas of erythema***

Source: © Dr P. Marazzi/Science Photo Library/Alamy Stock Photo.

CONSIDERATION FOR PRACTICE

A specific type of folliculitis, called 'hot tub folliculitis', is caused by *Pseudomonas aeruginosa* and is characterised by follicular or pustular lesions that occur 1 to 4 days after being in a hot tub or public swimming pool.

Furuncles

Furuncles, often called *boils*, are also inflammations of the hair follicle. They often begin as folliculitis, but the infection spreads down the hair shaft, through the wall of the follicle and into the dermis. The causative organism is commonly *Staphylococcus aureus*. A furuncle initially presents as a deep, firm, red, painful nodule from 1 to 5 cm in diameter (see Figure 15.5) but can result in a painful cystic nodule. The cysts may drain substantial amounts of purulent drainage.

Contributing factors include poor hygiene, heat and humidity, trauma to the skin, areas of excessive moisture (including perspiration) and systemic diseases such as diabetes mellitus and haematological malignancies.

Carbuncles

A **carbuncle** is a group of infected hair follicles. The lesion begins as a firm mass located in the subcutaneous tissue and the lower dermis. This mass becomes swollen and painful and has multiple openings to the skin surface. Carbuncles are most frequently found on the back of the neck, the upper back and the lateral thighs. In addition to the local manifestations, the person may experience chills, fever and malaise. The contributing factors for carbuncles are the same as for furuncles. Both infections are more common in hot, humid climates.

Cellulitis

Cellulitis is a localised infection of the dermis and subcutaneous tissue. Cellulitis can occur in intact skin or be associated with a wound or furuncles or carbuncles. The infection spreads

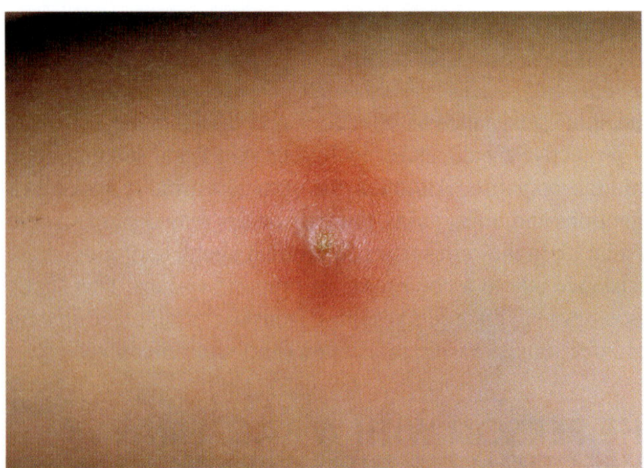

FIGURE 15.5 ***A furuncle (boil) is a deep, firm, red, painful nodule***

Source: © Dr P. Marazzi/Science Photo Library/Alamy Stock Photo.

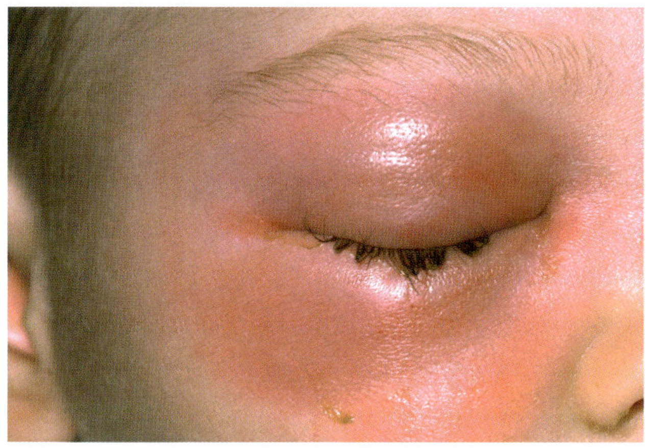

FIGURE 15.6 ***Cellulitis is a bacterial infection localised in the dermis and subcutaneous tissue. The involved area is red, swollen and painful***

Source: Mediscan/Alamy Stock Photo.

as a result of a substance produced by the causative organism, called spreading factor (hyaluronidase). This factor breaks down the fibrin network and other barriers that normally localise the infection. The area of cellulitis is red, swollen and painful (see Figure 15.6). In some cases, vesicles may form over the area of cellulitis. The person may also experience systemic signs and symptoms such as fever, chills, malaise, headache and swollen lymph glands.

Erysipelas

Erysipelas is an infection of the skin most often caused by group A streptococci. Chills, fever and malaise are prodromal symptoms, occurring from 4 hours to 20 days before the skin lesion appears. The initial infection appears as firm red spots that enlarge and join to form a circumscribed, bright red, raised, hot lesion. Vesicles may form over the surface of the erysipelas lesion. The area usually is painful, itches and burns. Erysipelas most commonly appears on the face, ears and lower legs.

Impetigo

Impetigo is frequently referred to as 'school sores' as it is common in infants and children. It is a skin infection caused by staphylococci or group A beta-haemolytic streptococci. Lesions commonly occur on the face but can affect any anatomical site. The lesions appear as vesicles or pustules; when they rupture, the lesion discharges serous exudate that forms yellowish crusts as it dries on the skin. Pruritus and excoriations may result from scratching, and cross-infection can occur. Impetigo is usually treated topically with mupirocin or, in extensive cases, oral antibiotics (Grossman & Porth, 2014).

INTERPROFESSIONAL CARE

The diagnosis of a bacterial infection of the skin is made by assessing the appearance of the lesion and by identifying the causative organism. Antibiotics specific to the organism are used in treatment.

Diagnosis

Wound aspirate or swab is collected and sent to pathology for microbiological culture and sensitivity to identify the causative organism and determine the most effective antibiotic. People who experience repeated bacterial skin infections or who provide care for others who exhibit infections may have a culture taken from the external nares to determine whether they are carriers of bacteria (e.g. MRSA) and are reinfecting themselves or others.

Medications

The primary treatment for bacterial infections of the skin is an antibiotic specific to the organism. The antibiotic is usually taken orally, but for extensive or severe infections, antibiotics may be administered intravenously. Multiple furuncles and carbuncles may be treated with cloxacillin (a penicillinase-resistant penicillin); the cephalosporins also are often effective. Topical antibiotics are not commonly prescribed as overuse can increase the risk of antibiotic resistance. However, prudent use of antiseptic-impregnated dressings can restore bacterial balance in the tissue without undue tissue toxicity or the use of systemic antibiotics (see Box 15.12).

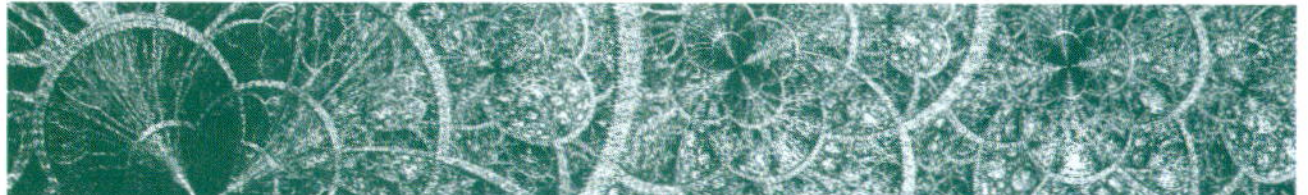

Nursing care

Nursing care focuses on preventing the spread of infection and restoring normal skin integrity. Most people provide self-care at home, but the incidence of secondary bacterial infections in the inpatient population is great enough to warrant their inclusion in planning and implementing care.

Nursing diagnoses and interventions

Potential risk of infection related to ineffective infection control practices by healthcare personnel

- Practise good personal hygiene and hand hygiene and teach their importance to all people.
- Teach the person and their family how to identify the signs and symptoms of localised and spreading infection. Local signs and symptoms include pain, swelling, erythema, heat and purulent or increased exudate. Signs of spreading infection may be manifested systemically by fever, tachycardia, chills and malaise.
- Prudent preventive use of modern antiseptic dressings such as cadexomer iodine (Iodosorb™), wound honey preparations, silver or polyhexamethylene-biguanide-impregnated dressings may be warranted in the treatment of these wounds.

Community-based care

Person and family teaching focuses on facilitating tissue healing and eliminating the infection. Address the following topics:

- the importance of maintaining good nutrition
- the importance of maintaining cleanliness through careful hand hygiene, and proper handling and disposal of dressings or contaminated materials
- preventing the spread of infection in the home by not sharing bed linen and towels, and washing clothing and linen in hot water
- the importance of not squeezing or trying to open a bacterial lesion
- avoiding plucking of nasal hair or picking nose
- the importance of taking the full course of prescribed antibiotics on a regular schedule until the prescribed supply is finished
- showering daily and using an antibacterial soap or lotion if warranted when bacterial skin infections exist.

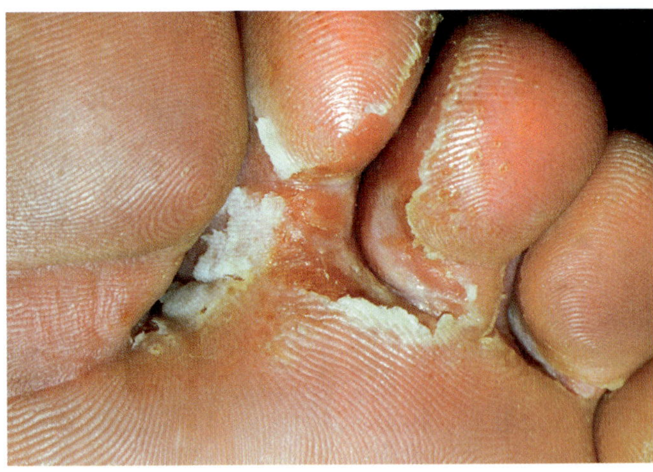

FIGURE 15.7 ***Tinea pedis (athlete's foot) is a fungal infection that often occurs between the toes***

Source: Science Photo Library/Alamy Stock Photo.

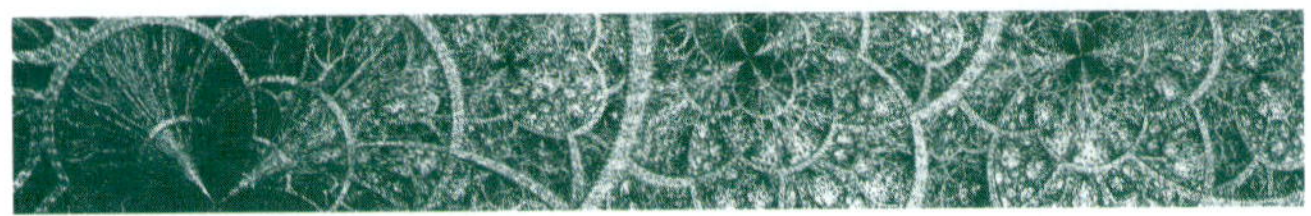

THE PERSON WITH A FUNGAL INFECTION

Fungi are free-living plant-like organisms that live in the soil, on animals and on humans. The fungi that cause superficial skin infections are called dermatophytes. In humans, the dermatophytes live on keratin in the stratum corneum, hair and nails. Fungal disorders are also called *mycoses*.

Pathophysiology

Fungal infections include dermatophytoses (tinea or ringworm) and candidiasis (yeast) infections.

Dermatophytoses (ringworm or tinea)

Superficial fungal infections of the skin are called **dermatophytoses** or, more commonly, *ringworm* or *tinea*. Fungal infections occur when a susceptible host comes in contact with the organism. The organism may be transmitted by direct contact with animals or other infected people or by inanimate objects such as combs, pillowcases, towels and hats. The most important factor in the development of the infection is moisture; the onset and spread of the fungal infection is greatest in areas where moisture content is high, such as within skin folds, between the toes and in the mouth. Other factors that increase the risk of a fungal infection include the use of broad-spectrum antibiotics that kill off normal skin or mucosal flora and allow the fungi to grow, and conditions such as diabetes mellitus, immunodeficiencies, nutritional deficiencies, pregnancy, increasing age and iron deficiency. Fungal infections of the skin are more common in warm, humid climates. The dermatophyte infections are named by the body part affected, as follows:

- *Tinea pedis* is a fungal infection of the soles of the feet, the space between the toes, and/or the toenails (see Figure 15.7). More often called *athlete's foot*, this is the most common tinea infection. The lesions vary from mild scaliness to painful fissures with drainage and they are usually accompanied by pruritus and a foul odour. The infection is often chronic, absent in winter but reappearing in hot weather when perspiring feet are encased in shoes.
- *Tinea capitis* is a fungal infection of the scalp. The primary lesions are grey, round, bald spots, often accompanied by erythema and crusting. The hair loss is usually temporary. Tinea capitis is seen more often in children than in adults.
- *Tinea corporis* is a fungal infection of the body. It can be caused by several different fungi and the lesions vary according to the causative organism. The most common lesions, often called *ringworm*, are large circular patches with raised red borders of vesicles, papules or pustules. Pruritus and erythema are also present.
- *Tinea versicolour* is a fungal infection of the upper chest, back and sometimes the arms. The lesions are yellow, pink or brown sheets of scaling skin. The patches do not have pigment and do not tan when exposed to ultraviolet light.
- *Tinea cruris* is a fungal infection of the groin that may extend to the inner thighs and buttocks. Often called 'jock itch', it is often associated with tinea pedis and is more common in people who are physically active, are obese and/or wear tight underclothing.

Candidiasis

Candidiasis infections are caused by *Candida albicans*, a yeast-like fungus. This fungus is normally found on mucous membranes, on the skin, in the vagina and in the gastrointestinal tract. The fungus becomes a pathogen when the following factors encourage its growth:

- a local environment of moisture, warmth or altered skin integrity
- the administration of systemic antibiotics
- pregnancy
- the use of birth control pills
- poor nutrition
- the presence of diabetes mellitus, Cushing's disease or other chronic debilitating illnesses
- immunosuppression
- some malignancies of the blood.

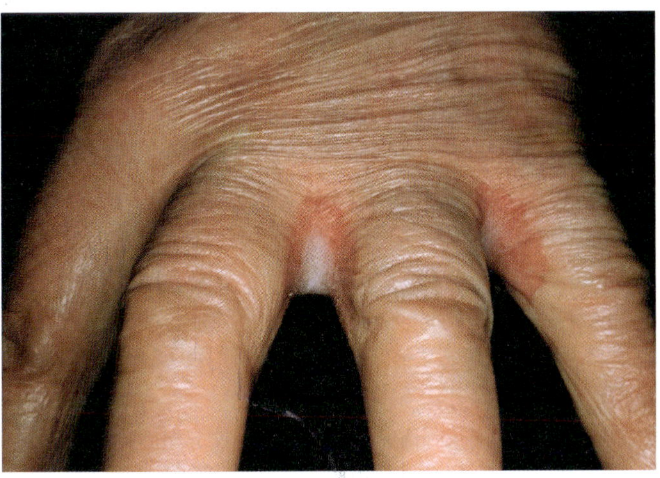

FIGURE 15.8 Candida albicans, *a fungus, causes a skin infection characterised by erythema, pustules and a typical white substance covering the area*

Source: © CNRI/Science Photo Library.

Candidiasis affects the outer layers of the skin and mucous membranes of the mouth, vagina, uncircumcised penis, nails and deep skin folds (under large breasts or an abdominal pannus). The first sign of infection is a pustule that extends under the stratum corneum. The pustule has an inflamed base and often burns and itches. As the infection spreads, the accumulation of inflammatory cells and shedding of surface cells produce a white to yellow curd-like substance that covers the infected area (see Figure 15.8). Satellite lesions (maculopapular areas found outside the clearly demarcated border of the original infection) are characteristic of candidiasis. The appearance of the infection differs by location, as summarised in Table 15.2.

INTERPROFESSIONAL CARE

Fungal infections are primarily diagnosed in outpatient settings and treated at home but may also occur in hospitalised people. The treatment is the same, regardless of the setting.

Diagnosis

Diagnostic tests are conducted to determine the causative fungi and may include cultures of skin scrapings and examination of the skin with ultraviolet light (Wood's lamp). See the chapter 'Assessing the integumentary system' for further information.

Medications

Fungal infections of the skin are treated by topical or systemic antifungal medications. Nursing implications for these medications are described in the 'Medication administration' box.

- Candidiasis infections are treated, depending on the location, with antifungal oral medication, powder or vaginal suppositories.

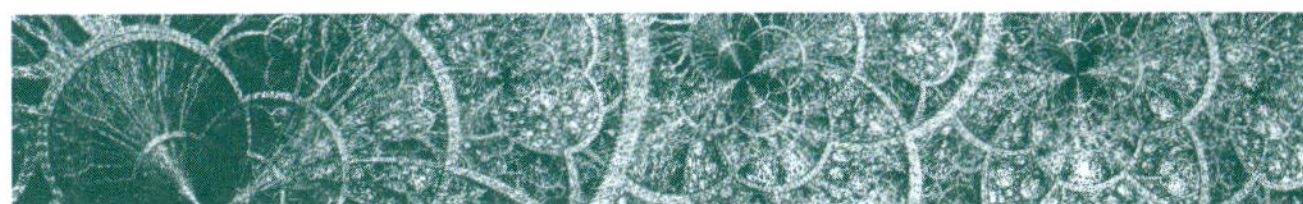

Nursing care

Many people treat themselves with over-the-counter antifungal medications. It is recommended, however, that the person be professionally diagnosed, especially if the infection is ongoing or repetitive. The interventions discussed for nursing care of the person with a bacterial infection are also appropriate for the person with a fungal infection. Teaching topics specific to fungal infections are as follows:

- Fungal diseases are contagious. Do not share linen or personal items with others.
- Use a clean towel and washcloth each day.
- Carefully dry all skin folds, including those under the breasts, arms, abdominal pannus and between the toes.
- Wear clean cotton underclothing each day.
- Fungi grow in moist environments, such as on sweaty feet. To prevent further infections:
  - Do not wear the same pair of shoes every day.
  - Wear socks that permit moisture to wick away from the skin surface.
  - Do not wear rubber- or plastic-soled shoes.

TABLE 15.2 Characteristics of candidiasis infections by location

LOCATION	CHARACTERISTICS
Skin folds (under breasts, in groin, axillae, anus, umbilicus, abdominal pannus and between toes or fingers)	Erythematous lesions can be either dry or moist. The lesions have clear borders and satellite lesions are present.
Nails	Nail bed is red, swollen and painful.
Mouth (thrush)	Mucous membranes are red and may be swollen; surface is covered with white, creamy material. Eroded areas may be present over the tongue and the oral cavity.
Penis (balanitis) (glans and shaft)	The penis is covered with small, red, clearly demarcated lesions that are painful and itch. The lesions may be covered with a white plaque.
Vagina	Red mucous membranes contain brighter red, demarcated, oozing lesions. The cervix may be covered with white plaque. A white, cheesy, foul-smelling vaginal discharge is present, accompanied by itching and burning. The vaginal and labial membranes may be swollen; the infection may extend to the anus and groin.

MEDICATION ADMINISTRATION Antifungal agents

Examples:

Nystatin (Mycostatin™, Nilstat™)

Itraconazole (Sporanox™)

Miconazole (Daktarin™)

Ketoconazole (Nizoral™)

Fluconazole (Diflucan™)

Amphotericin B (Fungilin™)

Griseofulvin (Fulcin™)

Terbinafine hydrocholoride (Lamisil™)

Antifungal medications are prepared in a variety of forms, depending on the specific drug: powders, creams, shampoos, suspensions, troches, vaginal suppositories and oral tablets. Some drugs interfere with the permeability of the fungal cell membrane; others interfere with DNA synthesis. Most of these medications are fungistatic, but in large doses they may be fungicidal.

NURSING RESPONSIBILITIES

- When taking the health history, ask about known hypersensitivity reactions to these agents; document carefully.
- Assess for side effects: skin rash, local irritation, gastrointestinal symptoms (if given orally) and cognitive status.
- Administer ketoconazole with food to minimise gastrointestinal irritation.
- Shake suspensions well before administration and ask the person to swish them around the mouth before swallowing.
- If advised by the manufacturer, advise the person to allow oral tablets to dissolve in the mouth.

HEALTH EDUCATION FOR THE PERSON AND FAMILY

- Therapy usually continues over a long period of time, but regular use of medications for the recommended period is necessary. Do not miss doses and do complete the full treatment.
- *For griseofulvin*: take with meals or foods high in fat (such as ice-cream) to avoid stomach upset and help with absorption. Avoid alcohol (which may cause rapid pulse and flushing) and exposure to sunlight (this drug causes increased sensitivity).
- *For nystatin*: dissolve lozenges completely in the mouth. Hold suspensions in the mouth and swish throughout the mouth as long as possible before swallowing. Insert intravaginal medication high in the vagina. Continue with intravaginal applications throughout the menses.
- *For antifungal shampoo*: use two times a week for 4 weeks, allowing at least 3 days between each shampoo. Wet hair, apply shampoo to produce lather, leave in place for 1 minute, then rinse. Apply shampoo a second time, lather, leave in place for 3 minutes, then rinse thoroughly.
- *For topical application*: rub well into the affected areas, but do not get the medication in your eyes.
- *For vaginal candidiasis infections*: treatment with antifungal creams and pessaries can weaken condoms, so apply after sexual intercourse. Also, use plenty of lubricant during sexual intercourse as thrush can cause discomfort.
- A sexual partner will need to be treated at the same time so that you do not pass the infection back and forth to each other.

- For vaginal *Candida albicans* infection:
  - Avoid tight clothing, such as jeans and pantyhose.
  - Wear cotton or cotton-crotch underwear.
  - Shower more frequently and dry the genital area well.
  - Treat the sexual partner at the same time to avoid passing the infection back and forth to each other.

CONSIDERATION FOR PRACTICE

Recommend the person with repeated skin infections have a blood glucose test because this may indicate diabetes mellitus.

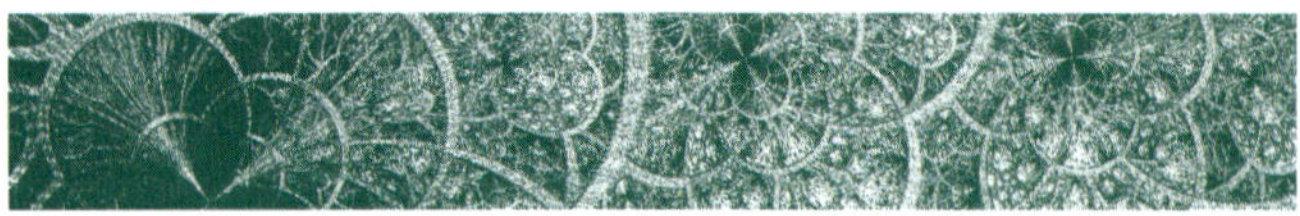

THE PERSON WITH A VIRAL INFECTION

Viruses are pathogens that consist of an RNA or DNA core surrounded by a protein coat. They depend on live cells for reproduction and so are classified as intracellular pathogens. The viruses that cause skin lesions invade the keratinocyte, reproduce and either increase cellular growth or cause cellular death.

An increase in the incidence of viral skin disorders has been attributed to a variety of causes. Some commonly used drugs, such as birth control medications and corticosteroids, are known to have immunosuppressive properties that allow the viruses to multiply. Other drugs, such as antibiotics, kill off normal skin bacteria that would otherwise serve as defence against viral infections.

Pathophysiology

Viral infections cause many different kinds of skin disorders, including warts, and herpes simplex and herpes zoster infections.

Warts

Warts, or *verrucae*, are lesions of the skin caused by the human papillomavirus (HPV). More than 60 types of HPVs have been found on the human skin and mucous membranes (Bullock & Hales, 2019). Warts may be found on non-genital skin or genital skin and mucous membranes. Non-genital warts are benign lesions; genital warts may be precancerous. Warts are transmitted through skin contact. Wart lesions may be flat, fusiform (tapered at both ends) or round, but most are round and raised and have a rough, grey surface. There are many different types of warts; the location and appearance of

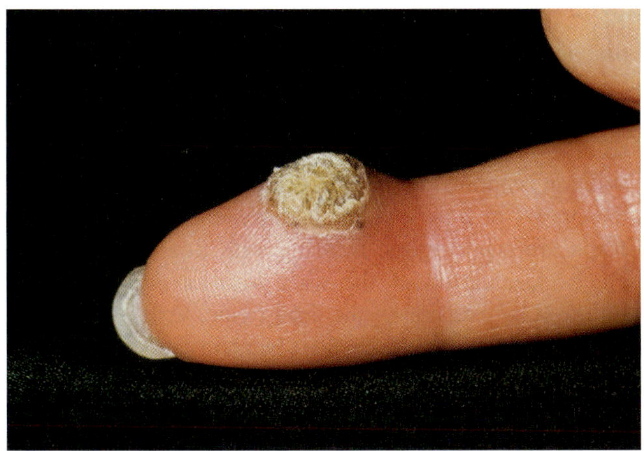

FIGURE 15.9 ***The common wart, caused by a virus, appears as a raised, dome-shaped lesion***

Source: Dr P. Marazzi/Science Photo Library/Alamy Stock Photo.

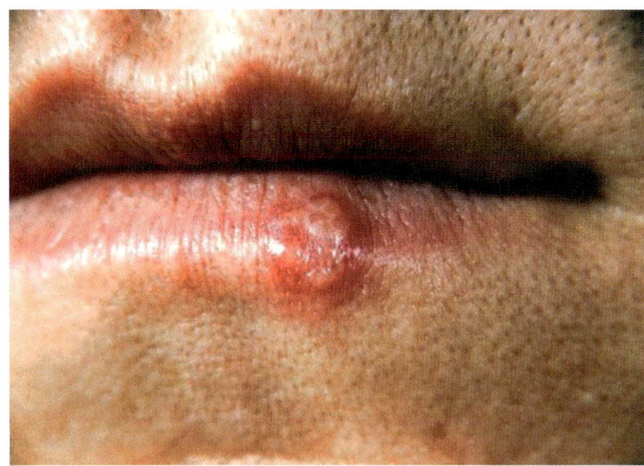

FIGURE 15.10 ***Herpes simplex is a viral infection of the skin and mucous membranes***

Source: CDC/Dr Hermann.

the warts depend on the causative virus. Those most common are as follows:

- A common wart (*verruca vulgaris*) may appear anywhere on the skin and mucous membranes of the body, but it most commonly appears on the fingers. Common warts grow above the skin surface and may be dome-shaped with ragged borders (see Figure 15.9).
- Plantar warts occur at pressure points on the soles of the feet. The pressure of shoes and walking prevents these warts from growing outwards, so they tend to extend deeper beneath the skin surface than common warts do. Plantar warts are often painful.
- A flat wart (*verruca plana*) is a small flat lesion, usually seen on the forehead or the dorsum of the hand.
- *Condylomata acuminata*, also called HPV or venereal warts, occur in moist areas, along the glans of the penis, in the anal region and on the vulva and cervix. They are usually cauliflower-like in appearance and have a pink or purple colour.

Warts resolve spontaneously when immunity to the virus develops. This response may take up to 5 years.

Herpes simplex

Herpes simplex (also called a *cold sore*) virus infections of the skin and mucous membranes are caused by two types of herpes virus: HSV-1 and HSV-2. Most infections above the waist are caused by HSV-1, with herpes simplex lesions most often found on the lips, face and mouth. (Genital herpes infections, which result from either HSV-1 or HSV-2, are classified as sexually transmitted infections. They are discussed in the chapter 'Nursing care of people who have sexually transmitted infections'.) The virus may be transmitted by physical contact, oral sex or kissing.

The infection begins with a burning or tingling sensation, followed by the development of erythema, vesicle formation and pain (see Figure 15.10). The vesicles progress through pustules, ulcers and crusting until healing occurs in 10 to 14 days.

The initial infection is often severe and accompanied by systemic manifestations, such as fever and sore throat; recurrences are more localised and less severe. The virus lives in nerve ganglia and may cause recurrent lesions in response to sunlight, menstruation, injury or stress. Oral aciclovir (Zovirax™) may be used prophylactically to prevent reoccurrences and to treat recurrent outbreaks.

Herpes zoster

Herpes zoster, also called *shingles*, is a viral infection of a dermatome section of the skin caused by varicella zoster (the herpesvirus that also causes chickenpox). The infection is believed to result from reactivation of a varicella virus remaining in the sensory dorsal ganglia after a childhood infection of chickenpox. When reactivated, the virus travels from the ganglia to the corresponding skin dermatome area.

Herpes zoster most often affects adults over the age of 60 (Grossman & Porth, 2014). People with Hodgkin's disease, certain types of leukaemia and lymphomas are more susceptible to an outbreak of the disease. Herpes zoster is more prevalent in immunocompromised people, such as those with human immunodeficiency virus (HIV) infections, those receiving radiation therapy or chemotherapy, and those who have had major organ transplants. The appearance of the lesions in people with HIV infections may be one of the first manifestations of immunocompromise. The herpes eruption lasts for about 2 to 3 weeks and usually does not recur.

Herpes zoster lesions are vesicles with an erythematous base. The vesicles appear on the skin area supplied by the neurons of a single or associated group of dorsal root ganglia (although they may occur beyond this area in immunosuppressed people). The lesions usually appear unilaterally on the face, trunk and thorax (see Figure 15.11). New lesions continue to erupt for 3 to 5 days, then crust and dry. Recovery occurs in 2 to 3 weeks. The person often experiences severe pain for up to 48 hours before and during eruption of the lesions. The pain may continue for weeks to months after the lesions have disappeared. The older adult is especially sensitive to the pain and often experiences more severe outbreaks of herpes zoster lesions.

Eruption of vesicles over a single dermatome usually only occurs one time. Generalised herpes zoster may indicate an associated immunocompromised disease, such as Hodgkin's

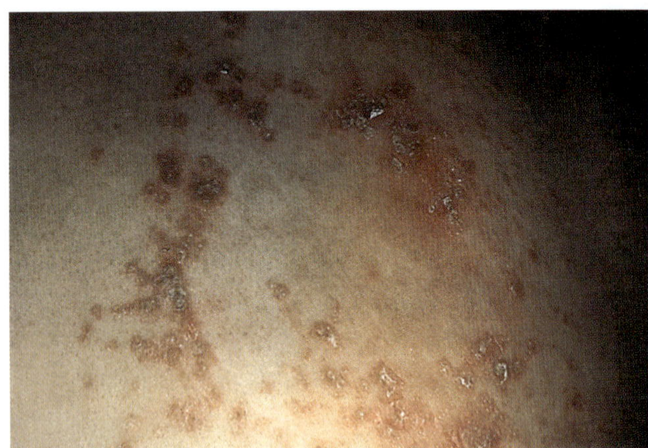

FIGURE 15.11 ***Herpes zoster is a viral infection of a dermatome section of the skin. The typical lesions are painful vesicles lying along the path of the nerve***

Source: CDC/Dr Dancewiez.

disease or HIV infection. People infected with HIV are 20 times more likely to develop herpes zoster (Papadakis et al., 2018).

Complications of herpes zoster include post-herpetic neuralgia (a sharp, spasmodic pain along the course of one or more nerves) and visual loss. The neuralgia, described as burning or stabbing, results from inflammation of the root ganglia. This complication is more common in people over the age of 55 (Papadakis et al., 2018). Permanent loss of vision may follow occurrence of lesions that arise from the ophthalmic division of the trigeminal nerve. The disease may disseminate in immunocompromised people, causing lesions beyond the dermatome, visceral lesions and encephalitis. This serious complication may cause death.

INTERPROFESSIONAL CARE

The treatment for viral skin infections focuses on stopping viral replication and treating the person's responses, such as itching and pain.

Diagnosis

Although diagnosis is usually based on manifestations and appearance of the lesions, laboratory tests may be necessary to differentiate herpes zoster from impetigo, contact dermatitis and herpes simplex. The laboratory tests include a Tzanck smear that identifies the herpes virus but does not distinguish herpes zoster from herpes simplex. Cultures of fluid from the vesicles and antibody tests are used to make the differential diagnosis of herpes virus types. The HIV testing should be considered if the person has a history of HIV risk factors.

Medications

Most viral skin disorders are treated with antiviral medications, and other types of medications are used to relieve pruritus and pain in the person with herpes zoster.

- *Warts.* Depending on their size, location and any associated discomfort, warts may be treated with medications, cryotherapy or electrodesiccation and curettage. A common method of wart removal is acid therapy, using a colloidal solution of 16% salicylic acid and 16% lactic acid. The solution is applied to the wart every 12 to 24 hours; the wart disappears in 2 to 3 weeks. Other methods of eradicating warts are cryosurgery, freezing with liquid nitrogen and electrodesiccation of the wart with an electric current followed by excision of the dead tissue. Venereal warts are further described in the chapter 'Nursing care of people who have sexually transmitted infections'.
- *Herpes simplex.* Herpes simplex lesions are treated with topical aciclovir (Zovirax™), an antiviral agent. Aciclovir shortens the time of symptoms and speeds healing.
- *Herpes zoster.* Antiviral drugs are used to treat herpes zoster infections. Aciclovir interferes with viral synthesis and replication. Although it does not cure herpes infections, it does decrease the severity of the illness and also decreases pain. It may be administered topically, orally or parenterally. It is more effective if administration begins within the first 1 to 2 days after the first vesicles appear. Nerve blocks may be needed to treat initial pain. Narcotic and non-narcotic analgesics are prescribed for pain management and antihistamines may be administered for relief of pruritus. People with eye involvement are treated with topical steroid ophthalmic ointments and mydriatics.

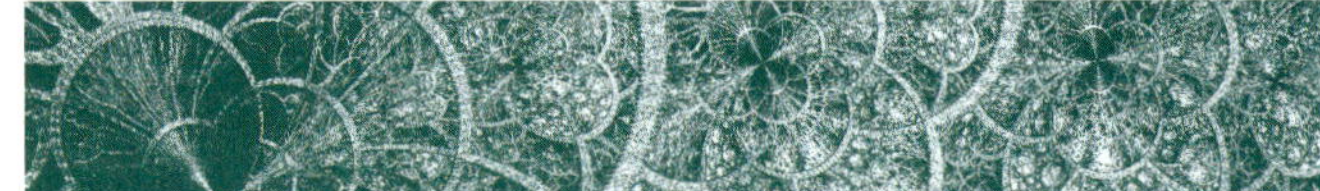

Nursing care

People with viral skin disorders require nursing care for infection, pruritus and pain. They also require teaching about preventing the spread of the virus to others. Of the viral disorders, herpes zoster is the most painful and debilitating. See the following nursing interventions that aim to relieve pain for the person with herpes zoster.

Nursing diagnoses and interventions

This section discusses the nursing care of the person with herpes zoster, focusing on the nursing diagnosis of *Acute pain* related to viral infection of herpes zoster.

Acute pain

The person with herpes zoster often experiences severe pain over the entire dermatome supplied by the affected nerve root. The pain is described as burning, tearing or stabbing. The person may avoid movement and does not want clothing or bed linen to touch the affected area.

- Monitor the location, duration and intensity of the pain.
- Explain the rationale for taking prescribed medications on a regular schedule.

- Teach measures to relieve pruritus:
  - Take prescribed antipruritic medications.
  - Topical application of amorphous hydrogels, especially those that contain tea tree oil, may soothe. Similarly, calamine lotion or wet compresses may be prescribed.
  - Keep the room temperature cool.
  - Use a bed cradle to keep sheets off affected areas of the body.
- Encourage the use of distraction (such as music) or a specific relaxation technique (such as progressive muscle relaxation or deep breathing).
- Pregabalin (anti-epileptic and co-analgesic medications) may be prescribed for post-hepatic neuralgia.
- Tea tree oil creams (Burn Aid®, Wound Aid®) are anti-inflammatory and topical application may provide relief.

CONSIDERATION FOR PRACTICE

Pregnant women must avoid exposure to people with herpes zoster because the herpes virus can cross the placental barrier.

Community-based care

Most people with viral infections are self-caring in their home environment. Provide the following information and instructions:

- Herpes zoster infections are usually self-limiting and heal completely. Second occurrences of herpes zoster are rare.
- Do not have social contact with children or pregnant women until crusts have formed over the blistered areas with herpes zoster, because the disease is contagious to people who have not had chickenpox.
- Use pain medications regularly.
- Follow suggestions to help reduce itching, scratching and pain: use medications as prescribed, wear lightweight cotton clothing, keep room temperatures cool, wear cotton gloves at night if scratching is a problem and practise relaxation and distraction activities.
- Report to your healthcare provider any increase in pain, fever, chills, drainage that smells bad and has pus or a spread in the blisters.

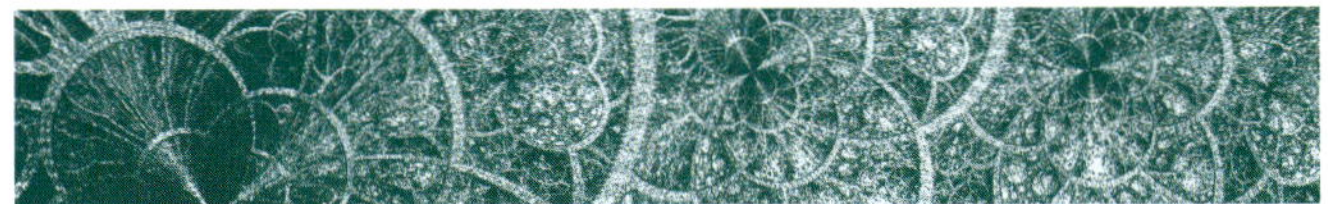

THE PERSON WITH A PARASITIC INFESTATION

Infestations of the skin by parasites are more common in developing countries but may occur in any geographical area of the world. They affect people of all social classes but are associated with crowded or unsanitary living conditions.

Pathophysiology

In Australia, two of the more common parasitic infestations of the skin are caused by lice and scabies. These parasites do not normally live on the skin but infest the skin through contact with an infested person or contact with clothing, linen or objects infested with the parasites.

Pediculosis

Pediculosis is an infestation with lice, parasites that live on the blood of an animal or human host. The louse is a 2 to 4 mm oval organism with a stylet that pierces the skin; an anticoagulant in its saliva prevents host blood from clotting while it eats. The female louse lays its eggs (small pearl-grey or brown eggs, called nits) on hair shafts. The louse within the egg hatches, reaches the adult reproductive stage and dies in 30 to 50 days (Bullock & Hales, 2019).

There are three types of human pediculosis:

1. Pediculosis corporis is an infestation with body lice. This type of infestation is more common in people who do not have access to facilities for bathing or washing clothes, such as the homeless. The lice live in clothing fibres and are transmitted primarily by contact with infested clothing and bed linen. The skin lesions occur at the site of a louse bite; macules appear initially, followed by wheals and papules. Pruritus is common and scratching often results in linear excoriations. Secondary infections cause hyperpigmentation and scarring. The lesions are most often seen on the shoulders, trunk and buttocks.
2. Pediculosis pubis is an infestation with pubic lice (often called crabs). This infestation is spread through sexual activity with someone already infested or by contact with infested clothing or linen. The lice are found in the pubic region and occasionally spread to the axillae or men's beards. The lice cause skin irritation and intense itching.
3. Pediculosis capitis is an infestation with head lice. The lice are most often found behind the ears and at the nape of the neck but may also spread to other hairy areas of the body: the eyebrows, pubic area or beard. The lice are transmitted by contact with an infected person or sharing combs, hairbrushes or hats. Manifestations of head lice include pruritus, scratching and erythema of the scalp. If untreated, the hair appears matted and crusted with a foul-smelling substance.

Scabies

Scabies is a parasitic infestation caused by a mite (*Sarcoptes scabiei*). The pregnant female mite burrows into the skin and lays two to three eggs each day for about a month. The eggs hatch in 3 to 5 days and the larvae migrate to the surface but burrow into the skin for food or protection. The larvae develop and the cycle repeats. Scabies infestation affects people of all socioeconomic classes. The infestation is found in webs between the fingers, the inner surfaces of the wrist and elbow, the axillae, the female nipple, the penis, the belt line and the gluteal crease. The lesions are small red-brown burrows, about 2 mm in length, sometimes covered with vesicles, which appear as a rash. Pruritus in response to the mite or its faeces is common, especially at night, and excoriations may develop. The excoriations predispose the person to secondary bacterial infections (Bullock & Hales, 2019).

INTERPROFESSIONAL CARE

Parasitic infestations are diagnosed by identifying the organism and are treated with medications that kill the lice or scabies.

Diagnosis

When a person has manifestations of pediculosis, the hair shaft and the clothing are examined to identify the lice or the nits. Microscopic examination of the parasite provides a positive diagnosis. Scabies is diagnosed by skin scrapings and microscopic examination for the mites or their faeces.

Medications

Lice are eradicated with agents that kill or mechanically remove (i.e. a fine-tooth comb) the parasite. Infestations of the body and pubic area are treated with topical medications that have a neurotoxic mode of action (permethrin, malathion, carbaril, spinosad) or a physical mode of action (demeicones, isopropyl myristate or herbal remedies). Ivermectin is the only oral treatment currently used as a pediculicide (Feldmeier, 2014). Mechanical removal methods involve wet fine-tooth combing to remove nits from the hair shaft.

Manufacturers' instructions are to be followed for use. Repeat applications may be required in some instances to kill newly hatched lice.

Scabies is treated with topical permethrin or lindane creams and the diligent treatment of other people who have been in close contact, as well as the laundry of contact linen and clothing to prevent reinfestation. Secondary skin infections are common with untreated scabies infestations or immunocompromised individuals.

The associated itching is treated with systemic or topical medications, including corticosteroids. Secondary bacterial infections are treated with the appropriate antibiotic.

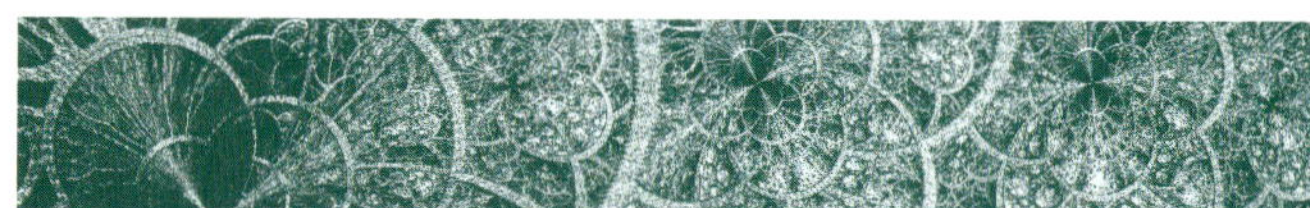

Nursing care

Nursing care for the person with a parasite infestation most often focuses on teaching to prevent infestation or to eradicate an existing infestation.

Education for the person and family is necessary to facilitate treatment at home, to prevent the spread of the infestation and to dispel the myth that lice infest only people with poor hygiene or in dirty living conditions. Specific information includes the following:

- Wash clothing and linen in soap and hot water or have them dry-cleaned.
- Ironing the clothes kills any lice eggs.
- Personal care items, such as combs or brushes, may be boiled to kill the parasites.
- All family members and sexual partners must also be treated.
- Avoid using the combs, brushes or hats of others.
- Lice and mites may infest anyone.

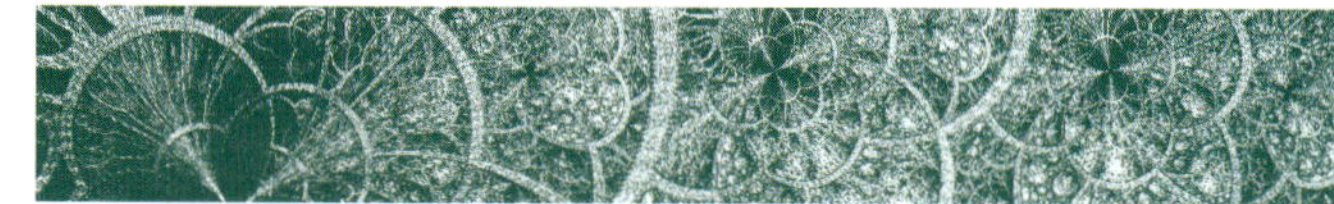

Inflammatory disorders of the skin

The inflammatory skin disorders discussed in this section are dermatitis and acne.

THE PERSON WITH DERMATITIS

Dermatitis is an inflammation of the skin characterised by erythema and pain or pruritus. Dermatitis may be acute or chronic.

Pathophysiology

In dermatitis, various exogenous and endogenous agents cause an inflammatory response of the skin. Different types of skin eruptions occur, often specific to the causative allergen, infection or disease. The initial skin responses to these agents or illnesses include erythema, formation of vesicles and scales, and pruritus (see Figure 15.12). Subsequently, irritation from scratching promotes oedema, a serous discharge and crusting. Long-term irritation in chronic dermatitis causes the skin to become thickened and leathery and darker in colour.

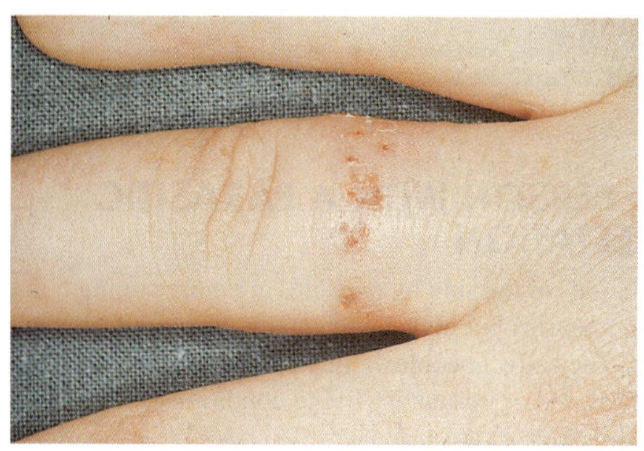

FIGURE 15.12 *Dermatitis may be a response to allergens, infections or chemicals. This person has contact dermatitis resulting from the metal salts in a ring*

Source: © Biophoto Associates/Science Source.

Contact dermatitis

Contact dermatitis is a type of dermatitis caused by a hypersensitivity response or chemical irritation. The major sources known to cause contact dermatitis are dyes, perfumes, certain plants (ivy, oak, sumac), chemicals, latex and metals (see Box 15.3).

Allergic contact dermatitis is a cell-mediated or delayed hypersensitivity to a wide variety of allergens. Sensitising antigens include microorganisms, plants, chemicals, drugs, metals or foreign proteins. On initial contact with the skin, the allergen binds to a carrier protein, forming a sensitising antigen. The antigen is processed and carried to the T cells, which in turn become sensitised to the antigen. The first exposure is the sensitising contact and the person does not experience manifestations, which then occur with subsequent exposures. The manifestations include erythema, swelling and pruritic vesicles in the area of allergen contact. For example, a person hypersensitive to metal may have lesions under a ring or watch.

Irritant contact dermatitis is an inflammation of the skin from irritants; it is not a hypersensitivity response. Common sources of irritant contact dermatitis include chemicals (such as acids), soaps and detergents. The skin lesions are similar to those seen in allergic contact dermatitis.

BOX 15.3 Common causes of contact dermatitis

- Acids
- Alkalis: soaps, detergents, household ammonia, lye, cleaners
- Bromide
- Chlorine
- Cosmetics: perfumes, dyes, oils
- Dusts of lime, arsenic, wood
- Hydrocarbons: crude petroleum, lubricating oil, mineral oil, paraffin, asphalt, tar
- Iodine
- Insecticides
- Fabrics: wool, polyester, dyes, sizing
- Latex: gloves, catheters (latex allergy is especially common among people with spina bifida (International Federation for Spina Bifida and Hydrocephalus (IFSBH), 2018)
- Metal salts: calcium chloride, zinc chloride, copper, mercury, nickel (common in costume jewellery and support bras), silver
- Plants: chrysanthemums, primula, tomato plants, grevillea, English ivy and rhus trees
- Colouring agents
- Rubber and leather products
- Soot

FAST FACTS

Latex allergy

- The increased use of latex gloves among healthcare providers has resulted in increased reporting of latex allergies. It is estimated that 10% to 17% of healthcare providers are allergic to latex (Gawchik, 2011).
- There is an increased risk of latex allergy among individuals with spina bifida due to their increased contact with latex as a result of healthcare procedures such as catheterisation (IFSBH, 2018).
- The most common type of allergic response to latex gloves is type IV, T-cell-mediated contact dermatitis.
- Type I, IgE-mediated hypersensitivity, manifested by urticaria, rhinoconjunctivitis, asthma or anaphylaxis, is far more serious than the T-cell-mediated type.
- The person with a latex allergy should be treated in a latex-free environment.
- Healthcare providers with severe allergic responses to latex may have to seek a different type of employment.

Atopic dermatitis

Atopic dermatitis is an inflammatory skin disorder that is also called *eczema*. The exact cause is unknown, but related factors include depressed cell-mediated immunity, elevated IgE levels and increased histamine sensitivity. The disorder is seen more often in children, but chronic forms persist throughout life.

People with atopic dermatitis have a family history of hypersensitivity reactions, such as dry skin, eczema, asthma and allergic rhinitis. Although up to one-third of people with atopic dermatitis also have food allergies, a positive correlation has not been found.

The dermatitis results when mast cells, T lymphocytes, monocytes and other inflammatory cells are activated and release histamine, lymphokines and other inflammatory mediators. The immune response interacts with the allergen to create a chronic inflammatory condition. In the adult form of atopic dermatitis, characteristic lesions include chronic lichenification, erythema and scaling, the result of pruritus and scratching (see Figure 15.13). The lesions are usually found on the hands, feet or flexor surfaces of the arms and legs. Scratching and excoriation increase the risk of secondary infections, as well as invasion of the skin by viruses such as herpes simplex. Serum studies may find elevated eosinophil and IgE levels.

Seborrhoeic dermatitis

Seborrhoeic dermatitis is a chronic inflammatory disorder of the skin that involves the scalp, eyebrows, eyelids, ear canals,

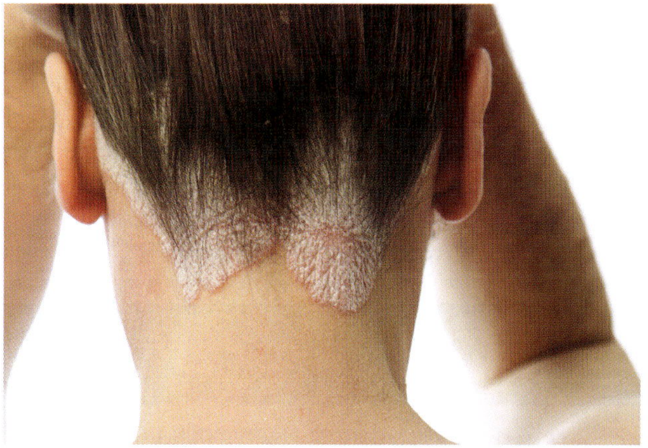

FIGURE 15.13 ***Atopic dermatitis or eczema causes pruritus, resulting in lichenification, erythema and scaling***

Source: Christine Langer-Pueschel/Shutterstock.

nasolabial folds, axillae and trunk. The cause is unknown. This disorder is seen in all ages, from the very young (called 'cradle cap') to the very old. People taking methyldopa (Aldomet™) for hypertension occasionally develop this disorder and it is a component of Parkinson's disease. Seborrhoeic dermatitis is also frequently seen in people with AIDS.

The lesions are yellow or white plaques with scales and crusts. The scales are often yellow or orange and have a greasy appearance. Mild pruritus is also present. Diffuse dandruff with erythema of the scalp often accompanies the skin lesions.

Exfoliative dermatitis

Exfoliative dermatitis is an inflammatory skin disorder characterised by excessive peeling or shedding of skin. The cause is unknown in about half of all cases, but a pre-existing skin disorder (such as psoriasis, atopic dermatitis, contact dermatitis or seborrhoeic dermatitis) is found in a majority of the cases (Papadakis et al., 2018). Reactions to medications, such as sulfonamides, account for 20% to 40% of cases. Certain cancers (such as lymphoma) may also cause exfoliative dermatitis.

Both systemic and localised manifestations may appear. Systemic manifestations include weakness, malaise, fever, chills and weight loss. Scaling, erythema and pruritus may be localised or involve the entire body. In addition to peeling of skin, the person may lose their hair and nails. Generalised exfoliative dermatitis may cause debility and dehydration. The impairment of skin integrity increases the risk of local and systemic infections.

INTERPROFESSIONAL CARE

The person with dermatitis is treated primarily with topical medications and therapeutic baths. If the dermatitis is due to hypersensitivity to an allergen, the person avoids exposure to environmental irritants and suspected foods. The person also discontinues as many medications as possible to determine whether the dermatitis is the result of a drug allergy.

Diagnosis

The diagnosis is often based on the manifestations of the disorder and on a history of exposure to a known allergen. Patch tests and intradermal tests are used to identify a specific allergen.

Medications

The medications used depend on the cause of the dermatitis and the severity of the manifestations. Minor cases are treated with antipruritic medications, whereas more severe cases are treated with oral antihistamines, oral and/or topical corticosteroids and wet dressings. Topical anti-infectives may be prescribed.

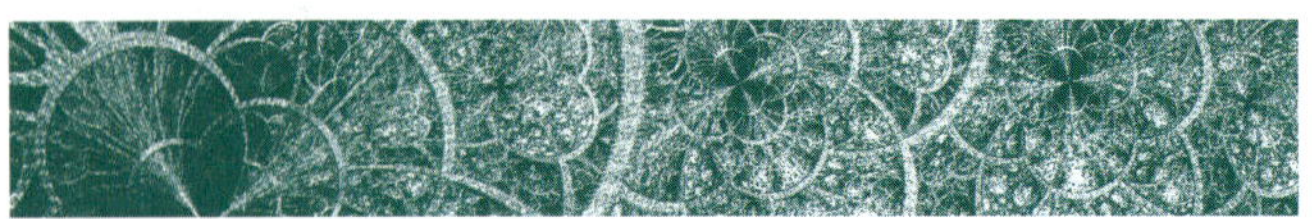

Nursing care

Nursing care of the person with dermatitis focuses primarily on providing information for self-care at home. The person is responsible for managing skin problems and requires education and support. The following topics should be addressed in the person's management plan:

- Medications and treatments do not cure the disease; they only relieve the symptoms.
- Dry skin increases pruritus, which stimulates scratching. Scratching may in turn cause excoriation, and excoriation increases the risk of infection.
- It may be necessary to change the diet or environment to avoid contact with allergens.
- When using steroid preparations, apply only a thin layer to slightly damp skin (e.g. after taking a bath). See Box 15.4 for information on dosage for steroid preparations.
- Occlusive dressings or wraps may enhance the effect of topically applied steroids.

BOX 15.4 Fingertip unit

It can be hard to know how much cream or ointment to apply to an area. If you apply too little, it may not work; too much, and you risk side effects (Pharmaceutical Society of Australia, 2018).

Dose of cream in a fingertip unit varies with age:

- adult male: one fingertip unit provides 0.5 g
- adult female: one fingertip unit provides 0.4 g
- children of 4 years: approximately one-third of adult amount
- infants 6 months to 1 year: approximately one-quarter of adult amount

Amount of cream used varies with body part:

- one hand: apply one fingertip unit
- one arm: apply three fingertip units
- one foot: apply two fingertip units
- one leg: apply six fingertip units
- face and neck: apply 2.5 fingertip units
- trunk, front and back: 14 fingertip units
- entire body: about 40 fingertip units (DermNet NZ, 2014).

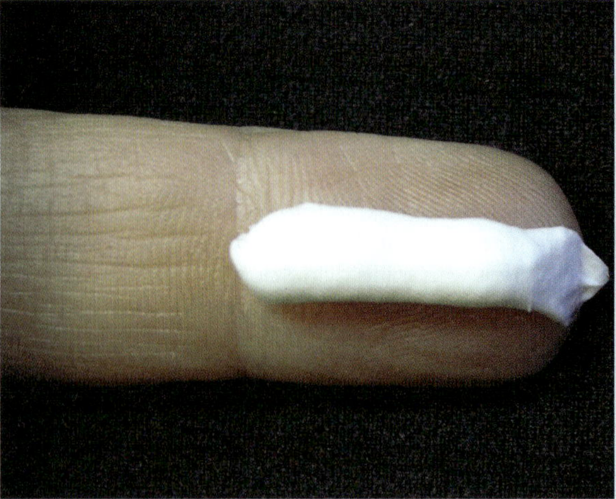

A fingertip unit describes the amount of cream squeezed out of its tube onto the end of the finger as shown

Source: © DermNetNZ.

- When using oral corticosteroids, never abruptly stop taking the medication. Rather, follow instructions to taper the dosage gradually.
- Antihistamines cause drowsiness. When using these medications, avoid alcohol and use caution when driving or working around machinery.

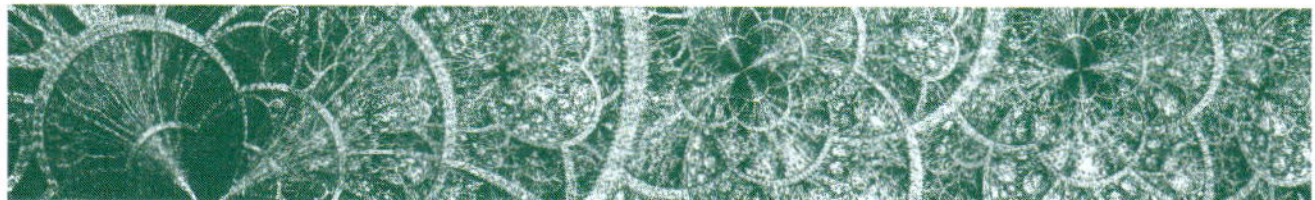

FAST FACTS

Acne vulgaris

- Acne vulgaris is the most common of all skin conditions.
- 12% of women and 3% of men over the age of 25 have acne vulgaris and the rate does not begin to decrease until after age 44 (Papadakis et al., 2018).
- Scarring may be a sequela of the disease or may result from the person picking and manipulating the comedones.

THE PERSON WITH ACNE

Acne is a disorder of the pilosebaceous (hair and sebaceous gland) structure, which opens to the skin surface through a pore. The sebaceous glands, which empty directly into the hair follicle, produce sebum, a lipid substance. Sebaceous glands are present over the entire skin surface except the soles of the feet and the palms of the hands, but the largest glands are on the face, scalp and scrotum. Sebum production is a response to direct hormonal stimulation by testicular androgens in men and adrenal and ovarian androgens in women.

Pathophysiology

Acne may be non-inflammatory or inflammatory. Non-inflammatory acne lesions are primarily **comedones**, more commonly called pimples, whiteheads and blackheads. Whiteheads are pale, slightly elevated papules categorised as closed comedones. Blackheads are plugs of material that accumulate in the sebaceous glands. They are categorised as open comedones. The colour is the result of the movement of melanin into the plug from surrounding epidermal cells. Inflammatory acne lesions include comedones, erythematous pustules and cysts (see Figure 15.14). Inflammation close to the skin surface results in pustules; deeper inflammation results in cysts. The inflammation is believed to result from irritation from fatty acid constituents of the sebum and from substances produced by *Propionibacterium acnes* bacteria, both of which escape into the dermis when the follicular walls of closed comedones rupture.

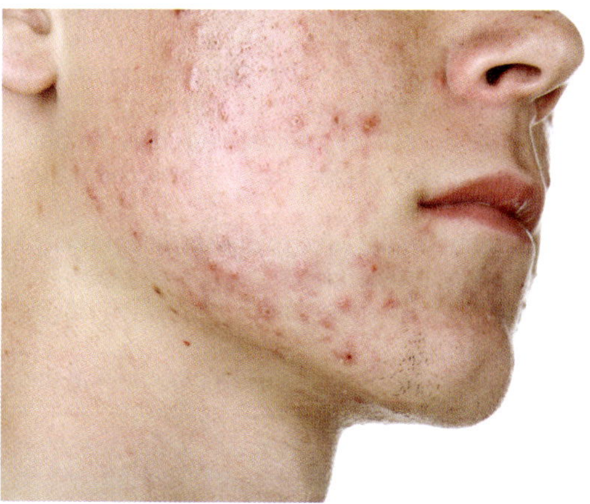

FIGURE 15.14 ***Acne vulgaris lesions include comedones, erythematous pustules and cysts***

Source: Suzanne Tucker/Shutterstock.

Several forms of acne occur at different periods of the lifespan. The most common are acne vulgaris, acne rosacea and acne conglobata.

Acne vulgaris

Acne vulgaris is the form of acne common in adolescents and young to middle adults. The actual cause of acne vulgaris is unknown. Possible causes include an androgenic influence on the sebaceous glands, increased sebum production and proliferation of the organism *P. acnes*. Many factors once thought to cause acne vulgaris, including high-fat diets, chocolate, infections and cosmetics, have been disproved (Bullock & Hales, 2019).

Mild cases may involve only a few scattered comedones, but severe cases are manifested by multiple lesions of all types. Most acne vulgaris lesions form on the face and neck, but they also occur on the back, chest and shoulders. Women in their thirties and forties, often with no prior acne, may develop papular lesions on the chin and around the mouth. The lesions are usually mildly painful and may itch. The complications of acne vulgaris, especially in severe cases, are formation of cysts, pigment changes in people with dark skin, severe scarring and lowered self-concept from the skin eruptions.

Acne rosacea

Acne rosacea is a chronic type of facial acne that occurs more often in middle and older adults. The cause is unknown. The lesions of acne rosacea begin with erythema over the cheeks and nose. Other skin lesions may appear. Over the years, the skin colour changes to dark red and the pores over the area become enlarged. The soft tissue of the nose may exhibit *rhinophyma*, an irregular bullous thickening.

Acne conglobata

Acne conglobata is a chronic type of acne of unknown cause that begins in middle adulthood. This type causes serious skin lesions. Comedones, papules, pustules, nodules, cysts and scars occur primarily on the back, buttocks and chest, but may occur on other body surfaces. The comedones have multiple openings and a discharge that ranges from serous to purulent with a foul odour.

INTERPROFESSIONAL CARE

The management of acne is similar, regardless of type. Because acne vulgaris is most common, the discussions of interprofessional and nursing care focus on that type. Treatment is based on the type and severity of the lesions.

Diagnosis

The disease is diagnosed by the typical location and appearance of lesions. If the person has pustules, a culture of the drainage is performed to differentiate viral or bacterial dermatitis from acne.

Medications

The treatment of acne is tailored to the individual and is based on the severity of the lesions. For acne with comedones, tretinoin or benzoyl peroxide preparations are prescribed. Azelaic acid may also be used. The administration of these vitamin A analogues is discussed in the 'Medication administration' box. Benzoyl peroxide preparations are found in over-the-counter medications, and these products are keratolytic and loosen the comedones.

Mild forms of papular inflammatory acne are treated with topical clindamycin, a bacteriostatic agent that decreases the amount of fatty acids on the skin surface. This medication may be combined with tretinoin therapy.

Moderate forms of papular inflammatory acne are treated with oral or topical antibiotics, such as tetracycline, erythromycin and minocycline. These anti-acne antibiotics are administered for 3 to 4 months; if the person's skin is clear, the dose is lowered gradually to a maintenance dose that will maintain clear skin.

Severe forms of papular inflammatory acne are treated with isotretinoin. This drug is effective but has serious side effects. Isotretinoin, with nursing responsibilities, is discussed in the 'Medication administration' box.

MEDICATION ADMINISTRATION Anti-acne retinoids

ANTI-ACNE RETINOIDS

Tretinoin

Isotretinoin

Tretinoin is a vitamin A derivative classified as an acne agent. This topical agent acts as an irritant to decrease the cohesiveness of follicular epithelial cells, thereby decreasing comedone formation while increasing the extrusion of comedones from the skin surface.

Isotretinoin is a vitamin A analogue classified as an acne product. It reduces the size of sebaceous glands, inhibits sebaceous gland differentiation to decrease sebum production and alters sebum lipid composition.

Nursing responsibilities

- Administer tretinoin with caution to pregnant women, because the effects of absorption on the developing fetus are not clearly defined.
- Isotretinoin is absolutely contraindicated for pregnant women or for women who want to become pregnant. The medication poses a high risk of major deformities in the infant if pregnancy occurs during use, even use that continues only for short periods.
- Do not administer to people with eczema or to those who are hypersensitive to the sun.

Health education for the person and family

Tretinoin

- Use the prescribed cream in a test area twice at night to test for sensitivity; if no reaction occurs, increase applications gradually to the prescribed frequency.
- A pea-sized amount of the cream is enough to cover the entire face.
- Apply the cream to clean, dry skin.
- Do not apply the cream to the eyes, mouth, angles of the nose or mucous membranes.
- Wash the face no more than two to three times a day, using a pH neutral cleanser or mild soap. Do not use skin preparations (such as aftershave lotion or perfumes) that contain alcohol, menthol, spice or lime; they may irritate your skin.
- The medication may cause a temporary stinging or warm sensation but should not cause pain.
- The skin where you apply the cream will be mildly red and may peel; if you experience a more severe reaction, consult your healthcare provider.
- The medication may cause increased sensitivity to sunlight; use sunscreens and wear protective clothing when outdoors.
- Acne may become worse during the first 2 weeks of treatment; this is an expected response.

Isotretinoin

- Take the prescribed medication with food.
- Acne may become worse during the initial period of treatment; this is an expected response.
- The medication causes dryness of the eyes, so the person will have trouble wearing contact lenses during and after treatment.
- Do not take vitamin A supplements; they will increase the effects of the medication.
- Avoid prolonged exposure to sunlight; use sunscreen and protective clothing when in the sun.
- Notify the doctor at once if abdominal pain, severe diarrhoea, rectal bleeding, headache, nausea or vomiting, or visual disturbances occur.
- Do not drink alcohol while taking this medication. (It causes an increase in triglycerides.)
- Night vision may become worse; use caution when driving at night.
- Do not donate blood while, or for 1 month after, taking this medication.
- (For *women*) Use two reliable forms of contraception simultaneously for at least 1 month before, during and at least 1 month after therapy with this medication. The medication may cause deformities in a baby conceived at this time.

Treatments

Acne scars may alter the individual's self-concept. They may be removed by dermabrasion and laser treatment. Dermabrasion of inactive acne lesions can improve the person's appearance, especially if the scars are flat. Laser excision of deep scars may also be performed.

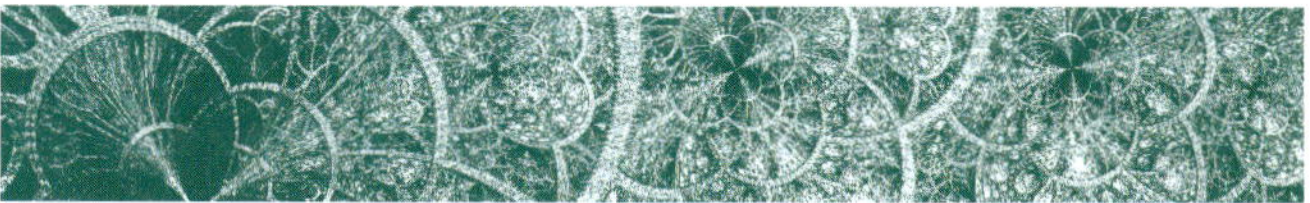

Nursing care

Nursing care is individualised to the person's developmental needs and is conducted primarily through teaching in clinics or the home setting. Regardless of the person's age or gender, it is important to remember that almost everyone with acne is embarrassed by and self-conscious about their appearance. Prior to teaching, establish rapport with the person and clarify beliefs; for example, the person may believe some myths such as the lesions result from poor hygiene, masturbation, use of cosmetics, eating the wrong types of foods or lack of sexual activity. It is critical to teach the person about the causes of and factors involved in acne prior to teaching self-care.

The teaching plan for the person with acne includes general guidelines for skin care and health, as well as specific guidelines for care of the acne lesions. The following topics should be addressed in the person's management plan:

- Wash the skin with a pH-neutral cleanser or mild soap and water at least twice a day to remove accumulated oils.
- Shampoo the hair often enough to prevent oiliness.
- Eat a regular, well-balanced diet. Foods do not cause or increase acne.
- Expose the skin to sunlight but avoid sunburn.
- Get regular exercise and sleep.
- Try to avoid putting your hands on your face.
- Do not squeeze a pimple. Squeezing forces the material of the pimple deeper into the skin and may cause the pimple to become larger and infected.
- The treatment for acne lasts months, and in some cases, for the rest of one's life. It is very important to take the medications each day for the prescribed length of time.

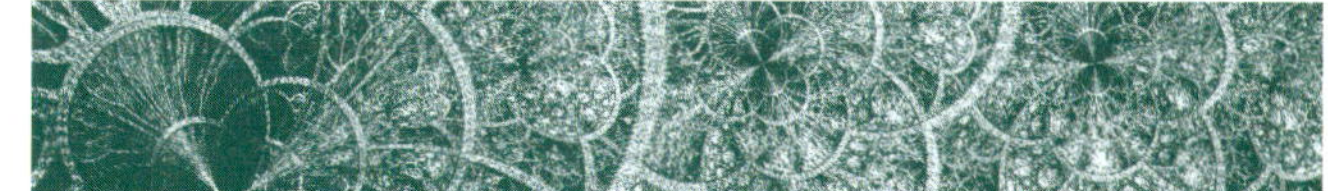

Malignant skin disorders

THE PERSON WITH ACTINIC KERATOSIS

Actinic keratosis, also called senile or solar keratosis, is an epidermal skin lesion directly related to chronic sun exposure and photo damage. The prevalence is highest in people with light-coloured skin; these lesions are rare in people with dark skin. Actinic keratosis may progress to squamous cell carcinoma. Fewer than 1% of early lesions become malignant, but many of those that persist progress to malignancy (Grossman & Porth, 2014). Because of this tendency, the lesions are classified as premalignant.

The lesions are erythematous rough macules a few millimetres in diameter. They are often shiny but may be scaly; if the scales are removed, the underlying skin bleeds. They occur in multiple patches, primarily on the face, dorsa of the hands, the forearms and sometimes on the upper trunk (see Figure 15.15). Enlargement or ulceration of the lesions suggests transformation to malignancy.

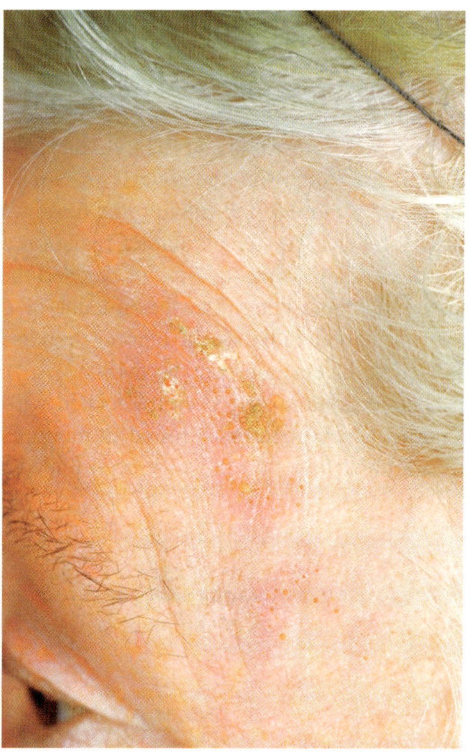

FIGURE 15.15 *The effects of long-term sun exposure are illustrated in this epidermal skin lesion, called actinic keratosis*

Source: Mediscan/Alamy Stock Photo.

THE PERSON WITH NON-MELANOMA SKIN CANCER

The skin, despite its ability to protect the internal body from external damage, is a fragile organ and is subject to damage from ultraviolet radiation and chemicals. Over time, this damage results in alterations in cellular structure and function, and malignancies of the skin occur. The common skin cancers found among Australians are non-melanoma skin cancers (NMSCs) such as basal cell carcinoma and squamous cell carcinoma, as well as malignant melanoma.

The health burden of non-melanoma skin cancer

The leading cause of death in Australia is cancer, and non-melanoma skin cancers are the most commonly diagnosed cancers (Cancer Council, 2021a). However, although other invasive cancers are reportable by law to cancer registries, there is no such requirement for NMSCs, and the scope of the health burden is determined from review of hospital and general medical practice records. Therefore, the full extent of the problem may be underreported. In Australia, basal cell carcinoma comprises about 70% and squamous cell carcinoma 30% of NMSC cases reported (Cancer Council, 2021b).

Risk factors

Multiple aetiological factors are involved in the development of non-melanoma skin cancer, including environmental factors and host factors.

Environmental factors

The environmental factors implicated in the non-melanoma skin cancers are ultraviolet radiation, pollutants, chemicals, ionising radiation, viruses and physical trauma.

Ultraviolet radiation (UVR) from the sun is believed to be the cause of most non-melanoma skin cancers. Sunlight contains both short-length rays (UVB) and long-length rays (UVA). The UVB rays are absorbed by the top layer of skin and cause sunburn. UVA rays penetrate deeper into the skin layers, causing tissue damage. Both types of rays are believed to cause DNA alterations and suppress T-cell and B-cell immunity. The amount of UVR reaching the earth is increasing, most likely from depletion of the ozone layer surrounding the planet (Diaz & Nesbitt, 2013).

Geographical, environmental and lifestyle factors affect the amount of exposure to the sun and the risk of NMSC. People who live in latitudes close to the equator and those who live at higher altitudes receive greater ultraviolet radiation exposure. The amount of clothing worn, the time of day and the amount of time in the sun also determine the amount of exposure. Exposure to ultraviolet radiation in tanning booths has also been implicated in the development of NMSC.

Certain chemicals have long been associated with NMSC. Polycyclic aromatic hydrocarbons, found in mixtures of coal, tar, asphalt, soot and mineral oils, have been linked with skin cancers. Psoralens, used in conjunction with UVA for treatment of psoriasis and cutaneous T-cell lymphoma, increase the risk of squamous cell carcinoma.

Other factors associated with NMSC are the use of ionising radiation, viruses and physical trauma. X-ray therapy for tinea capitis and the use of radium to treat other malignancies are risk factors. Human papillomavirus is implicated in the development of squamous cell carcinoma. Squamous cell changes can also occur in scar or chronic wounds and are referred to as Marjolin's ulcers (Wounds UK, 2020).

> **FAST FACTS**
>
> **Risk factors for non-melanoma skin cancer**
>
> - Fair skin, freckles, blue or green eyes, and blonde or red hair
> - Family history of skin cancer
> - Unprotected and/or excessive exposure to UV radiation (natural or artificial)
> - Radiation treatment
> - Occupational exposures to coal, tar, pitch, creosote, arsenic compounds or radium
> - Severe sunburn episodes as a child

Host factors

Certain host factors increase the risk of non-melanoma skin cancer. These include skin pigmentation, as well as the presence of premalignant lesions.

Skin pigmentation is an important factor in the development of NMSC. The amount of melanin pigment produced by the melanocytes determines a person's skin colour. The more melanin, the more the skin is protected from the damage produced by ultraviolet rays. Indigenous Australians, African Americans, Asians and people of Mediterranean descent have a much lower incidence of NMSC than people who have fair complexions and tend to freckle or sunburn easily, such as people of northern European ancestry.

A major risk factor in the development of NMSC is a change in an existing lesion or the presence of a premalignant lesion, such as actinic keratosis. Organ transplant recipients who undergo immunosuppression to prevent rejection are also at risk of the development of squamous cell carcinoma.

Pathophysiology

Basal cell carcinoma and squamous cell carcinoma arise from epithelial tissue but have different pathophysiology, classifications and manifestations.

Basal cell carcinoma

Basal cell carcinoma (BCC) is an epithelial tumour believed to originate either from the basal layer of the epidermis or from cells in the surrounding dermal structures. These tumours are characterised by an impaired ability of the basal cells of the epidermis to mature into keratinocytes, with mitotic division beyond the basal layer. This results in a bulky neoplasm that grows by direct extension and destroys surrounding tissue, including healthy skin, nerves, blood vessels, lymphatic tissue, cartilage and bone. Basal cell carcinoma is the most common but least aggressive type of skin cancer, rarely metastasising.

Basal cell carcinomas tend to recur. Tumours greater than 2 cm in diameter have a high recurrence rate. Predisposing factors for metastasis are the size of the tumour and the person's resistance to treatment with surgery or chemotherapy. Even though they rarely metastasise, untreated BCCs invade surrounding tissue and may destroy body parts, such as the nose or eyelid.

Basal cell carcinoma is classified into different types: nodular, superficial, pigmented, morpheaform and keratotic. These types are described here and are summarised in Table 15.3.

Nodular basal cell carcinoma is the most common type of BCC and most often appears on the face, neck and head. The tumour is made up of masses of cells that resemble epidermal

TABLE 15.3 Types and characteristics of basal cell carcinomas

TYPE	COMMON LOCATION	MANIFESTATION
Nodular	Face, neck, head	Small, firm papule; pearly, white, pink or flesh coloured; telangiectasis; enlarges; may ulcerate.
Superficial	Trunk, extremities	Papules or plaque that is flat, erythematous or scaling; pink colour; well-defined borders; may have shallow erosions and surface crusting.
Pigmented	Head, neck, face	Dark brown, blue or black colour; border is shiny and well defined.
Morpheaform	Head, neck	Looks like a flat scar; ivory or flesh coloured.
Keratotic	Ear	Small, firm papule; pearly, white, pink or flesh coloured; may ulcerate.

basal cells and grow in a bulky, nodular form from lack of keratinisation. In the early stages, the tumour is a papule that looks like a smooth pimple. It is often pruritic and continues to grow at a steady rate, doubling in size every 6 to 12 months. As the tumour grows, the epidermis thins, but it remains intact. The skin over the tumour is shiny and pearly white, pink or flesh coloured. Telangiectasis may be visible over the area of the tumour. As the tumour continues to increase in size, the centre or periphery may ulcerate and the tumour develops well-circumscribed borders. It bleeds easily from mild injury.

Superficial basal cell carcinoma, found most often on the trunk and extremities, is the second most common type of BCC. This tumour is a proliferating tissue that attaches to the undersurface of the epithelium. The tumour is a flat papule or plaque, often erythematous, with well-defined borders. The tumour may ulcerate and be covered with crusts or shallow erosions (see Figure 15.16).

Pigmented basal cell carcinoma, found on the head, neck and face, is less common. This tumour concentrates melanin pigment in the centre of the basal cancer cells, giving it a dark brown, blue or black appearance. The border of the tumour is shiny and well defined.

Morpheaform basal cell carcinoma, the rarest form of BCC, usually develops on the head and neck. The tumour forms finger-like projections that extend in any direction along dermal tissue planes. The tumour resembles a flat ivory or flesh-coloured scar. This form is more likely to extend into and destroy adjacent tissue, especially muscle, nerve and bone. It is often more difficult to diagnose because of its appearance.

Keratotic basal cell carcinoma (basosquamous) is found on the preauricular and postauricular groove. It contains both basal cells and squamoid-appearing cells that keratinise. Its appearance is much like that of nodular basal cell carcinoma. This type of BCC tends to recur locally and also is the type most likely to metastasise.

Squamous cell carcinoma

Squamous cell carcinoma (SCC) is a malignant tumour of the squamous epithelium of the skin or mucous membranes. It occurs most often on areas of skin exposed to ultraviolet rays and weather, such as the forehead, helix of the ear, top of the nose, lower lip and back of the hands. Squamous cell carcinoma may also arise on skin that has been burned or has chronic inflammation. This is a much more aggressive cancer than basal cell carcinoma, with a faster growth rate and a much greater potential for metastasis if untreated.

The tumours arise when the keratinising cells of the squamous epithelium proliferate, producing a growth that eventually fills the epidermis and invades the dermal tissue planes. Keratinisation of some cells is present and the formation of keratin 'pearls' is common. The keratin formation diminishes as the tumour grows. As the tumour grows, the tumour cells increase in number and rate of mitosis, forming odd shapes.

Squamous cell carcinoma begins as a small, firm red nodule. The tumour may be crusted with keratin products. As it grows, it may ulcerate, bleed and become painful. As the tumour extends into the surrounding tissue and becomes a nodule, the area around the nodule becomes indurated (hardened) (see Figure 15.17).

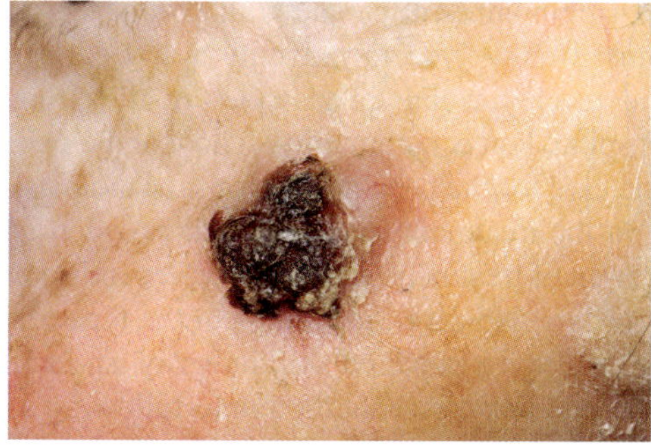

FIGURE 15.16 ***A superficial basal cell carcinoma is characterised by erythema, ulcerations and well-defined borders***

Source: Dr P. Marazzi/Science Photo Library/Alamy Stock Photo.

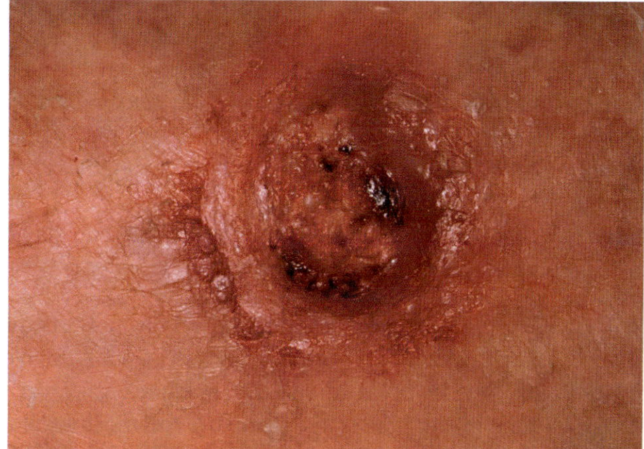

FIGURE 15.17 ***As a squamous cell carcinoma grows, it tends to invade surrounding tissue. It also ulcerates, may bleed and is painful***

Source: Dr P. Marazzi/Science Photo Library/Alamy Stock Photo.

Recurrent squamous cell carcinoma can be invasive, increasing the risk of metastasis. Invasive squamous cell carcinoma may arise from pre-existing skin lesions, such as scars and actinic keratosis, and extend into the dermis (called intraepidermal squamous cell carcinoma). This form appears as a slightly raised erythematous plaque with well-defined borders. Metastasis occurs most often via the lymphatics. The degree of risk of metastasis depends on the size and depth of penetration of the tumour.

INTERPROFESSIONAL CARE

Treatment of non-melanoma skin cancer focuses on removal of all malignant tissue using such methods as surgery, curettage and electrodessication, cryotherapy or radiotherapy. These modalities offer a greater than 90% cure rate. After the malignant tissue is removed, the person should have regular examinations for recurrence.

Diagnosis

Non-melanoma skin cancer is diagnosed by microscopic examination of tissue biopsied from the tumour. The biopsy is usually done in a medical practice or clinic under local anaesthesia. The types of biopsies used are shave, punch, incisional and excisional. See the chapter 'Assessing the integumentary system' for further information.

Treatments

Depending on the type, size and location of a non-melanoma skin cancer, it may be treated with surgical excision, Mohs surgery, curettage and electrodessication, or radiation.

SURGICAL EXCISION Both basal cell carcinomas and squamous cell carcinomas are excised surgically. The surgery may be minor or major, depending on the size and location of the tumour. Surgery for small tumours is most often performed in the outpatient surgery department or in the surgeon's office. Surgical excision allows rapid healing and yields good cosmetic results, but, as with any surgery, carries the risk of infection.

The goal of surgical excision is to remove the tumour completely, so some surrounding tissue is excised along with the tumour. If the tumour is on the face, the incision is made along normal wrinkle or anatomical lines so that the scars will be less obvious. The incision is closed in layers to leave the smallest possible scar. A pressure dressing is usually applied over the incision to provide support.

If a large tumour is removed, a skin graft or skin flap may be performed in hospital to cover the excised area.

MOHS SURGERY In Mohs surgery (also known as chemosurgery), thin layers of the tumour are horizontally shaved off. A frozen section of the tissue is stained at each level to determine tumour margins. This method is the most accurate in assessing the extent of non-melanoma skin cancer and the method that conserves the most normal tissue. It is often used in areas such as the nose, the nasolabial fold, the medial canthus and the ear.

CURETTAGE AND ELECTRODESICCATION Curettage and electrodesiccation are used to treat BCCs that are less than 2 cm in diameter, are superficial or recur because of poor margin control. They may also be used for primary SCCs that are less than 1 cm in diameter and have distinct borders. This type of treatment is most successful for tumours on anatomical sites over a fixed underlying surface, such as the ear, chest and temple.

Abnormal tissue is scraped away (curettage) within 1 to 2 mm of the margin and then a low-voltage electrode is used to abrade the tumour base (electrodesiccation). Tumour tissue is much softer and more friable than normal tissue. Therefore, curettage and electrodesiccation is not used for lesions where the dermis is thin (such as the eyelid) or where the tumour extends into the subcutaneous tissue.

Curettage and electrodesiccation provide good cosmetic results and preserve normal tissue. However, healing time is longer and it is difficult to ensure that all tumour margins have been removed.

Instead of a low-voltage electrode, some physicians use a carbon dioxide laser to vaporise the tumour. When used in conjunction with curettage, this treatment is effective on superficial basal cell carcinomas. Carbon dioxide vaporisation results in minimal thermal injury to adjacent cells, less pain and quicker healing.

RADIATION THERAPY Radiation is most often used for lesions that are inoperable because of their location (such as tumours on the corner of the nose, the eyelid, the canthus and the lip) or size (between 1 and 8 cm). Radiotherapy is also used for people who are older or of poor surgical risk. Radiation is painless and can be used to treat areas surrounding the tumour if necessary. However, the treatment—given over 3 to 4 weeks in a clinical facility—does not allow control of tumour margins and may itself cause skin cancer.

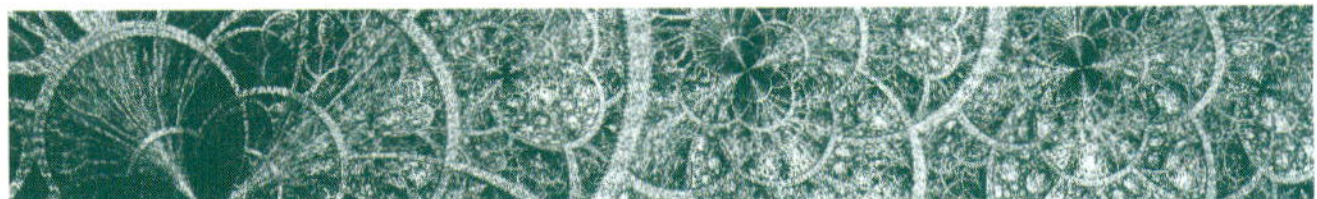

Nursing care

The increasing number of people with skin cancer means that nurses must be involved in prevention and early detection. Nurses can teach preventive behaviours in all settings, including the hospital, home, community, school and clinic.

Nursing care for the person with non-melanoma skin cancer depends on the treatment used. Surgical excision is the most common form of treatment; nursing care depends on the extent of the procedure. However, regardless of the type of treatment, the person will have impaired skin integrity, an increased risk of infection and anxiety about the future following a diagnosis of cancer. Interventions with rationales for the person with any type of skin cancer are discussed in the section on malignant melanoma.

BOX 15.5 Preventing skin cancer

- Minimise sun exposure between the hours of 10 am and 3 pm, when ultraviolet rays are the strongest.
- Cover up with a wide-brimmed hat, sunglasses, long-sleeved shirt and long pants made of tightly woven materials when in the sun.
- Apply a waterproof or water-resistant sunscreen with an SPF of 30 or higher at least 30 minutes before every exposure to the sun. If swimming or sweating heavily, reapply every hour.
- Apply sunscreen not only on sunny days but also on cloudy days (when ultraviolet rays can penetrate 70% to 80% of the cloud cover).
- Use sunscreen and protective clothing when you are on or near sand, snow, concrete or water (which can reflect more than 50% of the ultraviolet rays onto your skin).
- Commercial solariums are banned in Australia as they emit ultraviolet radiation, which increases risk of skin cancer (Cancer Council, 2016; SunSmart Cancer Council of Victoria, 2018).

Health promotion

It is well known that cumulative sun exposure positively correlates with non-melanoma skin cancers. Many skin cancers can be prevented by limiting exposure to risk factors. Primary prevention behaviours are outlined in Box 15.5. Information about sunscreens is listed in Box 15.6.

Nurses also provide person and family education for early detection of non-melanoma skin cancer. Numerous brochures describing the types of skin cancers, photographs of lesions and prevention behaviours are available from the Cancer Council, health education and support agencies, and pharmaceutical companies that manufacture sunscreen. Most of this literature is free.

The person or family at risk of or diagnosed with a skin cancer must be taught how to conduct a regular self-examination of the skin, described in Box 15.7. The use of a mirror or assistance from family members can help with areas that are hard to examine, such as the ears, scalp and back.

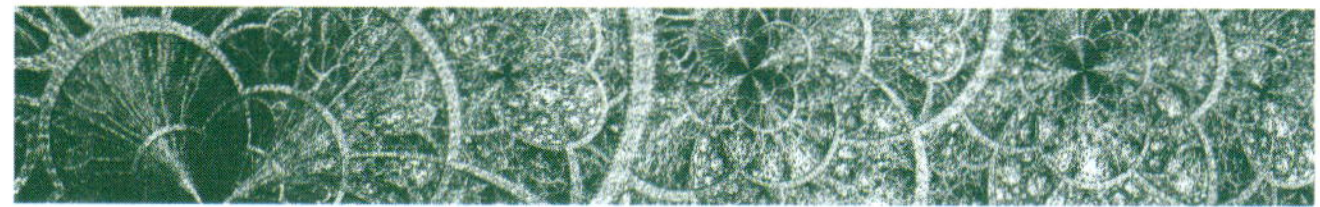

BOX 15.6 Sunscreen information

Types of sunscreen

Chemical

Chemical sunscreens absorb ultraviolet light and act as a radiation filter. Examples follow:

- *p*-Aminobenzoic acid (PABA)
- Anthranilates
- Benzophenones
- Salicylates

Physical

Physical sunscreens reflect and scatter ultraviolet light. Examples follow:

- Zinc oxide
- Ferric chloride
- Titanium dioxide
- Kaolin
- Magnesium silicate
- Ichthyol

Adverse reactions associated with sunscreens

Adverse reactions associated with sunscreens include contact and photocontact dermatitis. People with previous hypersensitivity reactions to benzocaine, procaine, sulfonamides or paraphenylenediamine may develop hypersensitivity responses to PABA. People who are also taking systemic thiazide diuretics or sulfonamides may develop eczematous dermatitis.

Sunscreen ratings

Sunscreens need to be used in conjunction with other methods of sun protection, such as protective clothing and eliminating sun exposure times. Sun protection factor (SPF) ratings are awarded to sunscreen products subject to the amount of ultraviolet light they filter. In Australia, the ingredients in sunscreens are regulated by the Therapeutic Goods Administration (Therapeutic Goods Administration, 2021). As well as preservatives, moisturisers, water, oils and emulsifiers, sunscreens contain agents that are described as either:

- chemical absorbers, which bind with the cells in the skin and absorb UV radiation and then release the energy as heat
- physical blockers, which reflect or scatter UV radiation (e.g. titanium dioxide and zinc oxide) (Therapeutic Goods Administration, 2018).

The SPF value is the ratio of the time required to produce minimal skin redness through a sunscreen product with the time required to produce the same degree of redness without the sunscreen. A person who can tolerate half an hour of sun without a sunscreen should be able to tolerate 3 hours of sun when a sunscreen of SPF 6 is applied to the skin. SPF values of sunscreens range from 2 to 50.

THE PERSON WITH MALIGNANT MELANOMA

Malignant melanoma arises from melanocytes. Although melanoma is less common than NMSC, it is the most serious form of skin cancer and Australia and New Zealand have the highest incidence and mortality rates in the world (Australian Institute of Health and Welfare (AIHW) and Australasian Association of Cancer Registries (AACR), 2016).

Incidence

In 2021, an estimated 16,878 new cases of melanoma, or 11% of all cancers, were diagnosed in Australia (Cancer Australia, 2021). This disease is more than 10 times more common in

BOX 15.7 Skin self-examination

1. Choose the same day each month (such as the first day) to conduct a thorough skin examination.
2. The best time to do the examination is after you take a bath or shower.
3. Examine yourself in a well-lit room in front of a full-length mirror. Have a hand mirror, a chair and a hair dryer available. If you have difficulty seeing your back and scalp (or any other parts of your body), ask someone to help you.
4. Follow the same pattern with each examination:

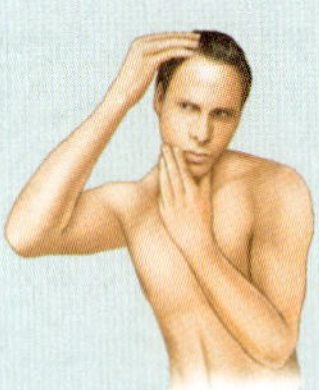

Examine head and face, using one or both mirrors. Use blow dryer to inspect scalp.

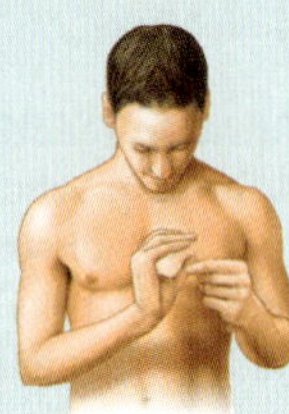

Check hands, including nails. In full-length mirror, examine elbows, arms, underarms.

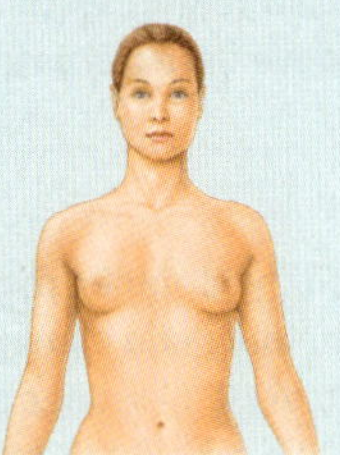

Focus on neck, chest, torso. Women: Check under breasts.

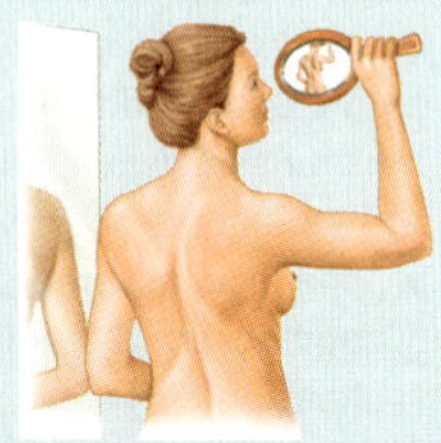

With back to the mirror, use hand mirror to inspect back of neck and back, including buttocks.

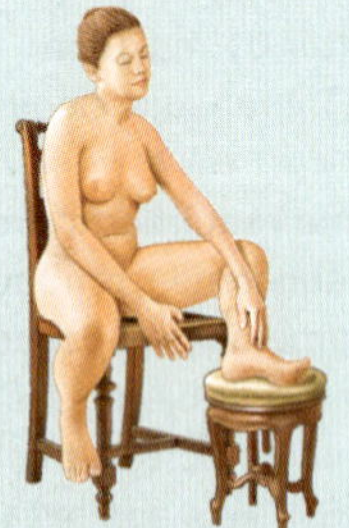

Sitting down, check legs and feet, including soles, heels and nails. Use hand mirror to examine genitals.

fair-skinned people than in dark-skinned people. As with the non-melanoma skin cancers, an increase in the incidence of malignant melanoma is believed to be related to the thinning ozone layer and increased exposure to ultraviolet rays. The incidence is highest in Caucasian upper-middle-class professionals who work indoors. This group of people often had severe sunburn with blistering during childhood and tend to holiday in areas of intense sun exposure. Malignant melanoma is also more common in people who live in sunny climates, burn easily and patronise tanning solariums. However, malignant melanoma may arise from already present lesions or from skin normally covered with clothing.

BOX 15.8 Risk factors for melanoma skin cancer

- A high number of moles or large moles
- Fair skin, freckling, blonde hair or blue eyes
- Close relative with the disease
- Men with gene changes from a family history of breast or ovarian cancer
- Treatment with medications that suppress the immune system
- Too much exposure to UV radiation from sunlight, tanning lamps or solariums
- Over age 50
- Xeroderma pigmentosus, a rare inherited disease in which people are less able to repair damage caused by sunlight
- Past history of melanoma

Risk factors

Although the exact cause of melanoma is unknown, it is known that certain risk factors are associated with the disease. The risk factors for melanoma are listed in Box 15.8.

Pathophysiology

Malignant melanomas arise from melanocytes, cells located at or near the basal layer (the deepest epidermal layer). These cells produce melanin, the dark skin pigment. Melanin is made in granules and transferred to keratinocytes, where it accumulates on the superficial side of each keratinocyte and forms a shield of pigment over the nucleus as protection against ultraviolet rays. Malignant melanomas can develop wherever there is pigment, but about one-third of them originate in existing naevi (moles).

Almost all malignant melanomas are more than 6 mm in diameter, are asymmetric and initially develop within the epidermis over a long period. While they are still confined to the epidermis, the lesions (called malignant melanoma in situ) are flat and relatively benign. However, when they penetrate the dermis, they mingle with blood and lymph vessels and are capable of metastasising. At this latter stage, the tumours develop a raised or nodular appearance and often have smaller nodules, called satellite lesions, around the periphery.

The prognosis for survival for people diagnosed with malignant melanoma is determined by several variables, including tumour thickness, ulceration, metastasis, site, age and gender. Younger people and women have a somewhat better chance of survival. Tumours on the hands, feet and scalp have a poorer prognosis; tumours of the feet and scalp are less visible and may not be diagnosed until they grow into the dermis.

Precursor lesions

The three specific precursor lesions for the development of malignant melanoma are congenital naevi, dysplastic naevi and lentigo maligna. A precursor lesion is also called a premalignant lesion, a name that indicates that the lesion's risk of becoming malignant is greater than normal.

CONGENITAL NAEVI Congenital naevi are present at birth. Some lesions are small; others are large enough to cover an entire body area. Their colour can range from brown to black. They are often slightly raised, with an irregular surface and a fairly regular border.

DYSPLASTIC NAEVI Dysplastic naevi are also called atypical moles. Although dysplastic naevi are not present at birth, they appear as normal naevi during childhood and become dysplastic (having abnormal development) after puberty. A person with classic dysplastic naevi has more than 100 naevi, at least one of which is larger than 8 mm in diameter, and at least one of which has the characteristics of malignant melanoma (asymmetry, irregular border, colour variegation and a diameter greater than 6 mm). A familial tendency to dysplastic naevi increases the risk of the development of malignant melanoma. However, it is not known whether people with dysplastic naevi and no family history of melanoma face a higher risk of melanoma.

Dysplastic naevi most often appear on the face, trunk and arms, but also are seen on the scalp, female breast, groin and buttocks. The pigmentation of the naevi is irregular, with mixtures of tan, brown, black, red and pink. An area of lighter pigmentation is surrounded by a papular area of deeper pigmentation (described as a 'fried egg appearance'). The borders of the naevi are irregular.

LENTIGO MALIGNA Lentigo maligna, also called Hutchinson's freckle, is a tan or black patch on the skin that looks like a freckle. It grows slowly, becoming mottled, dark, thick, and nodular. It is usually seen on one side of the face of an older adult who has had a large amount of sun exposure.

Classification

Malignant melanomas are classified into different types. The major types are superficial spreading melanoma, lentigo maligna melanoma, nodular melanoma and acral lentiginous melanoma. Each of these tumours is characterised by a radial and/or vertical growth phase. During the initial radial phase, which may last from 1 to 25 years (depending on the type), the melanoma grows parallel to the skin surface. During this phase, the tumour rarely metastasises and is often curable by surgical excision. However, during the vertical growth phase, atypical melanocytes rapidly penetrate into the dermis and subcutaneous tissue, greatly increasing the risk of metastasis and death.

SUPERFICIAL SPREADING MELANOMA Superficial spreading melanoma is the most common type, comprising about 70% to 80% of all melanomas (Bullock & Hales, 2019). The lesions are usually flat and scaly or crusty and are about 2 cm in diameter. They often arise from a pre-existing naevus. This type of melanoma is found on the trunk and back of men and on the legs of women. Superficial spreading melanomas occur more often in women than in men. The median age of occurrence is the fifties.

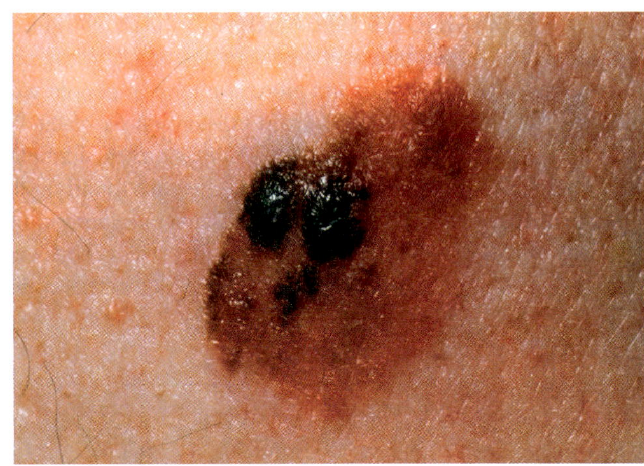

FIGURE 15.18 ***Malignant melanoma is a serious skin cancer that arises from melanocytes***

Source: Dr P. Marazzi/Science Photo Library/Alamy Stock Photo.

The radial growth phase lasts from 1 to 5 or more years. When the lesion enters the vertical growth phase, it grows rapidly and its colour changes from a mixture of tan, brown and black to a characteristic red, white and blue. The lesion also develops irregular borders and often has raised nodules and ulcerations (see Figure 15.18).

LENTIGO MALIGNA MELANOMA Lentigo maligna melanoma often arises from the precursor lesion, lentigo maligna. The lesions are large and tan with different shades of brown. This type of melanoma makes up 5% to 10% of malignant melanomas and is the least serious form (Bullock & Hales, 2019). It occurs on skin that has had long-term sun exposure, such as the face, neck and sometimes the dorsal surface of the hands and lower extremities. Lentigo maligna melanoma affects women more than men. It is typically diagnosed in people in their sixties and seventies.

Lentigo maligna melanoma is characterised by a proliferation of atypical melanocytes parallel to the basal layer of the epidermis. The radial growth phase may last from 10 to 25 years, with the lesion growing to as large as 10 cm. The lesion becomes malignant as soon as the melanocytes invade the dermis. In the vertical growth phase, raised nodules may appear on the surface of the lesion. The lesion tends to acquire a freckled or mottled appearance.

NODULAR MELANOMA Nodular melanoma lesions are raised, dome-shaped, blue-black or red nodules on areas of the head, neck and trunk that may or may not have been exposed to the sun. The lesions may look like a blood blister or they may ulcerate and bleed. The lesions arise from unaffected skin rather than from a pre-existing lesion. This type makes up 10% to 15% of malignant melanomas and is often diagnosed in people in their fifties (Bullock & Hales, 2019).

Nodular melanoma has only a vertical growth phase, but it grows aggressively during that phase. However, the absence of a radial growth phase makes this type more difficult to diagnose before it metastasises.

ACRAL LENTIGINOUS MELANOMA Acral lentiginous melanoma, also called mucocutaneous melanoma, is less common in people with fair skin and more common in people with dark skin. The lesions progress from tan, brown or black flat lesions to elevated nodules and are about 3 cm in diameter. The radial phase lasts from 2 to 5 years. They are found on the palms of the hands, soles of the feet, the mucous membranes and the nail beds. Acral lentiginous melanoma affects both men and women equally and is most often diagnosed in people in their fifties and sixties.

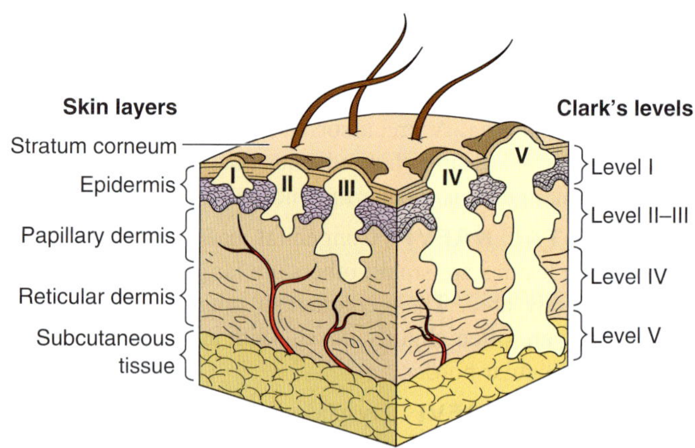

FIGURE 15.19 *Clark's levels for staging measure the invasion of a melanoma from the epidermis to the subcutaneous tissue*

INTERPROFESSIONAL CARE

The management of the person with malignant melanoma begins with identification, diagnosis and tumour staging. If treatable, the tumour is removed through surgical excision. Malignant melanoma is also treated with chemotherapy, immunotherapy and radiation therapy. Other therapies used with success include biological therapies with interleukin-2 and interferon, and therapeutic vaccines containing melanoma antigens.

Identification

Malignant melanoma can be found anywhere on the body and is most often found on the trunk of men and on the lower extremities of women. Nevertheless, it is important for the person to have a complete physical examination and total skin assessment. In addition to a visual examination of all skin surfaces, palpation of regional lymph nodes, the liver and the spleen is essential to assess for metastasis when a melanoma is suspected or found.

A change in the colour or size of a naevus is reported in 70% of people diagnosed with a malignant melanoma. The ABCD rule is used to assess suspicious lesions.

> **FAST FACTS**
>
> **The ABCD rule**
>
> Using the ABCD rule to assess for melanoma:
>
> - A = asymmetry (one half of the naevus does not match the other half)
> - B = border irregularity (edges are ragged, blurred or notched)
> - C = colour variation or dark black colour
> - D = diameter greater than 6 mm (size of a pencil eraser)

Diagnosis

In addition to biopsy of any suspicious lesion, diagnostic tests are conducted to determine whether the tumour has metastasised. Because malignant melanoma may metastasise to any organ or tissue of the body, a variety of tests may be conducted, including microscopic examination, biopsy and tests for metastasis (liver function tests and computed tomography (CT) scan of the liver, a complete blood count, serum blood chemistry profile, chest x-ray, bone scan and CT scan, or magnetic resonance imaging of the brain).

Microstaging

The term *microstaging* describes the assessment of the level of invasion of a malignant melanoma and the maximum tumour thickness. In the Clark system of microstaging, the vertical growth of the lesion is measured from the epidermis to the subcutaneous tissue to determine the level of invasion (Melanoma Research Alliance, n.d.) (see Figure 15.19).

However, variations in individual skin thicknesses and different anatomical sites can affect the accuracy of the measurement. In the Breslow system, an adaptation of the Clark system of assessment, the vertical thickness is measured from the granular level of the epidermis to the deepest level of tumour invasion (Melanoma Research Alliance, n.d.). This determination is important because as the thickness of the melanoma increases, survival rate decreases. After the thickness and depth of the tumour are determined, a clinical stage is assigned. The traditional three-stage system is still used, although it does not include tumour thickness.

Treatments

Surgical excision is the preferred treatment for malignant melanoma. Other methods of treatment are chemotherapy, immunotherapy and radiation therapy.

SURGERY If a biopsy identifies the lesion as a melanoma, a wide excision is performed that includes the full thickness of the skin and subcutaneous tissue. Because the risk of local recurrence for thin melanomas (those less than 0.76 mm) is quite low, margins of 0.5 to 1.0 cm of normal skin are excised around the tumour. Thick tumours require a 1 to 3 cm margin excision because they are at risk of local recurrence or satellite lesions.

Sentinel node biopsy is performed when a higher risk of primary melanoma has been diagnosed after an initial biopsy (melanoma 1.0 mm in depth, < 40 years, Clark level $\geq$ IV) (Keidan & Meyers, 2014). This will determine whether the melanoma has spread to the surrounding lymph nodes. This process starts with lymphatic mapping which will identify the first 'downstream' node—the sentinel node. This node is removed and sent to the pathologist to identify if malignant cells are present. Malignant cells are an indicator of the risk that melanoma may have spread to other parts of the body. Melanoma that has spread to sentinel nodes in the regional node groups in the armpits, neck or groin may linger before spreading to organs. In these cases, melanoma can sometimes be cured with surgery called regional lymph node clearance. Regional lymph nodes are the most common sites for metastasis of malignant melanoma. Standard surgical treatment for clinically suspicious lymph node involvement includes excision of the primary lesions as well as surgical dissection of the involved lymph nodes. Elective lymph node dissection (ELND) in the treatment of localised malignant melanoma remains controversial. Advocates of ELND believe that the procedure benefits people with intermediate-thickness tumours because approximately 20% of people whose lymph nodes were clinically negative at diagnosis show some metastasis on removal of the nodes. Those opposed to ELND believe the risks associated with the procedure are too high for the 80% of people who have no evidence of metastasis after removal of the nodes (Melanoma Institute Australia, 2022).

Surgery may be indicated for palliative management of isolated metastasis. Removal of metastatic tumours in the brain, liver, lung, gastrointestinal tract or subcutaneous tissue may relieve symptoms and prolong life.

IMMUNOTHERAPY Immunotherapy is a relatively new treatment modality for malignant melanoma. The role of the immunological response initially was recognised because of the numerous spontaneous remissions seen in people with melanoma—a higher occurrence than with any other adult tumour. In addition, researchers have recently identified tumour-specific antigen antibodies in people with melanoma. This also has stimulated an interest in immunotherapeutic interventions for the treatment of malignant melanoma (Melanoma Institute Australia, 2022).

Agents such as interferons, interleukins, monoclonal antibodies, bacille Calmette-Guérin, levamisole, transfer factors and tumour vaccines have been used to treat melanoma, with varying response rates. The effectiveness of these agents, used either alone, in combination with chemotherapy or in combination with each other, is under investigation.

RADIATION THERAPY Melanoma responds to higher-dose radiation, especially if the tumour is small. Response rates to radiation therapy depend on the site of the tumour, its thickness, the type of melanoma and the person's general health, but may range from 0% to 71%. Radiation frequently is used for palliation of symptoms resulting from metastasis to the brain, bone, lymph nodes, gastrointestinal tract, skin or subcutaneous tissue. Liver and lung metastases are not treated with radiation therapy because a loss of organ function may result (Melanoma Institute Australia, 2022).

NEW METHODS OF TREATMENT Melanoma skin cancer research is ongoing and directed towards more specific methods of diagnosis and treatment. Examples are as follows:

- *Gene therapy*: clinical trials are in progress to test the effectiveness of adding certain genes to the malignant cells.
- *Melanoma DNA research*: knowledge of how ultraviolet light harms DNA is increasing, providing support for referral for genetic counselling for people with a strong family history of melanoma.
- *Targeted therapy*: this involves the development of drugs that attack the gene changes in melanoma cells. These drugs work differently from standard chemotherapy drugs. Sometimes targeted drugs work when chemotherapy does not and they can have less severe side effects. These drugs are new and we are still learning about the best way to use these drugs to treat melanoma (American Cancer Society, 2015).
- *Immune therapy*: vaccines are being developed to make an individual immune to their own melanoma cells or to train the person's immune cells to fight the cancer.
- *Staging*: very sensitive new tests can better detect the spread of melanoma to lymph nodes and can possibly better identify people who could be helped by a treatment such as immunotherapy after surgery (Melanoma Institute Australia, 2022).

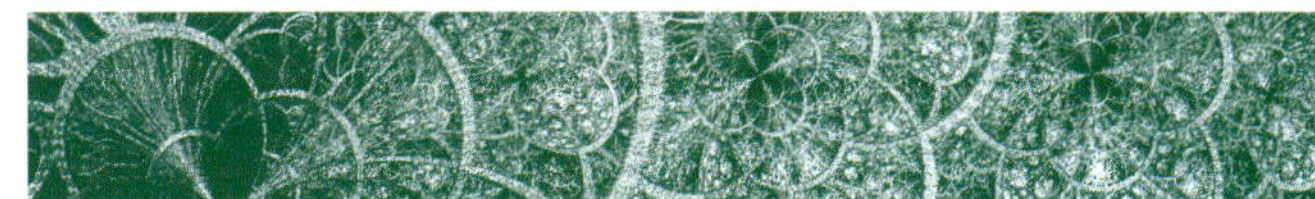

Nursing care

Nurses can assess the skin of people requiring care for many different health problems and may be the first healthcare provider to identify suspicious lesions. Wide excision and the high risk of metastasis from malignant melanoma usually require inpatient surgical treatment, with the nurse providing care and teaching.

Health promotion

The most important aspect of preventing malignant melanoma is identifying those at risk and performing regular skin assessments. Skin inspections should be performed monthly by those with actinic keratoses, at-risk individuals and those over 40 years of age. Mole clinics and summer beach skin inspection campaigns have become more popular and offer an alternative option for identification of sinister lesions. When self-assessing for melanoma, the person looks for a change in:

- colour, especially any lesion that becomes darker or variegated in shades of tan, brown, black, red, white or blue
- size, especially any lesion that becomes larger or spreads out
- shape, especially any lesion that protrudes more from the skin or begins to have an irregular outline
- appearance of a lesion, especially bleeding, drainage, oozing, ulceration, crusting, scaliness or development of a mushrooming outward growth
- consistency, especially any lesion that becomes softer or is more easily irritated
- skin around a lesion, such as redness, swelling or leaking of colour from a lesion into the surrounding skin
- sensation, such as itching or pain.

BOX 15.9 Nursing assessment for skin cancer

Interview questions

- Have any members of your family ever been treated for skin cancer?
- Have you had a skin cancer removed from any part of your body?
- Have you noticed any change in the size, shape or colour of a mole, wart, birthmark or scar?
- Do you have any moles, warts, birthmarks or scars that itch, are painful, have crusting or bleed?
- In what parts of the country or world have you lived?
- Have you ever been badly sunburned?
- Do you visit tanning solariums?
- Are you exposed to any hazardous chemicals in your job?
- Have you been taught how to examine your skin? If so, how do you do this examination? How often?

Physical assessment

1. Ensure privacy and provide a warm environment. Ask the person to remove all clothing and put on an examination gown. Ensure good light; natural, bright light is best for inspection of lesions. The person may sit, stand or lie down.
2. Inspect and palpate the skin. Stretching the skin tightly during assessment facilitates assessment of nodular and scaly lesions and lesions in the dermis. Assess for:
   a. obvious lesions
   b. visible swellings
   c. alterations in normal contour and borders of naevi
   d. enlarged lymph glands
   e. skin or mucosal discolourations
   f. areas of ulceration, scaling, crusting or erosion.
3. The order of assessment follows:
   a. head and neck: entire scalp, eyelids, external ear, auditory canals, external surface of the nose, internal surface of the nose, the oral cavity, facial skin, the facial glands (parotid, submaxillary, sublingual)
   b. thyroid and neck, including lymph glands
   c. chest and abdomen, with special attention under pendulous breasts, in skin folds and in areas covered with hair
   d. back and buttocks, with special attention to the area between the buttocks
   e. extremities, with special attention to the axillae, nail beds, webs between the fingers and toes and soles of the feet
   f. external genitals, with special attention to skin folds, mucous membranes and areas covered with hair.
4. Measure and record a description of all skin lesions on an anatomical chart. Take photographs (if possible) of any suspicious lesion and include them in the person's record for future reference.

Assessment

Skin assessment is discussed in the chapter 'Assessing the integumentary system'. Specific health history questions and assessments for skin cancer are outlined in Box 15.9.

Nursing diagnoses and interventions

Although many different nursing diagnoses may be appropriate for the person with a malignant melanoma, one potential diagnosis is as follows:

- *Impaired skin integrity* related to malignant melanoma.

Impaired skin integrity related to malignant melanoma

Malignant melanomas not only destroy skin layers but also invade body structures. Certain types of melanomas may ulcerate prior to diagnosis, and treatment typically involves some type of surgical biopsy and excision. Any open lesion or incision increases the risk of secondary infection.

- Monitor for manifestations of infection: fever, tachycardia, malaise, erythema, swelling, pain or drainage that increases or becomes purulent. *Intact skin is the first line of defence against infection; impaired skin integrity increases the risk of infection.*
- Keep the incision line clean and dry by changing dressings as necessary.
- Follow principles of medical and surgical asepsis when caring for person's incision. Teach family members and visitors the importance of careful handwashing. Maintain standard precautions if drainage is present.
- Encourage and maintain adequate kilojoule and protein intake in the diet. Suggest a consultation with the dietitian if the person's appetite is poor. *Adequate kilojoules and protein are necessary for proper healing.*

CONSIDERATION FOR PRACTICE

Nurses must use standard precautions with blood and body fluids to protect themselves from exposure to blood-borne viruses.

Community-based care

Health education for the person and family experiencing the diagnosis and treatment of non-melanoma and malignant melanoma involves self-care and ongoing self-monitoring. Education for the person and family is specific to the type of treatment. In addition to wound care for people who have had a surgical removal or lymph node dissection, they will need instructions on how to protect the extremity from bleeding, trauma and infection. People who have undergone lymph node dissection may develop lymphoedema and can benefit from manual lymph drainage therapy and compression therapy in the form of bandages and garments. Address the following topics:

- Schedule regular medical check-ups every 3 months for the first 2 years, every 6 months for the next 5 years and yearly thereafter.
- Proper self-care combined with regular medical care can help the person lead a fairly normal life.
- If assistance for home care is necessary, provide referrals to a community health or home care organisation. In addition,

refer the person to a local cancer support group if desired. Other resources are:

- Cancer Council: https://www.cancer.org.au
- Australian Melanoma Research Foundation: https://melanomaresearch.com.au/
- Melanoma Institute Australia: https://www.melanoma.org.au
- Australasian Lymphology Association: https://www.lymphoedema.org.au.

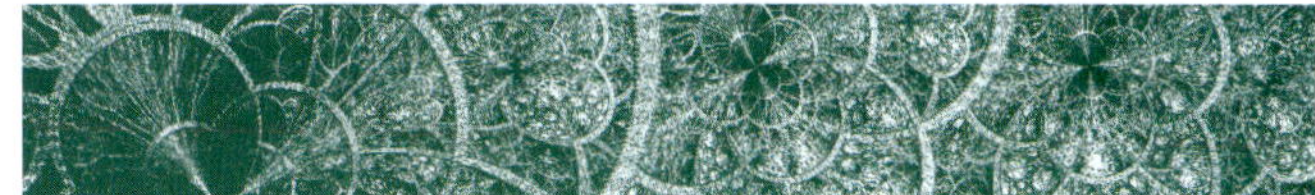

Skin trauma

Trauma to the skin can be unintentional or intentional (as in the case of surgery). Pressure, friction and shear are common causes of skin trauma and can result in pressure injuries, while shear and friction can result in skin tears. Pressure injuries and skin tears are the most common wounds found in the elderly, and both types of wounds are largely preventable (Mulligan, Prentice & Scott, 2011). Thermal, chemical, electrical or radiation-induced burns are discussed in the chapter 'Nursing care of people with burns'.

THE PERSON WITH A PRESSURE INJURY

Pressure injuries are synonymous with bed sores, decubitus ulcers and pressure ulcers, and are significant and preventable wounds. The term 'pressure injury' is the preferred term used in Australia (Australian Commission on Safety and Quality in Health Care (ACSQHC), 2021; Wounds Australia, 2012). A pressure injury is 'a localised damage to the skin and/or underlying tissue, as a result of pressure or pressure in combination with shear. Pressure injuries usually occur over a bony prominence but may also be related to a medical device or other object' (European Pressure Ulcer Advisory Panel (EUPAP), National Pressure Injury Advisory Panel (NPIAP) and Pan Pacific Pressure Injury Alliance (PPPIA), 2019).

Pressure injuries are ischaemic lesions of the skin and underlying tissue caused by external pressure or shear forces that lead to compression or distortion of tissues, resulting in impaired flow of blood and lymph (Martini, Nath & Bartholomew, 2018). The ischaemia causes tissue necrosis and eventual ulceration. Pressure injuries tend to develop over a bony prominence (such as the heels, greater trochanter, sacrum and ischia), but may appear on the skin of any part of the body subjected to external pressure, friction or shearing forces.

Pressure injuries in Australia

National data on prevalence and incidence of pressure injuries is difficult to benchmark due to inconsistencies in reporting, under-reporting and failure to publish (Strachan et al., 2007). Prevalence data collected from all 86 public hospitals in Western Australia in 2007 and 2009 reported prevalence of 11% respectively; two-thirds of these pressure injuries were hospital acquired (Mulligan et al., 2011; Strachan et al., 2007). Studies conducted by the Victorian Quality Council in 2003, 2004 and 2006 reported prevalence rates of 26.5% (16.6% hospital acquired), 20.8% (13.8 % hospital acquired) and 17.6% (11.9% hospital acquired) respectively (Victorian Department of Human Services, 2006). In New South Wales in 2018, prevalence surveys from 152 inpatient facilities, 67 public residential aged care facilities and 63 community/outpatient services reported prevalence rates of 7.9%, 8% and 9.4% respectively (Clinical Excellence Commission, 2019).

Pressure injuries substantially increase direct and indirect health expenditure for government and non-government agencies and individuals. In 2012–2013, the cost of treating pressure injuries across all Australian states and territories was estimated to be $983 million annually, which equated to 1.9% of all public hospital expenditure, or 0.6% of the public recurrent health expenditure (Nguyen & Chaboyer, 2015). The opportunity cost was valued at an additional $820 million annually based on 121,645 cases and a total number of 524,661 lost bed days (Nguyen & Chaboyer, 2015).

In 2016, the mean additional hospital stay in Australia for a pressure injury was estimated at 4.3 days, at a cost of $699 to $840 per bed day, which equated to $3,600 in preventable costs per patient with a pressure injury (Norman et al., 2016). The actual costs of treating (but not necessarily healing) 20 individuals with 23 pressure injuries in Australian aged care facilities in 2018 was $98,489 (Wilson, Kapp & Santamaria, 2019). Therefore, the financial costs of treating pressure injuries are substantial.

Pathophysiology

Pressure injuries develop from external pressure that compresses blood vessels or from friction and shearing forces that tear and injure vessels. The primary cause of pressure injuries is a sustained mechanical load that is applied to soft biological tissues, generally near a bony prominence. Pressure gradients that induce sustained deformation of skin and subdermal tissues must be present in order for tissue damage that characterises a pressure injury to occur. The magnitude of the mechanical load that will lead to tissue damage depends on the duration of time for which the pressure is applied. High pressure applied for a short period or low pressure applied for a longer period can lead to tissue damage. Recent evidence suggests that there are two physiologically events leading to tissue damage. One is a lower threshold of tissue tolerance to pressure and the other is the duration of pressure applied.

An increasing body of evidence suggests that the microclimate between skin and the supporting surface plays a role in the development of Stage I and II pressure injuries. Microclimate refers to the humidity and temperature between the person's skin and the surface they are lying on (EPUAP, NPIAP & PPPIA, 2019).

Links to National Patient Safety Standards

NSQHS: Comprehensive Care Standard

This standard dictates the need for 'integrated screening, assessment and risk identification processes for developing an individualised care plan, to prevent and minimise the risks of harm in identified areas' (ACSQHC, 2021). Pressure injuries are one such harm to be minimalised.

This standard will be achieved by the establishment of systems that ensure utilisation of best practice guidelines and risk assessment frameworks for pressure injury prevention and management. This includes implementation of processes that facilitate accurate identification and reporting, access to equipment and devices for prevention and treatment, and best practice for treatment and monitoring. Meaningful communication regarding risk, prevention strategies and management should exist across all individuals involved in a person's care.

On admission, all patients, including children, should be screened for their risk of pressure injuries. Risk assessment, using a validated risk assessment scale, is conducted when screening indicates a patient is at risk of developing a pressure injury. Ongoing assessment and documentation should form part of the comprehensive nursing plan.

Source: ACSQHC (2021). *National Safety and Quality Health Service Standards* (2nd ed.). Sydney: ACSQHC. © Australian Commission on Safety and Quality in Health Care.

TRANSLATION TO PRACTICE Pressure injury risk assessment and prevention

Nurses need to understand pressure injury risk assessment and preventive strategies. It is nurses who assess and manage patients' skin daily. Unfortunately, knowledge deficits have been identified among Australian nurses (Lawrence, Fulbrook & Miles, 2015), as they have in other countries (Chianca et al., 2010; Gunningberg et al., 2015). To address this deficit, the *Prevention and Treatment of Pressure Ulcers/Injuries: Clinical Practice Guideline* (2019), which was produced by the European Pressure Ulcer Advisory Panel (EPUAP), the National Pressure Ulcer Advisory Panel (NPUAP) (now called the National Pressure Injury Advisory Panel (NPIAP)) and the Pan Pacific Pressure Injury Alliance (PPPIA—Australia, Hong Kong, New Zealand and Singapore), includes dedicated chapters with recommendations for implementation of best practice guidelines; advancing health professional, consumer and caregiver education; and detailing quality indicators for monitoring guideline implementation and translation in the healthcare setting. This document can be accessed from www.internationalguideline.com. See Box 15.10.

The increase in humidity and temperature can make the skin less tolerant to pressure and shear force. The greater the body surface area in contact with the support surface, the lower the uniform pressure. The lesser the body surface area in contact with a support surface, the higher the point pressure (Lachenbruch et al., 2013). This principle can be clearly appreciated when one rests the knuckle of the index finger on a table and compares the level of discomfort to that experienced when one rests the whole palm against the same surface. When the body is in the supine position, the body's weight applies pressure to the sacrum, heels, scapula and occiput. The same amount of pressure causes more damage when it is applied to a small area such as the heels than when it is distributed over a large surface.

External pressure that is greater than capillary closing pressure and arteriolar pressure interrupts blood flow in capillary beds. Capillary closing pressure is frequently quoted to be 32 mmHg, as determined more than 80 years ago by Landis (1930). However, capillary closing pressure will differ greatly between individuals and be subject to underlying comorbidities or factors that impact on vascularity and perfusion, body mass index, nutrition and hydration status.

Shearing forces result when tissue slides over another surface. The stretching and bending of blood vessels cause injury and thrombosis. People in bed are subject to shearing forces when the head of the bed is elevated and the torso slides down towards the foot of the bed. Pulling the person up in bed or against a chair also subjects the person to shearing forces (for this reason, repositioning devices such as hoists and slide sheets should be used). Friction, particularly in the presence of moisture, causes the skin and superficial fascia to remain fixed to the bed sheet or chair, while the deep fascia and bony skeleton slides in the direction of body movement. The rubbing of heels against bedding surfaces is a common cause of friction.

When a person lies or sits in one position for an extended length of time without moving, pressure on the tissue between a bony prominence and the external surface of the body distorts capillaries and interferes with normal blood flow. The healthy, sensate and mobile individual will respond to the discomfort and alter their position. The immediate physiological response to relieved pressure is reactive hyperaemia. Reactive hyperaemia is a compensatory physiological response to tissue hypoxia and is evident when there is a transient increased blood flow or erythematous flush to the tissue. An area of reactive hyperaemia will blanch when pressure is applied (EPUAP, NPIAP, PPPIA, 2019). However, if the pressure continues, the capillaries become more permeable and metabolic wastes and oedema accumulate in the interstitial spaces. Oedema in the interstitial spaces inhibits perfusion to the skin. Platelets aggregate in the endothelial cells surrounding the capillaries and form microthrombi. These microthrombi further impede blood flow, resulting in ischaemia

BOX 15.10 The International Pressure Ulcer Classification System

Stage 1: Non-blanchable erythema

- Intact skin with non-blanchable redness of a localised area usually over a bony prominence.
- Darkly pigmented skin may not have visible blanching; its colour may differ from the surrounding area.
- The area may be painful, firm, soft, warmer or cooler compared to adjacent tissue.
- May be difficult to detect in individuals with dark skin tones.
- May indicate 'at-risk' people (a heralding sign of risk).

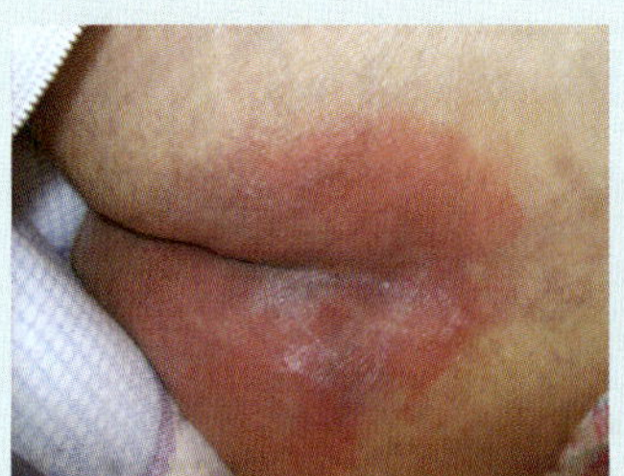

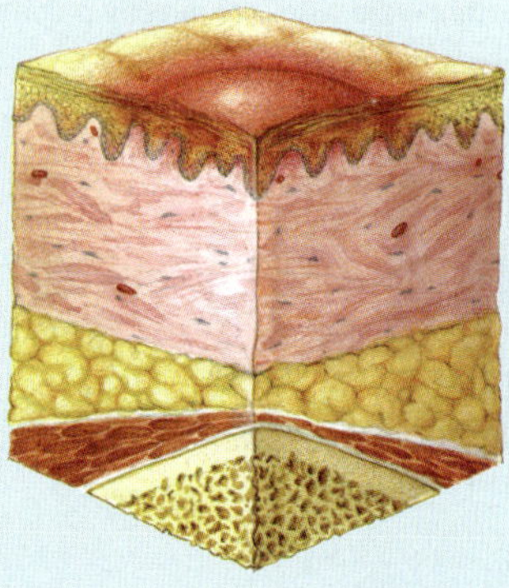

Stage 2: Partial-thickness skin loss

- Partial-thickness loss of dermis presenting as a shallow open ulcer with a red-pink wound bed, without slough.
- May also present as an intact or open/ruptured serum-filled blister. Presents as a shiny or dry shallow ulcer without slough or bruising (bruising indicates suspected deep tissue injury).
- Stage 2 should not be used to describe skin tears, tape burns, perineal dermatitis, maceration or excoriation.

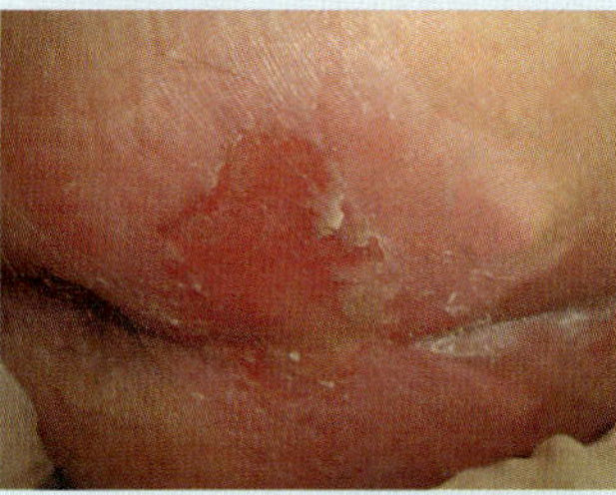

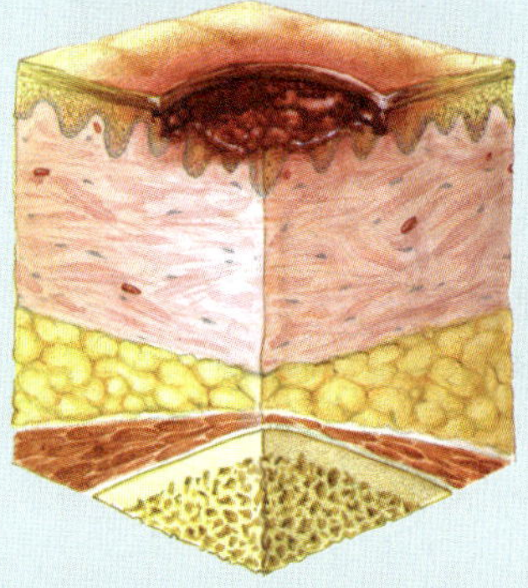

Stage 3: Full-thickness skin loss

- Full-thickness tissue loss. Subcutaneous fat may be visible but bone, tendon or muscle are not exposed. Slough may be present but does not obscure the depth of tissue loss. May include undermining and tunnelling.
- The depth of a Stage 3 pressure ulcer varies by anatomical location. The bridge of the nose, ear, occiput and malleolus do not have subcutaneous tissue and Stage 3 ulcers can be shallow. In contrast, areas of significant adiposity can develop extremely deep Stage 3 pressure injuries. Bone/tendon is not visible or directly palpable.

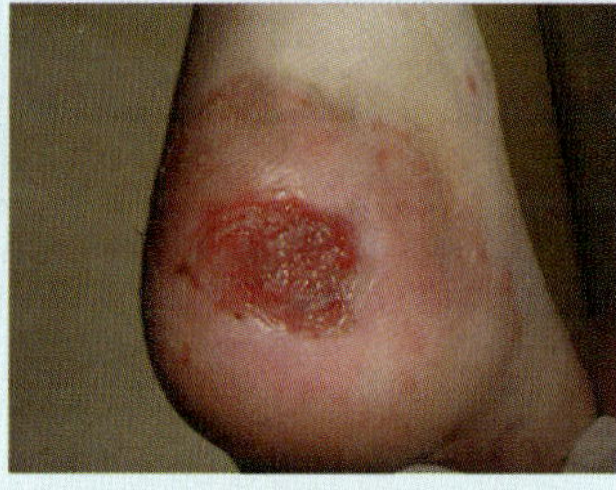

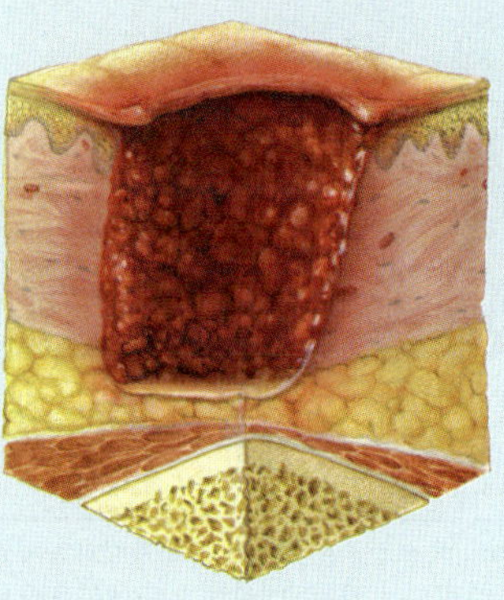

(continued)

BOX 15.10 The International Pressure Ulcer Classification System (continued)

Stage 4: Full-thickness tissue loss

- Full-thickness tissue loss with exposed bone, tendon or muscle. Slough or eschar may be present on some parts of the wound bed. Often include undermining and tunnelling.
- The depth of a Stage 4 pressure injury varies by anatomical location. The bridge of the nose, ear, occiput and malleolus do not have subcutaneous tissue and these ulcers can be shallow. Stage 4 injuries can extend into muscle and/or supporting structures (e.g. fascia, tendon or joint capsule) making osteomyelitis possible. Exposed bone/tendon is visible or directly palpable.

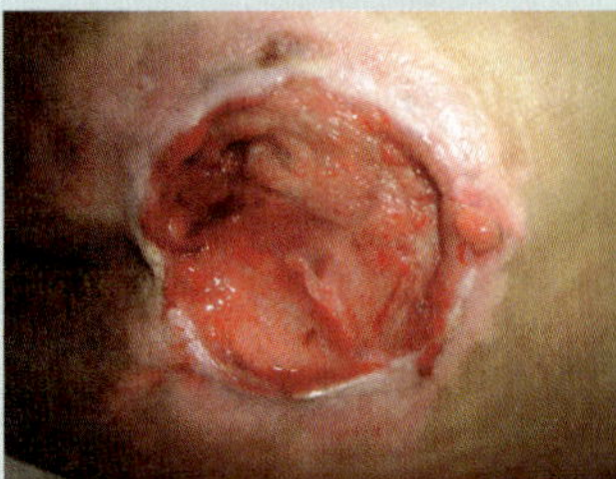

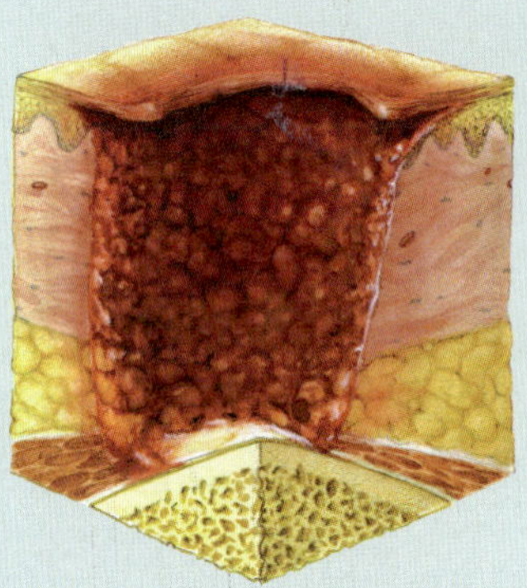

Unstageable: Depth unknown

- Full-thickness tissue loss in which the base of the ulcer is covered by slough (yellow, tan, grey, green or brown) and/or eschar (tan, brown or black) in the pressure injury bed.
- Until enough slough and/or eschar is removed to expose the base of the wound, the stage cannot be determined. Stable (dry, adherent, intact without erythema or fluctuance) eschar on the heels serves as 'the body's natural (biological) cover' and should not be removed.

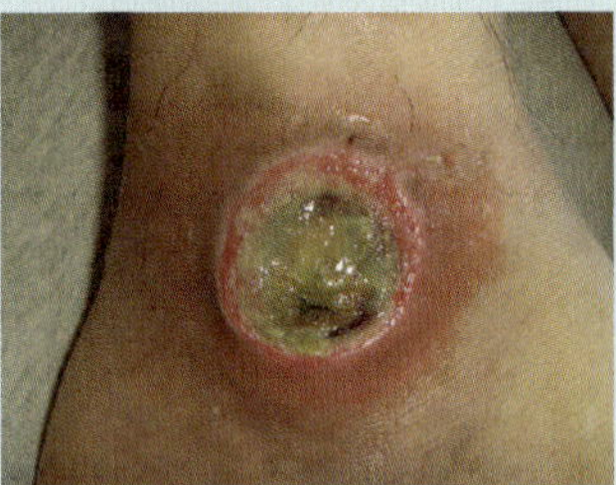

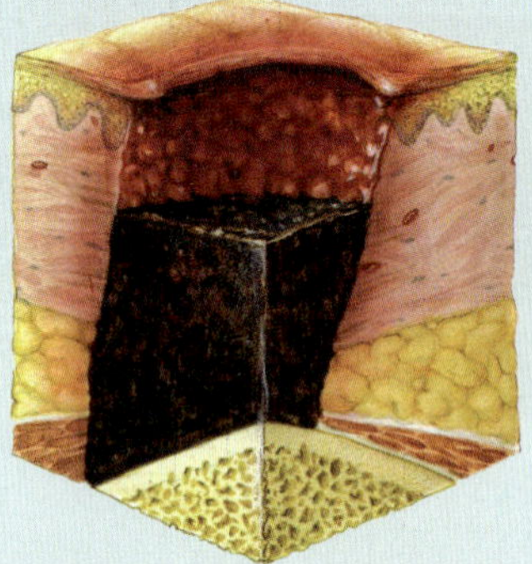

Suspected deep tissue injury: Depth unknown

- Purple or maroon localised area of discoloured intact skin or blood-filled blister due to damage of underlying soft tissue from pressure and/or shear. The area may be preceded by tissue that is painful, firm, mushy, boggy, warmer or cooler as compared to adjacent tissue.
- Deep tissue injury may be difficult to detect in individuals with dark skin tones.
- Evolution may include a thin blister over a dark wound bed. The pressure injury may further evolve and become covered by thin eschar. Evolution may be rapid exposing additional layers of tissue even with optimal treatment.

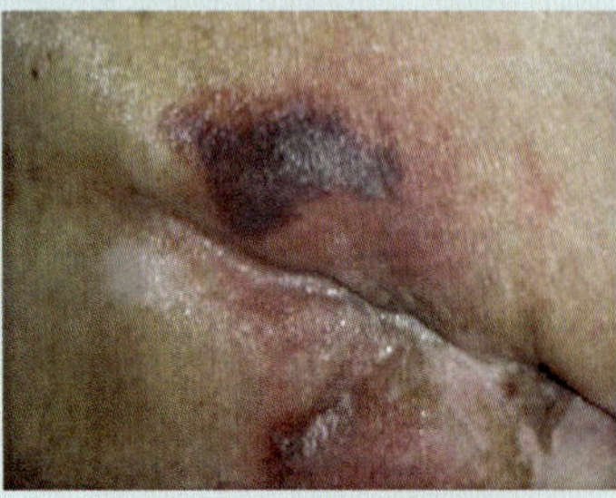

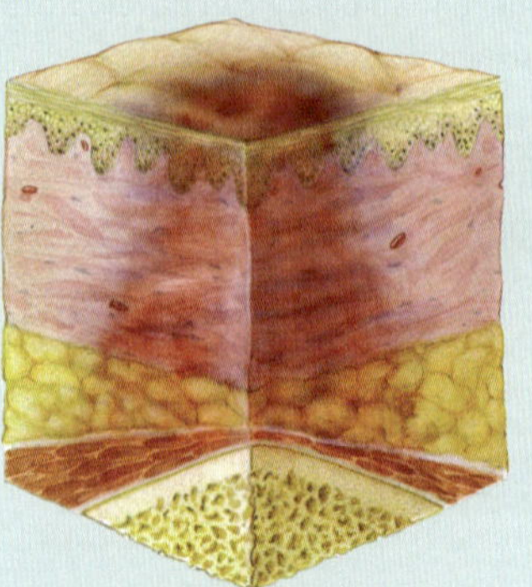

Source: Text as reproduced in EPUAP, NPIAP & PPPIA (2019). *Prevention and treatment of pressure ulcers/injuries: Clinical practice guideline*. Used with permission of the National Pressure Ulcer Advisory Panel. Images NPUAP copyright and used with permission.

and hypoxia of tissues. The skin may appear red; in darkly pigmented people, bluish or purple hues are evident. If the area of skin does not blanch when pressure is applied after relieving the pressure for 30 minutes, a Stage 1 pressure injury is present. Eventually, the cells and tissues of the immediate area of pressure and the surrounding area become necrotic. The 2019 international guideline outlines the pressure injury staging systems used in Australia (EPUAP, NPIAP, PPPIA, 2019).

Risk factors

Predisposing factors for pressure injuries are both intrinsic (pertaining to the individual) and extrinsic (pertaining to extracorporeal factors). Intrinsic factors include extremes in age (the very young or elderly), immobility, inactivity, malnutrition, dehydration, poor skin condition, impaired sensory perception and comorbidities that exacerbate these conditions, such as diabetes mellitus, malignancy, and renal, respiratory, vascular, lymphatic and hepatic disorders. Extrinsic factors include applied pressure, shear and friction forces, moisture (incontinence, wound exudate or perspiration) and contact with surfaces or devices such as plastic or vinyl which increase skin temperature.

The older immobile adult is at increased risk of the development of pressure injuries because of age-related skin changes that reduce the skin's tolerance to pressure, shear and friction.

The skin changes in the older adult include: a thinner dermis with decreased vascularity, decreased sebaceous gland activity, and decreased strength and elasticity. As a result, the thinner and less nourished dermal layer is more prone to shear and friction forces. Furthermore, wound healing is inhibited in the older adult due to a myriad of factors such as increased comorbidities, potential deficits in nutrition and hydration, polypharmacy and the effects of certain medications.

Since the early 1960s an increasing number of pressure injury risk prediction instruments have been developed to assist healthcare providers identify and assess the recognised clinical variables that contribute to pressure injury formation. The most commonly used instruments in Australia include the Braden Scale (1987), Norton Scale (1962) and Waterlow Score (1985), and Braden Q Scale (1996) or Glamorgan Scale (2007) for paediatric populations. Among these prediction instruments, there is no consensus on subscales assessed, scoring systems, methodological testing for reliability, sensitivity, specificity or predictive value rating, nor specific populations for use. However, when used in conjunction with informed clinical judgment they can increase the effectiveness of pressure prevention interventions.

INTERPROFESSIONAL CARE

For the person at risk of pressure injuries, the goal is prevention. An interprofessional and collaborative approach to the prevention and management of pressure injuries is required. The most contemporary evidence for prevention and treatment of pressure injuries which should be used by all health professionals is presented in the 2019 *Prevention and Treatment of Pressure Ulcers/Injuries: Clinical Practice Guideline* available at www.internationalguideline.com.

Table 15.4 summarises evidence-based pressure injury prevention recommendations described in the 2019 *Prevention and Treatment of Pressure Ulcers/Injuries: Clinical Practice Guideline*.

Pressure injury management

Pressure injuries are generally considered to be chronic wounds, as healing may be complicated by intrinsic and extrinsic factors that impact on the person, their wound and their healing environment. The principles of wound bed preparation were outlined in the original 'TIME' acronym

TRANSLATION TO PRACTICE Pressure injury risk assessment

The Prevention and Treatment of Pressure Ulcers/Injuries: Clinical Practice Guideline (EPUAP, NPIAP & PPPIA, 2019) outlines six recommendations for the risk assessment of pressure injuries. These recommendations are supported and upheld by the ACSQHC's NSQHS Standards. These recommendations are:

1 All patients should undergo a pressure injury risk assessment within 8 hours of admission. The risk assessment should be structured and incorporate the clinical judgment of the clinician.
2 The risk assessment should be performed as often as clinically required.
3 Risk should be reassessed if the patient's condition changes.
4 A comprehensive skin assessment should form part of every risk assessment.
5 Each risk assessment should be documented accurately so that changes to skin integrity can be detected and treated early.
6 A risk-based prevention plan should be developed for patients identified as being at risk of pressure injuries.

In addition, the guideline makes evidence-based recommendations for optimising nutritional status, repositioning and early mobilisation of individuals, and the use of support surfaces in the prevention and treatment of pressure injuries.

Source: Text as reproduced in EPUAP, NPIAP & PPPIA (2019). *Prevention and treatment of pressure ulcers/injuries: Clinical practice guideline*. Used with permission of the National Pressure Ulcer Advisory Panel. Images NPUAP copyright and used with permission.

TABLE 15.4 Pressure injury prevention

STRATEGY	DESCRIPTION
Skin care	• Avoid positioning patients on reddened areas of skin (erythema). • Keep the skin clean (using a pH-balanced skin cleanser) and dry. • Do not massage or rub skin at risk of pressure injuries. • Develop and implement an individualised continence plan. • Use a barrier method to protect skin from prolonged exposure to excessive moisture. • Use skin moisturisers judiciously to hydrate the skin (do not use dimethyl sulfoxides).
Microclimate control	• Use correct materials to alter the moisture absorption and heat dissipation depending on the client's need. • Do not apply heating devices directly on the skin or on a pressure injury.
Prophylactic dressings	• Apply multilayer silicone and polyurethane foam dressings to bony prominences on clients identified as being at high risk of pressure injuries. • Select the dressings paying consideration to the microclimate needs, ease of application and removal, ability to assess skin, anatomical location and correct sizing.
Fabrics and textiles	Use silk fabrics over cotton-based fabrics to reduce sheer and friction.
Electrical stimulation	Consider using electrical stimulation to areas at risk of pressure injuries on spinal cord injury patients.
Nutrition	• Screen all patients at risk of pressure injury with a validated screening tool and refer those identified as at risk of malnutrition to a dietician. • Assess each patient's weight status, ability to eat independently and adequacy of nutrient intake. • Develop an individualised care plan. • Ensure the patient's energy intake has been calculated according to their underlying pathology, weight needs and pressure injury risk. • Provide adequate protein for clients identified as being at risk of pressure injuries. • Provide adequate hydration and monitor for signs of dehydration. • Encourage a vitamin-rich intake or supplementation in patients at risk of pressure injuries.
Repositioning and early mobilisation	• Reposition all patients at risk of pressure injuries, unless contraindicated. • Take into consideration the patient's pressure redistribution support surface when determining the frequency of turns. • Reposition patients so that pressure is relieved or redistributed, avoiding bony prominences and shearing forces.
Support surfaces	• Use a high-specification reactive foam mattress for all patients at risk of pressure injuries. • Use an active support surface for all patients at *high* risk of pressure injuries.

(Schultz et al., 2003) and updated in 2012 (Leaper et al., 2012) (see Box 15.11).

TIME: TISSUE Wound debridement is the required intervention when assessment reveals the presence of non-viable or necrotic tissue. Chronic wounds may require ongoing debridement to remove necrotic tissue and reduce the levels of microbes and excessive proteases.

The methods of debridement include surgical sharp, conservative sharp, autolytic, mechanical, chemical, enzymatic and parasitic larvae. Surgical sharp debridement may lead to bleeding and may be performed by the medical practitioner, podiatrist or Nurse Practitioner. Conservative sharp wound debridement (CSWD)—the removal of loose avascular tissue without pain or bleeding—may be performed by the competent nurse when there are no contraindications such as:

- lack of access to sterile sharp instruments (Adson toothed forceps, scalpel or iris scissors)
- densely adherent necrotic tissue when the interface between viable and non-viable tissue cannot be clearly identified
- impaired clotting mechanism or the person is on anticoagulant or antiplatelet medications
- increased risk of bleeding—for example, malignant wounds
- a non-infected ischaemic ulcer covered with dry eschar when tissue oxygenation is insufficient to support infection control and wound healing—for example, a diabetic person with a dry or gangrenous foot ulcer (Carville, 2017).

The extent of debridement required and patient risk are outside the scope of practice.

Other methods of debridement such as autolytic, 'safe' chemical (using contemporary and non-cytotoxic antimicrobial agents), mechanical or parasitic debridement, may be employed when CSWD is inappropriate. At the time of publication there are no licensed enzymatic debridement agents available in Australia.

Dressings that hydrate the wound or maintain wound exudate at the wound interface and thus promote autolysis of eschar are used to promote autolytic debridement (see Table 15.5). Certain modern antiseptic dressings provide a means of autolytic and nontoxic chemical debridement and are commonly used when infection or the risk of infection is present (see Table 15.5). Mechanical debridement is the use of therapeutic cleansing

BOX 15.11 TIME acronym

T = Tissue, non-viable or deficit
I = Infection or inflammation
M = Moisture imbalance
E = Edge of wound on-advancing or undermined.

TABLE 15.5 Dressings for autolytic and 'safe' chemical debridement

AUTOLYTIC DEBRIDEMENT	AUTOLYTIC AND CHEMICAL DEBRIDEMENT
Hydrogel dressings	**Cadexomer iodine dressings**
Amorphous hydrogels	Iodosorb™ powder, paste and dressing
Intrasite™	**Wound honey (combines both autolytic and chemical properties)**
SoloSite™	MediHoney™
DuoDerm gel™	Activon™
Biatain gel™	Hypertonic saline-impregnated dressings
Solugel™	Mesalt™
Gel sheet hydrogels	**Polyhexamethylene Biguanide (PHMB)**
HydroTac™	Prontosan™ solution and gel (with Betaine)
Nu-Gel™	Octenidine dihydrochloride (Octenilin™ solution and gel)
Gel-impregnated gauze	
IntraSite Conformable™	
Hydrocolloid dressings	
Comfeel™	
DuoDerm™	

with wet gauze or commercially available debridement pads (Debrisoft® pad, Prontosan® pad, Alprep® debridement foam) or the use of wet to dry dressings.

Low frequency ultrasound debridement (LFUD) is another form of mechanical debridement. It uses low ultrasonic frequencies of 20 kHz to 100 kHz and converts electrical current to vibrations. As ultrasound does not travel easily through air, saline solution is used as a transducing media, which allows the ultrasound waves to travel from the probe into the tissues. The mechanical energy produced converts into acoustic energy, or a cavitation phenomenon, which is the creation and destruction of small bubbles within the saline fluid surrounding the probe (Shannon, Williams & Bloomer, 2012). During cavitation, the bubbles oscillate and expand and rapidly collapse, causing shockwaves and selective fragmentation or debridement of devitalised tissues (Conner-Kerr et al., 2010). An available example of an LFUD device is the SONOCA-185® (Soring).

The use of fly larvae therapy or maggots for debridement is attracting increased interest in Australia, and laboratory-raised 'sterile' *Lucilia sericata* (greenbottle fly) larvae are being produced at Westmead Hospital in Sydney for this purpose. Parasitic or larval debridement is also known as biosurgical or myasitic larval therapy and involves the deliberate infestation of laboratory-raised fly maggots into a necrotic wound. The L. sericata species is deemed to be the most suitable larvae as it secretes collagenases and trypsin enzymes and limits its interest to necrotic rather than healthy tissue (Polat et al., 2014). The enzymes facilitate liquidification of the necrotic tissue which is then digested by the larvae. Prior to application of the larvae, the periwound skin is best protected with a hydrocolloid dressing and the larvae entrapped under a semi-permeable film dressing which requires the insertion of small pin-pricked holes to facilitate air entry and survival of the maggots. Subject to the amount of necrotic tissue and the number of larvae, they are generally allowed to remain in the wound for 2 days or until they are engorged.

TIME: INFECTION OR INFLAMMATION The classic signs and symptoms of inflammation were noted by Celsus in the first century to be *tumor* (swelling), *rubor* (erythema), *calor* (heat) and *dolor* (pain) (Haeger, 1988). Inflammation can occur as a normal response to wound healing. It can also occur in response to wound infection with the added sign of purulence or increased malodorous exudate.

Contamination, which is defined as the presence of non-replicating bacteria in a wound, does not inhibit wound healing (Bullock & Hales, 2019). However, tissue hypoxia or necrosis is conducive to colonisation, which is defined as the presence of replicating bacteria, but with no host reaction. Skin commensals such as *Staphylococcus epidermis* and *Corynebacterium* flora are to be expected in the wound and, in fact, have been found at low levels to demonstrate a positive effect on healing (Moffatt, 2004). Local infection is either covert or overt and is defined as an increase in the bacterial burden of the wound in which healing is inhibited (International Wound Infection Institute (IWII), 2022). Local infection in chronic wounds may not portray the classic signs of infection, although the wound may demonstrate one or more of the following signs: static healing; increased exudate; hypergranulated, bright-red, friable granulation tissue that bleeds easily; tissue bridging; granulation pocketing in the base of the wound; and rolled edges (IWII, 2022).

There is a lack of international consensus as to whether local infection is a transitional stage between colonisation and overt infection or is indicative of chronic inflammation in the presence of a biofilm in the wound. Spreading infection is also referred to as cellulitis. Systemic infection can lead to sepsis and death. Figure 15.20 shows the IWII Wound Infection Continuum.

Bacteria react to threat in two ways: the development of resistance and the formation of biofilms. **Biofilms** are polymicrobial microbial communities that proliferate and are encased in a protective glycocalax matrix. The bacteria secrete glycocalyx, which forms a biofilm (an extracellular polysaccharide (ESP)) that protects the organisms from immune responses by phagocytes and from topical and systemic antibiotics. Biofilms have been found in 60% of chronic wounds compared to 6% of acute wounds but are suspected to be in all chronic wounds (James et al., 2008).

Biofilms form in the following manner:

1. Planktonic (free-floating) organisms attach to the surface of the wound.
2. Sessile (firmly attached) organisms communicate between microorganisms of the same or different species via a process referred to as quorum sensing. Quorum sensing is responsible for phenotypic diversity and some of the genotypic diversity seen in wound biofilms, and enhances the community's nutrient-gathering capacity, defence and reproductive abilities.
3. Firmly attached microorganisms secrete an extracellular polymeric substance (EPS) or protective matrix.
4. The EPS is comprised of polysaccharides, proteins, glycolipids and bacterial DNA.

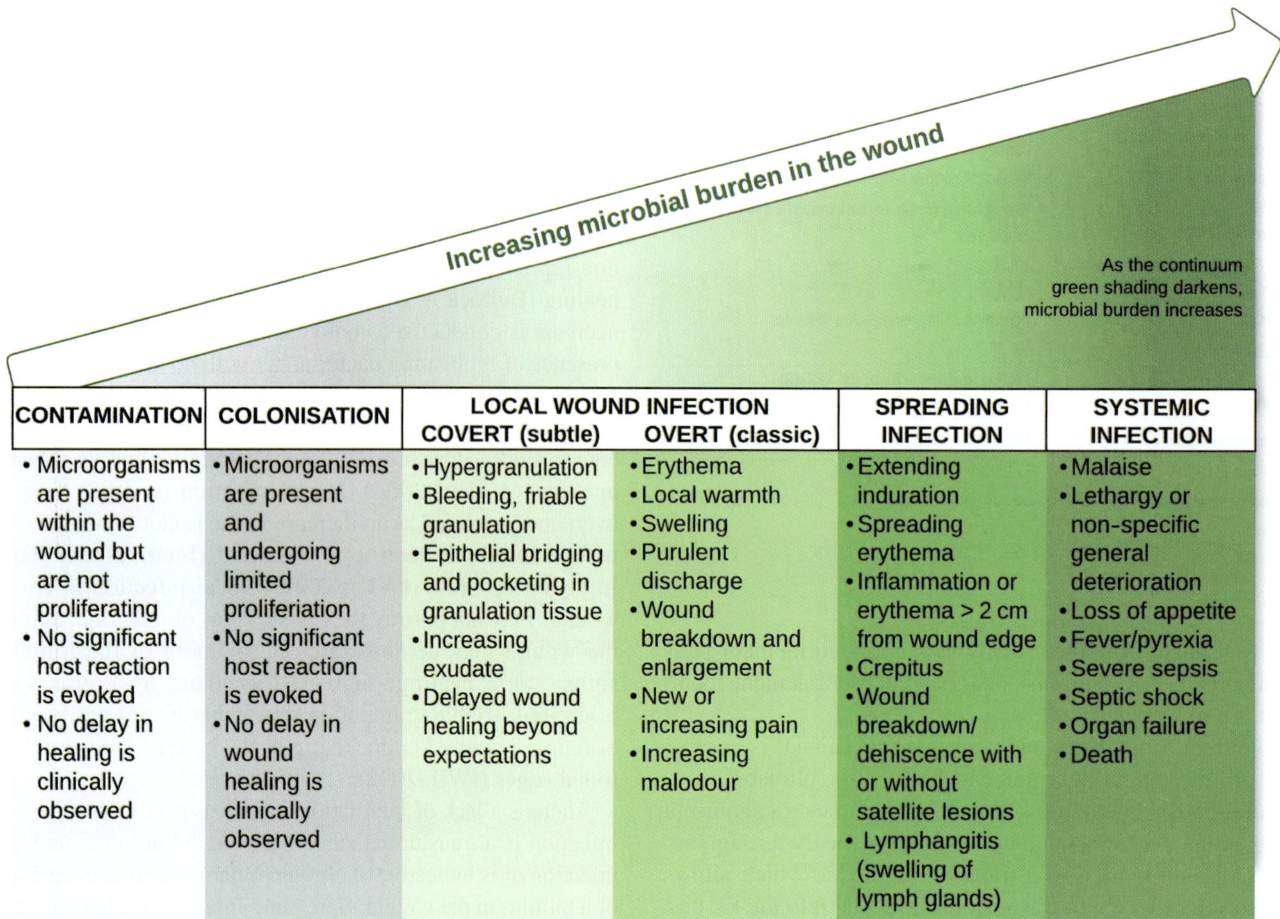

FIGURE 15.20 ***Wound Infection Continuum***

Source: IWII (2022). *Wound infection in clinical practice: Principles of best practice*. Wounds International. Retrieved from https://woundinfection-institute.com.

5. The mature biofilm releases planktonic bacteria, which disperse and attach to other parts of the wound, and the cycle is repeated (James et al., 2008; Phillips, Wolcott et al., 2010).

The prudent use of topical antiseptic dressings can restore the bacterial balance in the wound and there is some evidence that polyhexamethylene biguanide (PHMB) with a surfactant (betaine) (Andriessen et al., 2008; Forstner et al., 2013; Kaehn & Eberlein, 2009), cadexomer iodine (Phillips, Yang et al., 2010) and silver dressings with antibiofilm mechanisms such as EDTA (a chelating agent with broad-spectrum antimicrobial and antibiofilm activity, and benzethonium chloride, a surfactant) (IWII, 2022) can denature a biofilm. Because bacterial imbalance usually results in increased amounts of wound exudate, maintenance of moisture balance is an aligned goal (Carville, 2017). Examples of antiseptic dressings available for restoration of bacterial balance are outlined in Box 15.12.

BOX 15.12 Antiseptic dressings

Cadexomer-iodine dressings
Iodosorb™ paste, powder and dressing
Povidone-iodine-impregnated tulle gras
Inadine™
Wound honey
MediHoney™
Activon™
Silver-impregnated dressings
Acticoat™
Aquacel Ag™
Biatain Ag™
SilverCel™
Polyhexamethylene biguanide (PHMB)
Prontosan™ solution and gel (with Betaine)
AMD™ foam and gauze
Octenidine dihydrochloride
Octenilin™ solution and gel

TIME: MOISTURE IMBALANCE Desiccation of the wound inhibits epithelialisation, and excessive moisture leads to maceration and further breakdown of the tissues. Chronic wound fluid contains increased levels of matrix metalloproteases which have the potential to degrade much-needed extracellular matrix proteins such as fibronectin and vitronectin. Excessive fluid in chronic wounds can interfere

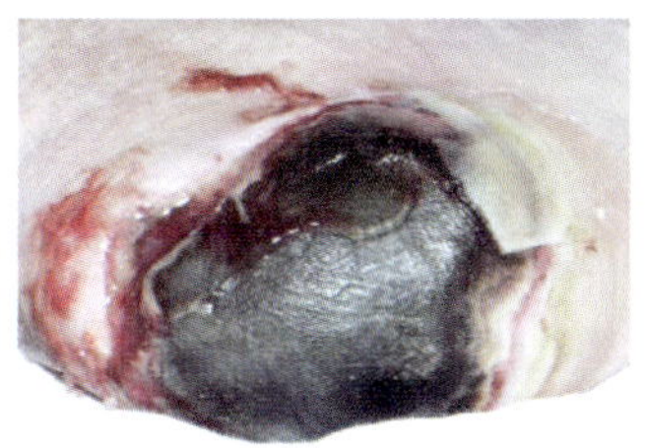

Dry

Dressing options:

- Hydrogels
- Hydrocolloids
- Interactive wet dressings

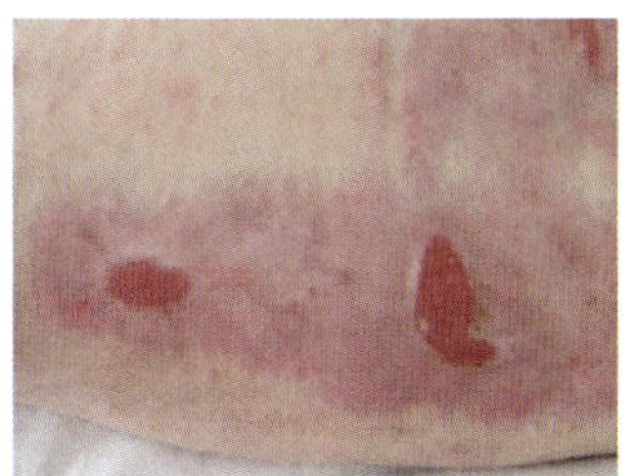

Low exudate

Dressing options:

- Semi-permeable films
- Hydrocolloids
- Calcium alginates

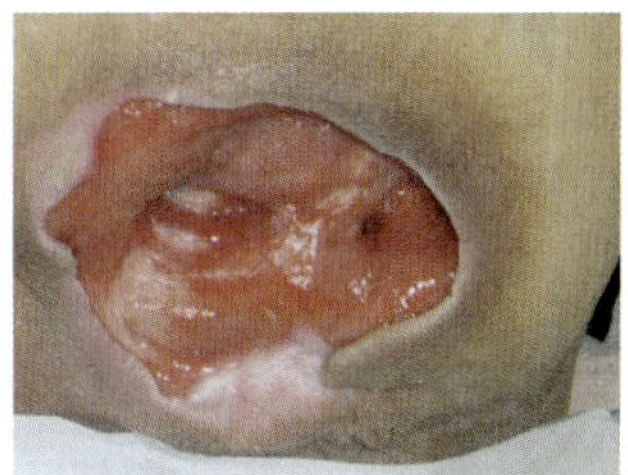

Moderate exudate

Dressing options:

- Calcium alginate
- Hydrofibre
- Foams

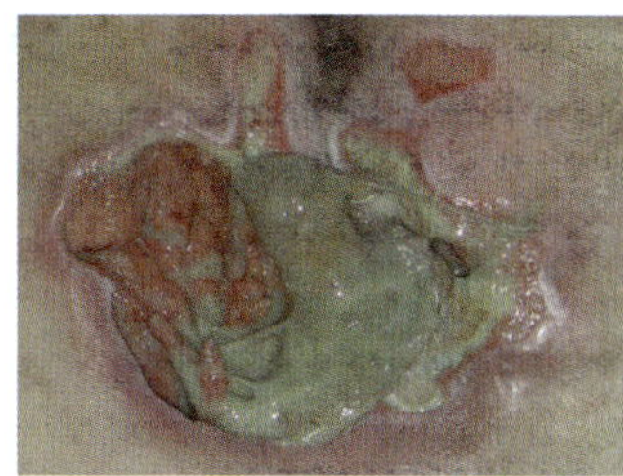

Heavy exudate

Dressing options:

- Hydrofibre dressing
- Foam sheet/cavity
- Super-absorbent dry dressings
- Wound/ostomy bag
- Topical negative-pressure therapy systems

FIGURE 15.21 ***Dressings for maintaining moisture balance in pressure injuries***

Source: Carville (2012). *Wound care manual* (6th ed.). Osborne Park, WA: Silver Chain Foundation. Images reproduced with permission of K. Carville.

with the activities of important cell mediators, such as growth factors (Dowsett, 2011). The goal is to maintain moisture balance while avoiding desiccation and maceration. Thus, dressing selection will be influenced by the assessment outcome, and the goal of care will be either to hydrate the wound bed or absorb excessive exudate. Cavity or sinus wounds such as Stage 3 and 4 pressure injuries will require a cavity-filling dressing to eliminate the dead space in the wound and facilitate controlled wound closure. Most generic groups of dressings (e.g. calcium alginates, gelling fibre, foams and hydrogel-impregnated gauzes) now come in forms suitable for filling cavity defects.

Dressing options for maintaining moisture balance in pressure injuries are outlined in Figure 15.21.

TIME: EDGES ADVANCING Assessment of wound edges is frequently overlooked, but coloured, raised, rolled or undermined wound edges can indicate delays in healing, abnormal pathologies or unrelieved pressure. Desiccation of the wound bed, hypergranulation and periwound debris (scale, scab or dried exudate) will inhibit epithelisation across the wound surface. Hypergranulation commonly results from bacterial imbalance or ongoing wound irritant trauma. Rolled or undermined edges can also indicate bacterial imbalance. Raised edges may indicate unrelieved trauma. However, further diagnostic investigations such as a wound biopsy may be indicated if the wound edge appearance indicates potential malignant changes. The use of negative pressure wound therapy (NPWT) for advancing wound closure is now a common intervention.

Surgical treatment

Surgical debridement may be performed by a medical practitioner when there is infection or extensive slough or eschar. Extensive pressure injuries may also require skin grafting or flap reconstruction to facilitate complete closure.

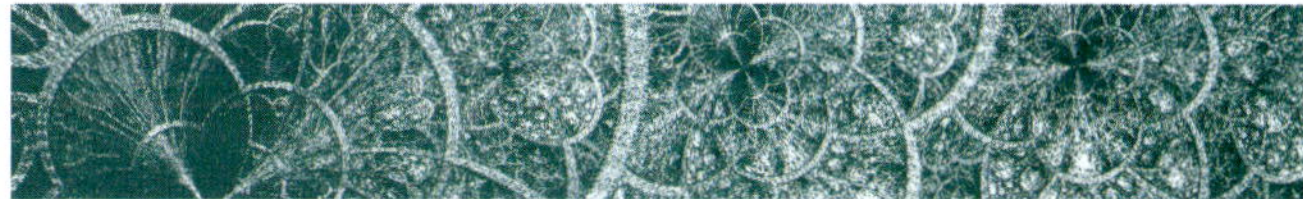

Nursing care

The person with a pressure injury not only has impaired skin integrity but also is at increased risk of other pressure injuries, infection, pain, decreased mobility and death. Pressure injuries prolong treatment for other health problems, increase health-care costs and diminish the person's quality of life. Therefore, pressure injury prevention is the optimal principle of care (see Box 15.13).

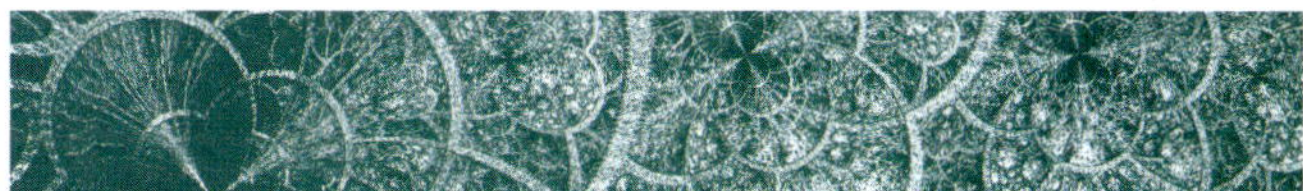

THE PERSON WITH A SKIN TEAR

A **skin tear** is defined as 'as trauma-induced partial or full thickness wounds which primarily occur on the extremities of older persons with age-related changes to the skin's structural and mechanical support properties, and are commonly associated with elastosis and/or ecchymosis' (Rayner, Carville & Leslie, 2019).

The International Skin Tear Advisory Panel (ISTAP) updated definition defines a skin tear as 'a traumatic wound caused by mechanical forces, including removal of adhesives. Severity may vary by depth (not extending through the subcutaneous layer)' (LeBlanc et al., 2018).

Skin tears are the most common wound found in elderly populations but they are also common in neonates and paediatric populations. Reasons for this are related to the changes that occur in immature and ageing skin and the increased incidence of knocks, falls and manual handling requirements (Carville, 2017). The risk factors associated with acquiring skin tears are

BOX 15.13 Nursing care of the person at risk of a pressure injury and the person with a pressure injury

Comprehensive recommendations for pressure injury prevention and management are to be found in the *Prevention and Treatment of Pressure Ulcers/Injuries: Clinical Practice Guideline* (EPUAP, NPIAP & PPPIA, 2019) at www.internationalguideline.com.

The principle interventions for pressure injury prevention and management are as follows:

Risk assessment

1. Conduct a comprehensive assessment for all people to identify pressure injury risk factors. A comprehensive assessment should include:
   - clinical history
   - pressure injury risk scale
   - skin assessment
   - mobility and activity assessment
   - nutritional assessment
   - continence assessment
   - cognitive assessment
   - assessment of extrinsic risk factors.
2. Use a validated pressure injury risk assessment scale in conjunction with a comprehensive risk assessment to determine the person's risk of pressure injury and to inform the development of a prevention plan.
3. Inspect the skin of all people on admission and at each repositioning to identify indications of pressure injury including:
   - erythema
   - blanching response
   - localised heat
   - oedema
   - induration
   - skin breakdown.

Prevention of pressure injuries

1. Implement preventative strategies to protect the person's skin.
2. Provide high-protein oral nutritional supplements in addition to an appropriate diet for people at a high risk of pressure injury who have been identified at risk of having malnutrition.
3. Use a high-specification, constant-low-pressure support mattress on beds, trolleys, operating theatre tables and chairs for people at high risk of pressure injury (refer to the International Guideline for information on characteristics of high-specification support surfaces).
4. Any device used to prevent heel pressure injuries should be selected and fitted appropriately to offload heel pressure.
5. Frequency of repositioning should consider the person's risk of pressure injury, comfort, functional level, medical condition and the support surface used.
6. Skin protection should include:
   - Individuals at risk of developing pressure injuries should have a comprehensive skin inspection at least daily for signs of impaired skin integrity.
   - The skin should be kept clean and free from all potentially irritating substances or those that substantially alter the skin pH.
   - All intrinsic and extrinsic factors that result in dryness or maceration of the skin should be eliminated or minimised by:
     a. treating dry, flaky or scaling skin with a topical moisturiser
     b. avoiding sustained or excessive contact with body fluids, and/or
     c. encouraging continence by employing interventions such as continence training or the use of continence aids.
7. Avoid extremes in skin temperature by avoiding skin contact with plastic support surfaces and ensuring that turning schedules do not exceed 2-hourly intervals for people at high risk.

Mechanical offloading and support surfaces

1. Alternating-pressure mattress replacements and overlays provide similar benefits to high-specification, constant-low-pressure support mattresses and could be used as an alternative in people at high risk of pressure injury.
2. Support surfaces should be used in conjunction with a comprehensive prevention strategy based on frequent observation and assessment, individualised turning regimens and measures to increase the tissues' tolerance to pressure.
3. Pillows and foam wedges can be used to avoid direct contact between bony prominences.
4. Avoid prolonged uninterrupted sitting in a chair or wheelchair. Repositioning or shifting of pressure points should occur as frequently as every 15 minutes to hourly depending on the tissues' tolerance to pressure.
5. Exposure to shear and friction should be reduced by:
   a. employing correct lifting and manual handling techniques
   b. protecting skin constantly exposed to friction with protective dressings or padding or medical-grade sheepskin
   c. elevating the foot of the bed to 20 degrees when sitting to prevent sliding
   d. maintaining the head of the bed at the lowest possible elevation consistent with the individual's medical condition and comfort.
6. Individuals who are bed-bound or have immobilised lower extremities should have total relief of pressure from their heels.
7. Individuals should be encouraged to maximise their activity and mobilisation consistent with their medical condition, ability and energy level.

Documentation

All individuals at risk of developing pressure injuries should have the following details recorded in the person's record on a regular, ongoing basis: risk assessment status (low, moderate or high); identified risk factors; management plan which includes interventions used such as turning schedules, support surface, referrals and the individual's response to treatment.

BOX 15.13 Nursing care of the person at risk of a pressure injury and the person with a pressure injury (continued)

Evaluation

1. Any pressure injury risk management program should be based on a demonstrable need, relevant to the healthcare setting and supported by a policy and protocol based on the best available research.
2. All pressure injury risk management programs should include the individual at risk and significant family members. The individual should be considered an active participant in the management plan and should be informed of the relevant risk factors and the strategies employed to minimise or eliminate the risk of pressure injury development.
3. A pressure injury risk management program should be supported by a continuing educational program and a multidisciplinary continuous improvement process that is able to monitor and compare the impact of interventions over time.

Source: Adapted from EPUAP, NPIAP & PPPIA (2019). *Prevention and treatment of pressure ulcers/Injuries: Clinical practice guideline*. The international guideline. Retrieved from https://www.internationalguideline.com.

NURSING CARE PLAN A person with a pressure injury

Mrs Sibitu is 85 years old and lives in a nursing home. Mrs Sibitu has been unable to walk since suffering a dense stroke 2 years ago. She requires full assistance to transfer and change her position in bed. She has a history of type II diabetes which is reported to be diet controlled, chronic obstructive pulmonary disease (COPD) and osteoarthritis. Her medications include preventative inhaled corticosteroids (beclomethasone) twice daily and non-steroidal anti-inflammatory agents (naproxen 500 mg) twice daily. In addition, she takes aspirin (Cardiprin) 100 mg daily as a preventive anticoagulant. Her weight is average, but she has had a recent weight loss of 4 kg. While her appetite was previously good, over the past month she has required a lot of assistance and encouragement with fluid and foods. A deterioration in her general condition has been noted and she is reportedly increasingly drowsy and reluctant to be repositioned regularly. She is incontinent of faeces and urine. Her incontinence is managed with incontinent pads. She normally sits out of bed for 4 to 6 hours a day in a recliner chair but otherwise spends the remainder of the day in bed.

ASSESSMENT

On routine skin inspection Mrs Sibitu was assessed to have a pressure injury measuring 3 cm by 4 cm over her sacrum. The wound bed was covered in a layer of yellow slough that inhibited assessment of the depth of the wound. There was a moderate amount of yellow-stained, slightly malodorous exudate. On palpation the surrounding skin is noted to be indurated and dark red. The edges of the wound are level with the surrounding skin, which is macerated due to contact with wound exudate and urine. Although she cannot articulate her pain level, Mrs Sibitu appears restless when the wound is touched or she is repositioned. A pressure injury risk assessment using the Braden Scale was performed and she was assessed as being at high risk of pressure injury.

DIAGNOSIS

- *Impaired skin integrity* related to pressure, friction and shear—an Unstageable sacral pressure injury.
- *Infection risk* due to contamination of pressure injury with faeces and urine.
- *Pain* related to the pressure injury.
- *Anxiety* related to alterations in cognition, mobility and activity.

PLANNING

- Assess Mrs Sibitu, her wound and her healing environment.
- Eliminate pressure, shear and friction.
- Control wound infection and manage the wound according to best evidence.
- Debride the slough.
- Manage urinary and faecal incontinence.
- Keep skin clean and dry.
- Optimise nutritional status with supplements.
- Manage pain.

Expected outcomes

- Mrs Sibitu's pressure injury will be assessed daily, managed and progress to healing.
- Mrs Sibitu will be free of further pressure injuries or extension of her existing injury with appropriate assessment and intervention.
- Mrs Sibitu will be free of wound infection from faecal and urine contamination based on appropriate infection prevention and control strategies.
- Mrs Sibitu will be free of pain based on accurate assessment and appropriate interventions.

IMPLEMENTATION

- Assess pain and request a medical review for pain management medications.
- Perform a skin assessment and a pressure injury risk assessment on admission and on altered change of condition, or as directed by her risk score and the organisation's protocol.
- Conduct a skin inspection daily and document outcomes.
- Increase repositioning times and use pillows or wedges to secure position and elevate heels from bed and position off sacrum.
- Optimise pressure offloading—utilise an active alternating-pressure replacement mattress on her bed for sleeping.
- Optimise pressure offloading—utilise a constant-low-pressure cushion when seated. The occupational therapist will be requested to review Mrs Sibitu's seating.

(continued)

NURSING CARE PLAN **A person with a pressure injury (continued)**

- Request a dietitian to review Mrs Sibitu's nutritional intake and determine a plan of care for regular nutritional supplements and increased oral fluids.
- Keep Mrs Sibitu's skin clean and dry and use protective moisturisers and barrier films to protect against maceration.
- Review incontinence management strategies and quality of incontinence pads used. Implement a regular toileting regimen and review her bowel management plan.
- Request the physiotherapist to review her activity and mobility and implement a program of passive and active exercise as appropriate.
- Document wound assessment outcomes including stage of pressure injury, wound bed appearance and dimensions, type and amount of exudate, presence of malodour, status of surrounding skin and wound edges, and pain score, using a validated instrument.
- Document an individualised care plan for pressure injury management with the aim of reducing pain and discomfort, debridement of the slough, the need to maintain a bacterial balance in the wound, promote wound healing and prevent further pressure injury development.
- Observe for clinical signs of overt infection (increased pain, heat, redness, swelling or purulence, elevated temperature, malaise) and report to the medical practitioner.

EVALUATION

Mrs Sibitu will require daily skin inspections and regular ongoing risk assessments for pressure injury risk. Ongoing wound assessments will be evaluated for healing progress and successful care planning. Her pain will be controlled. The occupational therapist will review Mrs Sibitu's seating on a regular basis and adapt it as appropriate. The alternating-pressure mattress will be checked each shift to ensure the correct pressure offloading is provided under her bony prominences. The dietitian will review the effectiveness of the nutritional plan. The physiotherapist will review the effectiveness of the exercise plan.

CRITICAL THINKING IN THE NURSING PROCESS

1 Consider Mrs Sibitu's risk factors for pressure injury development and why daily skin inspection of an 'at-risk' individual is of the utmost importance.
2 Use a validated risk assessment tool such as the Braden Scale, Norton Score or Waterlow Score to determine Mrs Sibitu's risk score.
3 What primary dressing would you most likely select to manage Mrs Sibitu's wound if your goal of care is bacterial balance and debridement?
4 What secondary dressing would you most likely select to control the moderate amount of exudate and protect against further contamination by body waste?

REFLECTION ON THE NURSING PROCESS

1 Outline what you have learned from Mrs Sibitu's situation that you will apply to your future practice.
2 What education strategies would you give to Mrs Sibitu and her family to prevent her developing further pressure injuries?

poorly studied but anecdotally are reported to be visual impairment, impaired mobility or balance, dementia and the use of certain medications such as steroids or anticoagulants (Crisp et al., 2020). Skin tears are all too frequently considered to be minor wounds, yet they can become extremely problematic and their treatment can be costly.

Until recently, skin tear prevalence was poorly reported in Australia. However, skin tears were found to be the third-largest group of wounds in Western Australia during surveys of all public hospitals conducted in 2007, 2008, 2009 and 2011 (Mulligan et al., 2011). Of particular concern was the fact that the majority of these injuries were hospital-acquired. In a Western Australian community setting, skin tears were found to comprise 20% of wounds in a population aged 70 years or older (Carville & Smith, 2004).

In 1990, Payne and Martin outlined a system for classification of skin tears. They refined this system in 1993, although the classification is poorly utilised in Australia. The Payne–Martin Skin Tear Classification (1993) lists three categories and two subcategories of injury; however, it does not take into account the presence of haematoma or ischaemic changes in the skin or flap (see Box 15.14).

The STAR Skin Tear Classification System (Carville et al., 2007) also lists three categories and two subcategories of skin injury and takes into account skin or flap colour changes that occur with haematoma or hypoxia (see Figure 15.22).

BOX 15.14 Payne–Martin Skin Tear Classification (1993)

Category 1: Able to approximate the wound borders within 1 mm, no tissue loss
A–linear tear
B–flap
Category 2: Varying amounts of tissue loss
Type A < 25% loss–scant
Type B < 25% loss–moderate
Category 3: Total loss of flap

The ISTAP Skin Tear Classification (LeBlanc & Baranoski, 2018) lists three categories:

1. No skin loss: linear or flap tear which can be repositioned to cover the wound bed.
2. Partial flap loss: cannot be repositioned to cover the wound bed.
3. Total flap loss: exposure of entire wound bed.

Preventing skin tears

Rayner, Carville, Leslie and Dhaliwal (2019, 2020) identified the following indicators as risk predictors in a study of elderly aged care residents in Australia: a history of skin tears in the previous 12 months; purpura ≤ 20 mm in size; a history of falls

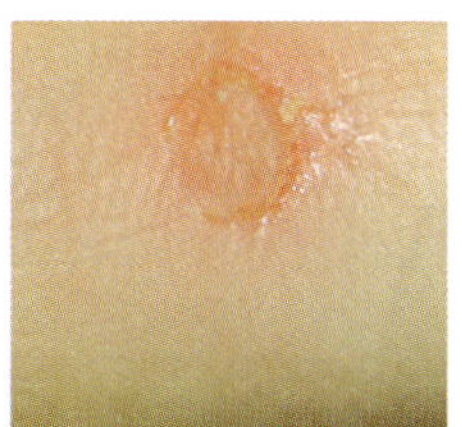

Category 1a
A skin tear where the edges can be realigned to the normal anatomical position (without undue stretching) and the skin or flap colour is not pale, dusky or darkened.

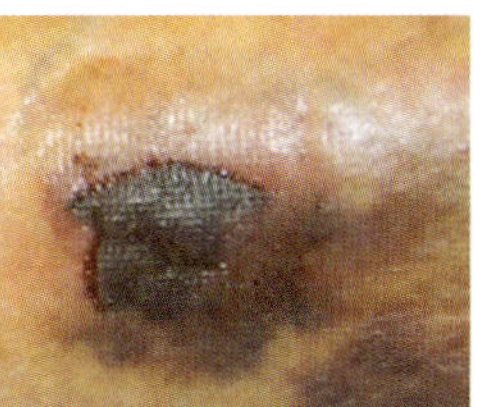

Category 1b
A skin tear where the edges can be realigned to the normal anatomical position (without undue stretching) and the skin or flap colour is pale, dusky or darkened.

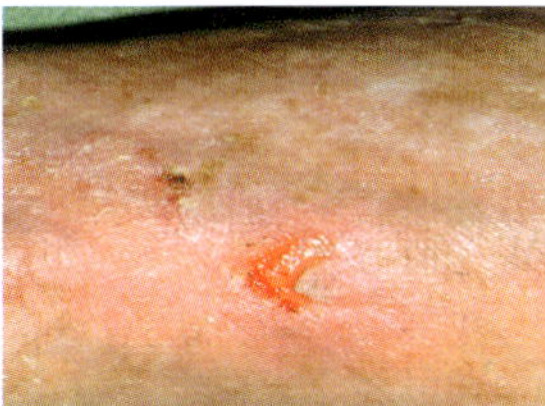

Category 2a
A skin tear where the edges cannot be realigned to the normal anatomical position and the skin or flap colour is not pale, dusky or darkened.

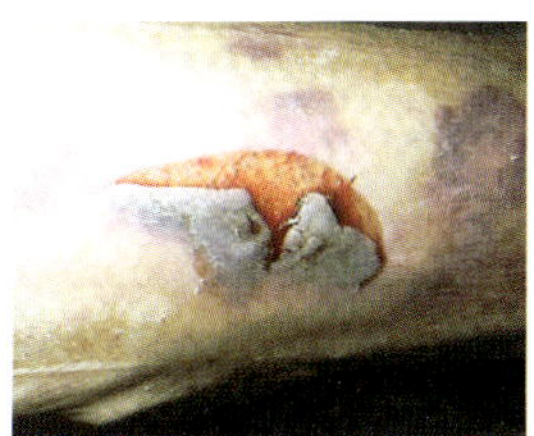

Category 2b
A skin tear where the edges cannot be realigned to the normal anatomical position and the skin or flap colour is pale, dusky or darkened.

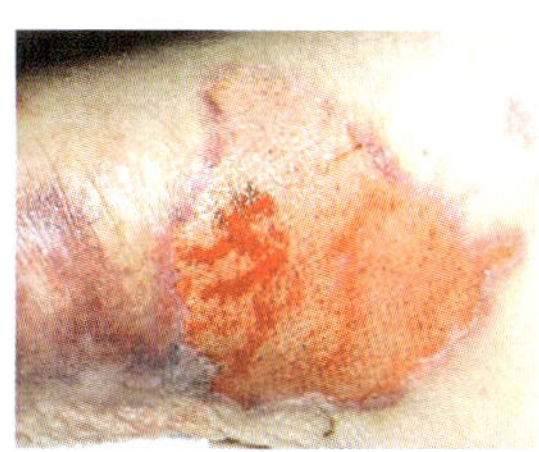

Category 3
A skin tear where the skin flap is completely absent.

FIGURE 15.22 ***STAR Skin Tear Classification System***

Source: Skin Tear Audit Research, Silver Chain Foundation and Curtin University. Reprinted with permission.

in the previous 3 months; clinical manifestations of elastosis; and male gender. However, individuals who require personal assistance with transfer or mobility, such as the frail, elderly or disabled, are at increased risk. Skin tears can also occur on any individual with the removal of adhesive agents such as tapes, dressings and devices, and due care must be taken during these procedures. A large, randomised control trial found that twice-daily moisturising of extremities of aged care residents with a pH-friendly, perfume-free moisturiser reduced skin tear incidence by 50% (Carville et al., 2014). Prevention of skin tears is a fundamental aspect of caring for these populations (see Box 15.15).

Skin tear management

The principles of skin tear management focus on control of any bleeding, restoration of skin flaps if present and provision of an environment that is conducive to healing and protection from further injury. Skin tears are commonly managed by dressings alone; stabilisation of the skin flap can be achieved via the use of silicone dressings (Prentice, Morey & Rodriguez, 2014). If the skin tear is deep or extensive, primary closure using sutures or tissue adhesives such as Histacryl™ may be required. The use of skin closure strips such as Steri-Strips™ are not recommended across flexures as they can compromise perfusion on flexing of tissues. If tape is required, the use of skin-protective barrier film prior to application and an adhesive remover prior to removal is advised (Prentice et al., 2014).

Selection of an appropriate dressing is subject to the ideal features and benefits, which should include the following:

- easy to apply
- provides a protective anti-shear barrier
- tissue friendly, moulds to contours, flexible
- maintains wound physiological balance—moisture, temperature, pH
- secure, but not aggressive retention
- extended wear time
- non-traumatic removal
- optimises quality of life and cosmesis
- cost-effective.

BOX 15.15 Skin tear prevention

- Assess for falls risk and implement prevention strategies.
- Use gentle and timely handling on transfer and repositioning.
- Use devices that reduce shear and friction.
- Moisturise the skin twice a day with a pH-friendly, perfume-free moisturiser.
- Cover vulnerable skin surfaces with protective clothing or devices.
- Maintain position with pillows and foam wedges to prevent shear. (Satin or silk covers will further reduce shear forces.)
- Avoid perfumed soaps that dry and alter the skin's pH.
- Cease smoking.
- Maintain adequate hydration and optimal nutrition.
- Avoid adhesive tapes and dressings on fragile skin in favour of roller or tubular bandages.
- Review medications and eliminate if possible those that alter the skin's integrity.
- Control any comorbidities that alter the skin's condition or risk of injury.
- Provide person and carer education on skin health and injury prevention.

Source: Carville (2012). *Wound care manual* (6th ed.). Osborne Park, WA: Silver Chain Foundation.

THE PERSON WITH A DISORDER OF THE HAIR

Racial characteristics and gender influence the amount and type of hair. Caucasians typically have more facial and body hair than Asians do. The latter usually have straight hair, those of African descent have wavy to curly hair and Caucasians have straight to curly hair. In addition, male hair growth characteristics (such as facial hair and hair on the lower extremities) are normal in certain women of some races and families.

The hair grows at various rates. Facial hair grows the most rapidly, followed by the hair of the scalp, axillae, thighs and eyebrows. Normally, an adult's hair grows at a rate of 10 to 12 mm per month; however, the growth rate is influenced by both the person's state of health and the environment. (Hair grows faster in hot climates, more slowly in cold climates.)

Pathophysiology

Hair colour, growth and pattern vary from person to person and are determined largely by genetic inheritance. However, changes do occur. For example, in some instances, hair loss recurs in successive generations of males in a family; in other cases, hair loss may be the result of chemotherapy. Excessive facial hair may be a response to certain endocrine disorders or to the loss of oestrogen after menopause. These changes may seem minor, but they may create psychosocial problems for the person experiencing the changes.

Hirsutism

Hirsutism, also called hypertrichosis, is the appearance of excessive hair in normal and abnormal areas of the body in women. Hirsutism most often occurs in a male distribution (that is, on the upper lip, chin, abdomen and chest) in women. The excess hair is primarily the result of an increase in androgen levels (especially testosterone), which may be due to any of the following:

- familial predisposition (considered normal)
- polycystic ovary syndrome
- ovarian, adrenal or pituitary tumours
- Cushing's syndrome
- central nervous system disorders
- medications, such as minoxidil, cyclosporin, phenytoin, certain progestins and anabolic steroids.

The manifestations of hirsutism include increased male pattern hair growth, acne and menstrual irregularities. If the androgen excess is great, defeminisation (a decrease in breast size and loss of normal adipose tissue) and virilisation (frontal balding, increased muscle mass, deepening of the voice and enlargement of the clitoris) may occur. Virilisation indicates the presence of an androgen-producing tumour.

Alopecia

Alopecia is loss of hair or baldness (see Figure 15.23). Alopecia can affect both men and women and may result from scarring, various systemic diseases or genetic predisposition. Scarring from trauma, radiation and severe bacterial, fungal or viral infections causes permanent and irreversible hair loss over the scarred area. Systemic diseases that may cause alopecia include systemic lupus erythematosus, thyroid disorders and pituitary insufficiency. The hair loss from these disorders may be reversible. Hair loss from androgenic causes may also occur in postmenopausal woman. Alopecia may be drug induced and is a side effect of a variety of medications (see Box 15.16).

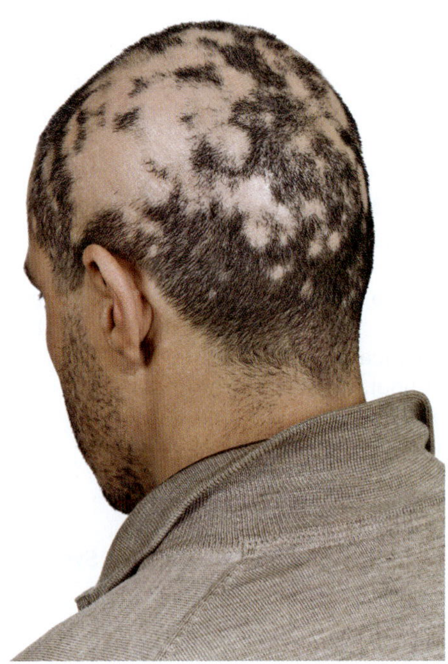

FIGURE 15.23 ***Alopecia (baldness) may be the result of scarring, disease or genetic predisposition***

Source: © Fresnel/Shutterstock.com.

Types of alopecia follow:

- Male pattern baldness is the most common cause of alopecia in men and is genetically predetermined. The hair loss begins at the temples, with recession of the hairline and baldness of the crown.
- Female pattern alopecia begins in women in their twenties and thirties, with progressive thinning and loss of hair over the central part of the scalp. Unlike men, women do not lose hair from the frontal hairline. Many of these women have elevated adrenal androgens.

BOX 15.16 Medications causing alopecia

- Thallium
- Retinoids
- Anticoagulants
- Antimitotic agents
- Antithyroid drugs
- Oral contraceptives
- Trimethadione
- Excessive use of vitamin A
- Allopurinol
- Propranolol
- Indomethacin
- Amphetamines
- Salicylates
- Levodopa
- Gentamicin
- Chemotherapy

- Alopecia areata is characterised by round or oval bald patches on the scalp, as well as on other hairy parts of the body. The cause is unknown. This type of alopecia is usually self-limiting and reverses without treatment, although it often recurs.
- Alopecia totalis is the loss of all hair on the scalp. This rare condition is irreversible.
- Alopecia universalis is the total loss of hair on all parts of the body.

INTERPROFESSIONAL CARE

Alopecia is diagnosed by assessing the appearance of the hair and hair loss, and by assessing the person for other systemic diseases and the use of medications that may cause hair loss. Various treatments are used to restore hair.

The person with hirsutism is examined for hormone levels and indications of other systemic illnesses. Hirsutism is treated by addressing the underlying systemic disorder and stopping medications that may be causing the problem.

Diagnosis

Diagnostic tests that may be ordered for the woman with hirsutism include serum testosterone levels and an adrenal CT scan. Testosterone levels greater than 200 ng/dL indicate the need for further tests, such as a pelvic examination and tests of ovarian function. Adrenal tumours, a possible cause of hirsutism, are identified with an adrenal CT scan.

Medications

Hirsutism is treated with medications specific to the underlying cause. Oral contraceptives containing oestrogen decrease ovarian androgen production and decrease free testosterone levels. Dexamethasone may be prescribed for people with high cortisol levels. Ketoconazole inhibits androgen production. Anti-androgenic medications cause congenital abnormalities in male infants and are therefore given only to non-pregnant women, who are cautioned to avoid pregnancy while taking the medications.

Male pattern baldness has been successfully treated with topical minoxidil. These drugs, which are vasodilators, stimulate vertex hair growth, probably by stimulating the epithelium of the hair follicle. These agents have been most successful in people who have a recent onset of alopecia or are less than 50 years of age. About 40% of people treated two times a day for a year are proposed to have moderate to dense regrowth of hair at the temples (Bullock & Hales, 2019).

Surgery

Hair transplant techniques are used to restore hair or reduce the size of areas of alopecia. Other types of surgical procedures include scalp reduction and flaps.

- Transplanting hairs as small hair plugs or single hairs taken from the back or sides of the scalp is an effective means of replacing hair to areas of alopecia. This procedure is done in an outpatient office or clinic.
- Scalp reduction is done by excising a portion of the affected scalp. In some cases, a tissue expander (such as a silicone balloon) is first implanted under the scalp to enlarge the hair-bearing scalp so that larger areas of alopecia can be removed.
- Flaps from hair-bearing areas of the scalp can be surgically transplanted from adjacent areas into areas of alopecia. This procedure may be done in stages.

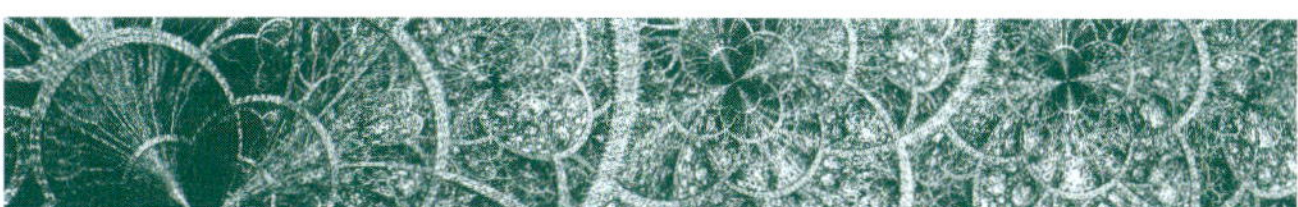

Nursing care

The person with either hirsutism or alopecia is often self-conscious about their appearance and tries a variety of over-the-counter treatments before seeking medical care. Nursing care for the person with hair disorders focuses on teaching them self-care and providing support during long-term care. Women with hirsutism are taught to use various means of removing unwanted hair, such as shaving, applying depilatories, waxing, undergoing electrolysis or having laser treatments. Women with mild hirsutism may bleach facial hair to make it less obvious. People with alopecia may wear hair pieces or wigs.

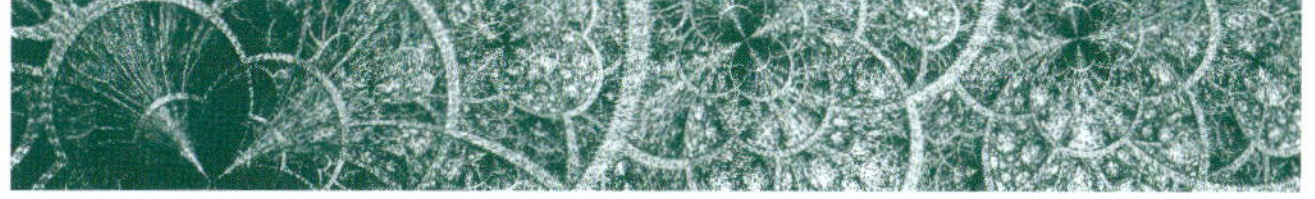

THE PERSON WITH A DISORDER OF THE NAILS

Nail disorders may be due to systemic diseases, trauma, allergies or irritants. They may also be congenital or genetic. Nails may be discoloured, multicoloured, malformed, infected or separated from underlying tissue.

Pathophysiology

The nail disorders discussed here are separation of the nail, infection and ingrown toenails:

- *Onycholysis* is the separation of the distal nail plate from the nail bed. It occurs most often in the fingernails. This disorder may result from many different factors, including excessive or prolonged exposure to water, soaps, detergent, alkalines and industrial keratolytic agents; *Candida* infections; nail hardeners; and thyroid disorders. Prolonged application of false fingernails may also cause this disorder.
- A *paronychia* is an infection of the cuticle of the fingernails or toenails. The disorder often follows a minor trauma and secondary infection with staphylococci, streptococci or *Candida*. The acute form begins with a painful inflammation that may progress to an abscess. The chronic form is seen most often in people who have frequent exposure to water. In the chronic form, the skin around the nail is painful, oedematous and infected. The nail plate may become ridged and discoloured.

- An *onychomycosis* is a fungal or dermatophyte infection of the nail plate. The nail plate elevates and becomes yellow or white. Psoriasis infections of the nail plate cause the nails to pit.
- An *ingrown toenail (unguis incarnatus)* results when the edge of the nail plate grows into the soft tissue of the toe. Pain and infection may occur. The infection, if untreated, may spread to the bone. This disorder is especially dangerous for the person with diabetes mellitus or peripheral vascular disease (Gebauer & Carville, 2022).

INTERPROFESSIONAL CARE

The treatments of disorders of the nail vary from pharmacological treatment to surgical removal. Infections of the nails are treated, depending on the causative agent, with antifungal or antibiotic medications. If the causative agent is a fungus or chronic dermatological disorder, treatment is difficult and may not be effective. Persistently painful and/or infected nails are in some cases surgically removed.

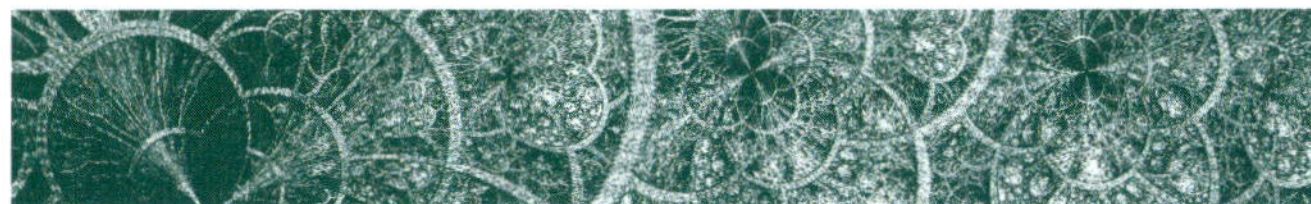

Nursing care

Nursing care of the person with a disorder of the nail focuses on teaching self-care. People with nail disorders that are caused by frequent exposure to water are taught to protect the hands or feet by wearing rubber gloves or boots, and to keep the nails as clean and dry as possible. People with ingrown toenails are cautioned not to cut into the lateral nail bed, but rather to soak the nail twice a day and insert a piece of cotton or gauze under the softened nail until the nail has grown out enough to trim.

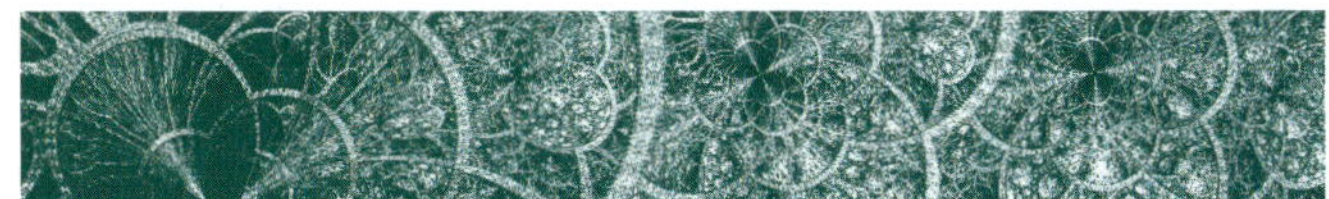

CHAPTER HIGHLIGHTS

- Pruritus (itching) accompanies dry skin (xerosis) and many skin disorders and may result in excoriation and infection as a result of scratching.
- Cysts, hypertrophic scars, keloids, naevi, angiomas, skin tags and keratoses are benign skin lesions. However, naevi should be monitored for changes indicating transformation into a malignant lesion.
- Psoriasis is a chronic immune skin disorder arising from keratinocytes. A variety of medications and treatments are used, with ultraviolet light therapy being most effective for generalised lesions.
- Skin disorders may be caused by a variety of bacterial infections, fungal infections, parasitic infestations and viral infections. The disorders are treated with a specific antibiotic, fungicide, antiviral agent or agents that kill the parasites. Herpes zoster, believed to follow a childhood infection with chickenpox, causes acute pain.
- Inflammatory disorders of the skin range from mild dermatitis to potentially lethal toxic epidermal necrolysis. Acne, a disorder of the hair and sebaceous glands opening to the skin surface, is characterised by comedones, pustules and cysts.
- Malignant skin disorders include actinic keratosis, non-melanoma skin cancer (basal cell carcinoma and squamous cell carcinoma) and malignant melanoma skin cancer. Skin cancer is the most common malignancy found in fair-skinned Australians. Prevention by avoiding sunburn, using sunscreen and maintaining monthly skin self-examination is critical in preventing loss of tissue or metastasis and death.
- Skin trauma may be intentional (as in the case of cutaneous and plastic surgery) or unintentional (as from trauma and pressure). Older adults with limited mobility, as well as people who are unable to move or are in critical care units, are at greater risk of pressure injuries and skin tears. Prevention is the goal of both interprofessional and nursing care.
- Disorders of the hair include alopecia (loss of hair) and hirsutism (excess hair in women). Nails may be discoloured, multicoloured, malformed, infected or separated from underlying tissue.

CONCEPT CHECK

1 You are caring for an elderly person with severe xerosis. What topic should be included in your teaching plan?
 1 Take a hot bath every day.
 2 Use fabric softeners when laundering clothing.
 3 Apply skin lotions after a bath.
 4 Maintain a warm environment.

2 Which of the following common skin lesions has the potential of becoming malignant?
 1 naevi
 2 angiomas
 3 skin tags
 4 keloids

3 You have been asked to teach a woman with generalised psoriasis about ultraviolet light therapy (UVB). What should be included in teaching?
 1 'The exact effect of UVB is unknown, but it decreases severe itching.'
 2 'When combined with hot baths, UVB is very effective.'
 3 'Treatments with UVB have to be given in the hospital to be safe.'
 4 'UVB slows the growth of epidermal cells and decreases keratosis.'

4 Which of the following people is at risk of the development of a candidiasis infection?
 1 an older adult with pruritus
 2 a young woman who is pregnant
 3 an older man with a premalignant skin condition
 4 a young man with multiple naevi

5 Which questions should be included in a health history of a person with a linear pattern of painful vesicles over the left thorax?
 1 Do you remember being sunburned as a child?
 2 Are you a regular patron of tanning booths?
 3 Have you ever been diagnosed with acne?
 4 Did you have chickenpox when you were young?

6 Which of the following statements is true of an infestation with lice?
1 Only dirty people have lice.
2 Anyone can have lice.
3 Lice do not like to live on humans.
4 Lice are a form of fungus.

7 Which assessments would indicate a greater risk to develop a non-melanoma skin cancer?
1 blonde hair, freckles, fair skin
2 alopecia, thin hair, itching
3 dark hair, dark skin, dry skin
4 tanned skin, dark hair, oedema

8 Of the following, which is most significant to the development of a malignant melanoma?
1 a change in the colour or size of a naevus
2 sexual contacts with a person who has a herpesvirus infection
3 inadequate knowledge about infection prevention
4 a dietary intake of high-kilojoule foods

9 The rationale for lifting, rather than pulling, a person up in bed is that:
1 lifting a person allows a brief period of increased capillary circulation
2 lifting a person prevents tissue injury from shearing forces
3 pulling a person up in bed decreases tissue ischaemia and hypoxia
4 pulling a person up in bed promotes capillary blood flow

10 What STAR Skin Tear Classification would you assign to a skin tear where the edges can be aligned to the normal anatomical position without undue stretching and the skin or flap is pale, dusky or darkened?

BIBLIOGRAPHY

American Cancer Society (2015). *Treating skin cancer. Melanoma: Targeted therapy for melanoma skin cancer*. Retrieved from https://www.cancer.org/

Andriessen, A. et al. (2008). Assessment of a cleansing solution in the treatment of problem wounds. *Wounds*, *20*(6), 171–175.

Australian Commission on Safety and Quality in Health Care (ACSQHC) (2021). *National Safety and Quality Health Service Standards* (2nd ed.). Sydney: ACSQHC.

Australian Institute of Health and Welfare (AIHW) and Australasian Association of Cancer Registries (AACR) (2016). *Skin cancer in Australia*. Cat no. 96. Canberra: AIHW.

Bullock, S. & Hales, M. (2019). *Principles of pathophysiology* (2nd ed.). Frenchs Forest, NSW: Pearson.

Cancer Australia (2021). *Melanoma of the skin statistics*. Retrieved from https://www.canceraustralia.gov.au/

Cancer Council (2016). *National cancer prevention strategy: Ultraviolet radiation. Effective interventions: Eradication of solariums*. Retrieved from https://www.cancer.org.au/

Cancer Council (2021a). *Understanding skin cancer*. Retrieved from https://www.cancer.org.au/

Cancer Council (2021b). *Skin cancer: Non-melanoma*. Retrieved from https://www.cancer.org.au/

Carville, K. (2012). *Wound care manual* (6th ed.). Osborne Park, WA: Silver Chain Foundation.

Carville, K. (2017). *Wound care manual* (7th ed.). Osborne Park, WA: Silver Chain Foundation.

Carville, K., Leslie, G., Osseiran-Moisson, R., Newall, N. & Lewin, G. (2014). The effectiveness of a twice-daily skin-moisturising regimen for reducing the incidence of skin tears. *International Wound Journal*, *11*, 446–453.

Carville, K., Lewin, G., Newall, N. et al. (2007). STAR: A consensus for skin tear classification. *Primary Intention*, 15(1), 18–28.

Carville, K. & Smith, J. (2004). A report on the effectiveness of comprehensive wound assessment and documentation in the community. *Primary Intention*, *12*(1), 41–49.

Chianca, T. C., Rezende, J. F., Borges, E. L., Nogueira, V. L. & Caliri, M. H. (2010). Pressure ulcer knowledge among nurses in a Brazilian university hospital. *Ostomy Wound Management*, *56*(10), 58–64.

Clinical Excellence Commission (2019). *2018 NSW pressure injury point prevalence survey report*. Sydney: Clinical Excellence Commission, NSW Health.

Conner-Kerr, T. et al. (2010). The effects of low-frequency ultrasound (35 khz) on methicillin-resistant *Staphylococcus aureus* (MRSA) in vitro. *Ostomy Wound Management*, *56*(5), 32–42.

Crisp, J., Douglas, C., Rebeiro, G. & Waters, D. (2020). *Potter and Perry's fundamentals of nursing* (6th ed.). Chatswood, NSW: Elsevier.

de Menezes, S. (2016). *Pruritus*. DermNet NZ. Retrieved from https://dermnetnz.org/

DermNet NZ (2014). *Fingertip unit*. Retrieved from https://dermnetnz.org/

Diaz, J. H. & Nesbitt, L. J. (2013). Sun exposure behavior and protection: Recommendations for travelers. *Journal of Travel Medicine*, *20*(2), 108–118.

Dowsett, C. (2011). Moisture in wound healing: Exudate management. *British Journal of Community Nursing*, S6–S12.

European Pressure Ulcer Advisory Panel (EPUAP), National Pressure Injury Advisory Panel (NPIAP) & Pan Pacific Pressure Injury Alliance (PPPIA) (2019). *Prevention and treatment of pressure ulcers/injuries: Clinical practice guideline*. The international guideline. Retrieved from https://www.internationalguideline.com

Feldmeier, H. (2014). Treatment of pediculosis capitis: A critical appraisal of the current literature. *American Journal of Clinical Dermatology*, *15*, 401–412.

Forstner, C., Leitgeb, J., Schuster, R., Dosch, V., Kramer, A., Cutting, K. F. & Assadian, O. (2013). Bacterial growth kinetics under a novel flexible methacrylate dressing serving as a drug delivery vehicle for antiseptics. *International Journal of Molecular Sciences*, *14*(5), 1582–1590.

Gawchik, S. M. (2011). Latex allergy. *Mount Sinai Journal of Medicine*, *78*(5), 759–772.

Gebauer, K. & Carville, K. (2022). Discoloured nails. *Wound Practice and Research*, *30*(1), 50–54.

Grossman, S. & Porth, C. (2014). *Porth's pathophysiology: Concepts of altered health states* (9th ed.). Philadelphia: Lippincott Williams & Wilkins.

Gunningberg, L., Mårtensson, G., Mamhidir, A. G., Florin, J., Muntlin Athlin, Å. & Bååth, C. (2015). Pressure ulcer knowledge of registered nurses, assistant nurses and student nurses: A descriptive, comparative multicentre study in Sweden. *International Wound Journal*, *12*(4), 462–468.

Haeger, K. (1988). *The illustrated history of surgery*. London: Harold Starke.

International Federation for Spina Bifida and Hydrocephalus (IFSBH) (2018). *Latex allergy*. Retrieved from https://www.ifglobal.org/

International Wound Infection Institute (IWII) (2022). *Wound infection in clinical practice: Principles of best practice*. Wounds International. Retrieved from https://woundinfection-institute.com

James, G., Swogger, E., Wolcott, R. et al. (2008). Biofilms in chronic wounds. *Wound Repair and Regeneration*, *16*(1), 37–44.

Kaehn, K. & Eberlein, T. (2009). Prontosan made easy. *British Journal of Nursing*, *18*(11), S4–S10.

Keidan R. & Meyers, A. (2014). *Sentinel lymph node biopsy inpatient with melanoma*. Medscape. Retrieved from http://emedicine.medscape.com/

Lachenbruch, C., Tzen, Y. T., Brienza, D. M., Karg, P. E. & Lachenbruch, P. A. (2013). The relative contributions of interface pressure, shear stress, and temperature on tissue ischemia: A cross-sectional pilot study. *Ostomy/Wound Management*, *59*(3), 25–34.

Landis, E. (1930). Microcirculation studies of capillary blood pressure in human skin. *Heart*, *15*, 209–228.

Lawrence, P., Fulbrook, P. & Miles, S. (2015). Nurses' knowledge of pressure injury/pressure ulcer management. *Journal of Wound, Ostomy and Continence Nursing*, *42*(5), 450–460.

Leaper, D., Schultz, G, Carville, K., Fletcher, J., Swanson, T. & Drake, R. (2012). Extending the TIME concept: What have we learned in the past 10 years? *International Wound Journal*, 9(Suppl 2), 1–19.

LeBlanc K. et al. (2018). *Best practice recommendations for the prevention and management of skin tears in aged skin*. Wounds International. Retrieved from www.woundsinternational.com

LeBlanc K. & Baranoski, S. (2018) Skin tears: The under-appreciated enemy of aging skin. *Wounds International*, 9(1), 6–10

Luo, A. (2014). *Koebner phenomenon*. DermNet NZ. Retrieved from https://www.dermnetnz.org/

Mar, V., Wolfe, R. & Kelly, J. W. (2011). Predicting melanoma risk for the Australian population. *Australasian Journal of Dermatology*, *52*(2), 109–116.

Martini, F. H., Nath, J. L. & Bartholomew, E. F. (2018). *Fundamentals of anatomy and physiology* (11th ed.). San Francisco: Pearson Education.

Melanoma Institute Australia (2022). *Melanoma treatment*. Retrieved from https://melanoma.org.au

Melanoma Research Alliance (n.d.). *Breslow Depth and Clark Level*. Retrieved from https://www.curemelanoma.org/

Metz, M., Wahn, U., Gieler, U., Stock, P., Schmitt, J. & Blume-Peytavi, U. (2013). Chronic pruritus associated with dermatologic disease in infancy and childhood: Update from an interdisciplinary group of dermatologists and pediatricians. *Pediatric Allergy & Immunology, 24*(6), 527.

MIMS Online (2022). Retrieved from https://www.mimsonline.com.au/

Moffatt, C. (2004). Wound bed preparation in practice. *European Wound Management Position Document*. London: MEP Ltd.

Monstrey, S., Middelkoop, E., Vranckx, J. J., Bassetto, F., Ziegler, U. E., Meaume, S. & Téot, L. (2014). Review: Updated scar management practical guidelines: Non-invasive and invasive measures. *Journal of Plastic, Reconstructive & Aesthetic Surgery, 67*(8), 1017–1025.

Mulligan S., Prentice J. & Scott, L. (2011). *WoundsWest: Wound prevalence survey 2011—State-wide overview report*. Perth: Ambulatory Care Services, Department of Health.

Nguyen, K. H & Chaboyer, W. J. (2015). Pressure injury in Australian public hospitals: A cost-of-illness study. *Australian Health Review, 39*(3), 329–336.

Norman, R., Gibb, M., Dyer, A. et al. (2016). Improved wound management at lower cost: A sensible goal for Australia. *International Wound Journal, 13*(3), 303–316.

Oakley, A. (2014). *Psoriasis*. DermNet NZ. Retrieved from https://dermnetnz.org/

Oakley, A. (2018). *Treatment of psoriasis*. DermNet NZ. Retrieved from https://dermnetnz.org/

Papadakis, M., McPhee, S. & Rabow, M. (2018). *Current medical diagnosis and treatment* (57th ed.). New York: Lange McGraw Hill Medical Publications.

Payne, R. & Martin, M. (1993). Defining and classifying skin tears: Need for a common language: A critique and revision of the Payne–Martin Classification System for skin tears. *Ostomy Wound Management, 39*(5), 16–20.

Pharmaceutical Society of Australia (2018). *Australian pharmaceutical formulary* (24th ed.). Canberra: Author.

Phillips, P., Wolcott, P., Fletcher, J. & Schultz, G. (2010). Biofilms made easy. *Wounds International, 1*(3). Retrieved from https://www.woundsinternational.com

Phillips, P., Yang, Q., Sampson, E. & Schultz, G. (2010). Effects of antimicrobial agents on an in vitro biofilm model of skin wounds. *Advances in Wound Care, 1*, 299–304.

Polat, E., Aksöz, İ., Arkan, H., Coşkunpinar, E., Akbaş, F. & Onaran, İ. (2014). Gene expression profiling of *Lucilia sericata* larvae extraction/secretion-treated skin wounds. *Gene, 550*, 223–229.

Prentice, J., Morey, P. & Rodriguez, L. (2014). Clinical edge: Skin tears understanding causation, prevention and management. *Medicus, 54*(6), 40–41. Retrieved from http://search.informit.com.au/

Rayner, R., Carville, K. & Leslie, G. (2019). Defining age-related skin tears: A review. *Wound Practice & Research, 27*(3), 135–143.

Rayner, R., Carville, K., Leslie, G. & Dhaliwal, S. S. (2019). A risk model for the prediction of skin tears in aged care residents: A prospective cohort study. *International Wound Journal, 16*(1), 52–63. https://doi.org/10.1111/iwj.12985

Rayner, R., Carville, K., Leslie, G. & Dhaliwal, S. S. (2020). Models for predicting skin tears: A comparison. *International Wound Journal, 17*(3), 823–830. https://doi.org/10.1111/iwj.13340

Schultz, G., Sibbald, R., Falanga, V. et al. (2003). Wound bed preparation: A systematic approach to wound management. *Wound Repair and Regeneration* (Supplement), *11*(2S), S1–S28.

Shannon, M. K., Williams, A. & Bloomer, M. (2012). Low-frequency ultrasound debridement (Sonoca-185) in acute wound management: A case study. *Wound Practice & Research, 20*(4), 200–205.

Stavrou, D., Weissman, O., Winkler, E. et al. (2010). Silicone-based scar therapy: A review of the literature. *Anaesthetics & Plastic Surgery, 34*, 646–651.

Strachan, V., Prentice, J., Newall, N., Elmes, R., Carville, K., Santamaria, N. & Della, P. (2007). *WoundsWest wound prevalence survey 2007 state-wide report*. Perth: Ambulatory Care Services, Department of Health.

SunSmart Cancer Council of Victoria (2018). *Solariums and tanning*. Retrieved from https://www.sunsmart.com.au

Therapeutic Goods Administration (2018). *Sunscreens: Information for consumers*. Author. Retrieved from https://www.tga.gov.au/

Therapeutic Goods Administration (2021). *About sunscreen regulation*. Retrieved from https://www.tga.gov.au/

Victorian Department of Human Services, V. Strachan (ed.). (2006). *PUPPS 3: Pressure ulcer prevalence report*. Melbourne: Clinical Epidemiology and Health Services Evaluation Unit, Melbourne Health. Retrieved from http://www3.health.vic.gov.au/

Watkins, J. (2012). Benign skin tumours part 1: Macular or slightly raised lesions. *Practice Nursing, 23*(3), 135–136.

Wilson, L., Kapp, S. & Santamaria, N. (2019). The direct cost of pressure injuries in an Australian residential aged care setting. *International Wound Journal, 16*, 64–70.

Witte, E. & Sabat, R. (2014). Genetics of psoriasis. In W. Sterry, R. Sabat & S. Philipp (eds), *Psoriasis: Diagnosis and management*. Chichester, UK: John Wiley & Sons, Ltd. doi: 10.1002/9781118661796.ch5

Wolz, M. & Burge, S. (2014). The itch-scratch cycle: Quality of life assessment and management of atopic eczema in children. *Pediatrics & Therapeutics, 4*(2), 1–4. doi: 10.4172/2161-0665.1000198

Wounds Australia (2012). *Pan Pacific clinical practice guideline for the prevention and management of pressure injuries*. Retrieved from https://www.woundsaustralia.com.au/

Wounds UK (2020). Understanding Marjolin's ulceration. *Wounds UK, 16*(2), 50–53.

Xander, C., Meerpohl, J., Galandi, D., Buroh, S., Schweizer, G., Antes, G. & Becker, G. (2013). Pharmacological interventions for pruritus in adult palliative care patients. *Cochrane Database Systematic Reviews, 9*(6).

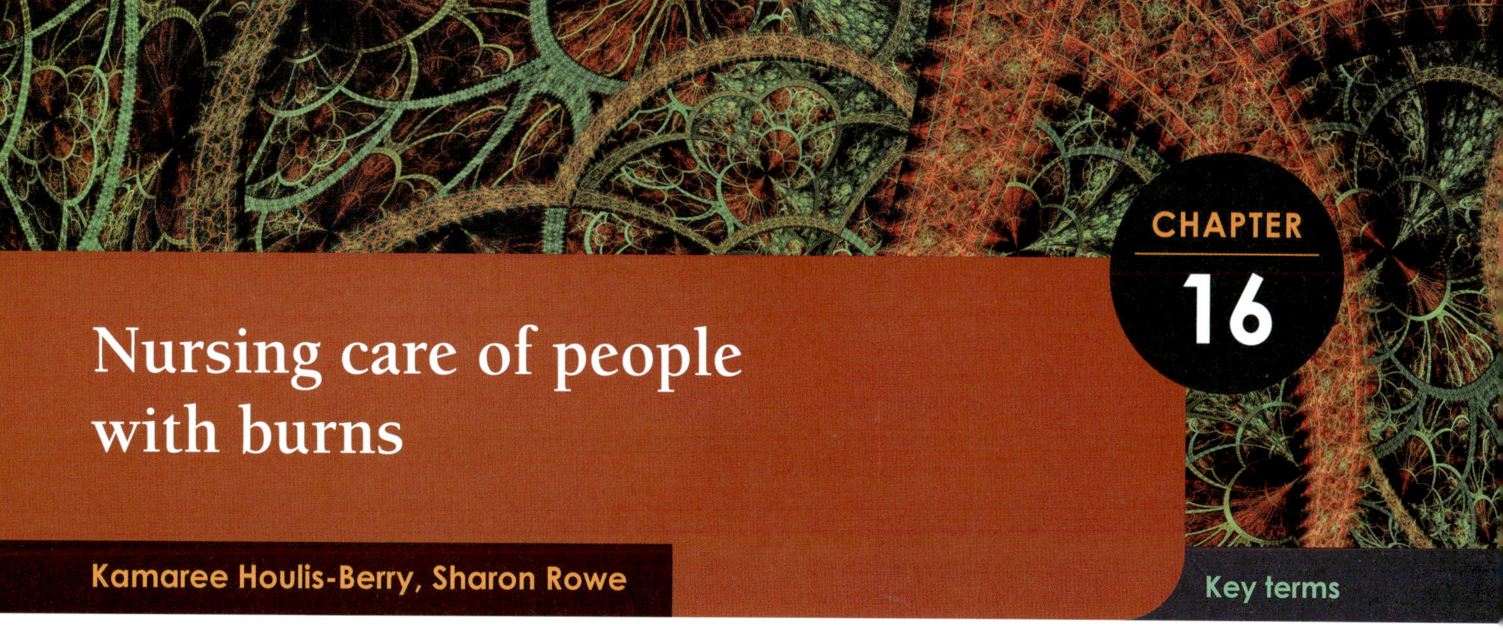

CHAPTER 16

Nursing care of people with burns

Kamaree Houlis-Berry, Sharon Rowe

Key terms

allograft 495
autograft 495
burn 474
burn shock 483
compartment syndrome 488
contracture 480
Curling's ulcers 490
debridement 497
eschar 480
escharotomy 494
fascial excision 495
fluid resuscitation 481
full-thickness burn 480
heterograft 495
homograft 495
hypertrophic scar 485
keloid 485
partial-thickness burn 479
superficial burn 478
surgical debridement 495
xenograft 495

Learning outcomes

- Discuss the types and causative agents of burns.
- Explain burn classification by depth and extent of injury.
- Describe the pathophysiology of a minor burn.
- Describe the pathophysiology of a major burn.
- Outline the role of the nurse as part of the interprofessional team in the provision of first aid, acute care and rehabilitation of a burned person.

Clinical competencies

- Assess the functional health status of people with burns and monitor, document and report abnormal manifestations.
- Use evidence-based research to plan and implement nursing care for people with burns.
- Determine priority nursing diagnoses, based on assessed data, to select and implement individualised nursing interventions for the person with burns.
- Administer medications knowledgeably and safely to people with burns.
- Integrate interprofessional care into care of people with burns.
- Provide teaching appropriate for prevention of burns.
- Revise plan of care as needed to provide effective interventions to promote, maintain or restore functional health status to people with burns.

A **burn** is an injury resulting from exposure to heat including friction, chemicals, radiation, cold injuries or electric current. A transfer of energy from a source of heat to the human body initiates a sequence of physiological events that in the most severe cases leads to irreversible tissue destruction. Burns range in severity from a minor loss of small segments of the outermost layer of the skin to a complex injury involving all body systems. Treatments vary from simple application of a topical wound dressing in an outpatient clinic or general practice to an invasive, multisystem, interprofessional team approach in the aseptic environment of a burn centre.

Over the past two decades, there have been worldwide improvements in the overall care of burns victims and, ultimately, an increased survival rate. These improvements include first aid, fluid resuscitation, nutrition, management of hypermetabolism, understanding of the post-burn immune response and technological advances in surgery and wound care products. All are a result of the continuous research into burns. In the 12 months to June 2021, 3,484 paediatric and adult patients with acute burn injury were admitted to Australian and New Zealand burn services—a decrease of 14% from the previous year. However, there were notable effects in admission times and length of stay due to the COVID-19 lockdowns experienced across the country.

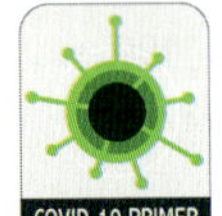

Furthermore, the rate of admission for the Aboriginal and Torres Strait Islander population (29.1% per 100,000) continues to be more than three times the rate of the non-Indigenous population (8.8% per 100,000) (Burns Registry of Australia and New Zealand (BRANZ), 2022).

Current data provided by the BRANZ (2022) highlighted that the most common burn injury among paediatric and adult patients were as follows:

- *Paediatric*: scalds 49% (common cause of injury across all age groups from 0 months to 15 years), contact 24%, flame 11% and friction burns 11%—data has remained consistent with previous reporting years
- *Adult*: flame 41% (common cause of injury in patients 16–79 years), scalds 28% (common cause of injury in patients over 80 years) and contact burns 17%.

These trends are consistent with data in other countries.

Geographically, 56% of burn injuries occurred in major cities, with 39% in regional Australia and 5% in remote areas. The rate per 100,000 people was higher in regional and remote areas than in the major cities and also higher in Indigenous people for each remoteness region, with the exception of very remote Australia (BRANZ, 2022).

Older adults and young children are more vulnerable to burn injuries because of their thinner skin. Burns in the older adult are complicated by comorbidities, lower threshold for infection, higher risk of pulmonary problems, a decrease in lean body mass, micronutrient deficiency or malnutrition. There is a higher proportion of older adults relative to the age distribution of the general population. It has been suggested that this may be due to older adults being more active than previously thought (Tracy et al., 2020). These factors all lead to an increased recovery time, and rebuilding of muscle tissue is slow. There is a thinning of the dermis in older adults and epidermal replacement is slowed.

FAST FACTS

High-risk populations

- Children
- Disabled
- Older adults
- Military

Scalds are the most common cause of burns in children, typically from hot tap water or from pulling a hot beverage onto themselves. Children are inquisitive and do not necessarily have a concept of danger, particularly if something looks interesting.

People in occupations involving work with chemicals, petrol and electricity, and those in military service, are at higher risk of burn injury. Burn and scald injuries caused by physical abuse to children or disabled or older people also occur. Abuse is suspected when a burn injury does not fit with the explanation of how it occurred; for example, scald burns show a clear line of demarcation, which could indicate deliberate immersion. The presence of small, circular burns may be the result of cigarette burns. Abused individuals may also present with poor personal hygiene status, evidence of malnutrition or behavioural problems. There may be associated soft tissue injury or fractures and old scars. In older adults, the burn may be a result of self-neglect rather than neglect by others (Herndon, 2018). Healthcare workers should be careful when using heat packs, heat lamps and electrical equipment when caring for older people or the young.

Older people are vulnerable to fire and burn injuries because of potentially impaired visual acuity, depth perception, sense of smell, hearing and mobility. All of these factors increase the risk of accidental burn injury and increased mortality.

Deaths due to a burn injury are considered uncommon in high-income countries such as Australia. Now, only 1% of patients die in hospital and the proportion of deaths increases with the increased size of the burn. Multisystem organ failure is the most common cause of death (43%), followed by burns shock (33%) (BRANZ, 2022).

Many burns can be prevented. Nurses can play a part in educating the public about prevention of burns, burns first aid and care of minor burn injuries at home. Box 16.1 identifies some common tips for preventing burns that nurses can advocate to the wider public.

FAST FACTS

The aims of early burn management are to:

1. preserve life
2. preserve quality of life: functional and cosmetic.

BOX 16.1 Burn prevention tips

- Store matches and lighters out of reach of children in a locked cupboard.
- Never leave children unattended around fire or in the bathroom or bathtub.
- Install and maintain smoke detectors in the home and regularly check that they are working. Change smoke detector batteries at the same time each year (check state/territory fire service recommendations). Create a fire escape plan and practise the plan with children, carers and all members of the household.
- Set the water heater temperature at 50°C or lower and always test the temperature of the bath water.
- Never smoke in bed.
- Never throw flammable liquids onto an already burning fire.
- Never use flammable liquids to start fires.
- Never remove a radiator cap from a hot engine.
- Watch for overhead electrical wires and underground wires when working outside.
- Use safety electrical switches in electrical boxes and never overload power outlets.
- Store cleaning solutions and paints in well-labelled containers away from naked flame and out of reach of children, or in a locked cupboard.
- Keep looking when cooking.
- Keep a working fire extinguisher and fire blanket in your home and workplace

For further information on injury prevention for children, see https://kidsafe.com.au

TYPES OF BURN INJURY

The types of burn injury are thermal, chemical, electrical, radiation, cold injury and friction. The extent of the injury is determined by the causative agent, length of time the tissue is exposed to the agent, body part involved and depth of burn.

Thermal burns

Thermal burns result from exposure to dry heat (flames) or moist heat (steam and hot liquids). Direct exposure to the source of heat causes cellular destruction, resulting in damage to the skin and underlying structures.

Immediate management of thermal burns

In the case of flames, the person should stop, drop and roll to extinguish the flames. Clothing should be removed where possible and first aid commenced. First aid is the application of cool running water for at least 20 minutes. Management of thermal burns is discussed in detail later in this chapter.

Chemical burns

Chemical burns are caused by direct skin contact with acids, alkaline agents or toxic organic compounds (see Box 16.2 for specific household agents). The chemical denatures tissue protein, leading to necrosis. Chemical elements may also have a systemic effect as their elements circulate through the injured person.

BOX 16.2 Household cleaning agents that may cause burns

- Drain cleaners
- Lye
- Industrial-strength ammonia
- Household ammonia
- Oven cleaners
- Toilet bowl cleaners
- Dishwasher detergents
- Bleach

Chemical burn severity is determined by the:

- strength or concentration of the agent
- type of agent
- duration of contact
- amount of body surface area involved
- mechanism of action of the agent.

Chemical agents are further classified according to the manner by which they structurally alter proteins. Chemical burns are classified according to six mechanisms of action: reduction, oxidation, corrosive agents, protoplasmic poison, vesicants and desiccants. Chemicals can also cause eye injuries, as well as other systemic problems. Burning chemicals and substances give off toxic gases that cause inhalation injuries.

Alkalis

Alkalis cause liquefaction of the skin, which allows the alkali to move deeper into the tissue. Examples of alkalis include lime, sodium hydroxide and potassium hydroxide. These are present in many household cleaning products and workplace chemicals. Cement is both an alkali and a desiccant. It can penetrate clothing and when combined with sweat causes an exothermic reaction.

Acids

Acids are found in many household agents and include oxalic acid, hydrofluoric acid and hydrochloric acid. Acids often cause hard, dry eschar to form. However, hydrochloric acid fumes can also cause inhalation injury (Bajraktarova-Valjakova et al., 2018). Hydrofluoric acid is a common industrial acid that causes coagulation necrosis and cellular death. The resultant chelating of calcium and magnesium causes a depletion of intracellular calcium, leading to death Calcium gluconate should be used as first aid; if not available, the area should have copious irrigation (Herndon, 2018).

Organic compounds

Organic compounds such as petroleum distillates cause damage by dissolving the lipid wall of cell membranes and may also cause renal and liver failure if absorbed. Some organic compounds such as phenols and petroleum products cause both a contact burn and systemic toxicity. Protoplasmic poisons, such as organic compounds, form salts with proteins, inhibiting calcium and other ions needed for cell viability.

Immediate management of chemical burns

Following a chemical burn, the most important first aid intervention is to remove the chemical from the skin. This should include removing all contaminated clothing and irrigation of the area with large amounts of tepid water. Care should be taken to prevent spread of the chemical on unaffected skin or on the person giving assistance. If there is dry alkali residue, it should be brushed off carefully prior to irrigation with cool running water that should be directed 'to the floor' or down a suitable drain, not in a bath where the chemical will spread to other areas of the body. The pH of the affected skin can be monitored with the use of pH indicator sticks to determine the efficacy of first aid measures. Remember to monitor for hypothermia as irrigation periods may be from 20 minutes to 2 hours (Chai et al., 2022). Irrigation should not be performed with elemental metals such as lithium, potassium, sodium and magnesium. Combining these metals with water produces an exothermic reaction causing thermal injury. The area should be soaked in mineral oil and the metallic pieces removed with forceps, or the area should be covered in gauze soaked in mineral oil (e.g. liquid paraffin).

The use of a neutralising agent (e.g. Diphoterine) is supported in the literature as being an effective first aid for chemical burns. Irrigation should not be delayed if a neutralising agent is not available or cannot be located. It is reported to resolve pH faster and decrease tissue necrosis. Irrigation with tepid water is still recommended following the use of a neutralising agent (Chai et al., 2022).

A person who has sustained a chemical burn should be directed to an emergency centre for prompt and appropriate care. At time of injury a chemical burn may not appear to have caused much damage. However, the damage can be ongoing. Wound management principles for chemical burns are the same as for thermal burns. General advanced trauma life support principles—that is, the ABCs of basic life support—should always be followed and include maintenance of haemodynamics.

Electrical burns

The severity of electrical burns depends on the type (alternating or direct current), duration of current, amount of voltage, resistance at point of contact and individual susceptibility. In Australia, electrical injuries are classified as low or high voltage. Low-voltage injuries are caused by electric currents below 1,000 volts; high-voltage injuries are caused by over 1,000 volts or up to 33,000 volts in high-tension cables. However, less than 12 volts—for instance, that produced by a car battery—can cause a burn due to a short circuit if the person is wearing a ring or a watch (Nischwitz et al., 2020). A high-voltage burn is associated with deep, underlying tissue damage similar to a crush injury. Low-voltage burns are usually more localised. Immediate death can occur as a result of current-induced ventricular fibrillation or asystole, or from respiratory arrest resulting from paralysis of the central respiratory control system and respiratory muscles (Nischwitz et al., 2020).

Electric current exists in two forms: alternating current (AC), in which the electrons move back and forth through a conductor in a cyclical fashion; and direct current (DC), in which the electrons flow in one direction. An AC current, like that found in conventional households, produces repeated electrical surges that lead to tetanic muscle contractions that can cause further injury through prolonged contact with the source or if the person is thrown. Loss of consciousness can also result in longer contact exposure. Any differences in potential injuries caused by AC and DC currents are in relation to low-voltage injuries, as high-voltage currents have a similar effect. The heart can be affected either by direct necrosis of the heart tissue or by arrhythmias. Cardiac complications are the most serious injuries associated with electrical burns and are fatal unless resuscitation measures are commenced. Respiratory arrest can occur as a result of injury to the respiratory control centre in the brain or as a result of muscle contractions causing a form of suffocation.

In addition to the injury caused by the electric current passing through vital organs, the person can receive an arc injury and a flame injury if clothing catches fire. Electric current follows the line of least resistance, and in the body this is along blood vessels and through organs, rather than through bone and fat. Deeper tissues retain the heat, and structures between bones sustain more damage than superficial structures (Herndon, 2018).

Direct current injury—for example, caused by lightning—exposes the body to very high voltage for a short period of time. Lightning is the result of the electrical difference between a thundercloud and the ground overcoming the insulating properties of the surrounding air. Lightning injuries can range from minor to major burns. Formation of cataracts is the most common permanent injury resulting from lightning strikes. Cardiac and respiratory arrest can occur, as can damage to tympanic membranes in the middle and inner ear.

Immediate management of electrical burns

Advanced trauma life support principles should be followed as soon as possible. The person should be transferred to a hospital with a burns unit. Initially, an electrical injury can look less severe than it actually is, as most of the damage is beneath the skin surface. A thorough history of the event may assist in determining the pathway of the current and the areas of injury. The person should be checked for any fractures that may have occurred and cervical spine precautions should be adhered to, particularly if the person was thrown or fell. Cardiac arrest, arrhythmias, metabolic acidosis and myoglobinuria are complications of electrical injury and need specialist medical treatment at a burn centre. The person should be monitored for cardiac complications and have an ECG performed. Pigments from muscle damage (myoglobin) and red blood cell damage (haemoglobin) can cause the urine to become dark. If untreated, myoglobinuria can lead to acute renal failure (Herndon, 2018) (see Figure 16.1). Urine output should be maintained at 1–2 mL/kg/hr (Australian and New Zealand Burn Association Ltd (ANZBA), 2018).

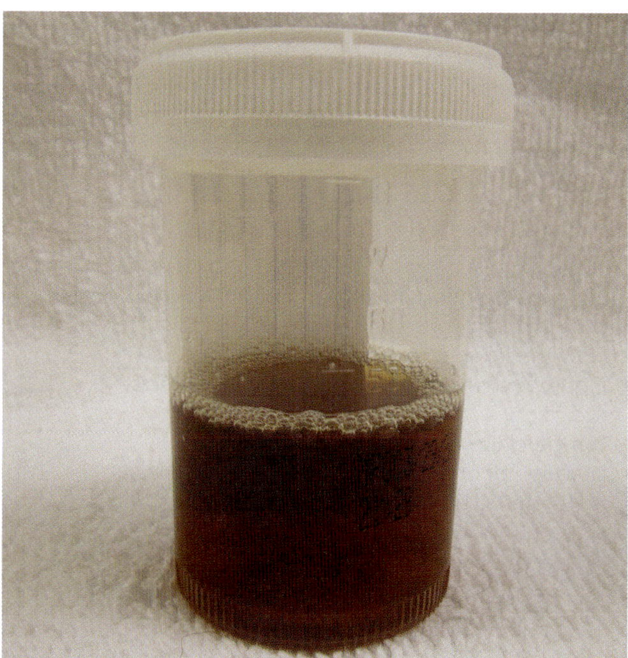

FIGURE 16.1 *Urine with myoglobinuria. Myoglobinuria turns the urine dark brown*

Source: Dr P. Marazzi/Science Photo Library/Alamy Stock Photo.

Radiation burns

Ionising radiation is mediated by energy transference. It can, for example, be the result of exposure to electromagnetic radiation, x-ray or particulate radiation (alpha and beta particles or neutrons). Exposure can be from small accidents occurring in a laboratory or x-ray in a hospital. Major accidents may stretch hospital resources, as in the case of multi-trauma from military detonation of nuclear devices.

The overall extent of damage depends on the dose of radiation exposure. Skin changes usually range from erythema to dry desquamation of epidermal cells. Partial-thickness burns may occur and are known as moist desquamation. Full-thickness burns can occur a few weeks to months after exposure. The most severe radiation injuries result from nuclear weapons and are a combination of thermal and radiation injuries

Sunburn tends to be superficial, involving only the epidermis; however, sunburned neonates, infants, children and older people can have significant injuries. Associated sunburn symptoms can include local discomfort, oedema, heat stroke and dehydration.

Immediate management of radiation burns

The management of radiation burns will differ subject to the cause (sunburn or exposure to radioactive substances) and local and systemic effects experienced. Management of relatively minor radiation burns involves removing patient from source, ABC of resuscitation procedures, removing contaminated clothing and copious irrigation to neutralise particles (Swain & Khan, 2019).

Management of radiation burns that occur following treatment for cancer tends to be subject to the policies of each radiotherapy unit.

Long-term effects of exposure to radiation include cancer and slow wound healing. Larger exposures or incidents can overwhelm hospital resources.

Cold injury

Cold-induced injury (also known as frostbite or localised hypothermia) is divided into two groups: peripheral cold injury and systemic hypothermia. Although peripheral cold injury is not common in Australia and New Zealand, prevalence is noted among homeless people, those with an interest in winter outdoor activities or individuals with alterations in cognition or perception due to dementia, high alcohol consumption or psychiatric disorders. Frostbite results when tissue temperatures fall below freezing and decreased blood flow causes tissue necrosis. Depth of injury from frostbite is classified similarly to burn injury. A cold injury can also be caused by the low boiling point of liquefied petroleum gas (LPG). This can result in a cold injury similar to frostbite. Tradespeople such as refrigeration mechanics are at risk of such an injury (ANZBA, n.d.).

If the exposure to freezing temperatures is limited, only the skin and subcutaneous tissues become involved; however, as exposure increases, deeper structures freeze. Frostbite is most common on exposed or peripheral areas of the body, such as the nose, ears, feet and hands.

As human tissues freeze, ice crystals form and increase intracellular sodium content. Small blood vessels initially vasoconstrict, but then vasodilate and become more permeable, causing cellular and tissue swelling. Continued exposure increases vasoconstriction, and increased viscosity of the blood causes infarction and necrosis of the affected tissue.

Superficial frostbite causes numbness, itching and prickling. The skin appears cyanotic, reddened or white. Deeper frostbite causes stiffness and paraesthesia. As the skin and tissues thaw, the skin becomes white or yellow and loses its elasticity. The person experiences burning pain. Oedema, blisters, necrosis and gangrene may present.

Immediate management of cold injuries

The biggest challenge in the field is to not cause further injury. Remove jewellery from affected area. Protect affected area from injury as the area is likely to be insensate.

Rapid thawing may significantly decrease tissue necrosis. General guidelines for re-warming areas of frostbite are:

- If outdoors, treat superficial frostbite by applying firm pressure with a warm hand or by placing frostbitten hands in the axillae. If the feet are frostbitten, remove wet footwear, dry the feet and put on dry footwear. Re-warming should not be commenced in the field unless there is certainty that the re-warming can continue uninterrupted.

Refreezing of affected parts causes further damage. Monitor person for hypothermia as well. Do not rub the areas with snow.

- In the hospital, rapidly re-warm affected areas in circulating warm water containing a mild antibacterial agent (such as povidine–iodine or chlorhexidine)—37–40°C to 40.5°C—for at least 30 minutes until complete thawing.

Following re-warming, the person is kept on bed rest with the affected parts elevated. Pain medications and anti-inflammatory agents are administered. Topical wound management is instigated subject to assessment outcomes. Recovery from frostbite is usually complete if the involved area has not become necrotic. Necrotic tissue may require debridement or amputation of affected digits or limbs. Fluid resuscitation is not required unless clinical dehydration is determined.

Inhalation injury

An inhalation injury occurs as a result of inhalation of toxic by-products of combustion or smoke inhalation. This is discussed later in this chapter.

Friction burns

Friction burns occur as a result of the heat caused when the body is moved across a hard surface, such as a road or grass. Depth can vary from an abrasion to a wound that has blistered. Examples of injuries that may cause a friction burn are a rope that is pulled through a person's hand or a fall from a bike onto a hard surface.

BURN CLASSIFICATION

Tissue damage following a burn is determined primarily by two factors: depth of the burn (the layers of underlying tissue affected) and extent of the burn (the percentage of body surface area involved). The assessment of the total body surface area and depth is then used to guide resuscitation and management protocols.

Depth of the burn

The depth of a burn injury is determined by the elements of the skin that have been damaged or destroyed. Burn depth results from a combination of the temperature of the burning agent and the length of contact. Burns are classified as superficial, partial-thickness or full-thickness burns. Characteristics of burns are outlined in Table 16.1 and illustrated in Figure 16.2.

FAST FACTS

Factors to be considered when determining the depth of burn include:

- How the injury occurred
- Causative agent (flame, chemical, electricity, radiation)
- Temperature of burning agent
- Duration of contact
- Age-related skin thickness
- Anatomical location of burn
- First aid measures employed

Superficial burns

A **superficial burn** involves only the epidermal layer of the skin (see Figure 16.3). This type of burn most often results from damage from sunburn, ultraviolet light, minor flash injury (from a sudden ignition or explosion) or mild radiation burn associated with cancer treatment. Because the skin remains intact, this degree of burn is not calculated into the estimates of burn injury. Due to the increased blood supply to the area, the erythema ranges from pink to bright red and there may be slight oedema over the burned area. Superficial burns involving large body surface areas may be accompanied by chills, headache, nausea and vomiting. The injury usually heals in 3 to 6 days, with dryness and peeling of the outer layer of skin. There is generally no scar formation as a result. Superficial burns are treated with analgesia and the application of non-perfumed moisturising ointments and lotions. Extensive superficial burns, especially in infants and older people, may require intravenous fluid treatment. Superficial burns can convert to partial-thickness wounds if inappropriate treatment is administered or infection and swelling are untreated.

TABLE 16.1 The characteristics of burns

	BURN DEPTH			
	Superficial	**Superficial partial**	**Deep partial**	**Full thickness**
Wound appearance	Involves the epithelium • Painful • Red or pink	Epidermis and superficial (papillary) dermis destroyed • Painful • Often blistered • Pink, moist • Blanches	Involves epidermis and reticular dermis • May blister • Mottled pink or white • Fairly dry > day 2 • Discomfort rather than pain • Slow or no capillary refill	Involves epidermis and dermis, and may include fat • Does not blanch • May be mottled, dry, translucent, black or pale in appearance • Full-thickness scalds may have red non-blanching appearance
Healing and scarring	Complete scarless healing within 7-10 days	Heals by epithelial migration within 2 weeks • Can convert to a deeper burn	Will take more than 3 weeks to heal • Will leave a scar if > 3 weeks to heal	Will require surgery unless very small wound • Will have a scar if left to heal without surgery • Early excision and grafting reduce scarring and contracture

Sources: T. McWilliams, Perth Children's Hospital, and S. Rowe, Fiona Stanley Hospital.

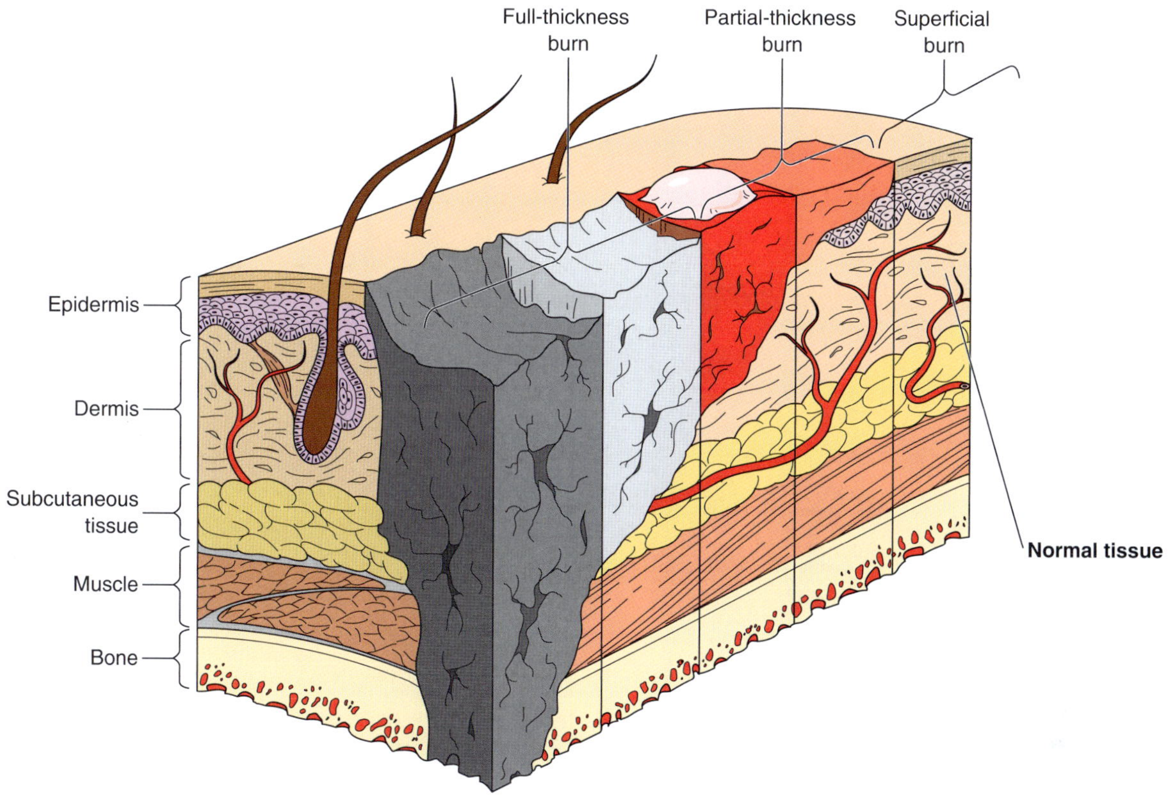

FIGURE 16.2 ***Burn injury classification according to the depth of the burn***

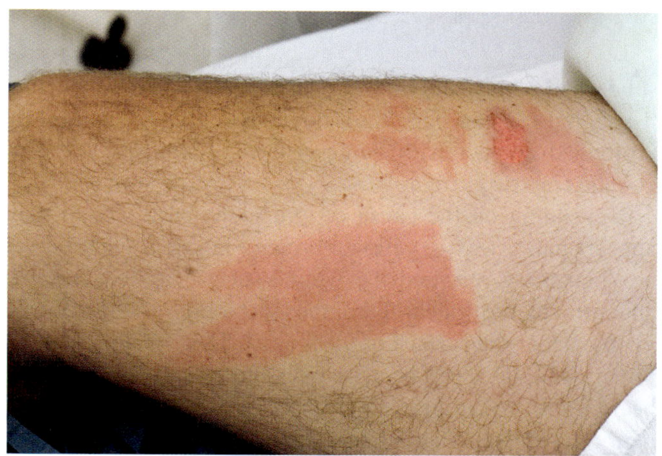

FIGURE 16.3 ***Superficial burn injury***

Source: Royal Perth Hospital.

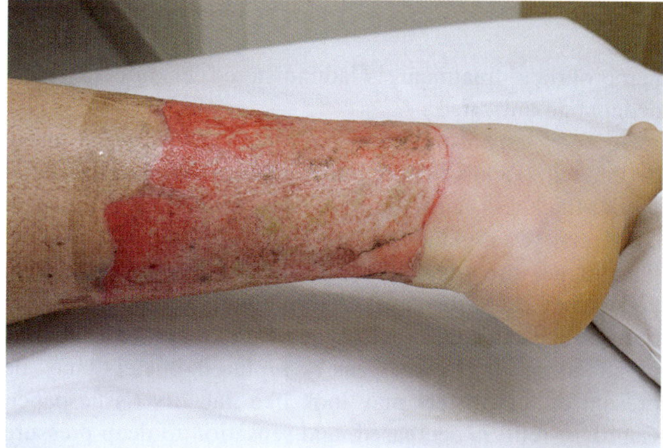

FIGURE 16.4 ***Mid-dermal or partial-thickness burn injury***

Source: Royal Perth Hospital.

Partial-thickness burns

Partial-thickness burns may be subdivided into superficial partial-thickness and deep partial-thickness burns. The classification depends on the depth of the burn.

A *superficial partial-thickness burn* involves the entire epidermis and the papillae of the dermis. Causes may include such injuries as brief exposure to a flash flame, dilute chemical agents or contact with a hot surface. This burn is often bright red, but has a moist, glistening appearance with blister formation (see Figure 16.4). The burned area will blanch on pressure, and touch and pain sensation remains intact. Pain in response to temperature and air is usually severe. These injuries heal within 14 days with minimal or no scarring, but pigment changes are common. Analgesics are administered and the wound will require a dressing. Superficial partial-thickness burns can convert to a deep partial if

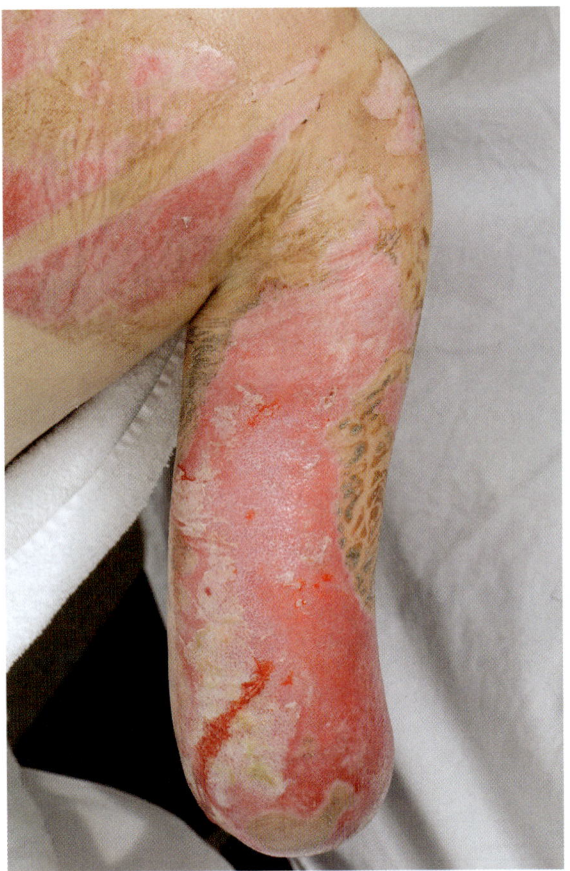

FIGURE 16.5 ***Deep partial-thickness burn injury***

Source: Royal Perth Hospital.

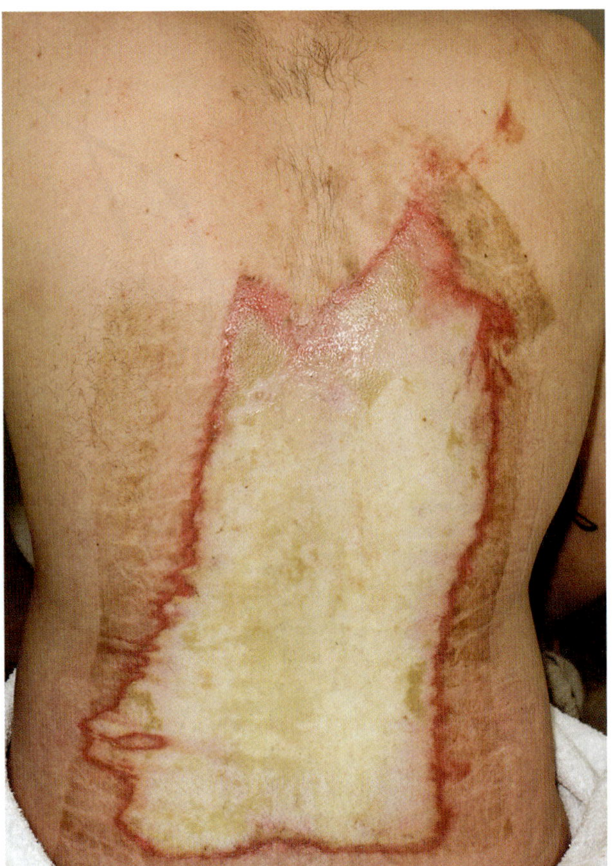

FIGURE 16.6 ***Full-thickness burn injury***

Source: Royal Perth Hospital.

inappropriate treatment is administered or infection and oedema go untreated.

A *deep partial-thickness burn* also involves the entire dermis but extends further into the dermis than a superficial partial-thickness burn. Hair follicles, sebaceous glands and epidermal sweat glands remain intact. Hot liquids or solids, flash flame, direct flame, intense radiant energy or chemical agents may cause this level of burn injury. The surface of the burn wound can appear pale, blotchy red or mottled, and may be moist or dry. Large, easily ruptured blisters may be present or the blisters may look like flat, dry tissue paper. Capillary refill is decreased, and sensation to deep pressure is present. The burn wound is less painful than a superficial partial-thickness burn, but areas of pain and areas of decreased sensation may be present. Deep partial-thickness burn wounds will take more than 21 days for healing and may convert to a full-thickness injury if necrosis extends the depth of the injury. **Contractures** are possible, as are hypertrophic scarring and functional impairment (see Figure 16.5). Excision and grafting may be necessary to decrease scarring and loss of function.

Full-thickness burns

A **full-thickness burn** involves all layers of the skin, including the epidermis, the dermis and the epidermal appendages (see Figure 16.6). The burn wound may extend to the subdermal level involving the subcutaneous fat, connective tissue, muscle and bone. Full-thickness burns are caused by prolonged contact with flames, steam, chemicals or high-voltage electric current.

Depending on the cause of injury, the burn wound may appear pale, waxy, yellow, brown, mottled, charred or non-blanching red, and the wound surface is dry, leathery and firm to the touch. Thrombosed blood vessels may be visible under the surface of the wound. There is no sensation of pain on light touch because pain and touch receptors have been destroyed, although there may be deeper discomfort or pain felt. Full-thickness burns require skin grafting to heal. In dark-skinned people, assessment of burned area should be done with gloved hands assessing for skin turgor and pain. The dead skin of the full-thickness burn wound is called **eschar** (Herndon, 2018).

Extent of the burn

Accurate assessment of the extent of burn injury is one of the most important aspects of initial care in the emergency treatment of burn injury. The extent of the burn injury is expressed as a percentage of the total body surface area (TBSA) or body surface area (BSA) and is determined according to validated guides (Rice & Orgill, 2021). Two of the most used guides to estimate TBSA and extent of burn wound are the Wallace (1951)

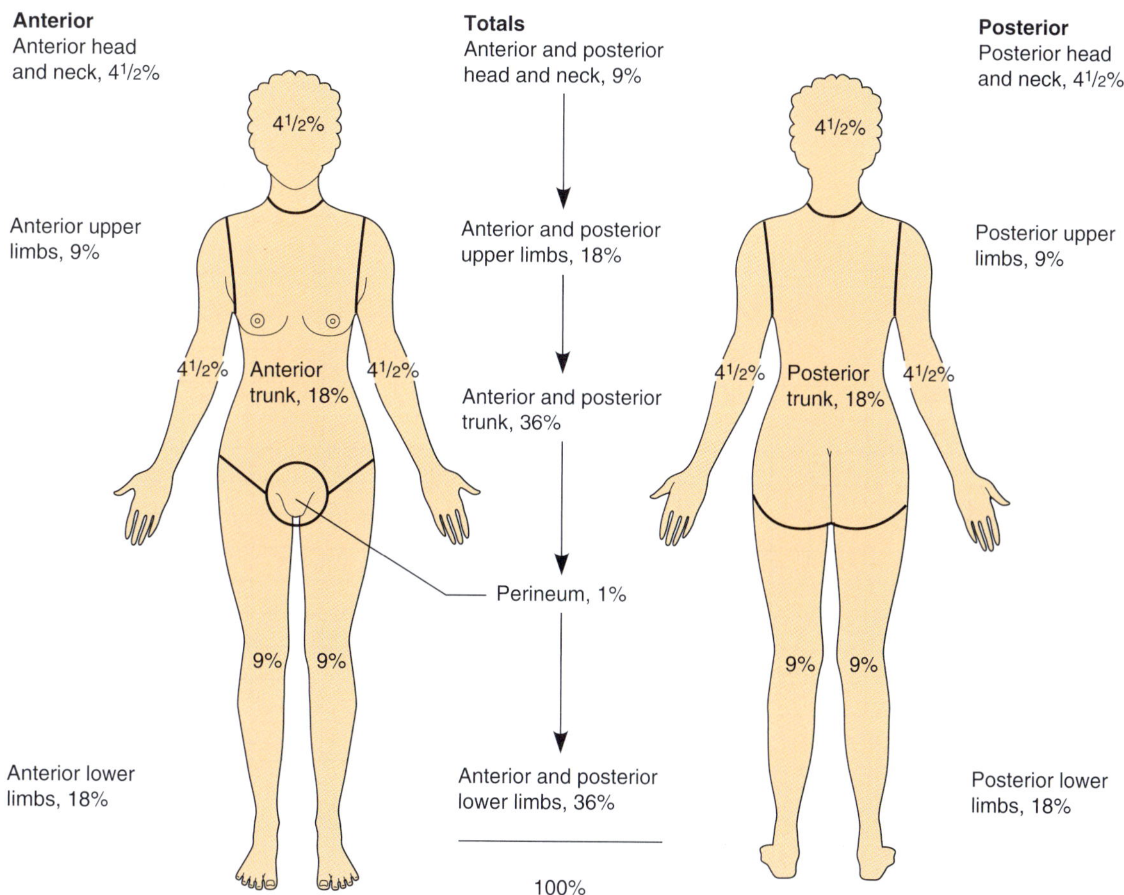

FIGURE 16.7 *The rule of nines (Wallace, 1951) is one method for quickly estimating the percentage of TBSA affected by a burn injury. Although useful in emergency care situations, the rule of nines is not accurate for estimating TBSA for adults who are short, obese or very thin, or for children*

rule of nines (see Figure 16.7) and the Lund and Browder (1944) burn assessment chart (see Figure 16.8).

Only partial-thickness and full-thickness burns are included in the estimation; superficial erythema is not classified as a percentage of TBSA. The rule of nines is adequate for initial assessment, but for irregularly shaped burns the palmar surface of the patient's hand (including fingers) is considered 1% TBSA. The percentage of TBSA is reassessed after oedema has subsided and demarcation of zones of injury has occurred. The rule of nines is relatively accurate in adults but is not suitable for children as children's body surface area proportions differ. Children have relatively large heads and smaller lower bodies than adults. Using the rule of nines on a child could lead to overestimation of TBSA and subsequent inaccurate **fluid resuscitation**. The Lund and Browder burn assessment chart is used for paediatric burn injuries.

The Wallace rule of nines

The Wallace rule of nines divides the surface area of the body into segments of 9%, 18% and 1%.

Head and neck	9% TBSA
Anterior torso	18% TBSA
Posterior torso	18% TBSA
Legs	18% TBSA
Arms	9% TBSA
Groin	1% TBSA

See Figure 16.7 for an example.

Lund and Browder burn assessment chart

Fluid loss in children is proportionally greater than in adults due to their body weight to body surface area ratio. Fluid loss is directly proportional to the burned surface area, so the rule of nines is inadequate in children under 16 years of age (ANZBA, 2018). Resuscitation fluid formulae for children are based on body surface area and account for age, height and weight. This formula was initially proposed by Lund and Browder (1944), and an assessment chart that takes these factors into account has been named after these practitioners (see Figure 16.8).

For example, a person with burns to the face, anterior right arm and anterior trunk has the following burn injury:

Face = 4.5%
Arm = 4.5%
Trunk = 18%
= 27% TBSA.

Area	Age (years)					% 1∞	% 2∞	% 3∞	% Total
	0–1	1–4	5–9	10–15	Adult				
Head	19	17	13	10	7				
Neck	2	2	2	2	2				
Ant. trunk	13	13	13	13	13				
Post. trunk	13	13	13	13	13				
R. buttock	2½	2½	2½	2½	2½				
L. buttock	2½	2½	2½	2½	2½				
Genitalia	1	1	1	1	1				
R.U. arm	4	4	4	4	4				
L.U. arm	4	4	4	4	4				
R.L. arm	3	3	3	3	3				
L.L. arm	3	3	3	3	3				
R. hand	2½	2½	2½	2½	2½				
L. hand	2½	2½	2½	2½	2½				
R. thigh	5½	6½	8½	8½	9½				
L. thigh	5½	6½	8½	8½	9½				
R. leg	5	5	5½	6	7				
L. leg	5	5	5½	6	7				
R. foot	3½	3½	3½	3½	3½				
L. foot	3½	3½	3½	3½	3½				
					Total				

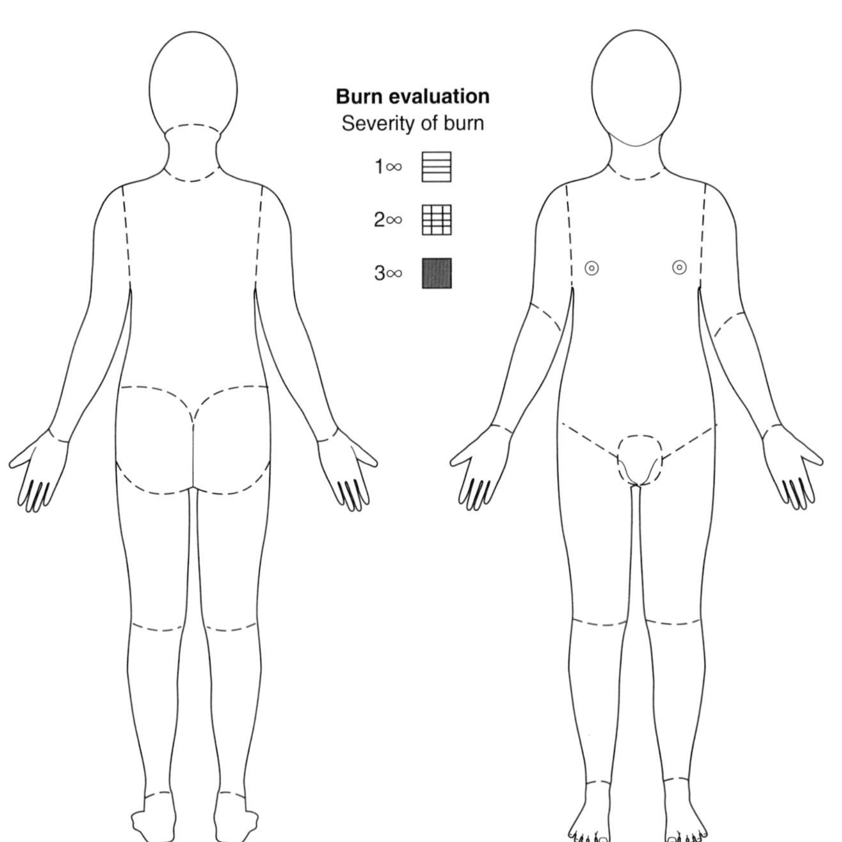

FIGURE 16.8 *The Lund and Browder (1944) burn assessment chart. This method of estimating TBSA affected by a burn injury is more accurate than the rule of nines because it accounts for changes in body surface area across the lifespan. As individual burn units may use a modified Lund and Browder chart, practitioners are advised to familiarise themselves with local assessment guidelines*

BOX 16.3 The Australian and New Zealand Burn Association referral criteria for transfer to a burns unit

- Burns greater than 10% total body surface area (TBSA)
- Burns greater than 5% TBSA in children
- Burns of specialised areas—face, hands, feet, genitalia, perineum and major joints
- Full-thickness burns greater than 5% TBSA
- Electrical burns
- Chemical burns
- Burns associated with inhalation injury
- Circumferential burns of the limbs and chest
- Burns in children and older adults
- Burns in people with pre-existing medical disorders that could complicate management, prolong recovery or increase risk of mortality
- Burn injury in pregnant women
- Burns with associated trauma
- Non-accidental burns

Source: ANZBA (2018). *Emergency management of severe burns*. Course manual (version 18). © Australian and New Zealand Burn Association Ltd. Reproduced with permission.

Phases of burn management

Burns are a traumatic event and as such clinicians need to follow the advanced trauma life support guidelines in addition to performing primary, secondary and tertiary surveys.

Management of burn injuries is divided into the resuscitative, acute and rehabilitative phases, although there is overlap of all phased interventions, particularly those involving wound management and rehabilitation. Rehabilitation starts on day 1 and may continue for months or years after wounds have healed.

1. Resuscitative phase:
   - First aid
   - Primary survey
   - Secondary survey.
2. Acute wound healing phase.
3. Rehabilitative phase.

The resuscitative phase begins at the time of injury and lasts until the fluid resuscitation phase is completed, which usually lasts 48 to 72 hours. The acute wound healing phase commences as part of the secondary survey. The rehabilitative phase commences on day one; all interventions from first aid through the continuum potentially impact on rehabilitation and may affect the long-term outcomes. The acute wound healing phase and the rehabilitative phase are discussed in depth later in the chapter.

Resuscitative phase

During this phase, first aid is administered, the percentage of TBSA is calculated, fluid resuscitation is initiated and lifesaving measures are implemented. Of primary concern is the onset of hypovolaemic or **burn shock** and the onset of oedema. The phase ends with the diuresis phase of burn fluid mobilisation. The person is assessed for signs of hypothermia, respiratory distress and shock. Intravenous access is obtained and the person may be prophylactically intubated if an inhalation injury is present. A decision should be made as to whether the person requires transfer to a specialist burn centre for complex care. A major burn injury should always be cared for by a specialist burn service (see Box 16.3).

Any concurrent injuries may need to take priority over the burn wound. Assess for concurrent injuries and treat as necessary. Communication is vital to the wellbeing of the injured person. All relevant information should be relayed to the receiving hospital, including circumstances surrounding the accident. This is especially important if the person was trapped in an enclosed space or there were chemicals involved or possible trauma (ANZBA, 2018).

FIRST AID At the scene of the burn, priority is given to removing the person from any danger, managing life-threatening conditions and cooling the burn. Rescuers must take care not to be injured as well. Table 16.2 outlines the procedures that must be undertaken at the scene of a burn. For large burns, it is not advisable to immerse the whole person in water for cooling as this will cause hypothermia. Never put ice in the water as this can cause cold injuries. Remove as much burned clothing as possible and replace with a clean sheet. Cover the person with a blanket to keep them warm.

TABLE 16.2 First aid procedures at the scene of a burn

Electrical burn	Switch off power. Remove the person from the source of electricity using a non-conducting object; preferably by a trained person. Put out flames if the person has sustained a flame injury as well. Begin primary survey. Protect cervical spine. Ensure rescuer safety. Remember high-voltage electricity will discharge through air.
Chemical burn	Brush residual dry chemical from person. Copious irrigation of area 'to the floor' with water. Ensure rescuer safety. Observe for signs of hypothermia. Begin primary survey.
Flame burn	Stop, drop and roll. Extinguish flames, remove clothing if possible and restrictive jewellery. Irrigate under cool, clean water for at least 20 minutes. If water for copious cool-water irrigation is not available, apply cool wet towels and change when they become warm. Observe for hypothermia. Ensure rescuer safety. Begin primary survey.
Scald	Remove clothing where possible. Irrigate with copious cool, clean water for at least 20 minutes. If water for copious cool-water irrigation is not available, apply cool wet towels and replace when they become warm. Observe for signs of hypothermia.

Source: ANZBA (2018). *Emergency management of severe burns*. Course manual (version 18). © Australian and New Zealand Burn Association Ltd. Reproduced with permission.

TABLE 16.3 Emergency resuscitative interventions—ABCDEF

PROBLEM	INTERVENTION
Airway	Check for patency, soot around mouth and nares, singed nasal hairs. Always use cervical spine precautions. Injuries above the clavicles or facial injuries can indicate spinal injuries.
Breathing and ventilation	Assess chest movement to ensure chest is rising equally. Administer humidified 100% oxygen. Ventilate with bag and mask if necessary; prepare for possible intubation. Assess for carbon monoxide poisoning (i.e. decreased conscious level, cherry red appearance). Respiratory rate of over 20/minute is not necessarily a good thing. Circumferential chest burns can restrict air entry. Non-circumferential full-thickness torso burns can also restrict air entry.
Circulation	Check for strength, regularity and presence of pulses. Capillary refill of nail beds should be 2 seconds. Longer capillary refill times could indicate hypovolaemia, hypothermia or the need for escharotomies. Stop any bleeding. Elevate any burned or oedematous limb above the level of the heart if not contraindicated. Electrical burns should be monitored for cardiac complications.
Disability and neurological status	Establish level of consciousness using Glasgow Coma Scale. Examine pupil reaction to light. Hypoxia and shock can cause restlessness and decreased level of consciousness.
Exposure and environment	Remove all jewellery and burned clothing. Prevent hypothermia. If clothing is stuck, trim loose pieces.
Fluid resuscitation	Insert two large-bore cannula into non-burned tissue. Take blood specimen for crossmatching. Commence intravenous fluids as per formula.

Sources: ANZBA (2018). *Emergency management of severe burns*. Course manual (version 18); Herndon (2018). *Total burn care* (5th ed.). New York: Elsevier Health.

PRIMARY SURVEY Life-threatening issues are identified and commencement of emergency management is done in this phase. The ABCDEF acronym (see Table 16.3) provides a guide to emergency resuscitative interventions (ANZBA, 2018).

SECONDARY SURVEY This phase is a head-to-toe examination commencing after any life-threatening conditions are dealt with. Secondary survey commences after the primary survey has been completed and the person is stabilised. It includes a comprehensive assessment of the person and records their allergies, medications, health history, the last time they ate and the events surrounding the incident. Identification of the mechanism of injury is vital, and the presence of any penetrating wounds or blunt trauma needs to be ascertained.

> **CONSIDERATION FOR PRACTICE**
>
> **Narcotics are always administered intravenously, rather than orally, subcutaneously or intramuscularly in the resuscitative or acute phase of a burn due to decreased circulation and absorption of medications.**

PREPARATION FOR TRANSFER TO A BURNS UNIT
Once the referral criteria for transfer to a specialised burns unit have been met (see Box 16.3), preparation of the stabilised person for transfer to that unit involves the following measures and interventions. The following points are covered as part of the primary and secondary survey:

1. *Respiratory system.* Establish and maintain airway; administer humidified 100% oxygen. Consider the need for endotracheal intubation (before transfer) if there is a possibility of upper airway obstruction. Transfer the person with their head elevated unless contraindicated (for instance, associated spinal injuries) as this will help decrease swelling and aid breathing
2. *Circulation.* Insert two large-bore intravenous cannula (size 16 for adults, size 20 for children) through non-burned skin where possible. Maintain resuscitation fluid as per formula for burn resuscitation. All limbs that are burned should be elevated where not contraindicated and cervical spine precautions maintained at all times.
3. *Urinary output.* Insert an indwelling catheter (IDC) for burns above 10% TBSA in children over 18 months of age and in children under 18 months of age with an 8% TBSA burn. An IDC should be inserted in adults with a 15% TBSA burn. An IDC should always be considered for burns of genitalia. Maintain urine output at:
   - adults 0.5–1 mL/kg/hr (1–2 mL/kg/hr in presence of electrical injury or confirmed inhalational injury)
   - children range 0.5–1 mL/kg/hr.
   - Accurate fluid balance monitoring is the most effective way of determining adequacy of fluid resuscitation measures. In the case of an electrical injury, urine should be maintained at 1.0–2.0 mL/kg/hr. Weighing of nappies for children is not an accurate assessment of urine output.
4. *Wound management.* Wash the burn area with an antibacterial/antiseptic soap or water and then cover with a silver-impregnated dressing. In remote Australian regions, time delays in transferring people to a burn unit may be prolonged. The use of cling wrap products is not advised as they can cause retention of heat in the burn and, if tied around a limb or digit, could cause a tourniquet effect. It is better to transfer with wet cloths which will continue the cooling of the burn.
5. *Analgesia.* Liaise with burns unit as to the preferred protocol for analgesia administration, particularly if children are involved. Oral analgesia is not recommended except in minor burns. Narcotic analgesia given intravenously is essential for the person's comfort. Monitoring of level of consciousness, respiratory status and effectiveness of analgesia should be maintained.
6. *Gastrointestinal system.* Insert a nasogastric or orogastric tube in a person who has sustained a burn of >15% TBSA in adults and >10% TBSA in children over 18 months. In a child under 18 months, one should be inserted for an 8%

TBSA burn. This is to decrease the risk of vomiting and potential aspiration, prevent translocation of gut bacteria which leads to infection, facilitate enteral feeding and prevent a Curling's ulcer.

7. *Tetanus status.* Tetanus prophylaxis is recommended for all people who sustain a burn injury. A correct history should be taken where possible to ascertain if a booster or immune globulin is required (Department of Health, 2022; Herndon, 2018).

Acute wound healing phase

The acute wound healing phase commences as part of the secondary survey and is discussed in depth later in the chapter.

Rehabilitative phase

The rehabilitative phase also commences on day one. All interventions from first aid through the continuum impact on rehabilitation. This is discussed later in the chapter.

BURN WOUND HEALING

Minor burns that heal via spontaneous regeneration and repair, while major burns will require surgical debridement, cultured epithelial autografts (CEAs), skin grafts or flaps. The healing process involves three phases: inflammation, reconstruction and remodelling. The degree of injury will influence the nature of healing and the amount of regeneration and repair that will occur (Norris, 2018).

- *Inflammation.* Immediately following the injury, platelets coming in contact with the damaged tissue aggregate. Fibrin is deposited, trapping further platelets and a thrombus is formed. The thrombus, combined with local vasoconstriction, leads to haemostasis, which inhibits bleeding.

  Local vasodilation and an increase in capillary permeability follow haemostasis. Neutrophils infiltrate the wound and peak in about 24 hours, and then monocytes predominate. The monocytes are converted into macrophages, which consume pathogens and dead cells and secrete various growth factors. These growth factors stimulate the proliferation of fibroblasts and the deposit of a provisional wound matrix.
- *Reconstruction.* Within 2 to 3 days post burn, fibroblasts are the major cell within the wound. Their number peaks at about 14 days after the injury. Granulation tissue begins to form, with complete re-epithelialisation occurring during this phase. Epithelial cells migrate to the centre of the wound, and contact inhibition and mitosis occur to form the 4 to 5 layers of epidermis. The proliferation phase lasts until complete re-epithelialisation occurs.
- *Remodelling*, or *maturation.* This phase may last for years. Collagen fibres, laid down during the proliferative phase, are reorganised to improve the tensile strength of the wound. Scars contract and fade in colour. In normal healing following a superficial minor burn injury, the newly formed skin closely resembles its neighbouring tissue. However, when a burn injury extends into the dermal layer of skin, two types of excessive scar may develop. A **hypertrophic scar** is an overgrowth of dermal tissue that remains within the boundaries of the wound. A **keloid** is a scar that extends beyond the boundaries of the original wound. People with dark skin, such as Indigenous Australians, Pacific Islanders and Asian, African and Middle Eastern populations, are at greater risk of hypertrophic scars and keloids.

The length of time a wound takes to heal influences scar formation. Time to healing is an outcome measure for treatment effectiveness, regardless of treatment choice. Healing after a 2-week period is known to be a predictor of hypertrophic scarring. Surgery may be needed to speed up healing time and to minimise scarring. All wound management decisions should focus on achieving re-epithelialisation within 2 weeks of the burn injury.

Post-burn itch

Although the exact cause of post-burn itch is not known, it is considered to be due to both peripheral and central mechanisms. Mediators that relay itch sensations peripherally are released when keratinocytes are damaged. These mediators include histamine, interleukins, protease-activated receptors and nerve growth factors. Itch is a common and disruptive part of burn injury. It can start in the first 2 weeks after the burn and can last for a long time. Itch can lead to further damage to fragile skin as the person scratches to relieve the itch. Consensus on successful treatment of the pruritus is scarce in the literature; however, there are a number of pharmacological and non-pharmacological treatments employed. Oral and topically applied antihistamines are commonly used. Non-pharmacological treatments include massaging the scar or healed burned area. Colloidal oatmeal baths and shower washes are also recommended, along with ice packs and instructions for keeping the area cool. Treatment of itch should be as much a priority as treatment of pain. Further research into the causes and treatment of post-burn itch is required (Chung, et al., 2020).

THE PERSON WITH MINOR BURNS

Minor burn injuries consist of superficial burns that are not extensive, and superficial partial-thickness burns that involve less than 10% of TBSA. However, the person as a whole must be taken into account rather than only the % TBSA when assessing burn severity. Minor burns can also be a small area of full-thickness eschar that is to be treated conservatively rather than with surgical debridement. Minor burn injuries are not associated with immunosuppression or hypermetabolism.

People with a minor burn injury are often treated as an outpatient. The goal of therapy is to promote wound healing, eliminate discomfort, maintain mobility and prevent infection.

Pathophysiology

Sunburn

Sunburns result from exposure to ultraviolet light. Such injuries, which tend to be superficial, are more commonly seen in people with lighter skin. Because the skin remains intact, the manifestations in most cases are mild and are limited to pain, nausea, vomiting, skin redness, chills and headache. Treatment is performed on an outpatient basis and generally consists of applying non-perfumed lotions, increasing fluid intake, administering mild analgesics and maintaining warmth. Older people and children should be monitored for evidence of dehydration. Proper use of sunscreen and limiting sun exposure to the less hazardous hours of the day can prevent sunburn.

Scald burn

Scald burns result from exposure to moist heat, and the depth of a scald depends on the temperature of the water, the thickness of the skin and the duration of contact. Water at 60°C from fluids such as hot coffee or soup can cause deep partial-thickness burns. Scalds in the young and old are often deep.

For scalds that are minor, the person can be treated as an outpatient with appropriate dressings and analgesia to allow for a full range of movement and to keep them comfortable. Tetanus toxoid prophylaxis is administered as appropriate.

Contact burn

Contact burns usually result from hot metals, plastics, hot footpaths or motorbike exhaust pipes. They are usually small in circumference but can be deep. Treatment may include dressings and/or surgery. Tetanus toxoid prophylaxis is administered as appropriate. Burns from sun-heated surfaces are not uncommon. Children and adults with diabetes are particularly susceptible. The focus for these kinds of burns should be on prevention and education of vulnerable people.

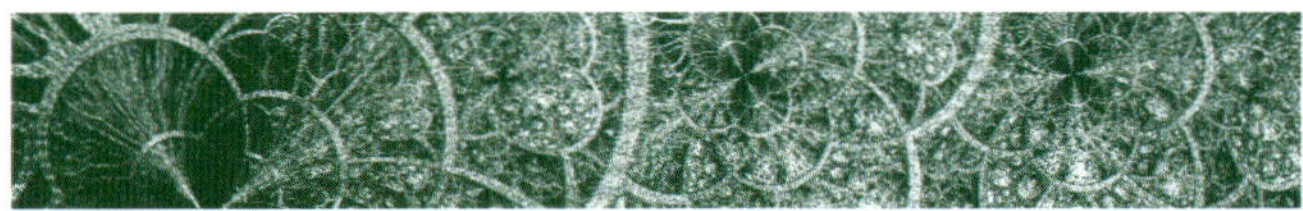

Nursing care

Management of a minor burn

Regardless of the care setting, the principles of management are the same. The aim is to promote wound healing and prevent infection while maintaining a full range of movement. Adequate analgesia should be prescribed to keep the person comfortable and to enable the person to maintain full range of movement. COVID-19 protocols will need to be followed.

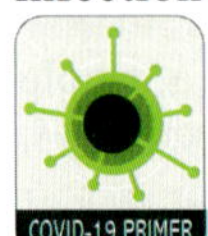

Nursing care includes taking a comprehensive history of the incident and health history, administration of prescribed analgesics, ongoing wound assessments, wound care planning, referrals for physiotherapy and/or occupational therapy and arranging follow-up appointments. Initially, the wound is washed using an antiseptic soap or wash. This varies between burns units. Remove any loose, non-viable skin with sterile scissors or while washing. Deroof blisters in accordance with hospital policy as blisters that extend over a joint can decrease function and movement. Blister fluid can also cause pressure over the wound bed, which compromises perfusion and increases pain.

Management for burn blisters >5 mm is deroofing (removal of skin and fluid) after adequate analgesia, while burn blisters ≤ 5 mm can be left intact. Clinical considerations include: (1) risk of infection/desiccation if removing blister skin when adequate facilities or resources are not available (e.g. in a remote area), and (2) consider leaving the blister intact if located on the hand or sole of the foot, as skin is much thicker, or if there is a risk of poor patient compliance and ongoing care (e.g. dementia etc.) (Agency for Clinical Innovation (NSW), 2019).

Once the burn has been cleaned and the non-viable tissue removed, a more thorough assessment can be made of the wound. Wounds with a pink wound bed, free of slough or eschar, are likely to be superficial or superficial partial thickness and should heal within 7 to 14 days and leave no permanent scarring. It should be noted that infection, poor dressing choice and oedema can cause the burn to convert to a deeper burn. Superficial burns where there is no skin loss may only require non-perfumed moisturising creams. A plethora of wound dressings are used in the treatment of burns, and individual health agencies and burn health professionals will have preferred protocols.

Hydrocolloids are a suitable choice for the low-to-moderate exudating superficial/partial-thickness wounds. A hydrocolloid is also suitable for a small area of full-thickness eschar. They are not suitable for wounds with a large amount of exudate as maceration may occur with the accumulation of exudate. Hydrocolloids are waterproof and for this reason a good choice for an outpatient. Dressing changes are required every 3–4 days depending on the amount of exudate.

Calcium alginates are useful for moderate-to-highly exudating wounds but require a secondary dressing. Alginates require dressing changes every 2–4 days, depending on the amount of exudate, and can be removed in the shower or bath if they have dried out.

Foams are a suitable choice for superficial/partial and deep partial burns if there are moderate-to-high amounts of exudate. Foams come in adhesive and non-adhesive forms, as well as silver-impregnated versions.

Hydrogels are a suitable choice for low-exudating wounds or wounds with dry eschar as they help to maintain a moist wound environment and assist in debridement of slough and eschar. Hydrogels are available in amorphous gels, or gel-impregnated gauzes or sheets.

Antimicrobial dressings will be required if infection is suspected or confirmed.

Community-based care

The nurse should address the following topics to facilitate self-care at home of minor burns.

- Educate the person and carer about the signs and symptoms of infection—that is, increase in pain, swelling and redness of the wound area. Provide instructions on:
  - how to care for the wound and dressing
  - how to take prescribed analgesia correctly and effectively
  - contact details for a clinic or a burns unit in case of any problems or concerns
  - how to change dressings if needed and equipment to do so
  - non-pharmacological pain-relieving measures—for example, elevation of the limb when sitting.

Asking an Indigenous patient if they have any 'questions or concerns' may be considered offensive as it could be thought disrespectful to ask questions. Instead, ask, 'Do you have any concerns or worries?'

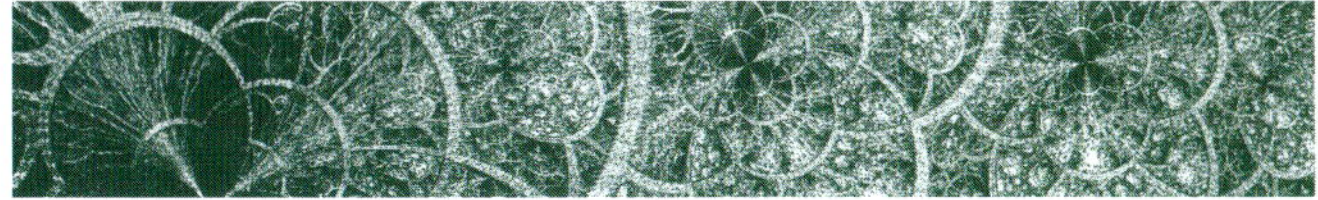

THE PERSON WITH MAJOR BURNS

The (ANZBA) identifies a major burn as above 15% to 20% TBSA in adults (15% TBSA in older adults or the infirm), above 10% TBSA in children over 18 months old and 8% TBSA in children under 18 months old. In addition, burns of certain anatomical sites, such as the perineum, hands or over joints, or those that occur because of certain agents, require specialised burn treatment and consultation should be sought (see Box 16.3).

Patients with pre-existing respiratory comorbidities and cardiovascular disease increase both the risk of intensive care unit admission and difficulties related to mechanical ventilation and mortality following a burn (Knowlin, Reid et al., 2018; Knowlin, Stanford et al., 2018).

Pathophysiology

There is a local and a general response to a burn injury. The local response is explained by Jackson's zones of burn injury model (1953) (see Figure 16.9). The general response is a multisystem response that requires specialised care to preserve life and result in the best possible outcome for the person.

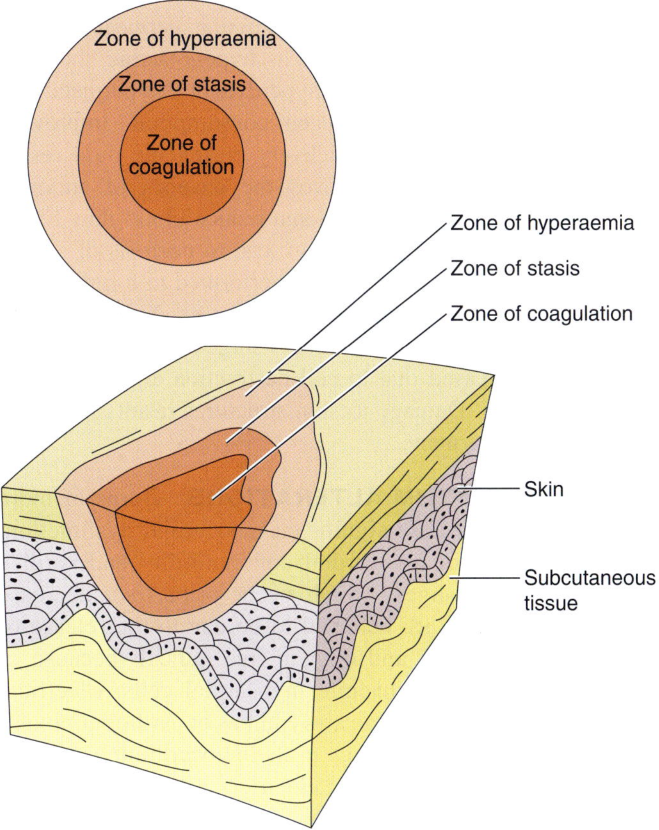

FIGURE 16.9 ***The Jackson zones of burn injury (Jackson, 1953)***

Source: Adapted from Jackson (1953). The diagnosis of the depth of burning. *British Journal of Surgery*, *40*(164), 588–596.

The pathophysiological changes that result from major burn injuries involve all body systems. Extensive loss of skin (the body's protective barrier) can result in infection, fluid and electrolyte imbalances, and hypothermia. Cytokines and other mediators are released into the systemic circulation causing a systemic inflammatory response. If the person inhales the products of combustion, an inhalation injury can result, thus compromising respiratory function. Cardiac arrhythmias and circulatory failure are potential complications of serious burn injuries. A hypermetabolic state dramatically increases kilojoule expenditure and nutritional deficiencies. The increase in metabolic rate can last for up to 1 year post injury (Holley et al., 2020). An alteration in gastrointestinal motility predisposes the person to developing paralytic ileus, and hyperacidity can lead to gastric and duodenal ulcerations. Translocation of gut bacteria due to increased permeability can lead to infection. The person is centrally dehydrated, so glomerular filtration rates and renal clearance of toxic wastes are less effective; this can result in acute tubular necrosis and renal failure.

Integumentary system

The loss of skin in burn injuries interrupts normal skin functions and its protective mechanisms (see the chapter 'Assessing the integumentary system'). Key mechanisms lost in burn injuries include the prevention of evaporative water loss, protection against bacteria and the maintenance of body warmth.

Heat transfer to skin is a complex phenomenon. If the microcirculation of the skin remains intact during burning, it cools and protects the deeper portions of the skin and cools the outer surface once the heat source is removed. When extensive burn injury occurs, the integrity of the microcirculation is lost and the burning process continues even after the heat source is removed.

JACKSON'S ZONES OF BURN INJURY Jackson (1953) proposed three concentric zones of burn injury. The zones are three dimensional and damage to the zone of stasis can lead to conversion to a deeper burn.

It is important to understand the pathophysiology of a burn in order to treat the person effectively (see Figure 16.9).

- The outermost zone of hyperaemia affects only the epithelium; there is no skin loss. In this zone, tissue perfusion is increased, giving rise to the reddened erythema appearance. This zone usually heals within 7 days unless there is trauma to the area, infection or oedema, which can cause a conversion to a deeper burn.
- The medial zone of stasis is initially moist, red and blistered, and blanches on pressure. Tissue perfusion is decreased in this zone. It may recover or become pale and necrotic because of inadequate fluid resuscitation, infection, trauma, oedema or poor wound management.
- The inner zone of coagulation is the area of most damage. There can be no reversal of necrosis. Proteins are coagulated and the burn has a 'leathery' appearance (Holley et al., 2020). The overall thickness of the dermis and epidermis varies considerably from one area of the body to another and is subject to the individual's age.

Similar temperatures produce different depths of injury to different body parts. For example, in the adult, skin covering the medial aspect of the forearm is thinner and more easily damaged than the skin covering the back of the same person. Skin dissipates heat maximally in areas of greatest vascularisation. When heat absorption exceeds the rate of dissipation, cellular temperatures rise and skin tissue is destroyed.

The deep burn injury results in the formation of necrotic skin and damage to subcutaneous tissue. During the acute phase of the injury a hard crust (eschar) forms which covers the wound. The eschar is characteristically leathery and rigid. Removal of the eschar is required if healing is to be facilitated. In a partial-thickness and deep partial-thickness wound, slough (moist non-viable tissue) covers the wound surface, which also needs to be debrided to facilitate healing.

Hypovolaemic shock

Fluid and electrolyte shifts in burn injury result in the movement of large amounts of fluid from the intracellular and intravascular compartments into the interstitial spaces. This results in hypovolaemia and oedema of the burn area. It is this fluid shift that causes hypovolaemic shock, which is also referred to as 'burn shock' (see Figure 16.10). Inflammatory mediators and stress hormones are released and start a cascade of events that, if left untreated, can lead to multi-organ failure.

Shock is the inability of the body to adequately deliver oxygen and nutrients to the body and remove cellular waste. Symptoms of hypovolaemic shock are similar to those of shock following haemorrhage: decreased blood pressure, cardiac output, urine output and plasma volume, and an increase in pulse rate along with an increase in systemic vascular resistance leading to decreased peripheral blood flow. Haematocrit and haemoglobin are elevated despite adequate fluid resuscitation due to the haemoconcentration of intravascular fluid. Red blood cells are haemolysed as a result of the burn and inflammatory mediators are released after a major burn injury. After fluid balance is restored, haematocrit levels usually return to normal.

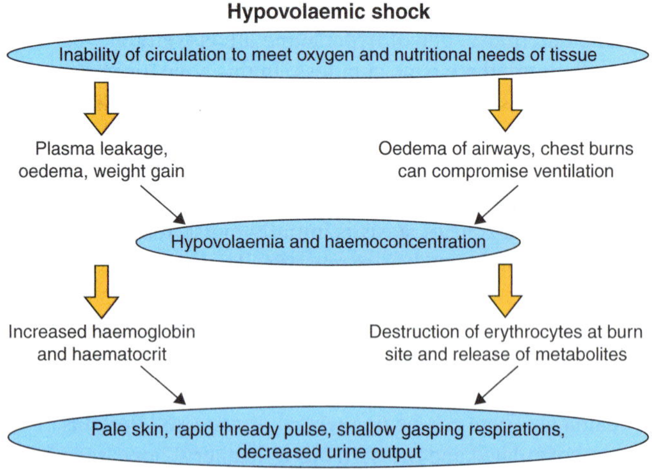

FIGURE 16.10 ***Hypovolaemic shock algorithm***

Source: Royal Perth Hospital.

Water, sodium and protein (albumin) leak through the less selectively permeable membranes of vessels to the interstitial spaces, causing oedema in non-burned tissue. There is also insensible fluid loss through the body surfaces that have been burned. Blisters and wound exudate are a result of this fluid shift. Potassium and sodium also move from the vessels and remain until the fluid shift resolves. Haemolysed red blood cells release potassium into the extracellular spaces (Nielson et al., 2017).

Towards the end of the resuscitative phase, as long as fluid replacement has been adequate, the membranes become selectively permeable again and leakage stops. Fluid is reabsorbed from the interstitial compartments into the intravascular compartment. The blood pressure rises as cardiac output increases and urinary output improves. This is usually around 24 hours post burn. This stage is known as the diuresis phase, with low specific gravity of urine. Potassium is slow to return to normal and hypokalaemia can occur, depending on the amount of potassium lost to the vascular space. Sodium can remain low due to sodium loss via the urine. The person is discouraged from drinking water and further depleting their sodium levels. During the diuresis phase the extra cardiac workload may predispose the older person or the person with cardiovascular disease to fluid volume overload. It is essential that the person is monitored and intravenous fluid is decreased and titrated to urine output and specific gravity.

Cardiovascular system

Major burns are manifested by widespread effects on the cardiovascular system. Increased vascular permeability and myocardial dysfunction as well as hypovolaemic shock, if left untreated, can result in a hyperdynamic/hypermetabolic state with an increased oxygen consumption. Improving cardiac output and oxygen delivery during the fluid resuscitation phase greatly improves the chances of survival. Circumferential burns and oedema reduce blood flow to the extremities and if not treated can lead to necrosis of a limb or digit. An escharotomy may be performed to a limb or the torso when there are circumferential burns. This should be done in consultation with the burns surgeon. Blood viscosity is initially increased due to cell destruction and fluid shifts within the body. Damage to skin structures results in microcirculation impairment.

CARDIAC RHYTHM ALTERATIONS Burns of more than 40% TBSA cause significant myocardial dysfunction, with a decrease in myocardial contractibility and cardiac output. These changes, which occur prior to a decrease in plasma volume, are believed to be due to the release of mediators, hormones and oxygen free radicals because of the burn and from ischaemic myocardial cells. Electrical burns often result in cardiac arrhythmias or cardiopulmonary arrest caused by heat damage to the myocardium or electrical interference with cardiac electrical activity (Nischwitz et al., 2020).

PERIPHERAL VASCULAR COMPROMISE Circumferential burns to the torso or extremities can result in **compartment syndrome** as a result of progressive development of arterial compression resulting in decreased blood supply to the area. Circulation to the extremities may be further impaired by oedema formation, inadequate fluid resuscitation and constrictive dressings or bandages. Limbs with circumferential burns should be elevated when not contraindicated and people with torso burns should be monitored for respiratory difficulties. Escharotomy may be required after consultation with the burn surgeon.

Respiratory system

Pulmonary damage may result from either direct inhalation injury or as part of the systemic response to the injury. The injury may range from mild respiratory inflammation to massive pulmonary failure, such as acute respiratory distress syndrome. Exposure to heat, toxic by-products of burned substances—for example, plastics—and smoke initiates the pathophysiological process associated with inhalation injury.

Inflammation occurs at localised sites within the airway and is manifested as hyperaemia. As a result, cells are destroyed and the bronchial cilia are rendered inactive. Because the mucociliary transport mechanism no longer functions, the person may develop bronchial congestion and infection.

Interstitial pulmonary oedema develops secondary to the escape of fluid from the pulmonary vasculature into the interstitial compartment of the lung tissue. Surfactant is inactivated, resulting in atelectasis and alveolar collapse. Sloughing of the damaged and dead lung tissue occasionally produces debris that may lead to complete airway obstruction.

Upper airway (above the level of the larynx) thermal injury results from the inhalation of hot gases, steam or vapours from chemicals dissolved in water. Generally, they occur when the person has been in an enclosed space. Inhalation injury is suspected when the person has singed facial, scalp or nasal hair. Physical findings include the presence of soot, charring, oedema, blisters and ulcerations along the mucosal lining of the oropharynx and larynx. The changes to tissue are the same as for thermal burn and severity is proportional to the length of exposure, type of chemical or temperature/pressure of steam. The resulting oedema in the airway may peak within 12 to 36 hours post injury (Holley et al., 2020). Signs of increasing respiratory distress include hoarseness, laboured breathing and stridor. Inflammatory mediators cause oedema and respiratory obstruction can develop. The oedema will occur despite adequate fluid resuscitation measures. If there is also skin burn to the neck, the swelling from this burn can further impede breathing.

The lower airway is protected very efficiently by laryngeal reflexes, so thermal injury below the larynx is not common and is usually only after exposure to extreme heat. However, when it does occur, it is typically associated with the inhalation of the products of combustion. Products containing sulfur, phosphorus or nitrogen, and compounds containing carbon, produce toxic by-products such as hydrogen chloride, hydrogen fluoride and ammonia. Acids and alkalis are released when these compounds come into contact with the moist respiratory mucosa, resulting in chemical burns. A classic finding is sputum containing soot or carbon particles which can damage alveoli (ANZBA, 2018; Reid & Ha, 2019).

TABLE 16.4 Carbon monoxide intoxication

CARBOXYHAEMOGLOBIN (%)	SYMPTOMS
0-15	None (smokers, long-distance truck drivers)
15-20	Headache, confusion
20-40	Nausea, fatigue, disorientation
40-60	Hallucination, ataxia, syncope, convulsions, coma
>60	Death

Source: ANZBA (2018). *Emergency management of severe burns*. Course manual (version 18). © Australian and New Zealand Burn Association Ltd. Reproduced with permission.

Carbon monoxide, a common asphyxiate, is a colourless, tasteless, odourless gas that has a 200 times greater affinity for haemoglobin than does oxygen. It displaces oxygen to bind with haemoglobin, forming carboxyhaemoglobin. As a result, the decrease in arterial oxyhaemoglobin produces tissue hypoxia. Carbon monoxide impairs both oxygen delivery and cellular oxygen use. The clinical manifestations of carbon monoxide poisoning range from mild visual impairment to coma and death (see Table 16.4). Carbon monoxide poisoning should be suspected if the burn was in an enclosed space and the person is unconscious (Victorian Government Department of Health, 2021).

Cyanide gas is released when plastics, polyurethane, nylon or silk are burned. The resultant production of cyanide gas affects cellular respiration. The brain and heart are most vulnerable to cyanide poisoning. Cyanide directly interferes with a cell's ability to utilise oxygen in metabolism. Cyanide poisoning should be suspected when the person shows signs of lactic acidosis regardless of adequate fluid resuscitation.

FAST FACTS

Manifestations of cyanide poisoning

- Headache
- Dizziness
- Seizures
- Tachycardia
- Fatal arrhythmias

Gastrointestinal system

Major burns cause a generalised response in the body that affects all organs, including the gastrointestinal tract (Murphy et al., 2021). Blood flow to the gut is decreased as part of the effect of hypovolaemic shock. Translocation of gut bacteria due to the disruption of the mucosa increases the risk of sepsis in the person with burns. This process is believed to be one of the mechanisms causing systemic sepsis and multiple-organ dysfunction syndrome (Nielson et al., 2017).

Other effects include malnutrition, hypermetabolism and splanchnic hypoperfusion as a result of intravascular fluid loss. Early enteral feeding can influence some of the gastrointestinal problems, including prevention of paralytic ileus and stress gastritis. The hypermetabolic response can lead to a catabolic state, which further decreases wound healing and increases the risk of infection. Maintaining blood flow to the gut is vital in preventing multi-organ failure. Maintaining the body's haemodynamics through fluid resuscitation is imperative to support gut blood flow (Nielson et al., 2017).

Stress ulcers, also known as **Curling's ulcers**, are acute ulcerations of the stomach or duodenum that may form following the burn injury. Abdominal pain, acidic gastric pH levels, haematemesis and melena may indicate a gastric ulcer. However, this is a less common presentation in contemporary medicine with the advances in burn management and the implementation of fluid resuscitation, early enteral feeding and antacids (Herndon, 2018).

Urinary system

During the early stages of the burn injury, renal blood flow and glomerular filtration rates are greatly reduced because of the decreased intravascular blood volume and the release of anti-diuretic hormone by the posterior pituitary. Urine output decreases and serum creatinine and blood urea nitrogen increase.

Dark-brown concentrated urine may indicate myoglobinuria or haemoglobinuria, the result of underlying muscle damage or the release of large amounts of dead or damaged erythrocytes after a major burn injury, particularly following an electrical injury. When large amounts of these pigments are released, the liver cannot keep pace with conjugation and the pigments pass through the glomeruli. The pigments can occlude the renal tubules and cause renal failure, especially when dehydration, acidosis or shock is also present. Adequate fluid resuscitation aims to prevent renal tubule damage as well as renal failure. An IDC is inserted to enable accurate monitoring of urine output.

The renal specialist team should be included for a patient with pre-existing kidney disease who may be having renal dialysis pre burn.

Immune system

Major burn injury can cause impairment of the immune system. The protection function of the skin is compromised, particularly in burns where there is a large TBSA. The amount of circulating immunoglobulin is decreased and the WBC function is also impaired. Part of the cascade of events that occurs following a major burn injury is the release of inflammatory cytokines. This release impedes the normal function of neutrophils, monocytes and lymphocytes. This series of events increases the person's risk of infection.

Metabolism

Major burns induce high energy expenditure, mediated by increased production of catecholamines, glucocorticoids and glycagon (Chourdakis et al., 2020). The body's high demand for energy cannot be fully reversed despite adequate nutrition and medical management. Hyperglycaemia is also common, with evidence suggesting that pharmacological management of elevated blood glucose levels is required.

Two distinct phases characterise the body's metabolic response to the burn injury. The ebb phase is manifested by decreased oxygen consumption, fluid imbalance, shock and inadequate circulating volume. The gut function also slows down.

A second phase, the flow phase, occurs when adequate burn resuscitation has been accomplished and is dependent on adequate metabolic response mediated by adrenal cortical steroids.

This phase is characterised by increases in cellular activity and protein catabolism, lipolysis and gluconeogenesis. Hypermetabolism persists until after wound closure has been accomplished and may reappear if complications occur.

CONSIDERATION FOR PRACTICE

An increased body temperature, without other manifestations of infection, is not indicative of infection in people with large burn wounds (in which the hypermetabolic response resets the core temperature to a higher level).

A thorough medical and surgical history should be obtained to determine any pre-existing medical problems as well as potential problems, such as COVID-19 in a person with a burn injury. Bariatric surgery is an effective weight-loss method but it does not always result in the patient being healthier or their nutritional requirements being optimised. Micronutrient deficiency as a result of not adhering to post-surgery multivitamin intake can affect recovery from a burn injury. Assessment of weight loss and micronutrients is important to aid recovery (Lupoli et al., 2017).

INTERPROFESSIONAL CARE

The burn team is composed of an interprofessional group of healthcare providers who together plan and implement the treatment of the burn-injured person during the acute and rehabilitative phases. The burn team consists of the nurse, physician and/or surgeon, physiotherapist, dietitian, occupational therapist, clinical psychologist and social worker. The team members meet regularly to discuss person progress and to determine collaboratively the most effective regimen of care and psychosocial support.

It is important to recognise that the process of burn injury is dynamic and that the clinical phase is not clearly delineated. Assessment and management of the burn-injured person are ongoing processes determined by the clinical picture; they last throughout the course of treatment.

Although many burn injuries are treated in local healthcare facilities, in many healthcare organisations throughout Australia there are guidelines for determining whether the person should be transported to a burns centre for interdisciplinary approaches to treatment and rehabilitation (see Box 16.3).

The resuscitative phase has been discussed previously. It includes pre-hospital care.

Acute wound healing phase

The acute phase begins on the day of the burn injury and has no defined end point as each person requires individual goal settings to determine progress. During this phase, wound care management, nutritional therapies and measures to control infectious processes are initiated. Excision and grafting of any wounds that require surgery is performed as soon as possible after injury. Enteral nutritional feeding to address kilojoule needs resulting from extensive energy expenditure are started in the resuscitative phase and continue through to discharge—and beyond, for some people. Measures to combat infection are implemented from the day of the burn injury and must continue until the wounds are healed.

Pain management constitutes a significant segment of the care plan throughout the clinical course of the burn-injured person. Adequate analgesia must be prescribed and given on a regular basis to maximise person comfort and to reduce the anxieties associated with wound debridement and intensive physiotherapy (Morgan et al., 2018).

Rehabilitative phase

The rehabilitative phase begins on the day of the burn injury and ends when the person returns to the highest level of health and function they can achieve. During this phase, the primary focus is the biopsychosocial adjustment of the person, specifically the prevention of contractures and scars. This phase includes significant others and family. The person's successful resumption of work, family and social roles is facilitated through physical, vocational, occupational and psychosocial rehabilitation. The person is taught to perform range-of-motion exercises to enhance mobility and support injured joints.

Behavioural disengagement, 'venting' and self-blame have been identified by Martin, Rea and Wood (2021) as being flags for the need for depression screening in patients following a burn injury. Their findings suggest that three main coping styles are associated with post-traumatic growth: positive reframing, religion and acceptance (Martin et al., 2022).

Fluid resuscitation formula

Fluid resuscitation is the administration of intravenous fluids to restore the circulating blood volume during the first 24 hours post burn injury. The ANZBA guidelines (2018) state that a burn injury of 20% TBSA and over results in a generalised sequestration of large amounts of fluid from the intravascular space to the interstitial spaces. Combined with oedema and insensible loss, plasma volume is depleted, resulting in intravascular hypovolaemia; left untreated, this can end in multi-organ failure. Some states will commence intravenous fluid resuscitation at 15% TBSA.

Several formulas may be used to replace fluid loss. The ANZBA (2018) recommends the use of the modified Parkland (Baxter) formula (see Box 16.4).

BOX 16.4 Calculation of Parkland formula

Formula

3 mL Hartmann's solution × kg (body weight) × % TBSA = total fluid requirements for first 24 hours after burn (commencing from time of injury)

(always check with the local burn service/hospital policy as to number of mL/kg recommended for administration)

Give:

½(50%) total over first 8 hours

¼(25%) total over next 8 hours

¼(25%) total over next 8 hours (makes a total of a 24-hour period)

Example

For a 70-kg person with a 50% TBSA burn

3 mL × 70 kg × 50% TBSA burn = 10,500 mL

= 10.5 L in 24 h

50% of total in first 8 h = 5,250 mL (656 mL/h)

25% of total in second 8 h = 2,625 mL (328 mL/h)

25% of total in third 8 h = 2,625 mL (328 mL/h)

- For adults the usual fluid maintenance of 2 L/24 hours will also be required (e.g. 2,000 mL ÷ 24 hours = 83 mL/h).
- This requires a total of 328 mL + 83 mL = 411 mL/h over the first 8 hours.
- Fluid resuscitation commences as soon as possible following injury and is calculated from time of injury, not time of arrival at the ED.

(Paediatric fluid maintenance requirements are determined subject to the child's weight.)

Enteral feeding volumes are taken into account when determining maintenance fluid volumes.

Formulas are guidelines. Fluid is administered at a rate to produce 0.5–1.0 mL/kg/h—that is, 30–50 mL of urine output per hour. In cases of an electrical burn, then urine output is maintained at 1–2 mL/kg/h.

Blood pressure and pulse rates should not be used in isolation to measure fluid resuscitation adequacy, as an adult with a major burn is in a hypermetabolic state and will probably be tachycardic, anxious and in pain.

All formula guidelines are used as starting points and fluids are titrated according to the person's physical response. Hourly urine output is often used as one indicator of effective fluid replacement. Specific gravity of the hourly urine should be monitored.

Source: Fiona Stanley Hospital Burn Service.

Respiratory management

On admission to the emergency department, COVID-19 protocols will need to be established and maintained along with several baseline assessments of respiratory status that must be obtained: chest x-ray study, arterial blood gases (ABGs), vital signs and carboxyhaemoglobin (COHb) levels, which should be ascertained from arterial blood. A portable breath analyser can be used to detect carbon monoxide levels. It is important to remember that high oxygen concentrations have usually been administered in transit and so accurate levels of COHb are difficult to assess. Preparation for possible intubation should always be done in case of airway obstruction. The primary treatment plan is oriented towards preventing atelectasis and maintaining alveolar oxygen exchange. The following interventions should be initiated:

- Maintain the head of the bed at 30 degrees or greater to maximise the person's ventilatory efforts (once cervical spine is cleared). Turn the person side to side every 2 hours to prevent hypostatic pneumonia.

- To keep airway passages clear, encourage the person to use incentive spirometry hourly and help them perform coughing and deep-breathing exercises regularly. Encourage expectoration of sputum. Monitor and document respiratory rate hourly depending on the person's condition. Measure oxygen saturation using pulse oximetry. In a person with high COHb levels the oxygen saturation will be inaccurate as no determination between oxygen and COHb can be made by the pulse oximeter.
- If respiratory status declines, prepare the person for intubation. Endotracheal or nasotracheal intubation may be used. If the person has suffered nasolabial burns, the endotracheal route may be preferred. Intubation is used for short-term ventilatory management. For long-term ventilatory management (i.e. greater than 3 weeks), a tracheostomy is performed.
- Humidified oxygen is administered to help prevent the drying of mucosa and tracheal secretions. Ambient air or oxygen flow is based on ABG results. The person may be placed on a face mask, steam collar, T-piece, mechanical ventilation with positive end-expiratory pressure, pressure-support ventilation or high-frequency jet ventilation. The person's room will be always maintained at an ambient temperature because hypothermia will delay wound healing, cause discomfort and affect consciousness. Breathing in warm air will assist the person to breathe comfortably. The goal of all therapies is to maintain adequate tissue oxygenation with the least amount of administered oxygen necessary.
- Medications to dilate constricted bronchial passages may be administered intravenously or by inhalation to control bronchospasms and wheezing. Mucolytic agents liquefy tenacious sputum and aid in expectoration.
- An arterial line may be inserted for continuous assessment of ABGs. Pulmonary artery pressure catheters may be inserted to measure pulmonary vascular resistance (PVR), pulmonary artery pressure (PAP), pulmonary artery wedge pressure (PAWP) and mixed venous oxygen saturation (SvO_2). The PVR and PAP rise in the presence of hypoxia. The SvO_2 is the average percentage of haemoglobin bound with oxygen in the venous blood and reflects overall tissue utilisation of oxygen. Pulse oximetry monitors arterial oxygen saturation levels. The person requiring this level of invasive monitoring may be in a critical care unit.
- Administer intravenous analgesia as ordered.

Intravenous analgesia is the preferred route of administration because of decreased gastric absorption. Intramuscular analgesia will not be absorbed from burned or oedematous areas and results in a build-up of analgesia in the tissues. In the diuresis phase. The analgesia is then released and the person could receive too much analgesia at once. Adjunct medications such as anxiolytics should be used to help calm the person.

After stabilisation in the emergency department, the person is transferred to the critical care unit or a specialised burns unit.

Diagnosis

The following diagnostic tests are used to evaluate the person's progress and to modify intervention strategies. The monitoring process should depend on the extent and depth of the burn, the presence of inhalation burn other injuries, comorbidities and age.

- *Urinalysis* indicates the adequacy of renal perfusion and the person's nutritional status. In catabolic states, nitrogen is excreted in large amounts into the urine. Nitrogen balance is a measure for nutritional support required and should be done in conjunction with serum protein measurements. Inactivity causes muscle wasting and an increased nitrogen excretion. An IDC is inserted and should be maintained until the person is medically stable and able to use a urinal or bedpan. During the resuscitative phase, hourly specific gravity tests should be done as a clinical indicator of fluid replacement adequacy.

  Monitoring of urine output should continue until after the diuresis phase and in conjunction with hospital protocols. Loss of plasma protein and dehydration lead to proteinuria and elevated urine specific gravity. Glycosuria is a transient development following major burn injury; it can indicate a need to adjust the nutritional program.
- *Myoglobinuria*, which manifests as a dark-brown or wine-coloured urine, signals the development of acute tubular necrosis. It usually occurs following an electrical injury, and intravenous fluid should be maintained to assist in clearing the myoglobinuria (see Figure 16.1).
- *The full blood count* is monitored regularly. Haematocrit is elevated secondary to haemoconcentration, haemolysis of RBCs and fluid shifts from the intravascular compartment. Haemoglobin is decreased secondary to haemolysis. Changes to leucocyte numbers occur in relation to the burn and further changes in response to medications or sepsis.
- *Serum electrolytes* are monitored regularly as clinically indicated during the resuscitation phase. They are a more accurate assessment of successful fluid resuscitation attempts than urine output. Frequency of tests should be done in accordance with the hospital policy. Sodium levels are decreased secondary to massive fluid shifts into the interstitium. Potassium levels initially are elevated during burn shock because of cell lysis and fluid shifts into the extracellular space. Potassium levels decrease after burn shock resolves, as fluid shifts back to intracellular and intravascular compartments.
- *Renal function* test results are closely monitored. Blood urea nitrogen (BUN) is elevated secondary to dehydration and if the enteral feeding is high in protein. Creatinine is elevated in the presence of renal insufficiency. It is used as an indicator of rhabdomyolysis following electrical injury.
- *Total protein, albumin, transferrin, prealbumin, retinol binding protein, alpha-1-acid glycoprotein* and *C-reactive protein* indicate protein synthesis and nutritional status. Because of the fluid shifts that occur during the early stages of the burn injury, they are more useful markers during the rehabilitative phase of care.
- *Creatine phosphokinase (CPK)* is elevated following an electrical burn, secondary to extensive muscle damage.
- *Serial ABGs* indicate the presence of hypoxia and acid–base disturbances and indicate the person's responses to changes

in oxygen therapies. The burn-injured person may demonstrate elevated or lowered pH, decreased PCO_2 and PO_2, and low to normal bicarbonate levels. Their ABGs are a more accurate estimation of COHb as pulse oximetry cannot distinguish between oxygen and carbon monoxide.

- *Pulse oximetry* allows continuous assessment of oxygen saturation levels.
- *Serial chest x-ray studies* document changes within the first 24 to 48 hours that may reflect the presence of atelectasis, pulmonary oedema or acute respiratory distress syndrome (ARDS), also referred to as severe pulmonary congestion.
- *Serial 12-lead electrocardiograms (ECGs)* are necessary to monitor the development of arrhythmias, especially those associated with hypokalaemic and hyperkalaemic states.

Medications

PAIN CONTROL Burns are painful. In the resuscitative phase of care, intravenously administered narcotics are the best means of managing pain. Intravenous narcotics must be administered subject to hospital policies. Burn treatments can also produce high levels of anxiety, necessitating the use of anxiolytic agents such as midazolam and lorazepam. Anxiolytics are especially useful when administered 1 hour before wound care. During the acute phase, narcotics are administered around the clock on a regular basis to decrease pain that occurs at rest (Morgan et al., 2018).

Patient-controlled analgesia (PCA) enhances the person's ability to cope with pain. The oral, subcutaneous or intramuscular route of administration should be avoided until haemodynamic stability and unimpaired tissue perfusion return. Some hospitals have access to specialty pain services and these should be involved to ensure the person receives the most appropriate analgesia to suit their needs. If the person has adequate analgesia at all times, they will be less anxious and more receptive to all care provided by occupational therapists, physiotherapists and nurses.

Alternative forms of pain and anxiety relief should be taught as an adjunct to pharmacological measures (Bermo et al., 2020). Distraction, self-hypnosis, guided imagery and relaxation techniques are helpful adjuncts in managing pain and coping with loss. See the chapter 'Nursing care of people in pain' for a discussion of strategies for managing pain.

On admission it is important to ascertain medications, either prescribed or illicit, taken by the person prior to the burn injury, as these may further complicate the treatment regimen. Drugs that affect any of the major body systems or cause mood alterations will need to be factored into the treatment plan.

TETANUS PROPHYLAXIS If the person's immunisation status is in doubt, tetanus toxoid is administered intramuscularly early in the acute phase of care to prevent *Clostridium tetani* infection. A thorough health history should be taken to ensure the person has had the primary three doses of tetanus vaccination. If not, or the last booster was 20 years or more ago, then they may require immunoglobulin, not a booster (Department of Health, 2022).

ANTIMICROBIAL AGENTS Systemic infection is a leading cause of death in people with major burns. Gram-positive organisms such as *Staphylococcus* and *Streptococcus* colonise the burn surface during the first week post burn; Gram-negative enteric organisms become more common with longer periods of hospitalisation. Prophylactic systemic antibiotics are not used in controlling burn wound flora because there may be poor delivery to the burn due to decreased blood flow. To aid in the prevention of infection the person is washed in an antibacterial soap Topical antimicrobial therapy in the form of wound dressings is used to manage the wound bioburden. Of the many antimicrobial agents available, bacteriocidal silver-impregnated dressings are recommended—for example, nanocrystalline silver-impregnated dressings may be used. Despite antimicrobial therapy, people with major burns have a greater risk of sepsis and septic shock. Systemic antibiotics are commenced when a definitive diagnosis of infection is made. A biopsy of the area may be taken to identify infective organisms. Surface swabbing for microbiology may not be accurate in determining the organism involved.

FAST FACTS

Local signs of burn wound infection

- Increased redness greater than 2 cm erythema around wound
- Increase in pain
- Increased sloughing of burn tissue
- Increased oedema
- Conversion of burn to a deeper burn
- Black or brown areas of discolouration

Systemic antimicrobial therapy is used on induction for surgery and may be administered postoperatively. The therapy is discontinued as soon as the person's haemodynamic status returns to normal, usually within the first 24 hours. In the long-term treatment of identified infectious processes, drug administration is limited to the least amount of time required to eradicate the infection.

Topical antimicrobial agents *Silver* Silver has a long history of use in wound care and is documented in use as early as the 19th century. It has a broad antibacterial activity. With the advent of antibiotics its use declined. It had a resurgence in the 1960s and again in current medicine, particularly in the use of burns. While there is a potential for resistance to silver in wounds, there has not been any definitive research to confirm resistance to silver-impregnated dressings (Haidari et al., 2020; Khansa et al., 2019).

Silver sulfadiazine Silver sulfadiazine (Flamazine™) is a silver and sulfonamide cream and has been used since the 1960s as a topical antimicrobial for burns. Silvazine™ (commonly called SSD) was originally used in Australia and contained chlorhexidine. This product is no longer available. Flamazine™ does not contain chlorhexidine. However, it has been shown to be effective against anaerobic and aerobic bacteria. The silver ion binds with the DNA of the bacteria. It is bactericidal and is easy to apply, and for some people it is soothing. However, it is contraindicated in instances of sensitivity to silver and sulfur drugs. It is not sustained release and therefore requires daily dressing changes (Haidari et al., 2020; Khansa et al., 2019).

Silver-impregnated dressings There is an increasing variety of silver-impregnated dressings and they all differ in the type and amount of silver they contain. In the management of burns, high-dose, sustained-release nanocrystalline silver formulations (Acticoat®) are preferred. Nanocrystalline silver dressings are bactericidal and have been shown to be effective against anaerobic and aerobic bacteria. Nanocrystalline silver dressings can leave a temporary blue staining of the skin. Water compresses or hydrogels are then placed over the dressing and they are secured with a roller bandage or tubular stretch bandage.

Research shows that the most effective topical agents are those that act against the major pathogens responsible for causing burn wound infection, achieve levels of concentration sufficient to decrease microbial colonisation, are rapidly excreted or metabolised, are non-toxic and are easy to use (Nherera et al., 2017).

Role of the nurse

The nurse will be the person who spends most time with the patient during the admission and afterwards in outpatients. The role of the nurse in the care of the burn-injured person encompasses all aspects of general nursing care and wound management, during which the nurse will focus on the following:

- administration of prescribed analgesia prior to treatment
- adherence to hospital protocol regarding wound cleansing and wound treatments
- ongoing assessment of the wound and healing status
- education for the person and their family to promote optimal wound healing outcomes:
    - Indigenous-specific information sheets should be created, all patient information should be assessed for clarity of understanding and the language used should be appropriate for the age, culture and intellectual level of the patient.
    - Learn from that patient and family what is important to them and how to best aid their recovery and discharge from hospital. Family meetings are often a good source of giving and receiving information that can help guide care and ensure the patient and family feel included and heard.

HEALTH EDUCATION FOR THE PERSON AND FAMILY

- Discuss procedure with the burned person and strategies for maximising comfort at dressing changes.
- Advise the person to take prescribed analgesia prior to each dressing and on a regular basis to maintain comfort.
- Identify resources available for the patient at the discharge location. Rural and remote communities may not have the resources of big city hospitals.
- Involve the Indigenous liaison team, drug and alcohol team, pastoral care, community leaders and, if the patient consents, any other supportive resources where appropriate.
- Educate the person about the importance of physiotherapy and performing given range-of-motion exercises while wounds are healing.
- Educate the person about the importance of good nutrition, particularly protein and carbohydrates to aid healing.

Role of the surgeon

The goal of any wound closure surgery is to provide the best possible cosmetic and functional outcome for the burned person. The current practice of early excision and grafting has improved the outcome for burns and has decreased mortality. Surgery is done once the person has achieved cardiovascular stability and after the resuscitation period. Not all wounds require the same surgical intervention. A small burn may be excised and directly closed, requiring only suture line care. Surgical management of burn injuries includes escharotomy, debridement of non-viable tissue and harvesting of autologous (person's own) split skin grafts (SSGs). Full-thickness skin grafts (FTGs) are used on functional areas if skin is available. The FTGs contract less than SSGs and in some of the deeper burns a tissue flap may be required to repair the defect.

Surgeons are mindful of the scar left by the donor site and will select an area of low exposure and good colour match when possible. The scalp may be used when there is little skin available for harvesting as it heals quickly and hair regrowth covers the donor site. The development of dermal regeneration templates such as Integra® has allowed earlier debridement of large areas of full-thickness eschar. Cultured epithelial autografts (CEAs) are also used by some surgeons when there is limited skin available for harvesting or to improve the meshed appearance of the scar from a meshed graft

ESCHAROTOMY When the burn eschar forms circumferentially around the torso or extremities, it acts as a tourniquet, impairing circulation. Left unchecked, the affected body part becomes gangrenous.

To prevent circumferential constriction of the torso or extremity, an **escharotomy** is performed by the physician with a scalpel or by electrocautery (see Figure 16.11). A sterile

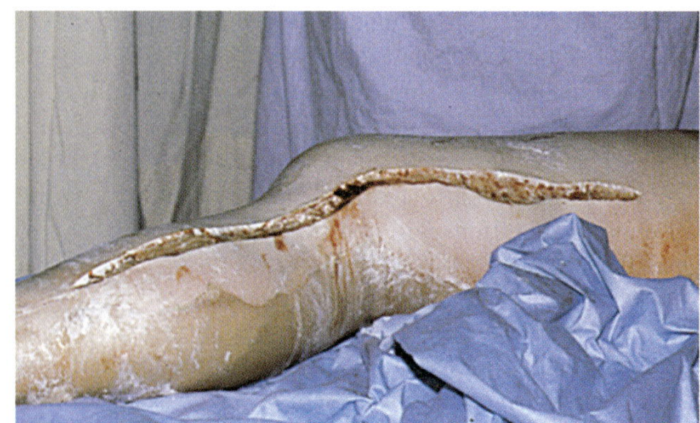

FIGURE 16.11 ***Escharotomy. The surgical procedure consists of making an incision through inelastic burned skin to relieve compartment pressure***

Source: Courtesy of Dr William Dominic.

BOX 16.5 Nursing implications for circumferential wound management

Care of the escharotomy wound

- Assess the extremity for reduced or absence of blood flow:
  a. Assess the extremity hourly for warmth, colour, sensation and capillary refill.
  b. Observe for evidence of numbness or tingling.
  c. Elevate the limb unless contraindicated.
  d. When dressing the escharotomy wound or limb with circumferential burns, leave fingertips and toes exposed for assessment purposes.
  e. Any applied bandages should not be tight.
- For circumferential burn wounds of the torso, assess for evidence of respiratory distress: elevate head of bed at least 30 degrees unless contraindicated.
- For circumferential burn wounds of the neck, assess for evidence of respiratory distress. Prepare the person for prophylactic intubation.
- Pack the escharotomy wound with calcium alginate dressings and dress the open wound with topical bactericidal silver dressing as ordered.

surgical incision is made longitudinally along the extremity or the trunk to release taut skin and allow for expansion caused by oedema formation. In the first 24 hours following the procedure, the incision should be gently packed with a calcium alginate dressing and covered with a nanocrystalline silver compress. After 24 hours, the site may be treated with a direct application of a topical bactericidal agent. See Box 16.5 for nursing implications for care of the person undergoing escharotomy.

SURGICAL DEBRIDEMENT **Surgical debridement** is conducted when there are full-thickness burns, extensive necrosis, infection or prior to skin grafting. Other methods of debridement are outlined in the chapter 'Nursing care of people with integumentary disorders'. The surgical technique is dictated by the depth of burn. The wound is excised to the level of fascia (**fascial excision**) in full-thickness skin injury, or sequential removal of thin slices of the burn wound to the level of viable tissue (tangential excision) is undertaken in partial-thickness skin injury. Because fascial excision sacrifices potentially viable fat and lymphatic tissue, its use is reserved for people with extensive or full-thickness burns. The most common technique used is electrocautery with cutting and coagulating current capabilities. Tangential excision is performed with the use of a dermatome. Shallow burns and some of moderate depth bleed briskly after one slice. If bleeding does not occur, the procedure is repeated until a viable bed of dermis or subcutaneous fat is reached. Following surgical debridement, haemostasis is vital to facilitate the repair of the wound surface. The debrided wound can be closed using traditional skin grafts in isolation or in association with tissue-engineered solutions. Once the wound has been dressed, the person is returned to the burn's unit and appropriately positioned and splinted, subject to the location of the injury and donor sites.

TYPES OF SKIN GRAFTS Autograft is the surgical removal of skin from one site on the individual (known as the donor site) and relocated to another site on the same individual. The donor site is allowed to heal by secondary intention.

Cultured epithelial autograft (CEA) Cultured epithelial **autografting** is obtained by taking a small piece of skin from the person with a burn injury. In some units, the piece of skin is sent to a laboratory for separation of the keratinocytes. This biopsy should be taken within 24 hours of the burn. The separated keratinocytes are then placed in a medium containing epidermal growth factor. Originally the technique involved placing the cells in a medium where, over a 5- to 7-day period, they expand to 50 to 70 times the size of the initial biopsies. The cells are again separated out and placed in a new culture medium for continued growth. With this technique, enough skin can be grown over a period of 3 to 4 weeks to cover an entire human body. The cells may be prepared as sheets attached to petroleum gauze backing, or in a suspension that is applied to the burn wound site. Problems with infection and lack of attachment have occurred. These problems have been reduced by using cells harvested at the time of the operation and immediately applying them to the wound. The skin cells undergo no laboratory expansion and adhere directly to the wound bed. The cells are ready to use within 15–20 minutes. The choice of technique is determined by the surgeon and availability of equipment. The CEA results in a smooth finish but is prone to shearing and blistering as cell layers are 10–15 cells thick (Manning et al., 2022).

Homograft, or **allograft**, is a temporary skin substitute and has some advantages when wound coverage is needed and for the body to behave as if it has skin. Human skin that has been harvested from cadavers is stored in a 'skin bank' until required. The development of methods to achieve prolonged storage of frozen, viable skin has increased the use of this dressing; however, its short supply, infection risk and expense still pose problems. It is manufactured as strips cut to the pattern of the burn and applied using sterile technique. Under normal circumstances, a homograft is rejected within 14 to 21 days following application.

Heterograft, or **xenograft**, is another kind of temporary wound coverage. Only heterograft from porcine dermis is available. Although fresh porcine heterograft is available at some centres, frozen heterograft is much more commonly used. Once applied, heterograft appears to undergo early softening and lysis from enzymatic action from the wound. As a result, frequent changes of the heterograft dressing are necessary. Because of the high infection rates associated with this dressing, silver-nitrate-treated porcine heterograft has been developed to retard microbial growth. Temporary skin coverage does not vascularise but the underlying wound bed may epithelialise. Amniotic membranes are also used, particularly for face burns, but they do not reduce healing times (Herndon, 2018).

Bioengineered tissue substitutes The multiple problems associated with the use of allograft and heterograft have driven the development of synthetic materials and composite material biological dressings. One such material is Biobrane®, a composite material consisting of nylon mesh bonded to silicone coated with bovine collagen, which has proved successful in the temporary coverage of partial- and full-thickness burns. Whereas Biobrane® adheres well to moderately clean wounds, it cannot adhere to grossly contaminated wounds. Biobrane® dressing is supplied in various sizes and is cut to fit the wound site and secured with staples or tape or skin closure strips (e.g. Steri-Strips®). It spontaneously separates from the wound when the underlying tissue heals.

If dermal thickness is lost, as in deep partial-thickness or full-thickness burns, several products can serve as a dermal replacement. Integra® is a synthetic dermal substitute made of bovine collagen and shark glycosaminoglycans, and Alloderm® is human cadaver allograft dermis processed such that it is non-immunogenic. These products are placed in the wound, and split-thickness autografts are then placed over the dermal replacement. These products are used to provide wound coverage, reduce pain and facilitate healing.

Dermal regeneration template (Integra®) Dermal regeneration template provides both dermal and epidermal characteristics. This is a manufactured template that, when placed onto a viable wound bed following debridement of full-thickness or deep partial-thickness burns, forms a matrix resembling dermis. It is of greatest use when autografting is not a possibility and is also used in scar revision. It has two layers and is secured with staples. The dermal layer is biodegradable and causes the body to regenerate a new dermal layer. The silicone layer stays intact for 3 weeks and then is removed and autologous grafting is done. This is a two-stage process. Integra® becomes infected easily, resulting in a non-viable product that must be removed immediately. Because of this, meticulous nursing care of Integra®-covered wounds is required to prevent infection and loss of graft. Integra® may be dressed daily with a silver-impregnated dressing (e.g. Acticoat®), or negative pressure wound therapy is applied in some hospitals while the silicone layer is separating. The silicone layer is removed prior to grafting. In some cases, cultured epithelial autograft (CEA) in the sheet or spray form (in conjunction with split skin grafts) will be used after the silicone layer is removed. Nursing care is specific for this template and shearing must be prevented, particularly in the first week post application.

Biodegradable temporising matrix (BTM) BTM is a recent product to the market. It is a synthetic product that does not contain any biological materials. It has been shown to be robust in the presence of infection. This is not done routinely, but rather when a burn is very deep and/or extensive and deep. Removing the eschar early can improve the injured person's chances of survival (Greenwood et al., 2020).

Split skin grafts Skin grafts can be split thickness (SSGs)—thin, intermediate or thick. They all contain epidermis and variable depths of dermis. Thin SSGs contract within the first few months. They contain no skin appendages,

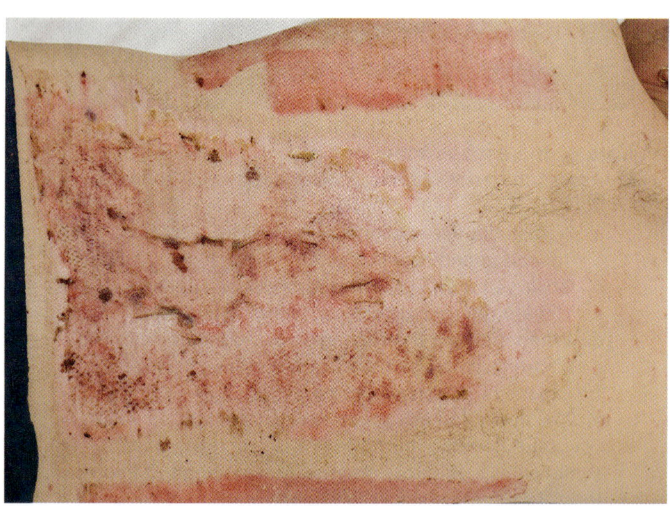

FIGURE 16.12 ***Split skin graft on a back***

Source: Courtesy of Tracy Levett-Jones.

and vascularisation occurs readily; while thick SSGs have less contraction and usually contain some hair follicles.

The SSG can be laid in sheet form or meshed to allow for a greater area to be covered. These grafts leave a 'meshed' scar pattern (see Figure 16.12) and in some instances surgeons will use cultured epithelial autograft (CEA) or spray-on skin cells to reduce the meshed look. Initially the graft is supplied by nutrients from the wound bed: the phase of imbibition. The graft will not take if the wound bed is insufficiently debrided, or slough, haematoma or excess exudate are present. Dressings must prevent shearing of the graft. Next, neovascularisation takes place; during this phase, blood vessels connect with capillaries in the graft. This is followed by the maturation phase when collagen forms between wound bed and graft. This last phase can take months to complete.

Full-thickness skin grafts Full-thickness skin grafts (FTGs) involve removal of the whole epidermis and the dermis. The thickness of the FTG depends on the thickness at the donor site from where it is harvested. The graft is sutured to the recipient wound bed. Care must be taken to ensure the graft is in contact with the wound bed or 'graft take' will not occur. Sometimes a 'tie over' dressing will be sutured over the top of the FTG to maintain the contact with the wound bed. The tie over is usually removed at the time of dressing change on about day 5 postoperatively or on the surgeon's instructions.

GRAFT CARE Grafts can be managed open with graft care attended to 1- to 4-hourly, depending on the surgeon's preferences or, more commonly, sealed under a bulky dressing for the first few days. The aim of graft care is to remove haematomas or exudate from beneath the graft to facilitate adherence. Small blisters are slit and exudate is expressed. Any wrinkles are flattened and edges prevented from rolling. Grafts can also be covered with paraffin gauze or silicone meshed dressings, which are then covered with a fluffed gauze filler to reduce any dead space in the wound defect and secured with a bandage system. This dressing is usually left sealed for at least 48 hours then removed. Ongoing burn wound management regimens are subject to the graft appearance. Grafts may also be sealed for up to 5 days with a negative pressure dressing.

DONOR SITE CARE A thin layer of donor skin is taken from the person with the use of a dermatome. Each surgical team has its preferred procedures for caring for donor sites and a range of dressings are used. Calcium alginate dressings are frequently used as they provide haemostatic and absorbent features. Donor sites generally take 2 weeks to re-epithelialise, and dressings are applied until healing.

FLAPS This procedure involves using a portion of skin with its intrinsic structures to repair a defect that is too extensive for an SSG or FTG. Flaps leave a scar at the point of injury, as well as the donor site scar. In burns, some flaps become non-viable due to decreased blood flow. There are many types of flaps; the surgeon decides which one to use depending on the defect and where it is located on the body.

Burn wound management

The outcomes of care for the person with a major burn depend in part on the prevention and treatment of infection. The goals of burn wound management are as follows alleviate pain

- control microbial colonisation and prevent burn wound infection
- prevent burn wound conversion to a deeper burn
- achieve burn wound coverage as early as possible
- promote function of healing skin
- preserve function of the body part.

Burn wound management decisions are delayed until primary survey and lifesaving measures have been established. After first aid, burn wound management involves washing and covering the burn with a clean sheet for transfer. Care decisions are dependent on assessment of the depth and appearance of the wound and the dressing products available for the healthcare professional to use. Various dressing products suitable for burn wounds are discussed later in the chapter.

DEBRIDING THE BURN WOUND Burned tissue releases chemical mediators that stimulate phagocytosis in an attempt to digest necrotic tissue. Necrotic tissue that remains despite phagocytic action slows healing and prolongs inflammation. **Debridement** is the process of removing all loose tissue, wound debris and eschar (dead tissue) from the wound. The methods of debridement commonly employed in burn care are surgical, mechanical (irrigation), and conservative sharp wound debridement (removal of loose non-viable tissue without pain or bleeding). Dressings that hydrate the wound will promote autolytic debridement.

During showering, non-viable tissue and slough can be removed while washing the burned area. Showers also promote a feeling of wellness for the person (Wound Healing and Management Node Group, 2017). The person should be encouraged to do as much of the showering themself as possible as this promotes independence and is good physical therapy. It may reduce the anticipation anxiety that arises when someone else is washing their burns. Hydrotherapy (in an immersion tank, a shower or on a spray table) is also used to cleanse the burn injury using a mild, non-perfumed, antimicrobial soap, to remove dead skin and separate eschar. The solution is then rinsed off with warm saline or tap water.

Body hair (except for eyebrows) may be shaved within the burn and to within 2.5 cm of the wound edges. This prevents debris building up around hair follicles, increasing the risk of infection. Shaving also allows for better washing of the burn and adherence of any dressing products. The edges of blisters or eschar are trimmed with sharp scissors. The wound is then covered with a topical antimicrobial agent according to hospital policy.

DRESSING THE BURN WOUND Once the burn wound has been cleaned and debrided, it will require a dressing. Moist wound healing principles and hospital policy on topical antimicrobials should be adhered to. Covering the burn helps to reduce the risk of infection and decreases pain.

All fingers and toes are wrapped separately. Dressings are held in place with roller bandages, retention tapes or tubular net. All care is taken not to restrict range of movement or circulation and to encourage person independence with activities of daily living.

TOPICAL NEGATIVE PRESSURE DEVICES Topical negative pressure devices consist of a foam or gauze dressing that is cut or folded to the wound shape and used to fill any defects. An occlusive, adhesive dressing seals the wound and tubing connects the dressing with the pump. Negative pressure systems reduce wound oedema, remove exudate, help stabilise SSG and promote granulation and epithelialisation (Lin et al., 2021). Single-use negative pressure wound therapy is now available. This is a comfortable therapy that distributes pressure evenly and manages wound fluid to prevent maceration. This device is smaller and therefore safer for the patient.

Role of the physiotherapist

Physiotherapists are primarily concerned with optimising the respiratory system and delivery of oxygen to healing tissues after a burn injury. Lung compromise may impede oxygen delivery to the wounded tissues, slow wound healing and increase the risk of wound infection (Haller et al., 2021; Niinikoski, Heughan & Hunt, 1971, 1972). To further facilitate oxygen transfer during the acute burn period, physiotherapists will focus on the reduction of oedema in order to improve the wound micro-environment (Finlay, Burrows, Burmaz et al., 2017). To prevent such long-term complications and assist with oedema reduction, the injured should be encouraged to exercise their burned and non-burned areas. As soon as possible following admission, the physiotherapist should prescribe and display active and self-assisted passive range-of-movement (ROM) exercises. The physiotherapist will perform passive ROM exercises and apply splints for those unable to move independently. Ideally, an active exercise program is initiated and reinforced by the multidisciplinary team members. The program must involve a warm-up and simple functional tasks, as well as specific exercises. Early ambulation is also part of the plan of care to reduce the risk of respiratory and circulatory complications. It is imperative that the person receives regular multimodal analgesia and pressure bandage support to facilitate these activities (Ryan, Parry & Richard, 2017).

After a burn, people must be maintained in positions that prevent or reduce the risk of contractures that reduce their quality of life (Finlay, Burrows, Kendell et al., 2017). As flexion is the natural resting position of joints and extremities, early physiotherapy includes maintaining and correcting anti-deformity positions. Splints immobilise body parts and may have a role to play in preventing joint contractures, particularly if the person is unconscious in the critical care unit. Splints, if required, should be applied soon after the injury and removed according to schedules prescribed by the therapist.

Physiotherapists facilitate postoperative recovery of the burned patient to prevent long-term loss of movement. The person should be encouraged to move all limbs and walk normally unless contraindicated following surgery. It is better that the patient continues to move while the wounds are healing, rather than waiting until their wounds are healed. Postoperative movement changes depending on the surgery type and the specialist's preferences.

Role of the occupational therapist

Occupational therapists who work with burn-injured people have two core areas of focus: function and scar management.

The World Health Organization (2018) *International Classification of Functioning, Disability and Health* represents the *functional impact* of illness and injury. It defines function and disability in terms of the whole person rather than by illness or injury and looks beyond the medical to include other aspects of disability. It specifically addresses body structure and function, the activities people engage in, the interests they have and the environmental and personal factors that affect those experiences. This framework has a very useful application to the person who has sustained a burn injury, as return to function must include the physical, psychological, relational and social impacts of the injury.

The return to functional independence is a journey that starts the day after injury. The contractile properties of the healing burn dictate early mobilisation to avoid scar contracture, and this is achieved through both specific exercise programs and the early resumption of self-care tasks. The occupational therapist will design a functional retraining program which graduates the resumption of these tasks to enable the individual to gradually improve in independence. Standardised assessments may be used to measure a person's ability to personally care for themself, but also include return to work, return to leisure and the resumption of social and relational roles.

One of the greatest long-term impacts of a burn injury is scarring. If healing is delayed beyond 21 days post injury, evidence suggests that this will result in an adverse scar outcome, as will an injury that has required surgical intervention. Hypertrophic scarring is an aberrant form of the normal processes of wound healing but is commonly associated with burn injury (Ogawa, 2021; Teot et al., 2020) and is defined as red, raised, firm and itchy. It carries the very real risk of joint contracture, which has the potential to severely impact function as well as being aesthetically unacceptable Since the 1970s, compression therapy has been the main form of treatment for hypertrophic scarring. This compression therapy is primarily delivered through the form of tight-fitting elastic garments (pressure garments). Compression should be commenced as soon as the healing skin is able to tolerate the pressure) and withstand the shearing forces of donning and removing the garment. Occupational therapists 'prescribe' the most appropriate pressure garment for the patient, selecting from a range of ready-to-wear and custom-made garments, and taking into account the patient's individual needs and lifestyle. Pressure garments are to be worn 23 hours a day for a period of up to 18 months (Ogawa, 2021; Teot et al., 2020).

Several other modalities that are employed to assure a positive scar outcome include:

- daily scar massage—in conjunction with the application of moisturisers. Massage therapy aims to discourage the formation of fibrotic tissue and to realign the collagen fibres
- contact media—silicone products (gel sheets, gels 'in a tube', putty) and hydrocolloid dressings which are used in conjunction with compression therapy to improve hydration in the scar, reduce pain and itch, reduce vascularity and scar height, and improve pliability
- splinting—contracting scars may need either dynamic splinting (splints with moving components to apply a pull against the scar) or static splints to be worn at night to maintain an anti-contracture position.

As the occupational therapist is concerned with both function and scar, there are two areas of the body that require additional specialist input. These areas, the hands and the face, carry the risk of significant psychosocial impact given their visibility and significant potential impact on independence and function. Specialised programs include splinting exercise and a range of scar management techniques unique to these areas, such as laser treatment, topical drug applications or transparent face marks (Kuehlmann et al., 2019).

Like many in the burns team, the intervention of the occupational therapist is prolonged. It starts at day 1 and accompanies the patient through the acute phase of burn injury, the stages of scar maturation and reintegration to life, work, independence and community.

Role of the dietitian

The role of the dietitian is to optimise the nutritional status of the burn-injured person. Goals may include assisting the patient to maintain weight within 5% to 10% of pre-injury weight, prescription of an enteral feed that meets estimated nutritional needs, coordination of a diet that meets the patient's nutritional and individual needs, prevention of signs and symptoms of micronutrient deficiency, and minimisation of the risk of complications such as hyperglycaemia, hyponatraemia and hypophosphataemia.

THE METABOLIC RESPONSE The person with a major burn is in a hypermetabolic and catabolic state Resting energy expenditure after severe burn injury can be elevated to twice normal levels (Phan, Nguyen & Nguyen, 2020). The mediators of the hypermetabolism include elevated levels of catecholamines, glucocorticoids and glucagon The extent of a person's hypermetabolism is directly proportionate to the size of the burn injury. Recent advances in medical and nursing care have blunted hypermetabolic response to burn injury; however, it cannot be fully reversed.

NUTRITION SUPPORT Careful nutrition assessment, planning, intervention and monitoring is required in order to ensure burns patients meet nutritional requirements. Adult patients with < 20% TBSA burns and paediatric patients with < 15% TBSA burns may be able to maintain nutritional status via a high-energy/high-protein diet and oral nutritional supplementation.

Early initiation of enteral nutrition may improve outcomes in adult patients with > 20% TBSA burns. Current recommendations suggest commencement of enteral nutrition (within 24–48 hours) for all adults with > 20% TBSA burns and children with > 15% TBSA burns. Early enteral feeding is promoted to offset hypermetabolism, improve nitrogen balance, decrease infection, maintain intestinal barrier function, prevent bacterial translocation and decrease length of hospital stay. As nasogastric feeding is usually well tolerated by people with burns, post-pyloric feeding is rarely required. People on enteral feeds are also encouraged to eat and drink, if possible. Parenteral nutrition is appropriate only for those patients who have prolonged intolerance to enteral feeds and who are unable to attain adequate protein and calorie intake with enteral nutrition (Romanowski, 2021). Examples where parenteral nutrition may be instigated include pancreatitis, bowel obstruction, paralytic ileus or intestinal perforation.

MONITORING AND EVALUATION As a patient's burn injury heals, they are usually able to tolerate larger amounts of oral diet and nutritional supplements. Patients with major burns will usually progress from complete nutrition via enteral feeds to overnight feeds, and then enteral feeding will cease. The decision as to when to progress the patient is made by the team. Considerations include adequacy of oral intake, consumption of oral nutritional supplements and healing stage of the wounds. Nutrition-related monitoring may include food-intake charts, weekly weights, biochemical indices (renal function, liver function, Mg, PO_4^{3-}, BSL), maintenance of muscle stores (e.g. handgrip strength), bowels and fluid balance.

DISCHARGE PLANNING Hypermetabolism related to a major burn can persist for up to 2 years after the injury (Berger, 2019). Patients with major burns should receive education prior to discharge about the importance of weight maintenance, adequate protein and following a general healthy diet. Evidence is scant about the long-term requirement for vitamins and minerals in burns patients. A daily multivitamin/multimineral supplement until wound healing is demonstrated may be useful to optimise vitamin and mineral intake.

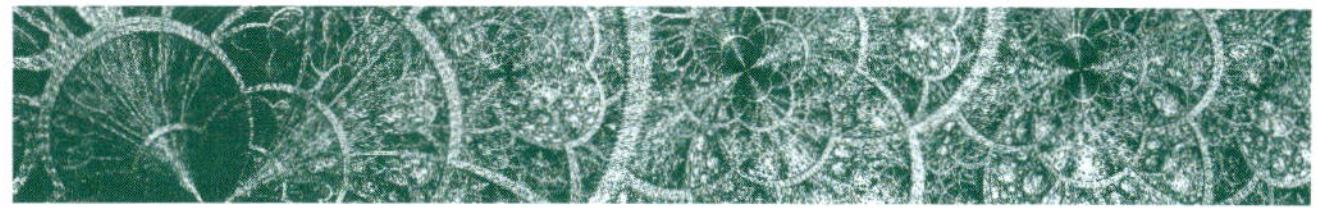

Nursing care

Health promotion

Although treatments have improved significantly during the past several decades, prevention remains the primary goal. The nursing profession is currently well positioned to collaborate with other disciplines to develop initiatives to reduce the number of burn injuries. For example, as advocates, nurses can alert political leaders to the need to pass legislation aimed at reducing the incidence of burns. Appropriate legislative themes might centre on safety in the workplace (e.g. requirements for smoke alarms and sprinkler systems), on the highways (e.g. regulations regarding the transportation of flammable liquids) and in the home (e.g. requirements for safety devices for water heaters and wood-burning stoves and for self-extinguishing cigarettes). As educators, nurses can develop teaching plans for families and communities to heighten awareness of the problem. As researchers, nurses can investigate conditions leading to burn injury and suggest methods to reduce its prevalence.

Nursing diagnoses and interventions

A major burn affects virtually every body system, as well as social, cultural, economic, psychological and spiritual wellbeing. Acute care is combined with ongoing rehabilitation that continues post discharge. Many nursing diagnoses are appropriate for the person with a major burn injury; they include *Impaired skin integrity*, *Deficient fluid volume*, *Acute pain*, *Risk of infection*, *Impaired physical mobility*, *Imbalanced nutrition: less than body requirements* and *Powerlessness*. The nursing care within a multidisciplinary team has been discussed with regard to the first six of these nursing diagnoses and the concept of *Powerlessness* is discussed.

CONSIDERATION FOR PRACTICE

An increased body temperature, without other manifestations of infection, is not indicative of infection in people with large burn wounds (in which the hypermetabolic response resets the core temperature to a higher level).

CONSIDERATION FOR PRACTICE

Assess all people, but especially the older person, for indications of pressure injury formation under a splint.

CONSIDERATION FOR PRACTICE

Narcotics are always administered intravenously, rather than orally, subcutaneously or intramuscularly in the resuscitative or acute phase of a burn due to decreased circulation and absorption of medications.

NURSING CARE PLAN A person with a major burn

Craig Howard is a 35-year-old coal miner from Queensland. Craig was driving home after a late shift when his 4-wheel drive veered off the road, rolled and caught on fire. He was freed from his vehicle by a passing motorist, who in turn summoned help and called police. The passing motorist stayed with Craig until the aerial rescue team arrived and transported him to the nearest metropolitan hospital emergency department. The hospital has a burns unit. Craig's wife, Mary, and twin daughters, Jessica and Jane, aged 10, were notified of the accident by police.

ASSESSMENT

On his admission to the emergency department, Craig was diagnosed with deep partial-thickness and full-thickness burns of the anterior chest, and circumferential full-thickness burns of the arms and hands. An initial quick assessment based on the rule of nines estimates the extent of his burn injury at 36% of TBSA. His vital signs were as follows: T 35.6°C, P 140, R 40 and BP 98/60. At the scene, the paramedics inserted two large-bore cannulae and started the rapid infusion of Hartmann's solution. Craig is receiving 100% humidified oxygen via a face mask. Initial ABGs are: pH 7.49, PO_2 60 mmHg, PCO_2 32 mmHg and bicarbonate 22 mEq/L. Lung sounds indicate inspiratory and expiratory wheezing, and a persistent cough reveals sooty sputum production. An IDC was inserted into his bladder and initially drained a moderate amount of dark, concentrated urine. A nasogastric tube was inserted. Craig is alert and oriented and complains of severe pain associated with the burn injuries. The burns unit is notified and Craig is transferred there. Craig's condition is serious. There are several nursing diagnoses that could be developed.

DIAGNOSIS

- *Impaired skin integrity* related to major burns injury.
- *Acute pain* related to major burns injury.
- Potential for *Infection* related to *Impaired skin integrity.*
- *Deficient fluid volume* related to major burns injury.
- *Impaired physical mobility* related to major burns injury.
- Potential for pressure injuries related to *Impaired physical mobility.*
- Potential for *Imbalanced nutrition* related to excess body requirements associated with burns injury.

PLANNING

- Ensure room is set up prior to Craig's arrival; i.e. assemble all equipment required to weigh, shower and dress him, administer IV fluids and nasogastric fluids, measure and test urine, correct documentation, analgesia ordered.
- Ensure all staff are aware a major burn is being admitted and that an appropriate staff member is allocated to Craig.
- Warm the room.
- Prepare for possible prophylactic nasotracheal or endotracheal intubation to maintain airway patency.
- Prepare Craig and his family when they arrive with an explanation of protocols and procedures. This may help reduce anxiety and help with compliance.

Expected outcomes

- Craig maintains an effective airway and vital signs are within normal limits. He has clear breath sounds and no evidence of cyanosis. Mental status is within normal limits.
- Craig does not suffer from hypothermia as evidenced by warm peripheries, conscious level and vital signs.
- Craig demonstrates adequate fluid volume by maintaining appropriate urine output and urea and electrolytes and other laboratory findings within normal limits.
- Craig demonstrates understanding of instructions and orientation to person, time and place through conversation and compliance with requests and treatment.

IMPLEMENTATION

- *Maintain effective airway clearance,* as there is potential for increased lung congestion secondary to smoke inhalation and torso burns.
- *Maintain adequate fluid volume,* as abnormal fluid loss is possible secondary to burn injury.
- *Monitor for adequate tissue perfusion* (peripheral), as peripheral constriction secondary to circumferential burn wounds of the arms is a possibility.
- Weigh Craig.
- Once cervical spine injury has been cleared, elevate head of bed to improve lung expansion and ventilation.
- Administer humidified 100% oxygen at prescribed amount.
- Educate Craig on the importance of deep breathing and sitting upright to improve his breathing.
- Monitor for expectoration of sooty sputum, stridor, increase in wheezing.
- Elevate both arms on one or two pillows to reduce swelling.
- Perform neurovascular observations ½–1 hourly depending on neurovascular status and hospital protocol—that is, colour, warmth, movement, sensation and capillary refill.
- Remove dressings from fingertips to enable neurovascular observations to be done.
- Administer intravenous analgesia as ordered for pain.
- Observe for any signs of respiratory distress or decrease in respiratory status.
- Observations to be performed ½–1 hourly depending on Craig's condition and hospital protocol—that is, respiratory rate, blood pressure and pulse. Temperature 1 hourly as Craig is hypothermic on admission. Oxygen saturations should be monitored continuously.
- Explain to Craig all procedures and protocols to help reduce anxiety and encourage compliance with treatment. This may need to be done on more than one occasion.
- Initiate fluid resuscitation therapy using the Parkland (Baxter) formula to calculate intravenous fluid rate for the first 24 hours post burn. Review original calculations based on real weight, not estimated weight, and ensure fluid resuscitation time is from time of injury.
- Insert nasogastric tube and commence enteral feeding as instructed. Discourage Craig from drinking water.
- Measure urine output 1-hourly and record specific gravity hourly.
- Document all observations, input and output accurately.
- Arrange for blood tests to be taken according to hospital burn resuscitation protocol and ensure the results are reviewed.
- Craig maintained his respiratory status and did not require intubation. He was continued on humidified oxygen sitting in an upright position in bed or chair with his arms elevated.
- Hourly urine outputs indicate adequate fluid resuscitation. Urine output has been maintained at 50 mL/h and is a straw colour; specific gravity is 1020. Blood pressure has increased to 100/64. He has remained tachycardic at 100, and his respiratory rate on humidified oxygen is 28. His temperature is now 37°C.

NURSING CARE PLAN A person with a major burn (continued)

- To improve tissue perfusion of both arms, the physician has performed bilateral escharotomies and the wounds are packed with alginate and covered in a silver antimicrobial dressing, such as Acticoat®. Colour, warmth, movement, sensation and capillary return have improved, indicating escharotomies have been successful.

EVALUATION

- Craig Howard demonstrated a patent airway, as evidenced by clear breath sounds; absence of cyanosis; and vital signs, chest x-ray findings and ABGs within normal limits.
- Adequate fluid volume and electrolyte balance demonstrated, as evidenced by urine output, vital signs, mental status and laboratory findings within normal limits.
- Adequate tissue perfusion demonstrated, as evidenced by palpable pulses, warm extremities, normal capillary refill and absence of paraesthesia.

CRITICAL THINKING IN THE NURSING PROCESS

1 Explain the rationale for the immediate insertion of an IDC and nasogastric tube.
2 An escharotomy was performed on both arms. Why was this procedure necessary in Craig Howard's case?
3 What is the rationale supporting the intravenous administration of narcotics to control Craig's pain?
4 Explain the sequence of events that led to a fluid and electrolyte shift during the first 24 to 48 hours after Craig sustained his injury.

REFLECTION ON THE NURSING PROCESS

1 Outline what you have learned from this case study that you will apply to your future practice.
2 Which communication and person-centred education strategies would you use when caring for people with major burns such as Craig's?

Powerlessness

Usually, the person with a major burn injury endures a lengthy hospital stay involving many treatments and care protocols that are beyond their control. During the early stages, much of the care regimen involves pain. Further, the foreign environment of the burns unit makes it difficult for the people to relate to the immediate surroundings. The person's body image is often altered, depending on the extent and location of the burn injury.

- Involve the person in their own care. Encourage independence with activities of daily living. Encourage the person to participate in showering and toileting and physiotherapy. Encourage the person to verbalise their feelings. *Powerlessness derives from the belief that one is unable to influence the outcome of a situation.*
- Keep needed items within reach, such as call bell, urinal, water pitcher and tissues, *to reinforce the person's feelings of control.*
- Encourage the person to express feelings. *The nurse can help the person cope by therapeutically listening, displaying a caring presence, clarifying misconceptions and providing positive feedback.*
- Involve the person in setting realistic goals to suit their level of recovery, but also encourage them to aim for improvement, not stasis, in rehabilitation. *Rehabilitation starts the day the person is admitted, not when healed. Small incremental gains are easier to achieve and allow for frequent positive reinforcement.*

Community-based care

Education for the person with burns and their family is an important component of all phases of burn care. As treatment progresses, the nurse encourages family members to assume more responsibility in providing care. From admission to discharge, the nurse teaches the person and family to assess all findings, implement therapies and evaluate progress. The following topics should be addressed when preparing the person and family for home care:

- The long-term goals of rehabilitation care, which are to prevent soft tissue deformity, protect skin grafts, maintain physiological function, manage scars and return the person to an optimal level of independence.
- Avoiding exposure to people with colds or infections and following aseptic techniques meticulously when caring for the wound.
- The need for progressive physical activity.
- How to apply splints, pressure support garments and other assistive devices.

NURSING CARE OF THE OLDER PERSON Burns in the older person

Older people are at greater risk of burns of all degrees of severity. Most burns are accidental, the result of slower reaction times, decreased mobility, visual deficits, a decreased sense of smell, forgetfulness and impaired sensation. Many older people are burned by stoves, hot water, hot food, irons, cookware and heating pads. Older people with cognitive impairments or dementia may start fires by leaving cooking foods unattended.

The care of older people with burns often presents unique challenges. They may delay seeking treatment, thus increasing the risk of infection and burn wound conversion. Their care may be complicated by the presence of other chronic illnesses. They may live alone and have no one to care for them during rehabilitation. Even small burns have the potential to become serious in older people.

Burn prevention strategies for older adults are as follows:

- Check the smoke detector battery once a month.
- Wear close-fitting clothing when cooking.
- Use a cooking timer with a loud alarm.
- Never lay anything over a heating device.
- Install anti-scald devices in bathroom plumbing.
- Encourage no smoking in the house.

TRANSLATION TO PRACTICE Evidence-based practice: a person with a major burn

In 2020, the American Burn Association (ABA) created a multidisciplinary committee to develop and maintain current clinical practice guidelines for burn care. The purpose of the guidelines was to provide recommendations on early rehabilitation and mobilisation interventions in critically ill burn patients (Cartotto et al., 2022).

People with major burn injuries are at risk of pressure injuries due to deficient fluid volume, inadequate nutrition, pain and immobility. Healthy, intact skin can experience damage from pressure, friction and shearing forces, posing a second area of risk of pressure injuries. Pressure injuries result from continuous, unrelieved pressure that causes reduced blood flow to vulnerable areas of the skin, resulting in tissue damage, particularly in patients with prolonged bedrest/immobilisation.

Contributing factors to the development of pressure injuries in people with burn injuries include inadequate dietary intake, increased age, altered level of consciousness, isolation and, potentially, the inability to communicate.

Mobilisation interventions including resistance exercises, active side-to-side turning, standing and walking (where appropriate) assist in the decrease in inflammation in affected areas and therefore in decreasing pressure injuries.

IMPLICATIONS FOR NURSING

Nurses and all members of the burn team assume an integral role in preventing pressure injuries. To prevent pressure injuries, nurses must constantly monitor the person with major burn injuries for signs of skin damage and conduct regular and frequent skin inspections. The chapter 'Nursing care of people with integumentary disorders' discusses interventions for pressure injury prevention, assessment and management.

CRITICAL THINKING IN PERSON-CENTRED CARE

1 The person's head must be elevated to 30 degrees when nasogastric tube feedings are implemented. What strategies would you recommend to prevent inhalation of nasogastric feeds?
2 How could splints that are being used to prevent contractures be modified as the person's amount and extent of oedema fluctuates?
3 Develop a teaching plan for instructing nursing assistants on how to move, position and transfer people in a burns centre unit. Include in the teaching plan the proper technique for cleansing unburned skin.

- Dietary requirements with required kilojoules.
- Alternative pain control therapies, such as guided imagery, relaxation techniques and diversional activities.
- Care of the graft and donor sites.
- Referral for social service, clergy and/or psychiatric services as appropriate.
- Helpful resources and websites:
  - Australian and New Zealand Burn Association (ANZBA): https://anzba.org.au
  - Burn Foundation Australia: www.burnfoundation.org.au
  - Burn Prevention Network: www.burnprevention.org
  - Burn Survivors Network: https://kidsfoundation.org.au/injury-recovery/burn-survivors-network
  - Burns Clinical Practice Guidelines, Royal Children's Hospital Melbourne Victoria, Australia: https://www.rch.org.au/clinicalguide/guideline_index/Burns/
  - Burns Support Foundation: http://burnssupportfoundation.org.au
  - Changing Faces: https://www.changingfaces.org.uk
  - Fiona Wood Foundation: https://www.fionawoodfoundation.com
  - International Society for Burn Injuries: www.worldburn.org
  - K.I.D.S Foundation: https://www.kidsfoundation.org.au
  - Wounds Australia https://www.woundsaustralia.com.au/.

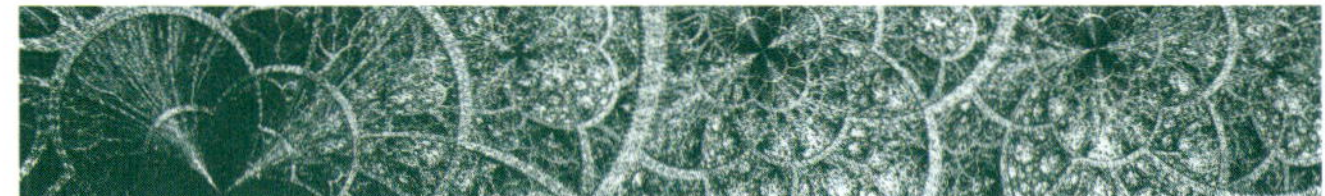

CHAPTER HIGHLIGHTS

- **Four types of burn injuries are thermal, chemical, electrical and radiation. The depth of the burn injury determines whether it is classified as a superficial, partial-thickness or full-thickness burn.**
- **The Wallace (1951) rule of nines, age-dependent burn graphs and the palmar surface assessment are all used to estimate the extent of a burn by assigning percentages to different parts of the body.**
- **Major burns involve multi-organ pathophysiological alterations. Most critical is the fluid shift from the intracellular and intravascular compartments into the interstitium, resulting in a type of hypovolaemic shock called burn shock. Other pathological processes include an impaired immune system, disturbed functions of the skin, inhalation injury, gastrointestinal ulcerations and ileus, renal failure and hypermetabolism.**
- **Interprofessional care focuses on managing the person during the resuscitative, acute and rehabilitative phases. To counter the effects of burn shock, fluid resuscitation using guidelines such as the Parkland (Baxter) formula are initiated to replace fluid and electrolyte losses.**

- Additional management for the person with major burns includes preventing atelectasis, maintaining respiratory function, controlling pain, preventing infection and Curling's ulcer, promoting nutrition and providing wound care.
- Extensive eschar of an extremity or the torso, called circumferential wounds, can potentially occlude arterial flow or decrease respiratory function. An escharotomy is used to release tension, preventing additional complications.
- Surgical management of burn wounds includes debridement and skin grafting. Biological and biosynthetic dressings provide temporary covering and prepare the wound for permanent autografts.
- Continual psychological support of the person and family is essential throughout convalescence and rehabilitation.

CONCEPT CHECK

1 During the resuscitative phase of burn management, what diagnostic test result should the nurse expect to find?
1 increased haematocrit
2 increased serum albumin
3 decreased serum potassium
4 decreased blood urea nitrogen (BUN)

2 A person is admitted with severe burns to the face and chest. The injured skin is dry and leathery, with no pain sensations present. The nurse recognises that this burn is classified as:
1 superficial
2 superficial partial-thickness
3 deep partial-thickness
4 full-thickness

3 Which of the following people is at greatest risk of developing burn shock?
1 a 21-year-old with 90% superficial burn from a tanning bed
2 a 30-year-old with 10% TBSA from a gasoline explosion
3 a 39-year-old with radiation burns following treatment for cancer
4 a 48-year-old with > 50% TBSA from a high-voltage electrical accident

4 A person with full-thickness burns over 50% of the body arrives in the emergency department. The person weighs 70 kg. Using the Parkland (Baxter) formula, calculate the amount of fluid replacement that the nurse should deliver in the first 8 hours.
1 3,500 mL
2 7,000 mL
3 10,500 mL
4 14,000 mL

5 For a person with a major burn, which of the following evaluation criteria indicate that fluid resuscitation is effective during the first 24 hours of care?
1 urine output of 30 to 50 mL/h
2 central venous pressure of 18
3 heart rate of 130 beats per minute
4 blood pressure 96/70

6 A person has deep partial-thickness burns to the entire left arm and left side of the back. What finding should be reported to the physician immediately?
1 fluid-filled vesicles on the left arm
2 pain in the left arm
3 blanching when pressure is applied to the left hand
4 decreased left radial pulse

7 A person received deep partial-thickness burns to the anterior trunk, perineum, and left arm anterior and posterior. Using the Wallace (1951) rule of nines, what is the percentage of total body surface area (TBSA) that was burned?
1 18%
2 28%
3 36%
4 40%

8 Which of the following topics should be included in a presentation on burn prevention at a senior citizens centre? (Select all that apply.)
1 Wear close-fitting clothing when cooking.
2 Use a solar-powered night light.
3 Check smoke detectors annually.
4 Install anti-scald devices in bathroom plumbing.
5 Have a neighbour routinely check for the odour of gas.

9 A person has possible carbon monoxide poisoning secondary to smoke inhalation. What manifestation should the nurse expect to find in a person with a 15% carbon monoxide level?
1 dark red skin colour
2 drowsiness
3 dizziness
4 hypotension

BIBLIOGRAPHY

Agency for Clinical Innovation (NSW) (2019). *Minor burn blister management*. Retrieved from https://aci.health.nsw.gov.au/

Australian and New Zealand Burn Association Ltd (ANZBA) (2018). *Emergency management of severe burns*. Course manual (version 18). Albany Creek, Qld: ANZBA.

Australian and New Zealand Burn Association (ANZBA) (n.d.). *First aid of LPG (cold) burns for clinicians: Fact sheet*. Retrieved from https://anzba.org.au/

Bajraktarova-Valjakova, E., Korunoska-Stevkovska, V., Georgieva, S., Ivanovski, K., Bajraktarova-Misevska, C., Mijoska, A. & Grozdanov, A. (2018). Hydrofluoric acid: Burns and systemic toxicity, protective measures, immediate and hospital medical treatment. *Open Access Macedonian Journal of Medical Sciences*, *25*(11), 2257–2269.

Berger, M. M. (2019). Nutrition determines outcome after severe burns. *Annals of Translational Medicine*, *7*(Suppl. 6), S216. doi: 10.21037/atm.2019.08.57

Bermo, M. S., Patterson, D., Sharar, S. R., Hoffman, H. & Lewis, D. H. (2020). Virtual reality to relieve pain in burn patients undergoing imaging and treatment. *Topics in Magnetic Resonance Imaging*, *29*(4), 203–208. doi: 10.1097/RMR.0000000000000248

Burns Registry of Australia and New Zealand (BRANZ) (2022). *Annual report 2020/21*. Melbourne: Department of Epidemiology and Preventive Medicine, Monash University. Retrieved from https://anzba.org.au/

Cartotto, R., Johnson, L., Rood, J. M. et al. (2022). Clinical practice guideline: Early mobilization and rehabilitation of critically ill burn patients. *Journal of Burn Care & Research* (irac008). https://doi.org/10.1093/jbcr/irac008

Chai, H., Chaudhari, N., Kornhaber, R., Cuttle, L., Fear, M., Wood, F. & Martin, L. (2022). Chemical burn to the skin: A systematic review of first aid impacts on clinical outcomes. *Burns* (online, May 2022). https://doi.org/10.1016/j.burns.2022.05.006

Chourdakis, M., Bouras, E., Shields, A. B., Stoppe, C., Rousseau, A. F. & Hayland, D. K. (2020). Nutritional therapy among burn injured patients in the critical care setting: An international multicenter observational study on 'best achievable' practices. *Clinical Nutrition*, *39*(12), 3813–3820.

Chung, B. Y., Kim, H. B., Jung, M. J. et al. (2020). Post burn pruritus. *International Journal of Molecular Sciences*, *21*(11). doi: 10.3390/ijms21113880

Department of Health (2022). *The Australian immunisation handbook*. Retrieved from https://immunisationhandbook.health.gov.au/

Finlay, V., Burrows, S., Burmaz, M., Yawary, H., Lee, J., Edgar, D. W. & Wood, F. M. (2017). Increased burn healing time is associated with higher Vancouver Scar Scale score. *Scars, Burns & Healing, 3*. doi: 10.1177/2059513117696324

Finlay, V., Burrows, S., Kendell, R., Berghuber, A., Chong, V., Tan, J., Edgar, D. W. & Wood, F. (2017). Modified Vancouver Scar Scale score is linked with quality of life after burn. *Burns, 43*(4), 741–746. doi: 10.1016/j.burns.2016.11.007

Greenwood, J., Damkat-Thomas, L., Schmitt, B. & Dearman, B. (2020). Successful proof of the 'two-stage strategy' for major burn wound repair. *Burns Open, 4*, (3). 121–131. https://doi.org/10.1016/j.burnso.2020.06.003

Haidari, H., Garg, S., Vasilev, K., Kopecki, Z. & Cowin, A. J. (2020). Silver-based wound dressings: Current issues and future developments for treating bacterial infections. *Wound Practice and Research, 28*(4), 173–180. https://doi.org/10.33235/wpr.28.4.173-180

Haller, H. L., Sander, F., Popp, D. et al. (2021). Oxygen, pH, lactate, and metabolism: How old knowledge and new insights might be combined for new wound treatment. *Medicina, 57*(11). https://doi.org/10.3390/medicina57111190

Herndon, D. N. (ed.). (2018). *Total burn care* (5th ed.). New York: Elsevier Health.

Holley, A. D., Reade, M. C., Lipman, J. & Cohen, J. (2020). There is no fire without smoke! Pathophysiology and treatment of inhalational injury in burns: A narrative review. *Anaesthesia and Intensive Care, 48*(2), 114–122. https://doi.org/10.1177/0310057X20913282

Jackson, D. M. (1953). The diagnosis of the depth of burning. *British Journal of Surgery, 40*(164), 588–596. https://doi.org/10.1002/bjs.18004016413

Khansa, I., Schoenbrunner, A. R., Kraft, C. T. & Janis, J. E. (2019). Silver in wound care—Friend or foe? A comprehensive review. *International Open Access Journal of the American Society of Plastic Surgeons, 7*(8) e2390. doi: 10.1097/GOX.0000000000002390

Knowlin, L. T., Reid, T., Williams, F. et al. (2018). Burn mortality in patients with preexisting cardiovascular disease. *Burns, 43*(5), 949–955. doi: 10.1016/j.burns.2017.01.026

Knowlin, L. T., Stanford, L. B., Cairns, B. A. & Charles, A. G. (2018). The effect of preexisting respiratory co-morbidities on burn outcomes. *Burns, 43*(2), 366–373. doi: 10.1016/j.burns.2016.08.029

Kuehlmann, B., Stern-Buchbinder, Z., Wan, D. C., Friedstat, J. S. & Gurtner, G. C. (2019). Beneath the surface: A review of laser remodeling of hypertrophic scars and burns. *Advances in Wound Care, 8*(4). https://doi.org/10.1089/wound.2018.0857

Lin, D. Z., Kao, Y. C., Chen, C., Wang, H. J. & Chiu, W. K. (2021). Negative pressure wound therapy for burn patients: A meta-analysis and systematic review. *International Wound Journal, 18*(1), 112–123. doi: 10.1111/iwj.13500

Lund, C. & Browder, N. (1944). Estimation of areas of burns. *Surgery, Gynecology & Obstetrics, 79*, 352–358.

Lupoli, R., Lembo, E., Saldalamacchia, G., Avola, C. K., Angrisani, L. & Capaldo, B. (2017). Bariatric surgery and long-term nutritional issues. *World Journal of Diabetes, 8*(11), 464–474. doi: 10.4239/wjd.v8.i11.464

Manning, L., Ferreira, I. B., Gittings, P. et al. (2022). Wound healing with 'spray-on' autologous skin grafting (ReCell) compared with standard care in patients with large diabetes-related foot wounds: An open-label randomised controlled trial. *International Wound Journal, 19*, 470–481. https://doi.org/10.1111/iwj.13646

Martin, L., Andrews, S., Rea, S. & Wood, F. (2022). Motivating patients towards better recovery after burn: The development of a booklet to reframe perspectives. *Burns, 1*, S0305-4179(21)00368-5. doi: 10.1016/j.burns.2021.12.011

Martin, L., Rea, S. & Wood, F. (2021). A quantitative analysis of the relationship between post traumatic growth, depressions and coping styles after burn. *Burns, 47*(8), 1748–1755. doi: 10.1016/j.burns.2021.05.019

Morgan, M., Deuis, J. R., Frosig-Jorgensen, M., Lewis, R. J., Cabot, P. J., Gray, P. D. & Vetter, I. (2018). Burn pain: A systematic and critical review of epidemiology, pathophysiology and treatment. *Pain Medicine, 19*, 708–734.

Murphy, C. V., Zhelezny, R., Porter, K. et al. (2021). Clinical outcomes following a burn injury across the continuum of chronic glycemic control. *Burns, 47*(5), 1059–1065. doi: 10.1016/j.burns.2020.10.018

Nherera, L., Trueman, P., Roberts, C. & Berg, L. (2017). Silver delivery, approaches in the management of partial thickness burns: A systematic review and indirect treatment comparison. *Wound Repair and Regeneration, 25*, 707–721.

Nielson, C. B., Duethman, N. C., Howard, J. M., Moncure, M. & Wood, J. G. (2017). Burns: Pathophysiology of systemic complications and current management. *Journal of Burn Care and Research, 38*, e469–e481.

Niinikoski, J., Heughan, C. & Hunt, T. K. (1971). Oxygen and carbon dioxide tensions in experimental wounds. *Surgery, Gynecology & Obstetrics, 133*(6), 1003–1007.

Niinikoski, J., Heughan, C. & Hunt, T. K. (1972). Oxygen tensions in human wounds. *The Journal of Surgical Research, 12*(2), 77–82.

Nischwitz, S. P., Luze, H., Kotzbeck, P. & Kamolz, L. P. (2020). Electrical burns and their consequences. *Burns, 46*(4), 982–984. doi: 10.1016/j.burns.2020.04.015

Norris, T. L. (2018). *Porth's pathophysiology: Concepts of altered health states* (10th ed.). Philadelphia: Lippincott Williams & Wilkins.

Ogawa, R. (ed.). (2021). *Total scar management*. Singapore: Springer Verlag.

Phan, K. Q., Nguyen, L. N. & Nguyen, A. H. (2020). Profile and factors influencing resting energy expenditure in adult burn patients. *International Journal of Burns and Trauma, 10*(3), 55–59.

Reid, A. & Ha, J. F. (2019). Inhalational injury and the larynx: A review. *Burns, 45*(6), 1266–1274. https://doi.org/10.1016/j.burns.2018.10.025

Rice, P. L. & Orgill, D. P. (2021). *Assessment and classification of burn injury*. Retrieved from https://www.uptodate.com/

Romanowski, K. S. (2021). *Overview of nutrition support in burn patients*. Retrieved from https://www.uptodate.com/

Ryan, C. M., Parry, I. & Richard, R. (2017). Functional outcomes following burn injury. *Journal of Burn Care and Research, 38*(3), e614–e617. doi: 10.1097/BCR.0000000000000537

Swain, C. & Khan, M. (2019). Surgical management of focal ionising radiation burns. *Journal of the Royal Army Medical Corps, 165*(6). doi: 10.1136/jramc-2018-000967

Teot, L., Mustoe, T. A., Middelkoop, E. & Gauglitz, G. G. (2020). *Textbook on scar management*. New York: Springer.

Tracy, L. M., Singer, Y., Schrale, R. et al. (2020). Epidemiology of burn injury in older adults: An Australian and New Zealand perspective. *Scars, Burns & Healing, 6*. doi: 10.1177/2059513120952336

Victorian Government Department of Health (2021). *Could it be carbon monoxide (CO) poisoning?* Retrieved from https://www2.health.vic.gov.au

Wallace, A. B. (1951). The exposure treatment of burns. *The Lancet, 3*(1)(6653), 501–504. doi: 10.1016/s0140-6736(51)91975-7

World Health Organization (2018). *International classification of functioning, disability and health*. Retrieved from https://www.who.int/

Wound Healing and Management Node Group (2017). Evidence summary: Wound management—Chlorhexidine. *Wound Australia Journal, 25*(1), 49–51. Retrieved from https://journals.cambridgemedia.com.au/

UNIT 4 BUILDING CLINICAL COMPETENCE

Responses to altered integumentary structure and function

Clinical scenario

You have been assigned to work with the following four people for the 0700 shift on a medical–surgical unit. Significant data obtained during report are as follows:

- Mr Johnson is a 46-year-old who has been hospitalised for surgery to release contractures at his elbows which resulted from a flash burn from a grill fire 3 years ago. He is scheduled for surgery at 0800 and needs vital signs, preoperative medication and the preoperative checklist completed.
- Mrs Carter is a 35-year-old who was hospitalised 2 days ago with cellulitis in the right calf. Vital signs are T 38°C, P 80, R 20, BP 116/76. She is complaining of a headache and pain in the right calf. She was last medicated for pain at 0300.
- Mr Jenkins is an 86-year-old with herpes zoster. He was admitted 4 days ago with lesions on his left neck and trunk. Vital signs are T 37.2°C, P 88, R 26, BP 158/90. He is complaining of burning pain across his back and is requesting a nurse to check his back for new lesions.
- Mr Ugandi is a 34-year-old Indigenous Australian male who has AIDS. He was transferred from the burn critical care unit to the medical–surgical unit at 0600 after being treated for toxic epidermal necrolysis for the past month. He is ready to begin discharge teaching.

Critical-thinking questions

1 In what order would you visit these people after report?

1.
2.
3.
4.

2 What top two priority nursing diagnoses would you choose for each of the people presented above? Can you explain, if asked, the rationale for your choices?

	Priority Nursing Diagnosis #1	Priority Nursing Diagnosis #2
Mr Johnson		
Mrs Carter		
Mr Jenkins		
Mr Ugandi		

3 Mr Johnson received partial-thickness and full-thickness flash burns on both anterior and posterior arms and his anterior trunk from the grill fire. Using the rule of nines, what is the percentage of total body surface (TBSA) burned? ________%

4 Morphine sulfate is the drug of choice for pain. Which manifestation requires immediate nursing intervention following morphine administration?

1. vomiting once after medication is administered
2. respiratory rate below 8 breaths per minute
3. blood pressure of 110/70 after a baseline blood pressure of 120/80
4. peripheral pulse of 68 after a baseline pulse of 78

5 A diet high in protein and iron may help prevent pressure injuries on the person who is on prolonged bed rest. Which foods should the nurse encourage the person to eat to help prevent pressure injuries?

1. eggs and chicken
2. broccoli and oranges
3. oatmeal and bananas
4. wholegrain bread and kidney beans

6 Mr Jenkins is being discharged to home. Which statement does the nurse need to teach Mr Jenkins about herpes zoster on discharge?

1. 'Continue taking the antiviral medication to cure the herpes zoster.'
2. 'You can attend church functions because herpes zoster is not contagious.'
3. 'Use narcotic pain medications only for severe pain so you do not become addicted to the medication.'
4. 'Wear cotton clothing and keep room temperatures cool to decrease the pain and itching from the herpes zoster lesions.'

7 Mrs Carter was admitted with cellulitis in the right calf. Which manifestations would the nurse assess on admission?

1. redness, oedema, and pain in the right calf
2. purulent drainage, pale skin, and pain in right calf
3. rash, redness, and swelling in right calf
4. itching, rash, and pain in right calf

8 The nurse applies mafenide acetate (Sulfamylon®) to Mr Ugandi's open skin wounds caused by toxic epidermal necrolysis. Which hypersensitivity reactions would require the nurse to discontinue the drug?

1. tachycardia and tachypnoea
2. nausea and vomiting
3. facial oedema and pruritus
4. diarrhoea and candidiasis

9 Which serum laboratory values are decreased with inadequate nutritional intake, such as in a person with severe burns? (Select all that apply.)

1. protein
2. potassium
3. iron
4. full blood cell count
5. glucose
6. calcium

10 When a person is admitted to the burns unit for treatment of severe burns, it is most important for the nurse to monitor the person for:

1. acute pain
2. nausea and vomiting
3. hypothermia
4. fluid and electrolyte imbalance

11 Which of these people is most at risk of skin breakdown leading to pressure injuries?

1. a 70-year-old who had a stroke with left-sided paralysis
2. a quadriplegic admitted to the hospital with pneumonia
3. a 56-year-old on dialysis three times a week
4. an 84-year-old in traction for a hip fracture

12 Health teaching for skin cancer includes which interventions? (Select all that apply.)

1. Wear long-sleeved shirts and a wide-brimmed hat in the sun.
2. Apply sunscreen once a day.
3. Avoid tanning booths or prolonged exposure to the sun.
4. Minimise exposure to the sun between 1 pm and 4 pm.
5. Apply sunscreen before and after swimming.

Case study

Ms Rachel Chelen is a 23-year-old who is admitted to the medical–surgical unit for observation and treatment after being exposed to the sun for a prolonged period of time. On admission, Ms Chelen stated she fell asleep lying on her stomach while sunbathing at the beach. Her vital signs are T 39°C, P 94, R 26, BP 116/76. Her height is 167 cm and weight is 87 kg. Assessment findings are that her back is red and slightly oedematous with an area approximately 6 cm by 3 cm between the scapula that is beginning to develop blisters. The backs of her arms and legs and soles of her feet are red and slightly oedematous. She is complaining of pain on her back, arms, legs and feet. She stated that she feels chilled, is nauseated and has a headache. Blood is drawn for a full blood count and electrolytes for baseline assessment. IV therapy is instituted to maintain hydration. The burn areas are washed with soap and water and an antibacterial dressing (e.g. Acticoat®) with moisturiser is applied to the erythema. A mild analgesic is administered as ordered. Ms Chelen is covered to prevent further chilling and to prevent burned areas being exposed to air.

She is diagnosed with superficial and superficial partial-thickness burns. Using the rule of nines, the partial-thickness burn on her back is classified as approximately 5% total body surface area. The superficial burns over the rest of the reddened areas are not classified.

Superficial burns involve the epidermis layer of the skin. Superficial partial-thickness burns involve the entire epidermis and the papillae of the dermis. The pathophysiological effects of the superficial and partial-thickness burns are the result of exposure to the sun for a prolonged time. Inflammation occurs in response to tissue injury. Platelets aggregate at the burn injury site, fibrin is deposited, and a thrombus is formed. The thrombus, along with vasoconstriction, walls off the burn injury site. Then vasodilation occurs with increased capillary permeability, which leads to redness and oedema. Injury to the dermis results in a moist, glistening appearance as blisters form. The burned area will blanch on pressure. There is pain in response to touch and temperature changes. The burned area should heal within 7–14 days, depending on how much dermis is involved, with minimal scarring, but may have pigment changes. Manifestations of superficial and superficial partial-thickness burns are skin redness, blister formation, local pain, headache, chills, nausea and vomiting. Complications of superficial and superficial partial-thickness burns are infection, hypothermia, dehydration and fluid and electrolyte imbalances.

Due to the severity of tissue injury from the burns, the priority nursing diagnosis of *Impaired skin integrity* is appropriate for guiding nursing care.

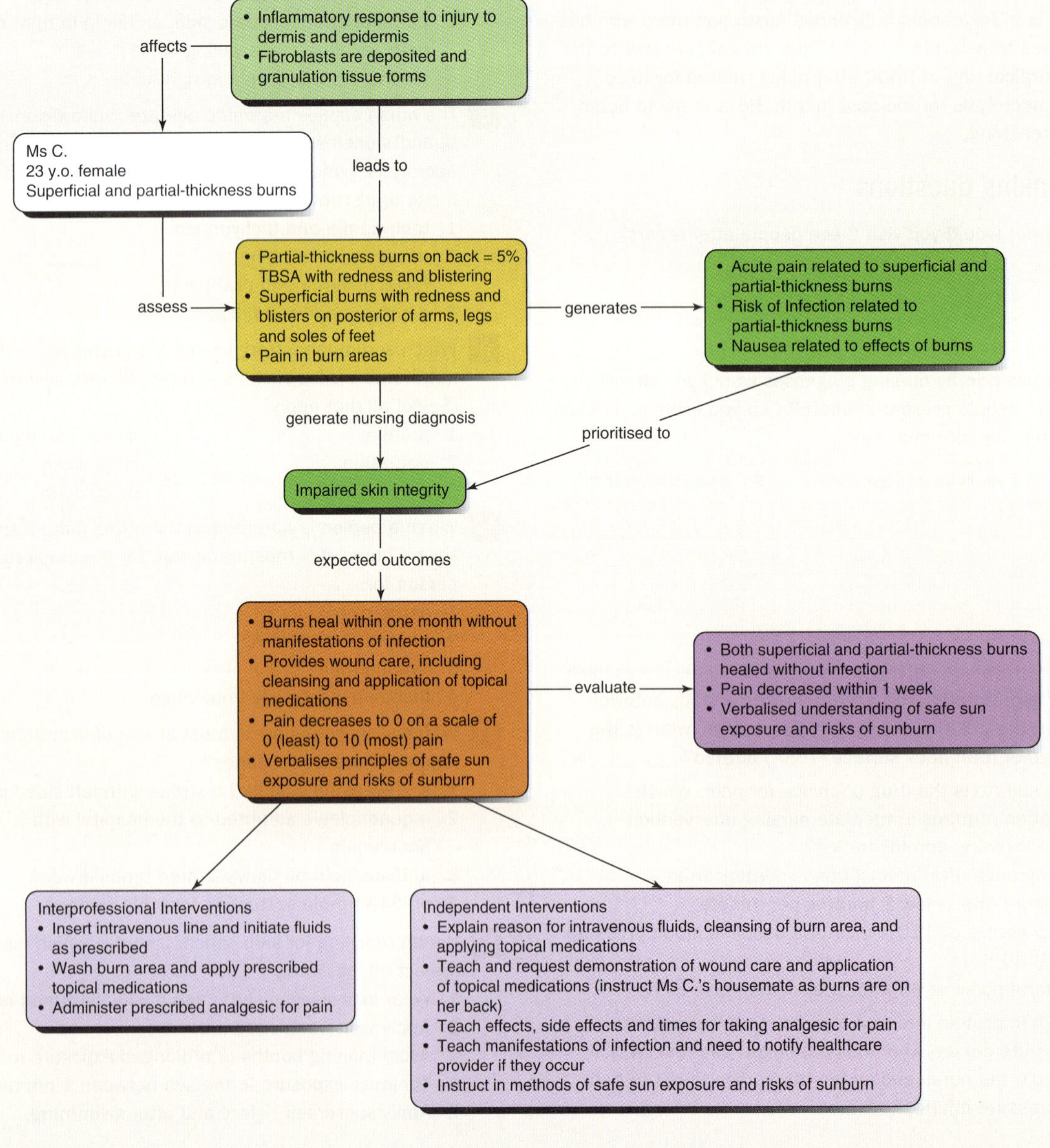

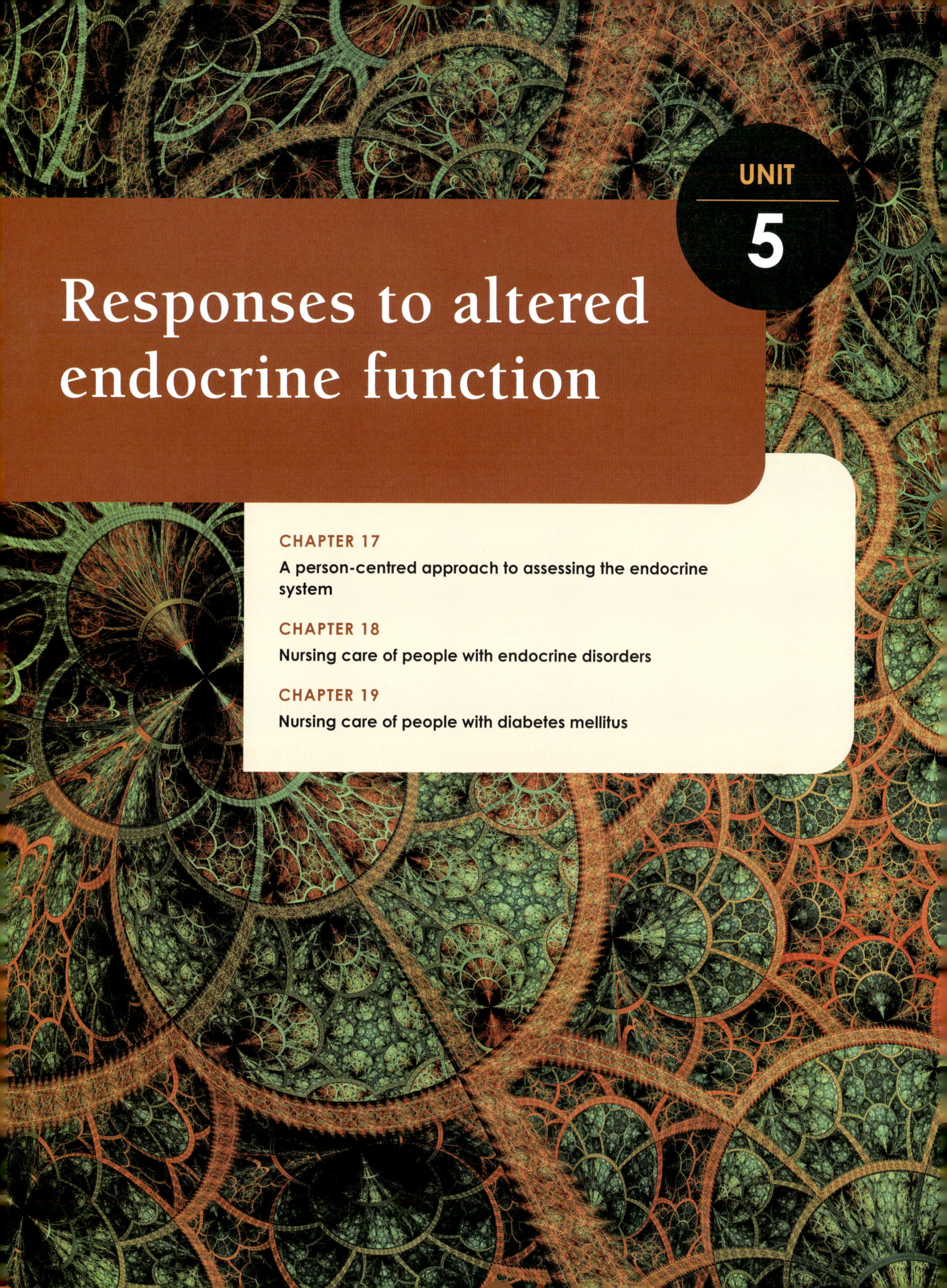

UNIT 5

Responses to altered endocrine function

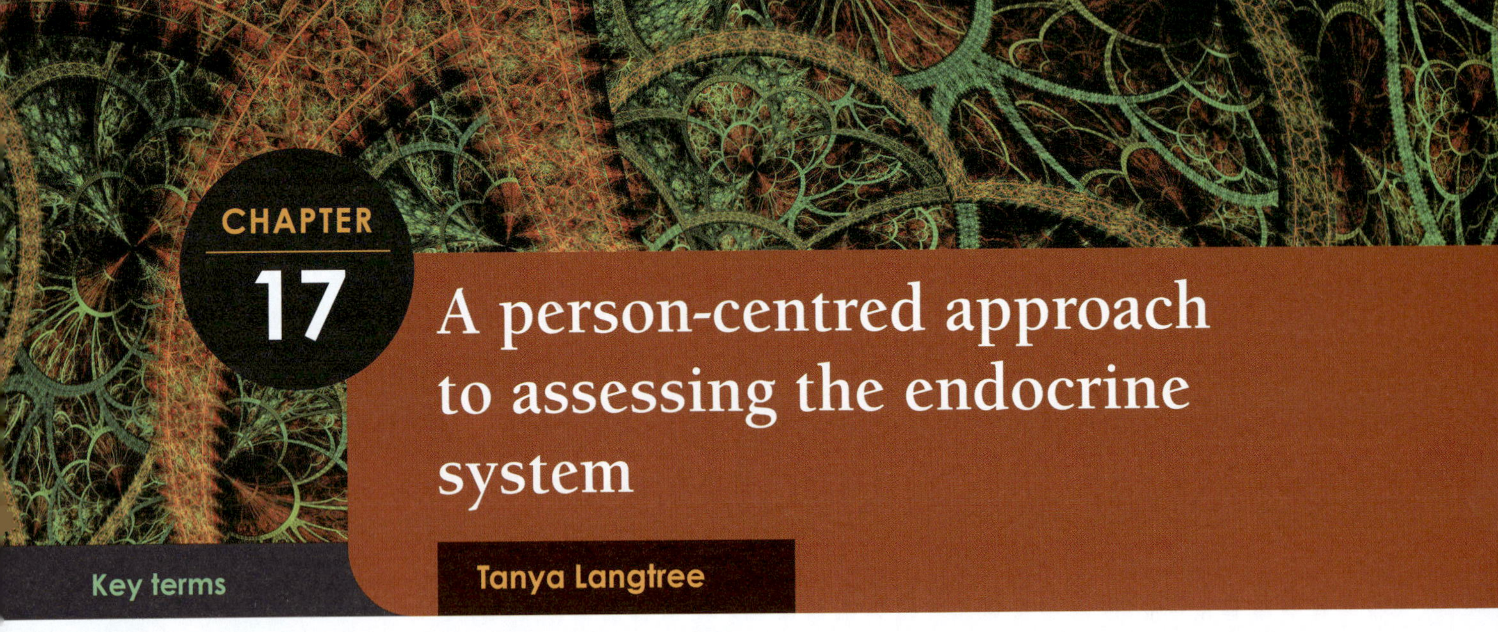

A person-centred approach to assessing the endocrine system

Tanya Langtree

Key terms

acromegaly 522
bitemporal homonymous hemianopia 523
carpopedal spasm 524
Chvostek's sign 524
diplopia 522
dwarfism 524
exophthalmos 522
gigantism 524
goitre 523
photophobia 522
tetany 524
thyroid gland 511
Trousseau's sign 524

Learning outcomes

- Describe the anatomy and physiology of the endocrine glands.
- Explain the functions of the hormones secreted by the endocrine glands.
- Identify key assessment areas including lifespan considerations that should be assessed during a health history interview with the person who has altered endocrine function.
- Explain the nursing implications for a range of diagnostic tests associated with the endocrine glands.

Clinical competencies

- Conduct and document a health history for the person who has or is at risk of alterations in the structure or function of the endocrine glands.
- Monitor the results of diagnostic tests and report abnormal findings.
- Conduct and document a physical assessment of the structure of the thyroid gland and the effects of altered endocrine function on other body structures and functions.

Equipment needed

- Tendon hammer
- Single-use neurological examination pin, cotton ball, containers with hot and cold water, tuning fork
- Snellen chart
- Sphygmomanometer
- Stethoscope

The endocrine system plays an integral part in the regulation of the body's internal environment. Through hormones secreted by its glands, the endocrine system regulates such varied functions as growth, reproduction, metabolism, fluid and electrolyte balance, and gender differentiation. It also helps the body adapt to constant alterations in the internal and external environment.

Anatomy, physiology and functions of the endocrine system

The major endocrine organs are the pituitary gland, thyroid gland, parathyroid glands, adrenal glands, pancreas and gonads (reproductive glands). The locations of these glands are illustrated in Figure 17.1. Table 17.1 summarises the functions of the endocrine organs and their hormones. Specific information about the ovaries and testes is found in the chapters 'A person-centred approach to assessing the male and female reproductive systems', 'Nursing care of men with reproductive system and breast disorders' and 'Nursing care of women with reproductive system and breast disorders'.

PITUITARY GLAND

The pituitary gland (hypophysis) is located in the skull beneath the hypothalamus of the brain (see Figure 17.2). It often is called the 'master gland' because its hormones regulate many body functions. The pituitary gland has two parts: the anterior pituitary (or adenohypophysis) and the posterior pituitary (or neurohypophysis). The anterior pituitary is glandular tissue, whereas the posterior pituitary is an extension of the hypothalamus.

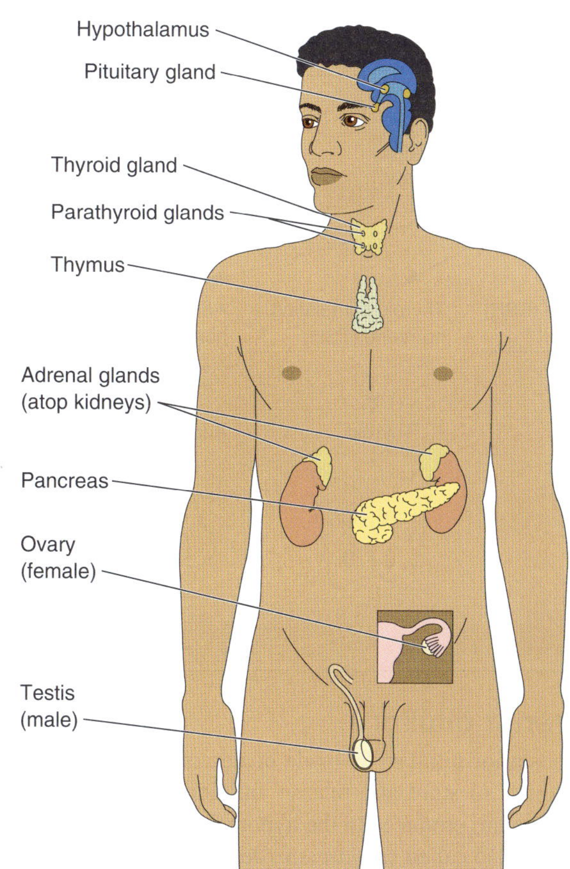

FIGURE 17.1 *Location of the major endocrine glands*

Anterior pituitary

The anterior pituitary has several types of endocrine cells and secretes at least six major hormones (see Figure 17.3).

- Somatotropic cells secrete growth hormone (GH) (also called *somatotropin*). GH stimulates growth of the body by signalling cells to increase protein production and by stimulating the epiphyseal plates of the long bones.
- Lactotropic cells secrete prolactin (PRL). Prolactin stimulates the production of breast milk.
- Thyrotropic cells secrete thyroid-stimulating hormone (TSH). TSH stimulates the synthesis and release of thyroid hormones from the thyroid gland.
- Corticotropic cells secrete adrenocorticotropic hormone (ACTH). ACTH stimulates release of hormones, especially glucocorticoids, from the adrenal cortex.
- Gonadotropic cells secrete the gonadotropin hormones, follicle-stimulating hormone (FSH) and luteinising hormone (LH). These hormones stimulate the ovaries and testes (the gonads). In women, FSH stimulates the development of ovarian follicles and induces the secretion

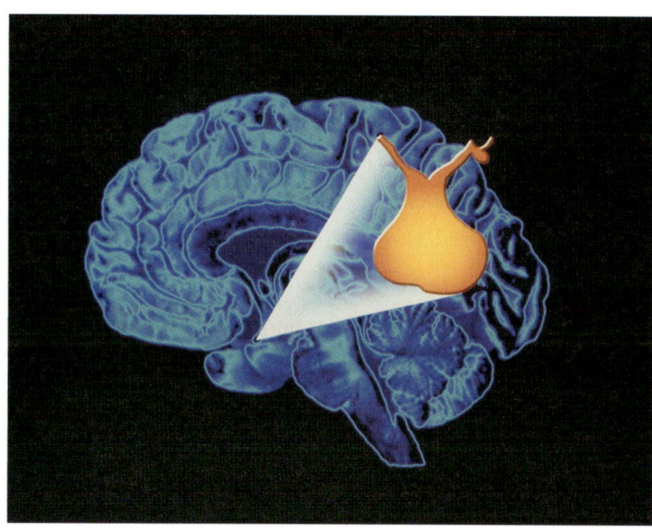

FIGURE 17.2 *Location of the pituitary gland*

Source: Alfred Pasieka/Science Photo Library/Alamy Stock Photo.

TABLE 17.1 Organs, hormones, functions and feedback mechanisms of the endocrine system

ENDOCRINE ORGAN	HORMONE SECRETED	TARGET ORGAN AND FEEDBACK MECHANISM
Thyroid gland	Thyroid hormone (TH): thyroxine (T_4) is the major hormone secreted by the thyroid gland. It is converted to triiodothyronine (T_3) at the target tissues.	Maintains metabolic rate and the growth and development of all tissues. T_3 and T_4 are secreted in response to thyroid-stimulating hormone (TSH).
	Calcitonin	Maintains serum calcium levels by decreasing bone resorption and decreasing resorption of calcium in the kidneys whenever levels of plasma calcium are elevated. Works together with parathyroid gland to regulate calcium levels.
Parathyroid gland	Parathyroid hormone (PTH)	Maintains serum calcium levels by stimulating bone resorption and formation and by stimulating kidney resorption of calcium in response to falling levels of plasma calcium.
Adrenal cortex	Mineralocorticoids (e.g. aldosterone)	Promotes renal tubule reabsorption of sodium and water and excretion of potassium in response to elevated levels of potassium and low levels of sodium, thereby increasing blood pressure and circulating blood volume.
	Glucocorticoids (e.g. cortisol)	Help to regulate metabolism of carbohydrates, fats and proteins. Activate anti-inflammatory responses to stressors. Low cortisol levels stimulate hypothalamic secretion of corticotropin-releasing hormone (CRH), which stimulates the anterior pituitary gland to release ACTH, which in turn stimulates the adrenal cortex to secrete cortisol.
	Gonadocorticoids (androgens and small amounts of oestrogen and progesterone)	The quantity of sex hormones produced here is minimal and the mechanism is not well understood.
Adrenal medulla	Catecholamines (adrenaline and noradrenaline)	Secreted in response to physical or psychological stress; catecholamines stimulate the heart, constrict blood vessels, inhibit visceral muscles, dilate bronchioles, increase respiration and metabolism, and promote hyperglycaemia.
Anterior pituitary (adenohypophysis)	Growth hormone (GH)	Promotes growth of body tissues by enhancing protein synthesis and promoting use of fat for energy and thus conserving glucose. Release is stimulated by growth-hormone-releasing hormone (GHRH) in response to low GH levels, hypoglycaemia, increased amino acids, low fatty acids and stress.

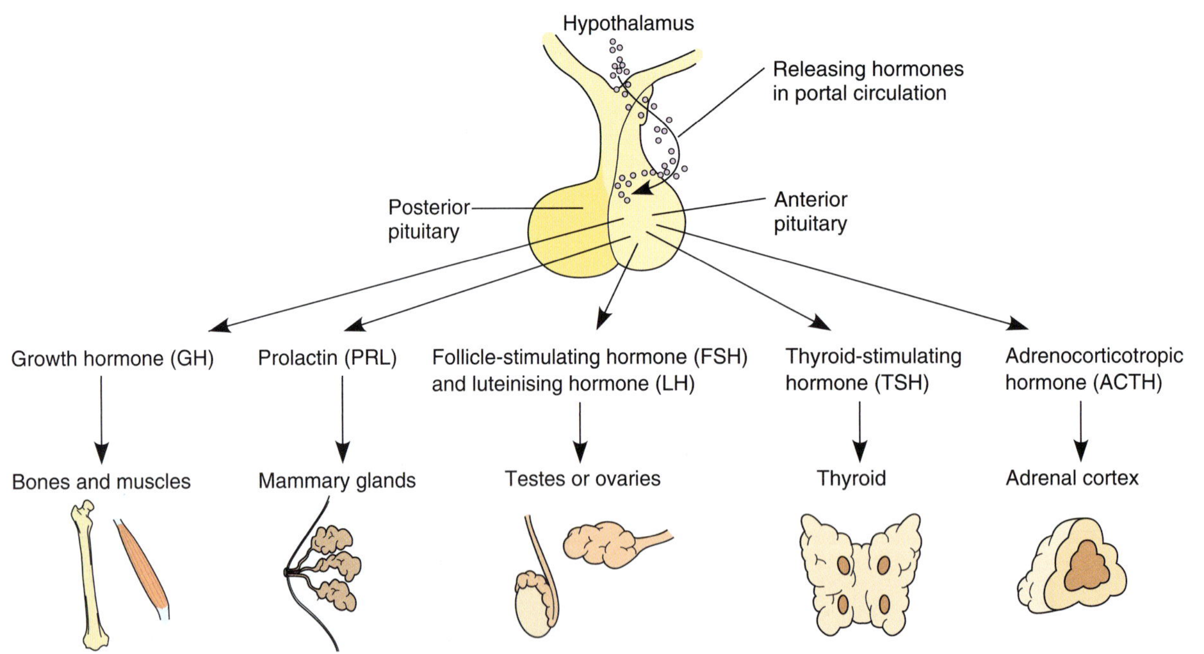

FIGURE 17.3 *Actions of the major hormones of the anterior pituitary*

of oestrogenic female sex hormones. Increasing levels of LH work together with FSH to lead to ovulation and the formation of the corpus luteum from an ovarian follicle. In men, FSH is involved in the development and maturation of sperm. LH in men is called the interstitial cell-stimulating hormone (ICSH), which stimulates the interstitial cells of the testes to produce male sex hormones.

Posterior pituitary

The posterior pituitary is made of nervous tissue. Its primary function is to store and release antidiuretic hormone (ADH) and oxytocin, produced in the hypothalamus.

- ADH, also called *vasopressin*, decreases urine production by causing the renal tubules to reabsorb water from the urine and return it to the circulating blood volume.

- Oxytocin induces contraction of the smooth muscles in the reproductive organs. In women, oxytocin stimulates the myometrium of the uterus to contract during labour. It also induces milk ejection from the breasts.

THYROID GLAND

The **thyroid gland** (see Figure 17.4) is anterior to the upper part of the trachea and just inferior to the larynx. This butterfly-shaped gland has two lobes connected by a structure called the isthmus.

The glandular tissue consists of follicles which produce the glycoprotein thyroglobulin. A jelly-like colloid substance containing a thyroglobulin–iodine complex is stored within the lumen of each follicle. Cells within the follicles secrete thyroid hormone (TH), a general name for two similar hormones: thyroxine (T_4) and triiodothyronine (T_3). The primary role of thyroid hormones in adults is to increase metabolism. TH secretion is initiated by the release of TSH by the pituitary gland and is dependent on an adequate supply of iodine.

The thyroid gland also secretes calcitonin, a hormone that decreases excessive levels of calcium in the blood by slowing the calcium-releasing activity of bone cells. Yet, when the thyroid gland is totally removed and thyroid hormone is replaced, calcium homeostasis and bone density remain relatively unchanged without replacing calcitonin.

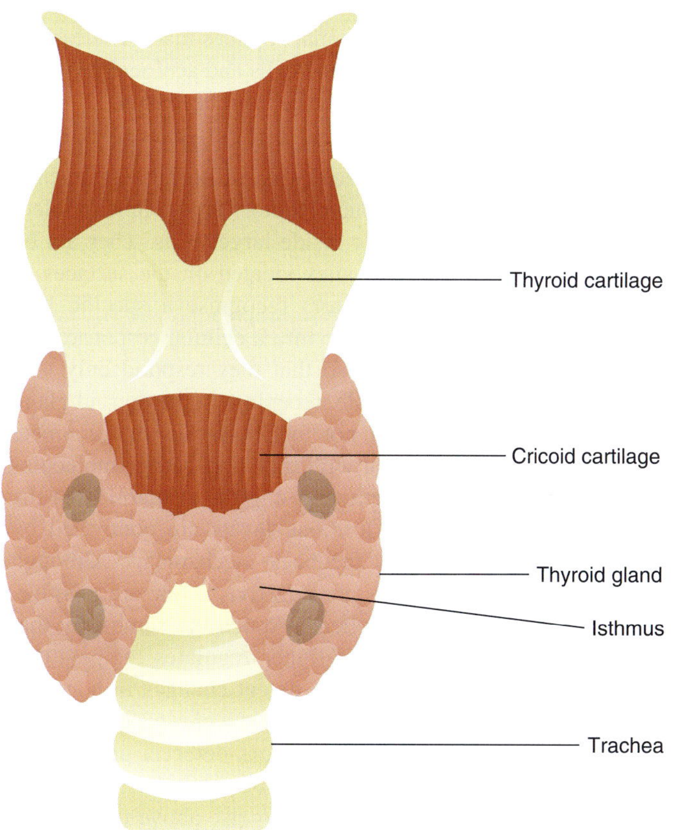

FIGURE 17.4 ***The thyroid gland***

Source: Zuzanae/Shutterstock.

Parathyroid glands

The parathyroid glands (usually four to six in number) are embedded on the posterior surface of the lobes of the thyroid gland. They secrete parathyroid hormone (PTH), or *parathormone*. When serum calcium levels fall, PTH secretion increases. PTH also controls phosphate metabolism. It acts primarily by increasing renal excretion of phosphate in the urine, by decreasing the excretion of calcium and increasing bone reabsorption to cause the release of calcium from bones. Normal levels of vitamin D are necessary for PTH to exert these effects on bone and the kidneys.

ADRENAL GLANDS

The two adrenal glands are pyramid-shaped organs that sit on top of the kidneys (see Figure 17.5). Each gland consists of two parts, which are distinct organs: an inner medulla and an outer cortex.

The adrenal medulla produces two hormones (also called catecholamines): adrenaline (epinephrine) and noradrenaline (norepinephrine). These hormones are similar to substances released by the sympathetic nervous system and thus are not essential to life. Adrenaline increases blood glucose levels and stimulates the release of ACTH from the pituitary; ACTH in turn stimulates the adrenal cortex to release glucocorticoids. Adrenaline also increases the rate and force of cardiac contractions; constricts blood vessels in the skin, mucous membranes and kidneys; and dilates blood vessels in the skeletal muscles, coronary arteries and pulmonary arteries. Noradrenaline increases both heart rate and the force of cardiac contractions. Noradrenaline also causes vasoconstriction of blood vessels throughout the body.

The adrenal cortex secretes several hormones, all corticosteroids. They are classified into two groups: mineralocorticoids and glucocorticoids.

An enzyme named renin primarily controls the release of mineralocorticoids. When a decrease in blood pressure or sodium is detected, specialised kidney cells release renin to

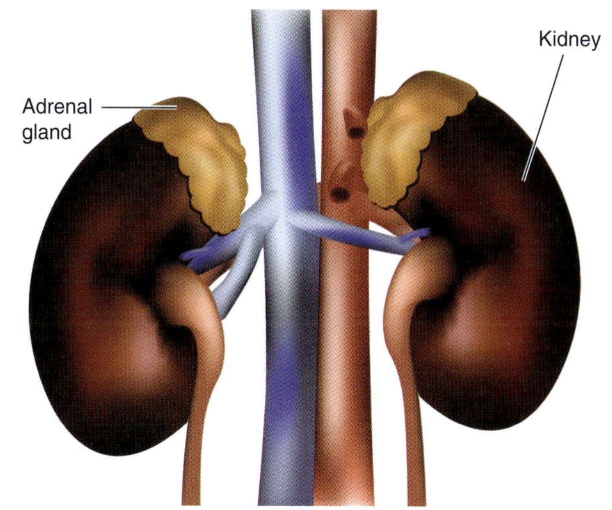

FIGURE 17.5 ***Location of the adrenal glands***

Source: GRei/Shutterstock.

act on a substance called angiotensinogen, manufactured by the liver. Renin modifies angiotensinogen to form angiotensin I, which is converted to angiotensin II by the angiotensin-converting enzyme. Angiotensin II stimulates the secretion of aldosterone from the adrenal cortex, which prompts the distal tubules of the kidneys to release increased amounts of water and sodium back into the circulating blood volume to increase blood pressure. This system (the renin–angiotensin–aldosterone system (RAAS)) is further described in the chapter 'Nursing care of people with altered fluid, electrolyte and acid–base balance'.

The glucocorticoids include cortisol and cortisone. These hormones affect carbohydrate metabolism by regulating glucose use in body tissues, mobilising fatty acids from fatty tissue and shifting the source of energy for muscle cells from glucose to fatty acids. Glucocorticoids are released in times of stress. An excess of glucocorticoids in the body depresses the inflammatory response and impairs the immune system's efficacy.

PANCREAS

The pancreas, located behind the stomach between the spleen and the duodenum, is both an endocrine gland (producing hormones) and an exocrine gland (producing digestive enzymes). This chapter focuses on the pancreatic hormones; however, the digestive enzymes produced by the pancreas are discussed in the chapter 'A person-centred approach to assessing the gastro-intestinal system'.

The endocrine cells of the pancreas produce hormones that regulate carbohydrate metabolism. They are clustered in bodies called pancreatic islets (or islets of Langerhans) scattered throughout the gland. Pancreatic islets have at least four different cell types:

1. Alpha cells produce glucagon. Glucagon decreases glucose oxidation and promotes an increase in the blood glucose levels by signalling the liver to release glucose from glycogen stores.
2. Beta cells produce insulin. Insulin facilitates the uptake and use of glucose by cells and prevents an excessive breakdown of glycogen in the liver and muscle. Consequently, insulin decreases blood glucose levels. Insulin also facilitates lipid formation, inhibits the breakdown and mobilisation of stored fat, and helps amino acids move into cells to promote protein synthesis. Generally, the actions of glucagon and insulin oppose one another and, in doing so, help to stabilise blood glucose levels.
3. Delta cells secrete somatostatin. Somatostatin inhibits the secretion of glucagon and insulin by the alpha and beta cells.
4. F cells secrete pancreatic polypeptide. Pancreatic polypeptide is believed to inhibit the exocrine activity of the pancreas.

GONADS

The gonads are the testes in men and the ovaries in women. These organs are the primary source of steroid sex hormones in the body. The hormones of the gonads are important in regulating body growth and promoting the onset of puberty.

In men, androgens (primarily testosterone) produced by the testes maintain reproductive functioning and secondary sex characteristics. Androgens also promote the production of sperm. In women, the ovaries secrete oestrogens and progesterone to maintain reproductive functioning and secondary sex characteristics. Progesterone also promotes the growth of the lining of the uterus to prepare for implantation of a fertilised ovum.

HORMONES

Hormones are chemical messengers secreted by the endocrine organs and transported throughout the body, where they exert their action on specific cells called target cells. Hormones do not cause reactions directly, but rather regulate tissue responses. They may produce either generalised or local effects.

Hormones are transported from endocrine gland cells to target cells in the body in one of four ways:

1. Endocrine glands release most hormones, such as TH and insulin, into the bloodstream. Some hormones require a protein carrier.
2. Neurons release some hormones, such as adrenaline, into the bloodstream. This method of transport is called the neuroendocrine route.
3. The hypothalamus releases its hormones directly to target cells in the posterior pituitary by nerve cell extension.
4. With the paracrine method, released messengers diffuse through the interstitial fluid. This method of transport involves a number of hormonal peptides that are released throughout various organs and cells and act locally. An example is endorphins, which act to relieve pain.

Hormones that are released into the bloodstream circulate as either free, unbound molecules or as hormones attached to transport carriers. Hormone receptors are complex molecular structures, located on or inside target cells. They act by binding to specific receptor sites located on the surfaces of the target cells. These receptors recognise a specific hormone and translate the message into a cellular response. The receptor sites are structured so that they respond only to a specific hormone. For example, receptors in the thyroid gland are responsive to TSH but not to LH. Drugs that compete with a hormone for binding with transport carrier molecules increase hormone action by increasing the availability of the free, unbound hormone. Hormone levels are controlled by the pituitary gland and by feedback mechanisms. Although most feedback mechanisms are negative, a few are positive. Negative feedback is controlled in much the same way that the thermostat in an air conditioner regulates temperature. Sensors in the endocrine system detect changes in hormone levels and adjust the level of hormone secretion to maintain normal body levels. When the sensors detect a decrease in hormone levels, they begin actions to cause an increase in hormone levels; when hormone levels rise above normal, the sensors cause a decrease in hormone production and release. For example, blood glucose levels rise after eating a meal. The increased blood glucose levels are detected by the beta cells in the pancreas, which are stimulated to secrete insulin into the blood. The resulting increased insulin levels cause glucose to move into the cells, which in turn reduces blood glucose levels. This reduction in blood glucose levels is identified by the beta cells in the pancreas and it stops releasing insulin (see Figure 17.6).

In positive feedback mechanisms, increasing levels of one hormone cause another gland to release a hormone. For example, the increased production of oestradiol (a female ovarian hormone) during the follicular stage of the menstrual cycle in turn stimulates increased FSH production by the anterior pituitary gland. Oestradiol levels continue to increase until the ovarian follicle disappears, eliminating the source of the stimulation for FSH, which then decreases.

Stimuli for hormone release may also be classified as hormonal, humoral or neural (see Figure 17.7). In hormonal release, hypothalamic hormones stimulate the anterior pituitary to release hormones. Fluctuations in the serum level of these hormones in turn prompt other endocrine glands to release hormones. In humoral release, fluctuations in the serum levels of certain ions and nutrients stimulate specific endocrine glands to release hormones to bring these levels back to normal. In neural release, nerve fibres stimulate the release of hormones.

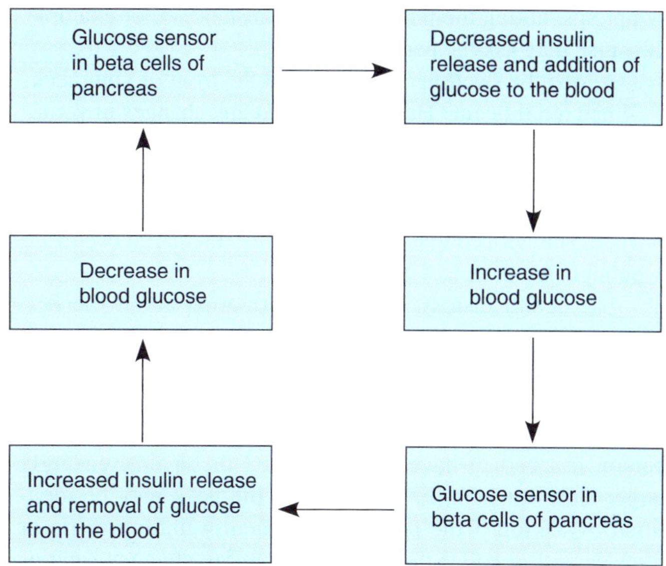

FIGURE 17.6 *Negative feedback*

ASSESSING ENDOCRINE FUNCTION

The function of the endocrine glands is assessed by findings from a health assessment interview to collect subjective data, a physical assessment to collect objective data and diagnostic tests. Hormones affect all body tissues and organs and manifestations of dysfunction are often non-specific, making assessment of endocrine function sometimes more difficult than assessment of other body systems.

Health assessment interview

A health assessment interview to determine problems with the endocrine system may be part of a health screening or total health assessment, or it may focus on the individual's presenting problem such as reports of increased urination or changes in energy levels. If the person has a problem with endocrine function, the nurse analyses its onset, characteristics and course, severity, precipitating and relieving factors, and any associated

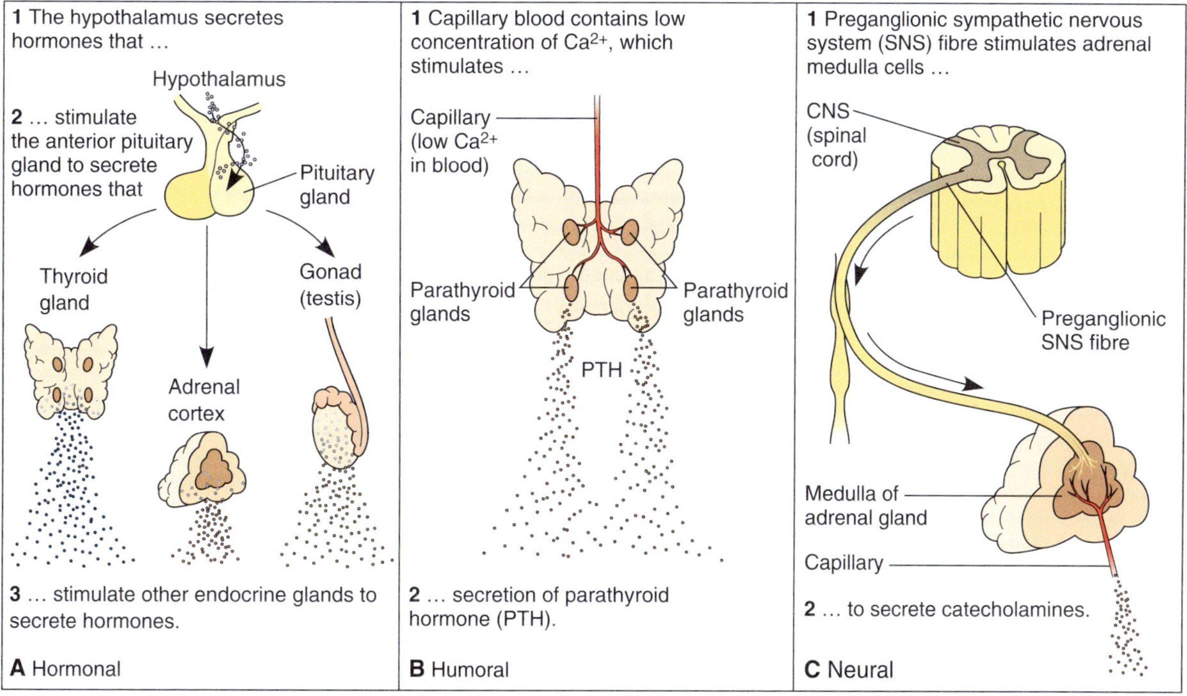

FIGURE 17.7 *Examples of three mechanisms of hormone release: A, hormonal; B, humoral; C, neural*

symptoms, noting the timing and circumstances. For example, the nurse may ask the person:

- Describe the swelling you noticed at the front of your neck. When did it begin? Have you noticed any changes in your energy level?
- When did you first notice that your hands and feet were getting larger?
- Have you noticed that your appetite has increased even though you have lost weight?

The health history includes information about the person's medical history, family history and social history. Ask the person about any changes in normal growth and development, as well as in height and weight. Changes in the size of extremities can often be detected by asking whether the person has had to have rings enlarged or buy increasingly larger shoes or hats. Enlargement of the neck may be identified by asking if the person has difficulty finding shirts or blouses with a collar that fits. Also explore changes such as difficulty swallowing; increased or decreased thirst, appetite and/or urination; visual changes; sleep disturbances; altered patterns of hair distribution (e.g. increased facial hair in women); changes in menstruation; changes in memory or ability to concentrate; mood changes; and changes in hair and skin texture. Ask the person about if they have experienced any recent head injuries and what medications they are currently taking (especially focusing on a history of using steroids or hormonal therapy). The nurse should also gather data about the person's previous hospitalisations and if they have previously received chemotherapy or radiation therapy (especially to the neck).

The nurse also asks about the person's occupational and social history. Include questions about the person's satisfaction with occupation, personal relationships and lifestyle. Other areas of assessment include the person's usual means of coping; use of alcohol, smoking or drugs (including anabolic steroid use); diet (including weight gain or loss); and exercise and sleep patterns. Although the person may not recognise changes in behaviour, family members may be able to provide important information.

Interview questions categorised by functional health patterns are listed here.

FUNCTIONAL HEALTH PATTERN INTERVIEW Endocrine system

FUNCTIONAL HEALTH PATTERN	INTERVIEW QUESTIONS AND LEADING STATEMENTS
Health perception–Health management	■ Describe your overall state of health, rating it on a scale of 1 to 10 with 10 being the best health you have had.
	■ Describe any problems you have had with an endocrine gland (pituitary, thyroid, parathyroid, adrenal, pancreas, ovaries, testes).
	■ If you had a problem with any of these glands, how was it treated (e.g. medications, surgery, diet, hormone replacement)?
	■ Has any relative experienced any problems with an endocrine gland (pituitary, thyroid, parathyroid, adrenal, pancreas, ovaries, testes)?
	■ Do you smoke, drink alcohol, and/or use recreational drugs? If so, how much and what kind?
	■ Have you ever been tested for high or low blood sugar?
Nutritional–Metabolic	■ Describe what you eat and how much (and what type of) fluid you drink in a 24-hour period.
	■ Do you take any nutritional supplements, herbs or vitamins?
	■ Have you noticed any recent changes to your hunger or thirst levels?
	■ Has your weight changed? If so, by how many kilograms and over what time period?
	■ Have you noticed any change in your energy level? If so, explain.
	■ Have you noticed any change in your ability to tolerate heat or cold?
	■ Have you noticed any difficulty swallowing? Explain.
	■ Have you noticed any changes in the texture of your skin? If so, what were they?
Elimination	■ Have you noticed any change in your urine colour, odour or amount or in the frequency of urination? If so, describe it.
	■ Have you ever had kidney stones? If so, how were they treated?
	■ Has there been a change in your bowel elimination (such as diarrhoea or constipation)? If so, explain the change.
Activity–Exercise	■ Describe the physical activities you undertake during a usual day.
	■ Has your energy level increased or decreased? Explain.
	■ Do you regularly undertake exercise? If yes, what type of exercise do you normally perform and how often? Have you had to make any changes to your exercise habits lately?

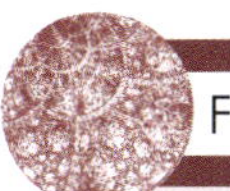

FUNCTIONAL HEALTH PATTERN INTERVIEW Endocrine system (continued)

FUNCTIONAL HEALTH PATTERN	INTERVIEW QUESTIONS AND LEADING STATEMENTS
	■ Do some activities make you very tired? Explain how you feel.
	■ Do you experience fatigue that is not related to exertion?
Sleep–Rest	■ How many hours of sleep do you get each night?
	■ Do you feel nervous and unable to rest?
	■ Do you sweat at night?
	■ Do you experience nightmares? If yes, is this new?
Cognitive–Perceptual	■ Have you noticed any problem with your memory?
	■ Do you feel restless, anxious or confused?
	■ Have you noticed any change in your voice?
	■ Have you noticed any change in the colour or condition of your skin and hair (e.g. a change in colour, dryness/oiliness, increased bruising)?
	■ Have you experienced any headaches, memory loss, sensation changes or mood swings recently? If so, describe them.
	■ Have you noticed any change in your vision? If so, describe them.
	■ Have you had any heart palpitations? What is it like? Does it occur at certain times during the day?
	■ Have you had any abdominal pain? What is it like and where is it located?
	■ Have you had any pain or stiffness in your muscles and joints?
Self-perception–Self-concept	■ Have you noticed any changes in your physical appearance lately? Are you concerned by these changes?
	■ Have you noticed you have needed to increase your hat or shoe size recently? Have you noticed your rings or collars are tighter?
	■ Are you concerned by your weight?
	■ How does this condition make you feel about yourself?
	■ How do you feel about taking medications?
Role–Relationships	■ How does this condition affect your relationships with others?
	■ What roles do you normally fulfil in and outside the home? How does having this condition affect your ability to undertake your roles?
	■ Does anyone in your family have an endocrine disorder? If so, when did it begin and how does it affect them? What family member is affected and at what age did it begin?
Stress tolerance	■ Does stress seem to make your condition worse? In what ways?
	■ Has this condition created stress for you? Can you explain how?
	■ Describe what you do when you feel stressed.
Value–Belief	■ Tell me about how specific relationships or activities help you cope with this condition.
	■ Describe specific cultural beliefs or practices that affect how you care for and feel about this condition.
	■ Are there any specific treatments that you would not use to treat this condition?
Sexuality–Reproductive	
Men	■ Have you noticed any difficulties in being aroused/maintaining an erection?
	■ Are you trying for children but have not conceived?
Women	■ When was your last menstrual period? How would you describe your period in terms of pattern and flow? Have you noticed any changes recently?
	■ Do you have any children?
	■ If yes, did you experience any difficulties falling pregnant? Were you told you had gestational diabetes while pregnant?
	■ If no, are you trying for children but have not conceived?
	■ Are you menopausal? How long have you been experiencing menopausal symptoms?

TABLE 17.2 Age-related endocrine changes

AGE-RELATED CHANGE	SIGNIFICANCE
Pituitary: ↓ production of ACTH, TSH, FSH	• Decreased secretion of glucocorticoids, 17-ketosteroids, progesterone, androgen and oestrogen (and thus lower levels on diagnostic tests)
Thyroid: ↑ in fibrosis and nodularity, ↓ in gland activity	• Lower basal metabolic rate • Increased incidence of hypothyroidism • Palpable nodules on palpation
Adrenal medulla: ↑ secretion and level of noradrenaline, increased plasma noradrenaline level, however ↓ beta-adrenergic response to noradrenaline	• Decreased response to beta-adrenergic and receptor blockers medications • May contribute to increased incidence of hypertension
Pancreas: calcification of blood vessels and distension and dilation of pancreatic ducts	• Decreased production of lipase with reduced fat absorption and digestion, leading to intolerance of fatty foods and indigestion • Decreased absorption of fat-soluble vitamins
Pancreas: delayed and decreased insulin release; believed accompanied by decreased sensitivity to circulating insulin	• Decreased ability to metabolise glucose with higher and more prolonged blood glucose levels may contribute to increased incidence of type 2 diabetes mellitus with ageing

Physical assessment

Physical assessment of the endocrine system may be performed as part of a total health assessment or may be a focused assessment of the person with known or suspected problems with endocrine function.

The only endocrine organ that can be palpated is the thyroid gland; however, other assessments that provide information about endocrine problems include inspection of the skin, hair and nails; facial appearance; and the musculoskeletal system. Changes to the person's visual fields and deep tendon reflexes should also be monitored. Measuring and monitoring trends in height and weight and vital signs also provide clues to altered endocrine system function.

The person may sit during the examination. Prior to the examination, the nurse collects the necessary equipment and explains the techniques to the person to decrease anxiety. Additional techniques for assessing hypocalcaemic tetany—a complication of endocrine disorders or surgery—are included in the examination sequence. Normal age-related changes in assessment findings are described in Table 17.2.

Diagnostic tests

The results of diagnostic tests of the endocrine system are used to support the diagnosis of a specific disease, to provide information to identify or modify the appropriate medication or therapy used to treat the disease, and to help nurses monitor the person's response to treatment and nursing care interventions. Diagnostic tests to assess the structure and function of the glands of the endocrine system are described in the 'Diagnostic tests' box. The normal reference values for all blood/urine tests vary slightly between laboratories due to the use of different test kits. More information is included in the discussion of specific disorders in the chapters 'Nursing care of people with endocrine disorders' and 'Nursing care of people with diabetes mellitus'.

Regardless of the type of diagnostic test, the nurse is responsible for explaining the procedure and any special preparation needed, for assessing medication use that may affect the outcome of the tests, for supporting the person during the examination as necessary, for documenting the procedures as appropriate and for monitoring the results of the tests.

DIAGNOSTIC TESTS The endocrine system

PITUITARY TESTS

NAME OF TEST Growth hormone (GH), Human growth hormone (hGH), somatotropin

PURPOSE AND DESCRIPTION In this blood test, GH levels (affected by food, stress and activity) are measured to identify GH deficiency (dwarfism) or GH excess (gigantism, acromegaly). Acromegaly may be indicative of a pituitary tumour.

Dynamic testing (either GH stimulation testing or GH suppression testing) are normally indicated due to the limited value of an isolated test.

Normal value:
$\geq$ 20 mU/L excludes a GH deficiency.

RELATED NURSING CARE Inform the person not to eat or drink 10–12 hours (usually overnight fasting) prior to having blood taken. The person is then given either an oral glucose solution to suppress GH or intravenous insulin under medical supervision. Repeat blood samples are then drawn at every 30 minutes for 3 hours.

Have the person sit down for 30 to 60 minutes before blood is taken.

DIAGNOSTIC TESTS The endocrine system (continued)

NAME OF TEST IGF-1 (Insulin-like growth factor 1 or somatomedin C)

PURPOSE AND DESCRIPTION The results of this blood test are used to identify diseases or conditions caused by hyper/hyposecretion of growth hormone (e.g. acromegaly/gigantism or Laron dwarfism) and to evaluate the function of the pituitary gland.

Normal value:
Adult: 13–50 nmol/L
Levels are increased in acromegaly and decreased in Laron dwarfism.
Results vary by age for children

RELATED NURSING CARE None; overnight fasting is preferred but not necessary.

NAME OF TEST Water deprivation test (Anti-diuretic hormone stimulation)

PURPOSE AND DESCRIPTION This combination blood and urine test is used to identify causes of polyuria (increased urine output), including central diabetes insipidus (DI), neurogenic diabetes insipidus, syndrome of inappropriate antidiuretic hormone (SIADH) and psychogenic polydipsia. ADH or vasopressin is given intramuscularly (IM) or subcutaneously (SC). In people without pathology, there is no change in urine and plasma osmolality. Urine osmolality increases in central diabetes insipidus and decreases in nephrogenic diabetes insipidus.

RELATED NURSING CARE Diuretics need to be withheld for 12 hours prior to the test. The recommended fluid restriction prior to this test is dependent on the person's current urine output.

The person needs to be admitted to hospital for this testing. Nil oral or parenteral fluids are provided while testing is undertaken.

Plasma and urine samples are taken hourly until the osmolality plateaus ($<$ 30 mmol/kg increase over a 1-hour period) or the person loses $>$ 3% of their body weight. Desmopressin (DDAVP) is then administered and urine osmolality is measured 30 to 60 minutes later.

Inform the person that the test may take up to 8 hours. Every hour for ordered length of test: assess weight, take postural BP (lying and standing measures separated by 2 minutes), collect blood and urine samples for laboratory analysis. Following the test, the person needs to be rehydrated with oral fluids and have their vital signs monitored.

NAME OF TEST Magnetic resonance imaging (MRI)

PURPOSE AND DESCRIPTION A radiographic study used to identify tumours of the hypothalamus or pituitary gland.

RELATED NURSING CARE Inform the person of need to lie still during the examination. Remove any metallic objects (e.g. hair clips, jewellery, piercings) and assess for any metallic implants (e.g. pacemakers, implantable cardioverter defibrillators, temporary transvenous pacing leads, metallic intraocular foreign bodies, implantable neurostimulation systems). If present, the test is not performed due to the danger caused by the magnetic field from the machine.

THYROID TESTS

NAME OF TEST Thyroid-stimulating hormone (TSH)

PURPOSE AND DESCRIPTION In this blood test, TSH and T_4 levels are measured to differentiate pituitary from thyroid causes of hypothyroidism. A decreased T_4 level and a normal or increased TSH level can indicate a thyroid gland disorder. A suppressed TSH level is indicative of hyperthyroidism, whereas an increased TSH level may be indicative of hypothyroidism. A decreased T_4 level combined with a decreased TSH level can indicate a disorder of pituitary origin.

Normal value:
0.4–4.0 mIU/L (dependent on method).

RELATED NURSING CARE Inform the person to avoid shellfish for several days prior to the test. Evaluate medications: TSH value may be increased by aspirin, amiodarone, iodides, steroids, dopamine and heparin; and decreased by lithium and potassium iodide.

NAME OF TEST Free thyroxine (Free T_4; T_4)

PURPOSE AND DESCRIPTION This blood test is paired with TSH testing to evaluate thyroid function and aid in the diagnosis of hyperthyroidism and hypothyroidism.

Free T_4 is elevated with hyperthyroidism and normally depressed in hypothyroidism.

Normal value:
Adult: 10–25 pmol/L (dependent on method)

RELATED NURSING CARE Assess medications: T_4 may be decreased by cortisone, amiodarone, chlorpromazine phenytoin, heparin, lithium, sulphonamides, testosterone and propranolol. Values may be increased by aspirin, amiodarone, iodine, oral contraceptives and oestrogens.

(continued)

DIAGNOSTIC TESTS The endocrine system (continued)

NAME OF TEST Free T_3 (T_3; free triiodothyronine, triiodothyronine, FT_3)

PURPOSE AND DESCRIPTION This blood test is used as an adjunctive to diagnose hyperthyroidism and to compare T_3 with T_4 for diagnosis of thyroid disorder. It is rarely used for the diagnosis of hypothyroidism due to being less reliable. It is useful in monitoring the effectiveness of thyroid replacement and suppressive therapy.

Normal value: 4.0–8.0 pmol/L (dependent on method)

RELATED NURSING CARE Evaluate medications: value can be decreased by amiodarone, propylthiouracil, lithium, phenytoin, propranolol, large doses of aspirin, steroids and sulfonamides. Values can be increased by oestrogens, progestins, oral contraceptives, amiodarone and methadone; it will also be increased during pregnancy.

NAME OF TEST Triiodothyronine resin uptake (T_3RU)

PURPOSE AND DESCRIPTION This blood test is an indirect measure of free thyroxine (T_4). The person's blood is mixed with radioactive T_3 and synthetic resin, and the radioactive T_3 will bind with available thyroid-binding globulin sites. The unbound radioactive T_3 is added to resin for T_3 uptake. In hyperthyroidism, there are few binding sites left; more T_3 is taken up by the resin and a high T_3 resin uptake results. The opposite occurs in hypothyroidism.

Normal value:
24–35% uptake

RELATED NURSING CARE No special preparation is needed.

NAME OF TEST Thyroid antibodies (TA)

PURPOSE AND DESCRIPTION A blood test used to identify thyroid autoimmune disease (Graves' disease, chronic thyroiditis, Hashimoto's thyroiditis).

Normal values:
Antithyroglobulin: negative to titre $< 1{:}20$
Antimicrosomal: negative to titre $< 1{:}100$

RELATED NURSING CARE Assess for family history of thyroid disease and ask about recent viral infection (which could trigger autoimmune disease). No specific preparation needed.

NAME OF TEST Thyroid scan

PURPOSE AND DESCRIPTION This radiological study evaluates thyroid size, structure, function and nodules. Radioactive isotopes are given orally or intravenously and a scanner is passed over the thyroid to make a graphic record of the radiation emitted. A normal thyroid scan has a homogeneous pattern of radiation with symmetric lobes. Benign lesions usually appear as warm spots (take up more radiation); malignant tumours usually appear as cold spots (less radiation taken up).

RELATED NURSING CARE No special preparation is needed. This test is contraindicated during pregnancy. Encourage the person to increase their intake of water to aid in the elimination of the radioactive isotopes following the test.

PARATHYROID TESTS

NAME OF TEST Parathyroid hormone (PTH)

PURPOSE AND DESCRIPTION A blood test done to identify hypoparathyroidism or hyperparathyroidism; also used to monitor response to PTH therapy.

In hyperparathyroidism, the PTH level is increased or at a high normal level, along with the person being hypercalcaemic.

A low PTH level is associated with hypothyroidism.

Normal value:
1.0–7.0 pmol/L (method dependent)

RELATED NURSING CARE PTH levels peak at 0200 hours. Blood sampling normally takes place in the morning as PTH levels vary during the day. They are normally ordered with a fasting serum calcium level so advise the person to avoid eating and drinking for 8 hours before the test. Evaluate medications: value can be decreased by propranolol and cimetidine. Values can be increased by phosphates, anticonvulsants, steroids, rifampin, lithium, steroids and isoniazid.

NAME OF TEST Calcium (Ca)

PURPOSE AND DESCRIPTION This blood test is used to check for serum calcium excess or deficit in parathyroid and bone disorders, and to monitor calcium levels.

Normal value:
Adults: Total Ca: 2.1–2.6 mmol/L
Corrected Ca: 2.1–2.6 mmol/L (corrected for albumin)
Ionised Ca: 1.16–1.30 mmol/L

RELATED NURSING CARE Assess for manifestations of tetany, including positive Chvostek's and Trousseau's signs, if hypocalcaemia is present.

DIAGNOSTIC TESTS The endocrine system (continued)

ADRENAL TESTS

NAME OF TEST Cortisol

PURPOSE AND DESCRIPTION A blood test that measures the amount of total cortisol in the blood and evaluates adrenal cortex function. It is decreased in Addison's disease and hypothyroidism and is increased in Cushing's syndrome and hyperthyroidism.

A saliva sample or 24-hour urine test may also be conducted to measure free (unbound) cortisol.

Normal plasma value:
Morning peak: 200–650 nmol/L
Trough level (at 2000 hours): $\leq$ 50% of morning peak levels.

Higher levels may be seen in people who are stressed or in women taking oral contraceptives.

Blood is taken prior to meals and the person may be required to rest before sample collection.

Normal urine value:
100–300 nmol/24 hours

RELATED NURSING CARE Instruct the person how to save urine for a 24-hour period, to eat a low-sodium diet before the test and to avoid stressful situations and physical activity for at least 24 hours prior to the test. You do not need to measure each urine specimen. Ensure the urine specimen is kept refrigerated. Assess medications: values may be increased by spironolactone, hydrocortisone and oral contraceptives.

NAME OF TEST Aldosterone

PURPOSE AND DESCRIPTION This blood test is taken to identify hyperaldosteronism and to compare blood and urine levels with other lab data to evaluate overhydration with increased sodium and adrenal malfunction.

A 24-hour urine test is considered a more reliable measure of aldosterone than a random aldosterone test.

Normal plasma value:
Men: 0.17–0.61 nmol/L
Women: 0.14–0.80 nmol/L

Normal urine value:
6–72 nmol/L/24 hours

RELATED NURSING CARE Usually the person must sit upright for a period of 2 hours prior to the test. The person should be instructed to follow a diet with normal levels of sodium for 2 weeks prior to the test. Assess diet and lab results: levels are increased by hyponatraemia, hyperkalaemia and a low-salt diet. Assess medications: values are increased by diuretics, hydralazine, nitroprusside and oral contraceptives. Values are decreased by propranolol, ACE inhibitors and liquorice.

NAME OF TEST Adrenocorticotropic hormone (ACTH)

PURPOSE AND DESCRIPTION This blood test is taken to determine if a decreased plasma level of cortisol is due to adrenal cortex hypofunction or pituitary hypofunction.

Normal value:
$<$ 10 pmol/L (dependent on the time the sample was taken)

RELATED NURSING CARE This blood test needs to be taken at a hospital that has laboratory facilities to immediately process it. The blood sample is normally collected between 0800 and 0900 hours. Advise the person that food and fluids may be restricted and to eat a low-carbohydrate diet for 24 hours prior to the test. Assess medications: ACTH values may be increased by metyrapone, vasopressin and insulin; and decreased by steroids, oestrogen, amphetamines and alcohol.

(continued)

DIAGNOSTIC TESTS The endocrine system (continued)

NAME OF TEST ACTH stimulation test (Synacthen test)

PURPOSE AND DESCRIPTION Performed to check for pituitary hypofunction. The drug (tetracosactide (tetracosactrin)) acts like ACTH to stimulate the adrenal gland to produce more cortisol. The rise in serum cortisol levels is measured through a series of blood tests.

This test is used to assess the presence of Addison's disease and pituitary functioning. A normal rise in cortisol levels confirms normal adrenal and pituitary functioning. If the rise in cortisol levels is low or absent, Addison's disease or a pituitary ACTH deficiency is suspected.

Normal value:
Adrenocortical function is normal if plasma cortisol level $\geq$ 200 nmol/L above the initial level or the plasma cortisol level $>$ 500 nmol/L.

RELATED NURSING CARE: The person will have a peripheral IV cannula inserted prior to the test for blood sampling. Baseline bloods are drawn prior to the person receiving 25 microg of Synacthen intramuscularly. A second sample is then collected after 30 minutes. A third sample may be collected after 60 minutes.

Let the person know that they may experience nausea, facial flushing or tachycardia post-Synacthen administration. Check for allergies or a history of asthma prior to administration.

NAME OF TEST ACTH suppression, Dexamethasone suppression test

PURPOSE AND DESCRIPTION Can be performed as an overnight test or as an inpatient 7-day test. Only the overnight test is described here. Performed to check the origin of the condition. The drug dexamethasone is given to suppress ACTH production. If the plasma cortisol continues to be high with ACTH suppression, the cause could be adrenal cortex hyperfunction (e.g. Cushing's syndrome).

RELATED NURSING CARE Advise the person to avoid caffeinated drinks and chocolates; no other food or fluid restriction is needed. Assess medications: false positives may be caused by phenytoin, barbiturates, meprobamate and carbamazepine. If dexamethasone causes gastric irritation, milk or antacids may be required.

In the overnight test, the person has a baseline cortisol level drawn at 0900 hours. The normal range for this baseline level is 200–650 nmol/L. At 2300 hours on the same day (day 1), the person is administered 1 mg oral dexamethasone. Cortisol levels are then taken at 0900 hours on day 2. The day 2 cortisol levels should be $<$ 50 nmol/L. If the day 2 result is $<$ 50 nmol/L, Cushing's syndrome is excluded. If the day 2 result is cortisol above 50 nmol/L, the cause could be adrenal cortex hyperfunction (e.g. Cushing's syndrome); however, other causes such as endogenous depression, stress, obesity and alcoholism also need to be excluded.

NAME OF TEST Computed tomography (CT) of the abdomen

PURPOSE AND DESCRIPTION This radiological study is used to assess for tumours (including size and metastasis).

RELATED NURSING CARE Determine if contrast medium will be used; if so, assess the person for an allergy to iodine (shellfish).

PANCREATIC ENDOCRINE TESTS

NAME OF TEST Glucose

PURPOSE AND DESCRIPTION This blood test is used to identify or confirm a diagnosis of diabetes mellitus.

Normal venous plasma or serum values:
Fasting: 3.0–5.4 mmol/L
2 or more hours post-prandial 'random':
3.0–7.7 mmol/L

Diabetes mellitus is indicated if the person has a fasting plasma glucose level of $\geq$ 7 mmol/L or $\geq$ 11.1 mmol/L 2 hours post prandial on two separate occasions.

An oral glucose tolerance test should be performed on people who are at high risk of diabetes and have a fasting plasma glucose level between 5.5 and 6.9 mmol/L or a random plasma glucose level $\geq$ 7.8 mmol/L.

RELATED NURSING CARE Advise the person not to eat or drink anything other than water for at least 8 hours before the test. Do not administer insulin or oral hypoglycaemic medications until blood specimen is taken. Assess medications: plasma glucose levels may be increased by cortisone, diuretics, ACTH, levodopa, some anaesthetics and phenytoin.

DIAGNOSTIC TESTS **The endocrine system (continued)**

NAME OF TEST (Oral) glucose tolerance test (OGTT or GTT)

PURPOSE AND DESCRIPTION Performed to diagnose diabetes mellitus if prior fasting plasma glucose findings are increased or inconsistent. It is also commonly used to diagnose gestational diabetes.

NURSING IMPLICATIONS The test should not be performed if the person: already has a diagnosis of diabetes mellitus; has symptoms of diabetes and a fasting plasma glucose ≥ 7.0 mmol/L or a random plasma glucose ≥ 11.1 mmol/L; has had recent surgery or trauma; or is taking certain medications such as corticosteroids or beta-adrenergic agonists.

RELATED NURSING CARE Advise the person that food, fluids (except water) and smoking are not allowed during the test or 8 hours prior to the test. Advise the person they must not exercise during the test. Assess medications: drugs that may increase OGTT levels are steroids, aspirin, lithium, tricyclic antidepressants, phenytoin, thiazide diuretics and oestrogens (oral contraceptives and hormone replacement therapy).

The person drinks a solution of glucose (adult 75 g, child 1.75 g/kg (maximum dose 75g)). Samples of blood are taken prior to the glucose 'challenge' (i.e. a fasting glucose level) and then at 60 and 120 minutes later.

Explain to the person that they may feel weak and may perspire during the test and that they should report these symptoms to the nurse. Although they usually are transitory, these symptoms may be manifestations of hyperinsulinism.

Reference values (non-pregnant) 2 hours post 75 g glucose challenge:
Normal glucose tolerance: 3.0 to 7.7 mmol/L
Impaired glucose tolerance: 7.8 to 11.0 mmol/L
Probable diabetes: fasting ≥ 11.1 mmol/L

If one or more criteria are met in pregnant women, gestational diabetes is diagnosed:
Fasting (pre-challenge): ≥ 5.1 mmol/L
At 1 hour: ≥ 10.0 mmol/L
At 2 hours: ≥ 8.5 mmol/L

NAME OF TEST Glycosylated haemoglobin (HbA1c)

PURPOSE AND DESCRIPTION This blood test is used to measure the effectiveness of treatment of diabetes mellitus. The results represent an average blood glucose level over the previous 3 months; an elevated level indicates uncontrolled diabetes mellitus and increased risk of complications.

Diagnosis of diabetes: HbA1c ≥ 6.5% (≥ 48 mmol/mol)

General target for person diagnosed with diabetes is < 7% (53 mmol/mol).

RELATED NURSING CARE Monitor findings: decreased levels can be caused by anaemias, long-term blood loss and chronic renal failure. Increased levels may result from hyperglycaemia, alcohol ingestion, pregnancy, haemodialysis and prolonged cortisone intake.

Genetic considerations

When conducting a health assessment interview and physical assessment, it is important for the nurse to consider genetic influences on the person's health. During the health assessment interview, ask about endocrine disorders in immediate family members, including the family member's age of onset and gender. Ask the person about a family history of diseases such as diabetes mellitus, thyroid disorders, growth problems, hypertension and obesity. Ask women about problems with pregnancy, menstruation and/or menopause.

During the physical assessment, assess for any manifestations that might indicate a genetic disorder (see the 'Genetic considerations' box). If data indicates genetic risk factors or alterations, ask about genetic testing and refer for appropriate genetic counselling and evaluation. The chapter 'Genetic implications of adult health nursing' provides further information about genetics in medical–surgical nursing.

GENETIC CONSIDERATIONS **Endocrine system**

- Type 1 and type 2 diabetes mellitus are classified as multifactorial inheritance disorders because both genetic and environmental factors are necessary for onset of the disorder.
- Pendred syndrome is an inherited disorder in which children develop progressive deafness and have a high chance of developing a thyroid goitre.
- Hashimoto's disease (chronic thyroiditis) is believed to have a genetic component.
- Multiple endocrine neoplasia is a group of rare diseases caused by genetic defects leading to hyperplasia and hyperfunction of two or more components of the endocrine system (especially the parathyroid, pancreas and pituitary glands).

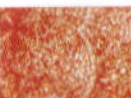

ENDOCRINE ASSESSMENTS

Technique/normal findings	Abnormal findings
Skin assessment	
Inspect skin colour. *Skin colour should be even and appropriate to the person's age and ethnicity.*	▪ Hyperpigmentation may be seen in people with Addison's disease or Cushing's syndrome. ▪ Hypopigmentation may be seen in people with diabetes mellitus, hyperthyroidism or hypothyroidism. ▪ A yellowish cast to the person's skin might indicate hypothyroidism. ▪ Purple striae over the abdomen and bruising may be present in the person with Cushing's syndrome.
Palpate the skin, assessing texture, moisture and the presence of lesions. *Skin should be appropriate to the person's ethnicity, smooth, warm, dry and intact without abnormal lesions.*	▪ Rough, dry skin is often seen in people with hypothyroidism, whereas smooth and flushed skin can be a sign of hyperthyroidism. ▪ Lesions (such as ulcerations) on the person's lower extremities might indicate diabetes mellitus.
Nails and hair assessment	
Assess texture, distribution and condition of nails and hair. *Hair should be of normal texture, appropriately distributed for gender; nail surfaces should have even colour with smooth surfaces.*	▪ Increased pigmentation of the nails is often seen in people with Addison's disease. ▪ Dry, thick, brittle nails and hair may be apparent in people with hypothyroidism; thin, brittle nails and thin, soft hair may be apparent in people with hyperthyroidism. ▪ Hirsutism (excessive facial, chest or abdominal hair) may be seen in people with Cushing's syndrome.
Facial assessment	
Inspect the symmetry and form of the face. *Face should be bilaterally symmetrical.*	▪ Variations of form and structure may indicate growth abnormalities such as **acromegaly** (continued growth of bone from growth hormone hypersecretion). ▪ A red, round face may be indicative of Cushing's syndrome.
Inspect position of eyes. *Eyes should be equal in position on both sides of the face. Eyelids should close over eyes.*	▪ **Exophthalmos** (protruding eyes) may be seen in people with hyperthyroidism.
Visual acuity and field assessments	
Assess the person's visual acuity. See the chapter 'A person-centred approach to assessing the eye and ear' for guidelines regarding visual acuity testing. *Nil changes to the person's visual acuity should be detected.*	▪ Blurred vision, **diplopia** (double vision) and **photophobia** (sensitivity to light) can be reported by people diagnosed with Graves' disease (see Figure 17.8).

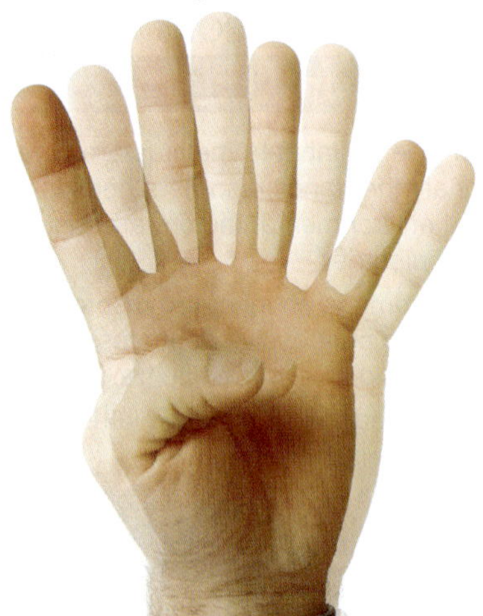

FIGURE 17.8 ***Example of diplopia***

Source: simply/123RF.

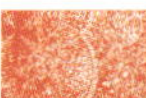

ENDOCRINE ASSESSMENTS (continued)

Technique/normal findings	Abnormal findings
Assess the person's visual fields. See the chapter 'A person-centred approach to assessing the eye and ear' for guidelines regarding visual field testing. *Nil changes to the person's peripheral vision should be detected.*	■ Pituitary adenomas can cause a **bitemporal homonymous hemianopia**—the loss of vision in each temporal visual field (outer half of vision) (see Figure 17.9). ■ This vision loss is due to the enlarged pituitary gland compressing the optic chiasm, the point where the optic nerves cross in the brain.

Bitemporal hemianopia

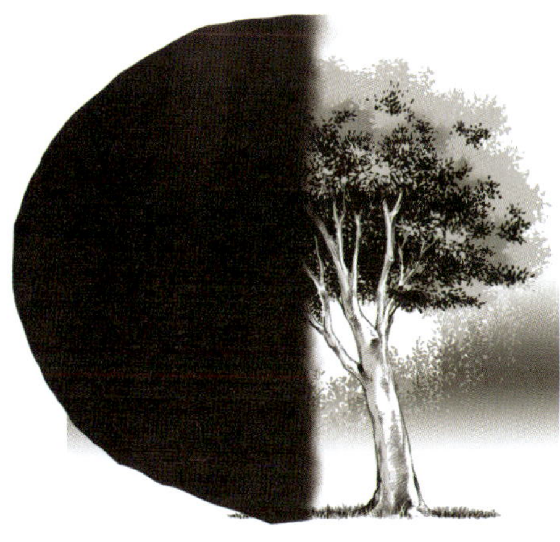

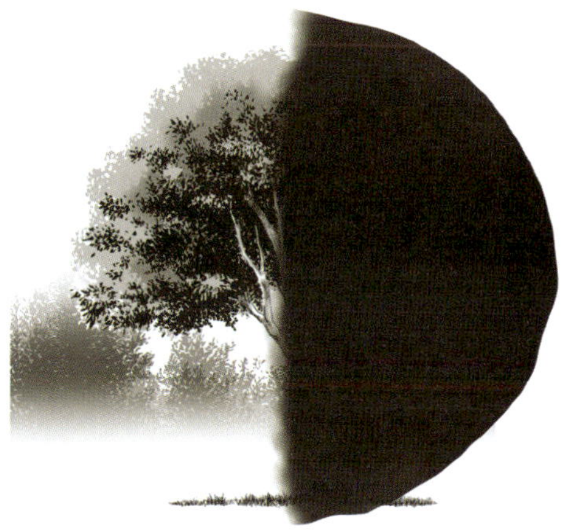

Left eye　　Right eye

FIGURE 17.9 *Example of vision with bitemporal homonymous hemianopia*

Source: Songkram Chotik-anuchit/Shutterstock.

Thyroid gland assessment

Technique/normal findings	Abnormal findings
Palpate the thyroid gland for size and consistency. Stand behind the person and place your fingers on either side of the trachea below the thyroid cartilage (see Figure 17.10). Ask the person to tilt their head to the right. Now ask the person to swallow. As the person swallows, displace the left lobe while palpating the right lobe. Repeat to palpate the left lobe. *Thyroid gland is not usually palpable. If it is, lobes should feel smooth, rubbery and free of nodules.*	■ The thyroid may be enlarged in people with Graves' disease or a **goitre** (enlarged thyroid gland). ■ Multiple nodules may be seen in metabolic disorders, whereas the presence of only one nodule may indicate a cyst or a benign or malignant tumour. ■ One enlarged nodule suggests malignancy.

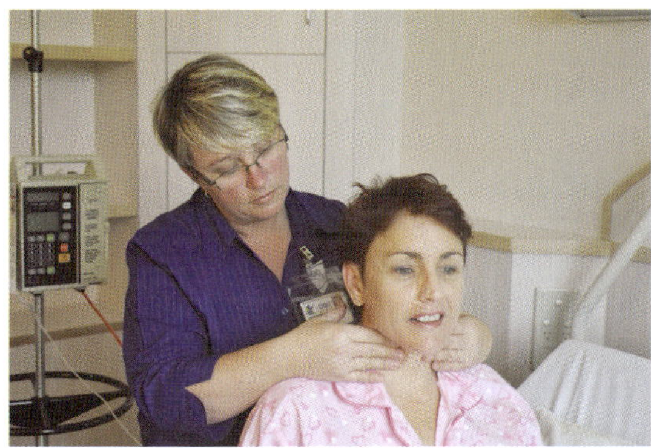

FIGURE 17.10 *Palpating the thyroid gland from behind the person*

Source: Courtesy of Tracy Levett-Jones.

(continued)

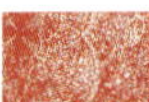

ENDOCRINE ASSESSMENTS (continued)

Technique/normal findings	Abnormal findings
Motor function assessment	
Assess the deep tendon reflexes. Deep tendon reflexes are assessed with the reflex hammer and include the biceps reflex, brachioradialis reflex, triceps reflex, patellar reflex and Achilles reflex. *Normal values range from 1+ (present but decreased) to 2+ (normal) to 3+ (increased). See the chapter 'A person-centred approach to assessing the nervous system' for guidelines and illustrations of deep tendon reflex assessment.*	■ Increased reflexes may be seen in people with hyperthyroidism; decreased reflexes may be seen in people with hypothyroidism.
Sensory function assessment	
Test the person's sensitivity to pain, temperature, vibration, light touch and stereognosis (the ability to identify an object merely by touch). Compare symmetrical areas on both sides of the body and compare the distal to the proximal regions of the extremities. Ask the person to close their eyes. *Sensory function should be bilaterally intact.* ■ **To test pain, use the blunt and sharp ends of a new neurological examination pin. Discard the pin after use.** ■ **To test temperature, use cups or other containers of cold and hot water.** ■ **To test vibration, use a tuning fork over one of the person's finger or toe joints.** ■ **To test light touch, use a cotton tip.** ■ **To test stereognosis, place in the person's hand a simple, familiar object, such as a rubber band, cotton ball or button. Ask the person to identify the object.**	■ Peripheral neuropathy and paraesthesias (altered sensations) may occur in people with diabetes, hypothyroidism or acromegaly.
Musculoskeletal assessment	
Inspect the size and proportions of the person's body structure. *Size and proportion of body structures should be bilaterally equal.*	■ Extremely short stature may indicate **dwarfism**, which is caused by insufficient growth hormone. ■ Extremely large bones may indicate acromegaly, which is caused by excessive growth hormone. ■ Excessive growth hormone in childhood or adolescence may result in **gigantism**.
Assessing for hypocalcaemia	
Assess for Trousseau's sign (a test for hypocalcaemia) with resulting tetany (tonic muscle spasms) by inflating a sphygmomanometer cuff above the antecubital space to 20 mmHg greater than the person's systolic blood pressure for 2–5 minutes. Trousseau's sign is discussed in relation to hypocalcaemia in the chapter 'Nursing care of people with altered fluid, electrolyte and acid–base balance'. *A normal finding would be no carpopedal spasm in response to compression of the arm by the blood pressure cuff.*	■ Decreased calcium levels cause the person's hand and fingers to flex and contract (**carpopedal spasm**).
Assess for Chvostek's sign (a test for hypocalcaemia) by tapping your finger in front of the person's ear at the angle of the jaw. A positive Chvostek's sign causes facial grimacing due to repeated contractions of the facial muscle. Chvostek's sign is discussed and illustrated in relation to hypocalcaemia in the chapter 'Nursing care of people with altered fluid, electrolyte and acid–base balance'. *A normal finding would be no facial grimacing in response to tapping the person's face in front of the ear.*	■ Decreased calcium levels cause the person's lateral facial muscles to contract.

CHAPTER HIGHLIGHTS

- The endocrine system comprises several glands: the pituitary gland, thyroid gland, parathyroid glands, adrenal glands, pancreas and gonads (reproductive glands).
- The endocrine system is essential to the regulation of the body's internal environment and affects a wide variety of human functions.
- Endocrine glands release most hormones, including thyroid hormone and insulin, into the bloodstream. Hormone receptors are located on or inside target cells. They recognise a specific hormone and translate the message into a cellular response.
- A targeted health history and physical assessment as well as various diagnostic tests help to diagnose endocrine disorders.

CONCEPT CHECK

1 What physiological response is expected if the pituitary gland produces an increased amount of ADH?
1 increased output of urine
2 decreased output of urine
3 increased facial hair growth in women
4 decreased production of testosterone

2 Which assessment might be performed to identify low calcium levels?
1 Save urine to measure cortisol levels.
2 Assess skin turgor.
3 Conduct a Trousseau's sign test.
4 Observe the colour of the person's skin.

3 Excessive amounts of glucocorticoids, produced by the adrenal cortex, potentially result in which health problem?
1 an impaired immune response
2 an increased response to glucagon
3 a delayed onset of puberty
4 a decreased metabolic rate

4 When conducting a health history focused on the endocrine system, which of the following questions should be included?
1 'When did you first notice the pain in your abdomen?'
2 'Do your children have problems with urination?'
3 'Have you noticed a change in your thirst?'
4 'How did you get this scar on your leg?'

5 What assessments are made when palpating the thyroid gland?
1 oedema and movement
2 size and consistency
3 character and texture
4 pain level and carotid pulse rate

6 A diagnosis of diabetes mellitus can be made after how many occasions where a person has an elevated plasma glucose level?
1 This diagnosis can be made after a single elevated result.
2 This diagnosis can be made if the elevated result occurs within 1 hour of lunch.
3 This diagnosis can be made after elevated results on two separate occasions.
4 Never. A glycosylated haemoglobin test is more accurate.

7 Which of the following tests is the most accurate indicator of thyroid function?
1 GH
2 GTT
3 aldosterone
4 TSH

8 Which is the only endocrine organ that can be palpated during physical assessment?
1 pancreas
2 liver
3 thyroid gland
4 pituitary gland

9 You are caring for a person with newly diagnosed hyperthyroidism. What might you find in an assessment?
1 increased thick hair growth
2 exophthalmos
3 decreased deep tendon reflexes
4 rough, dry skin

10 What endocrine disorder might be assessed by testing deep tendon reflexes?
1 Cushing's syndrome
2 acromegaly
3 tetany
4 hyperthyroidism

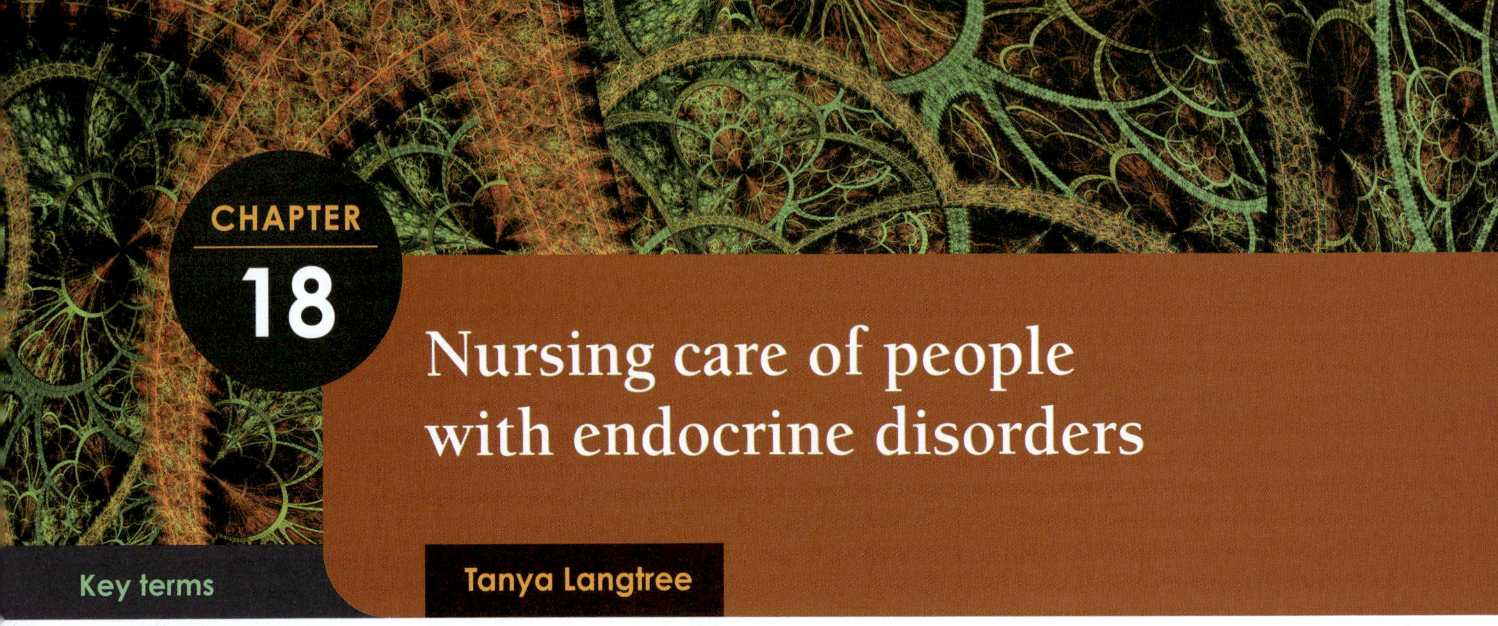

CHAPTER 18

Nursing care of people with endocrine disorders

Tanya Langtree

Key terms

acromegaly 553
Addisonian crisis 549
Addison's disease 548
bitemporal homonymous hemianopia 553
adrenal crisis 549
Cushing's disease 544
Cushing's syndrome 543
diabetes insipidus (DI) 554
euthyroid 530
exophthalmos 527
gigantism 553
goitre 527
Graves' disease 527
Hashimoto's thyroiditis 537
hyperparathyroidism 541
hyperthyroidism 527
hypoparathyroidism 543
hypothyroidism 535
myxoedema 535
myxoedema coma 537
pheochromocytoma 552
pretibial myxoedema 527
proptosis 527
subacute thyroiditis 529
syndrome of inappropriate ADH secretion (SIADH) 554
thyroid storm or crisis 529
thyroidectomy 530
thyrotoxicosis 527
toxic multinodular goitre 529

Learning outcomes

- Compare and contrast the manifestations of disorders that result from hyper- and hypofunction of the thyroid gland.
- Describe the pathophysiology, manifestations and nursing care of the person with hyper- and hypofunction of the parathyroid glands.
- Discuss common disorders of the adrenal glands, incorporating pathophysiology, manifestations and associated nursing care.
- Compare and contrast common disorders of the pituitary gland, resulting manifestations and associated nursing care.

Clinical competencies

- Assess the functional health status of people with endocrine disorders and monitor, document and report abnormal manifestations.
- Provide appropriate education regarding medication management for people living with endocrine disorders.
- Determine priority nursing diagnoses, based on assessed data, to select and implement individualised nursing interventions for people with endocrine disorders.
- Monitor for airway patency and respiratory function after a thyroidectomy.
- Monitor for latent tetany following parathyroid removal—planned or inadvertent.
- Anticipate and recognise the effects of adrenal hormones.
- Revise the plan of care as needed to provide effective interventions to promote, maintain or restore functional health status to the person with endocrine disorders.

The thyroid, parathyroid, adrenal and pituitary glands are part of the endocrine system. Disorders of the structure and function of these glands alter normal hormone levels and the way body tissues use those hormones. When hormone production increases or decreases, people experience alterations in health.

People with disorders of the endocrine glands discussed in this chapter require nursing care for multiple problems. Nursing care is directed towards meeting physiological needs, providing education and ensuring psychological support for the person and family. A holistic approach to the complex needs of people with these endocrine disorders is an essential component of nursing care.

Disorders of the thyroid gland

The thyroid uses iodine to secrete thyroid hormone (TH). TH is of vital importance for both the development and the maintenance of brain function and other major organ systems (Wouters et al., 2020).

Thyroid disorders—both hyperthyroidism and hypothyroidism—are among the most common endocrine disorders. Thyroid disease is the second most common endocrine condition in women of childbearing age. The prevalence of thyroid disease among Australians ranges from 0.5 to 12%, with the incidence of these conditions increasing with age (Walsh, 2016).

PEOPLE WITH HYPERTHYROIDISM

Hyperthyroidism, or **thyrotoxicosis**, is a disorder caused by excessive functional activity of the thyroid gland which results in an increased production of thyroid hormone (TH). Because the primary effect of TH is to increase metabolism and protein synthesis, hyperthyroidism is characterised by increased basal metabolism, weight loss despite an increased food intake and alterations of the autonomic nervous system. Cardiovascular manifestations such as hypertension, sinus tachycardia and increased cardiac output may also be present (Doubleday & Sippel, 2020).

Pathophysiology and manifestations

Hyperthyroidism results from different factors, including autoimmune thyroid stimulation as in Graves' disease (Hughes & Eastman, 2021); excess secretion of thyroid-stimulating hormone (TSH) by the pituitary gland; thyroiditis; non-malignant neoplasms such as toxic multinodular goitre (TMNG); and an excessive intake of thyroid medications. The most common aetiologies of hyperthyroidism in Australia are Graves' disease and TMNG.

The person with hyperthyroidism typically has an increased appetite, yet loses weight, and may have increased bowel motility without diarrhoea. Additional manifestations related to hypermetabolism include increased nervousness or irritability, heat intolerance, insomnia, palpitations and increased sweating. Muscle weakness or tremors may be observed and there is an increased risk of fractures (Blum et al., 2015). The skin is smooth and warm to touch, hair may become fine and hair loss in the scalp, eyebrow, axillary or pubic areas of the body is common. Emotional lability is also common. See 'Multisystem effects of hyperthyroidism'.

Graves' disease

Graves' disease is the most common cause of hyperthyroidism and is estimated to affect 1% of the population (Du et al., 2021). It is caused by a defect in immunoregulation in genetically predisposed individuals, leading to thyroid hyperplasia and an increased production of thyroid-stimulating hormone receptor antibodies (Cheetham & Boal, 2019).

Graves' disease is seen five times more often in women than in men and occurs most frequently between the ages of 20 and 40. It is seen worldwide, with the incidence often correlated with the amount of iodine in the diet. Increased iodine intake (such as from radiocontrast dyes used in diagnostic tests, ingestion of supplemental iodine tablets or medications such as amiodarone that contains 39% iodine by weight) have been associated with this disorder. Smoking, psychological stress and the postpartum period are also associated with the development of Graves' disease.

People with Graves' disease have an enlarged diffuse thyroid gland (**goitre**) and manifestations of hyperthyroidism (as shown in Table 18.1). Goitre may be present as a consequence of both iodine deficiency and excess and consequently may be evident in either hyperthyroidism or hypothyroidism (Zimmermann & Boelaert, 2015).

The common ophthalmopathy of Graves' disease (Graves' ophthalmopathy) is manifested as proptosis and visual dysfunction. **Proptosis** (forward displacement) of the eyeball occurs in about one-quarter of cases (Topilow et al., 2020). The forward protrusion (**exophthalmos**) results from an accumulation of inflammation by-products in the retro-orbital tissues. Often the sclera is visible above the iris. The upper lids are often retracted and the person has a characteristic unblinking stare (see Figure 18.1). In some cases, proptosis may involve only one eye. Due to stretching or compression of the optic nerve, the person may experience blurred vision, diplopia, eye pain, lacrimation and photophobia. The inability to close the eyelids completely over the protruding eyeballs increases the risk of corneal dryness, irritation, infection and ulceration. Infiltration of the muscles that move the eye and of the optic nerve leads to paralysis and vision loss. The treatment of Graves' disease generally does not reverse these changes in the eyes.

A rare characteristic dermopathy of Graves' disease is **pretibial myxoedema**, which occurs in 1% to 4% of people with the disease. Plaques and nodules develop bilaterally over the shins and dorsal surface of the feet. These plaques are oedematous, erythematous and sometimes hyperpigmented.

Multisystem effects of hyperthyroidism

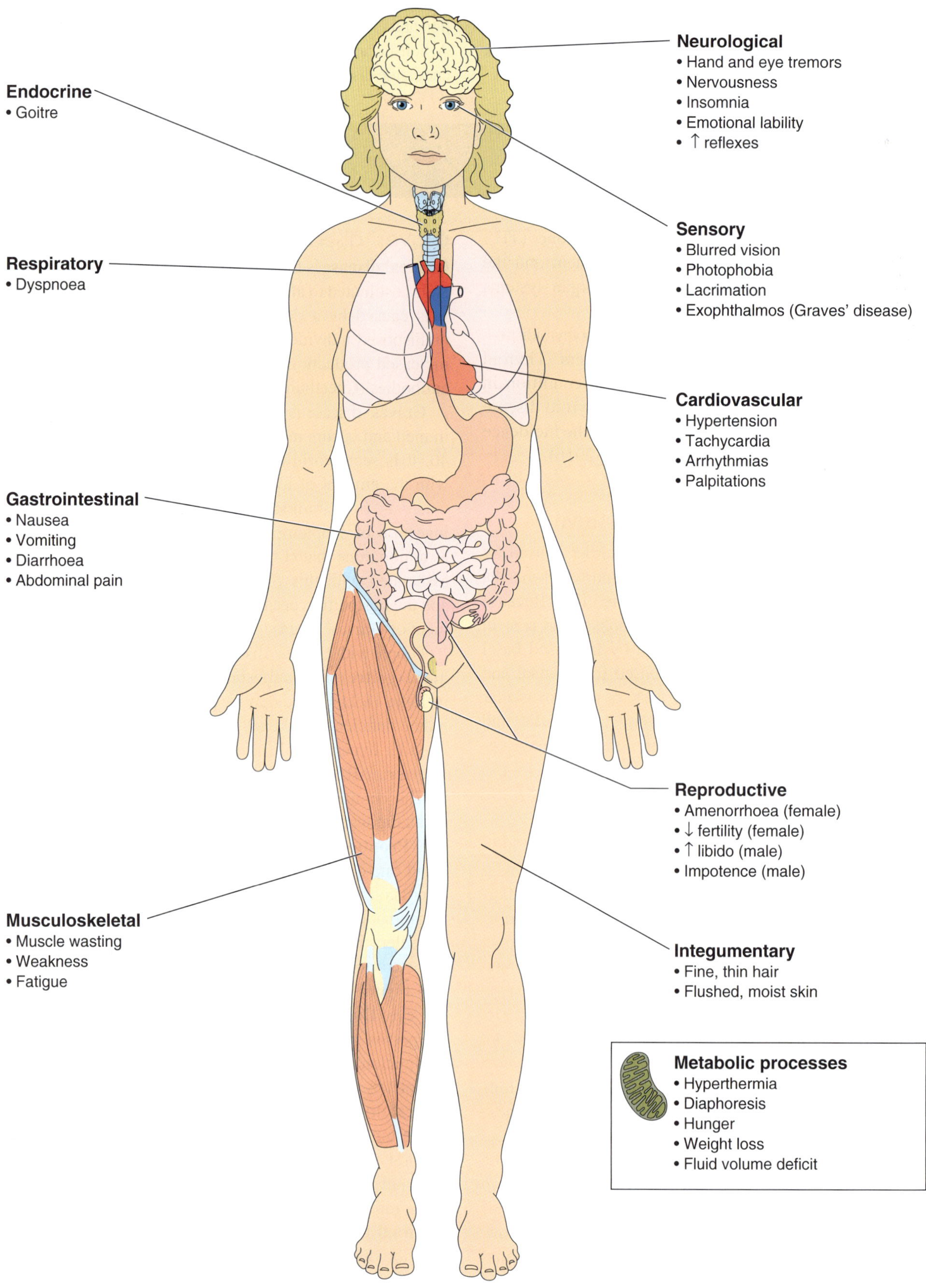

TABLE 18.1 Laboratory findings in hyperthyroidism

TEST	NORMAL VALUES	FINDINGS
Serum TA	≤ 1:20 titre	Normal to increased
Serum TSH (sensitive assay)	0.4–4.0 mIU/L	Decreased in primary hyperthyroidism
Serum T_4	Total 10–25 pmol/L	Normal to increased
Serum T_3	4–8 pmol/L	Normal to increased

Source: Adapted from The Royal College of Pathologists of Australasia (RCPA) (2015). *RCPA manual* (7th ed.). Retrieved from https://www.rcpa.edu.au/Manuals/RCPA-Manual.
mIU = milli-International units; pmol = picomoles.

Like the ophthalmopathy, the skin changes often persist despite successful treatment (Ramos et al., 2015).

Other manifestations include anaemia, vomiting, jaundice, fatigue, difficulty sleeping, hand tremors, increased bowel movements and changes in menstruation ranging from decreased flow to amenorrhoea. Twenty per cent of older people may present with atrial fibrillation, angina or congestive heart failure as a result of pulmonary hypertension.

Toxic multinodular goitre (TMNG)

Toxic multinodular goitre (see Figure 18.2) is a non-malignant tumour characterised by small, discrete, independently functioning nodules in the thyroid gland that secrete excessive amounts of TH. The aetiology includes a suspected genetic mutation of follicle cells as well as a deficiency of iodine (Zimmermann & Boelaert, 2015). People with this type of hyperthyroidism are usually women, aged between 60 and 80, who have had a goitre for several years.

Excess TSH stimulation

Overproduction of TSH by the pituitary usually stimulates the thyroid gland to produce excess TH. The elevation in TSH secretion often results from a pituitary adenoma. This secondary form of hyperthyroidism is rare.

Subacute thyroiditis

Subacute thyroiditis (inflammation of the thyroid gland) is most often the result of a viral infection of the thyroid gland such as influenza or mumps. The symptoms of subacute thyroiditis are those of inflammation and increased TH. Subacute thyroiditis may become chronic, resulting in a hypothyroid state as repeated infections destroy gland tissue. See the discussion of Hashimoto's thyroiditis later in this chapter.

Thyroid crisis

Thyroid crisis (also called **thyroid storm**) is an extreme state of hyperthyroidism that is rare today because of improved diagnosis and treatment (Nasrullah et al., 2022). Those affected usually have had untreated hyperthyroidism (most often Graves' disease) or have been receiving therapy but have experienced an acute stressor, such as an infection, trauma, myocardial infarction, diabetic ketoacidosis (DKA) or manipulation of the thyroid gland during surgery. Thyroid crisis is a life-threatening condition.

The rapid increase in metabolic rate results in manifestations including hyperthermia, with body temperatures ranging from 39°C to 41°C; cardiovascular abnormalities (tachycardia, atrial fibrillation, systolic hypertension, congestive heart failure) and gastrointestinal symptoms (abdominal pain, nausea, vomiting and increased bowel motions). Agitation, restlessness

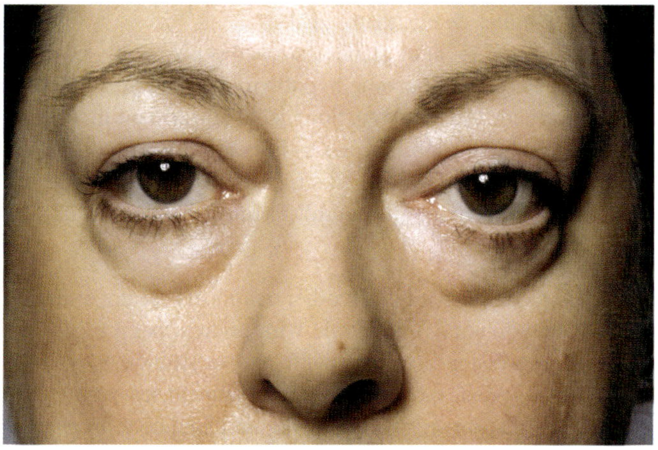

FIGURE 18.1 ***Exophthalmos in a person with Graves' disease. The disorder causes oedema of fat deposits behind the eyes and inflammation of the extraocular muscles. The accumulating pressure forces the eyes outward from their orbits***

Source: Mediscan/Alamy Stock Photo.

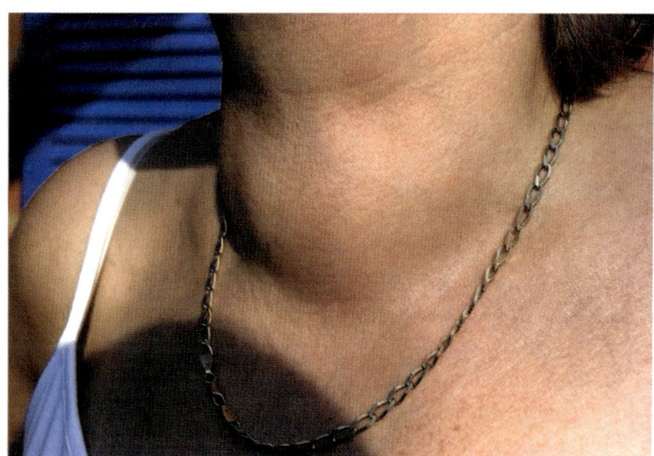

FIGURE 18.2 ***Toxic multinodular goitre. The formation and growth of numerous nodules in the thyroid gland cause the characteristic massive enlargement of the neck***

Source: Chris Pancewicz/Alamy Stock Photo.

and tremors are common, progressing to confusion, psychosis, delirium and seizures. The estimated mortality rate is between 8% and 50% (Nasrullah et al., 2022). Rapid treatment of thyroid crisis is essential to preserve life. Intensive care treatment includes cooling without aspirin (which increases free TH) or inducing shivering; replacing fluids, glucose and electrolytes; relieving respiratory distress via mechanical ventilation; stabilising cardiovascular function through the administration of beta-blockers (Doubleday & Sippel, 2020); and reducing TH synthesis and secretion.

INTERPROFESSIONAL CARE

Treatment of hyperthyroidism focuses on reducing the production of TH, thus establishing a **euthyroid** (normal thyroid) state, and preventing or treating complications. Depending on the person's age and physical status, oral antithyroid medications, radioactive iodine therapy or surgery may be used.

Diagnosis

Hyperthyroidism is diagnosed according to the manifestations of the specific disorders causing excessive TH and by diagnostic test results. Elevated levels of TH (both T_3 and T_4) and increased radioactive iodine (RAI) uptake are diagnostic criteria of hyperthyroidism. Laboratory findings in hyperthyroidism were shown in Table 18.1.

The following diagnostic tests may be ordered:

- *TSH receptor antibodies.* This test is useful to establish the diagnosis of Graves' disease, especially when a radionuclide thyroid scan is not able to be performed, as in pregnancy or lactation. Thyroid peroxidase and thyroglobulin autoantibodies may be useful in the diagnosis of subacute thyroiditis or autoimmune chronic lymphocytic thyroiditis.
- *TSH test (sensitive assay).* Serum TSH levels are measured and compared with thyroxine (T_4) levels to differentiate pituitary from thyroid dysfunction. The best indicator of primary hyperthyroidism (such as in Graves' disease) is suppression of TSH below 0.27 mIU/L. When the sensitive TSH is not suppressed, the hyperthyroidism is caused by a TSH-secreting pituitary tumour.
- *T_4 test, total.* Serum tetraiodothyronine (thyroxine) levels are measured to determine TH concentration and to test thyroid gland function. Levels are elevated in hyperthyroidism and acute thyroiditis.
- *T_3 test, free.* Serum triiodothyronine (T_3) is the active form of TH. T_3 is measured by radioimmunoassay (T_3RIA), which measures bound and free forms of this hormone. T_3 levels may be elevated in hyperthyroidism and thyroiditis. T_3 decreases in acute illness and starvation and is affected by medications such as amiodarone, propranolol and steroids.
- *T_3 uptake test.* T_3 uptake (T_3RU) is measured by an in vitro test in which the person's blood is mixed with radioactive T_3; the results are elevated in hyperthyroidism and in metastatic neoplasms.
- *Thyroid scan.* This scan measures the uptake of intravenous sodium pertechnetate, a radiopharmaceutical, in the thyroid gland. After 15 to 20 minutes, a scintillation camera (a camera that detects gamma rays) is used to take a series of images of the thyroid gland to determine its function, size and shape. The entire process takes 40 to 60 minutes.
- *Thyroid suppression test.* RAI and T_4 levels are measured first. The person then takes TH for 7 to 10 days, after which the tests are repeated. Failure of hormone therapy to suppress RAI and T_4 indicates hyperthyroidism.
- *Fine-needle biopsy.* Any suspicious enlargement of the thyroid gland should undergo biopsy with expert cytological examination.

Medications

Hyperthyroidism can be treated by administering antithyroid medications that reduce TH production. See the 'Medication administration' box.

Radioactive iodine therapy (RAI)

Because the thyroid gland takes up iodine in any form, radioactive iodine (^{131}I) concentrates in the thyroid gland and damages or destroys thyroid cells so that they produce less TH. The person is placed on a low-iodine diet for at least 1 week prior to therapy to facilitate uptake (Doubleday & Sippel, 2020).

Most RAI recipients show a response to treatment in 1 to 2 months, with hypothyroidism being induced between 3 to 6 months. In most instances, the person is not hospitalised during treatment and does not require radiation precautions. Women of childbearing age should delay becoming pregnant for 6 months and men should allow 4 months for sperm turnover production (Poppe et al., 2021). A repeat RAI treatment may be necessary in some individuals. RAI therapy can exacerbate pre-existing ophthalmopathy in people with Graves' disease or may lead to the development of *de novo* (new onset) Graves' ophthalmopathy (Taïeb, 2020). Therefore, RAI may not be a suitable treatment for people with significant thyroid eye disease. Prophylactic corticosteroids may also be administered at the time of RAI therapy to decrease the risk of ophthalmopathy (Hughes & Eastman, 2021).

Because the amount of gland destroyed is not readily controllable, the person may become hypothyroid and require lifelong TH replacement. Adverse reactions include transient thyrotoxicosis and cardiac instability due to liberation of stored thyroid hormone in the gland, sialadenitis (inflammation of the salivary gland) and xerostomia (dry mouth) (Padda & Nguyen, 2022).

Surgery

Surgery is recommended when other treatments are not effective in younger individuals; in people with goitres that are causing tracheal compression; in people with large or suspicious nodules (e.g. toxic or TMNG); for people with treatment-resistant/recurrent Graves' disease; for women who are planning a pregnancy in the next 6 to 12 months; or if rapid resolution of symptoms is required (Kane & Shore, 2020). A total **thyroidectomy** is normally performed to treat TMNG or Graves' disease. A partial resection (e.g. a hemithyroidectomy) may be appropriate for the person who has an asymmetrical goitre or has been diagnosed an isolated thyroid adenoma. The latter must be confirmed via ultrasound prior to surgery. The need for postoperative thyroid

MEDICATION ADMINISTRATION **Hyperthyroidism**

IODINE SOURCES

Sodium iodide (^{131}I) therapy

This radioactive medication is used in the treatment of hyperthyroidism. It can also be used for the ablation of residual functioning thyroid tissue in differentiated thyroid cancer. It is available in a capsule form and as an oral solution. Both are stored in a glass vial and lead container. The dose administered is dependent on the treatment goal (e.g. the dose to treat thyrotoxicosis is 150–600 megabecquerels).

Nursing responsibilities

- The person should be managed in a single room to limit radiation exposure to others.
- Only a doctor who specialises in radioisotopes should administer the dose.
- Disposable gloves and a cup with water should be given to the patient prior to removing the sodium iodide from its lead container.
- Give the person water following the administration of the dose.
- The equipment used during administration (i.e. gloves worn by the staff and recipient; vial, stopper and cap; and cup) must be treated as radioactive waste.
- Monitor for hyponatraemia and increased bleeding tendencies if the person is also taking anticoagulants.

Health education for the person and family

Pre-administration

- Instruct the recipient to restrict iodine in their diet for at least 1 week prior to receiving the sodium iodide or as instructed by the endocrinologist.
- Antithyroid drugs should be withheld for 3 days prior to receiving the treatment.
- Thyroxine sodium should be withheld for 4 weeks prior to receiving the treatment.
- Women of childbearing age should undertake a pregnancy test prior to receiving the treatment.

Post-administration

- Encourage the person to drink copious fluids before and after the solution and to void as often as possible to reduce the radiation dose to the stomach, kidneys and bladder.
- Instruct the recipient to use contraception for the time period prescribed by the treating doctor.
- Instruct the recipient to avoid kissing for at least 10 days following administration as the drug is secreted in saliva.
- Encourage the recipient to double flush the toilet and undertake regular hand hygiene.
- The recipient will require lifelong follow up with their treating doctor.

ANTITHYROID DRUGS

Carbimazole (Neo-Mercazole) and Propylthiouracil (PTU)

Antithyroid drugs, also known as thionamide medications, inhibit the incorporation of iodine into thyroglobulin, thus lowering TH production. They do not affect already formed hormones; therefore, several weeks may elapse before the person experiences therapeutic effects. Carbimazole is converted to methimazole in the body. This oral medication is given in divided doses according to the severity of the hyperthyroidism, from 15 mg/day up to 60 mg/day in severe cases. Once symptoms are controlled, the dosage can be tapered to a long-term maintenance dose. Carbimazole use in pregnancy can lead to birth defects; therefore, it should only be used cautiously when propylthiouracil is unsuitable. The dose for use in pregnant women should not exceed 15 mg twice daily and it must be ceased 3 to 4 weeks prior to birth. A course of supplemental iodine will then be prescribed.

Propylthiouracil is taken in divided doses two to four times daily until the person becomes euthyroid. The initial daily dose is 200 to 400 mg daily. However, individuals with severe hypertension may require a daily dose of up to 1,200 mg. The maintenance dose is normally between 50 to 800 mg daily divided into two to four doses. Propylthiouracil is the preferred medication for use prior to conception and during the first trimester of pregnancy.

Nursing responsibilities

- Monitor for side effects: life-threatening agranulocytosis evidenced by reduced neutrophil count and fever, hypothyroidism, pruritus rash, periorbital oedema, anorexia or vomiting, loss of taste, menstrual irregularities.
- Severe hepatocellular injury occurs with propylthiouracil in 0.1% of patients. Women under 30 years are at particular risk of propylthiouracil-induced hepatotoxicity, especially in the first 3 months of therapy. Monitor for evidence of jaundice.
- Administer drugs at the same time and dosing intervals each day with meals to maintain stable blood levels.
- Monitor for symptoms of hypothyroidism: fatigue, weight gain, bradycardia.

Health education for the person and family

- Instruct the person to watch for unusual bleeding, redness, swelling, nausea, loss of taste or epigastric pain.
- Educate the person that it may take up to 12 weeks before the full effects of the drugs are experienced.
- Encourage the person to take the medication exactly as prescribed and to not discontinue abruptly.
- Encourage the person to keep medical appointments during the initial stages of treatment.

hormone replacement is largely dependent on the amount of thyroid that was removed during the surgery.

Before surgery, the person should be in as nearly a euthyroid state as possible. Antithyroid drugs may be given to reduce hormone levels and iodine preparations to decrease the vascularity and size of the gland, which also reduces the risk of haemorrhage during and after surgery. Postoperative complications include laryngeal nerve palsy or hypocalcaemia due to removal of or damage to the parathyroid glands (Quérat et al., 2015).

NURSING CARE OF THE PERSON undergoing a thyroidectomy

PREOPERATIVE CARE

- Administer ordered antithyroid medications and iodine preparations and monitor their effects. *Antithyroid drugs are given before surgery to promote a euthyroid state. Iodine preparations are given before surgery to decrease vascularity of the gland, thereby decreasing the risk of haemorrhage.*
- Teach the person preoperatively to support the neck by placing both hands behind the neck when sitting up in bed, while moving about and while coughing. *Placing the hands behind the neck postoperatively provides support for the suture line.*
- Answer questions and allow time for the person to verbalise concerns. Because the incision is made at the base of the throat, people (especially women) are often concerned about their appearance after surgery. *Explain that the scar will eventually be only a thin line and that jewellery or scarves may be used to cover the scar.*
- Teach the person to expect postoperative hoarseness due to generalised swelling at the suture line. *Postoperative hoarseness will diminish with healing and is not caused by laryngeal nerve damage.*

POSTOPERATIVE CARE

- Ensure safety equipment (i.e. suction equipment, oxygen delivery device, suture cutter and a mini-tracheostomy kit) is located at the bedside as per local policy. Check that suction and oxygen is working at the commencement of each shift. *Airway obstruction is a known postoperative complication of thyroidectomies due to the formation of a haematoma at the surgical site. This equipment must be available for immediate use if airway obstruction is observed.*
- Perform focused assessments to observe airway patency and to monitor for complications such as sudden swelling at the suture line and respiratory distress. Assess the person's respiratory rate, rhythm, depth and effort as per local policy. Maintain humidification as ordered. Assist the person with deep breathing and coughing. *Respiratory distress may result from haemorrhage and oedema, which may compress the trachea; from tetany and laryngeal spasms resulting from removal or damage to the parathyroid glands; and from damage to the laryngeal nerve, causing spasms of the vocal cords. Stridor is heard in acute airway obstruction.*
- Assess for signs of haemorrhage. Frequently observe the dressing for signs of strikethrough and the area under the person's neck and shoulders for bleeding. Ask the person if their neck dressing feels tight and inspect the edges of dressing for increase tautness. Monitor drain patency (if present) and record drainage volume, colour and consistency. Monitor the person's blood pressure and pulse as well as other signs and symptoms of hypovolaemic shock. Document all assessment findings to enable a baseline for future observations, thereby enabling the prompt detection of possible haemorrhaging. *The vascularity of the gland increases the risk of haemorrhage. The location of the incision and the position of the person may cause the drainage to run back and under the person's neck. Haematoma formation may increase the person's neck circumference. The danger of haemorrhage is greatest in the first 6 to 12 hours after surgery.*
- Monitor for pain and provide comfort measures: administer analgesia as ordered and monitor their effectiveness; place the person in a semi-Fowler's position after recovery from anaesthesia; support the person's head and neck with pillows. *Analgesic medications reduce acute pain and physical stress during the postoperative period. Positioning the person in a semi-Fowler's position and supporting the head and neck decreases strain on the suture line.*
- Monitor for signs of laryngeal nerve damage through assessing the person's voice quality and tone, swallow reflex and respiratory status. *The location of the laryngeal nerve increases the risk of damage during thyroid surgery. Although hoarseness may be due to oedema or the endotracheal tube used during surgery and will subside, permanent hoarseness or loss of vocal volume is a potential danger. Dysphagia and/or an ineffective cough are also signs of possible laryngeal nerve damage.*
- Assess for signs of secondary hypoparathyroidism including tetany (involuntary muscle contraction) due to decreased circulating calcium levels. Observe for neuromuscular irritability (i.e. numbness or tingling of toes, fingers and lips; muscular twitches; positive Trousseau's and Chvostek's signs; seizure activity). Evaluate for cardiac dysrhythmias and assess deep tendon reflexes as indicated. Ensure calcium gluconate or calcium chloride is available for immediate intravenous use. *The parathyroid glands are located in and near the thyroid gland; surgery of the thyroid gland may injure or remove parathyroid glands, resulting in hypocalcaemia and tetany. Tetany may occur up to 7 days after a thyroidectomy.*
- Monitor for possible wound infection including assessing the wound site and person's temperature regularly, observing for any malodourous discharge on the wound dressing and reviewing the person's white cell count. Administer prophylactic antibiotics as ordered. *Postoperative wound infections are uncommon in thyroidectomy patients. However, an elevated temperature and white cell count, changes in the temperature and appearance of the wound and the presence of malodourous discharge warrants further investigation.*

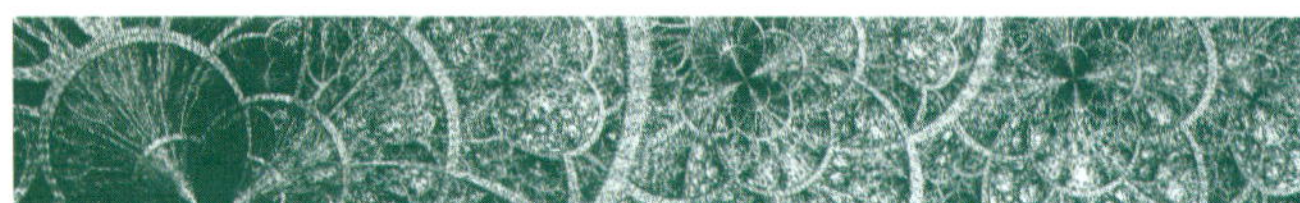

Nursing care

Assessment

The following data are collected through the health history and physical examination (see the chapter 'A person-centred approach to assessing the endocrine system'). Further focused assessments are described with nursing interventions.

- *Health history*: inquire about the following when conducting a health interview with the person: other known medical conditions; whether there is a family history of thyroid disease; the characteristics, commencement and severity of presenting symptoms; routine dietary intake of iodine; regular medication regimens; menstrual history; recent changes in weight; and normal elimination pattern.

- *Physical assessment*: assess the following when performing a physical assessment on the person: muscle strength, tremors, vital signs, cardiovascular and peripheral vascular systems, integument, the size of thyroid, the presence of a bruit over the thyroid, eye appearance and positioning and the presence of visual disturbances.

Nursing diagnoses and interventions

In planning and implementing nursing care for the person with hyperthyroidism, the nurse considers the person's responses to the systemic effects of the disorder. Although each person may have different needs, nursing diagnoses discussed in this section focus on the most common problems: cardiovascular problems, visual deficits, altered nutrition and body image disturbance. See the accompanying 'Nursing care plan'.

Risk of increased cardiac output

Excess TH directly affects the heart, resulting in an increased rate and stroke volume. There are also increases in the metabolic demands and oxygen requirements of the peripheral tissues and the demands on the heart. Resultant clinical manifestations include fatigue, dyspnoea, systolic hypertension, angina, dysrhythmias and congestive cardiac failure. The risk of complications is greater in people with pre-existing cardiovascular disorders.

- Monitor for signs of cardiovascular compromise. Regularly assess the person's blood pressure, pulse rate and rhythm, respiratory rate, oxygen saturation levels and breath sounds. Assess for peripheral oedema, jugular vein distension and increased activity intolerance. *Increased TH increases heart rate, stroke volume and tissue demand for oxygen, causing stress on the heart.*
- Keep the environment as cool and calming as possible. Decrease the person's stress by explaining interventions, providing reassurance and teaching relaxation techniques. *A physically comfortable and psychologically calm environment can reduce stimuli and stressors. Stress increases circulating catecholamines, which further increase cardiac workload.*

Disturbed visual perception related to exophthalmos

Exophthalmos can result in diminished visual acuity and increased risk of corneal infections and abrasions.

- Monitor the person's visual acuity. Ask the person if they are experiencing photophobia or diplopia. Decrease overhead lighting for people with photophobia. Apply an eye patch to one eye to decrease the effects of diplopia. Encourage the person to promptly report any pain or changes in their vision. *Thyroid eye disease can result in several visual disturbances including photophobia (sensitivity to light) and diplopia (double vision). These disturbances can be reduced through these simple interventions.*
- Assess the integrity of the person's cornea and their ability to close their eyes. Apply lubricating eye drops at regular intervals as ordered. Ask the person if they feel their eyes are dry. Consider using an eye bubble or a sheet of plastic wrap ('Gladwrap') placed over the impacted eye(s) while sleeping. *The cornea is at risk of dryness, injury, conjunctivitis and corneal infections including exposure keratopathy due to the person being unable to close their eye(s). Such corneal injuries and infections can result in further loss of visual acuity due to ulceration and scarring. The use of eye bubble or 'Gladwrap' forms a moisture chamber for the eye and acts as a physical barrier, thereby decreasing the risk of corneal injury or infections.*
- Teach additional measures for protecting the eye from injury and maintaining visual acuity including:
  - Use tinted glasses or shields as protection.
  - Use cool, moist compresses to relieve irritation.
  - Elevate the head of the bed to 45 degrees to promote periorbital fluid decrease.
  - Encourage the person to quit smoking as smoking exacerbates exophthalmos.

Imbalanced nutrition: less than body requirements related to gastrointestinal hypermotility

The hypermetabolic state that occurs in hyperthyroidism causes gastrointestinal hypermotility. Although the person may have an increased appetite and eat more than usual, weight loss continues.

- Ask the person to weigh themself weekly and keep a record of results. *The inability to meet metabolic demands results in loss of body weight. Regular monitoring detects continued weight loss.*
- In collaboration with a dietitian, teach the person the need for a diet high in carbohydrates and protein and including between-meal snacks. Six small meals a day may be more desirable than three large meals. Energy intake may need to be increased to 16,700 kilojoules/day if weight loss exceeds 10% to 17% for height and frame. *Increased nutrients as part of a well-balanced diet are necessary to meet metabolic demands. People are often better able to increase food intake by eating frequent, small meals. A 0.45 kg weight gain requires approximately 14,650 extra kilojoules.*
- Monitor nutritional status through results of laboratory data. Serum albumin, transferrin and total lymphocyte counts are commonly lower than normal in nutritional deficits. *A negative nitrogen balance signifies a catabolic state in which protein is lost and metabolic demands are not being met.*

Potential for disturbed body image related to physical changes common in hyperthyroidism

Physical changes common in hyperthyroidism include exophthalmos, goitre, tremors, hair loss, increased perspiration, loss of strength, fatigue, weight loss and changes in reproductive and sexual function (amenorrhoea in women, impotence in men and decreased libido in both men and women). In addition, the person often has mood changes and insomnia and is constantly nervous and anxious. There may even be periods of

NURSING CARE PLAN A person with Graves' disease

Mrs Juanita Martin is a 33-year-old mother of four small children. She is a second-year university student completing the requirements for an education degree. For the past 3 months, Juanita has been constantly hungry and has eaten more than usual, but she has still lost 6.8 kg. She has multiple bowel movements each day and often feels nauseated. Her hands shake, she can feel her heart beating rapidly and she finds herself laughing or crying for no apparent reason.

Juanita makes an appointment with her family doctor. The nurse at the GP clinic completes a health history and physical assessment. When asked how she has been feeling, Juanita replies, 'Well, I don't know what's wrong with me—but I keep losing weight and I cry at the drop of a hat. I am also just so hot all the time and I've never had that problem before. I hope I find out what's wrong and it's nothing serious.'

ASSESSMENT

The health history indicates that although her appetite has increased, Juanita has lost 6.8 kg. She states that she has had increased bowel movements, nausea, palpitations, heat intolerance and mood changes. Physical assessment findings include the following: T 38.3°C, P 110, R 24 and BP 162/86 mmHg. Her skin is moist and warm, her hair thin and fine. She has visible tremors in her hands. Her eyeballs protrude and she is unable to close her eyelids completely. Her thyroid is enlarged and palpable. Diagnostic tests reveal the following abnormal results: Free T_3, 18 pmol/L (normal range: 4.0–8.0 pmol/L), Total T_4, 30 pmol/L (normal range: 10–25 pmol/L). A thyroid scan demonstrates an enlarged thyroid with increased iodine uptake. The medical diagnosis of Graves' disease is made and Juanita is commenced on the antithyroid medication propylthiouracil, 150 mg orally every 8 hours.

DIAGNOSES

- *Risk of imbalanced nutrition: less than body requirements* related to hyperthyroid state and increased metabolism as evidenced by weight loss of 6.8 kg with present weight 10% less than normal for her height.
- *Increased bowel movements* related to increased food intake and peristalsis as evidenced by more than four loose stools per day.
- *Risk of disturbed visual perception* and/or *Risk of eye infection* related to an inability to close the eyelids completely.
- *Anxiety* related to a lack of knowledge about disease process.

PLANNING

- Request that she keep a record of weekly weight.
- Discuss adopting a high-kilojoule diet. Identify food likes and dislikes, before instituting a plan to increase her daily food intake.
- Request that she keep a stool chart, noting the time, type and precipitating factors for stools. Teach comfort measures for irritated anal area (clean washcloth and soap, no irritating ointment).
- Teach how to apply eye drops (artificial tears).
- Explain the need to elevate the head of the bed to 45 degrees at night and the trial of an eye bubble or 'Gladwrap' placed over impacted eyes before sleep.
- Teach about Graves' disease, the medication's effects and side effects, and the need for continued medical care.

Expected outcomes

- Gain at least 0.45 kg every 2 weeks.
- Regain normal bowel elimination patterns.
- Maintain normal vision (with no evidence of corneal damage and/or infection) and verbalise measures to protect her eyes.
- Verbalise medical treatment and self-care needs.
- Verbalise a decrease in anxiety.

IMPLEMENTATION

Juanita will:

- Adopt a high-kilojoule diet and increase her food intake.
- Maintain a weekly record of her weight.
- Monitor her bowel movements and adopt measures for anal comfort and hygiene.
- Regularly apply lubricating eye drops/ointment.
- Elevate her head at night and trial using an eye bubble or 'Gladwrap' at night.
- Have the contacts details for additional support organisations such as the Australian Thyroid Foundation and the clinic's contact details if she has any further queries or concerns.

EVALUATION

By her next visit, Juanita has gained 0.45 kg and has discussed her dietary needs with the nurse and her husband. She is having fewer bowel motions per day. She has safely applied the eyedrops and states that she is elevating her head at night using pillows. The practice nurse reviews the written and verbal information about Graves' disease and the medication prescribed. Mrs Martin verbalises her understanding, stating, 'I'll always take my medicine—I never want to feel like that again!' She also says that she feels much less anxious now that she understands what has happened.

CRITICAL THINKING IN THE NURSING PROCESS

1. What is the pathophysiological basis for Juanita's abnormal vital signs?
2. What is the rationale for having the person with exophthalmos elevate their head at night?

REFLECTION ON THE NURSING PROCESS

1. Can you think of at least three other strategies that you would add to the plan of education for Juanita and her family? Write the corresponding Expected outcomes and Implementation for your strategies.
2. Design an educational strategy to help teach Juanita about her nutritional requirements.

psychosis. These changes are frightening not only for the person but also for family members.

- Establish a trusting relationship; encourage the person to verbalise feelings about self and to ask questions about the illness and treatment. Provide reliable information and clarify misconceptions. *Establishing trust facilitates open sharing of feelings and perceptions.*

Community-based care

People with hyperthyroidism primarily provide self-care at home. Teaching is individualised to meet the person's needs. Address the following topics:

- The person taking oral medications must understand the need for lifelong treatment.
- The person who has a thyroidectomy requires information about postoperative wound care.
- The person having radioactive iodine therapy needs to know the symptoms of hypothyroidism.
- Depending on the age of the person and the support systems available, referral to community healthcare agencies may be necessary. In addition, suggest the following online resources:
  - Australian Thyroid Foundation: https://www.thyroidfoundation.org.au
  - Hormones Australia (Endocrine Society of Australia): https://www.hormones-australia.org.au/endocrine-diseases/hyperthyroidism/
  - Thyroid Federation International: www.thyroid-fed.org.

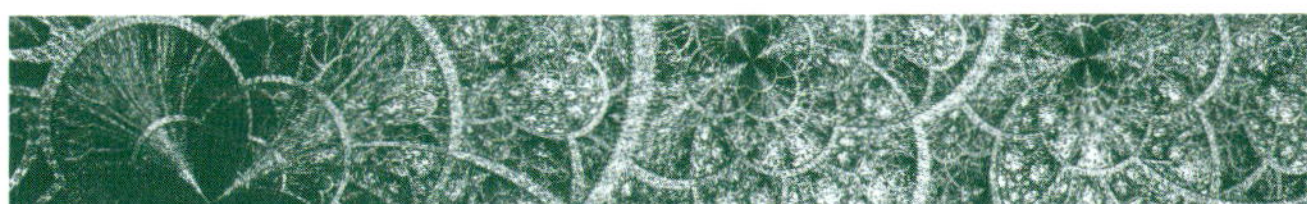

THE PERSON WITH HYPOTHYROIDISM

Hypothyroidism is a disorder that results when the thyroid gland produces an insufficient amount of TH. Because a decrease in TH levels decreases metabolic rate and heat production, hypothyroidism affects all body systems (see 'Multisystem effects of hypothyroidism'). Hypothyroidism is most common in women between ages 30 and 60; the incidence rises with age. It is also associated with an increase in morbidity and mortality due to cardiovascular involvement. Careful evaluation of symptoms is important in the older adult because manifestations of hypothyroidism are often thought to be the result of ageing instead of a pathological process.

Hypothyroidism occurs in about 5% of the adult population; most present with mild thyroid failure, characterised by raised serum TSH but normal free thyroxine or T_4. Worldwide, the most common cause of hypothyroidism is iodine deficiency. However, in Australia, the most common cause of hypothyroidism is autoimmune chronic lymphocytic thyroiditis characterised by raised levels of thyroid peroxidase antibody, also known as Hashimoto's thyroiditis (Hughes & Eastman, 2021).

Severe hypothyroidism is known as **myxoedema**. The term reflects the characteristic accumulation of non-pitting oedema in the connective tissues throughout the body. The face of a person with myxoedema appears puffy, the tongue is enlarged and the voice is hoarse and husky (Siskind et al., 2021). Proteinaceous fluid can also accumulate within body cavities. The most common sites are the pleural, peritoneal and pericardial cavities. This accumulation can result in serious complications such as the development of a pericardial effusion. The incidence of hypothyroid-induced pericardial effusions is estimated to be between 3% and 6% (Abrams et al., 2022).

Pathophysiology and manifestations

Hypothyroidism may be either primary or secondary. Primary hypothyroidism, which is more common, may be caused by congenital defects in the gland, loss of thyroid tissue following treatment for hyperthyroidism with surgery or radiation, antithyroid medications, thyroiditis or endemic iodine deficiency. Secondary hypothyroidism may result from pituitary TSH deficiency or peripheral resistance to thyroid hormones. Hypothyroidism has a slow onset, with manifestations occurring over months or even years. With treatment, the mental and physical symptoms rapidly reverse.

When TH production decreases, the thyroid gland enlarges in a compensatory attempt to produce more hormones. The goitre that results is usually a simple diffuse or non-toxic form. People living in certain areas of the world where the soil is deficient in iodine are more prone to become hypothyroid and develop simple goitre. The geriatric person has a decrease in T_4 production of approximately 30%, but serum levels are usually maintained because of the age-related decrease in T_4 degradation.

The person with hypothyroidism characteristically has manifestations of goitre, fluid retention and oedema, decreased appetite, weight gain, constipation, dry skin, dyspnoea, pallor, hoarseness and muscle stiffness. Many also have a decreased sense of taste and smell, menstrual disorders, anaemia and cardiac enlargement. The pulse is typically bradycardic (Siskind et al., 2021). Deficient amounts of TH cause abnormalities in lipid metabolism, with elevated serum cholesterol and triglyceride levels. As a result, the person is at increased risk of atherosclerosis and cardiac disorders. Decreased renal blood flow and glomerular filtration rate reduce the kidneys' ability to excrete water, which may cause hyponatraemia. Sleep apnoea is more common in people with hypothyroidism. A severe state of hypothyroidism is called *myxoedema coma.*

Iodine deficiency

Iodine deficiency may result from certain goitrogenic drugs (which block TH synthesis); lithium carbonate, used to treat bipolar disorders; and antithyroid drugs. Lack of iodine can cause hypothyroidism and goitre, but this is rare in developed countries. It can also have a devastating effect on the development of the fetus and newborn child. Insufficient iodine and thus TH during gestation and early childhood is known as the iodine deficiency disorder of congenital hypothyroidism, or cretinism.

Prior to 2009, there was an increase in iodine deficiency in Australia. This deficiency was due to changes in milk sterilisation processes, which no longer used iodides, combined with less consumption of iodised salt due to concerns about

Multisystem effects of hypothyroidism

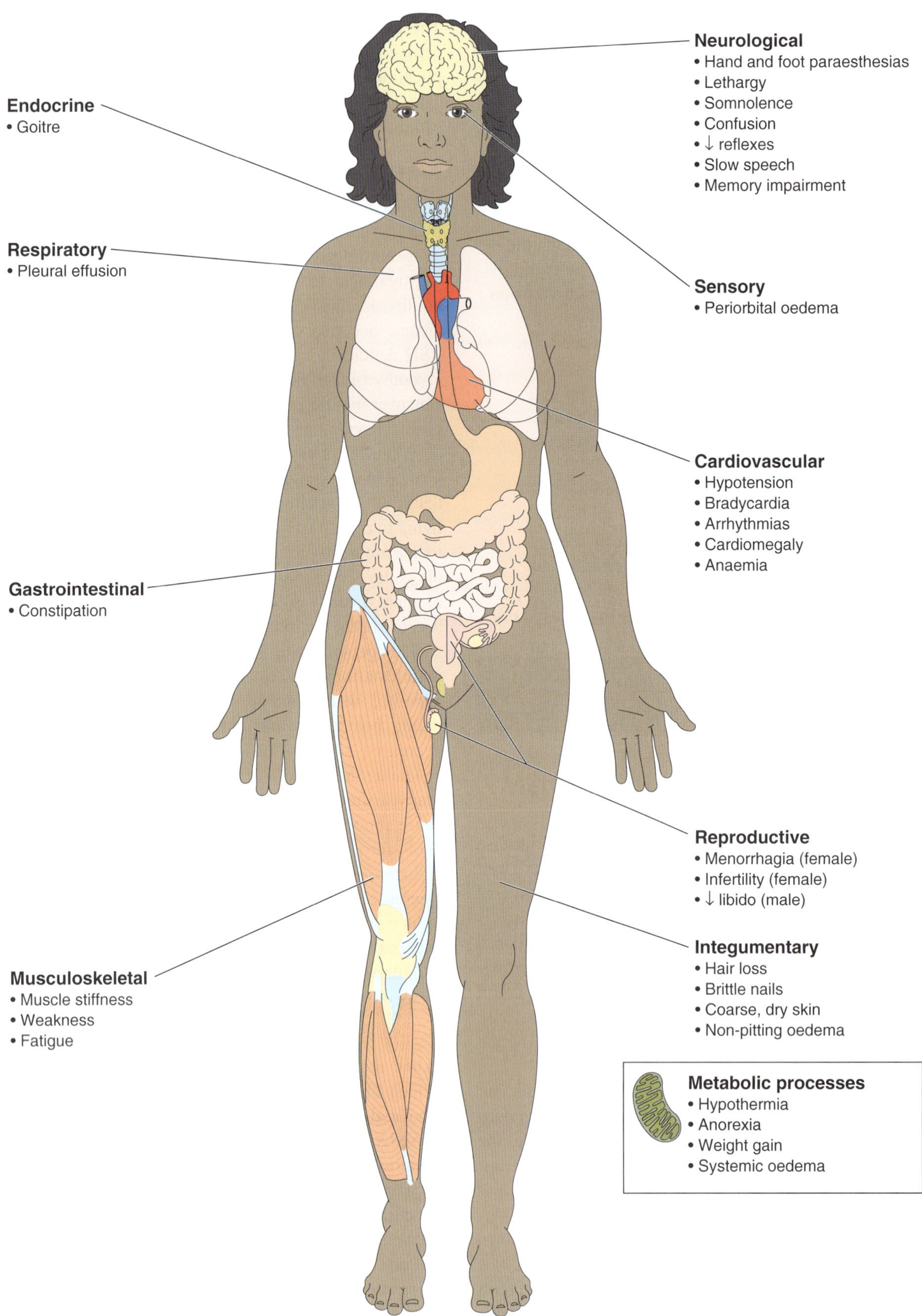

salt intake in general. Iodine deficiency in Australia has been addressed through mandatory fortification of iodised salt in bread. The recommended dietary intake of iodine for adults is 150 micrograms/day. Seafoods such as oysters are particularly rich in iodine. Pregnant and breastfeeding women need to include an oral iodine supplement so that they are consuming 220 micrograms and 270 micrograms respectively in total per day of iodine (Nutrition Australia, 2021).

Hashimoto's thyroiditis

Hashimoto's thyroiditis is the most common cause of goitre and primary hypothyroidism in Australia. In this autoimmune disorder, antibodies develop that destroy thyroid tissue. Functional thyroid tissue is replaced with fibrous tissue and TH levels decrease. In addition, decreasing levels of TH in the early stages of the disorder prompt the gland to enlarge to compensate, causing goitre. However, as the disease progresses, the thyroid gland becomes smaller. This disorder is more common in women and has a familial link.

Myxoedema coma

Myxoedema coma is a life-threatening complication of long-standing, untreated primary hypothyroidism usually triggered by an acute infection, the administration of thyroid-hormone-reducing medications or trauma. Five per cent occur as a result of hypothalamic or pituitary causes. It is characterised by severe metabolic disorders (hyponatraemia, hypoglycaemia and lactic acidosis), hypothermia (usually below 32.2°C), cardiovascular complications (hypotension, bradycardia, cardiac tamponade) and altered mental state such as confusion and coma (due to cerebral oedema, hypoxia and hypercarbia). Seizures may precede coma in 25% of people (Gupta, 2013).

The treatment of myxoedema coma addresses the precipitating factors and manifestations and involves maintaining a patent airway; maintaining fluid, electrolyte and acid–base balance; maintaining cardiovascular status; increasing body temperature; and increasing TH levels with intravenous thyroxine and corticosteroids. Despite aggressive treatment, the mortality rate for myxoedema coma remains up to 60% (Nasrullah et al., 2022).

INTERPROFESSIONAL CARE

The treatment of the person with hypothyroidism focuses on diagnosis, prevention or treatment of complications, and replacement of the deficient TH. With early and continued treatment, both appearance and mental function return to normal.

Diagnosis

Hypothyroidism is diagnosed by the clinical manifestations and by a decrease in TH, especially Free T_4 (see Table 18.2). TSH concentration often is increased because the negative hormonal feedback from TH is lost. The same laboratory and diagnostic tests used to diagnose hyperthyroidism are also used to diagnose hypothyroidism, with opposite results in most cases.

TABLE 18.2 Laboratory findings in hypothyroidism

TEST	NORMAL VALUES	FINDINGS
Serum TA	$\leq$ 1:20 titre	Increased
Serum TSH	0.4–4.0 mIU/L	Increased in primary hypothyroidism Decreased, secondary hypothyroidism
Serum T_4	Total 10–25 pmol/L	Normal to decreased
Serum T_3	Free 4–8 pmol/L	Normal to decreased
T_3 uptake (T_3RU)	25–35 %	Decreased

Source: Adapted from The Royal College of Pathologists of Australasia (RCPA) (2015). *RCPA manual* (7th ed.). Retrieved from https://www.rcpa.edu.au/Manuals/RCPA-Manual. mIU = milli-International units; pmol = picomoles.

Medications

Hypothyroidism is treated with medications that replace TH. Thyroxine is the preferred therapy. Medications commonly used to treat hypothyroidism and their nursing implications are shown in the 'Medication administration' box. In the geriatric person, an age-related decrease in serum albumin and renal excretion can increase the amount of available drug and cause an exaggerated pharmacological effect. Therefore, the older person may require less thyroid medication than a younger person.

Surgery

If the hypothyroid person has goitre large enough to cause respiratory difficulties or dysphagia, a thyroidectomy may be performed (see the 'Nursing care of the person: undergoing a thyroidectomy' box).

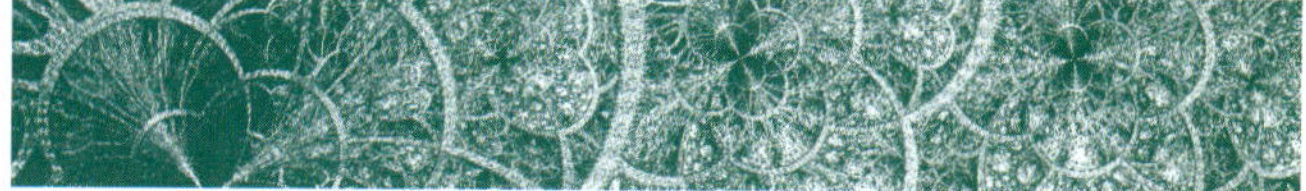

Nursing care

Health promotion

One of the most critical factors in preventing hypothyroidism is education of the public about the necessity of an adequate dietary intake of iodine. The mandatory fortification of bread with iodised salt in 2009 has reduced the prevalence of hypothyroidism in Australia.

Assessment

Collect data through the health history and physical examination (see the chapter 'A person-centred approach to assessing the endocrine system'). Further focused assessments are described with nursing interventions here. When assessing the older person, be aware of normal changes with ageing, outlined in the 'Nursing care of the older adult' box.

- *Health history*: inquire about the presence of any known pituitary disorders; when the person first began to experience symptoms, their characteristics and severity; whether the person has been previously treated for hyperthyroidism; if the person has previously had thyroid

MEDICATION ADMINISTRATION Hypothyroidism

THYROID PREPARATIONS

Thyroxine sodium (Oroxine, Eutroxsig, Eltroxin)

Replacement oral thyroxine is the preferred therapy for hypothyroidism. The dose is individualised according to the person's clinical response and plasma levels. A typical starting dose is 50 to 100 micrograms daily for adults. However, for adults $\geq$ 60 years or those with ischaemic heart disease, a lower dose of 25 to 50 micrograms/day is initiated. As required, the daily dose is gradually increased by 25 to 50 micrograms every 4 weeks, up to a maximum daily dose of 200 micrograms. In people with diabetes, the dose of insulin or hypoglycaemic drugs may need to be increased.

Specific responsibilities include:

- Administer thyroxine first thing in the morning on an empty stomach with water, at least 30 minutes before breakfast and preferably 60 minutes hours before taking other medications. *Absorption is promoted on an empty stomach.*
- Thyroid preparations potentiate the effects of anticoagulants. Monitor for bruising, bleeding gums and blood in the urine when the person is also taking an anticoagulant.
- Thyroid medications may reduce the clinical effects of digoxin.
- Monitor for symptoms of coronary insufficiency: angina, dyspnoea and tachycardia.
- During dose adjustment, assess the person's pulse before administering the drug. Report pulse readings of $>$100 bpm or if there is a noticeable change in the person's pulse rate or rhythm.
- Avoid switching between brands of levothyroxine as Eltroxin is not the bioequivalent on a same dose basis as Eutroxsig and Oroxine.
- Use whole tablets where possible (i.e. a 150 microgram dose should be given as one 100 microgram table and one 50 microgram tablet).

Health education of the person and family

- Opened and unopened packets of Oroxine and Eutroxsig tablets should remain refrigerated and in their original foil packaging until administration. The newer medication, Eltroxin, does not require refrigeration but should be stored below 25°C.
- These medications are lifelong therapy.
- Take thyroid preparation each morning to decrease the possibility of insomnia.
- Report symptoms indicative of excess thyroid hormone levels including weight loss, palpitations, leg cramps, nervousness or insomnia.
- Thyroid preparations increase the risk of iodine toxicity. Avoid using iodised salt or over-the-counter drugs containing iodine.
- If you are also taking an anticoagulant, monitor and report any signs of bleeding.
- Report any changes in menstrual periods.
- Closely monitor your blood pressure and pulse (especially with older adults).
- Avoid excessive intake of raw goitrogenic foods that are known to inhibit TH utilisation, such as kale, turnips, cabbage, carrots, spinach and peaches. Cooking such produce will partially destroys the goitrogenic enzymes.

Liothyronine sodium (Tertraxin)

Liothyronine sodium is a more potent, rapid thyroid replacement. It is used for people with severe and acute hypothyroidism (myxoedema) and in myxoedema coma. For myxoedema treatment, the person is normally started on 10 to 20 micrograms every 8 hours, with the dose increasing gradually until it reaches 60 micrograms daily in divided doses. The adult in a myxoedema coma will receive 60 micrograms via a naso- or oro-gastric tube, followed by 20 micrograms every 8 hours.

Specific responsibilities include:

- Liothyronine should be used cautiously in people with other endocrine disorders including diabetes mellitus. Adrenal deficiency should be corrected prior to administration.
- Treatment of myxoedema coma should occur in a critical care environment. ECG monitoring must be initiated when treating the person in a myxoedema coma with liothyronine.
- Liothyronine is contraindicated in people with a history of cardiovascular problems.
- Liothyronine potentiate the effects of anticoagulants. Monitor for bruising, bleeding gums and blood in the urine if the person is also taking an anticoagulant.

surgery or received radiation therapy for the treatment of head or neck cancer; the person's typical diet; their use of iodised salt; their normal elimination pattern and the presence of any respiratory difficulties.

- *Physical assessment*: focus on the following assessments when conducting a physical assessment on the person: their weight, muscle strength, deep tendon reflexes, vital signs and cardiovascular and peripheral vascular systems. Palpate the thyroid gland.

Nursing diagnoses and interventions

In planning and implementing care for people with hypothyroidism, the nurse needs to take into account that the disorder affects all body systems. Although many nursing diagnoses might be valid, this section focuses on problems related to an individual's cardiovascular function, elimination pattern and skin integrity. See the accompanying 'Nursing care plan'.

Decreased cardiac output related to decreased stroke volume, bradycardia and possible pericardial effusion

A TH deficiency causes a reduction in heart rate and stroke volume, resulting in decreased cardiac output. A history of coronary artery disease or the presence of a pericardial effusion may further compromise cardiac function.

- Monitor the person's blood pressure, heart rate and rhythm, respiratory rate and oxygenation saturation.

TRANSLATION TO PRACTICE

Evidence-based practice: thyroid nodules, benign or malignant? Common causes and a simple approach to diagnosis and management in the clinical setting

Thyroid nodules are common—up to 70% of adults have nodules visible on ultrasound and 5% of these also have palpable nodules. Between 7% and 15% of thyroid nodules are malignant (Wong, Farrell & Grossmann, 2018).

Thyroid nodules are more common in the older person, women, people with iodine deficiency and those who have had prior exposure to radiation. Significant symptoms, if present, may include dysphagia due to impingement of the goitre on the oesophagus, shortness of breath due to tracheal impingement and, less commonly, hoarseness of the voice due to possible laryngeal nerve compression.

Predictive factors that increase the likelihood of nodular malignancy include: an age < 20 or > 70 years, being male, a family history of thyroid cancer, childhood head and neck irradiation, exposure to ionising radiation, a nodule size > 4 cm and/or rapid nodule growth. Pain may not be present.

IMPLICATIONS FOR NURSING

Clinical assessment of the person and recognising abnormal thyroid signs and symptoms is within the scope of nursing. Clinical assessment of the thyroid gland includes *Inspection* for scars, goitre, movement when swallowing, prominent veins; *Palpation* by (i) positioning the person and examining from behind with the neck slightly flexed to relax sternomastoid muscles—feeling each lobe and the isthmus of the gland for characteristics of goitre or nodules and examining cervical lymph nodes, and (ii) in front of the person, examining characteristics of the nodules and position of the trachea, which may be displaced; *Percussion* over the manubrium, dullness may indicate goitre, although CT scan is a more common procedure; *Auscultation* as a bruit may occur in Graves' disease. *Pemberton's sign* is used to evaluate venous obstruction from goitres. Ask the person to raise the arms as high as possible and wait a few moments; signs of venous congestion such as redness of the face and breathlessness occur from retrosternal extension of the thyroid gland into the thorax (Matheus & Kowdley, 2021). Also look for signs of hyper- or hypothyroidism.

CRITICAL THINKING IN PERSON-CENTRED CARE

1 What is the prevalence of malignant thyroid nodules and who has a higher risk of developing them?
2 Most people with thyroid nodules do not have any significant symptoms. But, if present, which symptoms are important to notice and what do they indicate?
3 Which clinical assessments need to be attended when examining the thyroid gland of a person with suspected nodules? Which instructions would be given when assessing for the Pemberton's sign?

NURSING CARE OF THE OLDER ADULT

Variations in assessment findings—hypothyroidism

NORMAL CHANGES WITH AGEING

- The thyroid gland undergoes some degree of atrophy, fibrosis and nodule formation.
- Hair growth decreases.
- Nails are often thick, brittle and yellow.
- Facial skin sags and bones become more prominent.
- Deep tendon reflexes decrease.
- Response to questions may be slower.

Auscultate the person's heart and lungs. *Monopolysaccharide deposits in the pericardial sac may cause pericardial effusion, resulting in dysrhythmias and a decreased intensity of heart sounds. Monopolysaccharide deposits in the pleura space can result in pleural effusions. Dyspnoea or increased work of breathing may be present (McCance & Huether, 2019).*

- Administer supplemental oxygen as ordered. *Reduced cardiac output results in less oxygen being made available to the tissues.*
- Avoid cool temperatures, increase room temperature if necessary, use additional bed covers and avoid draughts. *Chilling increases metabolic rate and puts increased stress on the heart.*
- Explain the need to alternate activity with rest periods. Ask the person to report any breathing difficulties, angina, heart palpitations or dizziness. *Activity increases demands on the heart and should be balanced with rest. Symptoms of cardiac stress include dyspnoea, angina, palpitations and dizziness.*

Constipation

The hypothyroid person is likely to have a reduced appetite and decreased food intake, a diminished activity level because of muscle aches and weakness, reduced water absorption and reduced peristalsis to the point that faecal impaction may occur.

- Encourage an increased fluid intake. If kilojoule intake is restricted, ensure that liquids have no or low kilojoules. *Sufficient fluid intake assists stool consistency.*
- Discuss ways to maintain a high-fibre diet. *Diets high in fibre and fluid produce soft stools. Fibre that is not digested absorbs water, which adds bulk to the stool and assists in the movement of faecal material through the intestines.*
- Encourage activity as tolerated. *Activity influences bowel elimination by improving muscle tone and stimulating peristalsis.*

Risk of impaired skin integrity related to oedema, dry and rough skin

The person with hypothyroidism is at risk of impaired skin integrity related to the accumulation of fluid in the interstitial spaces and to dry, rough skin. Decreased peripheral circulation,

NURSING CARE PLAN A person with hypothyroidism

Jane Lee is a 60-year-old retired teacher living with her husband and daughter on a farm that has been in her Chinese family for four generations. Mrs Lee has gained 4.5 kg in the past few months, even though she is rarely hungry and eats much less than normal. She is always tired and weak—so tired that she has not even been able to help with the chores on the farm or do housework. She is concerned about her appearance and the way she sounds when she talks. Her face is puffy and her tongue always feels thick. Mr Lee convinces his wife to make an appointment at a health centre in a nearby town.

ASSESSMENT

Nurse Practitioner (NP) Brian Henning completes the health assessment for Mrs Lee at the health centre. He finds that she now weighs 68 kg, a 4.5 kg weight increase since her last visit 6 months earlier. Mrs Lee states that she always feels cold, tired and weak. She also states that she is constipated, has difficulty remembering things and looks different. Physical assessment findings include a palpable and bilaterally enlarged thyroid; dry, yellowish skin; non-pitting oedema of the face and lower legs; and slow, slurred speech. Diagnostic tests revealed the following abnormal findings: Free T_3, 1 pmol/L (normal range: 4–8 pmol/L); Total T_4, 8 pmol/L (normal range: 10–25 pmol/L); TSH increased. The medical diagnosis of hypothyroidism is made and Mrs Lee is started on levothyroxine 0.05 mg daily.

DIAGNOSES

- *Constipation* related to decreased peristalsis, as evidenced by hard, formed stools every 4 days.
- *Impaired verbal communication* related to changes in speech patterns and enlarged tongue.
- *Low self-esteem* related to changes in physical appearance and activity intolerance.

PLANNING

- Teach Mrs Lee to increase her fluids, bulk and fibre in the diet to help regain a normal bowel elimination pattern of a soft, formed stool every other day.
- Encourage Mrs Lee to take medication as prescribed and do not expect immediate reversal of symptoms affecting speech. It may take some time but need to continue with the treatment. Educate Mrs Lee to store the medication as per the manufacturer's recommendations.
- Educate Mrs Lee to plan her daily activities around regular rest periods. Encourage her husband and daughter to help with house cleaning and cooking.

Expected outcomes

- Regain normal bowel elimination patterns, having a soft, formed stool at least every other day.
- Experience improvement in verbal communication.
- Regain positive self-esteem as medication reduces physical changes and fatigue.

IMPLEMENTATION

- Mrs Lee will start consuming a diet with bulk and fibre as well as increase her fluid intake immediately.
- She will start and continue to take the prescribed medications and understand that it may take some time for the symptoms to improve.
- Mrs Lee will be resting and taking naps when required.
- She will seek appropriate advice from a healthcare practitioner if there are any issues or concerns.

EVALUATION

On return to the health centre 2 months later, Mrs Lee reports that she is no longer constipated and that she has increased her fluid intake and eats porridge every day. She no longer feels cold, is regaining her normal energy, and even feels well enough to plant her garden. Her speech is clear and easy to understand. As she leaves the examining room, Mrs Lee says: 'It's hard to believe that I have changed so much—now I look and feel like the "old" me!'

CRITICAL THINKING IN THE NURSING PROCESS

1. Which physical changes that normally occur with ageing are similar to the manifestations of hypothyroidism?
2. The person taking oral thyroid medications may become hyperthyroid. List the manifestations you would include in a teaching plan to signal this condition.

REFLECTION ON THE NURSING PROCESS

1. Which points have you learned from the case study that you will implement in your future nursing practice?
2. How will you plan an appropriate diet for Mrs Lee, taking into consideration her Chinese background as well as her likes and dislikes? Reflect on other people with different ethnic backgrounds in Australia.

decreased activity levels and slow wound healing further increase the risk. These interventions are outlined for the older person who is hospitalised for surgery or severe hypothyroidism.

- Monitor skin surfaces for redness or lesions, especially if the person's activity is greatly reduced. Use a pressure injury risk assessment scale (e.g. the Waterlow Pressure Ulcer Risk Assessment tool) to identify people at risk. *Hypothyroidism causes dry, rough, oedematous skin conditions that increase the risk of skin breakdown.*
- Provide or teach the immobile person measures to promote optimal circulation:
  - Implement a turning schedule if the person is on bed rest or teach the person to change their position every 2 hours.
  - Limit the person's time for sitting in one position; encourage them to shift their weight every 20 to 30 minutes.
  - Use pillows, pads or sheepskin or foam cushions for bed and/or chair.
- Teach and implement a schedule of range-of-motion exercises. *Prolonged pressure, especially in people with oedema and circulatory impairment, can occlude capillaries and cause hypoxic tissue damage.*
- Provide or teach the person measures to maintain skin integrity:
  - Take baths only as necessary; use warm (not hot) water.
  - Use gentle motions when washing and drying skin.
  - Use alcohol-free skin oils and lotions.

Dry skin and oedema increase the risk of skin breakdown. Hot water, rough massage and alcohol-based preparations may increase skin dryness, further impairing the body's ability to maintain skin integrity.

Community-based care

People with hypothyroidism require lifelong care, primarily at home. Address the following topics:

- the need to take medications for the rest of their life
- the correct storage of medications
- the need for regular periodic dosage reassessments (e.g. every 6 months)
- if the person is older or does not have a support system, advise about helpful community resources.

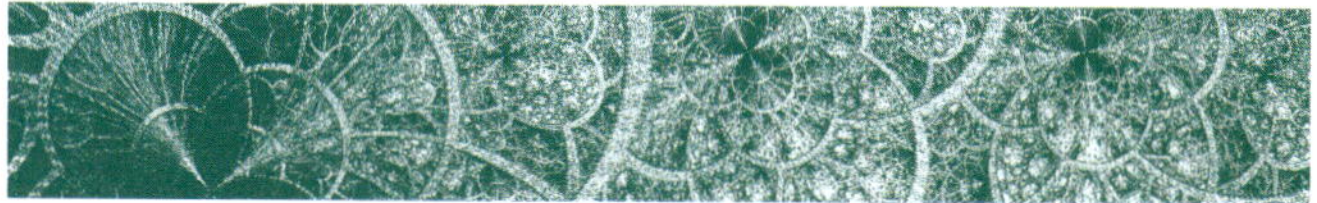

THE PERSON WITH CANCER OF THE THYROID

Thyroid cancer is the ninth most diagnosed cancer in Australia. The incidence of thyroid cancer has increased in Australia over the past two decades with approximately 3,830 new cases diagnosed in 2021 (Cancer Australia, 2022).

Risk factors associated with thyroid cancer include age, usually affecting people over the age of 35; gender, females having approximately three times the incidence of thyroid cancer than males; diet, either chronic iodine deficiency or chronically high iodine intake; history of thyroid disease; ionising radiation exposure; and family history and ethnicity, with a higher incidence in first-degree relatives. Obesity and smoking are also associated with increased risk (Lim et al., 2017).

There are several types of thyroid cancer:

- Papillary thyroid cancer (PTC) is the most common thyroid malignancy, accounting for approximately 85% of all cases (Wong et al., 2018). The cancer develops from the follicular cells in the thyroid. PTC is the least aggressive type, but can metastasise to the cervical lymph nodes and, less commonly, the lungs. The mortality rate of PTC is usually higher in the elderly.
- Follicular thyroid carcinoma (FTC) is the second most common thyroid malignancy and also arises with from the thyroid's follicular cells. FTC accounts for 12% of all thyroid cancer cases (Wong et al., 2018). FTC is more aggressive than PTC and has the potential for vascular invasion. It may also spread to the lungs and bone (Nguyen et al., 2015).
- Medullary thyroid cancer accounts for 2% of all thyroid cancers and originates from the parathyroid neuroendocrine cells of the thyroid. The person with a medullary thyroid cancer typically has a single mass and is in middle adulthood. This type of thyroid cancer can be linked to a genetic predisposition in about one-third of cases (Cabanillas et al., 2016).
- Anaplastic thyroid cancer accounts for 1% of all thyroid cancers and is most common in older adults. Most people with an anaplastic thyroid cancer will present with a rapidly growing, firm mass in their thyroid that is readily palpable.

The diagnosis is made by measuring thyroid hormones, performing thyroid scans and fine-needle biopsy. The usual treatment is subtotal or total thyroidectomy. TSH suppression therapy with levothyroxine may be conducted prior to surgery. Radioactive iodine therapy (^{131}I) and chemotherapy are additional therapeutic options. The 5-year survival rate, if the tumour has not metastasised, is 96.1% (Wong et al., 2018). Nursing care for the person with cancer is discussed in the chapter 'Nursing care of people with cancer'.

Disorders of the parathyroid glands

Disorders of the parathyroid glands—hyperparathyroidism and hypoparathyroidism—are not as common as those of the thyroid gland. Hypercalcaemia and hypocalcaemia (the primary results of alterations in parathyroid function) are discussed in the chapter 'Nursing care of people with altered fluid, electrolyte and acid–base balance'.

THE PERSON WITH HYPERPARATHYROIDISM

Hyperparathyroidism results from an increase in the secretion of parathyroid hormone (PTH), which regulates normal serum levels of calcium and phosphate. The four parathyroid glands that secrete PTH are located on the thyroid gland. The two upper parathyroid glands are located on the posterior aspect of the upper thyroid lobes and the two lower parathyroid glands are located in the lower thyroid lobes. Two per cent of people have parathyroid glands situated within the thyroid gland (Sung, 2015).

Pathophysiology and manifestations

Hyperparathyroidism occurs more often in older adults and is three times more common in women. The disorder itself is not common. The three types of hyperparathyroidism are as follows:

1. Primary hyperparathyroidism occurs when there is hyperplasia or an adenoma in one or more of the parathyroid glands, resulting in the unregulated overproduction of parathyroid hormone. The coexistence of thyroid nodules and primary hyperparathyroidism has been reported to range between 12% and 52% (Cinamon, Levy & Marom, 2015). This disorder interrupts the normal regulatory mechanism between serum calcium

levels and PTH secretion and increases the absorption of calcium through the gastrointestinal tract.

2. Secondary hyperparathyroidism is a compensatory response by the parathyroid glands to chronic hyperphosphataemia and hypocalcaemia. It is characterised by an increased secretion of PTH. Secondary hyperparathyroidism is found in people with early chronic kidney disease and vitamin D deficiency.
3. Tertiary hyperparathyroidism results from hyperplasia of the parathyroid glands and a loss of response to serum calcium levels. This disorder is most often seen in people with long-standing chronic kidney disease. Due to routine blood analysis of calcium, many people with hyperparathyroidism are identified prior to the development of symptoms. When symptoms occur, they are related to hypercalcaemia and various musculoskeletal, renal and gastrointestinal manifestations. Bone resorption results in pathological fractures, while elevated calcium levels alter neural and muscular activity, leading to muscle weakness and atrophy. Proximal renal tubule function is altered and metabolic acidosis, renal calculi formation and polyuria occur.

Manifestations of the effect of hypercalcaemia on the gastrointestinal tract include abdominal pain, constipation, anorexia and peptic ulcer formation. Hypercalcaemia also affects the cardiovascular system, causing dysrhythmias, hypertension and increased sensitivity to cardiotonic glycosides (e.g. digoxin). The manifestations of hyperparathyroidism are summarised in the 'Manifestations' box.

MANIFESTATIONS Hyperparathyroidism

MUSCULOSKELETAL SYSTEM
- Bone pain (back, joints and shins)
- Pathological fractures
- Muscle weakness
- Muscle atrophy

RENAL EFFECTS
- Renal calculi
- Polyuria
- Polydipsia

GASTROINTESTINAL SYSTEM
- Abdominal pain
- Peptic ulcers
- Pancreatitis
- Insulin resistance
- Nausea
- Constipation

CARDIOVASCULAR SYSTEM
- Dysrhythmias
- Hypertension
- Deposition of calcium and phosphate in arterial walls

CENTRAL NERVOUS SYSTEM
- Paraesthesia
- Depression
- Confusion
- Psychosis

METABOLIC EFFECTS
- Acidosis
- Weight loss
- Fatigue

INTERPROFESSIONAL CARE

Hyperparathyroidism is diagnosed by excluding all other possible causes of hypercalcaemia; by at least a 6-month history of symptoms; and by laboratory analysis of serum calcium and PTH levels. A parathyroid sestamibi (MIBI) nuclear medicine scan is also useful for determining hyperparathyroidism. Intravenous MIBI is administered prior to the scan. It will accumulate in an overactive gland but will not accumulate in healthy parathyroid glands. Bone mineral density is used to determine the extent, if any, of bone resorption.

Treatment of hyperparathyroidism focuses on decreasing the elevated serum calcium levels. People with mild hypercalcaemia are urged to drink fluids and keep active to prevent dehydration and reduce the risk of kidney stones. They should avoid prolonged immobilisation, thiazide diuretics, large doses of vitamins A and D, antacids containing calcium and calcium supplements. Gastrointestinal illness with vomiting and diarrhoea can cause serum calcium levels to rise. Severe hypercalcaemia requires hospitalisation and intensive treatment with intravenous saline. Medications to inhibit bone resorption and reduce hypercalcaemia or calcimimetic medications are the mainstay of secondary hyperparathyroidism. Calcitonin, a hormone produced by the thyroid gland, helps regulate calcium levels in the body by inhibiting bone resorption and increasing calcium excretion by the kidney. Bisphosphonates such as alendronate can be considered for those with symptomatic primary hyperparathyroidism who are unable to undergo surgery. Laser thermal ablation or radiofrequency ablation are other alternative therapies (Sung, 2015).

Surgical removal of the parathyroid glands affected by hyperplasia or adenoma treats all forms of hyperparathyroidism. The preoperative and postoperative nursing care is essentially the same as that for the person having a thyroidectomy. In some cases autotransplantation of one parathyroid to the forearm may assist in controlling postoperative calcium homeostasis.

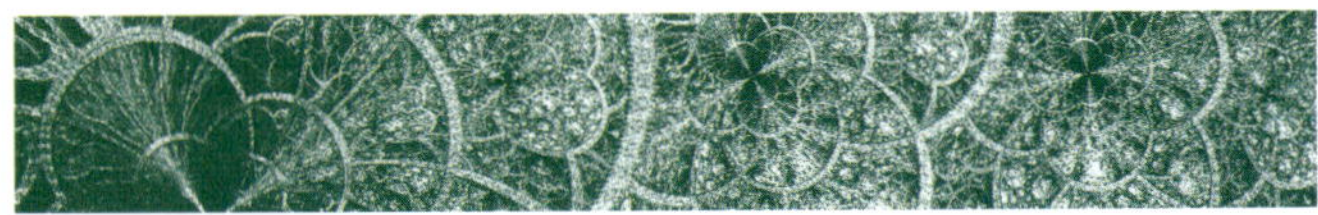

Nursing care

Nursing care of the person with hypercalcaemia is discussed in the chapter 'Nursing care of people with altered fluid, electrolyte and acid–base balance'.

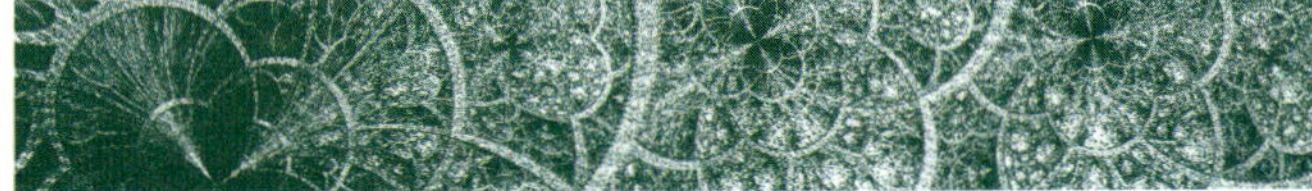

THE PERSON WITH HYPOPARATHYROIDISM

Hypoparathyroidism results from abnormally low PTH levels. The most common cause is inadvertent damage to or removal of the parathyroid glands during thyroidectomy.

Pathophysiology and manifestations

Due to reduced PTH, the ability to resorb calcium from the bone, and to regulate calcium reabsorption from the renal tubules, is impaired. Reabsorption of phosphate is increased in the renal tubules, causing hyperphosphataemia. The low calcium levels cause changes in neuromuscular activity, affecting peripheral motor and sensory nerves.

The neuromuscular manifestations that result from hypocalcaemia include numbness and tingling around the mouth and in the fingertips, muscle spasms of the hands and feet, convulsions and laryngeal spasms. Tetany, a continuous spasm of muscles, is the primary symptom of hypocalcaemia. In severe cases of tetany, death may occur. Assessments for tetany include Trousseau's sign (see the chapters 'Nursing care of people with altered fluid, electrolyte and acid–base balance' and 'A person-centred approach to assessing the endocrine system'). The manifestations of hypoparathyroidism are summarised in the 'Manifestations' box.

MANIFESTATIONS Hypoparathyroidism

MUSCULOSKELETAL SYSTEM
- Muscle spasms
- Facial grimacing
- Carpopedal spasms
- Tetany or convulsions

INTEGUMENTARY SYSTEM
- Brittle nails
- Hair loss
- Dry, scaly skin

GASTROINTESTINAL SYSTEM
- Abdominal cramps
- Malabsorption

CARDIOVASCULAR SYSTEM
- Dysrhythmias

CENTRAL NERVOUS SYSTEM
- Paraesthesia (affecting the lips, hands and feet)
- Mood disorders (irritability, depression, anxiety)
- Hyperactive reflexes
- Psychosis
- Increased intracranial pressure

INTERPROFESSIONAL CARE

Hypoparathyroidism is diagnosed by low serum calcium levels and high phosphorous levels in the absence of renal failure, an absorption disorder or a nutritional disorder.

Treatment of hypoparathyroidism focuses on increasing calcium levels. Intravenous calcium gluconate is given immediately to reduce tetany. Long-term therapy includes supplemental calcium, increased dietary calcium and vitamin D therapy.

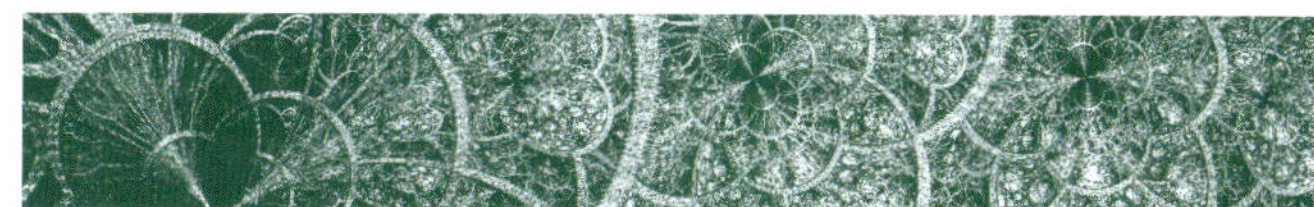

Nursing care

Nursing care for the person with hypocalcaemia is discussed in the chapter 'Nursing care of people with altered fluid, electrolyte and acid–base balance'.

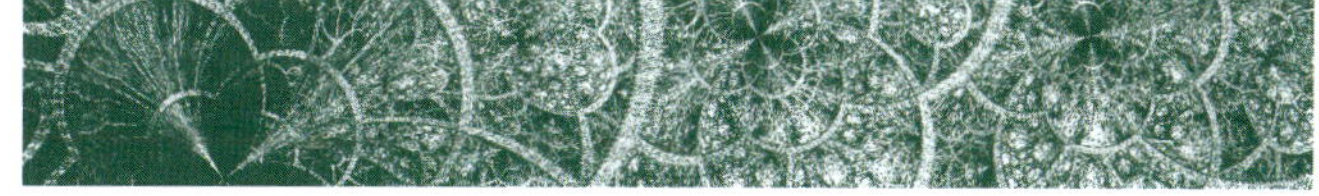

Disorders of the adrenal glands

Disorders of the adrenal cortex or adrenal medulla result in changes in the production of adrenocorticotropic hormone (ACTH). Hormones of the adrenal cortex are essential to life and maintain homeostasis in response to stressors. Disorders of the adrenal cortex result in complex physical, psychological and metabolic alterations. The disorders that occur are hyperfunction and hypofunction of the adrenal cortex or adrenal medulla.

THE PERSON WITH HYPERCORTISOLISM (CUSHING'S SYNDROME)

Cushing's syndrome is a chronic pathological disorder in which hyperfunction of the adrenal cortex produces symptoms associated with excessive amounts of circulating cortisol or ACTH (see Figure 18.3). Cushing's syndrome is more common in women, with the average age of onset between 30 and

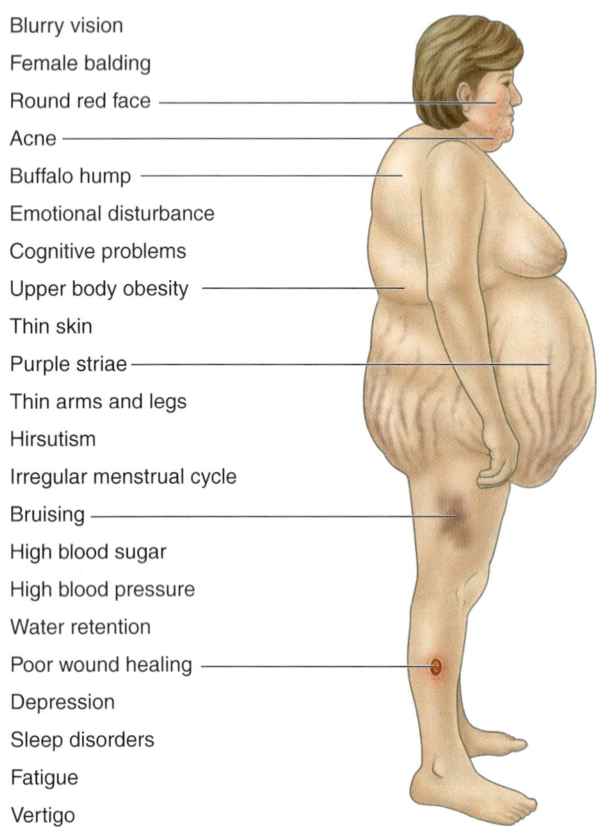

FIGURE 18.3 ***Characteristic features of a person with Cushing's syndrome***

50 years. However, the disorder may occur at any age, especially as the result of pharmacological therapy. People who take steroids (such as prednisone) for long periods of time are at increased risk of developing the disorder.

Pathophysiology

The most common aetiologies of Cushing's syndrome are as follows:

- The pituitary form, with ACTH hypersecretion by a tumour of the pituitary (called **Cushing's disease**). The pituitary adenoma results in a persistent but disorderly and random overproduction of ACTH (Lau, Rutledge & Aghi, 2015).
- The ectopic form, caused by ACTH-secreting tumours (usually of the lung or pancreas).
- The adrenal form, resulting from excessive cortisol secretion by a benign or malignant adrenal tumour. The excess secretion suppresses pituitary ACTH production, resulting in atrophy of the uninvolved adrenal cortex.
- Iatrogenic Cushing's syndrome, resulting from long-term therapy with potent pharmacological glucocorticoid preparations (steroids).

Manifestations

Excess cortisol results in a redistribution of body fat deposits in the abdominal region (central obesity), fat pads under the clavicle, a 'buffalo hump' over the upper back and a round 'moon face'. Changes in protein metabolism cause peripheral muscle weakness and wasting. Glucocorticoid excess inhibits fibroblasts, resulting in loss of collagen and connective tissue. Thinning of the skin, abdominal striae (reddish purple 'stretch marks'), easy bruising, poor wound healing and frequent skin infections result. Glucose metabolism is altered and type 2 diabetes mellitus may occur. Changes in calcium absorption result in osteoporosis, compression fractures of the vertebrae, fractures of the ribs and renal calculi. Hypokalaemia and hypertension occur as potassium is lost and sodium is retained. Inhibited immune responses increase the risk of infection and increased gastric acid secretion increases the risk of peptic ulcers. Emotional changes range from depression to overt psychosis. In women, increasing androgen levels cause hirsutism (excessive facial hair in particular), acne, menstrual irregularities and infertility. Men could suffer impotence (Lau et al., 2015). The manifestations and effects of Cushing's syndrome are grouped by body system in the 'Manifestations' box.

If the person undergoes a bilateral adrenalectomy as a treatment for Cushing's syndrome, an acute deficit of cortisol (Addisonian crisis) may result.

INTERPROFESSIONAL CARE

The treatment of Cushing's syndrome includes medications, radiation therapy or surgery, depending on the aetiological origin of the disorder.

Diagnostic tests

Cushing's syndrome is diagnosed through a variety of diagnostic tests. Findings are shown in Table 18.3 and summarised here:

- *Plasma cortisol levels* are measured. If Cushing's disease is present, test results show a loss of the normal diurnal variations of higher levels in the morning and lower levels in the afternoon.
- *Plasma ACTH levels* are measured to determine the aetiology of the syndrome. Normally, plasma ACTH levels are highest from 7 am to 10 am and lowest from 7 pm to 10 pm. In secondary Cushing's syndrome, ACTH is elevated; in primary Cushing's syndrome, ACTH is decreased.
- *24-hour urine tests* are conducted to measure free cortisol and androgens; these hormones are increased in Cushing's syndrome. Because synthesis and circulation of adrenal hormones are diurnal and episodic, 24-hour urine collections more correctly reflect total hormone than serum levels drawn intermittently.
- *Serum potassium, calcium and glucose levels* are measured to identify electrolyte imbalances.
- An ACTH suppression test may be conducted to identify the cause of the disorder. A synthetic cortisol (dexamethasone) is given to suppress the production of ACTH and plasma cortisol levels are measured. If an

MANIFESTATIONS Cushing's syndrome

MUSCULOSKELETAL SYSTEM
- Weakness
- Osteoporosis
- Peripheral muscle weakness and wasting

INTEGUMENTARY SYSTEM
- Thin, easily bruised skin ('tissue paper' skin)
- Skin infections
- Poor wound healing
- Ecchymosis
- Purple striae (around thighs, breasts, abdomen)
- Hirsutism

CENTRAL NERVOUS SYSTEM
- Emotional lability
- Psychoses

GASTROINTESTINAL SYSTEM
- Peptic ulcers

CARDIOVASCULAR SYSTEM
- Hypertension

RENAL EFFECTS
- Renal calculi
- Polyuria
- Polydipsia
- Glycosuria

METABOLIC EFFECTS
- Hypokalaemia
- Hypernatraemia
- Type 2 diabetes mellitus
- Truncal obesity
- 'Buffalo hump'

REPRODUCTIVE SYSTEM
- Oligomenorrhoea or amenorrhoea
- Impotence
- Decreased libido

extremely high dose of cortisol is necessary to suppress ACTH, the primary disorder is adrenal cortex hyperplasia. If there is an abnormal release of cortisol after a low-dose suppression test, an adrenal tumour that produces cortisol, a body tumour or a pituitary tumour that produces ACTH is suspected.

Medications

Cushing's syndrome that results from a pituitary tumour is treated by medications as an adjunct to surgery or radiation. Medical therapies are classified according to their site of action: at the pituitary gland by inhibiting ACTH secretion, at the adrenal gland by inhibiting steroidogenesis or at the target tissue by blocking the glucocorticoid receptor. Examples of some commonly prescribed drugs follow:

- Cabergoline, used to suppress lactation or Parkinson's disease, is a potent, long-acting dopamine-2 (D2) receptor agonist. Identification of D2 receptors in corticotroph tumours has led to clinical trials of cabergoline in Cushing's disease.
- Metyrapone directly suppresses activity of the adrenal cortex and decreases peripheral metabolism of corticosteroids by inhibition of steroidogenesis enzyme 11β-hydroxylase.
- There is growing literature that shows ketoconazole, a well-known antifungal, may be a useful treatment for adults and adolescents with endogenous Cushing's syndrome. Ketoconazole inhibits cortisol synthesis by the adrenal cortex, resulting in reduced production of adrenal steroids (Shirley, 2021).
- Pasireotide diaspartate is an analogue of somatostatin and is used to inhibit ACTH in people with pituitary tumours where surgery is not an option or where surgery has not been curative.

Surgery

When Cushing's syndrome is caused by an adrenal cortex tumour, an adrenalectomy may be performed to remove the tumour. Only one adrenal gland is usually involved; however, if an ACTH-producing ectopic tumour is involved, a bilateral adrenalectomy is performed. Lifelong hormone replacement is necessary if both adrenal glands are removed. Nursing care of the person having an adrenalectomy is discussed in the accompanying box.

Surgical removal of the pituitary gland (hypophysectomy) is indicated when Cushing's disease is the result of a pituitary tumour. Most tumours can be excised via the transsphenoidal route. However, a craniotomy is sometimes necessary. Immediate cure rates for neurosurgical resection are between 65% and 90% (Lau et al., 2015). Postoperatively, the person will normally receive desmopressin (DDAVP) to minimise the risk of developing and/or to treat diabetes insipidus. They may also be prescribed other hormone replacement therapy medications including cortisone acetate, thyroxine and testosterone. Nursing care for the person having cranial surgery is discussed in the chapter 'A person-centred approach to assessing the endocrine system'.

TABLE 18.3 Laboratory findings in Cushing's syndrome

	TEST	NORMAL VALUES	FINDINGS
Serum	Cortisol	Morning peak: 200-650 nmol/L Trough level (at 2000 hours): ≤ 50% of morning peak levels	Increased
	Urea	3.0-8.0 mmol/L	Normal
	Sodium	135-145 mmol/L	Increased
	Potassium	3.5-5.2 mmol/L	Increased
	Glucose (serum)	3.0-7.7 mmol/L	Increased

Source: Adapted from The Royal College of Pathologists of Australasia (RCPA) (2015). *RCPA manual* (7th ed.). Retrieved from https://www.rcpa.edu.au/Manuals/RCPA-Manual.

NURSING CARE OF THE PERSON **having a laparoscopic adrenalectomy**

PREOPERATIVE CARE

- Consider if the person requires a dietitian referral to assist them to maintain a high-protein, vitamin-rich diet. If hypokalaemia exists, encourage the person to consume foods high in potassium such as bananas or mangoes. *Glucocorticoid excess increases catabolism. Vitamins and proteins are necessary for tissue repair and wound healing following surgery.*
- Employ the principles of aseptic non-touch technique when providing care and procedures. *Cortisol excess increases the risk of infection.*
- Monitor electrolyte and glucose levels. *Electrolyte and glucose imbalances must be corrected prior to surgery.*
- Teach the person to turn, cough and perform deep-breathing exercises. *Although they are important for all surgical people, these activities are even more important for the person who is at risk of infection. Having the person practise and demonstrate the activities increases postoperative compliance.*

POSTOPERATIVE CARE

- Perform and document the person's vital signs, measure intake and output, and monitor electrolytes regularly, especially potassium during the first 48 hours after surgery. *Removal of an adrenal gland, especially a bilateral adrenalectomy, results in adrenal insufficiency. Addisonian crisis and hypovolaemic shock may occur. Cortisol is often given on the day of surgery and in the postoperative period to replace inadequate hormone levels. Intravenous fluids are also administered.*
- Assess the person's body temperature, white cell count levels and wound drainage. Change the person's dressings using aseptic non-touch technique. *Impaired wound healing increases the risk of infection in people with adrenal disorders. Using aseptic technique decreases this risk.*
- Regularly perform pain assessments and administer analgesia as ordered. *Adequate analgesia assists the person to undertake postoperative exercises including early ambulation. Such proactive measures can reduce the person's risk of complications.*

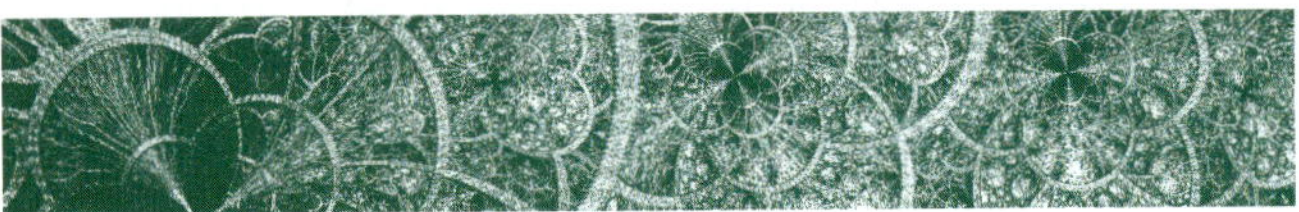

Nursing care

Health promotion

Stress the risk of developing Cushing's syndrome for people taking long-term steroids. The risk of adrenal crisis resulting from the abrupt discontinuation of steroid medications is an essential component of teaching. For a review of glucocorticoid administration, see the chapter 'Nursing care of people with infections'.

Assessment

Collect the following data through the health history and physical examination (see the chapter 'A person-centred approach to assessing the endocrine system'). Further focused assessments are described with nursing interventions here.

- *Health history*: inquire about the presence of any history of pituitary, adrenal, pancreatic or pulmonary tumour; frequent infections; gastrointestinal bleeding; stress fractures; pain, changes in weight distribution; change in height; fatigue; weakness; change in appearance; bruising; skin infections; menstrual history; sexual function.
- *Physical assessment*: the following focused assessments are recommended: vital signs, behaviour, appearance, fat distribution, face, skin, hair quantity and distribution, muscle size and strength, gait.

Nursing diagnoses and interventions

The nurse caring for the person with Cushing's syndrome must take a holistic approach to plan and implement interventions for a wide variety of responses, including problems related to fluid and electrolyte balance, injury, infection and body image. For additional information about people with alterations in fluid and electrolyte balance, see the chapter 'Nursing care of people with altered fluid, electrolyte and acid–base balance'. See the 'Nursing care plan'.

Fluid volume excess

The excess cortisol secretion associated with Cushing's syndrome results in sodium and water reabsorption, causing fluid volume excess. The person will have weight gain, oedema and hypertension.

- Ask the person to weigh themself at the same time each day and maintain a record of results. Body weight is an accurate indicator of fluid status. *One litre of fluid retention corresponds to about 1 kg of body weight.*
- Monitor blood pressure, rate and rhythm of pulse, respiratory rate and lung sounds. Assess for peripheral oedema and jugular vein distension. *Extracellular fluid volume excess resulting from sodium and water retention is manifested by hypertension and a bounding, rapid pulse. There may also be crackles and wheezes on lung auscultation, dependent oedema and venous distension.*
- Teach the person and family the reasons for the importance of limiting fluids as ordered. *Restricting fluid can help decrease the risk of fluid volume excess. Involving the person and family in the plan of care and teaching the rationale for interventions helps to achieve goals and minimise anxiety.*

Risk of injury related to decreased bone density

The person with Cushing's syndrome is at risk of injury from several causes. Excess cortisol causes increased absorption of calcium and demineralisation of bones, resulting in an increased risk of pathological fractures, particularly in the vertebra and ribs (Apaydin & Yavuz, 2021). Muscle weakness and fatigue are common, increasing the potential for falls.

- Teach the person and family to maintain a safe environment:
  - Keep unnecessary clutter and equipment out of the way and off the floor.
  - Ensure adequate lighting, especially at night.
  - Encourage the use of assistive devices for ambulation or to ask for help if needed.
  - If the person wears corrective lenses, be sure they are available and clean.
  - Encourage the use of non-slip slippers or shoes.
  - Monitor for signs of fatigue (e.g. increased work of breathing and pulse); encourage frequent rest periods.

A well-lit environment free of clutter decreases the risk of falls and injury. Sensory and motor deficits increase the risk of falls; corrective lenses, assistive devices and non-slip footwear can decrease this risk. Rest reduces the person's fatigue levels. To reduce energy expenditure, include alternating periods of rest and activity in daily schedules.

NURSING CARE PLAN A person with Cushing's syndrome

Lily Domico is a 30-year-old solicitor living in a major metropolitan area. Lily is single and shares her life with her black cat, Trevor. Her parents live in the same city. Lily has recently been diagnosed with Cushing's syndrome and is admitted for surgery for an adrenalectomy. Lily has been having increased muscle weakness, so much so that she has difficulty climbing the one set of stairs to her apartment. She has also had difficulty sleeping, irregular menstrual periods and hypertension.

ASSESSMENT

When Lily arrives at the hospital the morning of surgery, she is admitted by Registered Nurse Harley Sprengel. While performing Lily's physical assessment, Harley observes Lily has thin lower extremities, an enlarged abdomen, purple striae over the abdomen and buttocks, a round face and obvious facial hair. Lily's blood pressure is 160/96 mmHg. She tells Ann that she is always tired and that sometimes it 'just wears me out to walk from the bedroom to the kitchen'. Diagnostic tests conducted prior to admission reveal the following abnormal findings (all except cortisol levels are corrected before surgery):

Glucose: 16 mmol/L (normal range: 3.0–7.7 mmol/L)
Sodium: 152 mmol/L (normal range: 135–145 mmol/L)
Potassium: 3.2 mmol/L (normal range: 3.5–5.2 mmol/L)
Calcium: 2.10 mmol/L (normal range: 2.10–2.60 mmol/L)
Cortisol: 1,150 nmol/L (normal for am: 200–650 nmol/L)

DIAGNOSES

- *Fluid volume excess* related to sodium retention causing oedema and hypertension.
- *Risk of injury* related to generalised fatigue and weakness.
- *Risk of infection* related to impaired immune response and oedema.
- *Disturbed body image* related to physical changes secondary to Cushing's syndrome.

PLANNING

- Organise pre- and post-surgery education for Lily involving a specialist nurse, dietitian and other relevant allied health professionals.
- Develop a plan of pre-op care and recovery post surgery.
- Discuss the importance of monitoring and informing staff about intake and output of fluids as well as maintaining a record.
- Discuss about risks and risk prevention while hospitalised.
- Develop a written schedule of rest and activity periods.

Expected outcomes

- Regain a normal body fluid balance.
- Remain free of injury.
- Remain free of infection.
- Verbalise an understanding of the physical effects of the disease process and have realistic expectations of desired changes in appearance.

IMPLEMENTATION

- Weigh each morning, using the same scale.
- Maintain an accurate record of intake and output.
- Ensure adequate lighting in the room and wear glasses and shoes when getting out of bed.
- If possible, provide a private room and restrict visitors at this time after consulting with Lily.
- Use strict medical and surgical asepsis when providing care.
- Provide time for discussion of the disease and treatment; encourage verbalisation of feelings and identify successful coping mechanisms used in the past.
- Encourage turning, coughing and deep breathing, and/or incentive spirometry every 2–4 hours.

EVALUATION

Lily states that she is 'ready to have surgery and start feeling better'. She has not fallen or injured herself and she has remained free of infection. Although oedema is still present, she has lost 3.6 kg and her blood pressure has decreased. Lily has openly discussed her concerns about the way she looks and feels; she understands that symptoms will improve following surgery. She has strong religious beliefs and family support, both of which provide strength and help her cope with the effects of the disorder and the need for any further treatment.

CRITICAL THINKING IN THE NURSING PROCESS

1. When Lily was admitted to the hospital, several of her test results were abnormal. Describe the pathophysiological reason for those results.
2. List the assessments that nurses can make to determine body fluid balance.
3. Develop a plan of care for this person for the nursing diagnosis of *Fatigue*.

REFLECTION ON THE NURSING PROCESS

1. What have you learned from this scenario that you can incorporate into your future nursing practice?
2. Develop a discharge plan for Lily that takes into account the education and support she may need to ensure a safe discharge home.

Risk of infection

Elevated cortisol levels impair the immune response, increasing the risk of infection. Increased cortisol also affects protein synthesis, causing delayed wound healing, and inhibits collagen formation, which results in epidermal atrophy, further inhibiting resistance to infection. In addition, impaired blood flow to oedematous tissue results in altered cellular nutrition, which increases the potential for infection. The following interventions are outlined for the person with Cushing's syndrome who is hospitalised:

- Place in a private room, if possible, and limit visitors. *Such measures reduce the person's infection risk.*
- Monitor vital signs and verbalisations of subjective manifestations (for example, the person's response to 'How do you feel?') every 4 hours. *Increased body temperature and pulse are systemic indicators of infection; however, because Cushing's syndrome impairs the normal inflammatory response, the usual indicators of inflammation such as fever may not be present.*
- Pat skin dry gently after bathing. *Rough drying with towels increases risk of skin tears and skin infections.*
- Use principles of aseptic non-touch technique when performing procedures including wound care. *Impaired skin and tissues make aseptic techniques even more necessary to decrease the risk of infection. Intact, clean and dry skin is the first line of defence against infection.*
- If wounds are present, assess the colour, odour and consistency of wound drainage and look for increased pain in and around the wound. Document these findings in a wound assessment chart.
- Teach the importance of increasing oral intake of protein and vitamins C and A. *Protein, vitamin C and vitamin A are necessary for collagen formation; collagen helps support and repair body tissues.*

Disturbed body image

The person with Cushing's syndrome has obvious physical changes in appearance. The abnormal fat distribution, 'moon face', 'buffalo hump', thin skin, striae, acne and facial hair (in women) all contribute to disruptions in the way people with this disorder perceive themselves.

- Encourage people to express feelings and to ask questions about the disorder and its treatment. *The loss of one's normal body image may prompt feelings of hopelessness, powerlessness, anger and depression. Understanding the disease and adapting to changes from that disease are the first steps in regaining control of one's own body.*
- Discuss strengths and previous coping strategies. Enlist the support of family or significant others in reaffirming the person's worth. *Disturbances in body image are often accompanied by low self-esteem. Self-esteem derives from one's perception of competence and from appraisals of others.*
- Discuss signs of progress in controlling symptoms; for example, decreased facial oedema or increased activity tolerance. *Many physical changes from cortisol excess disappear with treatment. Clearly communicate this fact, because the person may believe changes are permanent.*

Community-based care

The person with Cushing's syndrome requires education about specific self-care responsibilities at home. Address the following topics:

- Safety measures to prevent falls if fatigue, weakness and osteoporosis are present.
- The prescribed medication regimen including information about possible side effects. People often require medications for the rest of their lives and dosage changes are highly likely.
- Having regular health assessments.
- Wearing a MedicAlert® bracelet indicating the person has Cushing's syndrome.
- Helping the older person with referrals to social services or community health services because of the complexity of the treatment and care required.
- Provide information about community-based support groups such as the Australian Pituitary Foundation (https://pituitary.asn.au).

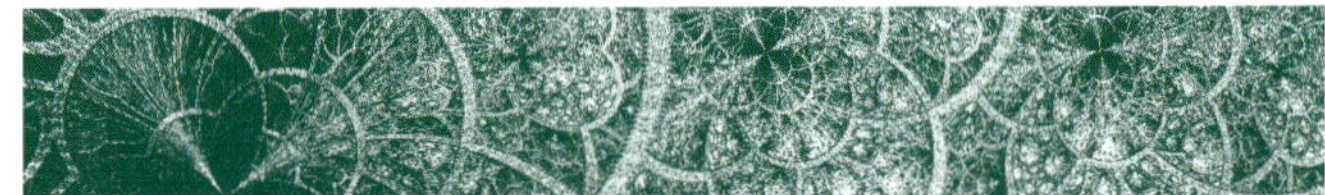

THE PERSON WITH ADRENAL INSUFFICIENCY

Primary adrenal insufficiency (PAI), also known as **Addison's disease**, is a rare endocrine disorder that affects about 2,500 Australians, with 100 new cases diagnosed annually (Hormones Australia, 2018). Adult-onset Addison's disease is typically diagnosed between 30 and 50 years of age and is more common in women. The disease is characterised by low serum cortisol levels which manifests as weight loss, muscle weakness, fatigue, low blood pressure and sometimes darkening of the skin in both exposed and unexposed parts of the body.

Pathophysiology

There are many possible causes of PAI including:

- Autoimmune destruction of the adrenals. Approximately 80% of all PAI cases in Western countries are due to this autoimmune destruction (Barthel et al., 2019). It may occur alone or may be part of an autoimmune polyglandular syndrome.
- The infiltration and destruction of adrenal tissue in infectious diseases such as tuberculosis, HIV/AIDS, cytomegalovirus, candidiasis and syphilis or in malignant diseases including colon, breast and lung cancers.
- Adrenal haemorrhage related to major trauma, surgery or sepsis.
- (Bilateral) adrenalectomy for the treatment of Cushing's syndrome or an adrenal tumour.

- Genetic diseases including adrenoleukodystrophy, an X-linked disorder characterised by an accumulation of very-long-chain fatty acids in the adrenal cortex, testes, brain and spinal cord, and congenital adrenal hyperplasia—the primary cause of Addison's disease in children.

Adrenocortical destruction initially causes a decrease in adrenal glucocorticoid reserves. Basal glucocorticoid secretion is normal, but does not increase in response to stress and surgery. As the destruction of the adrenal cortex continues, even basal secretion of glucocorticoids and mineralocorticoids is deficient. Decreasing plasma cortisol reduces the feedback inhibition of pituitary ACTH and plasma ACTH rises.

Secondary adrenal insufficiency occurs when there is an ACTH deficit resulting from damage to the pituitary or hypothalamus due to recent trauma, the presence of a pituitary tumour or the subsequent surgery or radiation to treat such tumours. Secondary adrenal insufficiency can also result from a person suddenly ceasing their corticosteroids after a prolonged period of use. Because of this sudden discontinuation, the hypothalamus and pituitary may not respond normally to the reduced level of circulating glucocorticoids. As a result, the person may develop manifestations of chronic adrenal insufficiency. Alternatively, an adrenal (Addisonian) crisis may ensue if the person is subject to additional stressors.

Manifestations

The onset of PAI is slow in most cases; the person experiences symptoms after about 90% of the function of the gland is lost. The primary manifestations are the result of elevated ACTH levels and decreased aldosterone and cortisol. Aldosterone deficiency affects the ability of the distal tubules of the nephron to conserve sodium. Sodium is lost, potassium is retained, extracellular fluid is depleted and the blood volume is decreased. Due to sodium loss, the person may have a craving for salt. Orthostatic hypotension and syncope are common and hypovolaemic shock may occur. The person may display dizziness, confusion and neuromuscular irritability due to hyponatraemia. In contrast, hyperkalaemia places the person at risk of developing cardiac dysrhythmias.

Cortisol insufficiency also causes decreased hepatic gluconeogenesis with hypoglycaemia. The person tolerates stress poorly and experiences weight loss, lethargy, weakness, anorexia, nausea, vomiting and diarrhoea. An increased production of α-melanocyte-stimulating hormone (αMSH) results in skin hyperpigmentation (Benner, Alsma & Feelders, 2019). In Caucasian people, the skin looks deeply suntanned or bronzed in both exposed and unexposed areas.

MANIFESTATIONS Adrenal insufficiency

INTEGUMENTARY SYSTEM
- Delayed wound healing
- Hyperpigmentation

CARDIOVASCULAR SYSTEM
- Orthostatic hypotension
- Dysrhythmias
- Tachycardia

CENTRAL NERVOUS SYSTEM
- Lethargy
- Tremors
- Emotional lability
- Confusion

MUSCULOSKELETAL SYSTEM
- Weakness
- Muscle wasting
- Joint pain
- Muscle pain

GASTROINTESTINAL SYSTEM
- Anorexia
- Nausea and vomiting
- Diarrhoea

REPRODUCTIVE SYSTEM
- Menstrual changes

METABOLIC EFFECTS
- Weight loss
- Hyperkalaemia
- Hyponatraemia
- Hypoglycaemia

Addisonian crisis

Addisonian, or **adrenal**, **crisis** is a rare, life-threatening response to acute adrenal insufficiency. Triggers include surgery, acute systemic illness, trauma or abrupt withdrawal of long-term corticosteroid therapy. The disorder is chronic after the acute episode resolves.

This response can occur in any person with Addison's disease; however, it is most commonly precipitated by major stressors, especially if the disease is poorly controlled.

The person with Addisonian crisis may have any of the manifestations of Addison's disease, but the primary symptoms develop rapidly: a high fever; weakness; severe, penetrating pain in the abdomen, lower back and legs; severe vomiting; diarrhoea; hypotension; and circulatory collapse, shock, seizures and coma.

Treatment of adrenal crisis is emergency resuscitation, restoring and maintaining circulating fluid, intravenous hydrocortisone, management of hypoglycaemia, and identification and treatment of precipitating factors. Admission to an intensive care unit may be necessary in most cases (Nasrullah et al., 2022).

INTERPROFESSIONAL CARE

The person with Addison's disease requires early diagnosis and treatment. Medical treatment includes cortisol replacement therapy.

Diagnostic tests

PAI is diagnosed through findings of decreased levels of cortisol and aldosterone. Dehydration may result in increased haematocrit and urea levels. Blood glucose levels are decreased and potassium is increased. A list of laboratory findings in Addison's disease is shown in Table 18.4. The following diagnostic tests are used:

- *serum cortisol levels*, which are decreased
- *blood glucose levels*, which are decreased
- *serum sodium levels*, which are decreased
- *serum aldosterone levels*, which are decreased
- *serum renin levels*, which are increased
- *serum potassium levels*, which are increased
- *serum urea levels*, which are increased
- *urinary cortisol levels*, which are decreased
- *plasma ACTH levels*, which are increased in primary adrenal insufficiency but decreased in secondary adrenal insufficiency
- *an ACTH stimulation test (synacthen test)*, showing a low or absent cortisol rise in primary adrenal insufficiency
- *CT scan* of the brain to identify any intracranial lesion impinging on the pituitary gland
- *CT scan of the adrenals* to determine the size of the adrenal glands.

Blood results for secondary adrenal insufficiency include low cortisol, low ACTH and low cortisol response to the synacthen and metyrapone tests.

Medications

Treatment of Addison's disease involves replacing the hormones that the adrenal glands are not making. Cortisol is replaced orally with oral hydrocortisone. Aldosterone is replaced with a daily oral dose of a mineralocorticoid, fludrocortisone acetate (Florinef). Aldosterone replacement therapy is usually accompanied with an increased salt intake. The doses of each of these medications are adjusted to meet the needs of each individual. During an Addisonian crisis, hypotension, hypoglycaemia and hyperkalaemia can be life threatening. Standard therapy involves intravenous saline or saline/glucose infusions to correct and maintain fluid status, the administration of intravenous glucocorticoids (e.g. hydrocortisone) to correct cortisol depletion, and as required, IV glucose to correct hypoglycaemia. When the person can take fluids and medications by mouth, the amount of hydrocortisone is decreased until a maintenance dose is achieved.

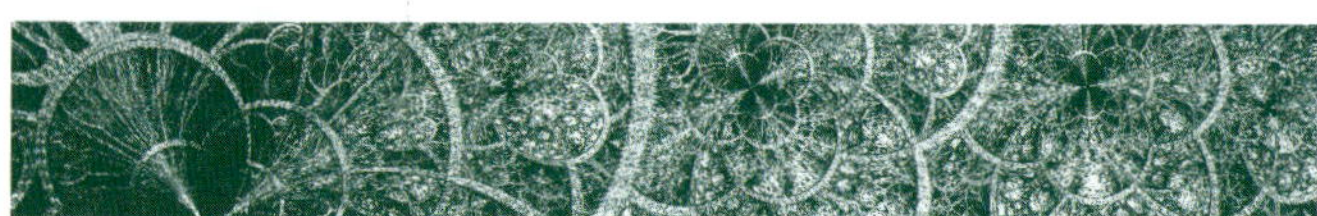

Nursing care

Health promotion

Health promotion interventions for the person with or at risk of Addison's disease focus on careful assessments during anticoagulant therapy and after major surgery and trauma treatments. If the disease is present, teaching to prevent or treat an Addisonian crisis is essential.

Assessment

Collect the following data through the health history and physical examination (see the chapter 'A person-centred approach to assessing the endocrine system'). Further focused assessments described with nursing interventions follow.

- *Health history*: inquire if the person has noticed/experienced any of the following: weight loss, changes in skin colour, nausea and vomiting, anorexia, diarrhoea, abdominal pain, weakness, amenorrhoea, decreased libido, confusion or stress intolerance.
- *Physical assessment*: assess the person's height and weight, vital signs, skin including observing for hyperpigmentation, hair quality and distribution, muscle size and strength.

Nursing diagnoses and interventions

The person with Addison's disease requires nursing care for a wide variety of responses to the decrease in cortisol levels. Nursing diagnoses discussed in this section are directed towards problems with fluid and electrolyte balance and adherence with lifelong self-care. See the accompanying 'Nursing care plan'.

Deficient fluid volume related to water and sodium loss

Fluid volume deficit in the person with Addison's disease results from loss of water and sodium, as well as from vomiting and diarrhoea. A decreased cardiac output, hypotension and hypovolaemic shock may occur, especially in crisis situations. Interventions for this diagnosis are outlined for the person who is hospitalised.

- Monitor intake and output and assess for signs of dehydration: dry mucous membranes; thirst; poor skin

TABLE 18.4 Laboratory findings in Addison's disease

	TEST	NORMAL VALUES	FINDINGS
Serum	Cortisol	Morning peak: 200–650 nmol/L Trough level (at 2000 hours): $\leq$ 50% of morning peak levels	Decreased
	Urea	3.0–8.0 mmol/L dL	Increased
	Sodium	135–145 mmol/L	Decreased
	Potassium	3.5–5.2 mmol/L	Increased
	Glucose (serum)	3.0–7.7 mmol/L	Decreased

Source: Adapted from The Royal College of Pathologists of Australasia (RCPA) (2015). *RCPA manual* (7th ed.). Retrieved from https://www.rcpa.edu.au/Manuals/RCPA-Manual.

turgor; sunken eyes; scanty or low, dark urine; increased urine specific gravity; weight loss; and increased haemoconcentration (increased haematocrit and urea levels). *Glucocorticoid and mineralocorticoid depletion causes fluid volume deficit. Fluid volume deficit may reach crisis levels if undetected, causing altered tissue perfusion and hypovolaemic shock.*

- Monitor cardiovascular status: take and record vital signs, assess character of pulses, monitor potassium levels and electrocardiogram (ECG). *Fluid volume deficit may lead to hypotension and a rapid, weak or thready pulse. As aldosterone levels fall, renal excretion of potassium decreases and causes hyperkalaemia.*
- Weigh the person daily at the same time and in the same clothing. *Dehydration is manifested by weight loss.*
- Encourage an oral fluid intake of 3,000 mL per day and an increased salt intake. Cortisol deficiency increases fluid loss, leading to extracellular fluid volume depletion. Oral fluid replacement is necessary to balance this loss. *An increase in dietary sodium can decrease the hyponatraemia characteristic of adrenal insufficiency.*
- Teach to sit and stand slowly and provide assistance as necessary. *Extracellular fluid volume deficit causes orthostatic hypotension, dizziness and possible loss of consciousness. These manifestations increase the risk of injury from falls.*

CONSIDERATION FOR PRACTICE

Hyperkalaemia causes changes in cardiac muscle function, which are reflected in ECG changes including peaked T waves, flattened P waves, a widening QRS complex and PR prolongation.

Adrenocorticosteroids are used for replacement therapy in acute and chronic adrenal insufficiency. These drugs have anti-inflammatory and immunosuppressant effects. They also facilitate coping with stress.

When these drugs are administered in small doses for replacement therapy, side effects are uncommon. Large doses or prolonged therapy may cause a Cushing's-like syndrome, with atrophy of the adrenal cortex. Older people, especially postmenopausal women, are more prone to develop hypertension and osteoporosis when undergoing glucocorticoid therapy. These drugs are used with caution in children and the older adult and are not usually administered to pregnant women.

Nursing responsibilities

- Establish baseline data, including the person's mental status, neurological function, vital signs and weight.
- Identify medications that might interact with corticosteroids such as oral hypoglycaemic medications, cardiac glycosides, oral contraceptives, anticoagulants and NSAIDs.
- Document and report increased any increases in blood pressure, oedema or weight gain, bleeding or bruising, weakness or manifestations of Cushing's syndrome.
- Administer oral forms of the drug with food to minimise its ulcerogenic effect. Discuss with the medical officer if additional gut protection is required (e.g. a proton pump inhibitor may be prescribed).
- Monitor electrolyte levels for hypernatraemia and hypokalaemia.
- Monitor capillary blood glucose for hyperglycaemia in the diabetic person. Regularly assess for glycosuria.

Health education for the person and family

- Take medications with food or milk and report any gastric distress or dark stools (melaena).
- Most people need to take the medications for the rest of their lives.
- Consume a diet that is low in potassium and higher in sodium and protein.
- Weigh yourself each day at the same time and report any consistent weight gain, which indicates fluid retention.
- Use safety measures in the home to prevent falls and injuries.
- Corticosteroids may impair the effectiveness of oral contraceptives.
- Take the medication regularly and continuously.
- Obtain and carry a MedicAlert® bracelet that says, 'Adrenal insufficiency—takes hydrocortisone'.
- Monitor for increased stressors (infection, dental work, personal crisis) and increase the dose as indicated by the doctor.
- Anticoagulant drugs or insulin may decrease the effectiveness of corticosteroids.
- Report signs of dizziness on sitting or standing, nausea and vomiting, pain, thirst, feelings of anxiety, malaise, infections to your doctor.

Community-based care

The person with PAI provides self-care at home. One of the most important components of caring for the person with Addison's disease is teaching both the person and family to provide care. Family stability, an awareness of the serious nature of the disease and treatment regimens promote effective management of the condition. In addition to the patient education aspects discussed earlier, the following topics should also be discussed:

- how to recognise the clinical manifestations of an impending adrenal crisis (i.e. hypotension, dizziness, nausea and vomiting, confusion, lethargy, muscle weakness and cramps)
- carry a medical treatment letter from the endocrinologist
- carry an emergency kit containing syringes, needles and injectable hydrocortisone at all times
- the importance of continuing medication regimens
- whether a referral to the social worker or other allied health professional may be necessary
- community support groups that offer additional education and support such as the Australian Addison's Disease Association (https://addisons.org.au).

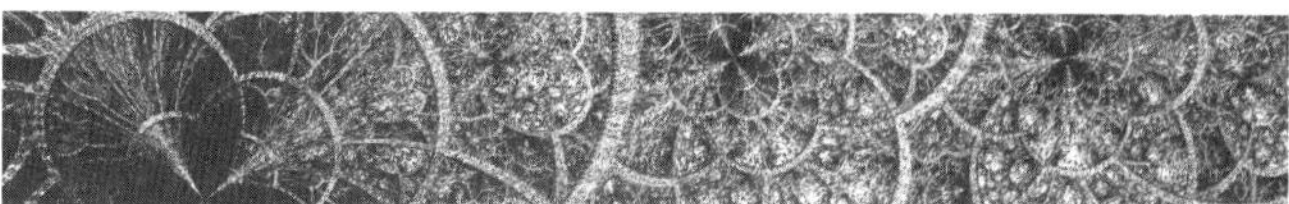

NURSING CARE PLAN A person with Addison's disease

A 51-year-old unemployed salesman, Mr Don Sardoff, is brought to the emergency department by his wife, Ellen, at 8 am. Mrs Sardoff tells the triage nurse that her husband has not been feeling well for the last week, but that when he got up this morning he was so weak he couldn't dress himself and didn't know where he was. Mrs Sardoff also tells the nurse that her husband has been taking a cortisone drug for treatment of his rheumatoid arthritis for the past 2 years, but stopped taking the medication as she notes, 'His script ran out awhile back and he hasn't made a GP appointment for a new script, despite me nagging him.'

ASSESSMENT

On admission to the emergency department, Mr Sardoff is dehydrated, with dry oral mucous membranes and tongue, poor skin turgor and sunken eyes. His blood pressure is 94/44 and his pulse is rapid and weak. He is lethargic, dizzy and disorientated to time and place. Diagnostic tests reveal the following abnormal findings at 0830 hours:

- ECG: peaked T waves, widening QRS complex and increased PR interval
- Sodium: 129 mmol/L (normal range: 135–145 mmol/L)
- Glucose: 2.9 mmol/L (normal range: 3.0–7.7 mmol/L)
- Potassium: 5.3 mmol/L (normal range: 3.5–5.2 mmol/L)
- Cortisol: 71 nmol/L (normal for am: 200–650 nmol/L)

The medical orders for Mr Sardoff include intravenous administration of 4% dextrose in 1/5 normal saline at 250 mL/h and hydrocortisone (Solu-Cortef) 200 mg. After the fluids and hydrocortisone are initiated, Mr Sardoff is admitted to the high-dependency unit.

DIAGNOSES

- *Deficient fluid volume* related to hypovolaemia secondary to adrenal insufficiency.
- *Ineffective peripheral tissue perfusion* related to fluid volume deficit.
- *Anxiety* related to lack of knowledge about the effects and treatment of adrenal insufficiency.

PLANNING

- Discuss a diet that is high in sodium, low in potassium and has an increased fluid intake (3,000 mL per day). Discuss the types of fluids desired and the best times for intake of increased fluids.
- Discuss and determine the need for and amount of intravenous therapy if the oral intake is not sufficient to restore circulating volume.
- Provide verbal and written instructions and encourage verbal feedback about the causes and effects of the disease, the effects of medications and the effects of not taking long-term cortisone drugs or abruptly stopping this medication.

Expected outcomes

- Regain normal fluid balance.
- Regain normal peripheral perfusion with blood pressure within normal range.
- Verbalise knowledge of the causes and effects of adrenal insufficiency.

IMPLEMENTATION

- Monitor intake and output closely.
- Take and record weight at the same time daily.
- Monitor blood pressure, pulses and skin turgor every 2 hours until stable, then four times a day.
- Monitor electrolytes and report abnormal results.
- Assist during activity to prevent falls.
- Ensure steroid medication is taken regularly or, if the medication is to stop, reduce the dosage in small doses over an extended period of time.

EVALUATION

Following treatment for acute adrenal insufficiency, Mr Sardoff is no longer dehydrated and his blood pressure has returned to his normal reading of 132/88 mmHg. He is alert and orientated and anxious to learn to care for himself at home. After dietary instructions and teaching for self-care that included his wife, Mr Sardoff verbalises an understanding of his illness and the need to take his medication carefully and accurately.

CRITICAL THINKING IN THE NURSING PROCESS

1. Adrenal insufficiency is often diagnosed only when the person becomes seriously ill in response to a stressor. Explain why this statement is or is not true.
2. Describe the physical assessments that are found in the severely dehydrated person.
3. Outline a teaching plan for Mr Sardoff with foods for a high-sodium, low-potassium diet.

REFLECTION ON THE NURSING PROCESS

1. Outline what you have learned from this case study and how you are going to apply this new knowledge to your future practice.

THE PERSON WITH PHEOCHROMOCYTOMA

A **pheochromocytoma** is a rare neuroendocrine tumour that develops in the adrenal medulla. While 40% of pheochromocytomas go undiagnosed, approximately 60% of these tumours produce catecholamines (adrenaline or noradrenaline) that stimulate the sympathetic nervous system (NeuroEndocrine Cancer Australia, 2020). Functioning pheochromocytomas tend to suddenly release hormones, which cause a sudden 'attack' or onset of symptoms. The signs and symptoms of pheochromocytoma include the classic triad of diaphoresis, severe headaches and palpitation. Other manifestations include flushing, pallor, nausea, weight loss, fatigue, hyperglycaemia and reports of panic and anxiety (Naranjo, Dodd & Martin, 2017). These symptoms may last for a few seconds to several hours. Attacks are often precipitated by stress, pain, position changes and abdominal manipulation.

A pheochromocytoma is diagnosed by increased catecholamine levels in the blood or urine and/or by imaging such as a CT scan, MRI, MIBG scan or PET scan. Surgical removal of the tumour(s) by adrenalectomy is the treatment of choice.

Disorders of the pituitary gland

The pituitary gland produces hormones that affect multiple body systems through regulation of endocrine function. Target tissues include the thyroid, adrenal cortex, ovary, uterus, mammary glands, testes and kidneys. Disorders result from an excess or deficiency of one or more of the pituitary hormones due to a pathological condition within the gland itself or to hypothalamic dysfunction.

Although disorders of the pituitary cause diverse and serious problems, they are not as common as disorders of other endocrine glands. Hyperpituitarism and hypopituitarism are discussed in this section.

THE PERSON WITH DISORDERS OF THE ANTERIOR PITUITARY GLAND

The most common cause of hyperpituitarism is a benign adenoma. The manifestations result from pressure on the optic nerve causing visual changes or an excess of growth hormone (GH), prolactin (PRL), ACTH or TSH. Typically, 70% to 90% of the anterior pituitary is damaged before clinical manifestations develop (Norris, 2018).

Conditions causing hypopituitarism include pituitary tumours (due to the resultant obstruction of hypothalamic releasing factors), surgical removal of the pituitary gland, radiation and pituitary infarction, infection or trauma.

Pathophysiology and manifestations

Growth hormone (also called somatotropin) is produced by cells in the anterior pituitary throughout life. GH is necessary for growth and also contributes to metabolic regulation. GH stimulates all aspects of cartilage growth, and one of its major effects is to stimulate the growth of the epiphyseal cartilage plates of the long bones. In addition, other body tissues respond to the metabolic effect of GH with increases in bone width and the growth of visceral and endocrine organs, skeletal and cardiac muscle, skin and connective tissue. Gigantism and acromegaly (discussed next) result from overstimulation of GH. Growth retardation and short stature result from deficient production of GH.

Hypersecretion of PRL affects reproductive and sexual function. Women may have irregular or absent menses, fertility problems and decreased libido. Men may be impotent and have decreased libido. A postpartum woman with PRL deficiency will be unable to lactate.

An excess secretion of ACTH overstimulates the adrenal cortex, which in turn increases secretion of adrenal hormones. The result is Cushing's syndrome. Deficiencies of TSH are uncommon, but cause hypothyroidism.

Gigantism

Gigantism occurs when GH hypersecretion begins before puberty and the closure of the epiphyseal plates. The person becomes abnormally tall, often exceeding 213 cm in height, but body proportions are relatively normal.

Acromegaly

Acromegaly, which literally means 'enlarged extremities', occurs when sustained GH hypersecretion begins during adulthood, most commonly because of pituitary tumours. As a result of constant stimulation, bone and connective tissue continue to grow. The forehead enlarges (frontal bossing), the maxilla lengthens, the tongue enlarges and the voice deepens (see Figure 18.4).

Other manifestations include enlargement of hands and feet, gaps between the teeth, barrel chest, oily skin, hair overgrow, hirsutism in women, obstructive sleep apnoea, cardiomyopathy, carpal tunnel syndrome, liver/spleen enlargement, skin tags and join pain (Inder & Jang, 2021). Headaches, visual disturbances—most commonly **bitemporal homonymous hemianopia**—impaired glucose tolerance and diabetes may also occur. However, sometimes the first thing the person with acromegaly notices is that they have needed to increase their hat, shoe or glove size for the first time since entering adulthood.

INTERPROFESSIONAL CARE

Acromegaly is treated by surgical removal or irradiation of the pituitary tumour. A transsphenoidal surgical procedure is most commonly used. Somatostatin analogues such as octreotide and pasireotide are used to suppress the anterior pituitary gland and decrease GH levels. Adverse effects of somatostatin analogues include abdominal cramping, flatulence and diarrhoea.

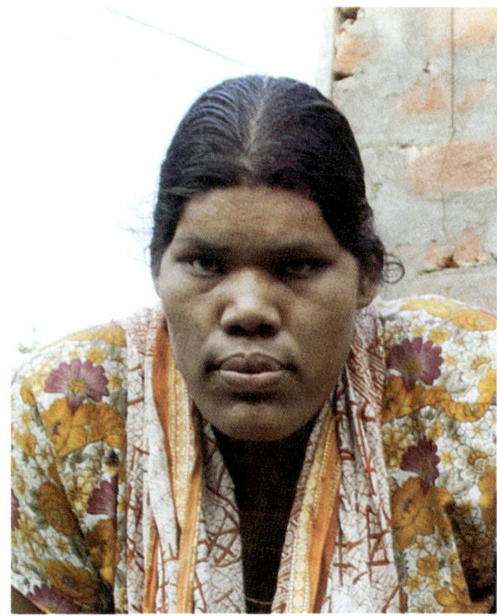

FIGURE 18.4 ***In acromegaly, progressive alterations in facial appearance include enlargement of the cheekbones and jaw, along with thickening of soft-tissue structures such as the nose, lips, cheeks and the flesh above the brows***

Source: © Barcroft Media/Splash News.

Prolonged use can lead to cholelithiasis. Consequently, a gallbladder ultrasound is recommended prior to the person commencing therapy. Repeat ultrasounds should then be performed every 6 to 12 months.

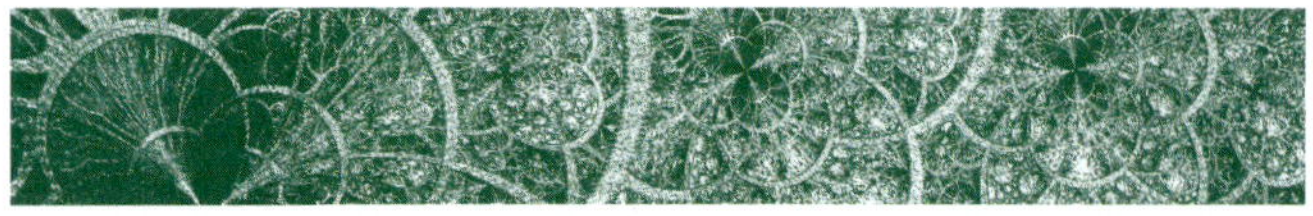

Nursing care

People with anterior pituitary disorders require interventions to help in coping with physical and emotional changes, as well as to prevent complications involving other organs and functions of the endocrine system. Nursing care for the person having cranial surgery is discussed in the chapter 'Nursing care of people with intracranial disorders'.

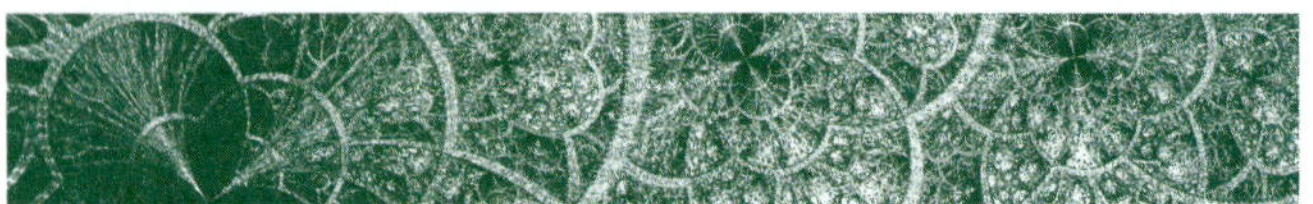

THE PERSON WITH DISORDERS OF THE POSTERIOR PITUITARY GLAND

Disorders of the posterior pituitary are related primarily to excessive or deficient antidiuretic hormone (ADH) secretion. The disorders discussed here are the syndrome of inappropriate ADH secretion and diabetes insipidus.

Pathophysiology and manifestations

Antidiuretic hormone is secreted in response to serum osmolality, which is monitored by osmoreceptors in the hypothalamus. When a condition of hyperosmolarity occurs, ADH secretion increases and renal water is reabsorbed. Hypoosmolality causes the suppression of ADH and renal water excretion increases.

Syndrome of inappropriate ADH secretion

The **syndrome of inappropriate ADH secretion (SIADH)** is characterised by high levels of ADH in the absence of serum hypoosmolality. SIADH causes include CNS disorders (e.g. infections, tumours, cerebral haemorrhage, neurotrauma), malignancy, especially bronchogenic carcinoma, pulmonary disorders (e.g. Legionella pneumonia, tuberculosis) and the use of some medications (e.g. barbiturates, general anaesthetics, chemotherapeutic agents) (Griffin, 2020).

Manifestations of SIADH occur as a result of excess water in relation to sodium in the extracellular fluid. Blood volume expands, but the plasma is diluted. Aldosterone is suppressed and, as a result, renal excretion of sodium increases. Water moves from the hypotonic plasma and the interstitial spaces into the cells.

Manifestations of SIADH (see the chapter 'Nursing care of people with altered fluid, electrolyte and acid–base balance', Table 9.6) are usually non-specific but are related to hyponatraemia and water intoxication. The resultant cerebral oedema causes neurological manifestations including headache, mental status changes, seizures, lethargy and irritability. A 5% to 10% weight gain results from the retention of fluid. However, usually no oedema is present because the water is distributed between the intracellular and extracellular spaces (Griffin, 2020).

Treatment addresses the low serum sodium and intracellular swelling. Nursing care involves teaching the person about restricting fluids to < 1,000 mL/day. Fluid restriction continues for 3 to 10 days until the source of excessive ADH secretion is addressed. The replacement of sodium via intravenous normal saline and/or hypertonic (3%) saline is administered slowly and carefully. The person is also prescribed a loop diuretic such as frusemide to promote diuresis.

> **NURSING ALERT**
>
> **Fluid restriction is contraindicated in individuals with SIADH post-subarachnoid haemorrhage as hypovolaemia will increase their risk of vasospasm. Vasospasm can lead to an ischaemic stroke.**
>
> **The rapid administration of hypertonic saline can cause the person to experience central pontine myelinolysis, also known as a 'locked in syndrome', due to the rapid correction of sodium levels. Ensure you follow the local institute's policy regarding its administration including the volume and rate of infusion.**

Diabetes insipidus

Diabetes insipidus (DI) is the result of ADH insufficiency, resulting in the affected person being unable to conserve water. The two types are as follows:

1. *Central (neurological) DI* results from a disruption or compression of the hypothalamus and pituitary gland. Causes of central DI include neurotrauma, cerebral haemorrhage, pituitary tumours and as a post-neurosurgery complication. However, 25% of cases are idiopathic (Griffin, 2020).
2. *Nephrogenic DI* is a disorder in which the renal tubules are not sensitive to ADH. This form of DI may be congenital in origin or the result of renal failure or drug toxicity (e.g. gentamicin, frusemide).

The ADH deficit results in the person excreting large amounts of dilute urine (polyuria), in some instances as much as 12 L/day. The person has extreme thirst and drinks large volumes of water (polydipsia). If they are unable to replace the water loss, the person becomes dehydrated and hypernatraemic. Even though hyperosmolarity is present, the urine is diluted (< 200 mOsm/L) and has a low specific gravity (1.001 to 1.005).

If this disorder is caused by cerebral injury, symptoms commonly appear 3 to 6 days after the initial injury and last for 7 to 10 days. If the increased intracranial pressure is relieved, symptoms of DI usually disappear. However, DI may also be a chronic illness requiring lifelong treatment and care.

INTERPROFESSIONAL CARE

SIADH is treated by correcting underlying causes, treating the hyponatraemia with a high-sodium diet, intravenous hypertonic saline and restricting the person's oral fluid intake to less than

1,000 mL/day. The person with SIADH must be placed on a fluid balance chart to monitor their intake and output.

DI is also treated by correcting underlying causes, if possible. Other medical interventions include administering intravenous hypotonic and isotonic fluids, increasing oral fluids and the administration of synthetic ADH, desmopressin acetate. Desmopressin acetate, also known as DDAVP, can be administered via the intranasal, oral, intravenous, intramuscular and sublingual routes. The person with DI's fluid status should be carefully monitored using a fluid balance chart as profound hypovolaemia may lead to cardiac arrest. Serum sodium levels should also be monitored as DDAVP administration can lead to hyponatraemia, thereby worsening the intracranial pressure of acutely unwell neurological patients.

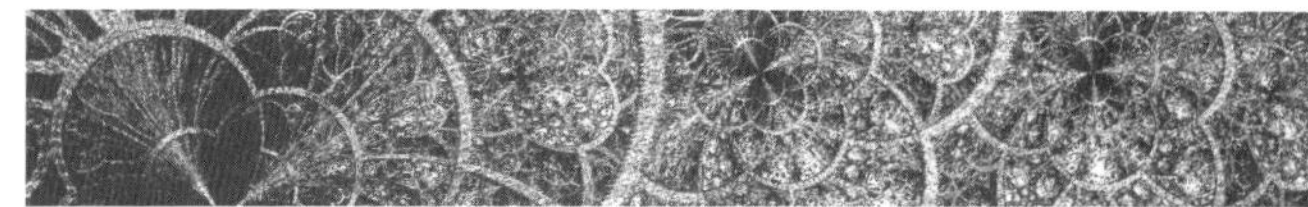

Nursing care

Nursing care for the person with SIADH and DI focuses on the person's problems with fluid and electrolyte balance, as discussed in the chapter 'Nursing care of people with altered fluid, electrolyte and acid–base balance'.

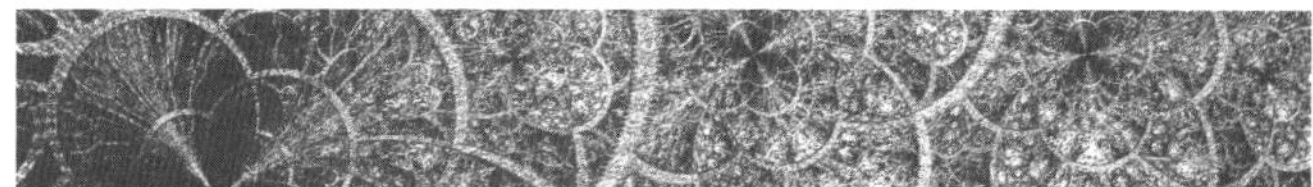

CHAPTER HIGHLIGHTS

- Hormones regulate growth, development and metabolism. Homeostasis is dependent on a balanced level of each type of hormone. Hormones not only affect organ function; they also interact and, when excesses or deficits occur, signs and symptoms are manifested.
- The pituitary gland, in conjunction with the hypothalamus, is the master gland of the body. Fifteen hormones and regulatory factors are synthesised in the anterior pituitary and hypothalamus; many are trophic hormones that stimulate the release of other hormones.
- Thyroid disorders are the most common endocrine disorders. Occurring mainly among women, these diseases change body image and impose challenges to energy levels, creating fatigue and exhaustion.
- Diagnostic tests and therapies are available to identify and treat thyroid disorders. Surgery, radiation therapy and medications support good quality of life, but the medications must be used throughout the lifetime.
- The parathyroid glands, which are located on thyroid tissues, provide parathyroid hormones that are essential for the maintenance of serum calcium, which is vital for cardiac function, bone stability, nerve conduction and muscle contraction.
- The adrenal glands regulate energy and fluid balance through corticosteroids and mineralocorticoids. Cushing's and Addison's diseases are polar opposites and treatment eliminates the signs and symptoms of one and creates the manifestations of the other. People with these disorders require education until they fully grasp the significance of the condition and the importance of adhering to the treatment plan.

CONCEPT CHECK

1 Graves' disease, the most common cause of hyperthyroidism, is categorised as what type of disorder?
   1 autoimmune
   2 infectious
   3 allergic
   4 genetic

2 What principle supports the treatment of hyperthyroidism with radioactive iodine?
   1 Radioactive iodine reduces the vascularity of the thyroid gland.
   2 Doses of radioactive iodine are too small to be hazardous to other body parts.
   3 The thyroid gland takes up iodine in any form.
   4 Irradiation of the thyroid gland decreases the risk of hypothyroidism.

3 You assess a person with newly diagnosed hypothyroidism as having a goitre. What physiological process cause a goitre?
   1 an excess of TH stimulates thyroid follicles
   2 an increased dietary iodine intake
   3 a compensatory effort to produce more TH
   4 tissue hypertrophy in response to increased TH

4 Mrs Jonah has taken cortisone for her rheumatoid arthritis for several years. What endocrine disorder is she most at risk of developing?
   1 hyperthyroidism
   2 hypothyroidism
   3 acromegaly
   4 Cushing's syndrome

5 Which statement illustrates that the person with Addison's disease understands your teaching?
   1 'I will be sure to stop taking my medications when I have an infection.'
   2 'I have purchased an emergency kit and keep it with me all the time.'
   3 'I know I should never alter my dose of medications.'
   4 'I wonder why I look suntanned all the time.'

6 Clinical manifestations of hyponatraemia found in SIADH include:
   1 weight loss
   2 irritability
   3 hyperkalaemia
   4 constipation

7 A community nurse is caring for a person with hyperparathyroidism and osteoporosis. Which nursing diagnosis has priority with this person?
   1 *Risk of fear*
   2 *Risk of injury*
   3 *Risk of isolation*
   4 *Risk of chronic low self-esteem*

8 A nurse is monitoring a person for signs of hypocalcaemia. Which of the following is a sign of hypocalcaemia?
1 oliguria
2 positive Trousseau sign
3 diminished bowel sounds
4 hyperactive deep tendon reflexes

9 A person with increased ACTH levels and Addison's disease is likely to manifest:
1 tremor
2 hair loss
3 gingival hyperplasia
4 dermal hyperpigmentation

10 People treated with glucocorticoids are at risk of Addisonian crisis due to:
1 rapid withdrawal of glucocorticoids
2 excessive ACTH
3 sodium retention
4 hypokalaemia

BIBLIOGRAPHY

Abrams, J. L., Fermi, D., Belligund, P. & McFarlane, S. I. (2022). Amiodarone-induced hypothyroidism related to pericardial effusion with tamponade physiology. *Curēus*, *14*(3), e22932. https://doi.org/10.7759/cureus.22932

Apaydın, T. & Yavuz, D. G. (2021). Assessment of non-traumatic vertebral fractures in Cushing's syndrome patients. *Journal of Endocrinological Investigation*, *44*(8), 1767–1773. https://doi.org/10.1007/s40618-020-01496-y

Barthel, A., Benker, G., Berens, K. et al. (2019). An update on Addison's Disease. *Experimental and Clinical Endocrinology & Diabetes*, *127*(2/03), 165–175. https://doi.org/10.1055/a-0804-2715

Benner, B. J. M., Alsma, J. & Feelders, R. A. (2019). Hyponatraemia and hyperpigmentation in primary adrenal insufficiency. *BMJ Case Reports*, *12*(3), e227200. https://doi.org/10.1136/bcr-2018-227200

Blum, M. R., Bauer, D. C., Collet, T.-H. et al. (2015). Subclinical thyroid dysfunction and fracture risk: A meta-analysis. *Journal of the American Medical Association*, *313*(20), 2055–2065.

Cabanillas, M. E. D., McFadden, D. G. M. D. & Durante, C. M. D. (2016). Thyroid cancer. *The Lancet*, *388*(10061), 2783–2795. https://doi.org/10.1016/S0140-6736(16)30172-6

Cancer Australia (2022). *Thyroid cancer*. Retrieved from https://www.canceraustralia.gov.au/

Cheetham, T. & Boal, R. (2019). Graves' disease. *Paediatrics and Child Health*, *29*(7), 316–320. https://doi.org/10.1016/j.paed.2019.04.006

Cinamon, U., Levy, D. & Marom, T. (2015). Is primary hyperparathyroidism a risk factor for papillary thyroid cancer? An exemplar study and literature review. *International Archives of Otorhinolaryngology*, *19*(1), 42–45.

Doubleday, A. R. & Sippel, R. S. (2020). Hyperthyroidism. *Gland Surgery*, *9*(1), 124–135. https://doi.org/10.21037/gs.2019.11.01

Du, J., Wang, X., Tan, G., Wei, W., Zhou, F., Liang, Z., Li, H. & Yu, H. (2021). Predisposition to Graves' disease and Graves' ophthalmopathy by genetic variants of IL2RA. *Journal of Molecular Medicine*, *99*(10), 1487–1495. https://doi.org/10.1007/s00109-021-02111-0

Griffin, L. (2020). Neuroendocrine disorders in neuroscience patients. In J. Hickey & A. Strayer (eds), *The clinical practice of neurological and neurosurgical nursing* (8th ed.; pp. 247–263). Philadelphia: Wolters Kluwer.

Gupta, K. J. (2013). Myxedema coma: A sleeping giant in clinical practice. *American Journal of Medicine*, *126*(12), e3–4.

Hormones Australia (Endocrine Society of Australia) (2018). *Adrenal insufficiency*. Retrieved from https://www.hormones-australia.org.au/

Hughes, K. & Eastman, C. (2021). Thyroid disease: Long-term management of hyperthyroidism and hypothyroidism. *Australian Journal for General Practitioners*, *50*, 36–42.

Inder, W. & Jang, C. (2021). Pituitary disease: An update. *Australian Journal of General Practice*, *50*(1–2). https://doi.org/10.31128/AJGP-10-20-5688

Kane, E. G. & Shore, S. L. (2020). Thyroidectomy. *Surgery*, *38*(12), 801–806. https://doi.org/10.1016/j.mpsur.2020.10.006

Lau, D., Rutledge, C. & Aghi, M. K. (2015). Cushing's disease: Current medical therapies and molecular insights guiding future therapies. *Neurosurgical Focus*, *38*(2), E11–E21.

Lim, H., Devesa, S. S., Sosa, J. A., Check, D. & Kitahara, C. M. (2017). Trends in thyroid cancer incidence and mortality in the United States, 1974-2013. *JAMA*, *317*(13), 1338–1348. https://doi.org/10.1001/jama.2017.2719

Matheus, M. V. & Kowdley, G. C. (2021). Pemberton's sign in a patient with multinodular goiter. *The American Surgeon*, *87*(12), 2003–2005. https://doi.org/10.1177/0003134820940289

McCance, K. & Huether, S. (2019). *Pathophysiology: The biologic basis for disease in adults and children* (8th ed.). Chatswood, NSW: Mosby.

Naranjo, J. D. O., Dodd, S. M. D. & Martin, Y. N. M. D. P. (2017). Perioperative management of pheochromocytoma. *Journal of Cardiothoracic and Vascular Anesthesia*, *31*(4), 1427–1439. https://doi.org/10.1053/j.jvca.2017.02.023

Nasrullah, A., Azharuddin, S., Young, M., Kejas, A. & Dumont, T. (2022). Endocrine emergencies in the medical intensive care unit. *Critical Care Nursing Quarterly*, *45*(3). Retrieved from https://journals.lww.com/

NeuroEndocrine Cancer Australia (2020). *Pheos and paras*. Retrieved from https://neuroendocrine.org.au/

Nguyen, Q. T., Lee, E. J., Huang, M. G. et al. (2015). Diagnosis and treatment of patients with thyroid cancer. *American Health Drug Benefits*, *8*(1), 30–40.

Norris, T. L. (2018). *Porth's pathophysiology: Concepts of altered health states* (10th ed.). Philadelphia: Lippincott Williams & Wilkins.

Nutrition Australia (2021). *Iodine*. Retrieved from https://nutritionaustralia.org/

Padda, I. S. & Nguyen, M. (2022). *StatPearls: Radioactive iodine therapy*. Retrieved from https://www.ncbi.nlm.nih.gov/books/NBK557741/

Poppe, K., Bisschop, P., Fugazzola, L., Minziori, G., Unuane, D. & Weghofer, A. (2021). 2021 European Thyroid Association guideline on thyroid disorders prior to and during assisted reproduction. *European Thyroid Journal*, *9*(6), 281–295. https://doi.org/10.1159/000512790

Quérat, C., Germain, N., Dumollard, J. M. et al. (2015). Surgical management of hyperthyroidism. *European Annals of Otorhinolaryngology, Head and Neck Diseases*, *132*(2), 63–66.

Ramos, L., Pertoti de Figueredo, G., Maia, A. & Romero, S. (2015). Pre-tibial myxedema: Treatment with intralesional corticosteroid. *Anais Brasileiros de Dermatologia*, *90*(3), 143–146.

Shirley, M. (2021). Ketoconazole in Cushing's syndrome: A profile of its use. *Drugs and Therapy Perspectives*, *37*(2), 55–64. https://doi.org/10.1007/s40267-020-00799-7

Siskind, S. M., Lee, S. Y. & Pearce, E. N. (2021). Investigating hypothyroidism. *British Medical Journal*, *373*, n993. https://doi.org/10.1136/bmj.n993

Sung, J. Y. (2015). Parathyroid ultrasonography: The evolving role of the radiologist. *Ultrasonography*, 34(4), 268–274.

Taïeb, D. (2020). Management of hyperthyroid patients following radioactive iodine therapy, with a specific emphasis on Graves' disease. *Médecine Nucléaire*, *44*(4), 284–286. https://doi.org/10.1016/j.mednuc.2020.06.003

The Royal College of Pathologists of Australasia (RCPA) (2015). *RCPA manual* (7th ed.). Retrieved from https://www.rcpa.edu.au/

Topilow, N. J., Tran, A. Q., Koo, E. B. & Alabiad, C. R. (2020). Etiologies of proptosis: A review. *Internal Medicine Review*, 6(3). https://doi.org/10.18103/imr.v6i3.852

Walsh, J. P. (2016). Managing thyroid disease in general practice. *MJA*, *205*(4), 179–184.

Wong, R., Farrell, S. G. & Grossmann, M. (2018). Thyroid nodules: Diagnosis and management. *Medical Journal of Australia*, *209*(2), 92–98. https://doi.org/10.5694/mja17.01204

Wouters, H. J. C. M., Slagter, S. N., Muller Kobold, A. C., van der Klauw, M. M. & Wolffenbuttel, B. H. R. (2020). Epidemiology of thyroid disorders in the Lifelines Cohort Study (the Netherlands). *PloS One*, *15*(11), e0242795–e0242795. https://doi.org/10.1371/journal.pone.0242795

Zimmermann, M. B. & Boelaert, K. (2015). Iodine deficiency and thyroid disorders. *The Lancet Diabetes Endocrinology*, *3*, 286–295.

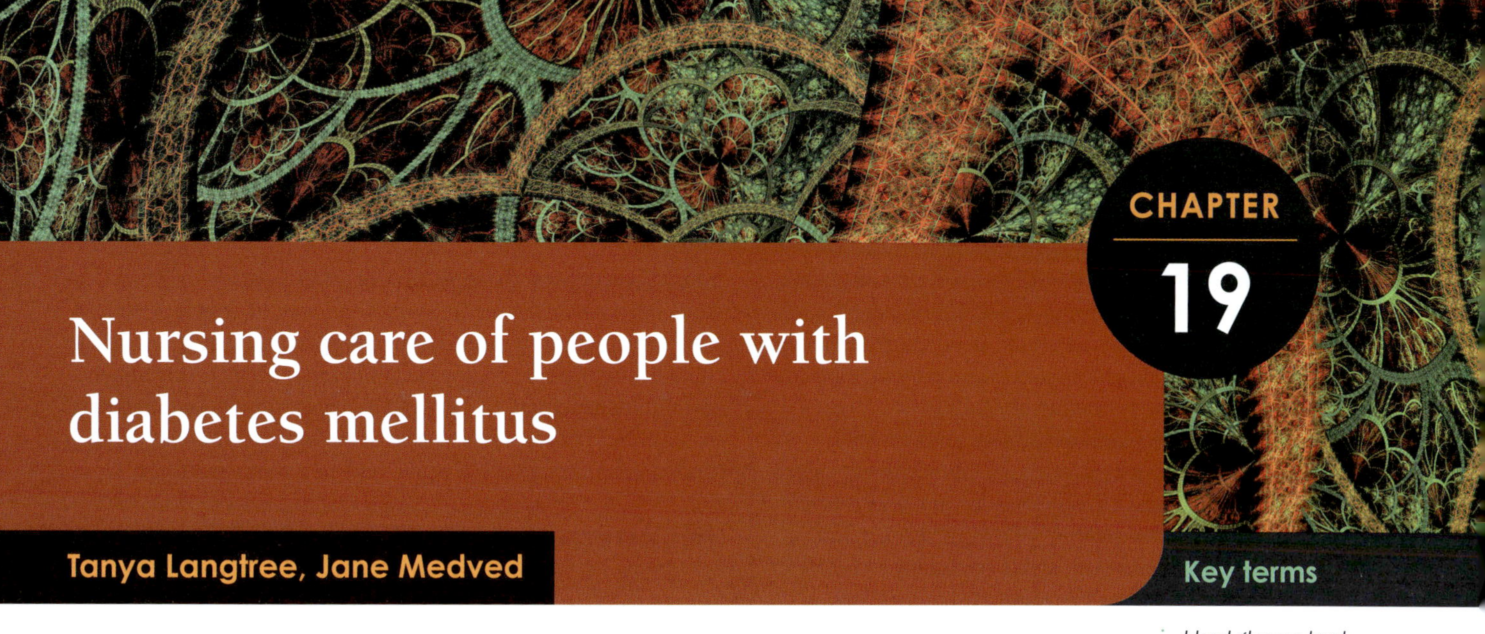

CHAPTER 19

Nursing care of people with diabetes mellitus

Tanya Langtree, Jane Medved

Learning outcomes

- Discuss the chronic condition diabetes mellitus (DM), identifying the prevalence and incidence of DM in Australia.
- Explain the pathophysiology, risk factors, manifestations and complications of type 1 and type 2 DM.
- Discuss the nursing implications for insulin and oral hypoglycaemic agents used to treat people with DM.
- Compare and contrast the manifestations and interprofessional care of hyperglycaemia, hypoglycaemia, diabetic ketoacidosis and hyperosmolar hyperglycaemic state.
- Identify and explain the chronic complications associated with DM.

Clinical competencies

- Assess blood glucose levels (BGLs) and patterns of hyperglycaemia and hypoglycaemia in people with DM.
- Recognise the importance of early diagnosis and control of BGLs to prevent complications.
- Determine priority nursing diagnoses, based on assessed data, to select and implement individualised nursing interventions for people with type 1 and type 2 DM.
- Administer oral and injectable medications used to treat type 1 and type 2 DM knowledgeably and safely.
- Provide skilled care to people with diabetic ketoacidosis and hyperosmolar hyperglycaemic states.
- Integrate interprofessional care into care of people with type 1 and type 2 DM, especially foot and eye care.
- Provide appropriate teaching to facilitate BGL monitoring, administration of oral and injectable hypoglycaemic medications, diabetic diet, appropriate exercise, and foot and eye care.
- Revise plan of care as needed to provide effective interventions to promote, maintain or restore normal BGL.
- Teach the relationship of hygiene, neuropathy and impaired microcirculation to infection; teach the principles and procedures of effective foot care.
- Assess the person's ability to read markings on syringes and to identify correct insulin and hypoglycaemics.

Key terms

Diabetes mellitus

Diabetes mellitus (DM) is a chronic disease affecting adults, adolescents and children, requiring continuing medical supervision and self-care education. However, depending on the type of DM and the age of the person, needs and nursing care may vary greatly. Consider the following examples:

- Cheryl Draheim is a 45-year-old school teacher. She developed type 1 DM at age 34 after a car accident caused severe pancreatic injuries. Cheryl has always been very careful about taking her insulin, following her diet and exercising regularly. However, she is beginning to notice that her vision is getting worse and that she is having increasing pain in her legs, especially after standing for long periods of time.
- Tom Chang is 63 years old. In his early forties, Tom was diagnosed with type 2 DM. Tom was provided education regarding type 2 DM, the importance of taking his oral medications, following a diet plan and exercising; however, he rarely did more than take his medication. Five years ago, Tom was hospitalised for hyperglycaemia and started taking insulin. Last year Tom had a stroke, leaving him paralysed on the left side of his body and unable to walk. He is now in hospital for treatment of gangrene of the big toe on his left foot.
- Grace Staples is an independent 82-year-old woman who lives alone and happily takes care of her two cats. She is slightly overweight. During Grace's annual eye examination, visual changes associated with DM were identified. Grace was referred to her general practitioner who diagnosed type 2 DM and prescribed oral medications. Grace follows her diet, walks a kilometre every day and plans to live to be 100.

These examples illustrate that DM is a group of chronic disorders of the endocrine pancreas affecting people across the lifespan, categorised under a broad diagnostic label. DM is characterised by inappropriate hyperglycaemia caused by a relative or absolute deficiency of insulin or by a cellular resistance to the action of insulin. Of the several classifications of DM, this chapter will focus on the two main types: type 1 DM and type 2 DM. **Type 1 DM** is the result of pancreatic islet cell destruction and a total deficit of circulating insulin; **type 2 DM** results from insulin resistance with a defect in compensatory insulin secretion.

DM has been recognised as a disease for centuries. *Diabetes* derives from a Greek word meaning 'to siphon', referring to the increased output of urine. *Mellitus* derives from a Latin word meaning 'sweet'. The two words together identify the disease as an outpouring of sweet urine. It was not until 1921 that techniques were developed for extracting insulin from pancreatic tissue and for measuring **blood glucose levels (BGLs)**. At the same time, researchers discovered that insulin, when injected, produces a dramatic drop in BGL. This meant that DM was no longer a terminal illness because hyperglycaemia could be controlled. Since then, oral hypoglycaemic drugs, human insulin products, insulin pumps, home BGL monitoring and transplantation of the pancreas or of pancreatic islet or beta cells have advanced the treatment and care of people with DM.

People with DM face lifelong changes in lifestyle and health status. Nursing care is provided in many settings for the diagnosis and management of DM and treatment of its complications. A major role of the nurse as part of the multidisciplinary team is that of educator in both hospital and community settings.

INCIDENCE AND PREVALENCE

According to Diabetes Australia (2022a), DM is one of the biggest health system challenges confronting 21st century Australia, with rates of diagnosis increasing daily. As of September 2022, there were over 1.4 million Australians living with diabetes and registered with the National Diabetes Services Scheme (NDSS). As this is a voluntary register, it is believed that numbers of new cases may be higher. The NDSS represents people diagnosed with any type of DM including type 1 DM (over 134,000), type 2 diabetes (over 1 million), gestational DM (GDM) (over 49,000 women) and other less common or unknown types of DM. There are over 300 registrations with NDSS every day in Australia (NDSS, 2022a).

Rates of DM are generally higher among males, the elderly, people born overseas, Aboriginal and Torres Strait Islander people and people living in remote and socioeconomically disadvantaged areas. Aboriginal and Torres Strait Islander people are almost three times more likely than non-Indigenous Australians to develop DM (Australian Institute of Health and Welfare (AIHW), 2022; Diabetes Australia, 2022a).

GDM is diagnosed through mandatory testing of pregnant women in the second trimester and affects between 12% and 14% of pregnant women. Once the baby is born, BGLs usually return to normal. However, some women will continue to have high BGLs after delivery. GDM is the fastest growing type of DM in Australia.

Diabetes is a National Health Priority Area with statistics revealing that it is the seventh leading cause of death by disease in Australia (Australian Bureau of Statistics (ABS), 2022). People with diabetes may develop heart disease 10 to 15 years earlier than people without diabetes. People with diabetes are also at higher risk of developing cardiovascular disease such as hypertension and renal impairment. Almost two-thirds of Australian adults with type 2 diabetes self-report some form of cardiovascular disease.

OVERVIEW OF ENDOCRINE PANCREATIC HORMONES AND GLUCOSE HOMEOSTASIS

Hormones

The endocrine pancreas produces hormones necessary for the metabolism and cellular utilisation of carbohydrates, proteins and fats. The cells that produce these hormones are clustered

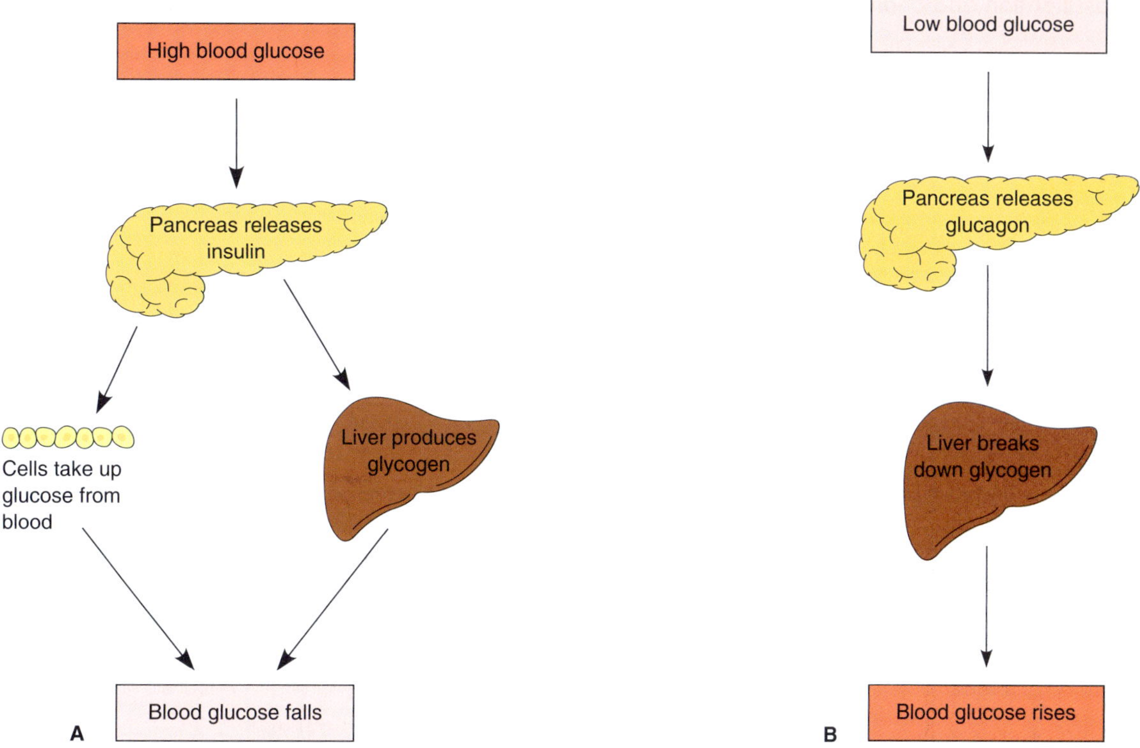

FIGURE 19.1 *Regulation (homeostasis) of blood glucose levels by insulin and glucagon. A, High blood glucose is lowered by insulin release. B, Low blood glucose is raised by glucagon release*

in groups of cells called the islets of Langerhans or pancreatic islets. These islets have three different types of cells:

1. Alpha (α) cells produce the hormone **glucagon**, which stimulates the liver to break down glycogen into glucose (**glycogenolysis**) and to synthesise glucose from lactic acid and non-carbohydrate molecules (**gluconeogenesis**).
2. Beta (β) cells secrete the hormone **insulin**, which reduces BGLs by facilitating the movement of glucose (and other simple sugars) across cell membranes into most body cells to be stored as glycogen, inhibiting the excessive breakdown of glycogen into glucose by the liver and preventing the breakdown of amino acids and stored fats that would increase plasma BGL.
3. Delta cells produce somatostatin, which is believed to be a neurotransmitter that inhibits the production of both glucagon and insulin.

Blood glucose homeostasis

All body cells require a constant supply of glucose for energy to maintain homeostasis or body regulation. However, not all tissues require insulin for glucose uptake. The brain, liver, intestines and renal tubules do not require insulin to transfer glucose into their cells, whereas insulin is necessary for the movement of glucose into the cells of skeletal muscle, cardiac muscle and adipose tissue. Any unused glucose is converted into fat (adipose tissue).

Insulin secretion by the beta cells is regulated by increasing when BGLs increase and decreasing when BGLs decrease. The liver and pancreas work in conjunction to influence the release of insulin. This is most evident in food consumption as insulin levels begin to rise in minutes, peak in 3 to 5 minutes and return to baseline levels in 2 to 3 hours (Norris, 2018). Through these actions, glucagon prevents BGLs from decreasing below a certain level (approximately 3.9 mmol/L) when the body is fasting or in between meals. Increased BGLs, amino acids and fatty acids stimulate pancreatic beta cells to produce insulin. As cells of skeletal muscle, cardiac muscle and adipose tissue take up glucose, plasma levels of nutrients decrease, suppressing the stimulus to produce insulin. If BGLs fall, glucagon is released to raise hepatic glucose output, raising BGLs. Adrenaline, growth hormone, thyroxine and glucocorticoids (often referred to as glucose counter-regulatory hormones) also stimulate an increase in glucose in times of hypoglycaemia, stress, growth or increased metabolic demand. The regulation of BGLs by insulin and glucagon is illustrated in Figure 19.1.

PATHOPHYSIOLOGY OF DIABETES

DM is a group of metabolic diseases characterised by hyperglycaemia resulting from defects in the secretion of insulin, the action of insulin or both. There are four main types of DM.

TABLE 19.1 Classification and characteristics of diabetes

	CLASSIFICATION	CHARACTERISTICS
Type 1 DM	Immune mediated (type 1A occurring in over 90% of people with type 1 DM)	Hyposecretion or hypoactivity of insulin due to destruction or damage to pancreatic beta cells. Markers to the immune destruction of beta cells include islet cell autoantibodies (ICAs) and insulin autoantibodies (IAAs). The rate of beta cell destruction is variable, usually more rapid in infants and children and slower in adults.
	Idiopathic (type 1B)	Has no known aetiological causes.
Type 2 DM		Insulin is present but ineffective. There is no immune destruction of beta cells. May range from predominantly insulin resistance with relative insulin deficiency to a predominantly secretory defect with insulin resistance. Initially, and in some cases for the entire life, insulin is not necessary. Most people with this form are obese or have an increased amount of abdominal fat. Risks for development include increasing age, obesity and a sedentary lifestyle. Occurs more frequently in women who have had gestational diabetes and in people with lipid disorders or hypertension. There is a strong genetic predisposition.
Other specific types	Genetic defects of beta cells	Hyperglycaemia occurs at an early age (usually before age 25). This type is referred to as maturity-onset diabetes of the young (MODY).
	Genetic defects in insulin action	Are genetically determined. Dysfunctions may range from hyperinsulinaemia to severe diabetes.
	Diseases of the exocrine pancreas	Acquired processes causing DM include pancreatitis, trauma, infection, pancreatectomy and pancreatic cancer. Severe forms of cystic fibrosis and haemochromatosis may also damage beta cells and impair insulin secretion.
	Endocrine disorders	Excess amount of hormones (e.g. growth hormone, cortisol, glucagon and adrenaline) impair insulin secretion, resulting in DM in people with Cushing's syndrome, acromegaly and pheochromocytoma.
	Drug- or chemical-induced	Many drugs impair insulin secretion, precipitating DM in people with predisposing insulin resistance. Examples are nicotinic acid, glucocorticoids, thyroid hormone, thiazides and phenytoin.
	Infections	Certain viruses may cause beta cells destruction, including congenital measles, cytomegalovirus, adenovirus and mumps.
Gestational diabetes mellitus (GDM)		Any degree of glucose intolerance with onset or first recognition during pregnancy.
Pre-diabetes		
Impaired fasting glucose/ impaired glucose tolerance	Metabolic stage between normal glucose homeostasis and diabetes	These states are risk factors for the development of DM and cardiovascular disease. Impaired fasting glucose is defined by a fasting glucose concentration of between 6.1 and 6.9 mmol/L

Type 1 DM was formerly called juvenile-onset diabetes or insulin-dependent diabetes mellitus (IDDM). Type 2 DM was formerly labelled non-insulin-dependent diabetes mellitus (NIDDM) or adult-onset diabetes. The other main types are gestational GM (GDM), with women who are diagnosed at higher risk of developing type 2 DM in the future (Diabetes Australia, 2020), and pre-diabetes. Pre-diabetes is characterised by an 'impaired fasting glucose' and is analogous to 'impaired glucose tolerance', indicating a metabolic stage between normal glucose homeostasis and diabetes. These states are risk factors for the development of diabetes and cardiovascular disease. An impaired fasting glucose is defined by a fasting glucose concentration of between 6.1 and 6.9 mmol/L. The classification and characteristics of the types of diabetes are described in Table 19.1.

Type 1 diabetes mellitus

Type 1 DM is a catabolic disorder that most often occurs in childhood and adolescence, but may occur at any age. DM is characterised by an absolute lack of insulin, **hyperglycaemia** (elevated BGLs), a breakdown of body proteins and the development of **ketosis** (an accumulation of ketone bodies produced during the oxidation of fatty acids). Type 1 DM begins with insulinitis, a chronic inflammatory process that occurs in response to the autoimmune destruction of pancreatic islet cells. This process slowly destroys beta cells, the only cells in the body that make insulin, with the onset of hyperglycaemia occurring when 80–90% of beta cell function is lost. This process usually occurs over a long pre-clinical period. It is believed that both alpha cell and beta cell functions are abnormal, with a lack of insulin and a relative excess of glucagon resulting in hyperglycaemia. When beta cells are destroyed, insulin is no longer produced. Although type 1 DM may be classified as either an autoimmune or idiopathic disorder, 90% of the cases are immune mediated.

Risk factors

Genetic predisposition plays a role in the development of type 1 DM. Genetic markers that determine immune responses—specifically, DR3 and DR4 antigens on chromosome 6 of the human leucocyte antigen (HLA) system—have been found in 95% of people diagnosed with type 1 DM. (HLAs are cell surface proteins, controlled by genes on chromosome 6.) Although the presence of these markers does not guarantee that the person will develop type 1 DM, they do indicate increased susceptibility (Norris, 2018).

Environmental factors are believed to trigger the development of type 1 DM. The trigger can be a viral infection (mumps, rubella or coxsackievirus B4) or a chemical toxin, such as those found in smoked and cured meats. As a result of exposure to the virus or chemical, an abnormal autoimmune response occurs in which antibodies respond to normal islet beta cells as though they were foreign substances, destroying them. The manifestations of type 1 DM appear when approximately 90% of the beta cells are destroyed. However, manifestations may appear at any time during the loss of beta cells if an acute illness or stress increases the demand for insulin beyond the reserves of the damaged cells. The actual cause and exact sequence are not completely understood, but research continues to identify the genetic markers of this disorder and to investigate ways of altering the immune response to prevent or cure type 1 DM.

Manifestations

The manifestations of type 1 DM are the result of a lack of insulin to transport glucose across the cell membrane into the cells (see Figure 19.2).

Glucose molecules accumulate in the circulating blood, resulting in hyperglycaemia. Hyperglycaemia causes serum hyperosmolarity, drawing water from the intracellular spaces into the general circulation. The increased blood volume increases renal blood flow and the hyperglycaemia acts as an osmotic diuretic. The resulting osmotic diuresis increases urine output. This condition is called **polyuria**. When the BGL exceeds the renal threshold for glucose—usually about 10 mmol/L—glucose is excreted in the urine, a condition called **glucosuria**. The decrease in intracellular volume and the increased urinary output cause dehydration. The mouth becomes dry and thirst sensors are activated, causing the person to drink increased amounts of fluid (**polydipsia**).

Because glucose cannot enter the cell without insulin, energy production decreases. This decrease in energy stimulates hunger and the person eats more food (**polyphagia**). Despite increased food intake, the person loses weight as the body loses water and breaks down proteins and fats in an attempt to restore energy sources. Malaise and fatigue accompany the decrease in energy. Blurred vision is also common, resulting from osmotic effects that cause swelling of the lenses of the eyes.

Thus, the classic manifestations of type 1 DM are polyuria, polydipsia and polyphagia, accompanied by weight loss, malaise and fatigue. Depending on the degree of insulin shortage, the manifestations vary from slight to severe. People with type 1 DM require **exogenous insulin** to maintain life.

Type 2 DM

Type 2 DM is a condition of fasting hyperglycaemia that occurs despite the availability of **endogenous insulin**. Type 2 DM can occur at any age, but it is usually seen in middle-aged and older people. Heredity plays a role in its transmission. The level of insulin produced varies in type 2 DM and despite its availability, its function is impaired by insulin resistance. Insulin resistance forces the pancreas to work harder and produce more insulin, but when demand exceeds supply, DM results. Whatever the cause, there is sufficient insulin production to prevent the breakdown of fats with resultant ketosis; thus, type 2 DM is characterised as a non-ketotic form of DM. However, the amount of insulin

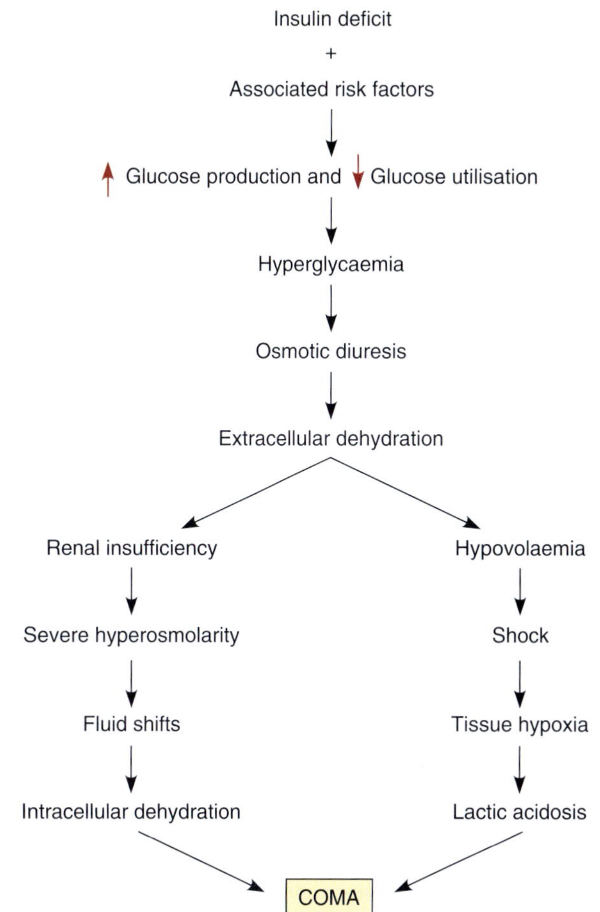

FIGURE 19.2 ***Pathophysiological results of type 1 DM***

available is not sufficient to lower BGLs through the uptake of glucose by muscle and fat cells. A major factor in the development of type 2 DM is cellular resistance to the effect of insulin. This resistance is increased by obesity, inactivity, illnesses, medications and increasing age. In obesity, insulin has a decreased ability to influence glucose metabolism and uptake by the liver, skeletal muscles and adipose tissue. Although the exact reason for this is not clear, it is known that weight loss and exercise may improve the mechanism responsible for insulin receptor binding or post-receptor activity (McCance & Huether, 2019). Hyperglycaemia increases gradually and may exist over time before diagnosis. According to the International Diabetes Federation (2021), DM remains seriously under-reported due to many people not being aware they have type 2 DM. Many people do not seek help until they have developed complications, usually many years after developing type 2 DM. Treatment usually begins with prescriptions for weight loss and increased activity. If these changes can be sustained, no further treatment will be necessary for many individuals. Hypoglycaemic medications are begun when lifestyle changes are insufficient. Often, a combination of insulin and hypoglycaemic medication is used to achieve the best glycaemic control in the person with type 2 DM.

Risk factors

The main risk factors for type 2 DM are as follows:

- History of DM in parents or siblings. Although there is no identified HLA linkage, the children of a person with type 2 DM have a 15% chance of developing type 2 DM and a 30% risk of developing glucose intolerance (the inability to metabolise carbohydrate normally).
- Obesity defined as being at least 20% over desired body weight or having a body mass index of at least 27 kg/m^2. Obesity, especially of the upper body, decreases the number of available insulin receptor sites in cells of skeletal muscles and adipose tissues, a process called *peripheral insulin resistance*. In addition, obesity impairs the ability of the beta cells to release insulin in response to increasing glucose levels.
- Physical inactivity.
- Race/ethnicity (see the 'Focus on cultural diversity' box).
- In women, a history of gestational DM, polycystic ovary syndrome or delivering a baby weighing more than 4.1 kg.
- Hypertension ($\geq$ 130/85 mmHg in adults), HDL cholesterol of $\geq$ 0.9 mmol/L, and/or a triglyceride level of $\geq$ 2.8 mmol/L.
- Metabolic syndrome is a connection between obesity and the development of type 2 DM and is thought to link cardiovascular disease with insulin resistance (Craft et al., 2019). Hypertension, abdominal obesity, dyslipidaemia, elevated C-reactive protein and fasting blood glucose (FBG) greater than 6.1 mmol/L increase the risk of type 2 DM, coronary heart disease and stroke (Diabetes Australia, 2022a; Norris, 2018).

Manifestations

The person with type 2 DM experiences a slow onset of manifestations and is often unaware of the disease until seeking healthcare for some other problem. The hyperglycaemia in type 2 DM is usually not as severe as in type 1, but similar symptoms occur, especially polyuria and polydipsia. Polyphagia is not often seen and weight loss is uncommon. Other manifestations are also the result of hyperglycaemia: blurred vision, fatigue, paraesthesia and skin infections. If available insulin decreases, especially in times of physical or emotional stress, the person with type 2 DM may develop diabetic ketoacidosis (DKA), but this occurrence is uncommon.

Diabetes in the older adult

Approximately 67% of all Australians with diabetes are aged 60 years or older (NDSS, 2022a). Although 90% of older adults with DM have type 2 DM, the improved survival rates for people with DM have resulted in an increased number of older adults with type 1. This is complicated by the fact that BGLs increase with age, beginning in the fifties. For this reason, it is more difficult to diagnose DM in the older adult; conversely, the older adult may be mistakenly diagnosed with the disease simply for exhibiting essentially normal age-related changes in glucose. The relationship between normal increases in glucose levels and the presence of DM is not yet understood.

The normal physiological changes of ageing may mask manifestations of the onset of DM. Signs can be dismissed and be considered as part of 'getting older'. Signs and symptoms of DM in older adults may not include the classic symptoms of polyuria and polydipsia. Conditions such as orthostatic hypotension, periodontal disease, infections, stroke, gastric hypotony, impotence, neuropathy, confusion, lethargy, gradual weight gain, leg cramps and glaucoma should be considered potential indicators of DM and may also increase the potential for complications from the disease or its treatment. Table 19.2 presents common problems in the older adult that make the diagnosis and management of DM more difficult. The older adult with DM also has a longer recovery period after surgery or serious illness, often requiring insulin to maintain BGLs. The benefits and risks of treatment to maintain glycaemic control, as well as blood pressure and lipid management, must be carefully balanced.

FOCUS ON CULTURAL DIVERSITY Diabetes in Aboriginal and Torres Strait Islander communities

Type 2 DM represents a serious public health problem for Aboriginal and Torres Strait Islander communities, occurring at a much higher rate than in the non-Indigenous population, and with a much earlier age of onset of the disease and its micro- and macrovascular complications. It is likely that type 2 DM is an important contributor to the considerably higher circulatory disease mortality rate among Aboriginal and Torres Strait Islander communities at younger ages. Thus, type 2 DM imposes significant financial and human costs on Australian society, which are disproportionately borne by Aboriginal and Torres Strait Islander communities.

The National Aboriginal and Torres Strait Islander Health Survey of 2018–2019 found that 8% of Aboriginal and Torres Strait Islander people reported they had DM (ABS, 2019), the most common being type 2 DM. The prevalence of DM is almost three higher in Aboriginal and Torres Strait Islander communities than in the rest of the population across all age groups. In 2021, diabetes was the second leading cause of death for Aboriginal and Torres Strait Islander people (ABS, 2022). The incidence of GDM in pregnancy is also two to three times higher among Aboriginal and Torres Strait Islander women than in the general Australian population. Living in remote areas also increases the prevalence rates for Aboriginal and Torres Strait Islander groups to six times higher than non-remote areas.

TABLE 19.2 Implications for nursing care of the older adult with diabetes

HEALTH PROBLEM/COMPLICATION	IMPLICATIONS FOR NURSING CARE
Urinary incontinence	Polyuria, a classic manifestation of DM, often is ignored. This problem also often leads to social isolation.
Increased thirst	Polydipsia, a classic manifestation of DM, often is ignored. This further increases the risk of dehydration and electrolyte imbalances.
Decreased hunger and weight loss	Polyphagia, a classic manifestation of DM, often is ignored. The ageing process, medications, depression or lack of socialisation may decrease hunger. Weight loss may be gradual and go unnoticed.
Fatigue	Fatigue is a common symptom of DM but may be blamed on increased age.
Hypoglycaemia	The older adult may have either very mild manifestations or none at all. As a result, hypoglycaemia is often ignored until it causes serious effects.
Peripheral neuropathy	Manifestations may be thought to be due to arthritis, and over-the-counter drugs often are used to self-medicate. The risk of falls increases, as does the risk of gangrene and amputation.
Peripheral vascular disease	May go undetected if the person does not get enough exercise to cause claudication. May also impair abilities to climb stairs and walk.
Diabetic retinopathy	May be undetected if the person has cataracts. The diabetic person also has an increased incidence of cataracts and glaucoma. Deficits in vision threaten independence, mobility and social interactions. Yellowing of the lens with age makes it difficult to read coloured test strips; numerical meters are preferable. Filling insulin syringes may be impossible for the person with macular degeneration or other causes of visual loss.
Hypertension	Treatment with diuretics may further impair glucose tolerance and result in electrolyte imbalances.
Arthritis	Older adults may believe the pain from arthritis to be more important than the DM management. Also, depression from chronic pain as well as inactivity and loss of appetite may interfere with DM self-care.
Parkinson's disease	The tremors and rigidity of this disease make self-care involving fine and gross motor skills difficult or impossible.
Medications	Older adults commonly take more than one type of medication and are at increased risk of problems relating to drug interactions.

Sources: Adapted from Haire-Joshu (1996). *Management of diabetes mellitus: Perspectives of care across the lifespan* (2nd ed.), pp. 755–830. St Louis, MO: Mosby; Eliopoulos (2005). *Gerontological nursing* (6th ed.). Philadelphia: Lippincott Williams & Wilkins.

INTERPROFESSIONAL CARE

Diagnosis

Diagnostic tests are conducted for screening purposes and to diagnose DM, and ongoing laboratory tests are conducted to evaluate the effectiveness of diabetic management. Definitions of normal BGLs vary in clinical practice, depending on the laboratory that performs the assay.

DIAGNOSTIC SCREENING According to the Royal College of General Practitioners (RACGP, 2020), DM is diagnosed if any of the following criteria are satisfied:

1. Glycosylated (glycated) haemoglobin (HbA1c $\geq$ 6.5% or 48 mmol/mol) is now an accepted method of diagnosing DM and is most useful in identifying macrovascular disease. The benefits of this test are it can be performed at any time of day, there is no pre-test preparation required and the testing is funded under Medicare. When interpreting HbA1c, it is important to consider any conditions that may affect red blood cells such as vitamin deficiency or anaemia.
2. Symptoms of diabetes (polyuria, polydipsia, unexplained weight loss) and random blood glucose (RBG; > 2 hours post prandial) $\geq$ 11.1 mmol/L.
3. Fasting blood glucose (FBG) $\geq$ 7.0 mmol/L.
4. Oral glucose tolerance test (OGTT) after 75 g glucose load, fasting plasma glucose $\geq$ 7.0 mmol/L or 2-hour plasma glucose result $\geq$ 11.1 mmol/L:
   a. Impaired glucose tolerance is diagnosed if a plasma glucose result 2 hours after a 75 g glucose load is between 7.8 and 11.0 mmol/L (inclusive).
   b. Impaired fasting glucose is diagnosed if a fasting plasma glucose result is between 6.1 and 6.9 mmol/L (inclusive).

In the absence of unequivocal symptoms, or if the BGL is borderline, diagnosis by criterion 2 or 3 should be confirmed by repeat testing on a separate day.

With regard to testing for FBG:

- People must fast from food and fluids for at least 8 hours prior to blood collection.
- The criteria apply to people who are otherwise well at the time of diagnosis. Physiological stress from infection, trauma or other illness, or the effect of some drugs, may cause false positive results. In general, the criteria should be applied to ambulant outpatients only.
- Samples for plasma glucose should be separated from red cells as soon as possible after collection. When there may be a delay greater than 1 hour prior to centrifugation, samples must be collected into fluoride-oxalate tubes (grey-top). Even with these tubes, a fall in plasma glucose of 0.1–0.2 mmol/L may occur.
- The criteria apply to venous plasma samples. Capillary or whole blood samples may require alternative decision points depending on the analysis method used.
- Home blood glucose meters are not appropriate methods for the diagnosis of diabetes.
- A fasting plasma glucose less than 5.5 mmol/L indicates a low probability of diabetes.

Who should be screened?

- People over the age of 40 should be screened for DM risk every 3 years using the Australian type 2 diabetes risk assessment tool (AUSDRISK). Those with a risk score of 12 or more should have a blood examination for FBG or HbA1c.

- Aboriginal and Torres Strait Islander people from 18 years of age.
- Anyone with symptoms suggestive of DM or who is in the high-risk category.
- Asymptomatic people of any age with impaired glucose tolerance (IGT), impaired fasting glucose (IFG) or cardiovascular disease should be screened annually for DM using FBG.

Interpretation of screening test If the FBG is:

- < 5.5 mmol/L—DM is unlikely; offer lifestyle advice as necessary and re-test in 3 years
- 5.5–6.9 mmol/L—DM is possible; may need OGTT
- ≥ 7.0 mmol/L—DM likely; confirm with repeat FBG on a separate occasion (RACGP, 2020).

DIAGNOSTIC TESTS TO MONITOR DM MANAGEMENT

The following diagnostic tests may be used to monitor DM management:

- *Fasting blood glucose (FBG).* This test is often ordered, especially if the person is experiencing symptoms of hypoglycaemia or hyperglycaemia. The FBG target range for people with DM is 4.0 to 7.0 mmol/L.
- *Glycated haemoglobin (c) (HbA1c or A1c).* This test determines the average BGL over approximately the previous 2 to 3 months. When glucose is elevated or control of glucose is erratic, glucose attaches to the haemoglobin molecule and remains attached for the life of the haemoglobin, which is about 120 days. HbA1c or A1c should be performed at the initial assessment and then every 3 to 6 months. The goal for most people with diabetes is an HbA1c of ≤ 7%, although this may need to be adjusted according to individuals (RACGP, 2020).
- *Urine glucose and ketone levels.* These are not as accurate in monitoring changes in blood glucose as blood levels. The presence of glucose in the urine indicates hyperglycaemia. Most people have a renal threshold for glucose of 10 mmol/L; that is, when the blood glucose exceeds 10 mmol/L, glucose is not reabsorbed by the kidney and spills over into the urine. However, this number varies between individuals. **Ketonuria** (the presence of ketones in the urine) occurs with the breakdown of fats and is an indicator of DKA; however, fat breakdown and ketonuria also occur in states of less-than-normal nutrition.
- *Albuminuria.* This is the presence of protein as albumin. If albuminuria is present, a 24-hour urine collection for creatinine clearance is used to detect the early onset of nephropathy.
- *Serum cholesterol and triglyceride.* These are indicators of atherosclerosis and an increased risk of cardiovascular impairments. Generally, people with DM have similar rates of HDL or 'good' cholesterol to the general population but, on average, people with DM have higher levels of triglycerides and LDL or 'bad' cholesterol. DM affects the balance between HDL and LDL in a number of ways.
- *Serum electrolytes.* Levels are measured in people who have DKA or hyperosmolar hyperglycaemic state (HHS) to determine imbalances.

SELF-MONITORING BLOOD GLUCOSE Self-monitoring blood glucose (SMBG) is a valuable tool for the person with DM and for their carer or health professional. Regularly monitoring one's own BGLs encourages good self-management and alerts carers and health professionals to possible issues in the management of DM. SMBG is a simple procedure which gives a result within seconds. In Australia, there are several types of blood glucose meters available for this purpose. Following are the requirements for self-blood glucose monitoring:

- Handwash with soap and water.
- Lancet device and lancets to perform a finger prick for obtaining a drop of blood.
- Test strips (check expiry date).
- A blood glucose meter appropriate for the person's individual needs. The manufacturer's instructions for use and maintenance of the meter must be followed correctly.
- Information on blood glucose monitoring and different blood glucose monitoring devices available in Australia can be found at https://www.ndss.com.au/type-1-blood-glucose-monitoring.

Blood glucose meters within the healthcare setting and in diabetes self-management are essential to obtaining BGLs to support good diabetes management. The Australian Diabetes Educators Association (2015) has developed guidelines to assist health professionals in choosing the appropriate device, training and education for use and quality control. This ensures timely and appropriate management of the person with diabetes, improved glucose control and better quality of life.

Flash glucose monitors (FGMs) or continuous glucose monitors (CGMs) are alternative glucose monitoring approaches. An FGM comprises a small electrode sensor that is inserted subcutaneously at the back of the arm for up to 2 weeks at a time (see Figure 19.3). The sensor measures the person's glucose level in interstitial subcutaneous fluid at 5 minutely intervals. The person then obtains their glucose level data by using a smartphone application or reader including information about the last 8 hours of glucose readings.

These readings can then be uploaded and retained so that they can be reviewed by the person's treating health professional. Another key advantage of FGMs is that they can trigger an alarm if the person's glucose levels fall outside their target range. However, it is important to note that FGMs do not completely replace the need for BGL monitoring as there is a 5–10-minute lag period between the person's blood and cellular glucose levels (Diabetes Australia, 2022b). Consequently, the person will still need to undertake traditional SMBG using a finger prick in certain circumstances, such as when glucose levels are more unstable (e.g. on sick days) or to confirm hypoglycaemia (NDSS, 2022b).

CGMs also consist of a subcutaneous sensor that is worn at the back of the arm. The sensor continuously measures the glucose levels of person's interstitial subcutaneous fluid. This continuous data is then transmitted to a receiver, smartphone application or insulin pump, enabling the early detection and management of the person's glucose levels in real time. Every 1 to 2 weeks, the CGM sensor is changed prior to being attached to the reusable transmitter. The person with CGM is

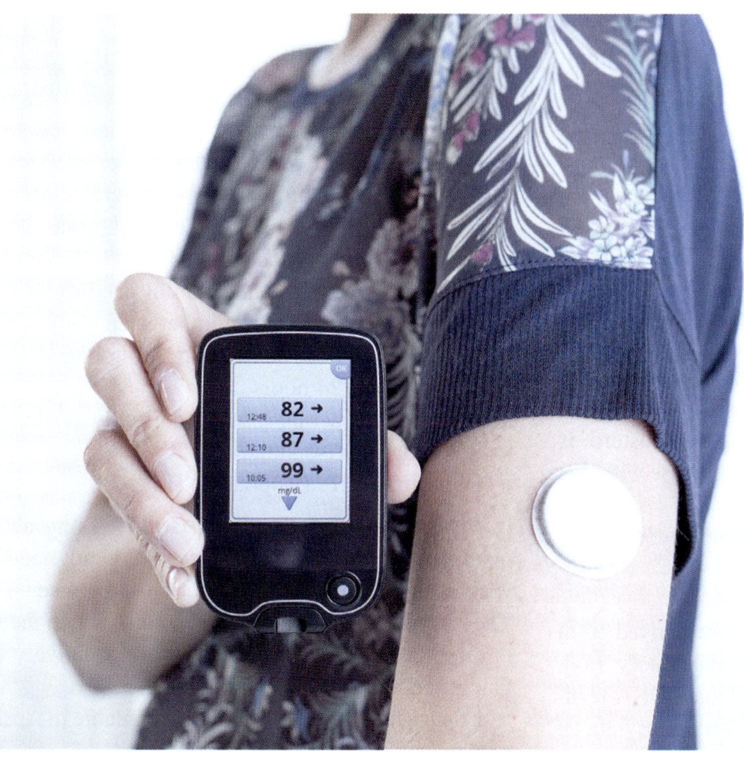

FIGURE 19.3 *An example of a flash glucose monitor*

Source: Click and Photo/Shutterstock.

required to conduct twice daily calibrations by performing SMBG to ensure the accuracy of the readings (Bruttomesso et al., 2019).

URINE TESTING FOR KETONES AND GLUCOSE Urine testing is recommended to monitor hyperglycaemia and keto-acidosis in people with type 1 DM who have unexplained hyperglycaemia during illness or pregnancy. Ketones may be detected through urine testing and reflect the presence of DKA. (See Procedure 19.1.)

HAEMATOCRIT People with higher haematocrit values will usually test falsely low in blood glucose and people with lower haematocrit will test falsely high. Anaemia and sickle cell anaemia are two conditions that can affect haematocrit values.

OTHER SUBSTANCES Overdoses of many medications will cause inaccurate results. Substances such as uric acid (a natural substance in the body that can be more concentrated in some people with diabetes), ascorbic acid (vitamin C) and a variation in haematocrit are known to interfere with glucose readings (American Diabetes Association, 2021). Check the package insert for each meter to find what substances might affect its testing accuracy. Furthermore, strips sometimes give inaccurate readings if they have not been stored properly; therefore, it is relevant that the maintenance and storage of blood glucose testing equipment is followed as per instructions.

Pharmacological treatment of diabetes mellitus

The pharmacological treatment for DM depends on the type of DM. People with type 1 DM must have insulin; those with

PROCEDURE 19.1 Testing urine for ketones and glucose

TO TEST THE URINE FOR KETONES AND/OR GLUCOSE

1. Wear appropriate personal protective equipment.
2. Collect a small amount of urine into a sample pot.
3. Remove a test strip from the container.
4. Dip the test strip into the urine sample.
5. Read desired test result at the specified time by comparing the colour change on the test strip with the standard colour range for your brand of test strip. The reference colour chart is usually printed on the container.

type 2 DM are usually able to control glucose levels with an oral hypoglycaemic medication, but they may require insulin if control is inadequate.

INSULIN The person with type 1 DM requires a lifelong exogenous source of the insulin hormone to maintain life. Insulin is not a cure for DM; rather, it is a means of controlling hyperglycaemia. Insulin is also necessary in other situations, such as these:

- people with type 2 diabetes who are unable to control BGLs with oral antidiabetic drugs and/or diet
- people with type 2 diabetes—or, in some cases, non-diabetics—who are experiencing physical stress (such as an infection or surgery) or who are taking corticosteroids
- women with GDM who are unable to control glucose with diet
- people with DKA or HHS
- people who are receiving high-kilojoule tube feedings or parenteral nutrition.

Sources of insulin Preparations of insulin are derived from animals (pork pancreas) or synthesised in the laboratory from either an alteration of porcine insulin or recombinant DNA technology, using strains of *Escherichia coli* to form a biosynthetic human insulin. Insulin analogues have been developed by modifying the amino acid sequence of the insulin molecule. Although different types are prescribed on an individualised basis, it is standard practice to prescribe human insulin.

Insulin preparations Insulin is classified according to how long it works in the body. There are five different types of insulin, ranging from short to long acting. Some insulins are clear in appearance, while others are cloudy.

Often people need varying amounts of both short- and longer-acting insulin. However, everyone is different and will respond differently to the insulin they take in the management of diabetes.

Types of insulin The five types of insulin are:

1. ultra-short-acting analogues
2. short-acting insulin
3. intermediate-acting insulin
4. long-acting analogue insulin
5. mixed insulin.

Ultra-short-acting analogue insulin Rapid-onset fast-acting insulin has a clear appearance. Their onset of action is within 5 to 15 minutes. Peak effect is 0.5 to 1.5 hours and their duration is between 3 and 5 hours. When people use this type of insulin, they must eat immediately after they inject.

Ultra-short-acting analogue insulin types currently available in Australia are:

- Fiasp® (faster-acting insulin aspart)
- NovoRapid® (insulin aspart)
- Humalog® (insulin lispro)
- Apidra® (insulin glulisine).

Short-acting insulin Short-acting insulins always look clear. The onset is 30 minutes. Food must be consumed within 30 minutes after injecting. Their peak effect is between 2 and 3 hours and their duration is between 6 and 8 hours. Short-acting insulin types currently available in Australia include:

- Actrapid® (insulin neutral, regular)
- Humulin R® (insulin neutral, regular).

Intermediate-acting insulin Intermediate-acting insulins appear cloudy. They have either protamine or zinc added to delay their action. These insulins need to be rolled between the hands before every use and do not need to be injected with a meal. Their onset of action is between 1 and 2.5 hours. Their peak action is between 4 and 12 hours. Their duration is between 16 and 24 hours.

Intermediate-acting insulins currently available include:

- Protaphane® (isophane)
- Humulin NPH® (isophane NPH).

Long-acting analogue insulin Long-acting analogue insulins have a clear appearance and do not need to be injected with a meal. Their onset of action is between 1 and 2 hours. They have no pronounced peak action, which means the insulin is released into the bloodstream at a relatively constant rate. One injection can last 24 hours.

Long-acting analogue insulins available in Australia include:

- Levemir® (insulin determir)
- Optisulin® and Toujeo® (insulin glargine).

Mixed insulin Mixed insulin always looks cloudy. It contains a pre-mixed combination of either a rapid-onset fast-acting or a short-acting insulin and intermediate-acting insulin. This makes it easier because two types of insulin can be given in one injection. If the insulin is '30/70', then it contains 30% of quick-acting and 70% of intermediate-acting insulin; '50/50' means 50% of each. Before injecting mixed or other cloudy insulin, the person must gently roll the vial or pen between the palms of their hands and/or rock it slowly to make sure the different strengths of insulin are evenly distributed.

The mixed insulins currently available include:

With ultra-short-acting insulin

- Humalog Mix25® (25% insulin lispro, 75% lispro protamine suspension)
- Humalog Mix50® (50% insulin lispro, 50% lispro protamine suspension)
- NovoMix 30® (30% insulin aspart, 70% aspart protamine suspension)
- Ryzodeg® (insulin aspart with degludec)

With rapid-acting insulin

- Humulin30/70® (30% insulin neutral regular, 70% isophane)

Other mixed insulins

- Mixtard 30/70® (30% insulin neutral regular, 70% isophane)
- Mixtard 50/50® (50% insulin neutral regular, 50% isophane) (Australian Medicines Handbook (AMH), 2022a; MIMS Online Australia, 2022).

Insulin regimens The appropriate insulin dosage is individualised by achieving a balance between insulin, diet and exercise. In the past, the tendency was to minimise the number of injections per day; however, most people with DM require two or more injections each day, often a mixture of rapid-acting and intermediate-acting insulins. People with DM across the lifespan are being treated with multiple daily injections or continuous infusion using insulin pumps in an attempt to mimic the body's insulin needs, similar to the way the pancreas works in people without diabetes. Timing of the injections depends on BGLs, food consumption, exercise and types of insulin used. The objective is to avoid daytime hypoglycaemia while achieving adequate blood glucose control overnight.

Box 19.1 shows how a combination regimen of insulin three times per day and four times per day is intended to work.

Insulin administration Nursing implications for administering insulin are outlined in the 'Medication administration' box and further discussion follows in the chapter. The considerations for administering insulin include routes of administration, syringe and needle selection, preparing the injection, sites of injection, mixing insulins and insulin regimens.

Routes of administration Only rapid-acting insulin is given by both subcutaneous and intravenous routes; all others are given only subcutaneously. If the intravenous route is not available, rapid-acting insulin may also be administered intramuscularly in an emergency situation.

Insulin delivery devices are available in a variety of forms according to the person's needs. These include insulin syringes, insulin delivery pens and insulin pumps.

Insulin syringes are only to be used with insulin vials. Insulin syringes available in Australia are 30 unit, 50 unit and 100 unit; the size depending on the insulin dose. Needles are usually already attached to the syringe. Insulin syringes are single use only and must be discarded. Syringes are free for people registered with the NDSS.

Insulin delivery pens provide convenience and portability for diabetics. There are a variety of shapes and sizes, but most are pen shaped. A standard insulin cartridge fits into the pen and is replaced once empty. Pen devices are also available prefilled with insulin and the whole device is disposed of once used. Needles are attached to the insulin delivery devices and vary in length and thickness. The higher the gauge, the finer the needle. It is recommended

BOX 19.1 Insulin regimens

Three times daily insulin injections

The diagram below shows how a combination is intended to work.

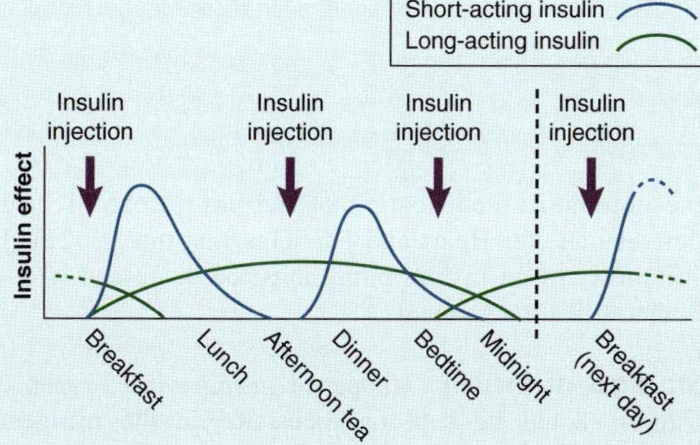

Figure showing an example of a 3 times per day injection pattern with injections at breakfast, afternoon tea and bed

In this routine people have:

- **Before breakfast: rapid- or short-acting insulin (meal bolus) plus long-acting insulin (basal insulin)**
- **Before afternoon tea: rapid- or short-acting insulin (meal bolus)**
- **Before bed: long-acting insulin (basal insulin).**

Four times daily injections (basal-bolus)

The diagram below shows how a combination is intended to work.

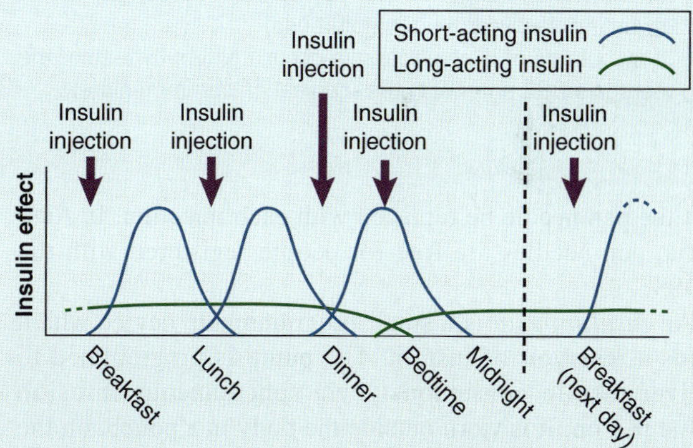

Figure showing a basal-bolus or MDI injection pattern

This routine is often referred to as a basal-bolus injection plan or multiple daily injections (MDI). Commonly about 40–50% of the insulin is given as long-acting insulin and the rest is divided up in the rapid- or short-acting doses. This offers very good flexibility for insulin adjustment and, when part of a comprehensive diabetes management plan, demonstrates advantages for diabetes control. It is the most common starting insulin plan for older children, adolescents and adults. It is also commonly used in younger children, although they will need assistance with injections, particularly at school.

Source: Ambler & Cameron (2010). *Caring for diabetes in children and adolescents* (3rd ed.), pp. 24–25. © Children's Diabetes Services. Reproduced with permission.

MEDICATION ADMINISTRATION Insulin

NURSING RESPONSIBILITIES

- Discard vials of insulin 30 days after opening or where expiration date has passed.
- Refrigerate, but do not freeze, extra insulin vials not currently in use.
- Store insulin in a cool place and avoid exposure to temperature extremes or sunlight.
- Store compatible mixtures of insulin for no longer than 1 month at room temperature or 3 months at 2°C to 8°C.
- Discard any vials with discolouration, clumping, granules or solid deposits on the sides.
- If the patient's meal is delayed, delay the administration of rapid-acting insulin.
- Monitor and maintain a record of BGL readings 30 minutes before each meal and bedtime (or as prescribed).
- Monitor food intake and notify the medical officer if food is not being consumed.
- Monitor electrolytes (especially potassium), blood urea nitrogen (BUN) levels and creatinine.
- Observe injection sites for manifestations of hypersensitivity, lipodystrophy and lipoatrophy.
- If symptoms of hypoglycaemia occur, confirm by testing the person's BGL and follow the healthcare facility's protocol for hypoglycaemia management; for example, administering an oral source of a fast-acting carbohydrate, such as a glass of juice or non-diet cordial, followed by a slow-acting carbohydrate such as a glass of milk or a piece of bread. Hypoglycaemic symptoms may vary but commonly include feelings of shakiness, hunger and/or nervousness, accompanied by sweating, tachycardia or palpitations.
- If symptoms of hyperglycaemia occur, confirm by testing the person's BGL and notify the medical officer immediately.

HEALTH EDUCATION FOR THE PERSON AND FAMILY

- Self-administration of insulin, with a return demonstration (see Boxes 19.2, 19.3 and 19.4).
- Follow instructions for mixing insulins (refer to Box 19.7).
- Always have an extra vial of insulin available.
- Be aware of the signs of hypersensitivity responses, hypoglycaemia and hyperglycaemia.
- Keep sweets or a sugar source available at all times to treat potential hypoglycaemia. Eat within 15 minutes of injecting rapid-acting insulins.
- Vision may be blurred during the first 6 to 8 weeks of insulin therapy; this is the result of fluid changes in the eye and should clear.
- Avoid alcoholic beverages which may cause hypoglycaemia.
- Follow these guidelines for sick days:
  a. Never omit insulin.
  b. Monitor BGLs and/or urine ketones at least every 2 to 4 hours.
  c. Drink plenty of fluids; try to drink at least one glass of water or other kilojoule-free, caffeine-free liquid each hour.
  d. Rest as much as possible.
  e. Contact the medical officer if there is persistent fever, vomiting, shortness of breath, severe pain in the abdomen, dehydration, loss of vision, chest pain, persistent diarrhoea, BGL above 14 mmol/L or ketones in the urine.
- Establish a plan for rotating injection sites and observe closely for changes in tissues, such as hardness, dimpling or sunken areas.

that the pen needle be replaced with each injection. In Australia, pen needles are free for people registered with the NDSS.

An *insulin pump* is a small programmable device which holds a reservoir of insulin. The pump is programmed to deliver insulin continuously via subcutaneous infusion to the person. It is worn outside the body in a pouch, on the belt or bra. The infusion set is a long, narrow tubing attached to a fine-needle or flexible cannula that is inserted just below the skin (usually on the abdomen) where it stays in place for 2 to 3 days. Only short- or rapid-acting insulin can be used in the pump. Whenever food is eaten, the pump is manually programmed to deliver an amount of insulin, similar to the way the pancreas does in people without diabetes. Between meals, a small and steady rate of insulin is delivered. There are several benefits associated with insulin pump therapy including that the person has improved BGL control, there is greater flexibility in the timing of meals and the person may experience fewer hypoglycaemic episodes. If the person also uses CGM, there is the option to use the hybrid-closed loop system, whereby the CGM system relays glucose data to the insulin pump, allowing for the automatic modification of the basal dose of insulin delivery (Baker Heart and Diabetes Institute, 2021). The suitability of an insulin pump must be discussed with the diabetes healthcare team.

Storage of insulin Unopened insulin vials or pen cartridges should be kept on their side in the refrigerator (between 2°C and 8°C) and away from the freezer or freezing coils. Once opened, insulin should be stored at or below 25°C or 30°C and discarded after 30 days, even if there is some insulin left. The expiry date and appearance of insulin must be checked prior to use. Discard any vials with discolouration, clumping, granules or solid deposits on the sides. Insulin is destroyed when exposed to direct sunlight, heat or if frozen, and should be discarded.

Disposal of used syringes Used syringes, pen needles and blood sampling lancets must be disposed of in a sharps container that meets Australian standards, is puncture proof and has a secure lid. These containers are usually yellow in colour and are available through pharmacies, councils and Diabetes Australia. Procedures to dispose of sharps containers vary between the states and territories. For information, contact Diabetes Australia in the relevant state or the state government department of health or the local council. These are also excellent sources of information about where to get help with insulin (see Box 19.5).

Hospitalised people with DM Hospitalised people with type 1 and type 2 diabetes require intense BGL monitoring and frequent adjustments that are responsive to glycaemic changes secondary to the admitting condition and its treatment, including surgery. Some individuals with type 2 diabetes cannot manage with oral medications alone during hospitalisation because additional risks, such as experiencing hypoglycaemia from anorexia or fasting, or the delayed response of these medications to correct hyperglycaemia. Hyperglycaemia is a serious and costly healthcare problem in hospitalised people today and is linked to increased morbidity, mortality and length of hospital stay. Hyperglycaemia is even seen in non-diabetic hospitalised people. Diabetic people with home insulin should be treated with an insulin regimen in hospital irrespective whether they have type 1 or type 2 diabetes. It is vital that BGLs are stable prior to elective

BOX 19.2 How to draw up a mixed dose of insulin from penfill cartridges

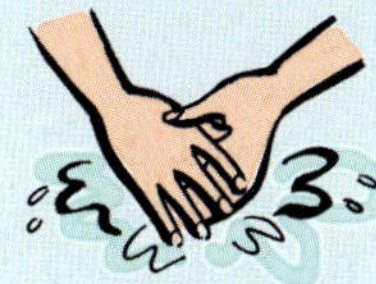

1. Wash hands.

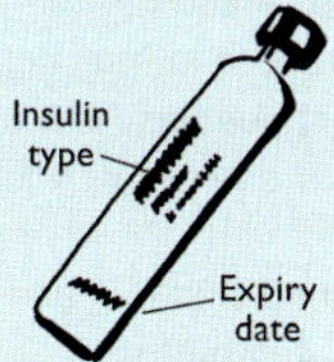

2. Check you have the correct insulin types. You will be drawing up the rapid- or short-acting insulin first.

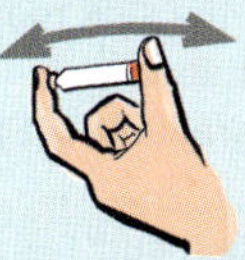

3. If your long-acting insulin is 'cloudy' insulin (e.g. Protaphane®, Humulin NPH®), mix by tipping the cartridge up and down 10 to 20 times. *Do not shake the cartridge* as this damages the insulin. Clear insulin does not need to be mixed.

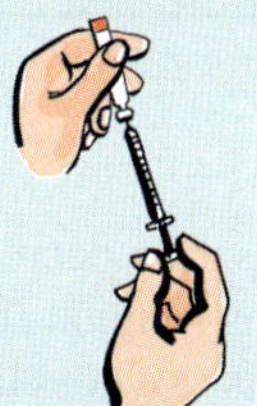

4. Open a new syringe. Make sure there is no air in the syringe by first pushing the plunger right down. Insert the needle into the cartridge of rapid- or short-acting insulin (e.g. Actrapid®, Humulin R®). Pull back the plunger of the syringe to draw up the dose required plus an extra 2 units, which allows you room to get rid of any air bubbles. The rubber stopper in the cartridge will gradually move down as you draw out the insulin and equalise the pressure.

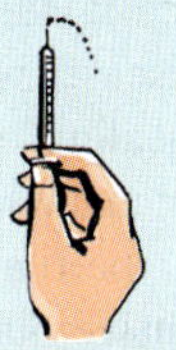

5. Remove the syringe from the bottle, hold it vertically and push the plunger gently to get rid of any air bubbles and any extra insulin to obtain the correct dose. It may help to tap the side of the syringe to remove all air bubbles.

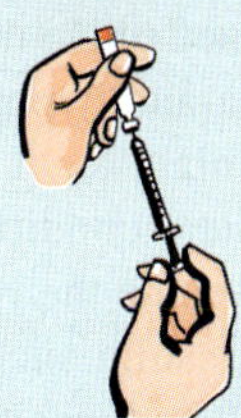

6. Insert the needle into the cartridge of long-acting insulin (e.g. Protaphane®, Humulin NPH®) and turn it upside down. Pull back the plunger to obtain the correct dose. If you draw back too much, you will have to discard the whole syringe and start again. *Do not push any insulin into the cartridge.*

7. Now you are ready to inject the insulin.

Source: Ambler & Cameron (2010). *Caring for diabetes in children and adolescents* (3rd ed.), p. 30. © Children's Diabetes Services. Reproduced with permission.

BOX 19.3 Giving insulin with a syringe

To give an injection with a syringe:

1. Draw up insulin as described in Box 19.2.
2. Take a small pinch of skin with the index finger and thumb. The pinch needs to be at least to the depth of the needle. This is especially important in lean people, otherwise the injection may go too deep into the muscle layer and hurt more and the insulin will act differently.
3. Insert the needle straight into the pinched up skin (i.e. at 90 degrees) to its full length and push the plunger slowly all the way down to push in the insulin. In very lean individuals, injecting at a 45-degree angle to the skin may be necessary to avoid the injection going too deep.
4. Leave the needle in for about 5–10 seconds, then gradually let go of the skin and pull out the needle.
5. Dispose of the syringe in an approved sharps container.

Source: Ambler & Cameron (2010). *Caring for diabetes in children and adolescents* (3rd ed.), p. 31. © Children's Diabetes Services. Reproduced with permission.

BOX 19.4 Giving insulin with a pen

1. Wash hands.
2. Check that you have the correct insulin pen (have your pens clearly marked) and that there is enough insulin remaining in the cartridge for the current injection. It is preferable to use a new needle for each injection.
3. If giving a cloudy long-acting or mixed insulin, be sure to mix the insulin well by inverting the pen 10 to 20 times. The cartridge contains a glass ball which mixes the insulin. Do not shake the pen as this will damage the insulin. Clear insulins do not need to be mixed.
4. Prime the pen (get rid of any air bubbles). Dial up a 2- to 4-unit dose and, holding the pen vertically, inject into the air to expel air bubbles (air shot) and to prime the pen. The pen is primed if drops of insulin without bubbles are coming from the needle. If not, keep repeating this procedure until a bubble-free stream of insulin is achieved with the air shot.
5. Dial up the required dose.
6. Select the injection site.
7. Steady the skin by taking a small pinch of skin with the index finger and thumb at the chosen site. The pinch needs to be at least to the depth of the needle. This is especially important in lean people, otherwise the injection may go too deep into the muscle layer and hurt more and the insulin will act differently. People who are not lean may not need to do a pinch, especially if using short needles (4, 5 or 6 mm), but only use a no-pinch technique if advised by your diabetes team.
8. Insert the needle straight into the pinched-up skin (i.e. at 90 degrees) to its full depth and push the pen button slowly all the way down to push in the insulin. In very lean individuals, injecting at a 45-degree angle to the skin may be necessary to avoid the injection going too deep.
9. Leave the needle in for 5–10 seconds, then gradually let go of the skin and pull out the needle.
10. Remove the needle from the pen after injection and dispose of it in an approved sharps container.

Source: Ambler & Cameron (2010). *Caring for diabetes in children and adolescents* (3rd ed.), p. 29. © Children's Diabetes Services. Reproduced with permission.

BOX 19.5 Where to get help with insulin

- Local doctor or general practitioner (GP)
- (Credentialled) diabetes educator
- Diabetes specialist
- Diabetes Australia: Tel. 1800 177 055 or website: https://www.diabetesaustralia.com.au/

surgery and, ideally, people dependent on insulin should be placed first on the morning list of surgery. Following the hospital protocol for medication administration is important in preventing hypoglycaemia or hyperglycaemia. If the person is undergoing major surgery, or hyperglycaemia develops, an insulin–glucose infusion should be commenced. Clinical practice guidelines for the management of perioperative diabetes recommend target BGLs of 5 to 10 mmol/L postoperatively. Clear written instruction regarding the management of the person's diabetes, including the frequency of BGL monitoring and their medication regimen, should be given preoperatively and again on discharge to prevent complications.

Maintaining normal BGLs during hospitalisation decreases the risk of postoperative infections and shortens hospital stays. Healing is impaired when haemoglobin is glycosylated (HbA1c); glycosylated haemoglobin has increased affinity for oxygen, putting tissues at risk of ischemia (McCance & Huether, 2019). Furthermore, DM leads to small-vessel disease, which impairs circulation and oxygenation of tissue for healing.

Intravenous insulin infusions are preferable for maintaining normal BGLs during hospitalisation, although their use is dependent on frequent BGL monitoring and intensive nursing care. Supplements of regular insulin following sliding-scale prescriptions (relative to monitored BGLs) are ineffective management protocols, risking both hyperglycaemia and hypoglycaemia. These supplements treat hyperglycaemia after it has occurred rather than preventing it. When medical conditions lead to observable periods of hyperglycaemia outside the ICU, it is preferable to provide basal subcutaneous insulin such as insulin glargine or short-acting insulin Actrapid® and mealtime supplements with rapid-onset fast-acting insulin or aspart insulin. Correctional doses can be added to the mealtime doses to keep serum glucose below 10.0 mmol/L.

Principles of insulin adjustment It is useful to think of three main types of insulin adjustments, and in this order:

1. *Long-term adjustments.* These are changes to regular doses based on patterns in blood glucose readings over several days or longer. This may occur:
   - when coming out of a honeymoon phase
   - as the young person with type 1 diabetes grows, and especially when they have their growth spurt with puberty or reach the end of puberty
   - when there is a general change in activity levels.
2. *Thinking-ahead adjustments.* These are temporary changes to some doses based on what is going to happen that day. Examples of this are:
   - reducing a dose or doses for sporting activity
   - reducing an evening dose of insulin after a very active day to avoid delayed hypoglycaemia
   - adjusting a dose to plan for eating more or less at a meal.
3. *Fix-up adjustments.* This is adjusting a dose or giving an extra dose to 'fix up' a blood glucose reading that is unexpectedly high or low. For example:
   - reducing a short-acting insulin dose after hypoglycaemia near to injection time
   - giving a little extra short-acting insulin when the BGL is found to be high before a meal
   - adjusting for sick days.

More detail on these three types of adjustment is given in the following sections. General points include:

- Insulin adjustments are generally based on the recognition of BGL patterns over several days, so enough blood glucose readings need to be done to allow this.
- At times of instability or illness it is necessary to do extra BGL readings to guide adjustment.
- Cautious adjustments in steps are made in insulin doses until BGLs in the target range are reached.
- Unexplained hypoglycaemia requires thinking about insulin doses without delay, and adjustment without waiting for a pattern to emerge may be justified.
- When adjusting, it is usually unwise to make changes to insulin doses every day, or to change too many doses at once, since this can lead to more instability and confusion.
- Frequent dose changes may be necessary when insulin needs are changing rapidly, in which case your diabetes educator or doctor should be aware and able to help.
- People on insulin are advised to adjust their dose in approximately 10% increments and observe the effects over several days before further changes.
- People on insulin pumps need to determine if changes need to be made to the basal or the bolus dose from their monitoring; increments of 5% to 10% are appropriate.
- Some people, children in particular, need variations in dose on a day-to-day basis to adjust for activity and exercise.
- Insulin adjustment also requires a knowledge of the insulin prescribed, particularly when it starts to work and how long it works/the effects last.

Preparing the injection Rapid-acting insulin is clear and therefore does not require mixing. Discard if this insulin is cloudy or discoloured. Other types of insulin, which appear cloudy, must be mixed to disperse the particles evenly throughout the solution. Mix the vial by gently rolling it between the hands—vigorous shaking causes bubble formation and frothing, which makes the dose inaccurate. It is critical that no air bubbles remain in the prepared dose, because even a small bubble can displace several units of insulin.

Sites of injection Theoretically, any area of the body with subcutaneous tissue can be used for injections of insulin, but certain sites are recommended (see Figure 19.4). The rate of absorption and peak of action of insulin differs according to the site. The site that allows the most rapid absorption is the abdomen, followed by the upper outer arm and then the thigh. Because of the rapid absorption, the abdomen is the recommended site. See Box 19.6 for techniques to minimise painful injections.

When administering insulin, aspiration to check for blood is not necessary. Do not massage the site after administering the injection, because this may interfere with absorption; pressure, however, may be applied for about 1 minute. Rotation of injection sites is recommended for people using porcine insulin; rotation within sites is recommended for people using human or purified porcine insulin. The distance between consecutive injections should be about 2.5 cm (avoiding the area within a 5 cm radius from the umbilicus). Insulin should not be injected into an area to be exercised (such as the thigh before a vigorous walk) or to which heat will be applied; exercise or heat may increase the rate of absorption and cause a more rapid onset and peak of action.

Lipodystrophy **Lipodystrophy** (hypertrophy of subcutaneous tissue) or **lipoatrophy** (atrophy of subcutaneous tissue) may result if the same injection sites are used repeatedly, especially with porcine and bovine insulins. The tissues become hardened and have an 'orange-peel' appearance. The use of refrigerated insulin may trigger the development of tissue

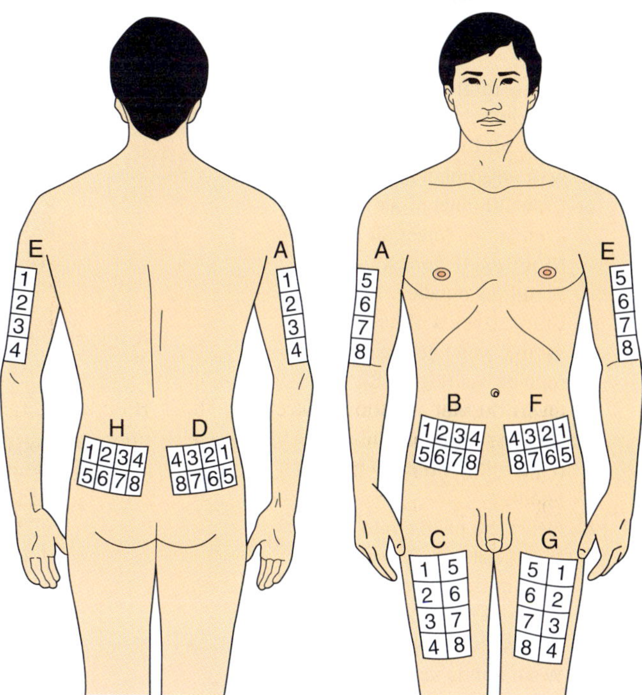

FIGURE 19.4 *Sites for insulin injections*

BOX 19.6 Techniques to minimise painful injections

- Inject insulin that is at room temperature.
- Make sure no air bubbles remain in the syringe before the injection.
- Although the use of alcohol to clean the skin prior to the insulin injection is not recommended for people who use insulin long term, if there is a need for its use due to a possible contamination risk in the skin then wait until alcohol on the skin completely dries before the injection.
- Relax muscles in the injection area.
- Penetrate the skin at 45 to 90 degrees with the needle quickly.
- Do not change the direction of the needle during insertion or withdrawal.
- Do not reuse needles. Always use a new needle with each injection.

Source: Adapted from Hirsch et al. (2010). Comparative glycemic control, safety and patient ratings for a new 4 mm × 32G insulin pen needle in adults with diabetes. *Current Medical Research and Opinion*, 26(6), 1531–1541.

atrophy or hypertrophy. These problems rarely occur with the use of human insulins. Lipodystrophy and lipoatrophy alter insulin absorption, delaying its onset or retaining the insulin in the tissue for a period of time instead of allowing it to be absorbed into the body. Lipodystrophy usually resolves if the area is unused for a minimum of 6 months.

Mixing insulins When a person with DM requires more than one type of insulin, mixing is recommended to avoid administering two injections per dose. Two different concentrations are administered, because a single dose of intermediate-acting or long-acting insulin rarely provides adequate control of BGLs. The procedure for mixing insulins is described in Box 19.7. Following are some general guidelines:

- Commercially mixed insulins are recommended if the insulin ratio is appropriate for the requirements of the person.
- Regular insulin may be mixed with all types of insulin except long-acting insulin or glargine; it may be injected immediately after mixing or stored for future use.
- Intermediate-acting insulin such as Protophane®, Humulin NPH®, HypurinIsophane® (porcine or bovine) may be mixed only with regular or short-acting insulin.
- Do not mix human and animal insulins.
- Always withdraw regular insulin first to avoid contaminating the regular insulin with intermediate-acting insulin.

Hypersensitivity responses When injected, insulin may cause local and systemic hypersensitivity responses. Manifestations of local reactions are a hardening and reddening of the area that develops over several hours. These result from a contaminant in the insulin and occur when less purified insulin products are used.

Systemic reactions occur rapidly and are characterised by widespread, red, intensely pruritic welts. Respiratory difficulty may occur if the respiratory system is involved. Systemic responses are due to an allergy to the insulin itself and are most common with

BOX 19.7 Mixing insulins: 10 units of regular or short-acting and 20 units of NPH® or intermediate-acting insulin

1. Wash hands.
2. Inspect regular insulin for clarity.
3. Gently rotate NPH® insulin to mix well.
4. Wipe off the top of both vials with an alcohol pad.
5. Draw 20 units of air into the syringe and inject air into the NPH® vial (Figure A). Withdraw needle.
6. Draw 10 units of air into the syringe and inject air into the regular vial (Figure B).
7. Invert the vial and withdraw 10 units of regular insulin (Figure C). Withdraw the needle.
8. Insert the needle into the NPH® vial and carefully withdraw 20 units of NPH® insulin (Figure D).
9. Administer the insulin.
10. Wash hands and dispose of the syringe and needle appropriately.

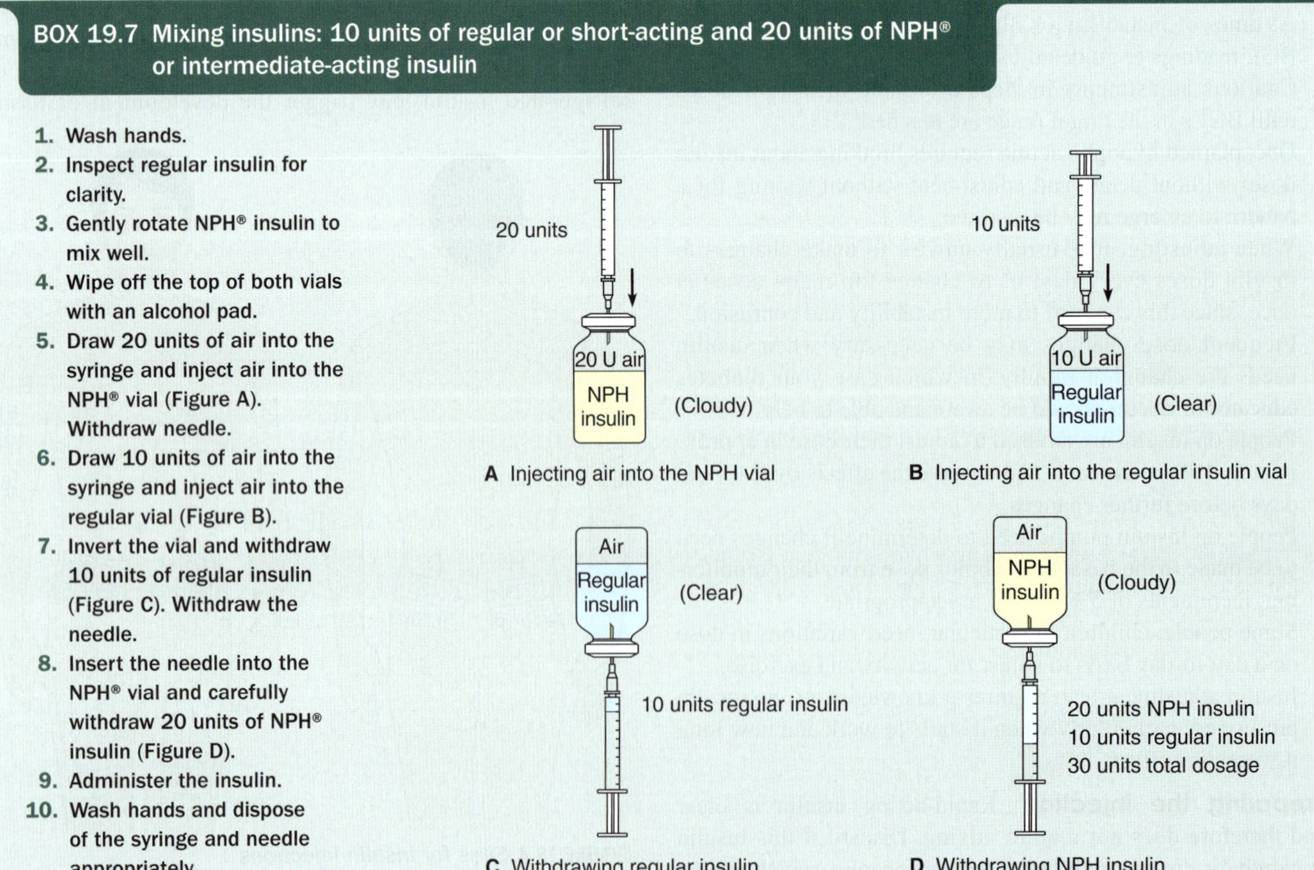

A Injecting air into the NPH vial

B Injecting air into the regular insulin vial

C Withdrawing regular insulin

D Withdrawing NPH insulin

bovine insulin (not commonly used in Australia). The person can be desensitised by administering small doses of purified porcine or human insulin, followed by progressively larger doses.

HYPOGLYCAEMIC AGENTS Oral hypoglycaemic agents are used to treat people with type 2 DM. The nursing implications for this category of drugs are discussed in the 'Medication administration' box. These medications lower BGLs by stimulating or increasing insulin secretion, preventing breakdown of glycogen to glucose by the liver and increasing peripheral uptake of glucose by making cells less resistant to insulin. Peripheral uptake refers to uptake by muscles and fat in the arms and legs, rather than in the trunk. Some oral hypoglycaemic agents keep BGLs low by blocking absorption of carbohydrates in the intestines.

Glucagon-like peptide-1 receptor agonists (GLP-1 RAs) are an alternative hypoglycaemic agent that are available as a subcutaneous injection. They are not a substitute for insulin and therefore are contraindicated in the management of type 1 diabetes and diabetes ketoacidosis. GLP-1 RAs work by mimicking the effects of the incretin (GLP-1) hormones, thereby increasing glucose-dependent insulin secretion and suppressing inappropriate glucagon secretion, delaying gastric emptying and reducing appetite. They are approved for use in Australia as a second- or third-line therapy to improve glycaemic control in people with type 2 DM who are already taking metformin but are not achieving adequate glycaemic control, are contraindicated or are not tolerated (RACGP, 2020). Currently, there are four GLP-1 RAs available in Australia: dulaglutide (Trulicity), liraglutide (Saxenda, Victoza), semaglutide (Ozempic) and exenatide (Byetta) (AMH, 2022b). Exenatide is administered twice daily while liraglutide is a once daily subcutaneous injection. Semaglutide and dulaglutide are longer-acting GLP-1 analogues and are required to be administered only once weekly.

The person receiving a GLP-1 RA will start with a low dose that is then gradually increased every month until the desired level of glycaemic control is achieved. Side effects include gastrointestinal symptoms such as nausea, vomiting and diarrhoea. GLP-1 RAs are contraindicated for use in pregnant women due to the limited data available about them.

LIPID-LOWERING MEDICATIONS People with DM are up to four times more likely to die from cardiovascular disease. Statins are often prescribed if the adult with type 2 diabetes has or is at high risk of developing cardiovascular disease, irrespective of their current lipid levels (RACGP, 2020). A fibrate may also be prescribed if the person's lipid levels remain suboptimal.

ANTIPLATELET THERAPY The increased risk of thrombotic cardiovascular events in people with diabetes is due to enhanced platelet activation and an alteration in the fibrin clotting properties (Parker, 2020).

The RACGP (2020) indicates that antiplatelet medications such as a daily dose of clopidogrel or low-dose aspirin may be given to reduce the atherothrombotic risk in people with diabetes who have history of cardiovascular disease. However, the benefits that result from taking these medications must first be assessed against the associated risks for each patient.

Nutrition The management of DM requires a careful balance between the intake of nutrients, the expenditure of energy and the dose and timing of insulin or oral antidiabetic agents. Although everyone has the same need for basic nutrition, the person with diabetes must eat a more structured diet to prevent hyperglycaemia. The goals for dietary management for adults with diabetes are outlined in Box 19.8.

CARBOHYDRATES AND THE GLYCAEMIC INDEX All carbohydrate foods break down to glucose during digestion. Glucose enters the bloodstream, raising the BGL, which reaches a peak 30 to 60 minutes later. As carbohydrate provides the body with fuel for energy, it should be a part of all diabetic meals and snacks. The quantity and types of carbohydrate-rich foods will affect BGLs. A very high carbohydrate intake may raise the BGLs too high. Foods with carbohydrates include bread, legumes, biscuits, rice, fruit, cakes, pasta, milk and yoghurt, sugar, grains, cereals and starchy vegetables such as potato, sweet potato and corn.

What does GI mean? The glycaemic index (GI) is a guide to how a carbohydrate food may affect the BGL. A low GI food breaks down to glucose more slowly and causes a slower rise

BOX 19.8 Goals for dietary management for adults with diabetes

- Control BGLs.
- Control weight.
- Improve cholesterol levels.
- Reduce the risk for heart disease.
- Improve general health and wellbeing.

The recommended dietary guidelines for Australian adults with diabetes include:

- meals should comprise high-fibre, low GI foods (e.g. wholegrain breads and cereals, legumes, vegetables and fruits) and lean meats, fish, poultry and/or alternatives
- drinking plenty of water and taking care to:
  - limit saturated fat and moderate total fat intake
  - choose foods low in salt
  - limit alcohol intake if the person chooses to drink
  - consume only moderate amounts of sugars and foods containing added sugars
  - eat regularly during the day and spread food over breakfast, lunch and dinner.

Adults with diabetes should aim to eat the following each day:

- 5 serves vegetables
- 2 serves fruit
- 3 to 6 serves of wholegrain breads and cereals
- at least 2.5 serves of low-fat dairy products
- 1 serve lean meat, chicken or fish, or a meat alternative such as lentils, beans or tofu.

People with higher energy needs may require more serves. A dietitian can offer guidance on the quantity of food that the person may need.

Sources: National Health and Medical Research Council (2013). *Eat for health educator guide: Information for nutrition educators*. Retrieved from https://www.eatforhealth.gov.au/sites/default/files/2022-09/n55b_educator_guide_140321_1.pdf; Diabetes Australia (2022c). *Healthy diet for diabetes*. Retrieved from https://www.diabetesaustralia.com.au/living-with-diabetes/healthy-eating/; Nutrition Australia (2021). *Diabetes*. Retrieved from https://www.diabetesaustralia.com.au/living-with-diabetes/healthy-eating/.

MEDICATION ADMINISTRATION Oral hypoglycaemic agents available in Australia

There are six classes of oral medications available in Australia to treat type 2 diabetes. They are prescribed alone or in combination.

1. Sulfonylureas
2. Biguanides
3. Alpha-glucosidase inhibitors
4. Thiazolidinedione
5. Dipeptidyl peptidase 4 (DPP-4) inhibitors
6. Sodium–glucose co-transporter 2 (SGLT2) inhibitors.

SULFONYLUREAS

Glibenclamide (Daonil)
Gliclazide ER (Diamicron MR, Glyade MR)
Glicazide (Glyade, Nidem)
Glimepiride (Amaryl, Glimepiride Sandoz)
Glipizide (Minidiab, Melizide)

Sulfonylureas act by stimulating the pancreatic cells to secrete more insulin and by increasing the sensitivity of peripheral tissues to insulin. The most common side effect is hypoglycaemia; therefore, it is important that the person eat regular meals while on this medication. A person should only be taking one type of sulfonylurea medication. These drugs are often suspended during hospitalisation. Other side effects that may be seen with these medications are weight gain, stomach upset, jaundice and possibly rash (but is rare).

BIGUANIDES

Metformin (Diabex, Diaformin, Formet, Glucobete)
Metformin ER (Diabex XR, Diaformin XR, Metex XR)

Biguanides decrease the overproduction of glucose by the liver, slow absorption of glucose in the small intestine and make the body more sensitive to insulin. Metformin is usually prescribed first for people with type 2 DM. Biguanides should be taken with meals and may help with weight loss and side effects including diarrhoea, nausea and metallic taste. If renal insufficiency develops, metformin must be discontinued. Because of an increased risk of metformin-induced lactic acidosis, it should be discontinued temporarily before and after using contrast media for diagnostic imaging and anaesthesia (AMH, 2022c).

ALPHA-GLUCOSIDASE INHIBITORS

Acarbose (Glybosay)

These agents inhibit the enzyme alpha-glucosidase, found in the brush-border cells that line the small intestine, which breaks down more complex carbohydrates into sugars. Because alpha-glucosidase inhibitors inhibit the breakdown and subsequent absorption of carbohydrates (dextrins, maltose, sucrose and starch) from the gut following meals, the impact of these drugs is on post-prandial hyperglycaemia. Acarbose should not be by women who are pregnant or breastfeeding, or by people with inflammatory bowel disease or malabsorption syndromes. Possible side effects are flatulence, bloating and diarrhoea.

THIAZOLIDINEDIONE

Pioglitazone (Actos, Vexazone)

This class of drugs acts by sensitising peripheral tissue to insulin, by enhancing insulin activity in both muscle and fat cells and, to a lesser extent, by inhibiting hepatic glucose production. Pioglitazone may also help by reducing cholesterol and triglyceride levels. They do not need to be taken with meals. Weight gain may occur due to fluid retention and increased fat tissue. People with heart failure or liver disease should avoid this medication. Liver function should be monitored regularly while on glitazones. An increased risk of small fractures in the arms, hands and feet have been reported in women taking this medication.

DIPEPTIDYL PEPTIDASE 4 (DPP-4) INHIBITORS

Alogliptin (Nesina)
Linagliptin (Trajenta)
Saxagliptin (Onglyza)
Sitagliptin (Januvia)
Vildagliptin (Galvus)

DDP-4 inhibitors reduce BGLs by inhibiting the enzyme DDP-4 and therefore prolong the action of the incretin hormones. These hormones work by reducing BGLs after meals by stimulating insulin production by the pancreas and by reducing the secretion of glucagon, which will decrease the release of glucose from the liver. Tablets need to be taken at the same time each day. People may develop headaches and nausea and have an increased risk of getting a cold. DPP-4 inhibitors should not be taken by pregnant or breastfeeding women and people under 18 years old. Caution must also be taken when administering to people with renal impairment (AMH, 2022d).

SODIUM–GLUCOSE CO-TRANSPORTER 2 (SGLT2) INHIBITORS

Dapagliflozin (Forxiga)
Empagliflozin (Jardiance)
Ertugliflozin (Steglatro)

Sodium–glucose co-transporter 2 (SGLT2) inhibitors work by inhibiting sodium–glucose co-transporter 2, a membrane protein responsible for glucose reabsorption in the kidney. This inhibition results in a reduction of glucose reabsorption in the kidney and therefore an increase of glucose excretion in the urine (AMH, 2022e). The efficacy of SGLT2 inhibitors is reliant on the person having adequate renal function; therefore, this should be checked prior to the initiation of this class of drug. Side effects include genital infections such as candidiasis and balanitis, urinary tract infections (UTIs), polyuria and euglycaemic ketoacidosis. Where possible, SGLT2 inhibitors should be ceased 3 days prior to surgery to limit perioperative risks such as dehydration and UTIs. SGLT2 inhibitors should be avoided for use in pregnant or lactating women because of increased risk for birth malformations.

COMBINATION ORAL HYPOGLYCAEMIC AGENTS

Alogliptin with metformin (Nesina Met)
Dapagliflozin with metformin (Xigduo XR)
Empagliflozin with linagliptin (Glyxambi)
Empagliflozin with metformin (Jardiamet)
Ertugliflozin with sitagliptin (Steglujan)
Linagliptin with metformin (Trajentamet)
Metformin with glibenclamide (Glucovance)
Saxagliptin with dapagliflozin (Qtern)
Saxagliptin with metformin (Kombiglyze)
Sitagliptin with metformin (Janumet)
Vidagliptin with metformin (Galvumet)

MEDICATION ADMINISTRATION **Oral hypoglycaemic agents available in Australia (continued)**

These medications provide the action of two classes of medications in only one tablet in order to achieve desirable glucose control.

Nursing responsibilities

- Assess people taking oral hypoglycaemic agents closely for the first 7 days to determine therapeutic response.
- Ensure strict compliance with medication regimen. Teach the person the importance of maintaining a prescribed diet and exercise program.
- Monitor for hypoglycaemia if the person is also taking non-steroidal anti-inflammatory agents (NSAIDs), sulfonamide antibiotics, ranitidine, cimetidine or beta-blockers; these drugs intensify the action of sulfonylureas.
- Monitor for hyperglycaemia if the person is also taking calcium channel blockers, oral contraceptives, glucocorticoids, phenothiazines or thiazide diuretics; these drugs decrease the hypoglycaemic responses to sulfonylureas.
- Do not administer these drugs to pregnant or lactating women.
- Assess for side effects.
- If the person is to have a thyroid test, determine whether a sulfonylurea has been taken; sulfonylureas interfere with the uptake of radioactive iodine.
- Monitor for hypoglycaemia with concurrent administration of an oral antidiabetic agent and insulin.

Health education for the person and family

- Maintain prescribed diet and exercise regimen.
- You may need insulin injections if you have surgery, trauma, fever or infection.
- Continue monitoring BGLs.
- Report illness or side effects to your healthcare provider.
- Undergo periodic laboratory evaluations as prescribed by your healthcare provider.
- Avoid alcohol intake, which may cause a reaction involving flushing, palpitations and nausea.
- The medication interferes with the effectiveness of oral contraceptives; other birth control measures may be required.
- Mild symptoms of hyperglycaemia may appear if a different agent is commenced.
- Take medications as prescribed—for example, once a day at the same time each day.

in the BGLs compared to a high GI food. Low GI carbohydrate foods should be chosen for a healthy diet. At least one low GI food should be included in each meal (see Table 19.3).

FIBRE A healthy meal plan contains foods high in dietary fibre. There are two types of fibre—soluble and insoluble. Eating soluble fibre helps to lower blood glucose and cholesterol levels. Insoluble fibre absorbs water and regulates the bowel. A variety of plant foods to get plenty of insoluble and soluble fibre should be included in the diet. The aim is to eat at least 30 g of fibre each day. Many of the low GI foods listed in Table 19.3 are also good sources of fibre.

SUGAR Small amounts of sugar can be included as part of a healthy meal—for example, 1–2 teaspoons of sugar added to porridge, or a teaspoon of jam or honey on multigrain toast. Savoury foods containing sugar, such as baked beans and tomato sauce, can also be eaten.

Foods which contain large amounts of sugar, such as soft drinks, regular jelly and confectionery, should be avoided. Some artificially sweetened foods are suitable, but some may be high in fat.

FATS Although BGLs are directly affected by carbohydrates, eating too much fat is also a problem. Fats provide energy and some vitamins, so a small amount is essential. However, too much fat leads to carrying excess body weight, which increases insulin resistance. There are different types of fats in food and some are worse than others. Saturated fat and trans fat increase the risk of heart disease by increasing blood cholesterol levels.

Saturated fat is found in animal products (e.g. butter, full-cream milk, cheese and yoghurt, fatty meats, processed meats, cream, lard), palm oil (often used in commercial snacks and baked products such as biscuits and pastries), takeaway foods and snacks (e.g. chips), and coconut oil, including coconut cream and milk.

Trans fat is found in a variety of foods manufactured with vegetable oils, such as biscuits, pastries and some margarines.

Ways to reduce saturated and trans fat intake are to eat less of the above-mentioned fats, trim any fat off meat before cooking, remove chicken skin, use low-fat dairy products, and use monounsaturated and polyunsaturated oils and margarine

TABLE 19.3 Foods with a low GI

Breads	Multigrain breads; pumpernickel; high-fibre, low GI white bread; wholemeal pita; Mission Lo GI wraps
Breakfast cereals	High-fibre breakfast cereals such as rolled oats, untoasted muesli, multigrain Weetbix
Pasta and noodles	Wheat pasta Most noodles, such as rice vermicelli, soba noodles, mung bean noodles
Rice	Long-grain rice such as Doongara and Basmati; wild, Moolgiri low GI, brown, black and red rice
Grains	Quinoa, barley, buckwheat, semolina and bulghur (cracked wheat), pearl couscous, Israeli couscous
Fruits	Fresh, dried and canned fruit, such as apples, pears, oranges, grapes, grapefruit, peaches, plums, kiwi fruit and bananas
Starchy vegetables	Sweet potato (orange), yam, corn, Carisma™ and Nicola potato *Note*: Most coloured vegetables are low in carbohydrate and have little effect on BGLs; e.g. salad, greens and orange
Legumes and pulses	All types (canned or dried) such as kidney beans, mixed beans, chickpeas, lentils and baked beans
Milk and yoghurt	Low-fat milk and yoghurt, soy milk and yoghurt, and almond milk
Crispbread	Vita-Weat soy and linseed, Vita-Weat pumpkin seed and grains, Ryvita multigrain

Source: Baker Heart and Diabetes Institute (2022). *Carbohydrates and glycaemic index (GI)*. Retrieved from https://baker.edu.au/health-hub/fact-sheets/carbohydrates-gi.

spreads. These foods may still be high in kilojoules; the amount should be minimised if weight control or weight loss is desired.

Monounsaturated fat is found in oils such as olive, canola, sunflower and peanut oil; in margarines made from monounsaturated vegetable oils such as olive or canola oil; in nuts such as peanuts, almonds and cashews; and in avocados and olives.

Polyunsaturated fat also helps to improve cholesterol levels. Polyunsaturated fat is found in oils such as sunflower, safflower and soybean oil, in margarines made from polyunsaturated vegetable oils such as sunflower or grapeseed oil, and in walnuts and fish.

Omega-3 fats (a type of polyunsaturated fat) improve heart health and have other health benefits. Eating fish (fresh or canned) at least twice a week can increase the intake of omega-3 fats. Fish such as salmon, sardines or tuna (including canned) are good sources of omega-3 fats.

Plant sterols are added to some foods, including margarine spreads such as Flora Proactiv™ and Meadow Lea Logicol™. These help to reduce cholesterol levels. The use of these products should be discussed with the health professional, as quantities are important and they are not suitable for everyone.

When used in small quantities, both monounsaturated fat and polyunsaturated fat can help to improve blood cholesterol levels. Monounsaturated fat can help improve cholesterol levels if it is used in place of saturated fat.

Cholesterol in food Cholesterol is found in foods such as eggs, offal (e.g. kidneys, liver and brain) and seafood. Although cholesterol in food can increase the blood cholesterol level, it is more important to limit foods high in saturated fat or trans fat.

PROTEIN Protein is used by the body for growth and repair and is found in foods such as meat, fish, eggs and dairy products. The body's requirements for protein are met by 2–3 serves of dairy foods and 1 serve of meat or fish each day. A higher protein intake is not necessary and many foods high in protein are also high in saturated fat (e.g. dairy foods, meat) so eating more protein may also increase saturated fat intake.

SALT A high salt (sodium) intake contributes to high blood pressure in some people. Reducing the amount of salt that is consumed may help reduce blood pressure.

ALCOHOL Alcohol is high in energy and therefore can contribute to weight gain. If taking insulin or medications for diabetes, alcohol may increase the risk of hypoglycaemia. To reduce the risk of hypoglycaemia, alcohol should not be consumed without having a meal or snack containing carbohydrates.

It is recommended that people with diabetes limit alcohol to no more than 2 standard drinks a day. One standard drink equals 285 mL of full-strength beer, a 100 mL glass of wine or a 30 mL nip of spirits.

SWEETENERS The diet plan for people with diabetes restricts the amount of refined sugars. As a result, many people use non-nutritive sweeteners and foods or drinks made with non-sweeteners. Commercially produced non-nutritive sweeteners are approved for use by the Food Standards Australia New Zealand (FSANZ). Although questions have been raised about the safety of these substances in laboratory animal studies, they are considered safe for use by humans. Included in this category of sweeteners are saccharin (Sweet & Low), aspartame or neotame (Nutrasweet®, Equal®), sucralose (Splenda®) and acesulfame potassium. The non-nutritive sweeteners have negligent amounts of or no kilojoules, do not produce dental caries and produce very little or no changes in BGLs.

People with diabetes can also use nutritive sweeteners, including fructose, sorbitol and xylitol. The kilojoule content of these substances is similar to that of table sugar (sucrose), but they cause less elevation in BGLs. Nutritive sweeteners are often included in foods labelled as 'sugar free'.

Researchers are continuing to study the safety and effectiveness of the sweeteners. When teaching people about diet, the nurse should include information about the kilojoule content of sweeteners and the meaning of such phrases as *sugar free* and *dietetic* on labels.

MEAL PLANNING Several different systems for meal planning are available to the person with diabetes. These systems include a consistent-carbohydrate diabetes meal plan, exchange lists, point systems, food groups, carbohydrate and kilojoule counting. No matter what system is used, however, it must take into account the person's individual eating habits, diet history, food values and special needs. Altering foods and meal patterns is often one of the most difficult parts of diabetes management; careful consideration of individualised preferences enhances compliance with the diet. Although dietitians provide nutrition information and advice, nurses must know what is prescribed and be able to reinforce teaching and answer questions.

For information on diabetes and healthy eating, refer to websites such as https://www.diabetesaustralia.com.au.

Diet plan for type 1 diabetes Diet and insulin prescription must be integrated for optimal energy metabolism and the prevention of hyperglycaemia or hypoglycaemia. The goals of the diet plan are to achieve optimal glucose and lipid levels, improve overall health and maintain reasonable body weight. To meet these goals, the following strategies must be implemented:

- Glucose regulation requires correlating eating patterns with insulin onset and peak of action.
- Meals, snacks and insulin regimens should be based on the person's lifestyle.
- Meal planning depends on the specific insulin regimen prescribed.
- Snacks are an important consideration in relation to the amount and timing of exercise.
- The diet plan must consider the availability of foods, while also incorporating the person's occupational, financial, religious and cultural beliefs and constraints.
- Self-monitoring of BGLs helps the person make adjustments for planned and unplanned changes in routines.

Diet plan for type 2 diabetes The goals of this diet plan are to improve BGLs, prevent or delay complications, and attain or maintain normal body weight. Weight loss is important as many people with type 2 DM are overweight. Weight loss will also facilitate achieving other goals.

There are no specific guidelines for the type 2 DM diet, but in addition to decreasing kilojoules, it is recommended that the person consume three meals of equal size, evenly spaced approximately 4 to 5 hours apart, with one or two snacks. The person with type 2 DM should also decrease fat intake.

Sick-day management When the person with DM is sick or has surgery, BGLs increase, even though food intake decreases. The person often mistakenly alters or omits the insulin dose, causing further problems. The guidelines for dietary management during illness focus on preventing dehydration and providing nutrition that promotes recovery. In general, sick-day management includes the following:

- monitoring BGLs at least four times a day throughout an illness
- testing urine for ketones if blood glucose is greater than 13mmol/L
- continuing to take the usual insulin dose or oral hypoglycaemic agent
- sipping 150 to 250 mL of fluid each hour
- consuming easily digested liquids or soft foods if solid foods are not tolerated (the substituted liquids and foods should be carbohydrate equivalents—e.g. ½ cup sweetened gelatine, ½ cup fruit juice, 1 ice block, ¼ cup sherbet and ½ cup regular soft drink)
- calling the healthcare provider if the person is unable to eat for more than 24 hours or if vomiting and diarrhoea last for more than 6 hours.

Diet plan for the older adult As well as following the same guidelines for type 2 DM, special consideration should be made for the older adult, including:

- dietary likes and dislikes
- who prepares the meals
- age-related changes in taste perception
- dental health
- transportation to buy foods
- available income.

Other factors to consider in planning the diet for the older adult include the age-related decline in kilojoule requirements, decline in physical activity due to age and/or chronic illnesses, and the onset or progression of other chronic illnesses. The older adult who is overweight should reduce kilojoule intake to ensure weight loss; but at the same time, careful monitoring for malnutrition is necessary. It is possible for the older adult to revert to normal glucose tolerance if their ideal body weight is regained.

Exercise

The third component of DM management is a regular exercise program. The benefits of exercise are the same for everyone, with or without diabetes, including improvements in physical fitness, emotional state, work capacity and weight control. In people with diabetes, exercise increases the uptake of glucose by muscle cells, potentially reducing the need for insulin. Exercise also decreases cholesterol and triglycerides, reducing the risk of cardiovascular disorders. People with DM should consult their primary healthcare provider before beginning or changing an exercise program.

The ability to maintain an exercise program is affected by many different factors, including fatigue and glucose levels. It is as important to assess the person's usual lifestyle before establishing an exercise program. Factors to consider include the person's usual exercise habits, living environment and community programs. The exercise that the person enjoys most is probably the one that they will continue with throughout life. People with diabetes should determine the best type of exercise for their individual needs and follow the recommendations and advice of their healthcare provider, diabetes educator and other professionals when engaging in any exercise program. Considerations include using proper footwear, inspecting the feet daily and after exercise, avoiding exercise in extreme heat or cold, and eating a snack prior to strenuous exercise to prevent hypoglycaemia.

ACUTE COMPLICATIONS OF DIABETES

The person with DM, regardless of type, is at increased risk of complications involving many different body systems. Alterations in BGLs, alterations in the cardiovascular system, neuropathies, and an increased susceptibility to infection and periodontal disease are common. In addition, the interaction of several complications can cause problems of the feet. The 'Multisystem effects of diabetes mellitus' illustration shows the progression from cardinal signs to acute and late complications for the person with diabetes. A discussion of each of these complications follows; related interprofessional care and nursing care are discussed later in the chapter.

Acute complications: alterations in blood glucose levels

The following section provides additional information about hyperglycaemia and hypoglycaemia. Table 19.4 compares DKA, HHS and hypoglycaemia.

Hyperglycaemia

The main problems resulting from hyperglycaemia in the person with diabetes are DKA and HHS. Two other problems are the dawn phenomenon and the Somogyi phenomenon.

The **dawn phenomenon** is a rise in blood glucose between 4 am and 8 am that is not a response to hypoglycaemia. This phenomenon may be due to an increase in counter-regulatory hormones such as growth hormone, cortisol and catecholamines which work against the action of insulin and cause morning hyperglycaemia.

The **Somogyi phenomenon** is a combination of hypoglycaemia during the night with a rebound morning rise in blood glucose to hyperglycaemic levels. The hypoglycaemia that occurs during the night stimulates counterregulatory hormones, including adrenaline, cortisol, glucagon and growth hormone, leading to the activation of gluconeogenesis and glycogenolysis while also inhibiting peripheral glucose use. This may cause insulin resistance for 12 to 48 hours (McCance & Huether, 2019).

Diabetic ketoacidosis

As the pathophysiology of untreated type 1 DM continues, the insulin deficit causes fat stores to break down, resulting in

Multisystem effects of diabetes mellitus

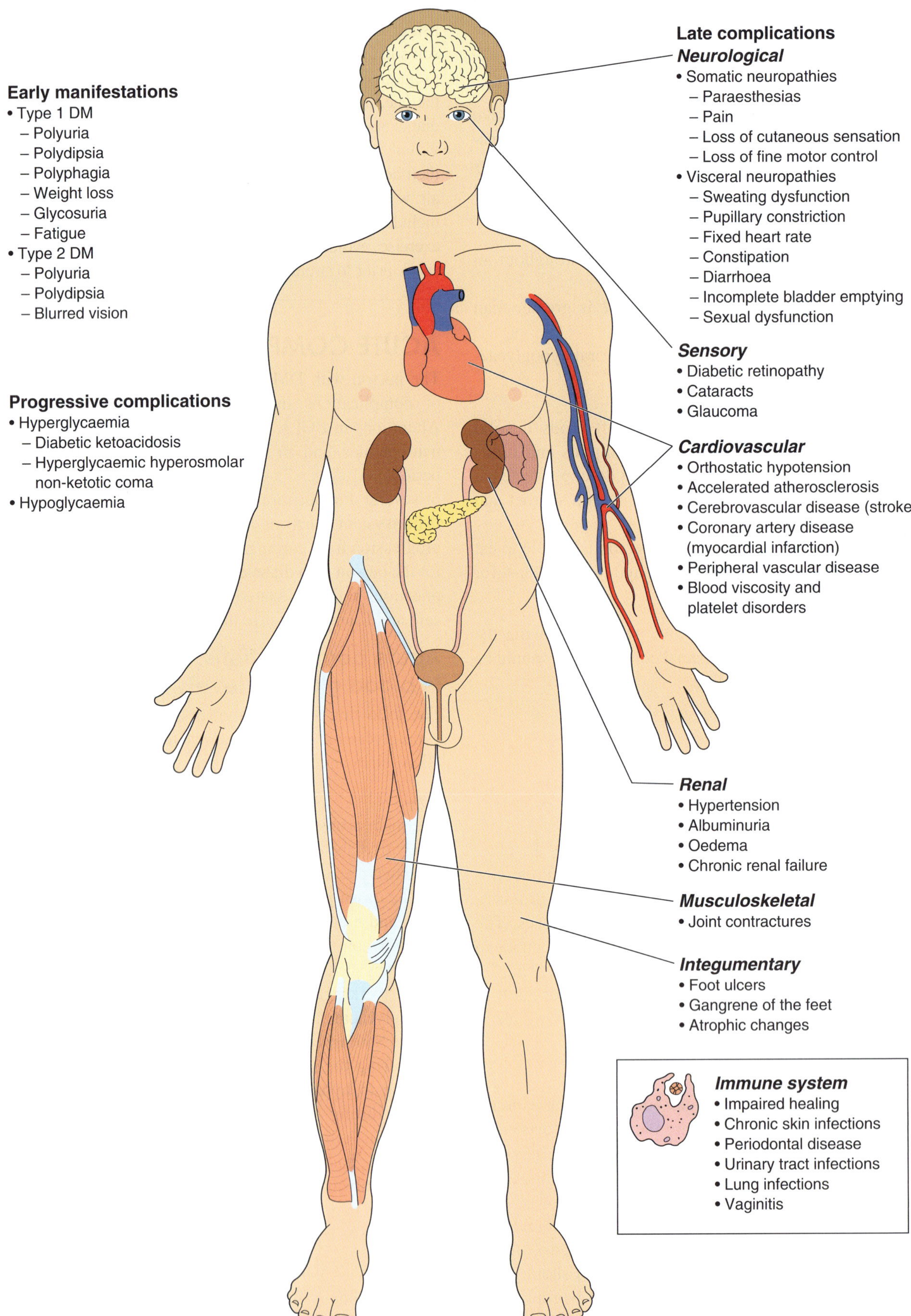

TABLE 19.4 DKA, HHS and hypoglycaemia comparison

		DKA	HHS	HYPOGLYCAEMIA
Diabetes type		Primary type 1	Type 2	Both
Onset		Slow	Slow	Rapid
Cause		↓ Insulin	↓ Insulin	↑ Insulin
		Infection	Older age	Omitted meal/snack
				Error in insulin dose
Risk factors		Surgery	Surgery	Surgery
		Trauma	Trauma	Trauma
		Illness	Illness	Illness
		Omitted insulin	Dehydration	Exercise
		Stress	Medications	Medications
			Dialysis	Lipodystrophy
			Hyperalimentation	Renal failure
				Alcohol intake
Assessments	Skin	Flushed; dry; warm	Flushed; dry; warm	Pallor; moist; cool
	Perspiration	None	None	Profuse
	Thirst	Increased	Increased	Normal
	Breath	Fruity	Normal	Normal
	Vital signs	BP ↓	BP ↓	BP ↓
		P ↑	P ↑	P ↑
		R Kussmaul's	R normal	R normal
	Mental status	Confused	Lethargic	Anxious; restless
	Thirst	Increased	Increased	Normal
	Fluid intake	Increased	Increased	Normal
	Gastrointestinal effects	Nausea/vomiting; abdominal pain	Nausea/vomiting; abdominal pain	Hunger
	Fluid loss	Moderate	Profound	Normal
	Level of consciousness	Decreasing	Decreasing	Decreasing
	Energy level	Weak	Weak	Fatigue
	Other	Weight loss	Weight loss	Headache
		Blurred vision	Malaise	Altered vision
			Extreme thirst	Mood changes
			Seizures	Seizures
Laboratory findings	Blood glucose	> 16.7 mmol/L	> 33.3 mmol/L	< 2.8 mmol/L
	Plasma ketones	Increased	Normal	Normal
	Urine glucose	Increased	Increased	Normal
	Urine ketones	Increased	Normal	Normal
	Serum potassium	Abnormal	Abnormal	Normal
	Serum sodium	Abnormal	Abnormal	Normal
	Serum chloride	Abnormal	Abnormal	Normal
	Plasma pH	< 7.3	Normal	Normal
	Osmolality	> 340 mmol/kg	> 340 mmol/kg	Normal
Treatment		Insulin	Insulin	Glucagon
		Intravenous fluids	Intravenous fluids	Rapid-acting carbohydrate
		Electrolytes	Electrolytes	Intravenous solution of 50% glucose

continued hyperglycaemia and mobilisation of fatty acids with a subsequent ketosis. **Diabetic ketoacidosis (DKA)** develops when there is an absolute deficiency of insulin and an increase in the insulin counter-regulatory hormones. Glucose production by the liver increases, peripheral glucose use decreases, fat mobilisation increases and ketogenesis (ketone formation) is stimulated. Increased glucagon levels activate the gluconeogenic and ketogenic pathways in the liver. In the presence of insulin deficiency, hepatic overproduction of beta-hydroxybutyrate and acetoacetic acids (ketone bodies) causes increased ketone concentrations and an increased release of free fatty acids. As a result of a loss of bicarbonate (which occurs when the ketone is formed), bicarbonate buffering does not occur and a metabolic acidosis occurs, called DKA. Depression of the central nervous system from the accumulation of ketones and the resulting acidosis may cause coma and death if left untreated (Norris, 2018). See Figure 19.5.

DKA also may occur in a person with diagnosed diabetes when energy requirements increase during physical or emotional stress. Stress states initiate the release of gluconeogenic hormones, resulting in the formation of carbohydrates from protein or fat. The person who is sick, has an infection, or decreases or omits their insulin doses is at a greatly increased risk of developing DKA.

DKA involves four metabolic problems:

1. hyperosmolarity from hyperglycaemia and dehydration
2. metabolic acidosis from an accumulation of ketoacids
3. extracellular volume depletion from osmotic diuresis
4. electrolyte imbalances (such as loss of potassium and sodium) from osmotic diuresis.

Manifestations of DKA result from severe dehydration and acidosis.

Hyperosmolar hyperglycaemic state (HHS)

People with type 2 DM are at risk of a serious, life-threatening metabolic condition called **hyperosmolar hyperglycaemic state (HHS)**. HHS is characterised by severe hyperglycaemia

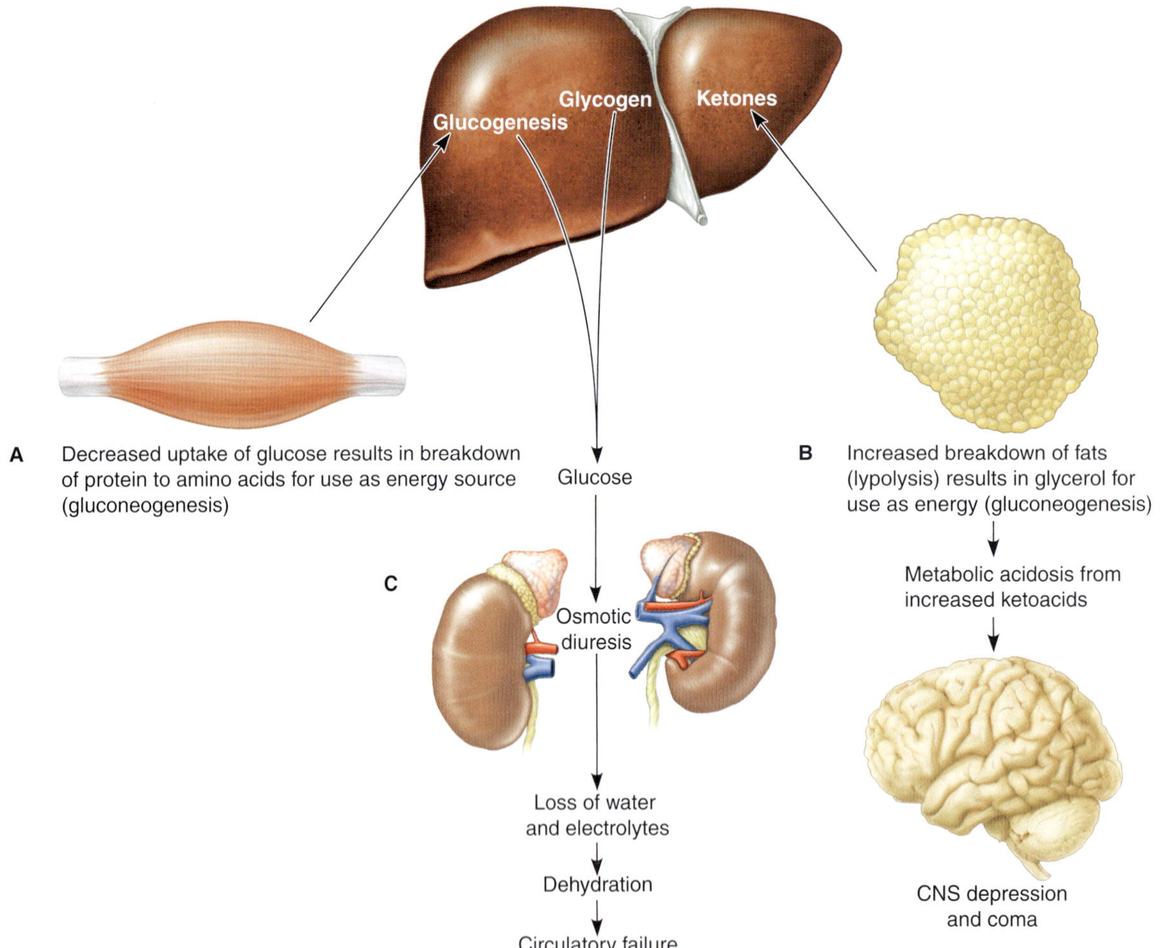

FIGURE 19.5 *In type 1 DM, without adequate insulin, muscle (A) and fat (B) cells are metabolised to provide sources of energy. Amino acids from skeletal muscle are converted to glucose in the liver; glycerol from fat cells is converted to glucose and fatty acids (ketoacids), which cause CNS depression and coma. Increased glucose (C) causes osmotic diuresis, leading to dehydration and decreased circulatory volume. These processes create the symptoms of diabetic ketoacidosis (DKA). The symptoms can be reversed with intravenous insulin to lower blood glucose. Blood pressure is raised to prevent circulatory failure by administering intravenous fluids; electrolytes are monitored and corrected*

(> 30 mmol/L, and often 55.5 to 111 mmol/L) resulting in an osmotic diuresis. Profound dehydration and hypovolaemia ensue, causing the person with HHS to have an altered level of consciousness and a plasma osmolality of 320 mOsm/kg (Willix, Griffiths & Singleton, 2019). HHS is a medical emergency and mortality is high, not only because of the severe metabolic changes, but because people with type 2 DM are usually older and have other medical conditions that either cause or are caused by HHS. The precipitating factors associated with the development of HHS include infection, therapeutic agents, therapeutic procedures, and acute and chronic illnesses (see Box 19.9). The most common precipitating factor is infection. The manifestations of this disorder may be slow to appear, with onset ranging from 24 hours to 2 weeks. The manifestations are initiated by hyperglycaemia, which causes increased urine output. With increased output, plasma volume decreases and glomerular filtration rate drops. As a result, glucose is retained and water is lost. Glucose and sodium accumulate in the blood, leading to an increased serum osmolality.

Serum hyperosmolality results in severe dehydration, reducing intracellular water in all tissues, including the brain. The person has dry skin and mucous membranes, extreme thirst and altered levels of consciousness (progressing from lethargy to coma). Neurological deficits may include hyperthermia, motor and sensory impairment, positive Babinski's sign and seizures. (Note: Metabolic acidosis is not part of the pathology; despite elevated blood glucose, sufficient insulin is present to prevent metabolism of fats with the resulting fatty acids and ketones of DKA.) Treatment is directed towards correcting fluid and electrolyte imbalances, lowering BGLs with insulin and treating underlying conditions.

BOX 19.9 Factors associated with the development of hyperosmolar hyperglycaemic state

Therapeutic agents
- Glucocorticoids
- Diuretics
- Beta-adrenergic blocking agents
- Immunosuppressants
- Chlorpromazine
- Diazoxide

Acute illness
- Infection
- Gangrene
- Urinary infection
- Burns
- Gastrointestinal bleeding
- Myocardial infarction
- Pancreatitis
- Stroke

Therapeutic procedures
- Peritoneal dialysis
- Haemodialysis
- Hyperosmolar alimentation (oral or parenteral)
- Surgery

Chronic illness
- Renal disease
- Cardiac disease
- Hypertension
- Previous stroke
- Alcoholism

INTERPROFESSIONAL CARE

Treatment of hyperglycaemia

DKA DKA requires immediate medical attention. Admission to the hospital is appropriate when the person has blood glucose of greater than 14 mmol/L, a decreasing pH and ketones in the urine. Priority management includes the assessment and management of the person's airway, breathing and circulation and the securement of two peripheral intravenous cannulas for fluid resuscitation. Routine bloods (i.e. a full blood count, urea and electrolytes, liver function tests and a venous blood gas) and blood cultures (to determine the presence of a septicaemia) should also be obtained within the first hour of the person's presentation with DKA. If the person's airway is compromised, intubation and ventilation may be required. If the person is hypoxic, oxygen therapy may be necessary. A nasogastric tube may also need to be inserted if the person has an altered level of consciousness and is at risk of aspiration or has protracted vomiting. Cardiac monitoring may also be implemented to monitor the development of hypokalaemic-related dysrhythmias.

The early assessment and correction of dehydration is essential. In the first 12 hours of treatment, adults usually require 8 to 10 L of intravenous fluid to replace losses from polyuria and vomiting. The initial fluid replacement may be accomplished by administering 0.9% sodium chloride solution at a rate of 500 to 1,000 mL/h. After 2 to 3 hours (or when blood pressure and perfusion is returning to normal), the administration of 0.9% sodium chloride at 250 to 500 mL/h may continue for several more hours. When the BGLs fall to < 14 mmol/L, 10% glucose is added to prevent any rapid decreases in BGLs; hypoglycaemia could result in fatal cerebral oedema.

Regular insulin is used in the management of DKA and may be given by various routes, depending on the severity of the condition. Mild ketosis may be treated with subcutaneous insulin, whereas severe ketosis requires intravenous insulin infusion. Nursing responsibilities for the person receiving intravenous insulin are described in the 'Medication administration' box.

The electrolyte imbalance of primary concern is hypokalaemia. Initially, serum potassium levels may be normal, but they decrease during treatment. In DKA (and from rehydration), the body loses potassium from increased urinary output, acidosis, catabolic state and vomiting or diarrhoea. Potassium replacement is begun early in the course of treatment, usually by adding

MEDICATION ADMINISTRATION **Intravenous insulin**

GENERAL GUIDELINES

- Regular insulin may be given undiluted directly into the vein or through a Y-tube or three-way stopcock.
- Insulin infusion is usually diluted in 0.9% sodium chloride.

Nursing responsibilities

- Monitor blood glucose levels hourly.
- Infuse the insulin solution separately from the hydration solution.
- Prime the intravenous tubing with the insulin infusion to saturate binding sites on the tubing before administering the insulin to the person; this step increases the amount of insulin delivered over the first few hours.
- Do not discontinue the intravenous infusion until subcutaneous administration of insulin is resumed as ordered.
- Monitor for manifestations of hypoglycaemia.
- Ensure that glucagon and/or 50% glucose is readily available as an antidote for insulin overdose or severe hypoglycaemia.
- Follow strict guidelines and protocols in relation to the administration, maintenance and titration of intravenous insulin infusions.

potassium to the intravenous fluids. Replacement is essential for preventing cardiac dysrhythmias secondary to hypokalaemia. Potassium levels must be monitored every 2 to 4 hours or more often, according to the severity of the person's condition. Often continuous cardiac monitoring is necessary.

HHS Treatment is similar to that of DKA: correcting fluid and electrolyte imbalances and providing insulin to lower hyperglycaemia. Treatment modalities include the following:

- establishing and maintaining adequate ventilation
- correcting hypovolaemic shock with adequate intravenous fluids
- instituting nasogastric suction or gastric drainage if comatose to prevent aspiration
- maintaining fluid volume with intravenous isotonic or colloid solutions
- administering potassium intravenously to replace losses
- administering insulin to reduce blood glucose, usually discontinuing administration when BGLs reach 14 mmol/L. (Because ketosis is not present, there is no need to continue insulin, as with DKA.)

Hypoglycaemia

Hypoglycaemia (low BGLs) is common in people with type 1 DM and occasionally occurs in people with type 2 DM who are treated with oral hypoglycaemic agents or insulin. This condition is often called insulin shock, **insulin reaction** or 'the lows' in people with type 1 DM. Hypoglycaemia results primarily from a mismatch between insulin intake (e.g. an error in insulin dose), physical activity and carbohydrate availability (e.g. omitting a meal). The intake of alcohol and drugs such as warfarin, monoamine oxidase inhibitors, probenecid, salicylates and sulfonamides can also cause hypoglycaemia.

The manifestations of hypoglycaemia (see the 'Manifestations' box) result from a compensatory autonomic nervous system (ANS) response coupled with an impaired cerebral function due to a decrease in glucose available for use by the brain. The manifestations vary, particularly in older adults. The onset is sudden and blood glucose is usually less than 2.5 to 3.3 mmol/L. Severe hypoglycaemia may cause death.

People who have had type 1 DM for 4 or 5 years fail to secrete glucagon in response to a decrease in blood glucose. They then depend on adrenaline to serve as a counter-regulatory response to hypoglycaemia. However, this compensatory response can become absent or blunted. The person then develops a syndrome called *hypoglycaemia unawareness*. The person does not experience symptoms of hypoglycaemia even though it is present. Because treatment is not initiated in the absence of symptoms, the person is likely to have episodes of severe hypoglycaemia.

MANIFESTATIONS **Hypoglycaemia**

MANIFESTATIONS CAUSED BY RESPONSES OF THE AUTONOMIC NERVOUS SYSTEM

- Hunger
- Shakiness
- Nausea
- Irritability
- Anxiety
- Rapid pulse
- Pale, cool skin
- Hypotension
- Sweating

MANIFESTATIONS CAUSED BY IMPAIRED CEREBRAL FUNCTION

- Strange or unusual feelings
- Slurred speech
- Headache
- Blurred vision
- Decreasing levels of consciousness
- Difficulty in thinking
- Inability to concentrate
- Seizures
- Change in emotional behaviour
- Coma

INTERPROFESSIONAL CARE

Treatment of hypoglycaemia

MILD HYPOGLYCAEMIA When mild hypoglycaemia occurs, immediate treatment is necessary. People experiencing hypoglycaemia should take about 15 g of a rapid-acting or simple sugar. This amount of sugar is found, for example, in three glucose tablets, ½ cup of fruit juice or a regular soft drink, five Life Savers® sweets, three large marshmallows or 3 teaspoons of sugar or honey. Sugar should not be added to fruit juice. Adding sugar to the fruit sugar already in the juice could cause a rapid rise in blood glucose, with persistent hyperglycaemia.

People with diabetes should have some source of carbohydrate readily available at all times so that hypoglycaemic symptoms can be quickly reversed. A meal, including complex carbohydrates, should be consumed immediately so that hypoglycaemia does not reoccur. If hypoglycaemia occurs more than two or three times a week, the diabetes management plan must be reviewed and adjusted.

SEVERE HYPOGLYCAEMIA People with diabetes who have severe hypoglycaemia are often hospitalised. The criteria for hospitalisation are one or more of the following:

- A BGL of less than 3.0 mmol/L and the prompt treatment of hypoglycaemia has not resulted in recovery of sensorium.
- The person has coma, seizures or altered behaviour.
- The hypoglycaemia has been treated, but a responsible adult cannot be with the person for the following 12 hours.
- The hypoglycaemia was caused by a sulfonylurea drug.

If the person is conscious and alert, 10 to 15 g of an oral carbohydrate may be given. If the person has altered levels of consciousness, parenteral glucose or glucagon is administered.

Glucose is administered intravenously as a 25–50% solution, usually at a rate of 10 mL over 1 minute by intravenous push or bolus, as the most rapid method of increasing BGLs.

Glucagon is an antihypoglycaemic agent that raises blood glucose by promoting the conversion of hepatic glycogen to glucose. It is used in severe insulin-induced hypoglycaemia and may be given in the recommended dose of 1 mg by the subcutaneous, intramuscular or intravenous routes. Glucagon has a short period of action; an oral carbohydrate (after the person becomes responsive) or an intravenous glucose infusion should be administered following the glucagon to prevent a recurrence of hypoglycaemia. If the person has been unconscious, glucagon may cause vomiting when consciousness returns.

Chronic complications

Alterations in the cardiovascular system

The macrocirculation (large blood vessels) in people with diabetes undergoes changes due to atherosclerosis; abnormalities in platelets, red blood cells and clotting factors; and changes in arterial walls. There is an increased incidence and an earlier age of onset of atherosclerosis in people with diabetes (although the reasons for this development are largely unknown). Other risk factors that contribute to the development of macrovascular disease of diabetes are hypertension, hyperlipidaemia, cigarette smoking and obesity. Alterations in the vascular system increase the risk of the long-term complications of coronary artery disease, cerebral vascular disease and peripheral vascular disease.

Alterations in the microcirculation in the person with diabetes involve structural defects in the basement membrane of smaller blood vessels and capillaries. (The basement membrane is the structure that supports and serves as the boundary around the space occupied by epithelial cells.) These defects cause the capillary basement membrane to thicken, eventually resulting in decreased tissue perfusion. Changes in basement membranes are believed to be due to one or more of the following: the presence of increased amounts of sorbitol (a substance formed as an intermediate step in the conversion of glucose to fructose), the formation of abnormal glycoproteins, or problems in the release of oxygen from haemoglobin (Norris, 2018). The effects of alterations in the microcirculation affect all body tissues but are seen primarily in the eyes and the kidneys.

Coronary artery disease

Coronary artery disease is a major risk factor in the development of myocardial infarction in people with diabetes, especially in the middle to older adult with type 2 DM. In 2020, coronary artery disease was the most common cause of death for people with diabetes in Australia (AIHW, 2022). Aboriginal and Torres Strait Islander people have a much higher incidence of death due to DM and ischaemic heart disease than non-Indigenous Australians. Diabetes is often reported as an associated cause of death when a person dies from ischaemic heart disease (see the chapter 'Nursing care of people with coronary heart disease'). Ischaemic heart disease and DM often occur concurrently, and DM can cause or exacerbate ischaemic heart disease.

Hypertension

Hypertension (blood pressure $\geq$ 140/90 mmHg) is a common complication of DM. It affects 20–60% of all people with diabetes and is a major risk factor for cardiovascular disease and microvascular complications such as retinopathy and nephropathy. Hypertension may be reduced by weight loss, exercise, and decreasing sodium intake and alcohol consumption. If these methods are not effective, treatment with antihypertensive medications is necessary.

Stroke

People with diabetes, especially older adults with type 2 DM, are two to six times more likely to have a stroke. Atherosclerosis of the cerebral vessels develops at an earlier age and is more extensive in people with diabetes due to high glucose levels over time leading to increased fat deposits in the blood vessel walls (Norris, 2018).

The manifestations of impaired cerebral circulation are often similar to those of hypoglycaemia or HHS: blurred vision, slurred speech, weakness and dizziness. People with these manifestations have potentially life-threatening health problems and require constant medical attention.

Peripheral vascular disease

Peripheral vascular disease of the lower extremities accompanies both types of DM, but the incidence is greater in people with type 2 DM. Atherosclerosis of vessels in the legs of people with diabetes begins at an earlier age, advances more rapidly and is equally common in both men and women. Impaired peripheral vascular circulation leads to peripheral vascular insufficiency with intermittent claudication (pain) in the lower legs and ulcerations of the feet. Occlusion and thrombosis of large vessels and small arteries and arterioles, as well as alterations in neurological function and infection, result in gangrene (necrosis or the death of tissue). Gangrene from diabetes is the most common cause of non-traumatic amputations of the lower leg. In people with diabetes, dry gangrene is most common, manifested by cold, dry, shrivelled and black tissues of the toes and feet. The gangrene usually begins in the toes and moves proximally into the foot.

Diabetic retinopathy

Diabetic retinopathy is the term used for the retinal changes that occur in the person with diabetes. The retinal capillary structure undergoes alterations in blood flow, leading to retinal ischaemia and a breakdown in the blood–retinal barrier. Retinopathy is a major long-term complication of diabetes, with approximately 40% people living with diabetes over the age of 40 having a degree of retinopathy (Watson et al., 2021). The development of retinopathy is strongly related to the length of time diabetes has been present and the degree of blood glucose control. Regular eye checks and treatment can help prevent retinopathy.

Retinopathy has three stages:

- *Stage I*: non-proliferative retinopathy. Dilated veins, microaneurysms, oedema of the macula and the presence of exudates characterise this stage.
- *Stage II*: pre-proliferative retinopathy. Retinal ischaemia causes infarcts of the nerve fibre layer, with characteristic 'cotton wool' patches on the retina. Shunts form between occluded and patent vessels.
- *Stage III*: proliferative retinopathy. As fibrous tissue and new vessels form in the retina or optic disc, traction on the vitreous humor may cause haemorrhage or retinal detachment.

After 20 years of diabetes, almost all people with type 1 DM and more than 60% of people with type 2 DM will have some degree of retinopathy, in most cases without vision loss. If exudate, oedema, haemorrhage or ischaemia occurs near the fovea, the person experiences visual impairment at any stage. In addition, the person with diabetes is at increased risk of developing cataracts (opacity of the lens) as a result of increased glucose levels within the lens itself. Screening for retinopathy is important, as laser photocoagulation surgery has proven beneficial in preventing loss of vision. Aboriginal and Torres Strait Islander people have an increased incidence (5.5% compared to 1.5% of non-Indigenous Australians) and rate of new cases of diabetes-associated retinopathy; therefore, this population needs to have culturally safe and appropriate resources allocated to improve the early detection, monitoring and treatment of diabetic retinopathy (Gilden, McKenzie & Anjou, 2022).

Diabetic nephropathy

Diabetic nephropathy is a disease of the kidneys characterised by the presence of albumin in the urine, hypertension, oedema and progressive renal insufficiency. Diabetes is the fastest-growing cause of renal failure. It is the leading cause of end-stage renal disease (ESRD). About 30% of people with diabetes will develop kidney disease.

Despite research, the exact pathological origin of diabetic nephropathy is unknown; it has been established, however, that thickening of the basement membrane of the glomeruli eventually impairs renal function. It has been suggested that an increased intracellular concentration of glucose supports the formation of abnormal glycoproteins in the basement membrane and mesangium. The accumulation of these large proteins stimulates glomerulosclerosis (fibrosis of the glomerular tissue). Glomerulosclerosis thickens the basement membrane and simultaneously makes it functionally leaky, allowing large molecules such as protein to be lost in the urine. *Kimmelstiel–Wilson syndrome* is a type of glomerulosclerosis found only in people with diabetes. In advanced nephropathy, tubular atrophy occurs and end-stage renal disease results. (Renal failure is discussed in the chapter 'Nursing care of people with kidney disorders'.)

The first indication of nephropathy is **microalbuminuria**, a low but abnormal level of albumin in the urine. Without specific interventions, people with type 1 DM with sustained microalbuminuria will develop overt nephropathy, accompanied by hypertension, over a period of 10 to 15 years. People with type 2 DM often have microalbuminuria and overt nephropathy shortly after diagnosis, because the diabetes has often been present but undiagnosed for many years. Because the hypertension accelerates the progress of diabetic nephropathy, aggressive antihypertensive management should be instituted. Management includes control of hypertension with an angiotensin-converting-enzyme (ACE) inhibitors or angiotensin receptor blocker (ARB), weight loss, reduced salt intake and exercise.

Alterations in the peripheral and autonomic nervous systems

Peripheral and visceral neuropathies are disorders of the peripheral nerves and the autonomic nervous system. In people with diabetes, these disorders are often called **diabetic neuropathies**. The aetiology of diabetic neuropathies involves: (1) a thickening of the walls of the blood vessels that supply nerves, causing a decrease in nutrients; (2) demyelinisation of the Schwann cells that surround and insulate nerves, slowing nerve conduction; and (3) the formation and accumulation of sorbitol within the Schwann cells, impairing nerve conduction. The manifestations depend on the locations of the lesions.

PERIPHERAL NEUROPATHIES The peripheral neuropathies (also called *somatic neuropathies*) include polyneuropathies and mononeuropathies. *Polyneuropathies*, the most common type of neuropathy associated with diabetes, are bilateral sensory disorders. The manifestations appear first in the toes and feet and progress upward. The fingers and hands may also be involved, but usually only in the later stages of diabetes. The manifestations of polyneuropathy depend on the nerve fibres involved.

The person with polyneuropathy commonly has distal paraesthesias (a subjective feeling of a change in sensation, such as numbness or tingling); pain described as aching, burning or shooting; and feelings of cold feet. Other manifestations may include impaired sensations of pain, temperature, light touch, two-point discrimination and vibration. There is no specific treatment for polyneuropathy.

Mononeuropathies are isolated peripheral neuropathies that affect a single nerve. Depending on the nerve involved, manifestations may include the following:

- palsy of the third cranial (oculomotor) nerve, with headache, eye pain and an inability to move the eye up, down or medially
- radiculopathy, with pain over a dermatome and loss of cutaneous sensation, most often located in the chest
- diabetic femoral neuropathy, with motor and sensory deficits (pain, weakness, dysreflexia) in the anterior thigh and medial calf
- entrapment or compression of the medial nerve at the wrist, resulting in carpal tunnel syndrome, with pain and weakness of the hand; the ulnar nerve at the elbow, with weakness and loss of sensation over the palmar surface of the fourth and fifth fingers; and the peroneal nerve at the head of the fibula, with foot drop.

VISCERAL NEUROPATHIES The visceral neuropathies (also called autonomic neuropathies) cause various manifestations, depending on the area of the ANS involved. These neuropathies may include the following:

- Sweating dysfunction, with an absence of sweating (*anhydrosis*) on the hands and feet and increased sweating on the face or trunk.
- Abnormal pupillary function, most commonly seen as constricted pupils that dilate slowly in the dark.
- Cardiovascular dysfunction, resulting in such abnormalities as a fixed cardiac rate that does not change with exercise, postural hypotension, and a failure to increase cardiac output or vascular tone with exercise.
- Gastrointestinal dysfunction, with changes in upper gastrointestinal motility (*gastroparesis*) resulting in dysphagia, anorexia, heartburn, nausea and vomiting, and altered blood glucose control. Constipation is one of the most common gastrointestinal symptoms associated with diabetes, possibly a result of hypomotility of the bowel. Diabetic diarrhoea is not as common, but it does occur and is often associated with faecal incontinence during sleep due to a defect in internal sphincter function.
- Genitourinary dysfunction, resulting in changes in bladder function and sexual function. Bladder function changes include an inability to empty the bladder completely, loss of sensation of bladder fullness and an increased risk of urinary tract infections. Sexual dysfunctions in men include ejaculatory changes and impotence. Sexual dysfunctions in women include changes in arousal patterns, vaginal lubrication and orgasm. Alterations in sexual function in people with diabetes are the result of both neurological and vascular changes.

Mood alterations

People with DM, both type 1 and type 2, endure the chronic strains of living with complex self-care and are at a somewhat increased risk of depression, which can negatively impact their management of DM. Diabetes Australia (2022d) reported that the risk of depression more than doubles in people with diabetes. Treating depression has been associated with better control of serum glucose, so screening for depression is an important part of assessing the individual's ability to manage the disease. Nurses can assist people with diabetes who are experiencing depression by referring the person to a mental health professional (e.g. a psychologist), correcting any misconceptions the person may have about depression, identifying individual strengths in person's management of their diabetes, acknowledging their negative feelings that may be expressed and suggesting problem-solving behaviours to better manage the disease.

Increased susceptibility to infection

The person with diabetes has an increased risk of developing infections. A combination of vascular insufficiency, neuropathies and systemic and local immunological dysfunction as well as hyperglycaemia and altered neutrophil function are believed to play a role in higher infection risks in people with diabetes (Berbudi et al., 2020; Norris, 2018).

The person with diabetes may have sensory deficits resulting in inattention to trauma and vascular deficits that decrease circulation to the injured area; as a result, the normal inflammatory response is diminished and healing is slowed. Nephrosclerosis and inadequate bladder emptying with retention of urine predispose the person with diabetes to pyelonephritis and urinary tract infections. Bacterial and fungal infections of the skin, nails and mucous membranes are common. Tuberculosis is more prevalent in people with diabetes than in the general population.

Periodontal disease

Although periodontal disease does not occur more often in people with diabetes, it does progress more rapidly, especially if the diabetes is poorly controlled. It is believed to be caused by microangiopathy, with changes in vascularisation of the gums. As a result, gingivitis (inflammation of the gums) and periodontitis (inflammation of the bone underlying the gums) occur.

Complications involving the feet

The high incidence of both amputations and problems with the feet in people with diabetes is the result of angiopathy, neuropathy and infection. People with diabetes are at high risk of amputation of a lower extremity, with increased risk in those who have had DM for more than 10 years, are male, have poor glucose control or have cardiovascular, retinal or renal complications.

Vascular changes in the lower extremities of the person with diabetes result in arteriosclerosis. Diabetes-induced

MANIFESTATIONS Peripheral vascular disease

- Loss of hair on lower leg, feet and toes
- Atrophic skin changes: shininess and thinning
- Cold feet
- Feet and ankles darker than leg
- Dependent rubor, blanching on elevation
- Thick toenails
- Diminished or absent pulses
- Nocturnal pain
- Pain at rest, relieved by standing or walking
- Intermittent claudication
- Patchy areas of gangrene on feet and toes

arteriosclerosis tends to occur at an earlier age, occurs equally in men and women, is usually bilateral and progresses more rapidly. The blood vessels most often affected are located below the knee. Blockages form in the large, medium and small arteries of the lower legs and feet. Multiple occlusions with decreased blood flow result in the manifestations of peripheral vascular disease (see the 'Manifestations' box). Peripheral vascular disease is discussed in the chapters 'A person-centred approach to assessing the cardiovascular and lymphatic systems' and 'Nursing care of people with vascular and lymphatic disorders'.

Diabetic neuropathy of the foot produces multiple problems. Because the sense of touch and perception of pain are absent, the person with diabetes may have some type of foot trauma without being aware of it. The person thus is at increased risk of trauma to tissues of the feet, leading to ulcer development. Infections commonly occur in traumatised or ulcerated tissue (see Figure 19.6).

Despite the many potential sources of foot trauma in the person with diabetes, the most common are cracks and fissures caused by dry skin or infections such as athlete's foot, blisters caused by improperly fitting shoes, pressure from stockings or shoes, ingrown toenails and direct trauma (cuts, bruises or burns). It is important to remember that the person with diabetic neuropathy who has lost the perception of pain may not be aware that these injuries have occurred. In addition, when a part of the body loses sensation, the person tends to dissociate from or ignore the part, so that an injury may go unattended for days or weeks. The injury may even be forgotten entirely.

Foot lesions usually begin as a superficial skin ulcer. In time, the ulcer extends deeper into muscles and bone, leading to abscess or osteomyelitis. Gangrene can develop on one or more toes; if untreated, the whole foot eventually becomes gangrenous. (Care of the feet, an essential part of health education for the person and family, is discussed later in the chapter.)

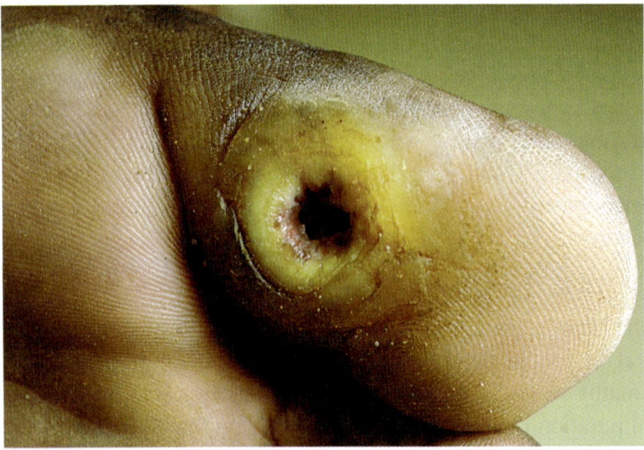

FIGURE 19.6 ***Ulceration following trauma in the foot of the person with diabetes***

Source: Medicshots/Alamy Stock Photo.

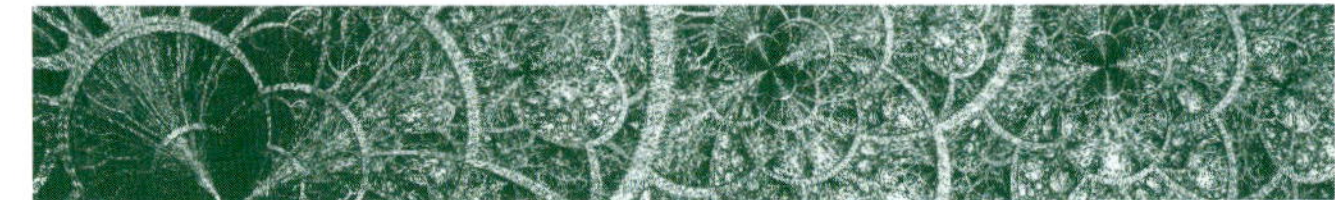

Nursing care

The responses of the person with diabetes to the illness are often complex and individual, involving multiple body systems. Assessments, planning and implementation differ for the person with newly diagnosed diabetes, the person with long-term diabetes and the person with acute complications of diabetes. The plan of care and content of teaching also differ according to the type of diabetes, the person's age and culture, and their intellectual, psychological and social resources. However, nursing care often focuses on teaching the person to manage the illness.

Health promotion

Health promotion activities primarily focus on preventing the complications of diabetes. Prevention of the disease has not been determined, although it is recommended that all people should prevent or decrease excess weight, follow a sensible and well-balanced diet, and maintain a regular physical exercise program. Blood glucose screening at 1–3-year intervals beginning at age 45 is recommended for those in the high-risk groups. These same activities, when combined with medications and self-monitoring, are also beneficial in reducing the onset of complications.

Assessment

The following data are collected through the health history and physical examination (see the chapter 'A person-centred approach to assessing the endocrine system'). Further focused assessments are described with nursing interventions in the following section. When assessing the older person, be aware of normal ageing changes in all body systems that may alter interpretation of findings.

- *Health history*: family history of diabetes; history of hypertension or other cardiovascular problems; history of any change in vision (e.g. blurring) or speech, dizziness, numbness or tingling in hands or feet; pain when walking; frequent voiding; change in weight, appetite, infections and healing; problems with gastrointestinal function or urination; or altered sexual function.

- *Physical assessment*: height/weight ratio, vital signs, visual acuity, cranial nerves, sensory ability (touch, hot/cold, vibration) of extremities, peripheral pulses, skin and mucous membranes (hair loss, appearance, lesions, rash, itching, vaginal discharge).

Nursing diagnoses and interventions

Although many different nursing diagnoses are appropriate for the person with diabetes, those discussed in this section address problems with skin integrity, infection, injury, sexuality, coping and health maintenance. The goals of care are to maintain function, prevent complications and teach self-management. See the accompanying 'Nursing care plan' for more information.

Risk of impaired skin integrity related to diabetic neuropathies

The person with diabetes is at increased risk of altered skin integrity as a result of decreased or absent sensation from neuropathies, decreased tissue perfusion from cardiovascular complications and infection. Impaired skin and tissue integrity, with resultant gangrene, may occur in the feet and lower extremities.

- Conduct baseline and ongoing assessments of the feet, including:
  - musculoskeletal assessment that includes foot and ankle joint range of motion, determining the presence of bone abnormalities (bunions, hammer toes, overlapping digits) or altered gait, the use of assistive devices for walking and abnormal wear patterns on shoes
  - neurological assessment that includes sensations of touch and position, pain and temperature

NURSING CARE PLAN A person with type 1 diabetes

Jim Meligrito, aged 24, is a third-year nursing student at a large university. Mr Meligrito also works 20 hours a week as an on-campus security guard. His working hours are 8 pm to midnight, 5 nights a week. He lives with his father, who is also a student. Neither of the two men like to cook and they usually eat 'whatever is handy'. Mr Meligrito has smoked 8 to 10 cigarettes a day for 5 years. He was diagnosed with type 1 DM at age 12. Although his insulin dosage has varied, he currently takes a total of 52 units of insulin each day, 8 units of Humalog (insulin lispro) three times per day, before each meal, and 28 units of Optisulin® (glargine insulin) at different times in the evenings or before bed. He monitors his blood glucose about three times a week. He feels that he is too busy for a regular exercise program and that he gets enough exercise at work and in weekend sports activities. He has not seen a healthcare provider for over a year.

One day during a 6-hour simulation intensive, Mr Meligrito notices that he is urinating frequently, is thirsty and has blurred vision. He is also very tired but blames all his symptoms on drinking a couple of beers and having had only 4 hours' sleep the night before while studying for an examination, and the stress he has been under lately from his studies and work. When he remembers that he had forgotten to take his insulin that morning, he realises he must have hyperglycaemia but decides that he will be all right until he gets home in the afternoon. Around noon, he begins having abdominal pain, feels weak, has a rapid pulse and vomits. When he reports his physical symptoms to his clinical facilitator, she sends him immediately to the hospital emergency department, accompanied by another student.

ASSESSMENT

As soon as Mr Meligrito arrives at the emergency department, his BGL is measured at 17.0 mmol/L. Urine samples and additional blood samples are sent to the laboratory for analysis. His venous BGL is 18.3 mmol/L and his pH is 7.1 with normal electrolyte levels. Mr Meligrito also has ketonuria. His vital signs are as follows: T 37.2°C, P 140 bpm, R 28 and BP 102/52 mmHg. An intravenous infusion of 1,000 mL normal (0.9%) saline with 40 mmol of KCl is started at a rate of 400 mL/h. Intravenous regular insulin at 5 units/h (diluted in 0.9% saline) is begun. Hourly blood glucose monitoring is initiated. Mr Meligrito is nauseated and lethargic but remains oriented. Five hours later, he has a BGL of 9.0 mmol/L and his pulse and blood pressure are normal. Now there are no ketones in the urine, his vital signs, including his glucose level, are within normal parameters and he has no signs of metabolic acidosis. He is discharged from the hospital the following day after seeing the hospital's diabetes nurse educator. When he meets with the diabetes educator, he says he no longer feels in control of the diabetes or his future goal to become an anaesthetic nurse.

DIAGNOSES

- *Powerlessness* related to a perceived lack of control of his diabetes due to present demands on time.
- *Deficient or poor knowledge* of self-management of diabetes.
- *Risk of ineffective role performance* related to uncertainty about capacity to achieve desired role as a Registered Nurse.

PLANNING

- Mutually establish specific and individualised short-term and long-term goals for self-management to control blood glucose.
- Assess his level of knowledge and establish his needs to develop a program of education in different aspects of diabetes.
- Determine the need and plan referrals to appropriate allied health professionals such as a diabetes educator, dietitian, exercise physiologist, psychologist, counsellor, etc.

Expected outcomes

- Identify those aspects of diabetes that can be controlled and participate in making decisions about self-managing care.

(continued)

NURSING CARE PLAN **A person with type 1 diabetes (continued)**

- Demonstrate an understanding of diabetes self-management through planned medication, diet, exercise and blood glucose self-monitoring activities.
- Explore and clarify Mr Meligrito's perceptions of his role as a student nurse, verbalising his ability to meet his expectations.

IMPLEMENTATION

- Provide opportunities for Mr Meligrito to express his feelings about himself and his illness.
- Explore Mr Meligrito's perceptions of his own ability to control his illness and his future and clarify these perceptions by providing information about resources and support groups.
- Facilitate Mr Meligrito's decision-making abilities in self-managing his prescribed treatment regimen.
- Provide Mr Meligrito with positive reinforcement for increasing involvement in self-care activities.
- Provide relevant learning activities about insulin administration, dietary management, exercise, self-monitoring of blood glucose and healthy lifestyle.

EVALUATION

After taking an active part in the weekly educational meetings for 2 months, Mr Meligrito has greatly enhanced his understanding of and compliance with self-management of his diabetes. He states that he finally understands how insulin, food and exercise affect his body, having previously thought they were 'just things I should do when I wanted to'. He decides to perform self-management activities 1 week at a time, rather than think too far into (and thereby feel overwhelmed by) the future. Both son and father have developed a workable meal schedule and weekly grocery list and they have begun eating breakfast and dinner together. Jim and a friend have arranged to walk 5 to 10 km three times a week on a hiking trail. To gain a sense of control over his illness, Mr Meligrito has also worked out a schedule that allows time for his university studies, work and self-care activities.

CRITICAL THINKING IN THE NURSING PROCESS

1 What is the pathophysiological basis for the changes in temperature, pulse, respirations and blood pressure that occurred on Mr Meligrito's admission to the hospital emergency department?
2 How can poor self-management of diabetes increase the risk of long-term complications?
3 Is powerlessness a common response to a chronic illness? Why or why not?
4 Consider that you are teaching Mr Meligrito and another person, Mr McDaniel (aged 75, newly diagnosed with type 2 DM). What components of your teaching plan would be the same and what components would be different?

REFLECTION ON THE NURSING PROCESS

1 List the aspects that you have learned from this scenario that you will apply to your future clinical practice when caring for a person with poorly controlled diabetes.
2 Detail how you would approach and communicate with a person who has poor management of their diabetes in order to provide advice and education.

  - vascular examination that includes assessment of lower extremity pulses, capillary refill, colour and temperature of skin, lesions and oedema
  - hydration status, including dryness or excessive perspiration
  - lesions, fissures between toes, corns, calluses, plantar warts, ingrown or overgrown toenails, redness over pressure points, blisters, cellulitis or gangrene.

  People with diabetes are at risk of lower-extremity gangrene. Peripheral neuropathies may result in alterations in the perception of pain, loss of deep tendon reflexes, loss of cutaneous pressure and position sensation, foot drop, changes in the shape of the foot and changes in bones and joints. Peripheral vascular disease may cause intermittent claudication, absent pulses, delayed venous filling on elevation, dependent rubor and gangrene. Injuries, lesions and changes in skin hydration potentiate infections, delayed healing and tissue loss in the person with DM.
- Teach foot hygiene. Wash the feet daily with lukewarm water and mild hand soap; pat dry and dry well between the toes. Apply a very thin coat of lubricating cream if dryness is present (but not between the toes). *Proper hygiene decreases the chance of infection. Temperature receptors may be impaired, so the water should always be tested before use.*
- Discuss the importance of not smoking if the person smokes. *Nicotine in tobacco causes vasoconstriction, further decreasing the blood supply to the feet.*
- Discuss the importance of maintaining BGLs through prescribed diet, medication and exercise. *Hyperglycaemia promotes the growth of microorganisms.*
- Conduct foot care teaching sessions as often as necessary (see the 'Meeting individualised needs' box). Include information about proper shoe fit and composition, avoiding clothing or activities that decrease circulation to the feet, foot inspections, care of toenails and the importance of obtaining medical care for lesions. If the person has visual deficits, is obese or cannot reach the feet, teach the caregiver how to inspect and care for the feet. Feet should be inspected daily. *Foot care is a priority in diabetes management to prevent serious problems. Many people with diabetes are unaware of lesions or injury until infection and compromised circulation are far advanced. The hows and whys of each component must be included in teaching. A variety of methods may be used, including demonstration, return demonstration, audiovisual aids and written lists. If the person is wearing shoes and socks, ask them to remove them to practise foot care effectively.*

Risk of infection

The person with diabetes is at increased risk of infection; this is believed to be due to vascular insufficiency that limits the inflammatory response, neurological abnormalities that

MEETING INDIVIDUALISED NEEDS Foot care teaching session

BUYING AND WEARING SHOES AND STOCKINGS

- Shoes that allow 1 to 2 cm of toe room are best; there should be room for toes to spread out and wiggle. The lining and inside stitching should be smooth and the insole soft. The sole should be flexible and cushion the foot. The heel should fit snugly and the arch support should give good support.
- Do not wear open-toed shoes, sandals, high heels or thongs; they increase the risk of trauma.
- Buy shoes late in the afternoon, when feet are at their largest; always buy shoes that feel comfortable and do not need to be 'broken in'.
- Shoes made of natural fibres (leather, canvas) allow perspiration to escape.
- Check the shoes before each wearing for foreign objects, wrinkled insoles and cracks that might cause lesions.
- Socks made of wool or cotton allow perspiration to dry.

INSPECTING THE FEET

- Check the feet daily for red areas, cuts, blisters, corns, calluses or cracks in the skin. Check between the toes for cracks or reddened areas.
- Check the skin of the feet for dry or damp areas.
- Use a mirror to check each sole and the back of each heel.
- If you are unable to inspect the feet daily, be sure that someone else does so.

CARE OF TOENAILS

- Cut the toenails after washing, when they are softer and easier to trim.
- Cut the nails straight across with a nail clipper and smooth edges and corners with an emery board.
- Do not use razor blades to trim the toenails.
- If you are unable to see well or to reach the feet easily, have someone else trim the nails. If the nails are very thick or ingrown, if the toes overlap or if circulation is poor, get professional care from a podiatrist.

GENERAL INFORMATION

- Never go barefoot. Wear slippers when leaving the bed during the night.
- Do not use commercial corn medicines or pads, chemicals (such as boric acid, iodine or hydrogen peroxide) or over-the-counter cortisone medications on the feet.
- Do not put heating pads, hot water bottles or ice packs on the feet. If the feet become cold at night, wear socks or use extra blankets.
- Do not allow the feet to become sunburned.
- Do not put tape on the feet.
- Do not sit with the legs crossed at the knees or ankles.

decrease their awareness of trauma and a predisposition to bacterial and fungal infections.

- Use and teach meticulous handwashing. *Handwashing is the single most effective method for preventing the spread of infection.*
- Monitor for manifestations of infection: increased temperature, pain, malaise, swelling, redness, discharge, cough. *Early diagnosis and treatment of infections can control their severity and decrease complications.*
- Discuss the importance of skin care. Keep the skin clean and dry, using lukewarm water and mild soap. *People with diabetes are more prone to develop furuncles and carbuncles; the infection often increases the need for insulin. Clean, intact skin and mucous membranes are the first line of defence against infection.*
- Teach dental health measures:
  - Obtain a dental examination every 4 to 6 months.
  - Maintain careful oral hygiene, which includes brushing the teeth with a soft toothbrush and fluoridated toothpaste at least twice a day and flossing as recommended.
  - Be aware of the symptoms requiring dental care: bad breath; unpleasant taste in the mouth; bleeding, red or sore gums; and tooth pain.
  - If dental surgery is necessary, monitor for need to make adjustments in insulin. All people with diabetes need to be taught proper oral hygiene, and about the risk of periodontal disease and the importance of obtaining dental care for symptoms of oral or dental problems.
- Teach women with diabetes the symptoms and preventive measures for vaginitis caused by *Candida albicans*. The symptoms are an odourless, white or yellow cheese-like discharge and itching. Sexual transmission is unlikely, but discomfort may cause the person to avoid sexual activity. *Diabetes is a predisposing factor for* Candida albicans *vaginitis, the most common form of vaginitis. Poor personal hygiene and wearing clothing that keeps the vaginal area warm and moist increase the risk of vaginitis. The infection may spread to the urinary tract, resulting in urinary tract infections; preventing and treating vaginitis decrease this risk.*

Risk of injury related to neuropathies, visual deficit, hyperglycaemia

The person with diabetes is at risk of injury from multiple factors. Neuropathies may alter sensation, gait and muscle control. Cataracts or retinopathy may cause visual deficits. Hyperglycaemia often causes osmotic changes in the lenses of the eye, resulting in blurred vision. In addition, changes in blood glucose alter levels of consciousness and may cause seizures. The impaired mobility, sensory deficits and neurological effects of complications of diabetes increase the risk of accidents, burns, falls and trauma.

- Assess for the presence of contributing or causative factors that increase the risk of injury: blurred vision, cataracts, decreased adaptation to the dark, decreased tactile sensitivity, hypoglycaemia, hyperglycaemia, hypovolaemia, joint immobility, unstable gait. *A knowledge base is necessary to develop an individualised plan of care. The risk of injury increases with the number of factors identified.*

- Reduce environmental hazards in the healthcare facility and teach the person about safety in the home and in the community.

IN THE HEALTHCARE FACILITY

- Orient the person to new surroundings on admission.
- Keep the bed at the lowest level.
- Keep the floors free of objects.
- Use a night-light.
- Check the temperature of the bath or shower water before the person uses it.
- Instruct the person to wear shoes or slippers when out of bed.
- Monitor BGLs regularly.
- Monitor for side effects of prescribed medications, such as dizziness or drowsiness.

IN THE HOME AND COMMUNITY

- Use a night-light, preferably one with a soft, no-glare bulb.
- Turn the head away when switching on a bright light.
- Avoid directly looking into headlights when driving at night.
- Test the temperature of the bath or shower water before use.
- Conduct a daily foot inspection.
- Wear shoes and slippers with non-skid soles.
- Do not use throw rugs.
- Install hand grips in the tub and shower and next to the toilet.
- Wear a seat belt when driving or riding in a car. *Strange environments and the presence of hazardous environmental factors increase the risk of falls or other accidents. Glare is often responsible for falls in people with visual deficits. The nurse can reduce factors that increase the risk of injury by implementing care and teaching safe practices during the activities of daily life.*
- Monitor for and teach the person and family to recognise and seek care for the manifestations of DKA in the person with type 1 DM: hyperglycaemia, thirst, headaches, nausea and vomiting, increased urine output, ketonuria, dehydration and decreasing level of consciousness. *BGLs increase if the insulin need is unmet or insufficiently met; the cellular use of fats for fuel results in ketosis. Osmotic diuresis increases urinary output, resulting in thirst and dehydration.*

CONSIDERATION FOR PRACTICE

Make frequent assessments to monitor for symptoms of HHS in the older adult who has had major surgery.

- Monitor for and teach the person and family to recognise and seek care for the manifestations of HHS in the person with type 2 DM: extreme hyperglycaemia, increased urinary output, thirst, dehydration, hypotension, seizures and decreasing level of consciousness. *HHS is a life-threatening condition requiring recognition and treatment.*
- Monitor for and teach the person and family to recognise and treat the manifestations of hypoglycaemia: low blood glucose, anxiety, headache, uncoordinated movements, sweating, rapid pulse, drowsiness and visual changes. Teach the person and family to carry some form of rapid-acting sugar source at all times. *Severe hypoglycaemia causes a decrease in the level of consciousness. The decrease in blood glucose most often results from too much insulin, too little food or too much exercise.*
- Recommend that the person wear a MedicAlert® bracelet or necklace identifying self as a person with diabetes. *In case of sudden, severe illness or accident, a medical alert bracelet can allow immediate medical attention for diabetes to be instituted.*

Risk of sexual dysfunction related to peripheral neuropathy

Sexuality is a complex and inseparable part of every person. It involves not only physical sexual activities but also a person's self-perception as male or female, roles and relationships, and attractiveness and desirability. Changes in sexual function and in sexuality have been identified in both men and women with diabetes.

Alterations in erectile ability occur in approximately 50% of all men with diabetes. The incidence of impotence increases with the duration of the diabetes and is often associated with peripheral neuropathy. Libido is usually unaffected, even when impotence is present.

CONSIDERATION FOR PRACTICE

Sexual function is a private matter and people rarely share concerns unless the nurse initiates the discussion.

Women with diabetes also have alterations in sexual function, although the reason is less clear. The problems reported by women involve decreased desire and decreased vaginal lubrication. Women with diabetes are also at increased risk of vaginitis and may avoid sexual intercourse in order to avoid pain.

- Include a sexual history as a part of the initial and ongoing assessment of the person with diabetes. A specific history form may be used that addresses sexual development, personal and family values, current sexual practices and concerns, and changes desired. Ask a non-threatening, open-ended question to elicit information, such as: 'Tell me about your experience with sexual function since you have been diagnosed with diabetes.' *Obtaining accurate information to assess the sexual health of a person is necessary before counselling can begin or referrals can be made.*
- Provide information about the actual and potential physical effects of diabetes on sexual function. Include the effect of poor control of blood glucose on sexual function as part of any teaching plan. *People benefit from basic information about male and female anatomy and the sexual response cycle and how diabetes can affect this part of the body. Changes in BGLs may not only cause changes in desire and physical response but may also alter sexual responses as a result of depression, anxiety and fatigue.*

- Provide counselling or make referrals as appropriate. The nurse is responsible for knowing about sexuality and sexual health throughout the lifespan and provides information based on knowledge of the effects of illness and treatment on sexual function. For example, men who are impotent may regain the ability to have sexual intercourse through penile implants, the use of a suction apparatus or sildenafil citrate (Viagra). Women with decreased vaginal lubrication can decrease painful intercourse by using vaginal lubricants (such as K-Y Jelly) or oestrogen creams. *The nurse may make specific suggestions to facilitate positive sexual functioning, referring the person to the appropriate healthcare provider as necessary for intensive therapy.*

Risk of ineffective coping related to the chronicity of diabetes

Coping is the process of responding to internal or environmental stressors or potential stressors. When coping responses are ineffective, the stressors exceed the individual's available resources for responding. The person diagnosed with diabetes is faced with lifelong changes in many parts of their life. Diet, exercise habits and medications must be integrated into the person's lifestyle and be carefully controlled. Daily injections may be a reality. Fear of potential complications and of negative effects on the future is common.

If the person is unable to cope successfully with these changes, emotional stress can interfere with glycaemic control. In addition, unsuccessful coping often results in non-compliance with prescribed treatment modalities, further impairing glycaemic control and increasing the potential for acute and chronic complications.

- Assess the person's psychosocial resources, including emotional resources, support resources, lifestyle and communication skills. *Chronic illness affects all dimensions of a person's life, as well as the lives of family members and significant others. A comprehensive assessment of strengths and weaknesses is the first step in developing an individualised plan of care to facilitate coping.*
- Explore with the person and family the effects (actual and perceived) of the diagnosis and treatment of diabetes on finances, occupation, energy levels and relationships. *Common frustrations associated with diabetes are the disease itself, the treatment modalities and the healthcare system. Effective coping involves maintaining a healthy self-concept and satisfying relationships, emotional balance and handling emotional stress.*
- Teach constructive problem-solving techniques. *Problem-focused behaviours include setting attainable and realistic goals, learning about all aspects of the problem, learning new procedures or skills that increase self-esteem and reaching out to others for support.*
- Provide information about support groups and resources, such as suppliers of products, journals, books and cookbooks for people with diabetes. *Sharing with others who have similar problems provides opportunities for mutual support and problem solving. Using available resources improves the person's ability to cope.*

Community-based care

Teaching the person and family to self-manage diabetes is a nursing responsibility. Even if a formal teaching plan is developed and implemented by advanced practice nurses, all nurses must be able to reinforce knowledge and answer questions. Teaching is necessary for both the person who is newly diagnosed and for the person who has had diabetes for years. In fact, the latter may need almost as much teaching as the newly diagnosed person. Products for diabetes care, especially insulins, have changed dramatically and knowledge about risk reduction to prevent complications has increased.

For the hospitalised person with diabetes, teaching should begin on admission. Prior to designing the teaching plan, the nurse makes an initial assessment of the person's and family's knowledge and learning needs, outlining past diabetes management practices and identifying physical, emotional and sociocultural needs. Educational level, preferred learning methods and style, life experiences and support systems are also assessed. Individuals who have been diagnosed with diabetes were shown to make a dramatic impact on the progression and development of their disease by being autonomous in their own care.

It is important that the nurse and person mutually establish goals based on the assessment data. It is equally important that family members understand that the responsibility for daily management lies with the person and that the primary role of the family is supportive. The person is the one who has the disease and who each day must take medications or inject insulin, test their blood or urine, manage their diet, exercise, adjust medications, inspect the body for injury and determine whether and when medical assistance is needed. However, family members require the same knowledge so that they can provide emotional support as well as physical care if necessary.

The following should be included in teaching the person and family about care at home.

- Information about normal metabolism, DM and how diabetes changes metabolism.
- Diet plan: how diet helps keep blood glucose in normal range; number of kilojoules required and why; amount of carbohydrates, meats and fats allowed, and why; and how to calculate the diet, integrating personal food preferences.
- Exercise: how it helps lower blood glucose; the importance of a regular program; types of exercise; integrating personal exercise preferences; how to handle increased activity.
- Self-monitoring of blood glucose: how to perform the tests accurately, how to care for equipment, what to do for high or low blood glucose.
- Medications:
  - Insulin: type, dosage, mixing instructions (if necessary), times of onset and peak actions, how to get and care for equipment, how to give injections, where to give injections.
  - Oral hypoglycaemic agents: type, dosage, side effects, interaction with other drugs.
- Manifestations of acute complications of hypoglycaemia and hyperglycaemia; what to do when they occur.
- Hygiene: skin care, dental care, foot care.

- Sick days: what to do about food, fluids and medications.
- Helpful resources:
  - Diabetes Australia: https://www.diabetesaustralia.com.au
  - Juvenile Diabetes Research Foundation Australia: https://www.jdrf.org.au
  - AIHW. *Diabetes: Australian facts*: https://www.aihw.gov.au/reports/diabetes/diabetes/contents/about
  - International Diabetes Federation: https://www.idf.org.

Teaching may have to be adapted to the special needs of the older adult. Because 40% of all people with diabetes are over the age of 65, considering the special needs of this population is essential. Uncontrolled diabetes in the older adult increases the potential for functional loss, social disengagement and increased morbidity and mortality. Education for self-care allows the older adult to be more actively involved in their diabetes management and decreases the potential for acute and long-term complications from the disease. Considerations for teaching the older adult with diabetes include the following:

- Changes in diet may be difficult to implement for many reasons. Favourite foods are difficult to give up. Balanced meals at regular intervals may not have been part of the person's lifestyle. Purchasing, storing and preparing foods may be a problem. Dentures may not fit well. Changes in taste sensation often cause the person to increase the use of salt and sugar.
- Exercise of any type may not have been part of the activities of daily living. Exercise must be individualised for any physical limitations imposed by other chronic illnesses, such as arthritis, Parkinson's disease, chronic respiratory diseases and/or cardiovascular diseases.
- The diagnosis of a chronic illness threatens independence and self-worth. After years of taking care of self, the older adult with diabetes may now have to depend on others for help in meeting self-care needs. This in turn often leads to withdrawal from social interactions with others.
- Money to purchase medications and supplies often must be taken out of a fixed income.
- Visual deficits make insulin administration difficult or impossible. Visual deficits also interfere with blood glucose monitoring, food preparation, exercises and foot care.

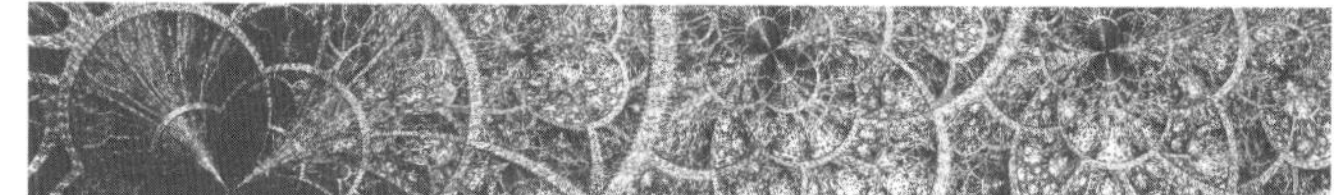

CHAPTER HIGHLIGHTS

- The incidence of type 2 DM is increasing in epidemic proportions in all racial and ethnic groups globally.
- Almost 1.5 million Australians have been diagnosed with diabetes.
- Type 2 diabetes represents a serious public health problem for Indigenous Australians, occurring at a much higher rate than in the non-Indigenous population.
- Type 2 DM has a hereditary link and is characterised by obesity and sedentary lifestyles. Unlike type 1 DM, in which the onset is often sudden, the development of symptoms that bring people to their healthcare providers for evaluation is slow; it is estimated that 50% of newly diagnosed type 2 DM people have already developed complications secondary to hyperglycaemia.
- Tighter, more intensive glycaemic control is increasingly the focus of care for hospitalised people with hyperglycaemia. Correcting hyperglycaemia is considered a benefit to diabetics and non-diabetics alike.
- New products for people with DM include insulins, non-insulin hypoglycaemics, insulin delivery devices such as pens and pumps, and blood glucose and ketone monitoring devices. Nurses must be familiar with these products and help people with diabetes become proficient in their use.
- Motivation for self-care by the person with diabetes continues to be a challenge because treatment commonly includes lifestyle changes. Through education and support, people can achieve control of DM and avoid complications.

CONCEPT CHECK

1 Increased susceptibility to the development of type 1 DM is indicated by which of the following?

1 genetic markers that determine immune response
2 persistent obesity throughout the adolescent years
3 delivery of a baby that weighs less than 2.7 kg
4 excessive amounts of plasma glucagon

2 Diabetic ketoacidosis is the result of which pathological process?

1 An excess amount of insulin drives all glucose into the cells.
2 A decreased amount of glucagon causes low protein levels.
3 A deficit of insulin causes fat stores to be used as an energy source.
4 An increase occurs in the breakdown of glucose molecules with hypoglycaemia.

3 Which of the following people would be most at risk of the development of type 2 DM?

1 a young adult who is a professional basketball player
2 a middle-aged man who maintains normal weight
3 a middle-aged woman who is the sole caretaker of her parents
4 a 70-year-old woman who is overweight and sedentary

4 You are assigned a person who has a nursing diagnosis of *Peripheral neurovascular dysfunction* involving both feet. Which of the following assessments would support this diagnosis?

1 The person reports normal sensation to touch.
2 There is a loss of normal reflexes.
3 The person states, 'I can't feel my feet any more.'
4 The person says, 'I have been having chest pain.'

5 Which of the following statements would indicate the person understands teaching about foot care at home?

1 'I will walk barefooted as long as I am in the house.'
2 'I always buy my shoes as soon as the stores open.'
3 'I will check my feet for cuts and bruises every night.'
4 'If I get a blister, I just put alcohol on it and bandage it.'

6 Lantus insulin, a long-acting insulin, has a unique insulin characteristic that increases the risk of administration error. The nurse understands that this long-acting insulin is:
1 combined with glucose to raise energy levels
2 subject to being inactivated by light
3 a clear solution like regular insulin, unlike intermediate and long-acting insulins
4 activated by vigorous agitation

7 The nurse is preparing an insulin infusion for a person in diabetic ketoacidosis (DKA). She is careful to select the only type of insulin that can be administered intravenously, which is:
1 Toujeo
2 Actrapid
3 Mixtard 30/70
4 Humalog Mix25

8 Severe hypoglycaemia is characterised by which of the following clinical signs and symptoms?
1 BGL $>$ 3 mmol/L, altered behaviour and thirst
2 BGL $<$ 3 mmol/L, altered behaviour, seizures and coma
3 BGL $<$ 4 mmol/L, seizures and coma
4 BGL $>$ 4 mmol/L, altered behaviour, seizures and coma

9 Subcutaneous injections of insulin can be made in several locations in the body. The nurse teaches the person that the most predictable absorption occurs in the:
1 hip
2 thigh
3 deltoid
4 abdomen

BIBLIOGRAPHY

Ambler, G. R. & Cameron F. J. (eds) (2010). *Caring for diabetes in children and adolescents* (3rd ed.). Children's Diabetes Services. Joint Project of the Children's Hospital at Westmead, NSW and the Royal Children's Hospital, Melbourne. Retrieved from video.rch.org.au/

American Diabetes Association (2021). 7. Diabetes technology: Standards of medical care in diabetes—2021. *Diabetes Care*, *44*(1), S85–S99. https://doi.org/10.2337/dc21-S007

Australian Bureau of Statistics (ABS) (2019). *National Aboriginal and Torres Strait Islander health survey*. Retrieved from https://www.abs.gov.au/

Australian Bureau of Statistics (ABS) (2022). *Causes of death, Australia*. Retrieved from https://www.abs.gov.au/

Australian Diabetes Educators Association (2015). *Use of blood glucose meters*. Retrieved from https://www.adea.com.au/

Australian Institute of Health and Welfare (AIHW) (2022). *Diabetes: Australian facts*. Retrieved from https://www.aihw.gov.au/

Australian Medicines Handbook (AMH) (2022a). *Insulins*. Retrieved from https://amhonline-amh-net-au.elibrary.jcu.edu.au/

Australian Medicines Handbook (AMH) (2022b). *Glucagon-like peptide-1 analogues*. Retrieved from https://amhonline-amh-net-au.elibrary.jcu.edu.au/

Australian Medicines Handbook (AMH) (2022c). *Metformin*. Retrieved from https://amhonline-amh-net-au.elibrary.jcu.edu.au/

Australian Medicines Handbook (AMH) (2022d). *Dipeptidyl peptidase-4 inhibitors*. Retrieved from https://amhonline-amh-net-au.elibrary.jcu.edu.au/

Australian Medicines Handbook (AMH) (2022e). *Sodium-glucose co-transporter 2 inhibitors*. Retrieved from https://amhonline-amh-net-au.elibrary.jcu.edu.au/

Baker Heart and Diabetes Institute (2021). *All about insulin pumps*. Retrieved from https://baker.edu.au/

Baker Heart and Diabetes Institute (2022). *Carbohydrates and glycaemic index (GI)*. Retrieved from https://baker.edu.au/

Berbudi, A., Rahmadika, N., Tjahjadi, A. I. & Ruslami, R. (2020). Type 2 diabetes and its impact on the immune system. *Current Diabetes Reviews*, *16*(5), 442–449. https://doi.org/10.2174/1573399815666191024085838

Bruttomesso, D., Laviola, L., Avogaro, A. et al. (2019). The use of real time continuous glucose monitoring or flash glucose monitoring in the management of diabetes: A consensus view of Italian diabetes experts using the Delphi method. *Nutrition, Metabolism, and Cardiovascular Diseases*, *29*(5), 421–431. https://doi.org/10.1016/j.numecd.2019.01.018

Craft, J., Gordon, C., Heuther, S., McCance, K., Brashers, V. & Rote, N. (2019). *Understanding pathophysiology* (3rd Australian and New Zealand ed.). Chatswood, NSW: Elsevier Australia.

Diabetes Australia (2020). *Position statement: Gestational diabetes in Australia*. Retrieved from https://www.diabetesaustralia.com.au/

Diabetes Australia (2022a). *Diabetes in Australia*. Retrieved from https://www.diabetesaustralia.com.au/

Diabetes Australia (2022b). *Blood glucose monitoring*. Retrieved from https://www.diabetesaustralia.com.au/

Diabetes Australia (2022c). *Healthy diet for diabetes*. Retrieved from https://www.diabetesaustralia.com.au/

Diabetes Australia (2022d). *Depression and mental health*. Retrieved from https://www.diabetesaustralia.com.au/

Eliopoulos, C. (2005). *Gerontological nursing* (6th ed.). Philadelphia: Lippincott Williams & Wilkins.

Gilden, R., McKenzie, R. & Anjou, M. D. (2022). Identifying best-practice features of diabetic retinopathy treatment models for Aboriginal and Torres Strait Islander Australians. *Australian Journal of Rural Health*. https://doi.org/https://doi.org/10.1111/ajr.12949

Haire-Joshu, D. (ed.) (1996). *Management of diabetes mellitus: Perspectives of care across the lifespan* (2nd ed.). St Louis, MO: Mosby.

Hirsch, L., Gibney, M., Albanese, J., Qu, S., Kassler-Taub, K., Klaff, L. J. & Bailey, T. S. (2010). Comparative glycemic control, safety and patient ratings for a new 4 mm × 32G insulin pen needle in adults with diabetes. *Current Medical Research and Opinion*, *26*(6), 1531–1541.

International Diabetes Federation (2021). *IDF diabetes atlas* (10th ed.). Retrieved from https://diabetesatlas.org/

McCance, K. L. & Huether, S. E. (2019). *Pathophysiology: The biologic basis for disease in adults and children* (8th ed.). Australia: Mosby.

MIMS Online Australia (2022). *Insulin*. Retrieved from https://www-mimsonline-com-au.elibrary.jcu.edu.au/

National Diabetes Service Scheme (NDSS) (2022a). *Snapshot: All types of diabetes as at 30 September 2022*. Retrieved from https://www.ndss.com.au/

National Diabetes Service Scheme (NDSS) (2022b). *Fact sheet: Flash glucose monitoring*. Retrieved from https://www.ndss.com.au/

National Health and Medical Research Council (2013). *Eat for health educator guide: Information for nutrition educators*. Retrieved from https://www.eatforhealth.gov.au/

Norris, T. L. (2018). *Porth's pathophysiology: Concepts of altered health states* (10th ed.). Philadelphia: Lippincott Williams & Wilkins.

Nutrition Australia (2021). *Diabetes*. Retrieved from https://www.diabetesaustralia.com.au/

Parker, W. A. E. (2020). Aspirin, clopidogrel and prasugrel monotherapy in patients with type 2 diabetes mellitus: A double-blind randomised controlled trial of the effects on thrombotic markers and microRNA levels. *Cardiovascular Diabetology*, *19*(1). https://doi.org/10.1186/s12933-019-0981-3

Royal Australian College of General Practitioners (RACGP) (2020). *Management of type 2 diabetes: A handbook for general practice*. East Melbourne, Vic.: RACGP. Retrieved from https://www.racgp.org.au/

Watson, M. J. G., McCluskey, P. J., Grigg, J. R., Kanagasingam, Y., Daire, J. & Estai, M. (2021). Barriers and facilitators to diabetic retinopathy screening within Australian primary care. *BMC Family Practice*, *22*(1), 239. https://doi.org/10.1186/s12875-021-01586-7

Willix, C., Griffiths, E. & Singleton, S. (2019). Hyperglycaemic presentations in type 2 diabetes. *Australian Journal for General Practitioners*, *48*, 163–167.

UNIT 5 BUILDING CLINICAL COMPETENCE

Responses to altered endocrine function

Clinical scenario

In the afternoon shift, you are looking after two people that were admitted to your ward earlier in the day:

- Mrs Kelly Ly is a 47-year-old Vietnamese woman who has limited English. She is accompanied by her husband and her son who are helping with English translation when necessary. Mrs Ly has been admitted from the emergency department with increased confusion, agitation, nausea and vomiting, tachycardia, hypertension and weight loss. She has a history of Graves' disease, diagnosed 2 years ago on her arrival to Australia from Vietnam. On your assessment her observations are T 38.9°C, P 119 bpm, R 30, BP 171/83 mmHg. Her blood glucose level is 3.7 mmol/L. She is anxious, agitated, her hands are shaking and she is complaining of abdominal pain and wanting to vomit. Her son told you that she is 'not herself' and she is 'confused'.
- Colin is 17 years old. He has had diabetes type 1 since he was 10 years old. He was transferred from the high dependency unit this morning. He is recovering from diabetic ketoacidosis (DKA) after falling ill with a severe chest infection. His vital signs are T 37.1°C, P 85 bpm, R14, BP 112/55 mmHg. His blood glucose level is 7.9 mmol/L 2 hours after lunch. Colin says that he is feeling better but still coughing. He has two cannulae for intravenous antibiotics. You performed a urinalysis that showed glucose + and ketones trace. Colin still has an indwelling catheter (IDC) and asks you when he can have it removed.

Critical-thinking questions

1. After your assessment and above findings, which person needs your immediate attention? Provide the rationale for your decision.
2. What do you think is occurring for Mrs Ly? Explain the signs and symptoms that she is showing and relate them to her diagnosis of Graves' disease.
3. Mrs Ly may be showing other significant signs and symptoms of hyperthyroidism. List them according to body systems.
4. What are the main nursing diagnoses for Mrs Ly? List your immediate actions.
5. Mrs Ly is very likely to be experiencing a thyroid crisis, which is a medical emergency. Thyroid crisis or thyroid storm can be defined as:
   1. extreme hypothyroidism
   2. excess production of parathyroid hormone (PTH)
   3. low production of thyroid hormone (TH)
   4. excess production of TH
6. Mrs Ly has been experiencing difficulty fully closing her eyelids for a few months. What is the possible cause for this?
   1. goitre
   2. pretibial myxoedema
   3. proptosis
   4. amenorrhoea
7. Mrs Ly has recovered with medication management and discharge planning is in progress as she may be discharged home tomorrow. Develop a discharge plan, taking into consideration her ethnic background and limited English. Include in your plan some education in relation to follow-up care, management and prevention of complications in Graves' disease.
8. Colin is upset because he feels that he has always done the best to manage his diabetes and he still got DKA. Explain DKA to Colin and how it occurred when he got the chest infection.
9. The medical officer has told Colin that he would like to leave the IDC in until there are no ketones present in the urine and this is likely to occur soon. What is the reason for ketones to be present in Colin's urine?
   1. Ketones are the product of glucose breakdown that is excreted in the urine.
   2. They are the product of fat breakdown excreted in the urine.
   3. Polyuria causes dehydration that leads to ketones in the urine.
   4. It is normal to have presence of ketones in the urine when there is glucose as well.
10. Colin presented to the hospital with a sugar level of 30 mmol/L. He was rehydrated, electrolytes were replaced and he was commenced on insulin and then dextrose intravenously. Why is it essential to reduce the blood sugar level slowly and gradually at that stage of DKA?
11. Colin's glycosylated haemoglobin or HbA1c is 9%. Explain glycosylated haemoglobin and what this result means.
12. If Colin has an episode of hypoglycaemia with a glucose level of 2.7 mmol/L, which signs and symptoms might he experience?
    1. bradycardia, nausea, vomiting
    2. polyuria, polydipsia, polyphagia
    3. diarrhoea, nausea, thirst
    4. hypotension, tachycardia, profuse sweating
13. Colin is preparing for dinner and needs to have his Humalog injection. When does he need to take his insulin?
    1. 30 minutes before he starts eating
    2. immediately after he finishes his meal
    3. immediately before he starts eating
    4. 1 hour before his meal

Case study

Mr Lewis is a 70-year-old Aboriginal male who was admitted with health problems of increased urination, increased thirst, fatigue, blurred vision and numbness in his feet. He states that he retired 9 months ago after 45 years as a construction worker. He now leads a sedentary lifestyle and doesn't have as much energy as he used to have. He has gained 14 kg since retirement. Upon assessment, Mr Lewis weighs 116 kg and is 180.5 cm tall. Vital signs are T 37°C, P 88 bpm, R 20 and BP 150/90 mmHg. Decreased pulses are palpated in dorsal pedalis and posterior tibial pulses. Both feet are cool to touch with slow capillary refill in toes. The following laboratory studies are ordered to confirm the diagnosis of type 2 diabetes mellitus: plasma glucose concentration, fasting blood glucose and oral glucose tolerance test.

Type 2 diabetes mellitus is a disease of fasting hyperglycaemia despite the production of some insulin by the beta cells of the pancreas. The level of insulin production varies, affecting the amount available for cellular metabolism.

With increased age, sedentary lifestyle and obesity, cells become resistant to insulin. The uptake of glucose by muscle and fat cells is not sufficient to lower the blood glucose. In obesity, insulin has a decreased ability to influence glucose metabolism and affect the uptake of glucose by cells in the liver, skeletal muscles and adipose tissue, resulting in a high blood glucose level.

The manifestations of type 2 diabetes mellitus include polyuria, polydipsia, blurred vision, fatigue, paraesthesias and skin infections. In times of physical or emotional stress, the person may develop a hyperosmolar hyperglycaemic state (HHS). Complications of type 2 diabetes mellitus include coronary heart disease (myocardial infarction), hypertension, stroke, peripheral vascular disease (atherosclerosis, vascular insufficiency, amputations), end-stage renal disease (nephropathy) and blindness (retinopathy).

Based on Mr Lewis's manifestations and weight gain, a priority nursing diagnosis of *Imbalanced nutrition: more than body requirements* is appropriate for guiding nursing care for this person.

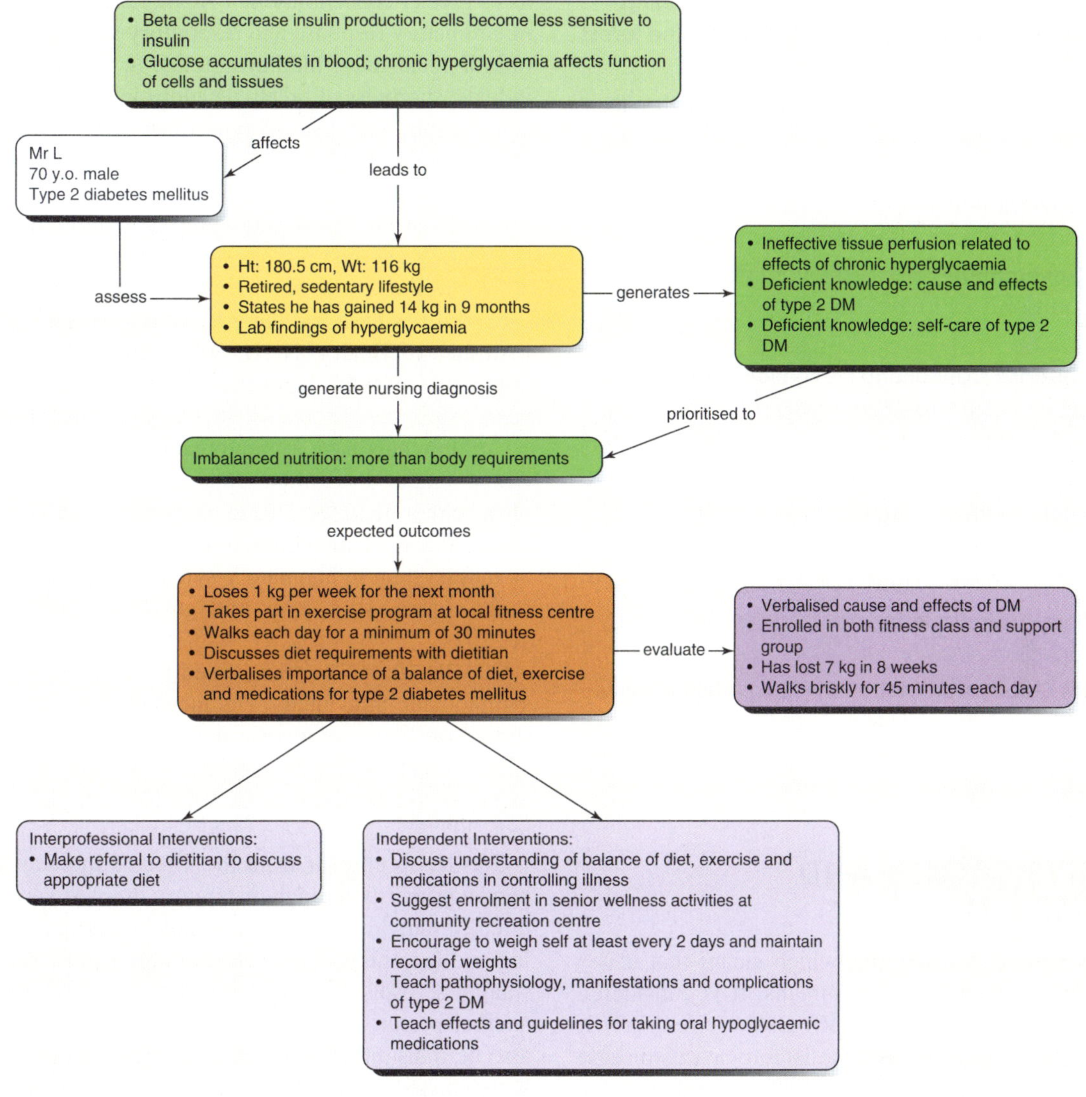

Appendix

Essentials for nurses: COVID-19

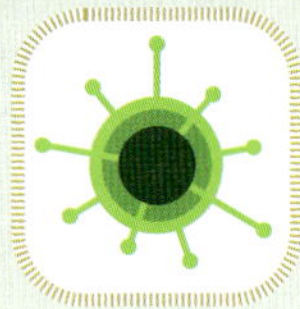

Stay current: knowledge about COVID-19 is changing daily. Check the following sources regularly for the latest information:

- **Australian Commission on Safety and Quality in Health Care:** https://www.safetyandquality.gov.au/covid-19-resources
- **Australian Government:** refer to relevant state or territory health departments for further details.
- **Australian Government:** refer to relevant state or territory health departments for further details on long COVID clinics.
- **Centers for Disease Control and Prevention (CDC):** https://www.cdc.gov/coronavirus/2019-ncov/index.html
- **Children and COVID-19:** refer to relevant state or territory children's hospitals for further details
- **Department of Health and Aged Care:** https://www.health.gov.au
- **Healthdirect:** https://www.healthdirect.gov.au/covid-19
- **Palliative Care Australia:** https://palliativecare.org.au/covid-19-updates/
- **Therapeutics Goods Administration (TGA):** https://www.tga.gov.au/
- **World Health Organization (WHO):** https://www.who.int/health-topics/coronavirus

PATHOPHYSIOLOGY AND TRANSMISSION

COVID-19 is a novel coronavirus, which means that it is a new virus not previously seen in humans. It is considered infectious and is caused by the SARS-CoV-2 virus (WHO, 2022a). The full name of this disease is coronavirus disease 2019. In the abbreviation COVID-19, *CO* represents *corona*, *VI* is *virus*, *D* is *disease* and *19* is *the year* it was identified (CDC, 2021a).

In the asymptomatic phase of COVID-19, the virus enters the nose and starts to replicate. In this stage, the person is infectious even though the viral burden is low. The virus is covered with spiked surface proteins that attach to receptors on cells, particularly in the lungs. It enters healthy cells through ACE2 receptors and destroys the cells. Over the next few days, the virus moves down the respiratory tract, which has a greater concentration of ACE2 receptors, and triggers an inflammatory response and respiratory symptoms. About 80% of individuals have mild symptoms. In the other 20% of individuals, shortness of breath develops in 5–8 days, followed by acute respiratory distress syndrome (ARDS) (Jackson et al., 2022; Mason, 2020).

Older adults and individuals with chronic illness are at greatest risk of developing symptoms and complications of COVID-19. At the time of writing, people aged 65 years and older and those who reside in aged care homes or long-term care facilities have had the greatest risk of mortality (National Institutes of Health (NIH), 2021). In Australia, the highest number of COVID-19 deaths was among those aged 80–89 years (85.2 years for males, 88.4 years for females).

Children may have asymptomatic infection or tend to experience similar, but milder, clinical manifestations that resemble a cold or flu (CDC, 2021a; Department of Health and Aged Care, 2022a). Some children develop a rare condition known as multisystem inflammatory syndrome that affects the heart, lungs, brain, skin, eyes and gastrointestinal tract (CDC, 2021b).

COVID-19 can be transmitted by both asymptomatic and symptomatic individuals. The incubation period for this virus (time from exposure to virus to onset of symptoms) is between 1 and 14 days, with a median onset of symptoms 5–6 days after exposure to a person with COVID-19 (CDC, 2021a; Healthdirect, 2022a).

COVID-19 spreads from the infected individual to another person primarily through respiratory droplets sprayed from the infected individual during coughing, sneezing, speaking, singing and breathing. The droplets range from large particles to smaller aerosols that may be inhaled into the lungs or land on another person's face, eyes, nose or mouth. The disease may also be transmitted by touching the face, mouth, nose or eyes with infected hands. The likelihood of transmission by droplets is greater when people are within 1.5–2 metres of each other (CDC, 2021c; Department of Health and Aged Care, 2022a; WHO, 2022a).

Viral shedding occurs when someone 'sheds' COVID-19 by breathing, sneezing, coughing or through their faeces and urine. It may occur up to several weeks after symptoms resolve. Some people continue to have non-infectious fragments which may still return a positive result when tested (CDC, 2021d; Department of Health and Aged Care, 2022a). The immune response and duration of immunity of individuals who have been infected with COVID-19 is not clearly understood and continues to be researched (CDC, 2021e).

At the time of writing, 13 variants of SARS-CoV-2 have been identified as causing COVID-19; however, only five (and their sub-variants such as XBB) continue to be classified as variants of concern—Alpha, Beta, Delta, Gamma and Omicron (Department of Health and Aged Care, 2022a; WHO, 2022a). Since 2019, the number of cases have risen significantly and continue to fluctuate due to these variants, which have caused severe illness in both vaccinated and unvaccinated people. It is thought that vaccinated people can carry and spread these variants to others. Although vaccinated people who contract one of these variants seem to have the same high amount of the virus, in most cases, they appear to have a milder case.

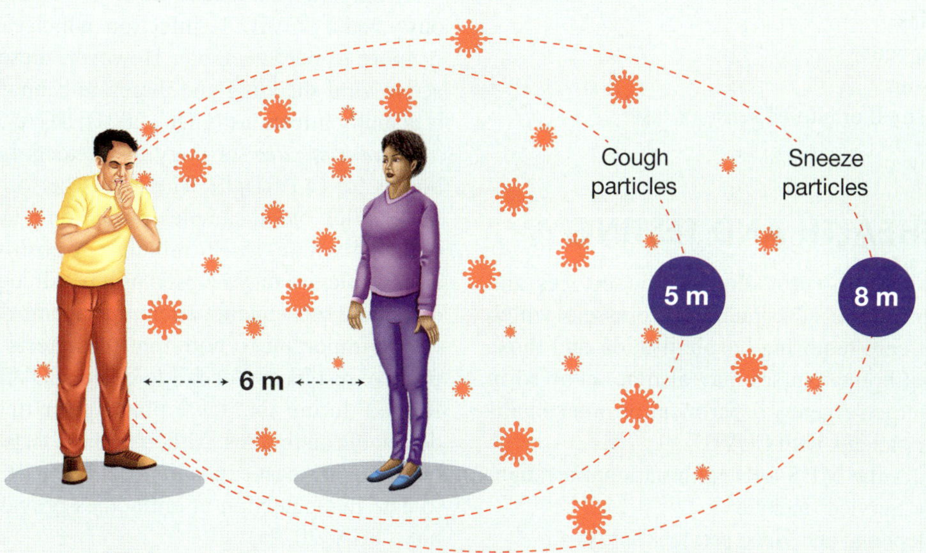

REDUCING AND PREVENTING SPREAD OF INFECTION

In the community: community spread of COVID-19 can be reduced or prevented by doing the following:

- placing at least 1.5 metres distance between people
- washing hands regularly with soap and water or hand sanitiser 70% + alcohol for a minimum of 20 seconds
- wearing a facemask in areas where it is a requirement, including healthcare settings, aged care facilities, doctors' surgeries and allied health clinics, public transport etc.
- sneezing or coughing into the elbow or a tissue if a mask is not being worn
- avoiding touching the face, eyes, nose and mouth
- receiving a vaccination against COVID-19
- disinfecting commonly touched surfaces and items.

In healthcare settings: spread of COVID-19 in healthcare settings can be reduced or prevented by:

- following policy for donning, doffing and disposing of PPE
- performing hand hygiene before entering a patient's room and/or donning PPE (gown, face shield or goggles and mask)
- correctly removing and disposing of PPE when leaving a patient's room followed by hand hygiene. (The Department of Health and Aged Care (2022b) and the Australian Commission on Safety and Quality in Health Care (ACSQHC) (2020) provide guidelines and resources about donning and doffing PPE in various healthcare settings.)
- avoiding touching the face and eyes
- washing hands frequently with soap and water for 20 seconds and/or using approved antimicrobial solutions
- taking breaks and eating food in designated areas away from the patient care unit.

In the home: nurses can reduce transmission of COVID-19 to family and others who share their living space by (American Nurses Association Enterprise, 2020):

- changing clothes and shoes before leaving work, if possible
- always washing hands before leaving work
- cleaning objects that are used at home and work, such as mobile phones, before leaving work
- removing shoes and clothing worn at work before entering the house and placing in a plastic bag or box
- washing hands before entering or immediately after entering the home
- washing scrubs/work clothes in hot soapy water and avoid mixing them with other clothing; discarding the plastic bag that held the contaminated items and washing hands
- leaving items such as stethoscope and pens at work.

SIGNS AND SYMPTOMS

Individuals with COVID-19 can present with various signs and symptoms; the most common are similar to cold and flu (CDC, 2021a; Department of Health and Aged Care, 2022a) including:

- fever
- coughing
- sore throat
- shortness of breath.

Other symptoms experienced include:

- runny nose or congestion
- headache or fatigue
- muscle or joint pains
- nausea or loss of appetite
- diarrhoea or vomiting
- temporary loss of smell or altered sense of taste.

TRIAGE, TELEHEALTH AND TESTING

Nurses are using telehealth (providing health services and information through the use of technology) to assess which patients need urgent care requiring hospitalisation and those who can be treated at home. Nurses may also be involved in triaging patients in the emergency department or other facilities set up to care for patients with COVID-19.

As of January 2022, the MBS telehealth national arrangements are permanent. Services include:

- a wide range of telephone and video services across a number of healthcare professionals (e.g. GPs, NPs, allied health, mental health, specialists)
- longer phone consultations for patients who have received a positive COVID-19 test (introduced in July 2022)
- electronic prescriptions.

All MBS telehealth services are informed by the relevant MBS Review Taskforce Principles in order to support safe and equitable services (Department of Health and Aged Care, 2022c). When using telehealth, it is important to:

- ***Prioritise!*** If the patient is experiencing a life-threatening emergency, advise the individual to call **000** and tell the operator if they have been in contact with or are experiencing symptoms of COVID-19 (Department of Health and Aged Care, 2022a).
- Ask patients if they have travelled to a place with a COVID-19 outbreak.
- Ask about vaccination status, signs and symptoms of the virus and any medical conditions that place individuals at high risk, such as chronic obstructive pulmonary disease (COPD), asthma, heart failure, diabetes, compromised/impaired immunity, liver disease, chronic kidney disease, obesity, neurological conditions and pregnancy.

The nurse will then direct patients to the appropriate level of care based on the severity of symptoms, other medical conditions and exposure. If patients are recommended to go to the hospital emergency department and/or a healthcare provider, they must review the relevant website and/or call to confirm any additional requirements prior to attending (e.g. face mask, RAT etc.).

A *polymerase chain reaction* (PCR) or *rapid antigen test* (RAT) may be performed to determine whether an individual currently has a COVID-19 infection. There are a variety of RATs available; their accuracy varies as they may not detect COVID-19 immediately. A PCR is recommended for confirmation (Department of Health and Aged Care, 2022c).

A number of laboratory-based serology immunoassay tests and point-of-care serology tests have also been approved by the TGA for use in Australia (TGA, 2022a).

An *antibody test* determines whether an individual has previously had a COVID-19 infection, which can take up to 2 weeks or more to be detectable. However, these tests do not detect active viral shedding and therefore cannot detect if the person is actually infectious (CDC, 2021f; TGA, 2022a).

A *point-of-care* serology test detects IgG and/or IgM antibodies for COVID-19. The test is performed from venous or finger prick blood samples placed on a test strip, with results obtained within 15–30 minutes. A positive test along with a clinical picture may be used as a possible positive diagnosis to determine subsequent patient management (TGA, 2022a).

It is important to note that these tests may produce false-positive results and/or fail to detect COVID-19 if they are performed during the acute phase prior to the development of detectable antibodies. Although these tests provide information on a person's past exposure to COVID-19, there is no evidence to date that detection of antibodies provides protective immunity (TGA, 2022a).

HOME CARE FOR PATIENTS WITH COVID-19

Individuals who are experiencing severe symptoms of COVID-19 should call **000**. Those who are experiencing mild symptoms should ideally speak to their healthcare professional and have either a telehealth or an in-person assessment (NIH, 2021). Suggested care for the patient with mild symptoms of COVID-19 includes the following:

- Stay home, even if no symptoms are present.
- Drink plenty of fluids to stay hydrated.
- Cough medicine may provide relief for dry and productive cough—take as per manufacturer recommendations.
- Take paracetamol for fever and/or pain as per manufacturer recommendations.
- Non-steroidal anti-inflammatory drugs (NSAIDs) such as ibuprofen (Nurofen) have also been reported to decrease signs and symptoms—take as per manufacturer recommendations.
- Continue to monitor for signs and symptoms that require calling **000**, including breathing difficulties, shortness of breath, pain or pressure in the chest that persists, confusion, inability to awaken and cyanosis (blue lips or face) (Department of Health and Aged Care, 2022a; CDC, 2021a).

- Monitor oxygen saturation (SpO_2) at home if a pulse oximeter is available. Advise the patient to use a warm finger and to notify their healthcare professional or **000** if the value is repeatedly (not one time) below 95% (NIH, 2021).
- Try resting in the prone (face-down) position if feeling short of breath (NIH, 2021).
- Stay away from other people as much as possible and wear a face mask when around others both in and outside the home.
- Wash hands often using soap and water or antimicrobial gel and disinfect common surfaces regularly.
- Do not share dishes and utensils.
- If possible, use a separate bathroom and bedroom. If this is not possible, improve ventilation such as by opening windows and disinfecting after use.

Nurses should educate patients staying at home about the signs and symptoms that require calling **000** and should provide or refer patients to the relevant federal, state or territory health department site for additional information.

HOSPITAL CARE FOR PATIENTS WITH COVID-19

The pandemic has and continues to have a profound impact on all private and public hospital activities including emergency departments, elective surgery and overall patient admissions (Australian Institute of Health and Welfare (AIHW), 2022).

The majority of people with COVID-19 will not require hospitalisation or any additional treatments, particularly if they have been vaccinated (AIHW, 2022). Individuals who are at high risk for serious COVID-19 and those with moderate to severe symptoms require close monitoring since there is a risk of them becoming critically ill and being admitted to ICU as soon as 1 week following the onset of symptoms (CDC, 2021d). However, where appropriate and available, individuals will be cared for on the ward in rooms with negative pressure or airflow that will lower the risk of transmission (Healthdirect, 2022b).

COVID-19 is a respiratory illness that weakens the immune system, causing inflammation, and leads to poor respiratory outcomes including pneumonia and secondary infections (Australian Bureau of Statistics (ABS), 2022).

The time taken to develop severe symptoms, such as dyspnoea and ARDS, and to be admitted to ICU varies among individuals depending on their current health, co-morbidities, vaccination status and other factors. At the time of writing, Australia had over 11 million total reported cases of COVID-19 and almost 18,000 deaths due to COVID-19, most of which had laboratory confirmation that they had died *with or from* the virus (ABS, 2022).

The Australian and New Zealand Intensive Care Society (ANZICS) has developed COVID-19 guidelines providing recommendations and suggestions to ensure the continued delivery of high-quality care in the ICU (adults and paediatric patients) and to its workforce (ANZICS, 2021).

LONG COVID OR POST-COVID CONDITIONS

The majority of people who contract COVID-19 will have symptoms for a short period of time and usually recover within a few weeks. However, some may continue to experience symptoms for weeks, months or sometimes years after diagnosis (WHO, 2022a).

A person is considered to have long COVID if symptoms have continued for more than 12 weeks after their initial infection (Healthdirect, 2022c). Although many long-term side effects remain unknown, common symptoms (Department of Health and Aged Care, 2022d, 2022e) include:

- extreme fatigue
- persistent cough, hoarse voice
- shortness of breath, heart palpitations, chest pains
- numbness, 'pins and needles' and joint or muscle pain
- issues with sleeping
- change in sense of taste or smell, reduced appetite and weight loss
- changes in mood such as anxiety, stress and depression
- cognitive dysfunction
- low-grade fever and rash
- headaches.

Research to date has identified that those who are at greater risk of long COVID varies and includes:

- those with underlying conditions (e.g. respiratory disease, diabetes, hypertension, chronic cardiovascular disease, chronic kidney disease, active cancer etc.)
- those who initially had mild illness which was managed at home
- those who suffered a severe illness during the initial phase of COVID-19
- those who were admitted to ICU
- those over 35 years of age
- females.

A Global Technical Network for Clinical Management of COVID-19 has been established by the WHO to undertake studies of patients in order to understand the proportion of patients experiencing long-term effects, how long they persist and why they occur in order to develop further guidance for patient care for both adults and children (WHO, 2022a).

At the time of writing, no specific treatment has been identified for long COVID. States and territories have opened long COVID clinics to specifically support those with ongoing symptoms, including personalised treatment plans requiring support from a range of healthcare professionals (Department of Health and Aged Care, 2022b, 2022c, 2022f; Healthdirect, 2022c).

DRUG THERAPY FOR COVID-19

According to the *Australian Guidelines for the Clinical Care of People with COVID-19*, treatment for patients is based on illness severity and monitoring of clinical progression markers (e.g. SpO_2, respiratory failure, sepsis etc.), particularly during days 5–10 of symptom onset (Department of Health and Aged Care, 2022g).

Patients with hypoxaemia despite increasing levels of oxygen supplementation may benefit from a trial of awake prone positioning. Careful positioning and protection are needed to avoid peripheral nerve and skin injury in the prone position (NIH, 2021). This position should not be used in patients who are haemodynamically unstable, in respiratory distress and who require imminent intubation (NIH, 2021).

In 2020 and 2021, the TGA provisionally approved the following drugs for the use in COVID-19 treatment:

- tixagevimab and cilgavimab (Evusheld)
- sotrovimab (Xevudy)
- remdesivir (Veklury).

In January 2022, the TGA also provided provisional approval for the first oral drug treatments—molnupiravir (Lagevrio®) and nirmatrelvir + ritonavir (Paxlovid®).

The Australian Guidelines provide a list of drug treatments recommended for use and those that are not recommended—detailed information is provided in the guidelines found at https://www.health.gov.au/health-alerts/covid-19/treatments/about.

The WHO continues to update and release new versions related to therapeutics and the role of medication management in COVID-19 patient treatment (Department of Health and Aged Care, 2022g; WHO, 2022b).

INDEPENDENT NURSING INTERVENTIONS

Nursing care for patients with COVID-19 focuses on supportive care, such as:

- monitoring vital signs, capillary refill and oxygen saturation levels (SpO_2)
- monitoring cardiac, respiratory, neurological, renal and other body systems for complications such as pneumonia, hypoxia, sepsis and septic shock, arrhythmias, cardiomyopathy, acute renal failure, thromboembolism and ARDS
- teaching patients to use a face mask when in contact with healthcare professionals
- turning and positioning patients, including the prone position
- providing psychosocial support to the patient and family
- providing care for patients requiring endotracheal intubation and mechanical ventilation.

Nurses are advocates for patients who are unable to express their own wishes and for family members who cannot be present with their loved ones. Nurses often create the technological connection between patients and families to say their goodbyes, explain care to families and provide both patients and families with end-of-life support. Nurses can also call on team members, such as chaplains and social workers, to provide patient and family support (Delgado, 2020; Palliative Care Australia, 2020).

Nurses who work with or need help having difficult conversations with patients and families may find the following resources useful:

- Palliative Care Australia, COVID-19 resources: https://palliativecare.org.au/covid-19-updates/
- VitalTalk, COVID-19 Ready Communication Playbook: https://www.vitaltalk.org/covid-resources/.

COLLABORATIVE CARE

Successfully dealing with any pandemic requires a multifaceted approach and strategies. This includes both clinical and non-clinical support as well as personal, cultural and socioeconomic mitigation measures (Lim et al., 2022; NIH, 2021) such as:

- administering supplemental oxygen, such as high-flow nasal cannula or non-invasive positive pressure ventilation
- administering medications, as prescribed, such as:
    - paracetamol for fever control
    - NSAIDs for pain relief
    - anticoagulants for thromboembolic prophylaxis
    - antibiotics for bacterial pulmonary infection
    - (See *Australian Guidelines for the Clinical Care of People with COVID-19* (Department of Health and Aged Care, 2022g) for recommended drug treatments: https://www.health.gov.au/health-alerts/covid-19/treatments/about.)
- consulting with healthcare providers and pharmacists before administering medications and treatments that are not yet TGA approved or are investigational/experimental to learn about factors such as indications, side effects and criteria to monitor
- assessing and managing fluid volume
- using prone position in patients with dyspnoea and mechanically ventilated patients with refractory hypoxaemia (NIH, 2021)
- using collaborative models and pathways of care that are supported by primary care and community organisations to alleviate pressure on hospitals so they can provide care for those with more severe illness or with risk factors for disease progression (Lim et al., 2022).

COVID-19 VACCINATIONS

There are currently four COVID-19 vaccines that are authorised by the TGA in Australia and recommended by the Australian Technical Advisory Group on Immunisation (ATAGI) for use (TGA, 2022b). See https://www.health.gov.au/our-work/covid-19-vaccines/advice-for-providers/clinical-guidance/doses-and-administration.

Viral vector, protein-based and mRNA vaccines work in different ways to protect against COVID-19. The *viral vector* vaccine uses recombinant viral vectors that do not replicate in the host but do induce an immune response. The *protein-based vaccine* contains part of the coronavirus spike protein. The immune system cells recognise the spike protein as a threat and begin building an immune response against it. The *mRNA* vaccine works by inserting fragments into the cells of the body to reprogram them to make antigens against the pathogen. The antigen then triggers an immune response (Department of Health and Aged Care, 2022h).

Common side effects that may occur following vaccination include pain, redness or swelling around the injection site. The person may also report fatigue, headache, muscle pain, chills, fever and nausea.

Side effects from the second dose may be more intense than following the first dose or there may be none at all (CDC, 2021g). The third booster dose and forth dose are recommended for those in high-risk categories—see ATAGI recommendations (TGA, 2022b).

Blood clots have been reported following viral vector vaccination (AstraZeneca). Severe allergic reaction (anaphylaxis) and myocarditis and pericarditis have been reported following protein-based vaccination (Novavax) (Department of Health and Aged Care, 2022i). Myocarditis and pericarditis have also been reported following mRNA vaccinations (Pfizer and Moderna), especially in adolescents and young adults (CDC, 2021h). These cases were predominantly in males aged 16 and older, within several days of being vaccinated, and often after the second dose. Be alert to shortness of breath, chest pain and palpitations in this age group following vaccination.

Children infected with the COVID-19 virus can become sick and can spread the virus to others. Please refer to ATAGI recommendations for further information regarding children and vaccine recommendations.

VACCINE HESITANCY

Many people have been hesitant to receive the COVID-19 vaccine and boosters. Reasons for this hesitancy include being against vaccines in general, believing the vaccines are not safe due to rushed production and lack of trust of authorities, government and science (Kaufman, Tuckerman & Danchin, 2022; Troiano & Nardi, 2021).

Other factors that may affect decisions about accepting the vaccine include cultural, social and political considerations (CDC, 2021c), along with potential allergic reactions (e.g. anaphylaxis) to any components or contraindications to the vaccines.

The first step in overcoming vaccine hesitancy is to listen to understand the person's concerns. Talk to the person who has vaccine concerns in an objective manner. Provide accurate and honest information to dispel the myths about the vaccines (CDC, 2021i; Department of Health and Aged Care, 2022j). There is a lot of misinformation in the media and online about the vaccines. Always choose a reliable source of information.

SELF-CARE FOR NURSES

This is an especially tough time for nurses and other healthcare professionals as they navigate the numerous stresses and detrimental impacts of the pandemic. Frontline healthcare workers have and continue to experience increased personal and professional challenges (Lewis et al., 2022; US Department of Veterans Affairs (DVA), 2020), including:

- risk in relation to the uncertainty and vulnerability of becoming infected and transmitting the virus to family and friends
- managing the strain of donning and doffing PPE over long periods of time
- managing the stress of restrictions and lockdowns
- mental and physical health issues such as anxiety, emotional distress and exhaustion, moral distress, palpitations, fatigue, burnout, feelings of anger and guilt, disruptions in usual self-care and coping strategies
- working with limited resources, both human and equipment, to ensure the delivery of safe, quality patient care.

Healthcare professionals have been faced with making difficult ethical decisions about who received care and who did not. Using an *egalitarian* approach, each patient has an equal chance to receive care. The *utilitarian* approach looks at who will benefit the most from receiving care. The *prioritarian* approach selects the sickest person first. These difficult and controversial decisions contribute to moral distress (Australian College of Nursing (ACN), 2020; Lewis, et al., 2022; US DVA, 2020).

There are significant challenges for healthcare organisations in recognising and supporting the wellbeing of frontline staff. Self-care actions that nurses who are engaged in patient care can take to manage stress and work demands (ACN, 2020; Lewis, et al., 2022) include:

- taking breaks, going outside and practising relaxation techniques (e.g. breathing exercises, meditation, short walks, listening to music)
- paying attention to bodily needs, such as using the bathroom, keeping hydrated and eating healthy food at regular intervals
- recognising strengths and maintaining strong boundaries to be more effective
- resting, engaging in regular exercise and enjoyable relaxation activities
- working as a team and supporting co-workers
- checking in regularly with colleagues (e.g. R U OK).

The following actions may be helpful to reduce the negative effects of moral distress (ACN, 2020; American Psychiatric Nurses Association, 2020; Greenberg et al., 2020):

- Engage in debriefing sessions to provide support and to help team members cope with the physical and emotional stress they are experiencing.
- Seek peer support and communicate with colleagues who can validate feelings.
- Engage in self-care activities such as journalling, meditating, breathing exercises and walking outside.
- Seek professional assistance to develop healthy coping mechanisms and process experiences.
- Check in regularly with colleagues on their mental wellbeing.

Discussion questions for nursing students

After you have read the news report and journal article, consider the following questions:

- Bernstein, L. & Gerberg, J. (2020). *A Brooklyn ICU amid a pandemic: Patients alone, comforted by nurses and doctors.* https://www.washingtonpost.com/national/health-science/in-the-icu-health-care-workers-with-little-to-offer-covid-19-

patients-soldier-on/2020/04/04/16face9e-74f3-11ea-a9bd-9f8b593300d0_story.html

- Raper, R. (2021). The implications of living with COVID-19 for intensive care in Australia. *Medical Journal of Australia, 215*(11), 511–512. doi: 10.5694/mja2.51332
- ***Discussion 1***: There are seven patients with COVID-19 in the emergency department who need a ventilator, but the hospital has only four available ventilators. Taking into consideration severity of COVID-19 symptoms, age, health, family role (e.g. mother of three young children), quality of life and other variables, how do you decide who receives ventilatory treatment?
- ***Discussion 2***: Think of the conversations you might have with patients and family members of those who will not receive ventilatory treatment due to lack of availability. Role-play these conversations with other group members.
- ***Discussion 3***: The intensive care unit at Best Hospital only has a 10-bed ICU capacity. Discuss ways to expand ICU capacity. What education and training will be necessary to make this change? Consider the changes that affect nurses as well as the interprofessional team.
- ***Discussion 4***: The nurses on a COVID unit are concerned about bringing the virus home to their families. Discuss measures that nurses can take to reduce virus spreading. Consider both your workplace and home resources and environment in your response.
- ***Discussion 5***: Experts are talking about a possible resurgence of COVID-19 infections in the next 1–2 years. Consider the resources in your workplace, community and at state/territory and federal levels and develop three changes that could be implemented as part of an overall plan to meet the predicted surge.
- ***Discussion 6***: You hear friends or family discussing their reluctance to be vaccinated against COVID-19 or hear them spreading misinformation about the disease. Think about how you will respond to these individuals. Practise role-playing your conversation with another student and have them give you feedback on your ability to listen and be objective.

Bibliography

American Nurses Association Enterprise (2020). *Keeping yourself and your family safe*. Retrieved from https://www.nursingworld.org/

American Psychiatric Nurses Association (2020). *Managing stress & self-care during COVID-19: Information for nurses*. Retrieved from https://www.apna.org/

Australian and New Zealand Intensive Care Society (ANZICS) (2021). *COVID-19 guidelines* (4th ed.). Retrieved from https://www.anzics.com.au

Australian Bureau of Statistics (ABS) (2022). *COVID-19 mortality in Australia, deaths registered to 31 January 2022*. Retrieved from https://www.abs.gov.au/

Australian College of Nursing (ACN) (2020). *Self-care resources*. Retrieved from https://www.acn.edu.au/

Australian Commission on Safety and Quality in Health Care (2020). Retrieved from https://www.safetyandquality.gov.au/

Australian Institute of Health and Welfare (AIHW) (2022). *Australia's hospitals at a glance*. Retrieved from https://aihw.gov.au/

Bernstein, L. & Gerberg, J. (2020). *A Brooklyn ICU amid a pandemic: Patients alone, comforted by nurses and doctors*. Retrieved from https://www.washingtonpost.com/

Centers for Disease Control and Prevention (CDC) (2021a). *Coronavirus disease 2019 (COVID-19). Frequently asked questions*. Retrieved from https://www.cdc.gov/

Centers for Disease Control and Prevention (CDC) (2021b). *For parents: Multisystem inflammatory syndrome in children (MIS-C) associated with COVID-19*. Retrieved from https://www.cdc.gov/

Centers for Disease Control and Prevention (CDC) (2021c). *Building confidence in COVID-19 vaccines*. Retrieved from https://www.cdc.gov/

Centers for Disease Control and Prevention (CDC) (2021d). *Interim clinical guidance for management of patients with confirmed coronavirus disease (COVID-19)*. Retrieved from https://www.cdc.gov/

Centers for Disease Control and Prevention (CDC) (2021e). *Clinical questions about COVID-19: Questions and answers*. Retrieved from https://www.cdc.gov/

Centers for Disease Control and Prevention (CDC) (2021f). *Testing for COVID-19*. Retrieved from https://www.cdc.gov/

Centers for Disease Control and Prevention (CDC) (2021g). *Possible side effects after getting a COVID-19 vaccine*. Retrieved from https://www.cdc.gov/

Centers for Disease Control and Prevention (CDC) (2021h). *Myocarditis and pericarditis following mRNA COVID-19 vaccination*. Retrieved from https://www.cdc.gov/

Centers for Disease Control and Prevention (CDC) (2021i). *How to talk to your patients about COVID-19 vaccination*. Retrieved from https://www.cdc.gov/

Delgado, S. (2020). End-of-life care during the COVID-19 pandemic. *AACN blog*. Retrieved from https://www.aacn.org/

Department of Health and Aged Care (2022a). *COVID-19 signs and symptoms*. Retrieved from https://www.health.gov.au/

Department of Health and Aged Care (2022b). *COVID-19—Donning and doffing personal protective equipment in primary care*. Retrieved from https://www.health.gov.au/

Department of Health and Aged Care (2022c). *Providing health care remotely during the COVID-19 pandemic*. Retrieved from https://www.health.gov.au/

Department of Health and Aged Care (2022d). *Getting help for long COVID*. Retrieved from https://www.health.gov.au/

Department of Health and Aged Care (2022e). *Long-term effects of COVID-19*. Retrieved from https://www.health.gov.au/

Department of Health and Aged Care (2022f). *Protect yourself and others from COVID-19*. Retrieved from https://www.health.gov.au/

Department of Health and Aged Care (2022g). *Treatments: Australian guidelines* (V65.2). Retrieved from https://www.health.gov.au/

Department of Health and Aged Care (2022h). *Approved COVID-19 vaccines*. Retrieved from https://www.health.gov.au/

Department of Health and Aged Care (2022i). *Nuvaxovid (Novavax)*. Retrieved from https://www.health.gov.au/

Department of Health and Aged Care (2022j). *Is it true? Get the facts on COVID-19 vaccines*. Retrieved from https://www.health.gov.au/

Greenberg, N., Docherty, M., Gnanaoragasam, S. & Wessely, S. (2020). Managing mental health challenges faced by healthcare workers during COVID-19 pandemic. *British Medical Journal*, *368*, m1211.

Healthdirect (2022a). *Symptoms of COVID-19 and when to seek medical advice*. Retrieved from https://www.healthdirect.gov.au/

Healthdirect (2022b). *Hospital and intensive care for COVID-19*. Retrieved from https://www.healthdirect.gov.au/

Healthdirect (2022c). *Understanding post COVID-19 symptoms and long COVID*. Retrieved from https://www.healthdirect.gov.au/

Jackson, C. B., Farzan, M., Chen, B. & Choe, H. (2022). Mechanisms of SARS-CoV-2 entry into cells. *Natural Review Molecular Cell Biology*, *23*, 3–20. https://doi.org/10.1038/s41580-021-00418-x

Kaufman, J., Tuckerman, J. & Danchin, M. (2022). Overcoming COVID-19 vaccine hesitancy: Can Australia reach the last 20 percent? *Expert Review of Vaccines*, *21*(2), 159–161. https://doi.Org/10.1080/14760584.2022.2013819

Lewis, S., Wills, K., Bismark, M. & Smallwood, N. (2022). A time for self-care? Frontline health workers' strategies for managing mental health during the COVID-19 pandemic. *SSM Mental Health*, *2*, 100053. doi: 10.1016/j.ssmmh.2021.100053

Lim, S. M., Allard, N. L., Devereux, J. et al. (2022). The COVID Positive Pathway: A collaboration between public health agencies, primary care and metropolitan hospitals in Melbourne. *The Medical Journal of Australia*, *216*(8), 413–419.

Mason, R. (2020). Pathogenesis of COVID-19 from a cell biology perspective. *European Respiratory Journal*, *55*. Retrieved from https://erj.ers-journals.com/

National Institutes of Health (NIH) (2021). *Coronavirus disease (COVID-19) treatment guidelines*. Retrieved from https://www.covid19treatmentguidelines.nih.gov/

Palliative Care Australia (2020). *Palliative care and COVID-19: Grief, bereavement and mental health*. Retrieved from https://palliativecare.org.au/

Raper, R. (2021). The implications of living with COVID-19 for intensive care in Australia. *Medical Journal of Australia*, *215*(11), 511–512. doi: 10.5694/mja2.51332

Therapeutic Goods Administration (TGA) (2022a). *COVID-19 testing in Australia—Information for health professionals*. Retrieved from https://www.tga.gov.au/

Therapeutic Goods Administration (TGA) (2022b). *Approved COVID-19 vaccines*. Retrieved from https://www.health.gov.au

Troiano, G. & Nardi, A. (2021). Vaccine hesitancy in the era of COVID-19. *Public Health*, *194*, 245–251.

US Department of Veterans Affairs (DVA) (2020). *Managing healthcare workers' stress associated with the COVID-19 virus outbreak*. Retrieved from https://www.ptsd.va.gov/

VitalTalk (2020). *COVID-19 Ready Communication Playbook*. Retrieved from https://www.vitaltalk.org/

World Health Organization (WHO) (2022a). *Coronavirus disease (COVID-19)*. Retrieved from https://www.who.int/

World Health Organization (WHO) (2022b). *Therapeutics and COVID-19: Living guideline*. Retrieved from https://www.who.int/

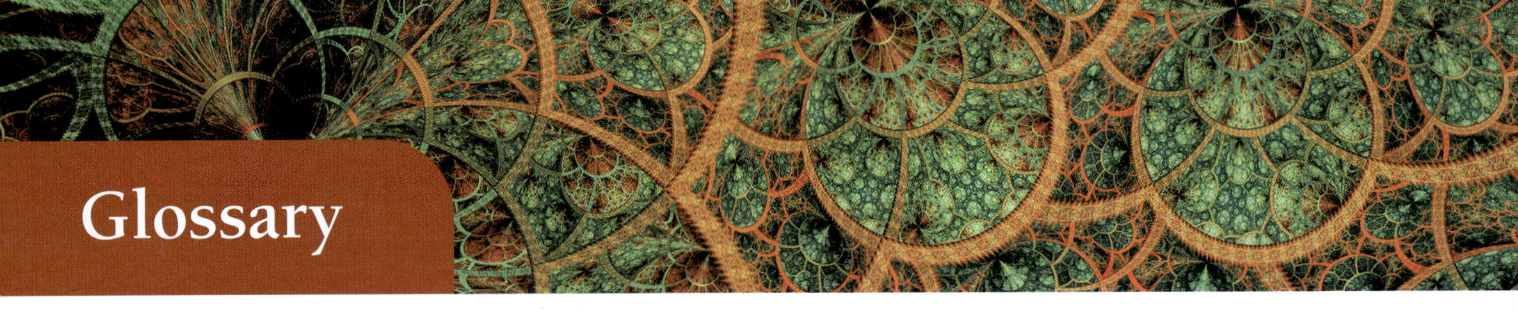

Glossary

abrasion Partial-thickness denudation of an area of integument, generally resulting from falls or scrapes.

accommodation The ability of the eye to adjust to variations in distance.

achalasia Absence of peristalsis of the oesophagus and high gastro-oesophageal sphincter pressure resulting in dilation and loss of tone in the oesophagus.

acidosis The condition in which the hydrogen ion concentration increases above normal (reflected in a pH below 7.35).

acid A substance that releases hydrogen ions in solution.

acne Disorder of the pilosebaceous (hair and sebaceous gland) structure, resulting in eruption of papules or pustules.

acoustic neuroma (schwannoma) Benign tumour of cranial nerve VIII.

acquired immune deficiency syndrome (AIDS) A specific group of diseases or conditions that are indicative of severe immunosuppression related to infection with the human immunodeficiency virus.

acromegaly Meaning literally 'enlarged extremities', this is a condition resulting from excessive growth hormone secretion during adulthood.

actinic keratosis Also called senile or solar keratosis, this is an epidermal skin lesion directly related to chronic sun exposure and photo damage.

active immunity Production of antibodies or development of immune lymphocytes against specific antigens.

active sense of self The development of meaning, purpose and direction in one's life.

active transport Movement of molecules across cell membranes and epithelial membranes against a concentration gradient; requires energy.

acute coronary syndrome (ACS) A general term used to describe the effects of coronary heart disease, including angina and myocardial infarction.

acute gastritis A benign, self-limiting disorder associated with ingestion of gastric irritants such as aspirin, alcohol, caffeine or foods contaminated with certain bacteria.

acute illness An illness that occurs rapidly, lasts for a relatively short time and is self-limiting.

acute inpatient unit A ward in a mental health facility that admits people who are generally very mentally unwell.

acute kidney injury (AKI) Kidney injury characterised by a rapid onset of symptoms that are potentially reversible with prompt intervention that addresses the initial cause of the injury.

acute myocardial infarction (AMI) Necrosis (death) of myocardial cells.

acute pain Usually temporary, localised and of sudden onset; it lasts for less than 6 months and has an identifiable cause, such as trauma, surgery or inflammation.

acute respiratory distress syndrome (ARDS) Non-cardiac pulmonary oedema and progressive refractory hypoxaemia.

acute tubular necrosis (ATN) A syndrome of abrupt and progressive decline in tubular and glomerular function.

adaptive immune response A specific and systemic immune response initiated by and directed against particular antigens.

addiction Dependency on a drug, which can be either physical or psychological.

Addisonian crisis A rare, life-threatening response to acute adrenal insufficiency; occurs in about 25% of patients.

Addison's disease A rare endocrine disorder wherein the adrenal glands produce insufficient steroid hormones.

adrenal crisis A constellation of symptoms that indicate severe adrenal insufficiency caused by insufficient levels of the hormone cortisol.

advance directive Also called a *living will*, this is a document in which a person formally states preferences for healthcare in the event that he or she later becomes mentally incapacitated, and names a person who has durable power of attorney to serve as a substitute decision maker to implement the patient's stated preferences.

afterload The resistance the ventricles must overcome to eject their blood volume; the pressure in the arterial system ahead of the ventricles.

agnosia The inability to recognise one or more subjects that were previously familiar; agnosia may be visual, tactile or auditory.

albuminuria Albumin (protein) in the urine.

alcohol An organic compound obtained by substituting a hydroxyl group for a hydrogen on a hydrocarbon.

alcoholic cirrhosis (Laënnec's cirrhosis) The end result of alcoholic liver disease.

alkalis Substances that accept hydrogen ions in solution.

alkalosis The condition where the hydrogen ion concentration decreases below normal (reflected in a pH above 7.45).

alleles Different forms of a gene or DNA occupying the same place on a pair of chromosomes; an allele for each gene is inherited from each parent.

allergy A hypersensitivity response to environmental or exogenous antigens.

allografts Grafts between members of the same species but who have different genotypes and HLA antigens. See also *homograft*.

alopecia Loss of hair; baldness.

Alzheimer's disease (AD) A form of dementia characterised by progressive, irreversible deterioration of the general intellectual functioning.

amenorrhoea Absence of menstruation.

amputation Partial or total removal of a body part.

anaemia An abnormally low number of circulating red blood cells, haemoglobin concentration or both.

anaesthesia State produced by medications given intravenously, intraspinally, subcutaneously or by inhalation to create temporary partial or total loss of sensation and consciousness in a person for invasive procedures such as surgery or painful diagnostic tests.

analgesic A medication that reduces or eliminates the perception of pain.

anaphylactic shock Shock resulting from a widespread hypersensitivity reaction (called *anaphylaxis*). The pathophysiology in this type of shock includes vasodilation, pooling of blood in the periphery and hypovolaemia with altered cellular metabolism.

anaphylaxis An acute systemic type I response that occurs in highly sensitive people following injection of a specific antigen.

anaplasia The regression of a cell to an immature or undifferentiated cell type.

anasarca Severe, generalised oedema.

androgens Hormones synthesised in the testes, ovaries and adrenal cortex that promote expression of male sex characteristics.

anergy Inability to react to specific antigens.

aneurysm Abnormal dilation of a blood vessel, commonly at a site of a weakness or tear in the vessel wall.

angina pectoris (angina) Chest pain resulting from reduced coronary blood flow that causes a temporary imbalance between myocardial blood supply and demand.

angioma (haemangioma) Benign vascular tumour.

anion gap The difference between the sum of two measured anions, chloride and bicarbonate, and the principal measured cation, sodium.

ankylosing spondylitis (AS) A chronic inflammatory arthritis that primarily affects the axial skeleton, leading to pain and progressive stiffening and fusion of the spine.

anorexia Loss of appetite.

anorexia nervosa An eating disorder characterised by a body weight less than 85% of expected for age and height, and an intense fear of gaining weight.

anorgasmia Absence of orgasm.

anosmia Inability to smell.

antibodies Immunoglobulin molecules that bind with an antigen to inactivate it.

antibody-mediated (humoral) immune response Activation of B cells to produce antibodies to respond to antigens such as bacteria, bacterial toxins and free viruses.

anticipatory grieving A combination of intellectual and emotional responses and behaviours by which people adjust their self-concept in the face of a potential loss.

antigen A substance capable of evoking a specific immune response; usually a protein, which the body recognises as foreign, causing an immune response to be stimulated.

anxiety An unpleasant feeling that is typically associated with uneasiness, apprehension, fear or worry.

aortic valve The semilunar valve between the left ventricle of the heart and the aorta in the heart. It prevents blood from flowing backwards into the ventricle.

aphasia Defective or absent language function.

apical impulse A normal, visible pulsation (thrust) in the area of the midclavicular line in the left fifth intercostal space. It can be seen on inspection in about half of the adult population.

aplastic anaemia A condition manifested by failure of the bone marrow to produce all three types of blood cells.

apnoea Cessation of breathing lasting from a few seconds to a few minutes.

appendicitis Inflammation of the vermiform appendix.

apraxia The inability to carry out a motor pattern (such as drawing a figure) even when strength and coordination are adequate.

arrhythmia Abnormal heart rate or rhythm.

arterial blood gas (ABG) A laboratory test used to evaluate acid–base balance and gas exchange.

arthritis Joint inflammation.

ascites Excess fluid in the peritoneal cavity.

asphyxiation Oxygen deprivation.

asthma Chronic inflammatory disorder of the airways that is characterised by recurrent episodes of wheezing, breathlessness, chest tightness and coughing.

astigmatism A condition that develops with abnormal curvature of the cornea or eyeball, causing the image to focus at multiple points on the retina.

ataxia Uncoordinated, irregular gait and muscle movement; weakness.

atelectasis Collapse of lung tissue following obstruction of the bronchus or bronchioles.

atherosclerosis A form of arteriosclerosis in which deposits of fat and fibrin obstruct and harden the arteries.

atrial natriuretic peptide (ANP) A hormone released by atrial muscle cells in response to distension from fluid overload.

atrioventricular block A block in the normal conduction pathways.

Australian College of Mental Health Nurses (ACMHN) Peak professional college for mental health nurses in Australia.

autograft Transplant of the person's own tissue; the most successful type of tissue transplant.

autoimmune disorder Failure of the immune system to recognise itself, resulting in normal host tissue being targeted by immune defences.

autonomic dysreflexia Exaggerated sympathetic response that occurs in people with spinal cord injuries at or above the T6 level.

autosome A single chromosome from any one of the 22 pairs of chromosomes not involved in sex determination (X or Y); humans have 22 pairs of autosomes.

B lymphocytes (B cells) Bursa-equivalent lymphocytes responsible for synthesising humoral antibody.

bacterial vaginosis Non-specific vaginitis.

bactericidal agent Capable of killing an organism without immune system intervention. These include the penicillins, cephalosporins and aminoglycoside antibiotics.

bacteriostatic agent Inhibits the growth of a microorganism, leaving its destruction to the host's immune system.

balloon tamponade The application of pressure to stop oesophageal bleeding using an inflatable balloon.

bariatric care The branch of healthcare that deals with the causes, prevention and treatment of obesity. The term *bariatrics* was created around 1965, from the Greek root *bar-* ('weight' as in barometer), suffix *-iatr* ('treatment' as in paediatrics) and suffix *-ic* ('pertaining to'). The field encompasses dieting, exercise and behavioural therapy approaches to weight loss, as well as psychotherapy, pharmacotherapy and surgery.

basal cell carcinoma (BCC) Epithelial tumour that is believed to originate either from the basal layer of the epidermis or from cells in the surrounding dermal structures. These tumours are characterised by an impaired ability of the basal cells of the epidermis to mature into keratinocytes, with mitotic division beyond the basal layer.

basal metabolic rate (BMR) The energy used when the body is at rest.

base excess (BE) A calculated value also known as buffer base capacity. Base excess reflects the degree of acid–base imbalance by indicating the status of the body's total buffering capacity.

bases (or alkalis) Substances that accept hydrogen ions in solution.

Bell's palsy (facial paralysis) Disorder of the facial nerve (seventh cranial nerve), characterised by unilateral paralysis of the facial muscles.

benign prostatic hyperplasia (BPH) Enlargement of the prostate gland.

benzodiazepines Minor tranquillisers belonging to the sedative–hypnotic group of drugs that have a CNS depressant effect through action at the gamma-aminobutyric acid (GABA) receptor sites.

bile A greenish, watery solution containing bile salts, cholesterol, bilirubin, electrolytes, water and phospholipids.

biliary colic A severe, steady pain in the epigastric region or upper right quadrant of the abdomen.

binge-eating disorder An eating disorder characterised by recurrent episodes of eating an excessive amount of food during a defined period of time, and a sense of lack of control over eating during binge episodes.

biofilms Polymicrobial microbial communities that proliferate and are encased in a protective glycocalax matrix.

biomedical model of health A model of health that mainly focuses on biological health determinants and broadly views health as the absence of disease. This model is also known as the medical model.

biopsychosocial model of health The biopsychosocial model of health broadly views health as individual holistic wellbeing.

biotherapy Treatment that modifies the biological processes that result in malignant cells, primarily through enhancing the person's own immune responses.

bitemporal homonymous hemianopia Loss of vision in each temporal visual field (outer half of vision) resulting from compression of the optic chiasm.

blood flow The volume of blood transported in a vessel, in an organ or throughout the entire circulation over a given period of time.

blood glucose levels (BGLs) The amount of glucose present in blood.

blood pressure The tension or pressure exerted by blood against arterial walls.

blunt trauma The type of trauma that occurs when there is no communication from the damaged tissues to the outside environment.

body mass index (BMI) Used to identify excess adipose tissue, BMI is calculated by dividing the weight (in kilograms) by the height (in metres squared, m^2).

bone marrow transplant (BMT) Infusion of bone marrow cells to restore bone marrow function after chemotherapy or radiation; allogeneic BMT uses donor bone marrow cells from a donor; autologous BMT uses the person's own bone marrow.

borborygmus Hyperactive high-pitched, tinkling, rushing or growling bowel sound.

botulism A severe, life-threatening form of food poisoning caused by *Clostridium botulinum*.

bradypnoea Abnormally low respiratory rate.

brain death The cessation of cerebral blood flow with global brain infarction and permanent loss of all brain function.

brain death criteria Clinical signs used to determine whether a comatose person is brain dead.

breakthrough pain A sudden flare or increase in pain despite comfort with or without baseline analgesia.

bronchiectasis Permanent abnormal dilation of one or more large bronchi and destruction of bronchial walls, usually accompanied by infection.

bronchitis Inflammation of the bronchi.

bruit An adventitious sound heard during auscultation; of venous or arterial origin.

buffer A substance that prevents major changes in pH by removing or releasing hydrogen ions.

bulimia nervosa An eating disorder characterised by recurring episodes of binge eating followed by purge behaviours such as self-induced vomiting, use of laxatives or diuretics, fasting or excessive exercise.

burn An injury resulting from exposure to heat, chemicals, radiation, cold injuries or electric current.

burn shock Hypovolaemic shock resulting from the shift of a massive amount of fluid from the intracellular and intravascular compartments into the interstitium following burn injury.

bursitis Inflammation of the bursa.

cachectic The state of very poor health and malnourishment in a person.

cachexia The wasted physical appearance characteristic of cancer and other chronic illnesses. It is characterised by rapid depletion of the body's protein, particularly in skeletal muscle, with less rapid loss of fat.

caffeine A bitter, white crystalline xanthine alkaloid that is a psychoactive stimulant drug.

calculi An abnormal concentration in the body, commonly called a stone; occur in the kidneys, ureters, bladder or urethra.

cancer A family of complex diseases with manifestations that vary according to body system and type of tumour cells involved; marked by uncontrolled growth and the spread of abnormal cells.

cancer pain A common condition of people suffering with advanced cancer, it is often persistent and arises from a number of factors.

candidiasis Infection of mucous membranes caused by *Candida albicans*, a yeast-like fungus.

cannabis The general name given to the psychoactive substances found in the marijuana plant, Cannabis sativa, the main active constituent being delta 9-tetra-hydrocannabinol (THC).

carbuncle A group of infected hair follicles.

carcinogen Cancer-causing agent.

carcinogenesis The production or origin of cancer.

cardiac arrest Sudden failure of the heart to pump.

cardiac index Cardiac output adjusted for body size.

cardiac output (CO) The amount of blood pumped by the ventricles into the pulmonary and systemic circulations in 1 minute.

cardiac rehabilitation A long-term program of medical evaluation, exercise, risk factor modification, education and counselling designed to limit the physical and psychological effects of cardiac illness and improve the person's quality of life.

cardiac reserve The ability of the heart to respond to the body's changing need for cardiac output.

cardiac tamponade Compression of the heart due to pericardial effusion, trauma, cardiac rupture or haemorrhage.

cardiogenic shock Shock that occurs when the heart's pumping ability is compromised to the point that it cannot maintain cardiac output and adequate tissue perfusion.

cardiomyopathy Primary abnormality of the heart muscle that affects its structural or functional characteristics.

cardiovascular disease (CVD) Generic term for disorders of the heart and blood vessels.

carpopedal spasm Involuntary flexion and contraction of the wrist and ankle joints.

carrier Any individual who carries a single copy of an altered gene or mutation for a recessive condition on one chromosome of a chromosome pair and an unaltered form of that gene on the other chromosome; a carrier generally is not affected by the gene alteration; on average, each person in the general population is a carrier of five or six gene mutations for recessive disorders.

catabolism Biochemical process involving the breakdown of complex structures into simpler forms.

cataract Opacification (clouding) of the lens of the eye.

cell cycle The four phases that occur during growth and development of a cell.

cell-mediated (cellular) immune response Direct or indirect inactivation of antigen by lymphocytes.

cellulitis A localised infection of the dermis and subcutaneous tissue.

central nervous system (CNS) depressants Drugs that can be used to slow down brain activity.

central obesity Obesity characterised by a waist-to-hip ratio of greater than 1 in men or 0.8 in women.

central pain Related to a lesion in the brain that may spontaneously produce high-frequency bursts of impulses that are perceived as pain.

cerebral oedema An increase in the volume of brain tissue due to abnormal accumulation of fluid.

cerumen Earwax.

chalazion Granulomatous cyst or nodule of the eyelid.

chancre Hard, syphilitic primary ulcer.

cheilosis Painful lesions at corners of mouth.

chemotherapy Cancer treatment involving the use of cytotoxic medications to decrease tumour size, adjunctive to surgery or radiation therapy, or to prevent or treat suspected metastases.

chlamydia A group of syndromes caused by *Chlamydia trachomatis*, a bacterium that behaves like a virus spreading within a host cell; spread by sexual contact and to the neonate by passage through the birth canal of an infected mother.

cholecystitis Inflammation of the gallbladder, usually associated with stones in the cystic or common bile duct.

cholelithiasis Formation of stones (calculi) within the gallbladder or biliary duct system.

chromosome Genetic material carried by each cell; found in the cell nucleus.

chronic bronchitis Excessive secretion of bronchial mucus characterised by a productive cough lasting 3 or more months in 2 consecutive years.

chronic condition A disease involving a long course in its development or its symptoms.

chronic gastritis Disorders characterised by progressive and irreversible changes in the gastric mucosa.

chronic hepatitis Chronic infection of the liver.

chronic kidney disease The presence of impaired or reduced kidney function that lasts longer than 3 months.

chronic obstructive pulmonary disease (COPD) Chronic airflow obstruction due to chronic bronchitis and/or emphysema.

chronic sorrow A cyclical, recurring and potentially progressive pattern of pervasive sadness experienced in response to continual loss, throughout the trajectory of an illness or disability.

chronic venous insufficiency A chronic disorder of inadequate venous return.

Chvostek's sign Contraction of the lateral facial muscles in response to tapping the face in front of the ear; caused by decreased blood calcium levels.

circulating nurse Assists scrub nurses and surgeons during surgery.

cirrhosis A progressive, irreversible disorder, eventually leading to liver failure; the end stage of chronic liver disease.

claudication Cramping, aching pain in the calves, thighs and buttocks that occurs with a predictable level of activity and is relieved by rest.

clinical governance A system of policies, processes and accountabilities that is directed at improving patient safety and the quality and effectiveness of patient care within a health service.

clinical pathway A healthcare plan designed to provide care with a multidisciplinary, managed-action focus; developed for specific diagnoses, usually those that are high volume, high risk and high cost.

clinical reasoning The process by which nurses (and other clinicians) collect cues, process the information, come to an understanding of a person's problem or situation, plan and implement interventions, evaluate outcomes, and reflect on and learn from the process.

cocaine An illegal drug extracted from a cocoa leaf that is white, odourless, and takes the form of a crystalline powder.

cognition The ability to process information and apply knowledge.

cold sore See *herpes simplex*.

colectomy Surgical removal of the colon.

collateral vessels Accessory pathways connected to the smaller arteries in the coronary system.

colostomy Ostomy made in the colon.

comedones Non-inflammatory acne lesions.

communication The exchange of information between two or more people, groups or entities. It involves verbal and written exchanges, as well as body language, attitude and tone.

community A collection of people who share some attribute of their lives.

community mental health nurse A nurse in mental health nursing who works with consumers who are living in the community. They are often involved in case management.

compartment syndrome Condition in which excess pressure constricts the structures within a compartment and reduces circulation to muscles and nerves.

concussion Injury resulting from a violent jar, shake or impact with an object.

conjunctivitis Inflammation of the conjunctiva.

consciousness A condition in which a person is aware of self and environment and is able to respond appropriately to stimuli; full consciousness requires both normal rousal and full cognition.

constipation The infrequent (two or fewer bowel movements weekly) or difficult passage of stools.

consultation liaison (CL) A specialist mental health nurse who is the interface between medicine and psychiatry.

consumer-directed care A model of service delivery designed to give more care choice and flexibility to consumers. This model provides consumers with more control over the types of care and services they access, and the delivery of those services, including who delivers the services and when they are delivered.

continuum of care The provision of ongoing quality healthcare in acute and community settings to optimise quality of life for people, underpinned by an interprofessional consultative team approach.

contractility The inherent capability of the cardiac muscle fibres to shorten.

contracture Permanent shortening of connective tissue.

contralateral deficit Manifestations of a stroke on the side of the body opposite the side of the brain that is damaged.

contusion Superficial tissue injury resulting from blunt trauma, such as a kick or blow from an object, that causes the breakage of small blood vessels and bleeding into the surrounding tissue.

convergence Moving inward of the eyes to see an object close to the face.

cor pulmonale Condition of right ventricular hypertrophy and failure that results from longstanding pulmonary hypertension.

corneal reflex Closure of eyelids (blinking) due to corneal irritation.

corneal ulcer Local necrosis of the cornea, may be caused by infection, exposure trauma or the misuse/overuse of contact lenses.

coronary heart disease (CHD) Heart disease caused by impaired blood flow to the myocardium.

coryza (rhinorrhoea) Profuse nasal discharge.

COVID-19 COVID-19 is a novel coronavirus, which means that it is a new virus not previously seen in humans. It is considered infectious and is caused by the SARS-CoV-2 virus.

crackles Discontinuous lung sound heard by auscultation; can be fine or coarse. Produced by air passing over airway secretions or the opening of collapsed airways.

creatinine The end product from the breakdown of creatine phosphate in muscles.

crepitation A grating sound heard on movement of a joint.

Creutzfeldt–Jakob disease (CJD, spongiform encephalopathy) Rare, progressive neurological disease that causes brain degeneration without inflammation.

critical thinking Self-directed thinking that is focused on what to believe or do in a specific situation.

Crohn's disease (regional enteritis) Chronic, relapsing inflammatory disorder affecting the gastrointestinal tract.

cultural competence Practising in a way that demonstrates the importance of social and cultural influences on patients' health beliefs and behaviours, and devising interventions that take these issues into account.

cultural safety The effective nursing practice of a person or family from another culture, as determined by that person or family.

culture A learned world viewpoint or paradigm shared by a population or group and transmitted socially. It influences values, beliefs, customs and behaviours, and is reflected in the language, dress, food, materials and social interactions of a group.

Curling's ulcers Acute ulcerations of the stomach or duodenum that form following a burn injury.

Cushing's disease One form of Cushing's syndrome caused by a functioning pituitary adenoma, leading to increased secretion of adrenocorticotropic hormone (ACTH), causing excessive cortisol levels.

Cushing's syndrome A chronic disorder in which hyperfunction of the adrenal cortex produces excessive amounts of circulating cortisol or adrenocorticotropic hormone (ACTH).

Cushing's ulcers Stress ulcers occurring as sequelae of head injury or central nervous system surgery.

cyanosis A bluish discolouration of the skin and mucous membranes due to oxygen deficiency.

cyst A sac containing fluid or semisolid fluid.

cystectomy Complete surgical removal of the urinary bladder and adjacent muscles and tissues.

cystic fibrosis (CF) Inherited disorder of the exocrine glands that results in the secretion of abnormal amounts of mucus.

cystitis Inflammation of the urinary bladder.

cytokines Hormone-like polypeptides produced primarily by monocytes, macrophages and T cells. Cytokines act as messengers of the immune system, facilitating communication between the cells to adjust or vary the inflammatory reaction or to initiate immune cell proliferation and differentiation.

dawn phenomenon A rise in blood glucose between 4 am and 8 am that is not a response to hypoglycaemia.

day surgery units/centres Facilities where surgery is performed and the person is discharged on the same day.

death Irreversible cessation of circulatory and respiratory functions or irreversible cessation of all functions of the entire brain, including the brainstem.

death anxiety Worry or fear related to death or dying.

debridement Process of removing dead tissue from a wound.

decerebrate posturing Abnormal posture with the neck extended; the jaw clenched; arms pronated, extended and close to the sides; legs extended and feet plantar flexed. Results from lesions of the midbrain, pons or diencephalons.

decorticate posturing Abnormal posture with the upper arms close to the sides; the elbows, wrists and fingers flexed; the legs extended and internally rotated; and the feet plantar flexed. Results from lesions of the corticospinal tracts.

deep venous thrombosis (DVT) Blood clot (thrombus) formation and inflammation within a deep vein, usually in the pelvis or lower extremities; a common complication of hospitalisation, surgery and immobilisation.

dehiscence An unintended separation of wound margins due to incomplete healing.

dehydration Loss of water.

delegation Assigning appropriate work activities to other members of the healthcare team. When the nurse delegates nursing care activities to another person, that person is authorised to act in the place of the nurse, while the nurse retains the accountability for the activities performed.

delusion A fixed false belief that is firmly sustained despite what constitutes incontrovertible and obvious proof or evidence to the contrary. The belief is not one ordinarily accepted by other members of the person's culture or subculture.

dementia A global impairment of cognitive function that usually is progressive and may be permanent; interferes with normal social and occupational activities.

dermatitis Acute or chronic inflammation of the skin characterised by erythema and pain or pruritus.

dermatophytoses Superficial fungal infection of the skin; also called *ringworm*.

determinants of health Factors that influence health in either a positive or a negative way. Some of these function on an individual level (e.g. health behaviours such as smoking or exercise, or our genetic make-up). Others function at a broader societal level, such as the availability of health services, vaccination programs or clean drinking water and healthy food.

diabetes insipidus (DI) The result of antidiuretic hormone insufficiency.

diabetes mellitus (DM) Group of chronic disorders of the endocrine pancreas, all categorised under a broad diagnostic label. The condition is characterised by inappropriate hyperglycaemia caused by a relative or absolute deficiency of insulin or by a cellular resistance to the action of insulin.

diabetic ketoacidosis (DKA) A form of metabolic acidosis induced by stress in a person with type 1 diabetes mellitus.

diabetic nephropathy A disease of the kidneys characterised by the presence of albumin in the urine, hypertension, oedema and progressive renal insufficiency.

diabetic neuropathies Disorders of the peripheral nerves and the autonomic nervous system manifesting one or more of the following: sensory and motor impairment, muscle weakness and pain, cranial nerve disorders, impaired vasomotor function, impaired gastrointestinal function and impaired genitourinary function.

diabetic retinopathy The collective name for the changes in the retina that occur in the person with diabetes. The retinal capillary structure undergoes alterations in blood flow, leading to retinal ischaemia and a breakdown in the blood retinal barrier.

***Diagnostic and Statistical Manual of Mental Disorders* (DSM)** A manual that is published by the American Psychiatric Association that provides common language and standard criteria for the classification of mental disorders.

dialysate Dialysis solution.

dialysis The diffusion of solute molecules across a semipermeable membrane from an area of higher concentration to one of lower concentration.

diaphoresis Copious production of sweat.

diarrhoea An increase in the frequency, volume and fluid content of the stool.

diastolic blood pressure The minimum pressure maintained by elastic arterial walls during diastole (cardiac relaxation) to maintain blood flow through capillary beds; averages 80 mmHg in a healthy adult.

differentiation A process occurring over many cell cycles that allows cells to specialise in certain tasks.

'differentness' Being different from another person or group of people.

diffuse oesophageal spasm Non-peristaltic contraction of oesophageal smooth muscle.

diffusion The process by which solute molecules move from an area of high solute concentration to an area of low solute concentration to become evenly distributed.

digital health A broad range of technologies that can be used to treat patients and collect and share a person's health information.

dilemma A choice between two unpleasant, ethically troubling alternatives.

diplopia Double vision.

disaster Event that requires extraordinary efforts beyond those needed to respond to everyday emergencies.

discharge planning A planned process beginning with the person's initial presentation, considering the needs of the unique individual, based upon the availability of, and access to, support and resources. This process ensures that these needs are met through ongoing assessment and consultation involving the relevant healthcare professionals, patient, family, carers and community services.

discovery Encompasses equality and respect. Equality is the belief that all people ought to be treated equally. Respect is esteem for, or a sense of the worth or excellence of, a person, a personal quality, ability or a manifestation of a personal quality or ability.

disease Literally meaning 'without ease', this term describes alterations in structure and function of the body or mind. Diseases may have mechanical, biological or normative causes.

dislocation Separation of contact between two bones of a joint.

dissection (aortic) A life-threatening emergency caused by a tear in the intima of the aorta with haemorrhage into the media.

disseminated intravascular coagulation (DIC) A disruption of haemostasis characterised by widespread intravascular clotting and bleeding; a syndrome that develops as a complication of many other disorders.

distal determinants Determinants of health that tend to be stable and concern historical, national, institutional, political, legal and cultural factors.

distributive shock Also called *vasogenic shock*, this includes several types of shock that result from widespread vasodilation and decreased peripheral resistance.

diverticulitis Inflammation in and around the diverticular sac; typically affects only one diverticulum, usually in the sigmoid colon.

diverticulosis Indicates the presence of diverticula.

DNA-based tests Tests that incorporate new, sophisticated technology that permits the examination of the DNA itself, obtained from blood, bone marrow, amniotic fluid, fibroblast cells of the skin or buccal cells from the mouth.

do-not-resuscitate (DNR) directive Usually written by the doctor for the person who has a terminal illness or is near death, this order is usually based on the wishes of the person and family that no cardiopulmonary resuscitation be performed for respiratory or cardiac arrest.

Down syndrome A human genetic disease caused by the presence of an extra chromosome 21; characterised by mental retardation and heart and respiratory defects.

dumping syndrome Complication of partial gastrectomy characterised by nausea, weakness, sweating, palpitation, syncope, sensation of warmth and occasionally diarrhoea.

duodenal ulcers Peptic ulcer disease affecting the duodenum.

dwarfism A medical disorder, the term being used to describe a person of short stature.

dysarthria Difficulty speaking.

dysfunctional uterine bleeding (DUB) Vaginal bleeding that is usually painless but abnormal in amount, duration or time of occurrence.

dysmenorrhoea Pain associated with menstruation.

dyspareunia Painful intercourse.

dysphagia Difficulty swallowing.

dysphonia Change in the tone of voice.

dysplasia The loss of DNA control over differentiation occurring in response to adverse conditions.

dyspnoea Difficult or laboured breathing.

dysuria Painful urination.

ecchymosis A flat, irregularly shaped lesion of varying size with no pulsation; caused by blood collecting under the skin.

ectopic beats Impulses originating outside normal conduction pathways of the heart.

ejection fraction (EF) The percentage of total blood remaining in the ventricle at the end of diastole (relaxation); normal is 50–70%.

electrolytes Substances that dissociate in solution to form charged particles called ions.

electronic medical records (EMRs) Electronic (digital) collections of medical information about a person that are stored on a computer. An electronic medical record includes information about a patient's health history, such as diagnoses, medicines, tests, allergies, immunisations and treatment plans. It can be seen by all healthcare providers who are taking care of a patient and can be used by them to help make recommendations about the patient's care. Also called EHR and electronic health record.

embolism Sudden obstruction of a blood vessel by debris.

emphysema Destruction of the walls of the alveoli, with resulting enlargement of abnormal air spaces.

empowerment Developing confidence in one's own capacities.

empyema Accumulation of purulent exudate in the pleural cavity.

encephalitis An acute inflammation of the parenchyma of the brain or spinal cord.

end-of-life care Care provided in the final weeks of life when death is imminent.

endocarditis Inflammation of the endocardium.

endogenous insulin The insulin the pancreas makes.

endometriosis A condition in which multiple, small implants of endometrial tissue develop throughout the pelvic cavity.

endotoxins Found in the cell wall of Gram-negative bacteria, endotoxins are released only when the cell is disrupted. They act as activators of many human regulatory systems, producing fever, inflammation and potentially clotting, bleeding or hypotension when released in large quantities.

end-stage kidney disease (ESKD) The final stage of chronic kidney failure in which the kidneys are unable to excrete metabolic wastes and regulate fluid and electrolyte balance adequately; characterised by a glomerular filtration rate of less than 5% of normal.

enduring power of attorney A document that can delegate the authority to make health, financial and/or legal decisions on a person's behalf. It must be provided in writing and state that the designated person is authorised to make healthcare decisions.

enophthalmos Sunken appearance of the eyes.

enteral nutrition Administration of liquid nutritional formulas to meet kilojoule and protein needs in people unable to consume adequate food; also called *tube feeding*.

enucleation Surgical removal of an eye.

epidemic A widespread occurrence of an infectious disease (biological), localised to a particular community, region or population.

epididymitis Infection or inflammation of the epididymis.

epidural haematoma (extradural haematoma) A collection of blood between the dura and the skull.

epilepsy Chronic seizure activity.

epistaxis Nosebleed.

erectile dysfunction Inability of the male to attain and maintain an erection sufficient to permit satisfactory sexual intercourse.

erosive gastritis Inflammation and superficial erosions of the gastric mucosa that may occur as a complication of other life-threatening conditions such as shock, severe trauma, major surgery, sepsis, burns or head injury.

erysipelas Infection of the skin most often caused by group A streptococci.

erythema A reddening of the skin.

erythropoiesis Red blood cell production.

eschar Hard, leathery crust that covers a burn wound and harbours necrotic tissue.

escharotomy Surgical removal of eschar from the torso or extremity to prevent circumferential constriction.

euthyroid The state of having normal thyroid gland function.

evisceration Protrusion of body contents through a surgical wound.

exogenous insulin The insulin people inject or infuse via an insulin pump.

exophthalmos Protrusion of the eyeballs.

exotoxins Soluble proteins secreted into surrounding tissue by the microorganism. Exotoxins are highly poisonous, causing cell death or dysfunction.

extracorporeal shock wave lithotripsy (ESWL, transcutaneous shock wave lithotripsy) Non-invasive technique for fragmenting kidney stones using shock waves generated outside the body.

faecal impaction A rock-hard or putty-like mass of faeces in the rectum.

family Two or more people who are emotionally involved with each other.

fascial excision (fasciectomy) Process of excising the wound to the level of fascia.

fasciculations Involuntary twitching.

fat embolism syndrome (FES) Characterised by neurological dysfunction, pulmonary insufficiency and a petechial rash on the chest, axilla and upper arms due to fat globules lodged in the pulmonary vascular bed or peripheral circulation.

fibrocystic changes (FCCs) Physiological nodularity and breast tenderness that increase and decrease with the menstrual cycle.

fibroid tumours (uterine leiomyomas) See *leiomyomas*.

fibromyalgia A common rheumatic syndrome characterised by musculoskeletal pain, stiffness and tenderness.

filtration The process by which water and dissolved substances (solutes) move from an area of higher hydrostatic pressure to an area of lower hydrostatic pressure.

flaccidity Decreased muscle tone in disease or trauma of the lower motor neurons.

flail chest Free-floating segment of the chest wall, resulting from two or more consecutive ribs fractured in multiple places.

flatus Gas in the digestive tract.

fluid resuscitation Replacement of the extensive fluid and electrolyte losses associated with major burn injuries.

fluid volume deficit (FVD) A decrease in intravascular, interstitial and/or intracellular fluid in the body.

fluid volume excess (FVE) Excess extracellular fluid resulting from retention of both water and sodium in the body.

focused assessment A physical assessment that concentrates on the part of the body that may be affected by disease or injury.

folliculitis Bacterial infection of the hair follicle, most commonly caused by *Staphylococcus aureus*.

forensic mental health A subspecialty of mental health in which scientific and clinical expertise is applied in legal contexts, combining civil, criminal, correctional and legislative matters.

fracture A break in a bone, usually due to trauma.

friction rub The sound heard when two dry surfaces are rubbed together.

full-thickness avulsion injuries Injuries that result in loss of all of the layers of the skin, causing fat and muscle to be exposed.

full-thickness burn A burn that involves all layers of the skin, including the epidermis, dermis and epidermal appendages.

fulminant hepatitis Hepatitis with a rapid and severe onset and course.

furuncle Often called a boil; an inflammation of the hair follicle.

gamma hydroxybutyrate (GHB) A dissociative anaesthetic agent; another of the newer drugs diverted to illicit use.

gastric mucosal barrier A protective barrier consisting of lipids, bicarbonate ions and mucous gel that protects the stomach lining from the damaging effects of gastric juices.

gastric outlet obstruction Obstruction of the pyloric region of the stomach and duodenum that impairs gastric outflow; a potential complication of peptic ulcer disease.

gastric ulcers Ulcers of the stomach lining, usually in the lesser curvature and antrum; more common in older adults.

gastritis Inflammation of the stomach lining.

gastroduodenostomy (Billroth I) Excision of the pylorus of the stomach with the anastomosis of the upper stomach to the duodenum; commonly used partial gastrectomy procedure.

gastroenteritis Inflammation of the gastrointestinal tract; not a specific disease, but a group of syndromes or a collection of related manifestations.

gastrojejunostomy (Billroth II) Subtotal excision of the stomach with closure of the duodenum and side-to-side anastomosis of the jejunum to the stomach; commonly used partial gastrectomy procedure.

gastro-oesophageal reflux Backward flow of gastric contents into the oesophagus.

gastro-oesophageal reflux disease (GORD) Causes heartburn, usually after meals, when bending over or reclining.

gene A sequence of DNA on a chromosome that represents a fundamental unit of heredity; occupies a specific spot on a chromosome (gene locus).

gene expression When the protein product of a gene is visible (e.g. through the presence of a body structure or identifiable through biochemical tests such as insulin or phenylalanine levels).

general anaesthesia Deep sedation, which includes analgesia and muscle paralysis. This type of anaesthesia requires respiratory maintenance without the aid of the person's respiratory musculature.

genetic locus The term used to describe a gene's location on a specific chromosome.

genetics The scientific study of heredity and hereditary variation.

genital herpes (herpes simplex genitalis) An infection of the external genitalia caused by herpes simplex genitalis; transmitted by vaginal, anal or oral–genital contact.

genital warts (*condyloma acuminatum*, venereal warts) A sexually transmitted condition caused by the human papillomavirus.

genomics The study of whole sets of genes and their interactions.

genotype The genes and the variations therein that a person inherits from his or her parents.

gigantism Occurs when growth hormone hypersecretion begins before puberty and the closure of the epiphyseal plates, leading the person to become abnormally tall.

gingivitis Inflammation of the gums, characterised by inflammation, redness and bleeding.

glaucoma Condition characterised by increased intraocular pressure of the eye and a gradual loss of vision.

glomerular filtration rate (GFR) The rate at which plasma is filtered through the glomeruli of the kidney.

glomerulonephritis Inflammation of the capillary loops of the glomeruli.

glossitis Inflammation of the tongue.

glucagon Hormone that stimulates the liver to breakdown glycogen into glucose and to synthesise glucose from lactic acid and non-carbohydrate molecules.

gluconeogenesis Formation of glucose from fats and proteins.

glucosuria Excessive glucose in urine.

glycogenolysis Breakdown of liver glycogen to glucose.

goitre An enlarged thyroid gland. Enlargement results from both inadequate and excessive synthesis of thyroid hormones.

gonorrhoea (GC, clap) An infection caused by *Neisseria gonorrhoeae* that is transmitted by direct sexual contact or by delivery of a neonate by an infected mother.

gout A syndrome that occurs from an inflammatory response to the production or excretion of uric acid resulting in high levels of uric acid in the blood (hyperuricaemia) and in other body fluids, including synovial fluid.

Graves' disease Caused by a defect in immunoregulation in genetically predisposed individuals, leading to production of thyroid-stimulating antibodies.

grief The emotional response to loss and its accompanying changes.

grieving The internal process the person uses to work through the response to loss.

Guillain–Barré syndrome (GBS) Acute demyelinating disorder of the peripheral nervous system characterised by progressive, usually rapid muscle weakness and paralysis.

gynaecomastia Breast enlargement in men.

haemangioma See *angioma*.

haematemesis Blood in the vomit.

haematochezia Blood in the stool.

haematopoiesis Blood cell formation.

haematuria Blood in the urine.

haemodialysis A procedure in which electrolytes, waste products and excess water are removed from the body by diffusion and ultrafiltration as blood passes by an artificial semipermeable membrane outside the body.

haemolysis The process of red blood cell destruction.

haemolytic anaemia Premature destruction (lysis) of red blood cells.

haemophilia A group of hereditary clotting factor disorders that lead to persistent and potentially severe bleeding.

haemoptysis Bloody sputum.

haemorrhage Rapid or excessive bleeding.

haemorrhagic stroke (intracranial haemorrhage) Cerebrovascular accident (CVA) occurring when a cerebral blood vessel ruptures.

haemorrhoids (piles) Clusters of dilated veins in swollen anal tissue.

haemostasis Control of bleeding.

haemothorax Blood in the pleural space.

halitosis (bad breath) A common condition caused by an increase in sulfur-producing bacteria in the oral cavity.

hallucination An alteration of sensory perception in the absence of a stimulus.

hallucinogens Drugs that produce hallucinations.

harm reduction A way of reducing the impact of drug- and/or alcohol-related harm to individuals and the community through a range of cost-effective public health policies, strategies and practices.

Hashimoto's thyroiditis An autoimmune disorder caused by the development of antibodies that destroy thyroid tissue.

health As defined by the World Health Organization, 'a state of complete physical, mental and social well-being, and not merely the absence of disease or infirmity'.

Health Care Home (HCH) A general practice that coordinates care for people with chronic and complex conditions.

health determinants Factors that affect the health of people.

health education Individualistic strategies to improve health, often by increasing knowledge or influencing attitudes to alter behaviours and lifestyle. Health education is often used interchangeably with health promotion although they are not the same.

health promotion Any activity undertaken for the purpose of achieving a higher level of health and wellbeing.

healthcare-associated infection (HAI) An infection contracted during residence in a hospital or extended care facility.

heart failure Inability of the heart to pump adequate blood to meet the metabolic demands of the body.

hemianopia The loss of half of the visual field of one or both eyes.

hemiparesis Weakness of the left or right half of the body.

hemiplegia Paralysis of the left or right half of the body.

hepatitis Inflammation of the liver, usually caused by a virus; may be acute or chronic.

hepatorenal syndrome Renal failure accompanied by azotaemia, sodium retention, oliguria and hypotension in people with cirrhosis and ascites.

hernia A defect in the abdominal wall that allows abdominal contents to protrude out of the abdominal cavity.

herpes simplex (fever blister, cold sore) Acute viral infections of the skin and mucous membranes caused by two types of herpes virus: HSV I and HSV II.

herpes zoster (shingles) Viral infection of a dermatome section of the skin caused by varicella zoster, the same herpes virus that causes chickenpox.

heterograft (xenograft) Skin obtained from an animal, usually a pig.

heterozygous Non-identical copies of a particular gene (different alleles) on the paired chromosomes.

hiatal hernia Protrusion of part of the stomach through the oesophageal hiatus of the diaphragm into the mediastinal cavity.

hirsutism Increased growth of coarse hair, usually on the face and trunk.

histocompatibility The ability of cells and tissues to survive transplantation without immunological interference by the recipient.

Hodgkin's disease Develops in a single lymph node or chain of nodes and spreads to adjoining nodes. Involved lymph nodes contain *Reed–Sternberg cells* (malignant cells) surrounded by host inflammatory cells. These malignant cells secrete inflammatory mediator substances, attracting inflammatory cells to the tumour site. They may invade almost any tissue in the body.

holistic healthcare Care in which all aspects of a person (physical, psychosocial, cultural, spiritual and intellectual) are considered as essential components of individualised care.

homeostasis The body's tendency to maintain a state of physiological balance in the presence of constantly changing conditions.

homograft (allograft) Human skin that has been harvested from cadavers.

homologous chromosomes Chromosomes that are members of the same pair and normally have the same number and arrangement of genes; usually one copy is from the mother and the other copy is from the father.

homozygous Identical copies of a particular gene (same alleles) on both paired chromosomes.

hope A belief in a positive outcome related to events and circumstances in one's life; the foundation of recovery from mental illness.

hordeolum (sty) Staphylococcal abscess that may occur on either the external or internal margin of the lid.

hospice care The delivery of care for terminally ill people either in healthcare facilities or in the person's home.

human genome The total amount of the DNA (genes) in an individual's cells.

human immunodeficiency virus (HIV) Virus responsible for AIDS.

Huntington's disease Progressive, degenerative, inherited neurological disease characterised by increasing dementia and chorea.

hydrocephalus An abnormal accumulation of cerebrospinal fluid within the cranial vault and dilation of the ventricles.

hydrocoele Fluid-filled mass within the scrotum.

hydronephrosis Distension of the urinary tract with urine behind an obstruction.

hyperglycaemia Elevated blood glucose levels (above 126 mg/dL), which causes osmotic diuresis and, if chronic, damages vessel epithelium and renal glomeruli.

hyperopia (farsightedness) The condition in which the eyeball is short, causing the image to focus behind the retina.

hyperosmolar hyperglycaemic state (HHS) A condition of very high blood glucose with adequate insulin to prevent ketosis, but which does cause diuresis.

hyperparathyroidism Results from an increase in the secretion of parathyroid hormone, which regulates normal serum levels of calcium and phosphate.

hyperplasia An increase in the number or density of normal cells.

hypersensitivity Exaggerated response of the immune system to an antigen.

hypertension Excess pressure in the arterial portion of systemic circulation.

hyperthyroidism A disorder caused by excessive delivery of thyroid hormone to the peripheral tissues. Also called thyrotoxicosis.

hypertrophic scar Overgrowth of dermal tissue that remains within the boundaries of the wound.

hyphaema Bleeding into the anterior chamber of the eye, possibly as the result of blunt eye trauma.

hypoglycaemia Low blood glucose levels; deficiency of blood sugar.

hypoparathyroidism A condition that results from abnormally low parathyroid hormone levels, causing hypocalcaemia and an elevated blood phosphate level.

hypothyroidism A disorder that results when the thyroid gland produces an insufficient amount of thyroid hormone.

hypovolaemic shock Shock caused by a decrease in intravascular volume of 15% or more. This form of shock is caused by the loss of whole blood, blood plasma or extracellular fluid.

hypoxaemia Decreased oxygen concentration in the blood, measured by PaO_2.

ileostomy An ostomy made in the ileum of the small intestine.

illness–wellness continuum A continuum representing health as a dynamic process, with high-level wellness at one extreme of the continuum and death at the opposite extreme.

illusion A distortion of the senses.

immunity The protection of the body from disease.

immunocompetent Possessing an immune system that can identify antigens and effectively destroy or remove them.

immunoglobulin (Ig) A protein that functions as an antibody.

immunosuppression Inability of the immune system to respond to an antigen. Occurs in response to disease or medications; may be intentional to prevent rejection of transplants or a side effect of some medications.

impetigo Infection of the skin caused by either *Staphylococcus aureus* or beta-haemolytic streptococci.

impotence Inability to achieve or maintain an erection.

impulse control The ability to control behavioural impetuosity.

increased intracranial pressure (IICP, intracranial hypertension) Sustained elevated pressure (10 mmHg or higher) within the cranial cavity.

Indigenous health A broad term which generally refers to the health status and health outcomes of the Aboriginal and Torres Strait Islander population of Australia.

infection Colonisation by and multiplication of an organism within a host. The host can be any organism capable of supporting the nutritional and physical growth requirements of the microorganism—for example, humans.

inflammation A complex, non-specific, adaptive response to injury that brings fluid, dissolved substances and blood cells into the interstitial tissues where the invasion or damage has occurred.

inflammatory bowel disease (IBD) Chronic inflammation of the bowel common to a group of conditions that includes Crohn's disease and ulcerative colitis.

influenza Highly contagious viral respiratory disease characterised by coryza, fever, cough and constitutional manifestations such as headache and malaise.

informed consent Disclosure of risks associated with the intended procedure or operation to the patient. The language of the document varies according to statutory and common law of each state.

innate immunity Specific and non-specific responses that prevent or limit the entry of invaders into the body, thereby limiting the extent of tissue damage and reducing the workload of the adaptive immune system.

insight The degree to which a person has an understanding of their illness or disorder.

instrument nurse The nurse primarily responsible for manual dexterity and in-depth knowledge of the anatomical and mechanical aspects of a particular surgery. The instrument nurse handles sutures, instruments and other equipment immediately adjacent to the sterile field.

insulin A hormone that facilitates entry of glucose into fat and muscle cells for energy.

insulin reaction Hypoglycaemia in people with type 1 diabetes mellitus.

intermediate determinants Determinants of health that concern community infrastructure, personal wealth or access to resources, natural, physical and built environments. This level also includes access to healthcare and health systems.

International Classification of Diseases (ICD) Classification of diseases, functioning and disability.

interprofessional care Care provided by an interprofessional team where two or more professions work together as a team with a common purpose, commitment and mutual respect (Freeth et al. 2005, cited in Dunston et al., 2009, p. 6).

intersectoral Working with more than one sector of society to take action on an area of shared interest, such as health.

intracerebral haematomas A collection of blood in the brain tissue, most often located in the frontal or temporal lobes.

intracranial aneurysm Saccular outpouching of a cerebral artery that occurs at the site of a weakness in the vessel wall.

intraoperative phase The time during surgery, from beginning to end.

iron deficiency anaemia The most common type of anaemia; results from inadequate iron for optimal red blood cell formation.

irritable bowel syndrome (IBS) A motility disorder of the gastrointestinal tract characterised by alternating periods of constipation and diarrhoea.

ischaemia Deficient blood flow to tissue.

ischaemic Deprived of oxygen.

isograft Tissue transplant where the donor and recipient are identical twins.

jaundice Yellow-to-orange colour visible in the skin and mucous membranes; most often the result of a hepatic disorder.

Kaposi's sarcoma (KS) A vascular malignancy (a tumour of the endothelial cells lining small blood vessels) that presents as vascular macules, papules or violet lesions affecting the skin and viscera. It is often the presenting symptom of AIDS.

keloid Elevated, irregularly shaped, progressively enlarging scar arising from excessive amounts of collagen in the stratum corneum during scar formation in connective tissue repair.

keratin A fibrous, water-repellent protein that gives the epidermis its tough, protective quality.

keratitis Inflammation of the cornea.

keratosis Any skin condition in which there is a benign overgrowth and thickening of the cornified epithelium.

ketamine A central nervous system depressant, best described as a dissociative anaesthetic agent.

ketonuria The presence of ketones in the urine.

ketosis An accumulation of ketone bodies produced during the oxidation of fatty acids.

kidney replacement therapy Therapy provided through haemodialysis, peritoneal dialysis or kidney transplantation.

kinaesthaesia The ability to perceive movement and sense of position.

Klinefelter's syndrome A syndrome in which males have an extra X chromosome in most of their cells (also known as the XXY condition).

knowledge resource base Ways in which knowledge is developed.

Korotkoff's sounds Sounds heard during auscultation of blood pressure.

kyphosis Exaggerated thoracic curvature of the spine common in older adults.

labyrinthitis Inflammation of the inner ear.

laceration Open wound that results from sharp cutting or tearing. Injuries to the integument are at risk of contamination from dirt, debris or foreign objects.

laminectomy Removal of the lamina of the vertebrae.

laparoscopic cholecystectomy Removal of the gallbladder using an endoscope.

laryngectomy Removal of the larynx.

laryngitis Inflammation of the larynx.

leiomyomas Solid, pedunculated benign tumours.

leucocytes Also called white blood cells, these are the primary cells involved in both non-specific and specific immune system responses. These cells isolate the infecting organism or injury, destroy pathogens and promote healing.

leucocytosis An increase in the number of leucocytes in the blood (above 10,000/mm^3), usually caused by infection.

leucopenia Abnormal decrease of circulating leucocytes, usually below 5,000/mm^3; occurs when bone marrow activity is suppressed, or when leucocyte destruction increases.

leucoplakia Formation of white patches or spots on the mucous membranes or tongue; these lesions may become malignant.

leukaemia ('white blood') A group of chronic malignant disorders of white blood cells (WBCs) and WBC precursors; characterised by replacement of bone marrow by malignant immature WBCs, abnormal immature circulating WBCs and infiltration of malignant cells into other tissues.

libido Instinctive drive associated with sexual desire.

life-limiting illness An illness where it is expected that death will be a direct consequence of the specified illness.

lipoatrophy Atrophy of subcutaneous tissue.

lipodystrophy Hypertrophy of subcutaneous tissue that may result if the same injection sites are used repeatedly, especially with porcine and bovine insulins.

lithiasis Stone formation.

lithotripsy Crushing of renal calculi.

liver transplantation Surgery to remove a diseased liver and transplant a healthy liver (whole or segment) from another person.

locked-in syndrome Person is alert and fully aware of the environment, but is unable to communicate through speech or movement as a result of blocked efferent pathways to the brain.

lordosis Increased lumbar curve.

loss An actual or potential situation in which a valued object, person, relationship, body part or emotion that was formerly present is lost or changed and can no longer be seen, felt, heard, known or experienced.

lung abscess Localised area of lung destruction or necrosis and pus formation.

lung compliance Distensibility of the lungs.

lymphadenopathy The enlargement of lymph nodes (over 1 cm) with or without tenderness. It may be caused by inflammation, infection or malignancy of the nodes or the regions drained by the nodes.

lymphocytes Account for 20–40% of circulating leucocytes. Lymphocytes are the principal effector and regulator cells of specific immune responses.

lymphoedema Extremity oedema due to accumulated lymph; may be primary or secondary, resulting from inflammation, obstruction or removal of lymphatic vessels.

lymphomas Malignancy of lymphoid tissue.

macrophages Monocytes mature into macrophages after settling into tissue. Macrophages are large phagocytes. They are important in the body's defence against chronic infections.

macular degeneration Destructive changes in the macula due to injury or gradual failure of the outer pigmented layer of the retina (the retinal layer adjacent to the choroid), which removes cellular waste products and keeps the retina attached to the choroid.

major trauma Serious single-system injury (such as the traumatic amputation of a leg) or multiple-system injuries. Also known as multiple trauma.

malabsorption A condition in which nutrients are ineffectively absorbed by the intestinal mucosa, resulting in their excretion in the stool.

malignant melanoma Skin cancer that arises from melanocytes.

malnutrition Inadequate nutrient intake to meet body needs; may include deficiency of major nutrients (kilojoules, carbohydrates, proteins and fats) or micronutrients such as vitamins and minerals.

man-made disasters Either accidental or intentional, they are complex emergencies, technological disasters, material shortages and other disasters not caused by natural hazards.

mass casualty incident (MCI) An event that generates more patients at one time than locally available resources can manage using routine procedures.

mastoiditis Bacterial infection of the mastoid process.

mean arterial pressure (MAP) The average pressure in the arterial circulation throughout the cardiac cycle; the product of cardiac output and systemic vascular resistance (SVR).

medical–surgical nursing The health promotion, healthcare and illness care of adults, based on knowledge derived from the arts and sciences and shaped by knowledge (the science) of nursing.

meiosis A modified type of cell division in sexually reproducing organisms consisting of two rounds of cell division but only one round of DNA replication. It results in cells with half the number of chromosome sets as the original cell.

melaena Black, tarry stool that contains blood.

melanin Skin pigment that forms a protective shield to protect keratinocytes and nerve endings in the dermis from the damaging effects of ultraviolet light.

memory The ability to store, retain and recall information.

Ménière's disease Chronic disorder of unknown cause characterised by recurrent attacks of vertigo with tinnitus and a progressive unilateral hearing loss.

meningitis Inflammation of the meninges of the brain and spinal cord.

menopause Permanent cessation of menses.

menorrhagia Excessive or prolonged menstruation.

menstrual cycle Cyclic build up of the uterine lining, ovulation and sloughing of the lining occurring approximately every 28 days in non-pregnant females.

menstruation Periodic shedding of the uterine lining in a woman of childbearing age who is not pregnant.

Mental Health Act Mental health legislation.

Mental Health Nurse Practitioner (MHNP) A specialist mental health nurse with qualifications at master's degree level.

mental state examination (MSE) A clinical assessment that describes the sum total of the examiner's observations at the time of the interview or interaction.

metabolic syndrome A cluster of manifestations often associated with type 2 diabetes. Includes insulin resistance, hypertension, low high-density lipoprotein cholesterol and high triglycerides.

metabolism The breakdown of complex structures into simpler forms to produce energy (catabolism) and the combination of simpler molecules to produce and maintain more complex structures necessary to living organisms (anabolism).

metaplasia A change in the normal pattern of differentiation such that dividing cells differentiate into cell types not normally found in that location in the body.

metastasis Secondary tumour; the process by which spreading of malignant neoplasms occurs; the transfer of disease from one organ or part to another not directly connected with it.

metrorrhagia Bleeding between menstrual periods; may be caused by hormonal imbalances, pelvic inflammatory disease, cervical or uterine polyps, uterine fibroids or cervical or uterine cancer.

microalbuminuria Protein in the urine.

micturition Releasing urine from the urinary bladder (voiding).

minor trauma Injury to a single part or system of the body, usually treated in the hospital or emergency department.

mitigation The action taken to prevent or reduce the harmful effects of a disaster on human health or property; it involves future-oriented activities to prevent subsequent disasters or to minimise their effects.

mitochondria Provide the energy a cell needs to move, divide, produce secretory products and contract.

mitosis A process of nuclear division in eukaryotic cells conventionally divided into five stages: prophase, prometaphase, metaphase, anaphase and telophase. Mitosis conserves chromosome numbers by allocating replicated chromosomes equally to each of the daughter nuclei.

mitral valve (bicuspid valve) Valve between the left atrium and ventricle in the heart; prevents blood from flowing backwards into the atrium.

monosomy (monosomic) When one member of the chromosome pair is missing—for example, in Turner syndrome (45, XO).

mood The way in which a person describes their feelings at a particular time.

morbid obesity Weight greater than 100% over ideal body weight.

motor neurone disease (MND) Progressive, degenerative neurological disease characterised by weakness and wasting of the involved muscles, without any accompanying sensory or cognitive changes; also called *Lou Gehrig's disease*.

mourning The actions or expressions of the bereaved, including the symbols, clothing and ceremonies that make up the outward manifestations of grief.

multifactorial Health conditions determined by multiple factors, including genetic and environmental factors, each having an additive effect.

multiple myeloma A malignancy in which plasma cells multiply uncontrollably and infiltrate the bone marrow, lymph nodes, spleen and other tissues.

multiple sclerosis (MS) A chronic demyelinating neurological disease of the CNS (brain, optic nerves and spinal cord), associated with an abnormal immune response to an environmental factor.

multiple trauma Most often the result of a motor vehicle crash, this type of trauma requires immediate intervention specifically focused on ensuring survival.

murmurs Sounds made by turbulent blood flow through the heart.

muscular dystrophy (MD) A group of inherited muscle diseases that cause progressive muscle degeneration and wasting.

myasthenia gravis Chronic, progressive neuromuscular disorder characterised by fatigue and severe weakness of skeletal muscles.

myocarditis Inflammatory disorder of the heart muscle.

myopia (nearsightedness) A condition in which the eyeball is elongated, causing the image to focus in front of the retina instead of on it.

myringotomy Incision of the tympanic membrane.

myxoedema An alternative term for severe or advanced hypothyroidism.

myxoedema coma A life-threatening complication of longstanding, untreated hypothyroidism usually triggered by an acute illness or trauma.

naevi (moles) Flat or raised macules or papules with rounded, well-defined borders.

natural disasters Disasters caused by acts of nature or emerging diseases. Some are unexpected, and some are predictable through advanced meteorological technologies.

natural killer cells (NK cells) Large, granular lymphocytes (found in the spleen, lymph nodes, bone marrow and blood) that provide immune surveillance and resistance to infection, and play an important role in the destruction of early malignant cells.

nausea An unpleasant sensation usually followed by vomiting.

neglect syndrome (unilateral neglect) A disorder of attention. In this syndrome, the person cannot integrate and use perceptions from the affected side of the body or from the environment on the affected side and, hence, ignores that part.

neoplasm A mass of new tissue (a collection of cells) that grows independently of its surrounding structures and has no physiological purpose.

nephrectomy Removal of the kidney.

nephrotic syndrome A condition marked by massive proteinuria, hypoalbuminaemia, hyperlipidaemia and oedema.

neurogenic bladder Dysfunctional urinary bladder due to lesion of central or peripheral nervous system.

neurogenic shock Shock resulting from an imbalance between parasympathetic and sympathetic stimulation of vascular smooth muscle. If parasympathetic overstimulation or sympathetic understimulation persists, sustained vasodilation occurs and blood pools in the venous and capillary beds.

neuropathic pain Pain caused by a lesion or dysfunction in the nervous system from the primary afferent conducting mechanism to the central nervous system.

nicotine An alkaloid found in the nightshade family of plants (*Solanaceae*) which constitutes approximately 0.6–3.0% of the dry weight of tobacco, with biosynthesis taking place in the roots and accumulating in the leaves.

nociception The physiological processes related to pain perception.

nociceptors Sensory nerve fibres that conduct pain impulses from the periphery to the central nervous system.

nocturia Voiding two or more times at night.

nondisjunction An error in meiosis or mitosis in which members of a pair of homologous chromosomes or a pair of sister chromatids fail to separate properly from each other.

non-Hodgkin's lymphoma (NHL) Lymphoid tissue malignancies that do not contain Reed–Sternberg cells.

non-union A state that exists when the ends of a fracture fail to heal together.

normal sinus rhythm (NSR) Normal heart rhythm, in which impulses originate in the sinus node and travel through normal conduction pathways without delay.

nursing process The series of critical-thinking activities nurses use as they provide care to patients; this logical approach to care ensures that patients receive comprehensive and effective care.

nutrients Substances found in food that are used by the body to promote growth, maintenance and repair.

nutrition The process by which the body ingests, absorbs, transports, uses and eliminates food.

nystagmus Rapid involuntary eye movements.

obesity An excess of body fat (adipose tissue).

obstructive shock Shock caused by an obstruction in the heart or great vessels that either impedes venous return or prevents effective cardiac pumping action.

occult bleeding Hidden bleeding.

oedema Accumulation of fluid in the body's tissues; an excess accumulation of fluid in the interstitial space.

oesophageal varices Enlarged, thin-walled veins that form in the submucosa of the oesophagus.

oesophagojejunostomy Removal of the entire stomach with anastomosis of the distal oesophagus to the jejunum.

oestrogen Hormone produced by the ovary.

oliguria Urine output of less than 400 mL in 24 hours.

oncogene Gene capable of triggering cancerous characteristics.

oncology The study of cancer.

opioid A chemical that works by binding to opioid receptors, which are found principally in the central nervous system and the gastrointestinal tract.

oral mucositis Inflammation and ulceration of the oral mucosa.

orchitis Infection or inflammation of the testicle.

orthopnoea Difficulty breathing when supine.

orthostatic hypotension A decrease in systolic blood pressure of more than 10 to 15 mmHg and a drop in diastolic blood pressure on standing.

osmosis The process by which water moves across a selectively permeable membrane from an area of lower solute concentration to an area of higher solute concentration.

ossification The process of bone formation.

osteoarthritis (OA) (degenerative joint disease) The most commonly occurring of all forms of arthritis. This disease is characterised by loss of articular cartilage in articulating joints and hypertrophy of the bones at the articular margins.

osteomalacia (adult rickets) Metabolic bone disorder characterised by inadequate mineralisation of bone matrix.

osteomyelitis Infection within the bone that can lead to tissue death and necrosis.

osteoporosis Literally defined as 'porous bones', a metabolic bone disorder characterised by loss of bone mass, increased bone fragility and an increased risk of fractures.

ostomy General term for an operation in which an artificial opening is created.

otitis externa Inflammation of the ear canal, commonly known as *swimmer's ear*.

otitis media Inflammation or infection of the middle ear.

otosclerosis Abnormal bone formation in the osseous labyrinth of the temporal bone causing the footplate of the stapes to become fixed or immobile in the oval window. The result is a conductive hearing loss.

ovarian cycle The female cycle that occurs from puberty until menopause in which the production of ova occur.

oxyhaemoglobin The combined form of haemoglobin and oxygen; found in arterial blood, it carries oxygen to body tissues.

pacemaker A pulse generator used to provide an electrical stimulus to the heart when the heart fails to generate or conduct on its own a rate that maintains the cardiac output.

$PaCO_2$ Partial pressure of carbon dioxide in arterial blood.

Paget's disease A skeletal disorder that results from excessive osteoclastic activity. Paget's disease is characterised by bone deformity, especially of the long bones of the lower limbs, the pelvis, the lumbar vertebrae and the skull.

pain tolerance The amount of pain a person can endure before responding to it.

palliative care An area of care that has evolved out of the hospice experience, but exists outside of hospice programs and is not restricted to the end of life. Palliative care is focused on the relief of physical, mental and spiritual distress for individuals who have an incurable illness and is used earlier in the disease experience than hospice care. The goal of palliative care is to prevent and relieve suffering by early assessment and treatment of pain and other physical, psychosocial and spiritual needs to improve the person's quality of life.

pallor Lack of colour; paleness of skin.

pancreatitis Inflammation of the pancreas.

pandemic The worldwide spread of a disease.

PaO_2 Partial pressure of oxygen in arterial blood.

paracentesis Aspiration of fluid from the peritoneal cavity.

paralytic ileus Impaired propulsion or forward movement of bowel contents.

paraplegia Paralysis of the lower portion of the body, sometimes involving the lower trunk.

parenchyma The key elements of an organ essential to its functioning, as distinct from the capsule that encompasses it and other supporting structures.

parenteral nutrition (PN) Intravenous administration of carbohydrates (high concentrations of dextrose), protein (amino acids), electrolytes, vitamins, minerals and fat emulsions.

Parkinson's disease (PD) Progressive, degenerative neurological disease characterised by non-intention tremor, bradykinesia and muscle rigidity.

paroxysmal nocturnal dyspnoea (PND) Attacks of acute shortness of breath that occur at night, waking up the person.

partial gastrectomy Removal of a portion of the stomach, usually the distal half to two-thirds.

partial-thickness burn Burn that involves the entire dermis and the papillae of the dermis (superficial partial-thickness burn) or extends into the hair follicles (deep partial-thickness burn).

passive immunity Temporary protection—provided by antibodies produced by other people or animals—against disease-producing antigens. Protection is gradually lost when these acquired antibodies are used up either by natural degradation or by combining with the antigen.

pathogens Virulent organisms rarely found in the absence of disease.

pediculosis An infestation with lice, parasites that live on the blood of an animal or human host.

pelvic inflammatory disease (PID) A term used to describe infection of the pelvic organs.

penetrance The percentage or likelihood that an individual who has inherited a gene mutation will actually express the disease signs and symptoms in his or her lifetime.

penetrating trauma Occurs when a foreign object enters the body, causing damage to body structures.

peptic ulcer An ulcer that occurs in any area of the gastrointestinal tract exposed to acid-pepsin secretions, including the oesophagus, stomach or duodenum.

peptic ulcer disease (PUD) A break in the mucous lining of the gastrointestinal tract where it comes in contact with gastric juice.

perforation Penetration of ulcer through mucosal wall.

pericarditis Inflammation of the pericardium.

perioperative nursing A highly skill, specialised area of nursing practice incorporating a number of sub-specialties.

peripheral obesity Obesity characterised by a waist-to-hip ratio of less than 0.8, more commonly seen in women.

peripheral vascular disease (PVD) Impaired blood supply to peripheral tissues, particularly the lower extremities.

peristalsis Alternating waves of contraction and relaxation of involuntary muscle.

peritoneal dialysis Procedure in which electrolytes, waste products and excess water are removed from the body by diffusion using the peritoneum surrounding the abdominal cavity as the dialysing membrane.

peritonitis Inflammation of the peritoneum.

pernicious anaemia Anaemia resulting from failure to absorb dietary vitamin B_{12} due to lack of intrinsic factor.

persistent (chronic) pain Ongoing and prolonged pain, not always associated with an identifiable cause but often arising from an acute cause.

persistent vegetative state (PVS) Condition of complete unawareness of self and the environment.

personal responsibility Admitting responsibility for choices made.

person-centred care A holistic approach to the planning, delivery and evaluation of healthcare that is grounded in mutually beneficial partnerships between healthcare professionals, patients and families. Person-centred care is underpinned by the principles of trust, empathy, dignity, autonomy, respect, choice, transparency and desire to help individuals lead the life they want.

pertussis (whooping cough) A highly contagious acute upper respiratory infection cause by the bacterium *Bordetella pertussis*.

phagocytosis A process by which a foreign agent or target cell is engulfed, destroyed and digested. Neutrophils and macrophages, known as phagocytes, are the primary cells involved in phagocytosis.

phantom limb syndrome (phantom pain) A confusing pain syndrome that occurs following surgical or traumatic amputation of a limb. The person experiences pain in the missing body part even though there is complete mental awareness that the limb is gone.

pharmacogenetics The study of how genetic factors influence drug action.

pharyngitis Acute inflammation of the pharynx.

phenotype The expression of a person's entire physical, biochemical and physiological make-up, as determined by the individual's genotype and environmental factors.

pheochromocytoma Tumours of chromaffi in tissues in the adrenal medulla. These tumours, which are usually benign, produce catecholamines (adrenaline or noradrenaline, also known as epinephrine and norepinephrine) that stimulate the sympathetic nervous system.

phimosis Constriction of the foreskin so that it cannot be retracted over the glans penis.

photophobia Sensitivity to light.

plasmapheresis (plasma exchange) Removal of the plasma component from whole blood.

pleural effusion Collection of excess fluid in the pleural space.

pleuritis Inflammation of the pleura.

pneumonia Inflammation of the lung parenchyma (the respiratory bronchioles and alveoli).

pneumothorax Results when air enters the pleural space due to blunt and penetrating injuries to the chest.

polycystic kidney disease (PKD) A hereditary disease characterised by cyst formation and massive kidney enlargement.

polycythaemia (erythrocytosis) Excess red blood cells characterised by a haematocrit higher than 55%.

polydipsia Excessive thirst.

polymorphisms DNA sequences that have many forms but give the genetic 'directions' for the same thing.

polymyositis A systemic connective tissue disorder characterised by inflammation of connective tissue and muscle fibres leading to muscle weakness and atrophy.

polyphagia Excessive eating.

polyuria A condition where increased blood volume increases renal blood flow and the hyperglycaemia acts as an osmotic diuretic, thereby increasing urine output.

portal hypertension Elevated pressure in the portal venous system that causes rerouting of blood to adjoining lower pressure vessels.

portal systemic encephalopathy Impaired consciousness and mental status due to the accumulation of toxic waste products in the blood (ammonia in particular) as blood bypasses the congested liver.

positioning Exposes the operative site in conjunction with access for anaesthesia administration. Proper positioning is imperative to prevent injury to the person.

postoperative phase Period when a procedure or surgery has been completed and the person is recovering from the stress associated with the surgery.

postpoliomyelitis syndrome A complication of a previous infection by the poliomyelitis virus.

preload The amount of cardiac muscle fibre tension or stretch that exists at diastole, just before ventricular contraction.

premenstrual syndrome (PMS) Complex of symptoms characterised by irritability, depression, oedema and breast tenderness preceding the monthly menses.

preparedness Having a comprehensive disaster plan in place that coordinates efforts among many people, agencies and levels of government.

preoperative phase Time when preparation of the person for surgery is conducted and completed.

presbycusis Age-related loss of the ability to hear high-frequency sounds; may occur because of cochlear hair cell degeneration or loss of auditory neurons in the organ of Corti.

presbyopia Impaired near vision resulting from a loss of elasticity of the lens related to ageing.

prescription medication misuse Non-medical use of pharmaceuticals or use for genuine medical purposes but without a valid prescription, or when prescribed in excessive quantities or frequencies, or when an iatrogenic dependence has developed.

pressure injury Ischaemic lesion of the skin and underlying tissue caused by external pressure that impairs the flow of blood and lymph.

pretibial myxoedema Also known as thyroid dermopathy, pretibial myxoedema refers to lesions of the skin resulting from the accumulation of hyaluronic acid, as a result of thyroid disease.

priapism Sustained, painful erection that lasts at least 4 hours and is not associated with sexual arousal.

primary care A clinical perspective that provides first contact services for individuals and families.

primary healthcare (PHC) Involves communities, public policy and social and environmental determinants of health.

primary hypertension (idiopathic, essential) A persistently elevated systemic blood pressure.

primary survey An initial assessment of a person to determine if there is serious compromise to airway, breathing or circulation.

procedural pain A type of breakthrough pain that is predictable because it is associated with movement such as turning or coughing.

progesterone Hormone produced by the ovary; works with oestrogen to control the menstrual cycle.

proptosis Forward bulging of one or both eyes.

prostatitis Inflammation of the prostate gland.

protein energy malnutrition (PEM) The state of decreased body pools of protein with or without fat depletion or a state of diminished functional capacity, caused at least partly by inadequate nutrient intake relative to nutrient demand, and/or which is improved by nutritional repletion.

proteinuria Abnormal proteins in the urine.

proximal determinants Determinants that have a more direct impact on health, and include lifestyle and behavioural factors as well as underlying health conditions.

pruritus Subjective itching sensation producing an urge to scratch.

psoriasis Chronic, non-infectious skin disorder that is characterised by raised, reddened, round circumscribed plaques covered by silvery white scales.

psychosis A mental health condition in which there is a loss of contact with reality.

psychostimulants A diverse group of natural and synthetic drugs with a wide range of psychological and physical effects, including euphoria, increased energy and irregular heartbeat.

ptosis Drooping of the eyelid.

pulmonary embolism Sudden occlusion of a pulmonary artery resulting in disruption of blood supply to the lung parenchyma.

pulmonary hypertension Condition in which the pulmonary arterial pressure is elevated to an abnormal level.

pulmonary oedema An abnormal accumulation of fluid in the interstitial tissue and alveoli of the lung.

pulmonic valve One of the semilunar valves, separating the ventricles from the great vessels.

pulse Rhythmic pressure waveform that can be felt over an artery.

pulse pressure The difference between the systolic and diastolic blood pressure.

puncture wound Wound that occurs when a sharp or blunt object penetrates the integument.

pupillary light reflex Reflex in which the pupil contracts in response to a bright light.

pyelonephritis Upper urinary tract inflammation affecting the kidney and renal pelvis.

pyuria (bacteriuria) Pus in the urine.

quadriplegia Injury to cervical segments of the cord thus impairing function of the arms, trunk, legs and pelvic organs.

rabies Viral (rhabdovirus) infection of the central nervous system transmitted by infected saliva that enters the human body through a bite or an open wound.

radiation therapy Therapy that uses radiation to kill a tumour, to reduce its size, to decrease pain or to relieve obstruction.

rapid cycling Having four or more mood episodes within a 12-month period.

Raynaud's disease Disorder characterised by episodes of intense vasospasm in the small arteries and arterioles of the fingers and possibly the toes; has no identifiable cause.

Raynaud's phenomenon Disorder characterised by episodes of intense vasospasm in the small arteries and arterioles of the fingers and possibly the toes; occurs secondarily to another disease.

reactive arthritis (Reiter's syndrome) An acute, non-purulent inflammatory arthritis that complicates a bacterial infection of the genitourinary or gastrointestinal tracts.

recovery The final phase of an emergency; the period when the emergency is under control and the community starts to rebuild.

Recovery A recognised and accepted paradigm, related to a personal journey, that has significant implications for people who have mental health problems, their carers, mental health professionals and mental health services.

referral Timely consultation and handing over of clinical care of people to the appropriate personnel and facility for ongoing management.

reflux, urinary Backflow of urine towards the kidneys.

refraction The bending of light rays as they pass from one medium to another medium of different optical density.

regional anaesthesia Anaesthesia that desensitises a particular area but does not involve the full central nervous system or cause sedation.

regional and remote health workforce A statistical representation of nurses working in identified regional and remote areas which includes the number of currently employed nurses, acknowledging their age, experience and qualifications.

regurgitation (valvular) Backflow of blood through an incompletely closed valve into the area it just left.

renal artery stenosis Narrowing of the renal artery.

renal colic Acute, severe, intermittent pain in the flank and upper outer abdominal quadrant generally associated with acute obstruction of a ureter and resulting ureteral spasm.

renal insufficiency Any condition in which the kidneys are unable to remove accumulated metabolites from the blood, leading to altered fluid, electrolyte and acid-base balance.

respiratory failure Inability of lungs to oxygenate the blood and remove carbon dioxide adequately to meet the body's needs, even at rest.

response Occurs in the emergency stage and after a disaster event has occurred.

retinal detachment Separation of the retina or sensory portion of the eye from the choroid.

retrieval Specialised transfer of people with needs exceeding the capacity of their current location to a clinical facility providing a higher level of specialised healthcare.

retrograde ejaculation Seminal fluid discharged into the bladder.

rheumatic disorders Refers to diseases of the muscles and bones as well as the joints.

rheumatic fever A systemic inflammatory disease caused by an abnormal immune response to pharyngeal infection by group A beta-haemolytic streptococci. The condition is characterised by acute inflammation, joint pain, fever and cardiac valve scarring.

rheumatic heart disease (RHD) Slowly progressive valvular deformity following acute or repeated attacks of rheumatic fever; characterised by rigid and deformed valve leaflets; fused valve commissures and fibrosis of chordae tendineae.

rheumatoid arthritis A chronic systemic autoimmune disease that causes inflammation of connective tissue, primarily in the joints.

rhinitis Inflammation of the nasal cavities.

rhinoplasty Surgical reconstruction of the nose.

risk factors Defined as individual or environmental variables that are related to the increased likelihood that a negative outcome will occur.

sarcoidosis Systemic disease characterised by granulomas in the lungs, lymph nodes, liver, eyes, skin and other organs.

scabies Parasitic infestation caused by the mite *Sarcoptes scabiei*.

schizophrenia A mental disorder characterised by abnormalities in the perception or expression of reality.

sciatica Pain over the sciatic nerve.

scleroderma Hardening of the skin; a chronic condition characterised by the formation of excess fibrous connective tissue and diffuse fibrosis of the skin and internal organs.

scoliosis A lateral curvature of the spine.

scope of practice The roles, functions, responsibilities, activities and decision-making capacity that nurses are educated, competent and authorised to perform.

sebum An oily substance secreted from sebaceous glands; softens and lubricates the skin and hair, and decreases water loss from the skin in low humidity. Sebum also protects the body from infection by killing bacteria.

secondary hypertension Elevated blood pressure resulting from an identifiable underlying process.

secondary survey A head-to-toe assessment of a person that includes all body systems.

seizure An episode of excessive and abnormal discharge of electrical activity within the central nervous system.

semen Contains sperm and fluids secreted by the male reproductive system glands.

septic arthritis Develops when a joint space is invaded by a pathogen.

septic shock One part of a progressive syndrome called systemic inflammatory response syndrome. Beginning with an infection, septic shock progresses to bacteraemia, then sepsis, then septic shock and finally multiple organ failure syndrome.

septicaemia Systemic disease associated with the presence of bacteria or their toxins in the blood.

seroconversion Antibody response to a disease or vaccine.

serum bicarbonate (HCO_3^-) Reflects the renal regulation of acid–base balance. It is often called the metabolic component of arterial blood gases.

severe acute respiratory syndrome (SARS) Lower respiratory illness of unknown aetiology; spread by close person-to-person contact.

sex chromosome A chromosome responsible for determining the sex of an individual.

sexually transmitted infection (STI, sexually transmitted disease, venereal disease) Any infection transmitted by sexual contact, including vaginal, oral and anal intercourse.

shingles See *herpes zoster*.

shock A clinical syndrome characterised by a systemic imbalance between oxygen supply and demand. This imbalance results in a state of inadequate blood flow to the peripheral tissues, causing life-threatening cellular dysfunction, hypotension and oliguria.

sickle cell anaemia A hereditary, chronic haemolytic anaemia characterised by episodes of sickling, during which red blood cells become abnormally crescent shaped.

sinusitis Inflammation of the mucous membranes of one or more of the sinuses.

Sjögren's syndrome An autoimmune disorder that causes inflammation and dysfunction of exocrine glands throughout the body.

skin tear A traumatic wound occurring principally on the extremities of older adults, as a result of friction alone or shearing and friction forces that separate the epidermis from the dermis (partial-thickness wound), or which separate both the epidermis and the dermis from underlying structures (full-thickness wound).

sleep apnoea Absence of airflow through the upper airways for 10 or more seconds.

social determinants of health The social factors that influence the health status and health outcomes of individuals and communities.

social model of health A model of health which views health as multifaceted, focusing on social rather than biological determinants of health. This model emphasises health equity and prevention of illness or injury, as well as collaboration and empowerment. The social model of health is also referred to as new public health or the social ecological model.

solvents Produce a depressant effect on the central nervous system and comprise a range of products producing vapours which, when inhaled through the nose or mouth, may cause an intoxicated feeling and lead to an altered state of consciousness.

somatic cell Any cell in the body that is not a sex cell (ova and sperm).

Somogyi phenomenon A morning rise in blood glucose to hyperglycaemic levels following an episode of nocturnal hypoglycaemia and a counter-regulatory hormone response.

spasticity Increased muscle tone in disease of the corticospinal motor tract.

spermatocoele A mobile, usually painless mass containing dead spermatozoa that forms in the epididymis.

spinal cord injury (SCI) Injury to spinal cord, usually due to trauma and classified according to systems.

spinal shock Temporary loss of reflex function below the level of injury.

sprain Tearing or stretching of a ligament that results from a twisting motion.

sprue A chronic primary disorder of the small intestine in which the absorption of nutrients, particularly fats, is impaired.

squamous cell carcinoma Malignant tumour of the squamous epithelium of the skin or mucous membranes.

starvation Inadequate dietary intake; the condition of being without food for long periods of time.

status asthmaticus Severe, prolonged asthma that does not respond to routine treatment. Without aggressive therapy, status asthmaticus can lead to respiratory failure with hypoxaemia, hypercapnia and acidosis.

steatorrhoea Greasy, frothy, yellow stools resulting from excess fat in the faeces.

stem cells (haemocytoblasts) Bone marrow precursor cells for all blood cells.

stem cell transplant (SCT) Infusion of donor stem cells to replace the recipient's blood cell lines (white blood cells, red blood cells and platelets).

stenosis Condition where valve leaflets fuse together and are unable to open or close fully.

steroids Often used illegally to build muscles and enhance exercise performance; also known as performance- and image-enhancing drugs (PIEDs).

stigma Severe social disapproval.

stoma Surface opening.

Strain Stretching injury to a muscle or a muscle–tendon unit caused by mechanical overloading.

stress-induced (erosive) gastritis See *erosive gastritis*.

striae A line above or below tissue that differs in colour and texture from surrounding tissue.

stridor High-pitched, harsh inspiratory sound indicative of upper airway obstruction.

stroke (brain attack, cerebrovascular accident, CVA) A condition in which neurological deficits occur as a result of decreased blood flow to a focal (localised) area of brain tissue.

stroke volume (SV) The amount of blood pumped into the aorta with each contraction of the left ventricle.

subacute thyroiditis Inflammation of the thyroid gland.

subdural haematoma A localised mass of blood that collects between the dura mater and the arachnoid mater.

subluxation Partial separation (or dislocation) of the bones of a joint.

substance dependence A severe condition occurring when the use of a chemical substance is no longer under an individual's control for at least 3 months. Continued use of the substance usually persists despite adverse effects on the person's physical condition, psychological health and interpersonal relationships (used interchangeably with 'addiction').

substance-induced disorder A reversible substance-specific syndrome related to the type of drug used.

substance-related disorder Maladaptive patterns of substance use leading to clinically significant impairment or distress.

substance use The use of any chemical in a fashion inconsistent with medical or culturally defined social norms despite physical, psychological or socially adverse effects.

substance use disorder A medical condition in which the use of one or more substances leads to a clinically significant impairment characterised by a range of mental, physical and behavioural symptoms that often cause problems related to one's personal life, relationships and work, as well as increasingly hazardous use, tolerance and withdrawal.

sudden cardiac death (SCD) Unexpected death occurring within 1 hour of the onset of cardiovascular symptoms.

sundowning A behavioural change in Alzheimer's disease characterised by increased agitation, time disorientation and wandering during afternoon and evening hours.

superficial burn Burn involving only the epidermal layer of the skin; most often results from damage from sunburn, ultraviolet light, minor flash injury (from a sudden ignition or explosion) or mild radiation burn associated with cancer treatment.

surfactant A lipoprotein produced by the alveolar cells; interferes with adhesion of water molecules, reducing surface tension and helping to expand lungs.

surgery An invasive medical procedure performed to diagnose or treat illness, injury or deformity. Although surgery is a medical treatment, the nurse assumes an active role in caring for the person before, during and after surgery.

surgical debridement The process of excising a wound to the level of fascia (fascial excision) or sequentially removing thin slices of a burn wound to the level of viable tissue (sequential excision).

syndrome of inappropriate ADH secretion (SIADH) Characterised by high levels of antidiuretic hormone (ADH) in the absence of serum hypo-osmolality, and most often caused by the ectopic production of ADH by malignant tumours.

synovitis Inflammation of the synovial membrane lining the articular capsule of a joint.

syphilis A sexually transmitted infection caused by a spirochaete that may invade almost any body tissue or organ. It enters the body through a break in the skin or mucous membranes and can be transferred to the fetus through the placental circulation.

systemic lupus erythematosus (SLE) A chronic inflammatory immune complex connective tissue disease.

systolic blood pressure This arterial pressure wave produced by ventricular contraction (systole) averages 120 mmHg in healthy adults.

T lymphocytes (T cells) Type of lymphocyte that matures in the thymus gland.

tachypnoea Abnormally rapid respiratory rate.

telehealth A broad term that refers to the use of technology to contribute to the provision of healthcare, usually at a distance.

tendonitis Inflammation of a tendon.

tension pneumothorax A condition in which an injury to the chest allows air to enter but not escape the pleural cavity.

terrorism An action, or threat of action, that causes harm or interference, and is made with the intention of advancing a political, religious or ideological cause.

test sensitivity How specifically a test identifies (positive test result) individuals who are affected and/or who have a disease phenotype.

test specificity How specifically a test does not identify (negative test result) individuals who are unaffected or do not have a disease phenotype.

testicular torsion Twisting of the testes and spermatic cord.

testosterone Male hormone produced in the testes.

tetanus Disorder of the nervous system caused by a neurotoxin elaborated by *Clostridium tetani*.

tetany Tonic muscular spasms.

thalassaemia An inherited disorder of haemoglobin synthesis in which either the alpha or beta chains of the haemoglobin molecule are missing or defective.

therapeutic relationship A relationship that aims to empower the person with the knowledge and ability to recover from their illness.

third spacing The accumulation and sequestration of trapped extracellular fluid in an actual or potential body space as a result of disease or injury.

thoracentesis Invasive procedure in which fluid (or occasionally air) is removed from the pleural space with a needle.

thought content The actual content of what a person is thinking.

thrill Palpable vibration over the precordium or an artery.

thromboangiitis obliterans (Buerger's disease) An occlusive vascular disease involving inflammation, spasm and clot formation in small and medium-sized peripheral arteries.

thrombocytopenia A platelet count of less than 100,000 per millilitre of blood.

thromboembolus A thrombus that breaks loose from the arterial wall.

thrombus A blood clot that adheres to a vessel wall.

thyroid crisis An extreme state of hyperthyroidism that is rare today because of improved diagnosis and treatment methods. Also called thyroid storm.

thyroid gland A gland situated at the front of the throat which secretes thyroid hormones (thyroxine (T_4) and triiodothyronine (T_3)) to regulate the body's metabolic process.

thyroid storm *See thyroid crisis.*

thyroidectomy A procedure performed to treat cancer of the thyroid.

thyrotoxicosis See *hyperthyroidism*.

tidal volume (TV) The amount of air (approximately 500 mL) moved in and out of the lungs with each normal, quiet breath.

tinnitus Perception of sound such as ringing, buzzing or roaring in the ears.

titrate To determine the concentration of (a solution) by titration or perform the operation of titration.

tolerance A cumulative state in which a particular dose of a chemical elicits a smaller response than before. With increased tolerance, the individual needs higher and higher doses to obtain the desired effect.

tonsillitis Acute inflammation of the palatine tonsils.

tophi Small white nodules in subcutaneous tissue composed of urate deposits resulting from gout.

total gastrectomy Removal of the entire stomach.

total peripheral vascular resistance (TPVR) The opposing forces or impedance to blood flow as the arterial channels become more and more distant from the heart.

toxic multinodular goitre A tumour characterised by small, discrete, independently functioning nodules in the thyroid gland tissue that secrete excessive amounts of thyroid hormone.

trachoma A chronic conjunctivitis caused by *Chlamydia trachomatis*, and a significant preventable cause of blindness worldwide.

transdermal Medication absorbed through the skin without injection.

transdisciplinary Transdisciplinary approaches in health involve partnerships and strategies that cross many health and other professional discipline boundaries to create a holistic approach, addressing multiple influences.

transfusion An infusion of blood or blood components.

transient ischaemic attack (TIA) Brief period of localised cerebral ischaemia that causes neurological deficits lasting for less than 24 hours.

transjugular intrahepatic portosystemic shunt (TIPS) Used to relieve portal hypertension and its complications of oesophageal varices and ascites.

translocation The joining of a part of or a whole chromosome to another separate chromosome.

trauma An injury to human tissues and organs resulting from the transfer of energy from the environment.

traumatic brain injury (TBI) A traumatic insult to the brain capable of causing physical, intellectual, emotional, social and vocational changes.

tremor Rhythmic movement.

triage Means 'sorting'. Triage is the process by which all people presenting to an ED for care are assessed and their care prioritised according to actual or potential severity of illness or injury.

triage in regional and remote areas Clinical determination of the acuity of the presenting health problems for people seeking healthcare in regional and remote areas.

trichomoniasis A sexually transmitted infection caused by a parasite passed from person to person.

tricuspid valve A valve between the right atrium and ventricle of the heart; prevents blood from flowing backwards into the atrium.

trigeminal neuralgia (tic douloureux) A chronic disease of the trigeminal cranial nerve (cranial nerve V) that causes severe facial pain.

triglycerides Molecules of glycerol with fatty acids used to transport and store fats in body tissues.

trisomy Possessing three chromosomes instead of the usual two, as in trisomy 21 or Down syndrome.

Trousseau's sign Contraction of the hand and fingers in response to occlusion of the blood supply by a blood pressure cuff; caused by decreased blood calcium levels.

tuberculosis (TB) Chronic, recurrent infectious disease caused by *Mycobacterium tuberculosis*; usually affects the lungs, although any organ can be affected.

tumour marker A protein molecule detectable in serum or other body fluids. This marker is used as a biochemical indicator of the presence of a malignancy.

Turner's syndrome A chromosomal abnormality in which all or part of one of the sex chromosomes is absent.

twilight sedation Anaesthesia that provides analgesia and amnesia, but in which the person remains conscious. People are able to breathe independently and are cardiovascularly stable.

tympanoplasty Surgical reconstruction of the middle ear.

type 1 diabetes mellitus The result of pancreatic islet cell destruction and a total deficit of circulating insulin.

type 2 diabetes mellitus Results from insulin resistance with a defect in compensatory insulin secretion.

ulcer A lesion of the skin or mucous membranes.

ulcerative colitis Chronic inflammatory bowel disorder of the mucosa and submucosa of the colon and rectum.

ultrafiltration Removal of excess body water using a hydrostatic pressure gradient.

uraemia Literally, 'urine in the blood'; the syndrome or group of symptoms associated with end-stage kidney disease.

urea An end product of protein metabolism and, along with water, the main constituent of urine.

ureteral (or ureteric) stent Thin catheter inserted into the ureter to provide for urine flow and ureteral support.

ureteroplasty Surgical repair of a ureter.

urgency A sudden, compelling need to urinate.

urinary calculi Calculi or 'stones' in the urinary tract.

urinary diversion Procedure to provide for urine collection and drainage following cystectomy. The most common urinary diversion is the ileal conduit.

urinary drainage system The ureters, urinary bladder and urethra.

urinary incontinence Involuntary urination.

urinary retention Incomplete emptying of the bladder.

urticaria Hives.

vaccine Suspensions of whole or fractionated bacteria or viruses that have been treated to make them non-pathogenic.

Valsalva manoeuvre Closing the glottis and contracting the diaphragm and abdominal muscles to increase intra-abdominal pressure to facilitate expulsion of faeces.

valvular heart disease Interference of blood flow to, within and from the heart.

varicocoele Dilation of the pampiniform venous complex of the spermatic cord.

varicose veins Irregular, tortuous veins with incompetent valves.

vasoconstriction Smooth muscle contraction that narrows the vessel lumen.

vasodilation Smooth muscle relaxation that expands the vessel lumen.

vasogenic shock See *distributive shock*.

venous stasis Occurs when venous blood collects and stagnates in the lower leg.

venous thrombosis (thrombophlebitis) Blood clot (thrombus) formation on the wall of a vein, accompanied by inflammation of the vein wall and obstructed venous blood flow.

vertigo Sensation of whirling or rotation.

very-low-kilojoule diet (VLKD) A protein-sparing modified fast (1,700 to 3,500 kilojoules/day or less) under close medical supervision that may be used to treat significant obesity.

vital capacity The sum of TV (tidal volume) 1 IRV (inspiratory reserve volume) 1 ERV (expiratory reserve volume); approximately 4,500 mL in healthy people.

vitiligo Abnormal loss of melanin in patches.

volatile acids Acids eliminated from the body as a gas.

Volkmann's contracture A common complication of elbow fractures; can result from unresolved compartment syndrome. Arterial blood flow decreases, leading to ischaemia, degeneration and contracture of the muscle.

voluntary assisted dying (VAD) The assistance provided to a person by a health practitioner to end their life.

vomiting The forceful expulsion of the contents of the upper gastrointestinal tract resulting from contraction of muscles in the gut and abdominal wall.

warts (verrucae) Lesions of the skin caused by the human papillomavirus.

weaning Process of removing the person from ventilator support and re-establishing spontaneous, independent respirations.

wheeze Continuous, musical sound caused by narrowing of the lumen in a respiratory passage.

wild-type gene The most common type of gene; designated as normal.

withdrawal Cessation of use of a substance to which an individual has become addicted.

xenograft A transplant from an animal species to a human.

xerosis Dry skin.

xerostomia Excessive dryness of the mucous membranes (due to chemotherapy or radiation).

X-linked dominant Any gene found on the X chromosome or traits determined by such genes; also refers to the specific mode of inheritance of such genes. One altered gene on an X chromosome in a male can produce disease, such as haemophilia.

X-linked recessive The result of an altered gene on the X chromosome.

Zollinger–Ellison syndrome Peptic ulcer disease caused by a gastrinoma, or gastrin-secreting tumour of the pancreas, stomach or intestines.

Index

Page numbers in **bold** indicate definitions of key terms.

O